Cardiac Pacing

Proceedings of the
VIIth World Symposium on Cardiac Pacing
Vienna, May 1st to 5th, 1983

Editor in Chief: K. Steinbach
Assistant Editors: D. Glogar, A. Laszkovics,
W. Scheibelhofer, H. Weber

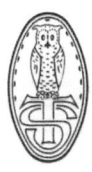

Steinkopff Verlag Darmstadt 1983

CIP-Kurztitelaufnahme der Deutschen Bibliothek

Cardiac pacing: proceedings ot the VIIth World Symposium on Cardiac Pacing / ed.: K. Stein-
bach . . . – Darmstadt: Steinkopff, 1983.
ISBN-13:978-3-642-72369-8   e-ISBN-13:978-3-642-72367-4
DOI: 10.1007/978-3-642-72367-4

NE: Steinbach, Konrad [Hrsg.]; World Symposium on Cardiac Pacing (07, 1983, Wien).

Editorial Assistance: Juliane K. Weller – Production: Heinz J. Schäfer

Preface

Proceedings of a congress serve the purpose to provide the reader with the latest knowledge in the specific field. They present at least for a limited time period a reference book that allows rapid access to the latest information for the medical profession and for an ongoing of future research.

This volume is addressed not only to the participants of the VIIth World Symposium on Cardiac Pacing but to everybody involved in diagnostic and therapeutic cardiac stimulation.

The experience has shown that proceedings of conferences of comparable size are usually published with a considerable time delay limiting its value as a source of prime information. The editors of this volume decided therefore, that their most important task was to guarantee the actuality of the publication.

Even if it seems desirable to include as many presentations of a conference as possible, the large number of excellent presentations at the VIIth World Symposium on Cardiac Pacing, 337 oral presentations and 236 posters, could not be published within an acceptable time period. The experience from previous conferences has shown that a book which includes all the papers can only be edited with a large delay, which reduces the value and actuality of the information.

The editors of such a book have to accept the responsibility for its quality and therefore it is their task to restyle or rewrite some of the papers. The selection of the oral presentations and posters for the scientific program of the VIIth World Symposium on Cardiac Pacing was performed by a review system which judged the quality of the papers in accordance to their originality, the methodology and their clinical as well as their scientific merits.

For publication we decided to select the 150 highest scored presentations and 29 contributions of the invited speakers. 148 authors have submitted their papers for publication. From these papers 95 contributions were accepted for publication without major changes. 13 papers were revised by the editors themselves, 28 papers were returned to the authors for rewriting and 12 papers had to be rejected.

The editors are confident that this revised form of editing a proceeding volume in comparison to previous conferences will be accepted by the readers and will be used for what it is ment for: as an information about the latest developments in diagnostic and therapeutic stimulation and as a reference book for scientists who are active in these fields.

We are proud to note that between the congress and the appearance of the book on the bookshelves it took not more than five months.

K. STEINBACH – Chief in Editor
D. GLOGAR, A. LACZKOVICS, W. SCHEIBELHOFER, H. WEBER – Assistant-Editors

November 1983

Contents

AV-Conduction – VA-Conduction

VIII

Influence of Physiological Pacing on Hemodynamics

New Generators

Leads

XIV

XV

Survey of Pacing Activities

Methods and Results of the Review Process

D. Glogar, G. Joskowics, H. Weber, K. Steinbach

Summary: The review committee for the VIIth World Symposium on Cardiac Pacing set up a selection process for the 964 submitted abstracts to guarantee a fair and evenhanded selection of the papers to be presented at the congress. Each abstract was reviewed by three internationally recognized specialists in their field using a scoring system. The individual reviewers had been trained prior to the review process by completing a test review. Among the 573 papers accepted for presentation 48.4% came from Western Europe, 27% from North America, 8.4% from Eastern Europe, the majority of the remaining abstracts from other developed nations all around the world. The acceptance ratios were similar for Western Europe and North America, the representation of lesser developed countries had to be guaranteed despite somewhat lower scores. Geographical differences revealed a slightly greater interest for clinical pacing in North America and in the Asian developed countries, while papers dealing with technology were represented in a larger portion from some of the rapidly growing Asian developed countries.

Introduction

The review committee of the VIIth World Symposium on Cardiac Pacing was confronted with a great number of papers to select from. To ensure a well balanced scientific program of high quality, the review committee decided to have each abstract assessed by three reviewers in a blinded fashion without knowledge of the author's name or institution. To avoid individual reviewers out-score because of unfamiliarity with the review process, we chose to have each reviewer initially complete our test review consisting of 20 test abstracts from a recent symposium, which were selected in random fashion. After completion of the test review, 60–70 abstracts were sent out for the actual review to each member of the review committee.

Methods

Each abstract had to be scored for (1) the originality of the study, (2) the study design and methodology and (3) the scientific value and/or its relevance. For each of the above categories up to 10 points could be given; therefore each abstract received a total of 0 to 30 points per reviewer or a total of 0 to 90 points along the review process.
Identification and origin of the reviewers, test review scores and abstract review scores as well as origin of the submitted abstracts were entered into a database for statistical analysis.

1

Results

A total of 965 abstracts were submitted from all around the world (Fig. 1). The greatest percentage of abstracts came from Western Europe (48.4%), approximately 27% from North America, while the representation of lesser developed countries was small (Fig. 1). Fig. 2 presents the comparison of the geographical distribution of accepted versus submitted abstracts.

The quality of submitted abstracts was similar for the different geographical regions as shown by their similar distribution curves (Fig. 3). The distribution curve of the Eastern European countries, however, was shifted somewhat to the left (Fig. 3). Thus, the selection process of the abstracts was based mainly on criteria of quality of abstracts and their suitability for the actual program.

The scientific committee was able to accommodate 573 papers out of the submitted abstracts for presentation. Using the review scores the following adaptions were made: (1) We attempted to exclude double entries. (2) We accepted a small number of lower scores to complete essential sessions. (3) We aimed for third world representation even as some of the submitted abstracts had somewhat lesser scores.

Considering those adjustements, how well did the scoring system hold up for the final selection? From the total of 965 submitted abstracts 55.7% were accepted. The distribution curves of accepted and rejected abstracts are shown in Fig. 4. We calculated a cut-off-point for acceptance of 51 points out of the total of 90 points. 75% of the abstracts received low or high scores and were rejected or accepted only on the basis of their review scores. One quarter of the abstracts was accepted or rejected for other reasons besides their review scores. 12.2% of the abstracts received higher scores than the cut-off-point, but had to be rejected for some of the reasons listed above, and 14.6% of the abstracts were accepted even though they received a somewhat lesser score.

The greatest number of submitted abstracts came from the United States with 241 abstracts submitted and 61% of these accepted, followed by Italy, the Federal Republic of

Fig. 1. Geographic distribution of submitted abstracts.

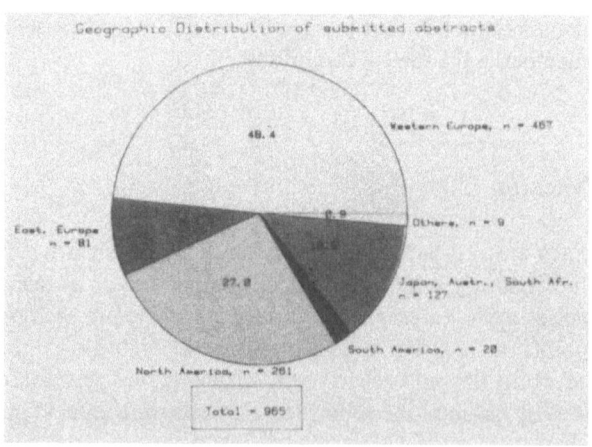

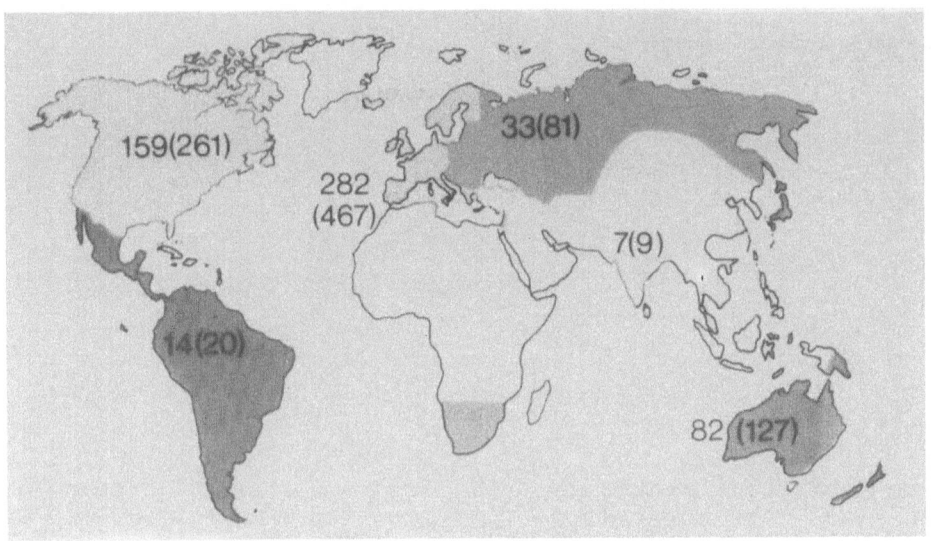

Fig. 2. Accepted versus submitted abstracts (in brackets). Geographical distribution.

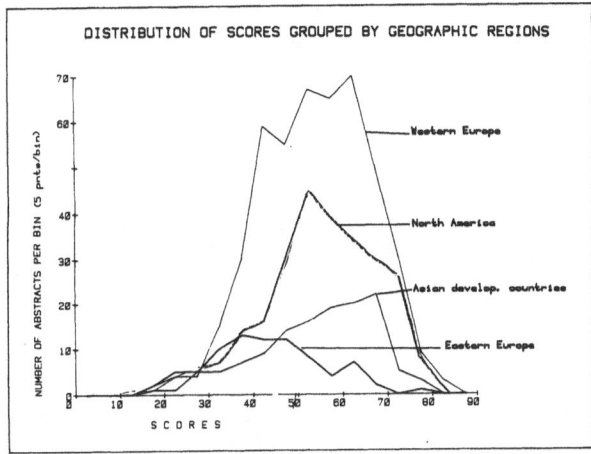

DISTRIBUTION OF SCORES GROUPED BY GEOGRAPHIC REGIONS

Western Europe

North America

Asian develop. countries

Eastern Europe

NUMBER OF ABSTRACTS PER BIN (5 pnts/bin)

SCORES

Fig. 3. Distribution of scores grouped by geographic regions.

Germany, Japan and France (Fig. 5). Among the countries with the greatest acceptance ratios were Switzerland, Austria and Japan with 92, 88 and 68 percent, respectively (Fig. 5).

The computer program allowed to explore possible regional differences in the topics of interest. The interest for arrhythmias appeared to be greatest in Japan and other Asian developed countries (37.8% of abstracts submitted) and lowest in North America (22.6% of abstracts submitted) (Fig. 6). However, clinical pacing seemed to attract the greatest interest in North America (Fig. 6). Technology papers were submitted more frequently from Western Europe. The percentage of the so called undefined topics, lacking a clear

3

Fig. 4. Histogram of scores from accepted and rejected abstracts.

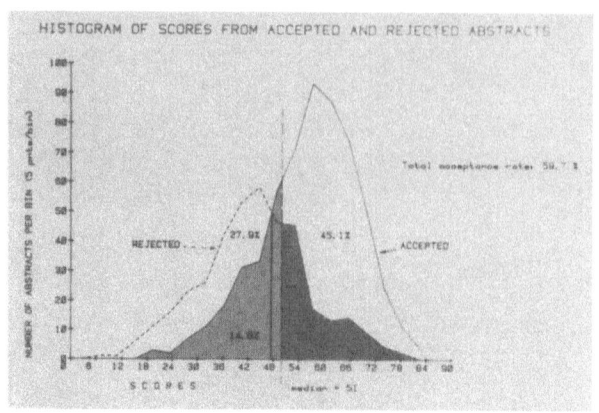

Fig. 5. Number of submitted papers and acceptance ratios for selected countries.

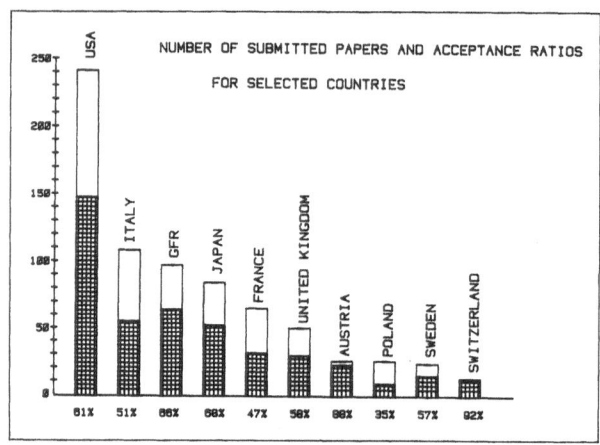

definition or overlapping the given major topics was greatest in Western Europe, while scientists from North America appeared to choose more clear-cut topics.

We further analyzed the mean scores and acceptance rates for the different major topics and grouped them according to their geographical distribution (Table 1). Among the papers dealing with clinical pacing the abstracts from North America received the highest scores and had the highest acceptance ratios, while papers dealing with technological topics received very similar scores from all geographical regions, with the highest acceptance ratios for the papers coming from the Asian-Pacific countries and from Eastern Europe.

Furthermore, we tried to analyse if the reviewers themselves, especially if their main interest had any significant effect on their judgement. The computer analysis revealed that surgeons scored highest and gave similar scores for all the major topics (Table 2). Rhythmonologists scored lowest; they were most critical in judging their own speciality

4

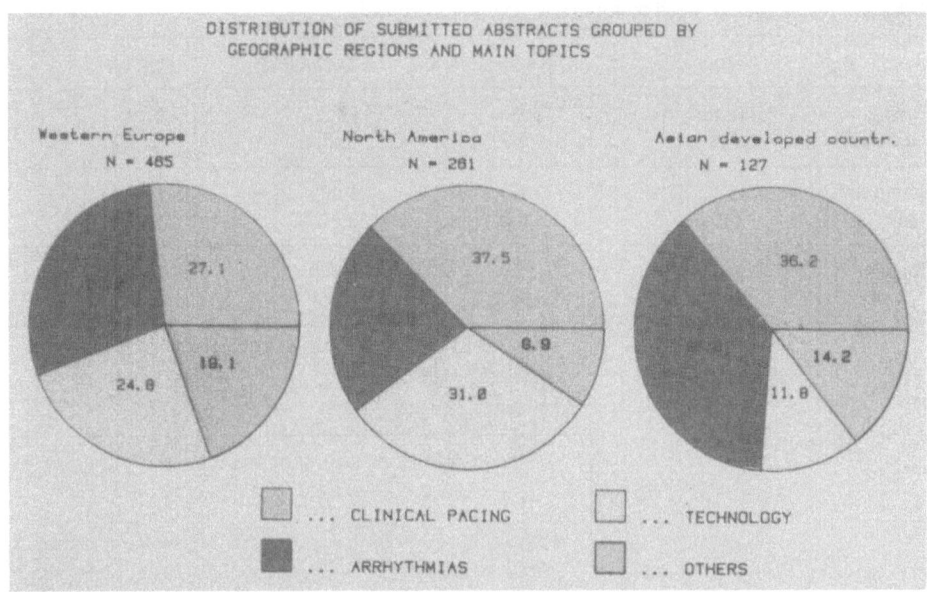

Fig. 6. Distribution of submitted abstracts grouped by geographic regions and main topics.

Table 1. Mean scores and acceptance rates for geographic regions.

TOPIC	West. Europe	North. Amer.	Asian devel.	East. Europe
Clin. Pacing	53.1 +/− 11.5	55.4 +/− 12.9	52.76 +/− 15.0	41.2 +/− 10.7
Accepted:	64.3%	66.3%	56.5%	45.5%
Rhythmology	55.4 +/− 10.8	59.7 +/− 9.2	54.9 +/− 11.8	44.5 +/− 12.5
Accepted:	60.7%	66.1%	70.8%	41.4%
Technology	52.0 +/− 12.5	50.6 +/− 13.8	52.1 +/− 13.4	52.4 +/− 11.5
Accepted:	52.2%	51.8%	60.0%	55.5%
Others	54.1 +/− 13.4	53.6 +/− 13.0	56.5 +/− 7.7	36.4 +/− 13.3
Accepted:	64.0%	56.5%	72.2%	28.6%
Totals:	53.8 +/− 12.1	54.7 +/− 12.9	54.0 +/− 12.8	42.4 +/− 12.9
Accepted:	61%	61%	65%	41%

rhythmonology as well as papers dealing with technology. Pacing specialists scored similarly to rhythmonologists for papers dealing with clinical pacing, but scored higher for papers dealing with technology and rhythmology (Table 2).

Another question of great importance to clarify was the value of the test review in determining or possibly correcting the abstract mean score. There was a very loose correlation between the reviewers' test scores and the actual abstract scores (Fig. 7). It is important to note that several reviewers gave very high scores in their test reviews, but scored rather low for their actual abstract review. If this phenomenon may indicate a learning process it cannot be determined for sure.

5

Table 2. Mean scores grouped by topic and reviewer's profession.

	Clinical Pacing	Rhythmonology	Technology	Others
Pacing specialist	18.8 ± 5.3	18.9 ± 5.3	18.2 ± 5.4	17.9 ± 6.0
Rhythmono-logist	18.6 ± 5.8	17.6 ± 6.2	16.2 ± 7.7	16.9 ± 5.8
Surgeon	20.1 ± 5.5	20.2 ± 4.5	20.6 ± 5.6	20.1 ± 6.0

Fig. 7. Abstracts versus test review.

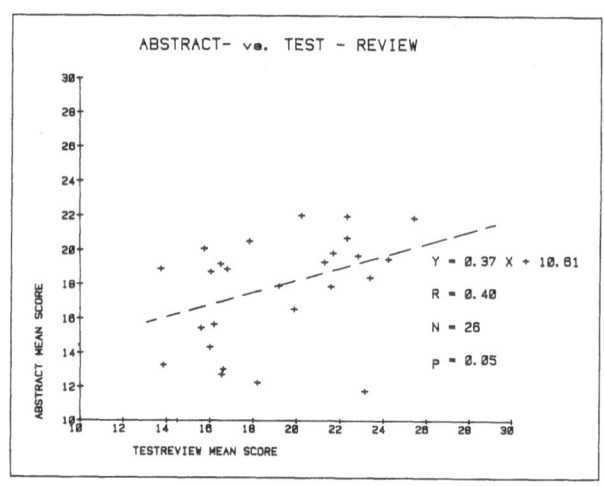

Was it realy important to have more than one reviewer for the abstracts? The review committee decided to have at least 3 reviewers score each abstract. Figure 8 presents the review groups with a high level of agreement (left panel) and the review groups with a high level of disagreement (Fig. 8, right panel). Surprisingly, acceptance ratios were quite similar between reviewer groups with a high degree of agreement and reviewer groups that disagreed to a greater extent. Only two reviewer groups with a large amount of disagreement (f-values of 82 and 34, respectively), that also had very low mean scores per group, had much lower acceptance ratios than all the other groups. Thus acceptance ratios are only influenced by an excessive amount of disagreement in groups with overall low scores.

Conclusion

The selection of abstracts to be read at a great conference with worldwide representation is an extremely difficult task. The scientific committee and the reviewers involved have

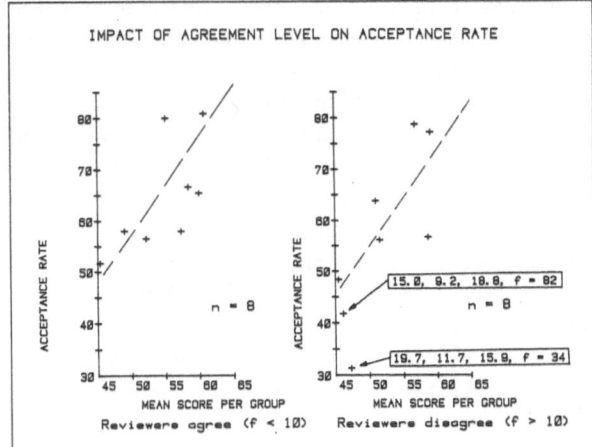

Fig. 8. Impact of agreement level on acceptance rate.

Fig. 9. Cartoon.

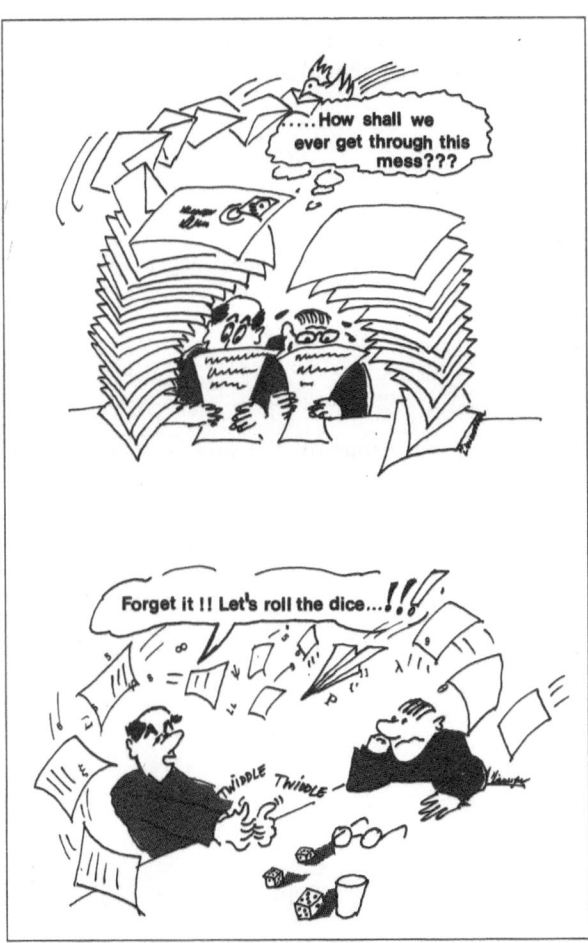

7

to insure the scientific quality of the papers actually represented, similarly to an editor-in-Chief for a medical journal. However, other factors like geographical distribution, the representation of topics that have to be presented and the exclusion of an excessive number of contributions for other topics are of similar importance. Like the editors of medical journals (1) we decided to have three internationally recognized reviewers judge the scientific standard of the papers. For this process we used a scoring system with a scale reaching from zero to 10. The scoring system held up for approximately three out of four papers discriminating them into the high quality papers to be accepted and into the lower quality papers to be rejected. One fourth of the papers had to be either selected or rejected because of other criteria like geographical reasons, technical reasons, over-representation by some authors, double or triple entries.

The review committee is confident that its selection process and its selection system, including test review and scoring system of three reviewers followed by statistical analysis, may hold up for other medical conferences to be used as a standard. This system appears to be fair in judging the great majority of papers; only on the occasions with excessive reviewers disagreement one should have more than 3 reviewers and should go into the process of possibly consulting a fourth or fifth reviewer prior to making the final judgement to avoid hardships (1).

At the onset of the review process the review committee was confronted with an enormous amount of high quality papers. Retrospectively should they have done it differently (Fig. 9)?

Acknowledgements

We gratefully acknowledge the secretarial assistance of Mr. Trude Haagen and Mrs. Ingrid Teufelhart.

Literature

1. Roberts William C: author-editor-reviewer: How the triumvirate is working at the AJC 51: A9–A10 (5), 1983.

Authors' address:
D. Glogar, M.D.
Kardiologische Univ. Klinik
Garnisongasse 13
A 1090 Wien, Austria

Coronary Circulation, Myocardial Energetics and Pumping Efficiency under Cardiac Pacing

D. Baller, H. J. Bretschneider, G. Hellige

Summary: To evaluate the effects of electrical stimulation of the heart on myocardial energetics 15 closed-chest experiments were carried out in anesthetized dogs.
Right atrial, right ventricular and AV-sequential pacing were intraindividually compared at identical rates over a wide range (70–220 beats/min) with special reference to catecholamine-induced variations of heart rate under maintained sinus rhythm. Myocardial blood flow was measured by a pressure difference catheter in the coronary sinus. Myocardial energy demand was calculated according to Bretschneider's equation from its hemodynamic determinants. Myocardial oxygen consumption (MVO_2) was markedly higher than the expected energy demand (E_t) under ventricular pacing. Compared to atrial pacing at identical rates MVO_2 was significantly ($p < 0.001$) higher with a mean oxygen wasting effect of 2.2 ml O_2/min 100 g. Under AV-sequential pacing MVO_2 was even higher as compared to ventricular pacing alone. Consequently cardiac efficiency was very low under ventricular pacing. It was markedly higher under atrial pacing with a mean increase of 63% over ventricular stimulation. Under AV-sequential pacing efficiency was only slightly increased as compared to ventricular pacing in spite of a higher cardiac output. Compared to atrial and sinus rhythm efficiency was, however, markedly decreased under sequential pacing.
The oxygen wasting effect of ventricular pacing and the deterioration of pumping efficiency under ventricular and sequential pacing probably result from the inhomogeneous contraction of the myocardium due to an abnormal spread of excitation.

Introduction

The hemodynamic effects of cardiac pacing have been extensively studied (1, 2).
It was the purpose of our study to evaluate the effects of three different modes of electrical stimulation of the heart on myocardial energetics.

Methods

Closed-chest experiments were carried out in 15 anesthetized dogs.
In the first group only ventricular pacing was used over a wide range of heart rates from 70 to 300 beats/min.
In the second group both atrial and ventricular pacing (70 to 220 beats/min) were intraindividually compared at identical rates with special reference to catecholamine-induced variations of heart rate under maintained sinus rhythm.
In addition, AV-sequential pacing was compared to both atrial and ventricular pacing in two experiments (90 to 200 beats/min) analysing 25 steady states.
Pacing rates were increased in steps of about 20 beats/min up to the maximally tolerated atrial rate of the AV-conduction system. Steady state conditions were accepted at hemodynamic, electrocardiographic and respiratory stability over five minutes. AV-sequential pacing was performed with an optimal AV-intervall leading to the highest cardiac output.

9

The observed effects were fully maintained during long-term pacing of two hours.

A transvenous pacing probe was advanced into the right atrium and into the apex of the right ventricle.

Myocardial blood flow was measured by a pressure difference catheter in the coronary sinus and was standardized on 100 gram left ventricular weight after autopsy.

Myocardial oxygen consumption (MVO_2) was calculated according to the Fick principle.

The expected energy demand of the heart was calculated from Bretschneider's equation which includes the major hemodynamic determinants of myocardial oxygen consumption such as heart rate, peak systolic pressure, peak rate of left ventricular pressure rise and an estimate of cardiac voume (3, 4).

Further details of the methods used have been described in previous papers (5, 6).

Although the coronary circulation was studied systematically under cardiac pacing in the normal and failing heart, this article focuses on the most interesting findings concerning myocardial energetics.

Results

In the first experimental group myocardial oxygen consumption markedly exceeded the expected energy demand calculated from its hemodynamic determinants under ventricular pacing. In contrast to this difference at unphysiologic origin and spread of excitation of the heart, at sinus rhythm a close correlation between calculated energy demand and directly measured O_2-consumption was obtained as demonstrated in previous studies.

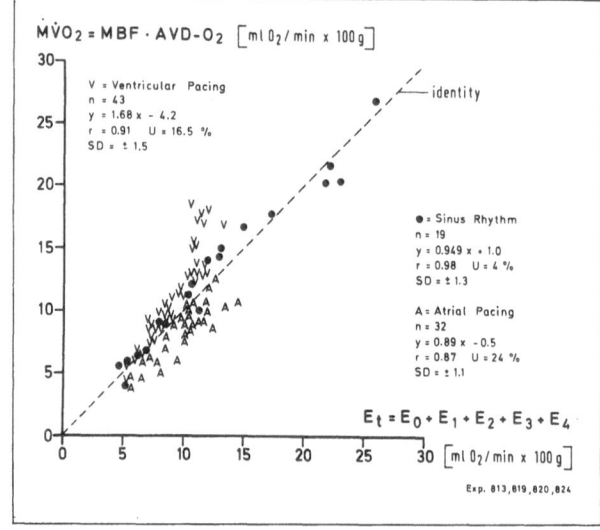

Fig. 1. Comparison of the effects of atrial and ventricular pacing on myocardial oxygen consumption (MVO_2) and myocardial energy demand calculated from its hemodynamic determinants. 32 intraindividual comparisons were analysed at identical rates. Sympathetic catecholamine stimulation served as a control group for the validity of the additive index E_t.
E_t: total energy demand of the left ventricle; E_0: basal energy demand of the artificially arrested heart in normothermia; E_1: energy demand of electrophysiologic processes; E_2: energy demand of maintenance of systolic wall tension; E_3: energy demand of tension development during isovolumetric contraction; E_4: approximated energy demand of inactivation of the contractile system. The mathematical equation has been described in previous papers (3, 4, 7).

At any heart rate under atrial pacing, however, actual O_2-consumption was significantly lower than the expected energy demand calculated from its hemodynamic determinants.

Fig. 1 summarizes the data on the comparison of ventricular and atrial pacing. During 32 steady states atrial and ventricular pacing were intraindividually compared at identical rates (2nd experimental group) including 11 data points at ventricular pacing alone with rates higher than 200 beats/min. Sinus rhythm points served as intraindividual controls for identity between measured and calculated energy demand.

These different effects of atrial and ventricular pacing on myocardial oxygen consumption could be demonstrated even without respect to its hemodynamic determinants as indicated in figure 2. Left ventricular oxygen consumption was significantly higher under ventricular pacing in this single experiment.

The different energetic effects of atrial and ventricular pacing are even more pronounced when considering external cardiac work and calculating myocardial pumping efficiency that is the ratio of O_2-equivalent of external work to myocardial oxygen consumption.

Cardiac efficiency was markedly higher under atrial pacing due to a higher cardiac output and a higher arterial pressure at simultaneously lower O_2-consumption. The mean value (22.5 ± 1%) was 63% higher under atrial pacing as compared to ventricular pacing (13.8 ± 1%). All differences between atrial and ventricular pacing were highly significant (p < 0.001).

Fig. 3 shows the effects of AV-sequential pacing on myocardial energetics. Directly measured O_2-consumption was again higher than expected energy demand under bifocal pacing. It was even higher as compared to ventricular pacing alone at identical rates due to increased left ventricular pressure and contractility resulting from the atrial contribution to left ventricular filling.

Cardiac efficiency was slightly increased under AV-sequential pacing as compared to ventricular pacing due to a higher cardiac output, but it was markedly decreased as com-

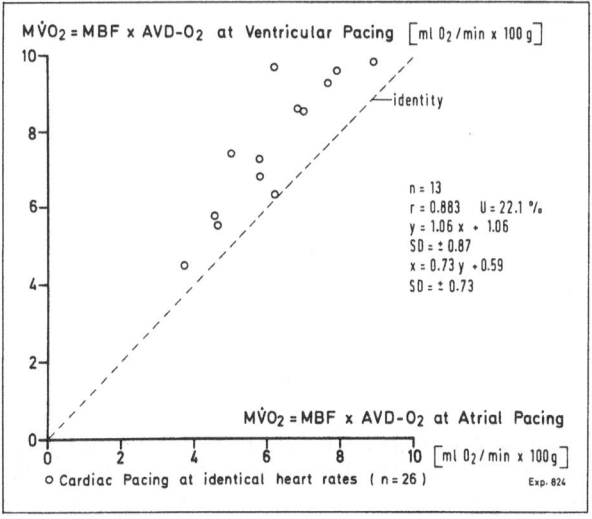

Fig. 2. Comparison of myocardial oxygen consumption ($M\dot{V}O_2$) under atrial and ventricular pacing at identical rates in a representative single experiment. Note that $M\dot{V}O_2$ is significantly higher under ventricular pacing.

Fig. 3. Comparison of measured O_2-consumption and calculated energy demand at atrial, ventricular and AV-sequential pacing. Note that $M\dot{V}O_2$ is higher during sequential pacing as compared to ventricular pacing alone (5 intraindividual comparisons). The 4 atrial pacing points have a lower O_2-consumption as compared to the other modes of cardiac excitation.

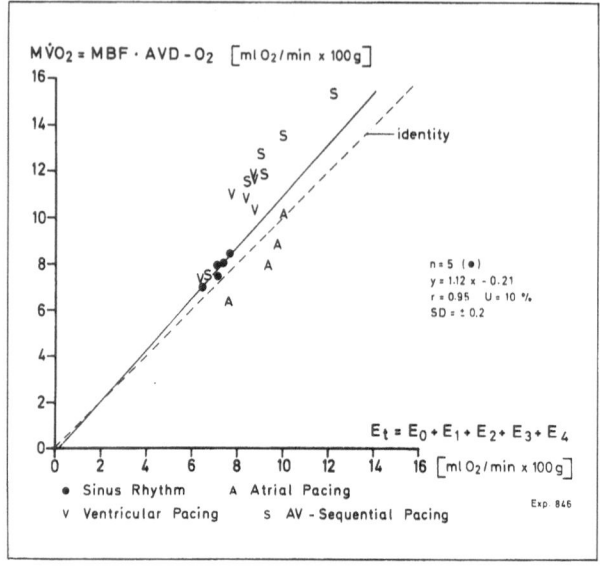

Fig. 4. Myocardial pumping efficiency is related to different pacing rates. Efficiency is marked lower under AV-sequential pacing as compared to atrial pacing and is only slightly higher as compared to ventricular pacing alone.

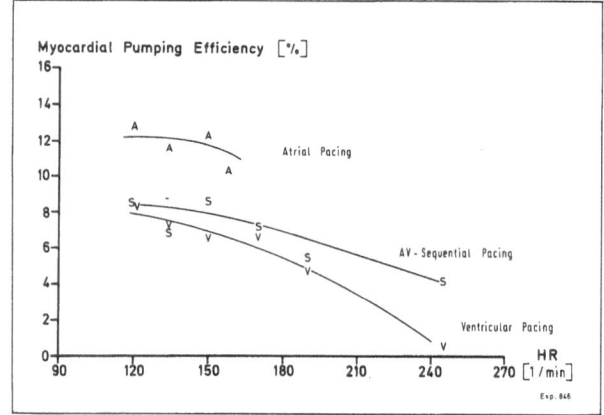

pared to atrial pacing due to markedly increased myocardial oxygen consumption as presented in fig. 4.

Discussion

Since little information is available on the effects of cardiac pacing on myocardial energetics, it was the specific aim of our study to evaluate the energetic effects of three different modes of electrical stimulation of the heart on myocardial oxygen consumption and

12

cardiac efficiency over a wide range of heart rates in an appropriate experimental model.

Conclusions:

1. Ventricular pacing exerts unfavorable effects on myocardial energetics due to an oxygen wasting effect as compared to atrial pacing and sinus rhythm (7).
2. Atrial pacing has beneficial effects on myocardial energy demand. It improves the relation of external cardiac work to myocardial oxygen consumption.
3. AV-sequential pacing seems to have unfavorable effects on myocardial energetics comparable to those of ventricular pacing alone.
4. The mechanism of the oxygen wasting effect under ventricular pacing is probably related to the inhomogeneous contraction of the myocardium due to an abnormal spread of excitation.

References

1. Sowton E: Haemodynamic studies in patients with artificial pacemakers. Brit Heart J 1964; 26: 737–746.
2. Samet P, Bernstein WH, Levine S, Lopez A: Hemodynamic effects of tachycardias produced by atrial and ventricular pacing. Amer J Med 1965; 39: 905–910.
3. Baller D, Bretschneider HJ, Hellige G: Validity of myocardial oxygen consumption parameters. Clin Cardiol 1979; 2: 317–327.
4. Baller D, Schenk H, Strauer BE, Hellige G: Myocardial oxygen consumption indices in man. Clin Cardiol 1980; 3: 116–122.
5. Baller D, Bretschneider HJ, Hellige G: A critical look at currently used indirect indices of myocardial oxygen consumption. Basic Res Cardiol 1981; 76: 163–181.
6. Baller D, Hoeft A, Korb H, Wolpers HG, Zipferl J, Hellige G: Basic physiological studies on cardiac pacing with special reference to the optimal mode and rate after cardiac surgery. Thoracic cardiovasc. Surgeon 1981; 29: 169–173.
7. Baller D, Wolpers HG, Zipfel J, Hoeft A, Hellige G: Unfavorable effects of ventricular pacing on myocardial energetics. Basic Res Cardiol 1981; 76: 115–123.

Authors' address:
Dr. D. Baller
Center of Physiology and Pathophysiology
Department of Experimental Cardiology
University of Goettingen
Humboldtallee 7
3400 Goettingen
West Germany

13

Effects of Alteration in Cardiac Pacemaker Site on Myocardial Contractile Response to Inotropic Stimulation and Exercise in Conscious Dogs

J. P. Vilaine, G. R. Heyndrickx, St. F. Vatner

Introduction

Normal cardiac excitation is followed by a rapid depolarization of the left ventricle through the Purkinje conduction system resulting in synchronized contraction. Previous work has shown that abnormal excitation of the left ventricle, such as occurs during ventricular pacing affects baseline hemodynamics, i.e. cardiac output and arterial pressure are depressed, while filling pressure rises (1,2). This depressant effect on myocardial performance has been attributed in part to the loss of atrial contribution to the filling of the left ventricle (3) and in part to a lack of synchronized ventricular contraction secondary to a delayed activation of muscle fibers during ventricular stimulation (4). In addition the myocardial work performed in the presence of ventricular pacing is less efficient compared to the same work performed during atrial pacing (5). The extent to which the abnormal ventricular activation will affect the left ventricular response to sympathetic stimulation is unknown. With this in mind, the goal of the present investigation was directed at comparing the myocardial contractile responses to sympathetic stimulation in the presence of a) spontaneous rhythm, b) atrial and c) ventricular pacing in conscious dogs.

Methods

Eight mongrel dogs wheighing between 25 and 35 kg were anesthetized with Na-pentobarbital 30 mg/kg i.v. Through a left thoracotomy in the fifth intercostal space, miniature pressure gauges were implanted within the left (L) ventricle (V) through a stab wound in the apex. Ultrasonic diameter transducers were implanted on opposing endocardial surfaces of the left ventricle and pacers were sutured to the right atrial appendage and right ventricle. Heparin filled catheters were implanted in the thoracic aorta (Fig. 1). Experiments were conducted 2 to 4 weeks postoperatively. While the conscious unsedated dogs rested quietly control records of left ventricular diameter and pressure, rate of change of diameter (dD/dt) i.e. the velocity of myocardial shortening, the rate of changes of pressures, dP/dt, arterial pressure and heart rate were obtained. These variables were continuously recorded during all interventions. Isoproterenol 0.2 μg/kg/min was infused intravenously. All animals were studied in spontaneous rhythm as well as with heart rate

Supported in part by Nationaal Fonds voor Wetenschappelijk Geneeskundig onderzoek, Grant 3.0012.81.

15

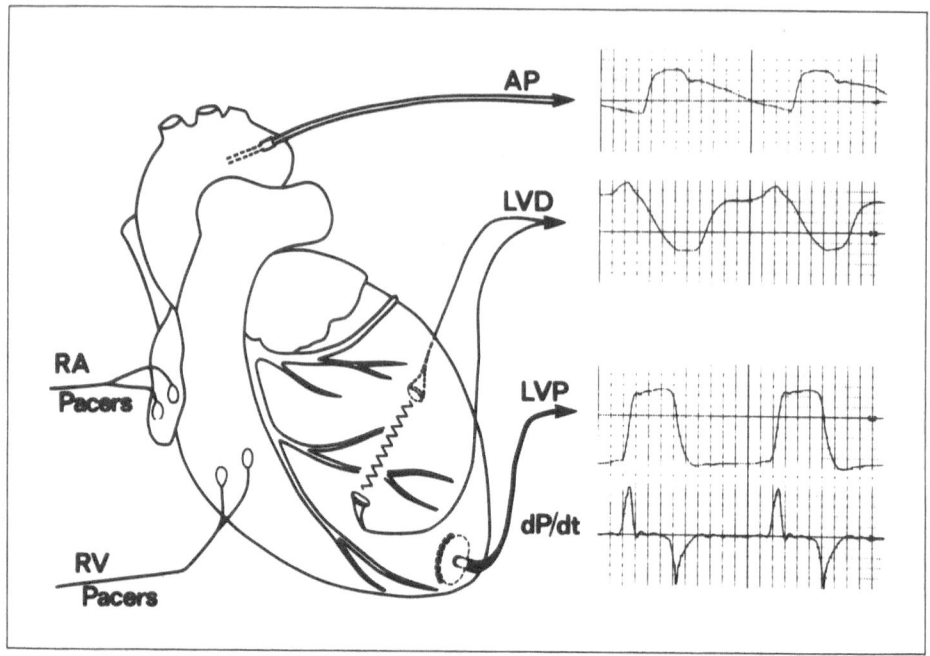

Fig. 1. Techniques used to measure left ventricular pressure and its first derivative and left ventricular diameter in conscious dogs.

kept constant using atrial or ventricular pacing at a rate similar as obtained during spontaneous rhythm.

In order to study the inotropic response to moderate exercise, all dogs were subjected to treadmill exercise, while all hemodynamic parameters were continuously monitored, again in spontaneous rhythm and with heart rate kept constant with either right atrial (RA) or right ventricular (RV) pacing. Data were recorded on a multichannel tape recorder and played back on a direct writing oscillograph at a paper speed of 100 mm/sec. The methods for measuring left ventricular diameter and pressure as well as for deriving dD/dt and dP/dt in conscious dogs have all been described in detail in previous publications (6).

Results

Inotropic response to isoproterenol during atrial and ventricular pacing

Isoproterenol infusion 0.2 μg/kg/min doubled heart rate and LV dP/dt while decreasing mean arterial pressure and LV end-diastolic diameter. During atrial stimulation by means of electrodes implanted on the right atrial appendage at a similar peak heart rate as obtained when heart rate was allowed to increase spontaneously with isoproterenol, mean arterial pressure and LV dP/dt were not different, but LV end-diastolic diameter fell due to a decreased time for ventricular filling. Under these conditions with isoproter-

16

enol about identical increases in LV dP/dt and decreases in mean arterial pressure were obtained, while LV end-diastolic diameter fell further. When right ventricular pacing was used to increase heart rate to the same level, mean arterial pressure was preserved but LV dP/dt fell and LV end-diastolic diameter was reduced to the same level as with atrial pacing. Isoproterenol still elicited a similar reduction in mean arterial pressure but the increase in LV dP/dt was markedly depressed. LV end-diastolic diameter fell similarly with isoproterenol in the presence of RV pacing as we observed with RA pacing (Fig. 2).

These data demonstrate markedly different responses of LV dP/dt to sympathetic stimulation by isoproterenol in the presence of abnormal RV depolarization as occurs with RV pacing as compared with either spontaneous rhythm or when RA pacing allowed relatively normal LV depolarization.

The difference could not be attributed to alteration in preload, suggesting that the atrial kick is of relative minor importance, and cannot explain the difference between inotropic response during atrial and ventricular pacing.

Inotropic response to exercise during atrial and ventricular pacing

To study a more physiological form of sympathetic stimulation, responses during exercise were compared.

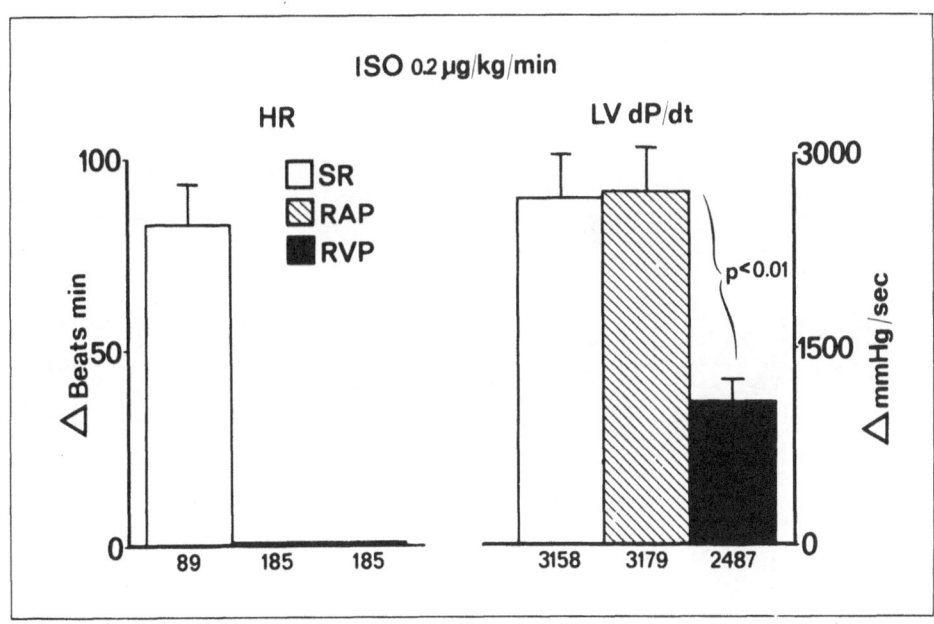

Fig. 2. During isoproterenol infusion 0.2 μg/kg/min left ventricular (LV) dP/dt and heart rate (HR) increased twofold in spontaneous rhythm. When heart rate was kept constant at peak heart response using atrial pacing LV dP/dt increased similarly. In contrast during RV pacing at the same rate increase in LV dP/dt during isoproterenol was markedly reduced.

During atrial pacing, at an identical rate as obtained during exercise with spontaneous rhythm, the increases in LV dP/dt were identical. In contrast, during ventricular pacing at a similar heart rate, the increases in LV dP/dt were considerably less (Fig. 3). Increases in mean arterial pressure did not differ in the three conditions.

Thus, the response of LV dP/dt with atrial and ventricular stimulation during exercise resembles the response observed during isoproterenol infusion.

Conclusion

Abnormal depolarization of the left ventricle during ventricular pacing results in an inappropriate inotropic response in terms of increase in LV dP/dt during isoproterenol infusion as well as during exercise. From these data it appears that the major cause for the decrease in the rate of pressure rise i.e. LV dP/dt is a delayed activation and subsequent lack of synchronized contraction rather than the loss of the atrial contraction.

References

1. Wiggers CF: Muscular reactions of the mammalian ventricles to artificial surface stimuli. Am J Physiol 1925: 73, 346–378.
2. Samet P, Bernstein WH, Levine S, Lopez A: Hemodynamic effects of tachycardia produced by atrial and ventricular pacing. Am J Med 1965: 39, 905–910.
3. Dagget WM, Bianco JA, Powell WJ Jr, Austen GW: Relative contributions of the atrial systole – ventricular systole interval and of patterns of ventricular activation to ventricualr function during electrical pacing of the dog heart. Circulation 1970: 27, 69–79.
4. Gilmore JP, Sarnoff SJ, Mitchell JH, Linden RJ: Synchronicity of ventricular contraction; Observations comparing hemodynamic effects of atrial and ventricular pacing. Brit Heart J 1963: 25, 299–307.

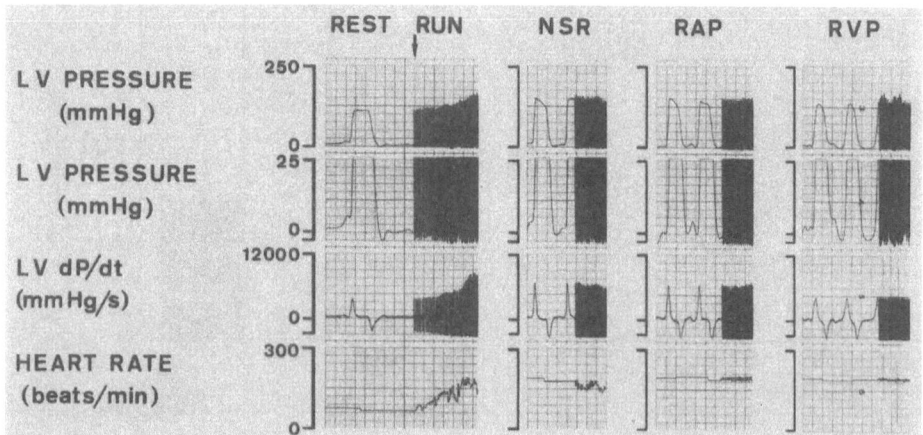

Fig. 3. During exercise with spontaneous rhythm the increase in LV dP/dt was comparable to the increase observed when heart rate was kept constant using atrial pacing (RAP). During right ventricular pacing (RVP) the increase in LV dP/dt during a similar exercise was markedly attenuated.

5. Baller D, Wolpers HG, Zipfel J, Hoeft A, Hellige G: Unfavourable effects of ventricular pacing on myocardial energetics. Basic Res Cardiol 1981: 76, 115–123.
6. Patrick TA, Vatner SF, Kemper WS, Franklin D: Telemetry of left ventricular diameter and pressure measurements from unrestrained animals. J Appl Physiol 1974: 37, 276–281.

Author's address:
Guy R. Heyndrickx, M.D.
Dept. of Cardiology
Akademisch Ziekenhuis
185 De Pintelaan
B-9000 Gent
Belgium

Effects of Reversible Cooling on Reentrant Tachycardia in Canine Infarction

N. El-Sherif, R. Mehra, W. B. Gough, R. H. Zeiler

Summary: Both sustained and nonsustained ventricular tachycardias were reproducibly induced in dogs 3–5 days following ligation of the left anterior descending coronary artery. Isochronal maps of ventricular activation were constructed from close bipolar electrograms recorded from the entire epicardial surface and selected intramural sites utilizing a computerized multiplexing technique. The induced tachycardias were due to reentrant activation in the surviving epicardial layer overlying the infarction. Cooling was applied to localized epicardial sites along the reentrant circuit to reversibly interrupt reentrant activation. The reentrant circuit could be consistently interrupted when cooling was applied to the distal part of the common reentrant wave front proximal to the site of earliest reactivation. Localized cooling of the site of earliest reactivation usually failed to interrupt reentry because the common reentrant wave front reactivated other sites close to the original reactivation site. Prior to interruption of reentry, cooling resulted in characteristic changes in conduction of the reentrant wave front. The study:
1. Fulfills Mines' criteria that circus movement reentry is the mechanism of the induced rhythms in this canine experimental model.
2. Identifies the critical site along the reentrant circuit where cryothermal ablation (or surgical interruption) of reentrant activation could be successfully accomplished.

Introduction

We have shown that ventricular arrhythmias induced by programmed stimulation in dogs 1 to 5 days post-infarction are due to reentrant circuits located in the surviving, although electrophysiologically abnormal, thin epicardial layer overlying the infarction (1, 2). These electrophysiological-anatomical correlative studies provide strong evidence for circus movement reentry. However to establish the reentrant mechanism, the reentrant circuit should be interrupted at one point resulting in termination of reentrant activation (Mines, 1914) (3). The present study was conducted to fulfill Mines criteria for proving the presence of circulating excitation as well as to identify the critical site along the reentrant circuit where interruption of reentrant activation could be successfully accomplished. For this purpose, we utilized reversible cooling of localized areas of the epicardial surface of the reentrant circuit.

Methods

In 18 mongrel dogs weighing 15–20 kg, the anterior descending coronary artery was ligated just distal to the anterior septal branch. Details of the surgical technique have been described (4). Three to five days following coronary artery ligation, the dogs were reanesthetized with sodium pentobarbital (30 mg/kg, iv) and maintained throughout the experiment with supplemental doses as required. The animal was ventilated with room air through an endotracheal tube using a Harvard positive pressure pump. A jugular vein was cannulated for the administration of fluids. Electrocardiographic lead II and femoral blood pressure were continuously monitored on an Electronics for Medicine DR10 electrophysiologic recorder. The heart was exposed through a left thoracotomy and cradled in the opened pericardium. Ventricular pacing was achieved via two fine Teflon-insulated stainless steel wires (0.005 inch in diameter) inserted by a 21-gauge hypodermic needle into the right ventricular wall. Both regular pacing and programmed premature stimulation were performed using a programmable digital stimulator (model DTU-101 MVA, Bloom Associates, Ltd.). Details of the stimulation protocol were described previously (2). In each experiment, a stimulation protocol was selected that resulted in the induction of a reproducible monomorphic ventricular rhythm.

Once a reproducible ventricular rhythm was established, 62 simultaneous bipolar electrode recordings were obtained utilizing a sock electrode. A higher density of electrodes (approximately 6–10 mm between pairs) covered the area of the infarction and the border zones and a lower density (approximately 15 mm), the remaining surface of the heart. In some experiments a patch electrode was also utilized to obtain epicardial recordings at closer interelectrode distance (4 mm). Intramural recordings were obtained with specially designed 21-gauge needles. Details of the recording techniques, the mapping system and the methods for construction of epicardial isochronal maps were previously reported (1–2). After termination of the electrophysiological study the anatomy of the infarction and the locations of intramural recording sites were determined and correlated with epicardial recording sites as previously reported (1–2).

Cryothermal techniques:

The cryothermal system was a Spembley-Amoils BMS 411 cryo unit (5). This apparatus regulates the flow of nitrous oxide through the tip of the cryoprobe. The cryoprobe utilized in the study (No. 7107) had a flat tip 12 mm in diameter. Local epicardial temperature could be measured by a thermocouple at the tip of the probe and intramural temperature by a needle thermistor. For reversible interruption of reentrant activation, the myocardial temperature at a localized epicardial site was reduced to between − 5 °C and + 5 °C for 10–30 seconds (6). Different epicardial sites were tested and the effects of transient epicardial cooling on ventricular activation patterns were analyzed. Sometimes transient cooling of two contiguous sites was performed in which case the probe was rapidly moved to the second site to achieve local cooling before the effects of cooling on the first site had expired. Alternatively, cryoablation was applied to one site and transient cooling to a contiguous site.

Results

A reproducible monomorphic ventricular rhythm could be induced by programmed stimulation in 16 of 18 dogs. In 3 dogs, the reentrant circuit could not be completely identified on the epicardial surface. In these dogs, cryothermal interruption of possible reentrant activations was not tried. In the remaining 13 dogs, isochronal mapping successfully identified an epicardial reentrant circuit. In these dogs, programmed stimulation reproducibly initiated a sustained monomorphic ventricular tachycardia (lasting for more than one minute) in 4 dogs and short runs of a monomorphic ventricular rhythm (2–10 beats)

22

in 9 dogs. The rate of the induced ventricular rhythms ranged from 240 to 360/min. Cryothermal interruption of the reentrant circuit could be consistently accomplished in each of the 13 dogs. The results from these experiments will be presented here.

Figure 1 illustrates electrocardiographic recordings from one of the experiments in which a sustained monomorphic ventricular tachycardia was reproducibly induced by programmed stimulation. Panel A shows the control recording. Pacing was applied to the base of the right ventricle at a basic cycle length (S_1–S_1) of 360 msec. Two premature stimuli (S_2 and S_3) were introduced at a coupling interval of 200 and 190 msec, respectively, and initiated a sustained ventricular tachycardia at a cycle length of 190–200 msec. Panel B illustrates reversible termination of the tachycardia by cooling and shows significant lengthening of the last cycle of the tachycardia prior to termination. Panels C and D illustrate the effect of cooling on the induction of the tachycardia. Panel C was obtained after localized epicardial cooling to 0 °C was applied for 20 seconds. Programmed premature stimulation could only initiate a single beat with markedly prolonged coupling compared to control. Panel D was obtained after 30 seconds of cooling at 0 °C and shows that programmed stimulation failed to initiate the reentrant tachycardia.

Figure 2 shows the control epicardial isochronal map and selected electrograms during ventricular tachycardia from the same experiment. The shaded area in the right upper panel represents the visible epicardial border of the infarction and the solid circles, the position of epicardial electrodes. The isochronal map in the right lower panel was drawn at 20 msec intervals. The reentrant circuit had a characteristic figure of 8 activation pattern (1, 2). It consisted of two separate arcs of functional conduction block (represented by the heavy solid lines) and two circulating wave fronts; one clockwise around the upper arc and the other, counterclockwise around the lower arc. The two wave fronts joined

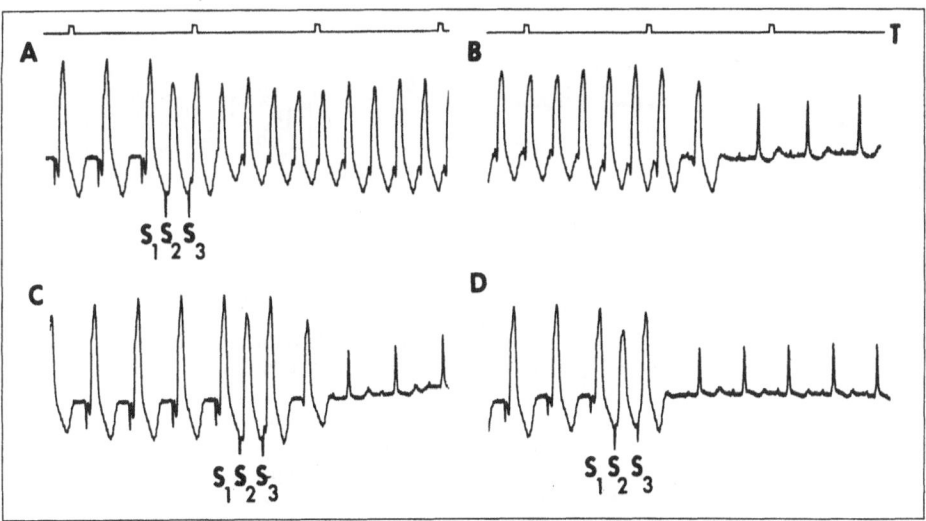

Fig. 1. Electrocardiographic recordings from an experiment in which a sustained monomorphic tachycardia was reproducibly induced by programmed stimulation. Panel A shows control recording. Panal B shows cooling induced termination of the tachycardia. Panels C and D show the effect of cooling on tachycardia induction. See Text for details.

23

into a common wave front that conducted slowly between the two arcs before reactivating an area on the septal border of the infarction. The left panel in figure 2 illustrates selected simultaneous electrograms from critical sites along the reentrant pathway. Specifically, electrograms recorded along the two arcs of functional conduction block as well as the common reentrant wave front are shown. The electrograms depict the presence of diastolic bridging between successive reentrant beats.

Figure 3 illustrates the effect of reversible cooling at two different epicardial sites along the reentrant circuit during ventricular tachycardia from the same experiment. Panel A of the figure illustrates the isochronal map of the control reentrant circuit and selected epi-

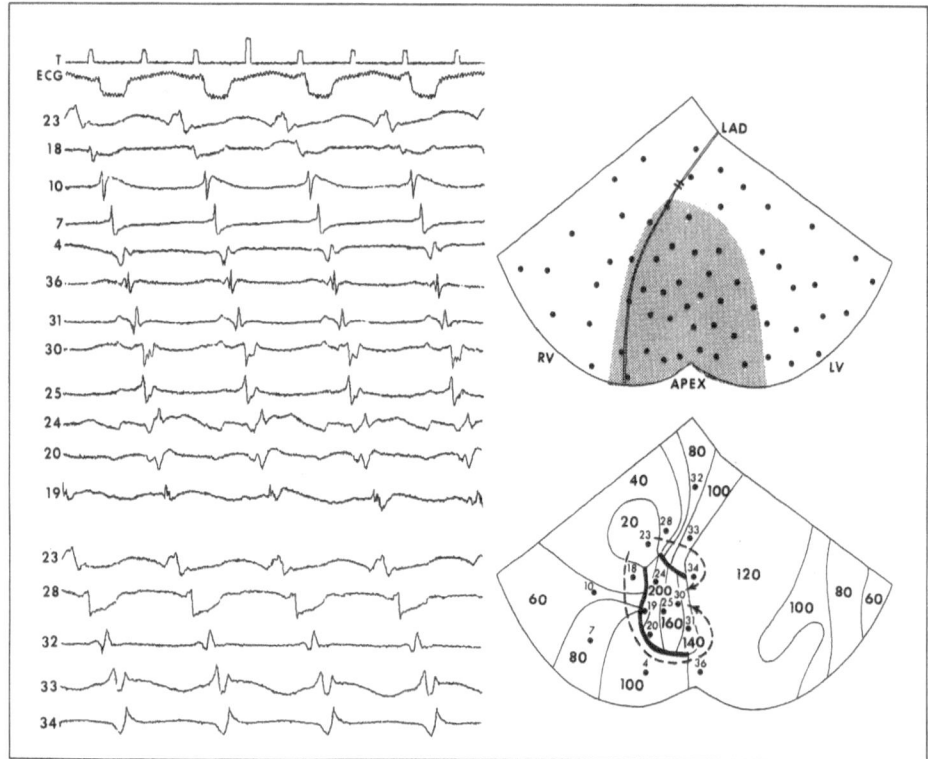

Fig. 2. Isochronal map of epicardial activation during the control ventricular tachycardia shown in Figure 1. The epicardial surface is depicted as if the ventricles were folded out after a cut was made from the crux to the apex. The top left and right borders represent the right and left atrioventricular junctions. The two curvilinear surfaces on the right and left are contiguous and extend from the posterior base to the apex of the heart. The double bar represents the site of left anterior descending coronary artery (LAD) ligation. The shaded area represents the visible epicardial border of the infarction and the solid circles, the position of epicardial electrodes. The isochronal map in the right lower panel was drawn at 20 msec intervals. The reentrant circuit has a characteristic figure of 8 activation pattern. See text for details. The left panel shows selected simultaneous electrograms recorded along the two arcs of functional conduction block (represented by the heavy solid lines) and the common reentrant wave front and depict the presence of diastolic bridging between reentrant beats. RV and LV = right and left ventricles, respectively.

cardial electrograms. The cryoprobe (shaded circles) was applied either to the site of earliest reactivation (panel B) or to the distal part of the common reentrant wave front (panel C). At the earliest reactivation site, represented by electrogram 23, the slow common reentrant wave front first reexcited myocardial zones on the other side of the arcs of conduction block. Electrogram 23 preceded the onset of surface QRS by 30 msec. Cooling resulted in conduction block between site 24, located along the distal part of the common reentrant wave front, and the early reexcitation site 23. Before cooling, electrogram 23 had two components, one, a low amplitude slow deflection approximately synchronous with the activation potential at site 24 and represented a passive far field or electrotonic potential. The second component was a larger, relatively sharp potential that represented the moment of local activation. When cooling induced conduction block between sites 24 and 23 the electronic potential was still recorded synchronous with the activation potential at 24. On the other hand, the activation potential at 23 was markedly delayed and occurred after the onset of the surface QRS. The isochronal map after cooling showed significant changes in the position of the upper arc of conduction block and the clockwise directed wave front. However, the common reentrant wave front still reexcited site 18 on the proximal border of the arc of block. This site was adjacent to the original site of early reactivation (site 23). Thus, cooling the original site of early reactivation did not interrupt the reentrant circuit but rather resulted in a shift of the early reexcitation site. Conduction of the common reentrant wave front to the new reexcitation site (site 24 to site 18) was slower compared to control (site 24 to site 23) and resulted in a 20 msec increase in the tachycardia cycle length.

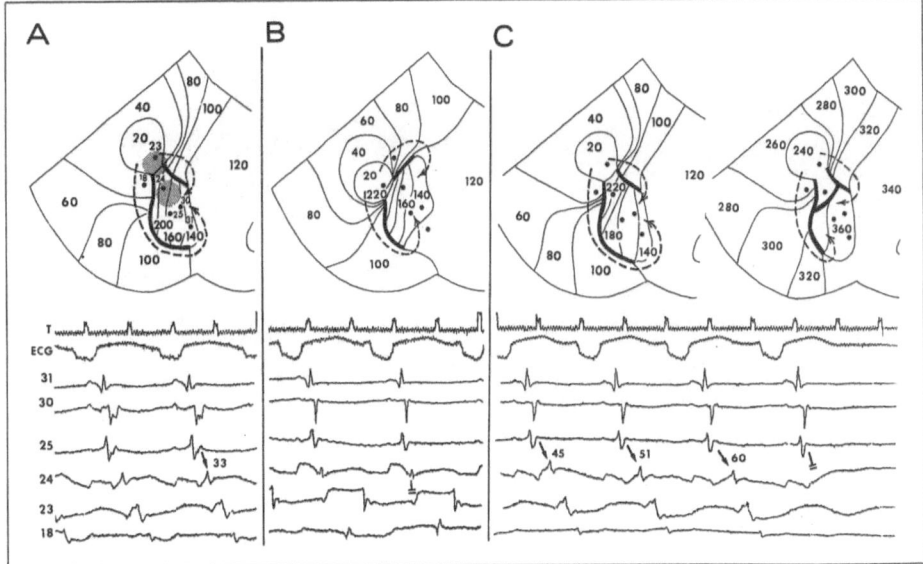

Fig. 3. The effects of reversible cooling when the cryoprobe (shaded circles) was applied either to the site of earliest activation (panel B) or to the distal part of the common reentrant wave front (panel C). Panel A shows control map. Selected epicardial electrograms are shown on the bottom. See text for details.

Panel C of Figure 3 shows that when cooling was applied to the distal part of the common reentrant wave front the reentrant circuit was interrupted. During control, the conduction time between proximal electrode site 25 and the more distal site 24 was 33 msec. Prior to termination of the tachycardia, an incremental beat to beat increase of the conduction time between sites 25 and 24 occurred associated with equal increases in the tachycardia cycle length. When conduction block developed between the two sites, the reentrant circuit was terminated and electrogram 24 recorded an electrotonic potential but no local activation potential. This was represented on the isochronal map by an arc of conduction block (heavy solid line) that joined the two separate arcs of conduction block into one.

Figure 4 was obtained from the same experiment and illustrates the effect of cooling of the distal part of the common reentrant wave front on the induction of the reentrant tachycardia. The isochronal maps in panels A to C represent, respectively, the epicardial activation pattern of the S_3 stimulated beat during control (A), following cooling at 0 °C for 20 seconds (B) and following cooling at 0 °C for 30 seconds (C). During S_3 stimulation, a continuous arc of functional conduction block developed with two circulating wave fronts, clockwise around the upper end of the arc and counterclockwise around the lower end. The two wave fronts joined into a slow common wave front that reactivated normal

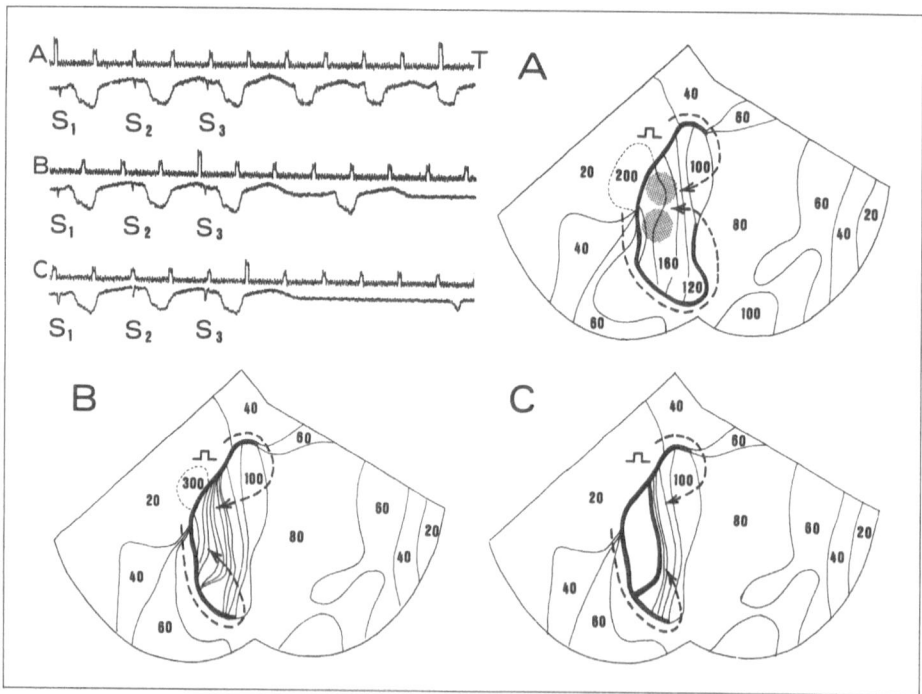

Fig. 4. The effects of reversible cooling on tachycardia induction. The isochronal maps in panels A to C represent, the epicardial activation pattern of the S_3 stimulated beat during control (A), following cooling at 0 °C for 20 seconds (B) and following cooling at 0 °C for 30 seconds (C). See text for details.

26

myocardial zones on the proximal side of the arc of block to initiate the first reentrant beat. The earliest reactivation zone is represented by the dotted line. Note that the arc of conduction block following S_3 stimulation was much longer compared to the arcs of block during subsequent reentrant beats. The common reentrant wave front was also much broader. As a consequence, cooling (shaded circles) has to be applied to a larger area of the distal part of the common reentrant wave front to prevent the induction of the tachycardia. In panel B, cooling resulted in marked slowing of conduction of the distal part of the common reentrant wave front. This accounted for the marked lengthening of the coupling interval of the reentrant beat. The subsequent turnaround of reentrant activation was blocked proximal to the area of markedly slowed conduction (not shown in the figure). This explained the occurrence of a single reentrant beat following S_3 stimulation. In panel C, following a longer period of cooling, S_3 failed to initiate the reentrant tachycardia due to block of conduction of the common reentrant wave front proximal to the cooled zone.

Discussion

During self-sustained reentrant activation, the wave front will move at the maximum velocity permitted by the state of recovery (i.e. the duration of the effective refractory period) of the myocardium (7). Any lengthening of the effective refractory period of a localized but critically located myocardial zone along the reentrant pathway will be directly reflected in changes in conduction. In the present study, cooling-induced lengthening of the effective refractory period (8) of localized zones of the epicardial layer where the common reentrant wave front was located did result in slowing of conduction and/or conduction block. Because the reentrant circuit was located in a 1–3 mm thick epicardial layer (1, 2) with reduced myocardial blood flow (9) overlying a core of necrotic myocardium, cryoprobe application to the epicardial surface resulted in sufficient cooling across the entire epicardial layer.

The present study has clearly demonstrated that reentrant activation could be successfully interrupted when cooling or cryoablation is applied to the part of the common reentrant wave front immediately proximal to the zone of earliest reactivation. At this site, the common reentrant wave front is usually narrow and is surrounded on each side by an arc of functional conduction block. On the other hand, localized cooling to the site of earliest reactivation commonly failed to interrupt reentry. The common reentrant wave front usually broke through the arc of functional conduction block to reactivate other sites close to the original reactivation site without necessarily changing the overall reentrant activation pattern. Usually, however, the reentrant cycle length increased by 10 to 30 msec.

Recent clinical studies advanced the notion of an earliest site of ventricular activation during possible reentrant rhythms. At this site, electrograms – mostly on the endocardial side – were recorded 2–48 msec before the onset of the surface QRS complex (10). Surgical excision of this site was reported to have resulted in termination of the ventricular tachycardia (11). In the present study, electrograms representing the earliest reactivation site preceded the surface QRS by 10–40 msec. However, cooling application to this site usually failed to interrupt reentrant activation. On the other hand, electrograms representing the distal portion of the common reentrant wave front from where the reentrant

27

circuit could be consistently interrupted preceded the surface QRS by 40 to 80 msec. It is possible that the anatomic-electrophysiologic characteristics of reentrant circuits in these clinical studies were significantly different from reentrant circuits in the present canine model. However, another plausible explanation is that the surgical excision in these studies was in fact extensive and included, in addition to the site of earliest reactivation, parts of the common reentrant wave front. Since the main advantage of cryoablation is that the resulting cryolesion is a localized and sharply demarcated homogeneous scar (12), it is obvious that in order to minimize the area of the cryolesion, precise localization of the site from which the reentrant circuit could be successfully interrupted must be accomplished.

The early studies of Mayer (13), Mines (3) and Garrey (14) have clearly established that circulating excitation could be initiated in simple rings of excitable tissue. The criteria for proving the presence of circulating excitation as established by Mines were (3):

1. An area of unidirectional block must be demonstrated.
2. The movement of the excitatory wave should be observed to progress through the pathway, to return to its point of origin, and then to again follow the same pathway.
3. "The best test for circulating excitation is to cut through the ring at one point. If impulses continue to arise in the cut ring, circus movement as a cause can be ruled out."

Suprisingly enough, no single arrhythmia in a mammalian heart has been demonstrated, to date, to fulfill all of Mines' three criteria for a definite proof of reentry (15). The present study by satisfying all of Mines' three criteria establishes, beyond any reasonable doubt, that circus movement reentry is the mechanism of the observed tachyarrhythmias. The study also demonstrates the fact that the configuration of the reentrant circuit in the mammalian ventricles (and most probably in the atria as well) is significantly different from that originally described in simple rings of excitable tissue. The reentrant circuit here, has a figure of 8 activation pattern whereby two circulating wave fronts advance in a clockwise and counterclockwise direction, respectively, around two zones (arcs) of unidirectional block. The two circulating wave fronts coalesce into a common reentrant wave front that conducts between the two zones of block before reexciting myocardium on the other side of the zones of block. The reentrant circuit could be successfully terminated only from localized areas along the common reentrant wave front. It should be emphasized that the localization of the reentrant circuit in a thin epicardial layer in the present study is only a reflection of the particular anatomy of this infarction. Depending on the distribution of myocardil pathology, reentrant circuits could also be expected to be located in the subendocardial and intramyocardial zones. However, irrespective of the anatomical localization of the circuit its configuration probably has to conform with the figure of 8 model.

References

1. El-Sherif N, Mehra R, Gough WB, Zeiler RH: Ventricular activation pattern of spontaneous and induced ventricular rhythms in canine one-day-old myocardial infarction. Evidence for focal and reentrant mechanisms. Circ Res 1982; 51: 152–166.
2. Mehra R, Zeiler RH, Gough WB, El-Sherif N: Reentrant ventricular arrhythmias in the late myocardial infarction period. 9. Electrophysiologic-anatomic correlation of reentrant circuits. Circulation 1983; 67: 11–24.

3. Mines GR: On circulating excitations in heart muscles and their possible relation to tachycardia and fibrillation. Trans Roy Soc Can Ser 3, Sect IV 1914; 8: 43–52.
4. El-Sherif N, Scherlag BJ, Lazzara R: Reentrant ventricular arrhythmias in the late myocardial infarction period. I. Conduction characteristics in the infarction zone. Circulation 1977; 55: 686–701.
5. Camm J, Ward DE, Spurrell RAJ, Reese GM: Cryothermal mapping and cryoablation in the treatment of refractory cardiac arrhythmias. Circulation 1980; 62: 67–74.
6. Gallagher JJ, Sealy WC, Anderson RW, Kasell J, Millar R, Campbell RW, Harrison L, Pritchett ELC, Wallace AG: Cryosurgical ablation of accessory atrioventricular connections. A method for the correction of the preexcitation syndrome. Circulation 1977; 55: 471–484.
7. Moe GK, Rheinboldt WC, Abildskov JA: A computer model of atrial fibrillation. Am Heart J 1964; 67: 200–220.
8. Wallace AG, Mignone RJ: Physiologic evidence concerning the re-entry hypothesis for ectopic beats. Amer Heart J 1966; 72: 60–70.
9. Hirzel HO, Nelson GR, Sonnenblick EH, Kirk ES: Redistribution of collateral blood flow from necrotic to surviving myocardium following coronary occlusion in the dog. Circ Res 1976; 39: 214–222.
10. Horowitz LN, Josephson ME, Harken AH: Epicardial and endocardial activation during sustained ventricular tachycardia in man. Circulation 1980; 6: 1227–1238.
11. Horowitz LN, Josephson ME, Harken AH: Ventricular resection guided by epicardial and endocardial mapping for treatment of recurrent ventricular tachycardia. N Engl J Med 1980; 302: 589–597.
12. Klein GJ, Harrison L, Ideker R, Smith WM, Kassell J, Wallace AG, Gallagher JJ: Reaction of the myocardium to cryosurgery: Electrophysiology and arrhythmogenic potential. Circulation 1979; 59: 364–372.
13. Mayer AG: Rhythmical pulsation in Scyphomedusae: II. Carnegia Inst Wash, Papers, Tortugar Lab. 1: 113–131, Carnegie Inst Wash Publ No 102, part VIII, 1908.
14. Garrey WE: The nature of fibrillary contractions of the heart. Its relation to tissue mass and form. Am J Physiol 1914; 33: 397–408.
15. Wit AL, Cranefield PF: Reentrant excitation as a cause of cardiac arrhythmias. In Levy MN, Vassalle M (eds): Excitation and Neural Control of the Heart, Bethesda, Maryland, American Physiological Society, 1982; pp 113–148.

Authors' address:
Nabil El-Sherif, M.D.
Brooklyn VA Medical College
Cardiology
800 Poly Place
Brooklyn, NY 11209
USA

Electropharmacology of Diltiazem in a Chronic Canine Myocardial Infarction, Ventricular Tachyarrhythmia Model

Masahito Naito, Makoto Miyairi, Tetsuyoshi Asato, Hideki Nagoshi, Masasada Honda, Eric L. Michelson, Leonard S. Dreifus

Summary: The electropharmacology of diltiazem was evaluated in 11 dogs with chronic myocardial infarction susceptible to the initiation of sustained ventricular tachyarrhythmias (VTs) using programmed pacing. Dogs were studied open chest under pentobarbital anesthesia both before and after either 0.2 (N = 5), 0.4 (N = 5) or 0.8 mg/kg (N = 5) intravenous diltiazem infused over 5 minutes. Two doses were studied in 4 dogs. The maximal changes in heart rate, AH, HV and QTc intervals, QRS duration and sinus node recovery time were determined. Mean transmyocardial conduction times from endocardium to epicardium, and excitability thresholds and ventricular refractory periods in both normal and infarct tissue were also determined. Although diltiazem had significant dose-related effects on the heart rate, AH interval and sinus node recovery time at these dosages, diltiazem had no significant effect on the transmyocardial conduction times, excitability thresholds or ventricular refractory periods of either normal or chronically infarcted myocardium. Correspondingly, diltiazem also failed to prevent the initiation of either ventricular tachycardia or fibrillation by programmed pacing in any of these 11 dogs.

Recently, chronic myocardial infarction models susceptible to the initiation of ventricular tachyarrhythmias have become available in which it is possible to evaluate the electropharmacologic properties of various antiarrhythmic agents including several investigational ones (1–4). However, the efficacy of various calcium-channel inhibitory agents in these models has not yet been fully evaluated. The objective of this study was to evaluate the electropharmacology of diltiazem in a chronic canine myocardial infarction, ventricular tachyarrhythmia model.

Methods

Eleven healthy adult dogs weighing 14 to 17 kg were studied open chest under pentobarbital anesthesia. The animals were studied 3 to 10 days after a two-stage, 2 hour occlusion and reperfusion of the mid left anterior descending coronary artery. At the time of study, plunge electrodes were placed in both endocardial and epicardial sites within the normal sites within the distribution of non-occluded vessels as well as the area of infarction.

Each of the dogs selected for this study was reproducibly susceptible to the initiation of sustained ventricular tachyarrhythmias using routine methods of programmed ventricular pacing with one, two or three ventricular extrastimuli. Ventricular pacing was done at a basic cycle length of 300 msec using unipolar cathodal stimulation both for tachyarrhythmia initiation and to determine strength-interval relations from measurements of excitability and refractoriness at each pacing site. Atrial pacing at a cycle length of 300 msec

31

was done to serially evaluate transmyocardial conduction times and various electrocardiographic parameters including the basic cycle length, PR, QRS, and QTc interval; AH and HV intervals as well as the sinus node recovery time.

After determining each dog's baseline susceptibility to arrhythmia initiation and measuring baseline electrophysiologic data, dogs received either 0.2 (N = 5), 0.4 (N = 5) or 0.8 (N = 5) mg/kg of diltiazem intravenously over 5 minutes. Two doses were studied in each of four dogs. At the completion of the infusion, all electrocardiographic and electrophysiologic parameters were again determined. Animals were then reevaluated to determine whether diltiazem prevented the re-initiation of sustained ventricular tachyarrhythmias using 1, 2 and 3 ventricular extrastimuli.

Results

Table 1 summarizes mean maximal change from baseline for several parameters following diltiazem infusion. After diltiazem was given, heart rate decreased, AH interval and sinus node recovery time increased, and the systolic blood pressure decreased transiently. These changes occurred in a dose-related manner. However, diltiazem had no significant effects on either the HV, QRS or QTc intervals at any of these dosages.

Typical strength-interval curves from normal tissue during pacing cycle length of 300 msec are shown in Fig. 1. The coupling interval in milliseconds is on the abscissa and the current of the extrastimulus in milliamps is on the ordinate. These curves were generated by shortening the coupling intervals of the extrastimuli with increasing the current of extrastimuli up to 10 mA. At this normal site, the excitability threshold was very low, 0.08 milliamps and there was a rapid and smooth transition to the effective refractory period (ERP) measured using 10 milliamps current, the maximum output of our isolator, The VRP, or ventricular refractory period measured using twice threshold current is also detailed.

As shown in this Figure 1, typically, at a normal site following diltiazem infusion, the strength-interval curve was displaced minimally to the right with no change in its overall configuration. However, changes in excitability threshold or ventricular refractory period were minimal.

Table 1. Mean Maximal Change from Baseline

Diltiazem mg/kg	HR (bpm)	BP (mmHg)	AH (msec)	HV	QRS	QTc	SNRT
0.2	−25*	−11	42*	6	0	0	88*
0.4	−34*	−18	80*	2	5	25	133*
0.8	−44*	−23	92*	1	0	17	156*
						(*p < 0.05)	

Abbreviations:
  BP: systolic blood pressure
  bpm: beats per minute
  HR: heart rate
  SNRT: sinus node recovery time

In Fig. 2, the typical strength-interval curves obtained from a mildly abnormal infarct site are shown. The excitability threshold at this infarct site was 0.16 milliamps, the ventricular refractory period was slightly prolonged compared to normal sites, and there were abnormal inflections in the strength-interval curves. After diltiazem was given, the strength-interval curve was again displaced to the right, and changes in excitability threshold and refractory periods were again minimal.

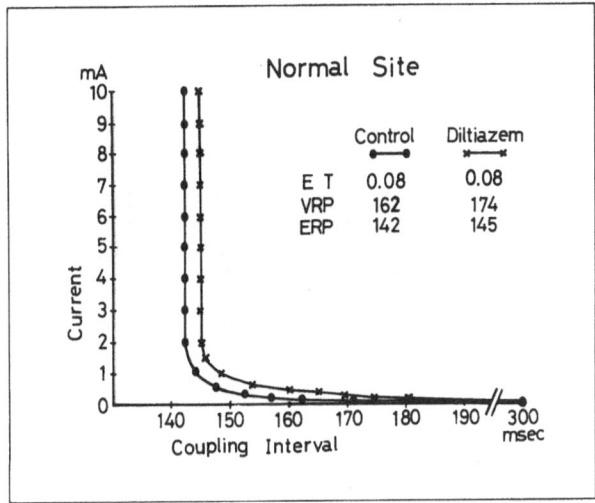

Fig. 1. Typical strength-interval curves obtained from normal tissue at a cycle length of 300 msec are shown. The excitability threshold (ET) was very low at this normal site and there was a rapid and smooth transition to the refractory period measured with 10 milliamps current. VRP is the twice threshold ventricular refractory period and ERP or effective refractory period is defined as the refractory period measured using the maximum output of the isolator, 10 milliamps. Following diltiazem infusion, the strength-interval curve was displaced to the right with no changes in its overall configuration and changes in ET or VRP were minimal.

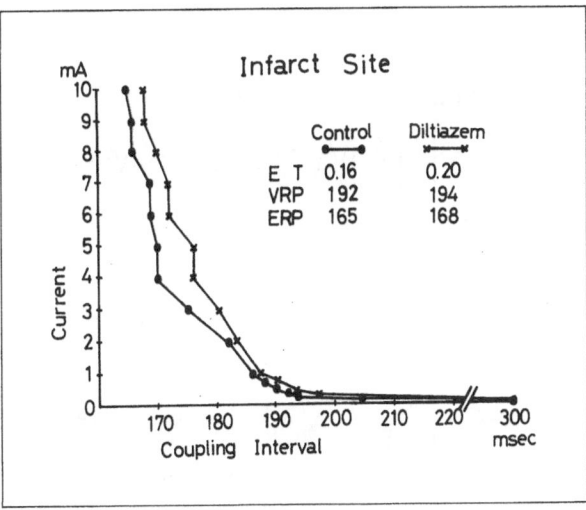

Fig. 2. These are typical strength-interval curves from a mildly abnormal infarct site. At this infarct site, the ET was 0.16 msec. The refractory periods were longer and there were abnormal inflections in the strength-interval curves. After diltiazem was given, the strength-interval curve was again displaced to the right, but changes in ET or refractory periods were minimal. Abbreviations are same as in Figure 1.

Table 2 demonstrates the mean maximal electrophysiologic effects of diltiazem both in normal and infarct tissue. Diltiazem had no significant effects on the conduction times, excitability thresholds or ventricular refractory periods of either normal or chronically infarcted myocardium.

Correspondingly, diltiazem showed no efficacy in preventing ventricular tachyarrhythmias in this chronic model. A typical example of arrhythmia inducibility both before and after diltiazem infusion is shown in Figure 3. In this example, ventricular fibrillation was initiated reproducibly with 3 extrastimuli at baseline and again after diltiazem infusion. Overall, 8 animals had ventricular fibrillation and 3 had ventricular tachycardia prior to diltiazem, but re-initiation of these ventricular tachyarrhythmias was not prevented in any of these 11 animals following the administration of diltiazem.

Table 2. Mean Maximal Electrophysiologic Effects of Diltiazem in Normal (N) and Infarct (I) Tissue

Diltiazem (mg/kg)	CTs (msec)		ET (mA)		VRP (msec)	
	N	I	N	I	N	I
0.2	2	3	0.01	0.01	11	11
0.4	0	0	0.04	0.01	6	4
0.8	0	0	0.02	0.02	5	8
N vs I	$p = NS$		$p = NS$		$p = NS$	

Abbreviations:
CTs: transmyocardial conduction times
ET: excitability threshold
I: infarct sites
N: normal sites
NS: statistically not significant
VRP: ventricular refractory period

Fig. 3. A typical example of arrhythmia inducibility both before and after diltiazem infusion is shown. S_1 is the pacing stimulus of basic drive, and S_2, S_3 or S_4 are those of extrastimuli. In this example, re-initiation of ventricular fibrillation (VF) was not prevented after diltiazem infusion.

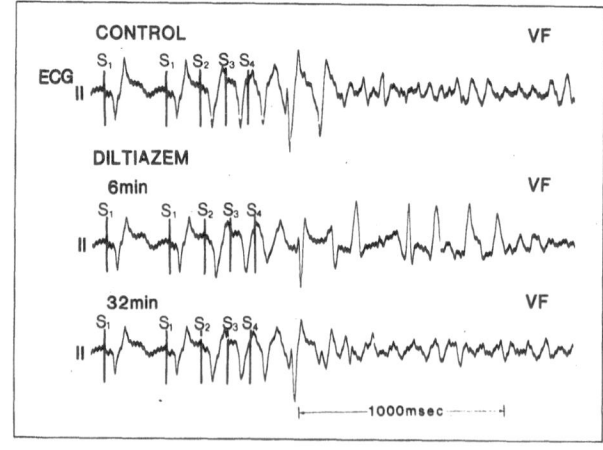

Discussion

Although this model is a rather severe one for testing antiarrhythmic agents, Michelson et al. (5, 6) have shown that procaine amide and meobentine sulfate prevented reinitiation of ventricular tachyarrhythmias. Notably, these drugs prolonged ventricular refractory periods within the area of chronically infarcted myocardium. However, lidocaine showed only minimal electrophysiologic changes in either normal or abnormal myocardium and almost no efficacy in preventing ventricular tachyarrhythmias (7). Garan et al. (4) found verapamil to be an ineffective antiarrhythmic agent in their model. Since diltiazem is an another calcium-channel inhibitory agent it was expected that the drug slowed heart rate, prolonged AH interval and sinus node recovery time as revealed in this study. But diltiazem did not show significant electrophysiologic alterations and thus was not effective in preventing the re-initiation of sustained ventricular tachyarrhythmias in this chronic canine myocardial infarction model.

As the effects of an antiarrhythmic agent in this model parallel those effects seen in patients studied in clinical electrophysiological laboratory with sustained ventricular tachyarrhythmias, the efficacy of diltiazem for ventricular tachyarrhythmias in patients with chronic myocardial ischemia is not promising.

References

1. Karagueuzian HS, Fnoglio JJ, Weiss MB: Protracted ventricular tachycardia induced by premature stimulation of the canine heart after coronary artery occlusion and reperfusion. Circ Res 1979; 44: 833.
2. Michelson EL, Spear JF, Moore EN: Electrophysiologic and anatomic correlates of sustained ventricular tachyarrhythmias in a model of chronic myocardial infarction. Am J Cardiol 1980; 45: 583.
3. Gibson JK, Lucchesi BR: Electrophysiologic actions of UM-272 (pranolium) on reentrant ventricular arrhythmias in postinfarction canine myocardium. J Pharmacol Exp Ther 1980; 214: 347.
4. Garan H, Fallon JT, Ruskin JN: Sustained ventricular tachycardia in recent canine myocardial infarction. Circulation 1978; 57: 845.
5. Michelson EL, Spear JF, Moore EN: Effects of procaineamide on strength-interval relations in normal and chronically infarcted myocardium. Am J Cardiol 1981; 47: 1223.
6. Michelson EL, Naito M, David D: Meobentine sulfate: Antiarrhythmic efficacy and mechanism of action in a chronic canine model of myocardial infarction susceptible to ventricular tachyarrhythmias. Am J Cardiol 1981; 47: 392.
7. Michelson EL, Spear JF, Moore EN: Description of chronic canine myocardial infarction models suitable for the electropharmacologic evaluation of new antiarrhythmic drugs. In: Morganroth J, Moore EN, Dreifus LS, Michelson EL, eds. The evaluation of new antiarrhythmic drugs. The Hague, The Netherlands: Martinus Nijhoff Publishers, 1980: 33.

Authors' address:
Dr. M. Naito
The 2nd Tokyo National Hospital
2-5-1, Higashigaoka Meguro-ku
Tokyo 151
Japan

"Late Potentials" and Delayed Intrinsic Deflections – A Comparative Study in Acute Regional Ischemia in Isolated Porcine Hearts[*)]

Ch. Naumann d'Alnoncourt, Ch. Eingartner, W. Zierhut, B. Lüderitz

Summary: Waveforms, occurring at the end of the QRS complex or during the ST segments, T wave, or diastolic intervals are defined as late potentials. Whether late potentials reflect delayed regional activiation is still under discussion. A correlation with electrophysiological parameters directly indicating delayed activation has yet not been done. – The present study was performed in isolated porcine hearts (n = 12) perfused according to the Langendorff method. An ischemic zone was produced by occluding the left anterior descending coronary artery. Unipolar electrograms were recorded by means of non polarizable electrodes using DC-amplifiers (0–1250 Hz) without signal averaging, filtering and high gain amplification. – We measured the intrinsic deflection of the ischemic zone electrogram, and compared it with deflections within the ST-segments of the normal zone. When the ischemic zone was activated more and more delayed, the intrinsic deflections and the deflections within the ST-segments were also progressively delayed. When 2 : 1 block into the ischemic zone occurred deflections within ST-segments showed the same sequence. When premature stimuli were applied both deflections could be delayed until they outlasted the ST-segment duration. If the delay was sufficient, ventricular tachycardia developed. – Our data demonstrate a definite correlation between late potentials and delayed intrinsic deflections and suggest, that late potentials in acute regional ischemia are due to extracellular current flow that might be sufficient to induce malignant ventricular dysrhythmia.

Late potentials are defined as waveforms occurring at the end of the QRS complex or during the ST segments, T wave or diastolic interval (1). The interest in late potentials is growing among cardiologists since experimental data accumulate, suggesting arrhythmogenic potency (2, 3, 4).

Late potentials recorded from the body surface or directly from the heart are thought to reflect delayed activation of a circumscript region of the heart (5, 6, 7). A correlation with electrophysiological parameters directly indicating delayed activation has yet not been done.

The aim of our study was to record delayed intrinsic deflections from the ischemic zone and correlate them with late potentials recorded from the normal zone in hearts with acute regional ischemia.

Methods

The experiments were carried out in isolated pig hearts (n = 12). The animals were anaesthetized by intravenous injection of sodium pentobarbitone. After intubation and du-

───────

*) Supported by the Deutsche Forschungsgemeinschaft.

ring artificial respiration the thorax was opened by a midsternal incision and the heart was rapidly removed, connected to a heart lung machine and perfused with the blood of the same pig according to the Langendorff technique. The temperature was 37 °C and the coronary flow was set at 200 ml/min. A region of delayed activation was produced by occluding the left anterior descending coronary artery. Occlusion periods lasted for less than 20 min. Unipolar epicardial electrograms were recorded by means of nonpolarizable cotton wick electrodes. The signals were amplified by means of a DC amplifier and were recorded on an ECG recorder with a range of 0–1250 Hz. The electrograms were recorded simultaneously from the ischemic zone and the normal zone. The distance between the recording points was 20 to 30 mm, the recording point at the normal zone was 5–10 mm away from the ischemic border zone. The hearts were paced at the atria or at the ventricles with a bipolar pacing electrode at one and a half times the diastolic threshold.

Results

ECG changes after LAD occlusion recorded from the ischemic zone consist in ST-elevation, negative T waves and delay of the intrinsic deflection. If the delay of the intrinsic deflection outlasts the duration of the QRS complex recorded from neighbouring normal myocardium an additional deflection is seen in the electrogram of the normal zone (Fig. 1). After LAD occlusion this additional deflection, a late potential, moves more and more into the ST segment.

T wave alternation is a common finding during the first minutes after LAD occlusion. 2 : 1 alternation in the electrogram of the ischemic zone reflects 2 : 1 propagation of the wavefront into the ischemic zone. If alternation occurs every second electrogram shows an intrinsic deflection, in case of conduction block the ECG is monophasic. The late potential in the electrogram of the normal zone shows the same sequence and appears simultaneously with the intrinsic deflection of the ischemic zone (Fig. 2).

The rate dependence of the delay of the late potential and the intrinsic deflection is shown in Table I. A good correlation between both is obvious.

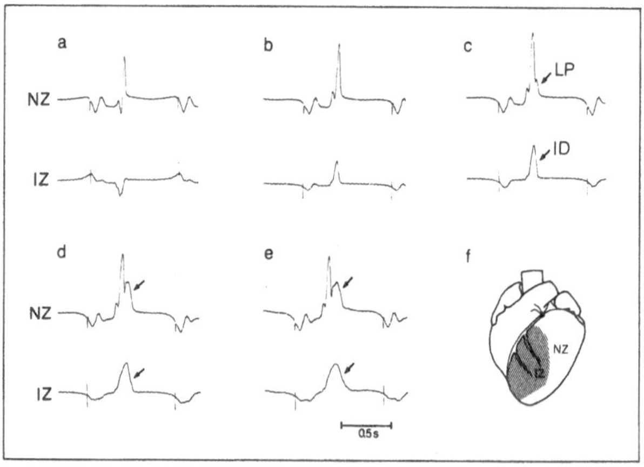

Fig. 1a–f. Correlation of intrinsic deflections (✓ ID) and late potentials (✓ LP). Epicardial electrograms from the normal zone (NZ) and the ischemic zone (IZ). a: control, b: 1 min after LAD occlusion, c: a late potential is seen 2 min after LAD occlusion and occurs simultaneously with the intrinsic deflection in the ischemic zone. d: 6 min after LAD occlusion, e: 12 min after LAD occlusion. f: isolated pig heart, ischemic zone after LAD occlusion.

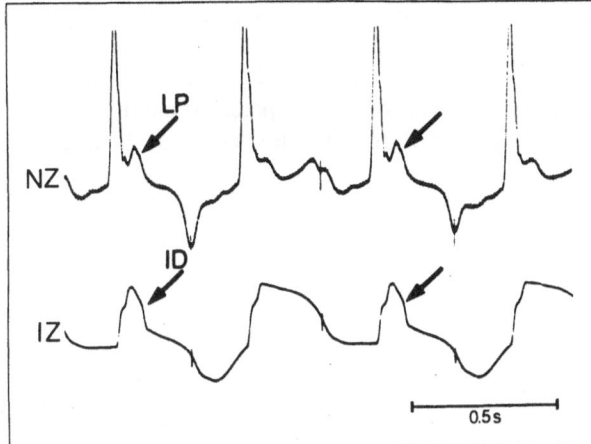

Fig. 2. At 2:1 block of the wave of activation into the ischemic zone intrinsic deflections (↙ ID) and late potentials (↙ LP) occur simultaneously.

Table 1. Correlation of the delays of late potentials (LP) and intrinsic deflections (ID) at different cycle lengths (CL) in 4 experiments.

CL	No 1 delay		No 2 delay		No 3 delay		No 4 delay	
	ID	LP	ID	LP	ID	LP	ID	LP
(ms)	(ms)	(ms)	(ms)	(ms)	(ms)	(ms)	(ms)	(ms)
600	30	28	30	30	33	33	40	50
575	40	38	33	33	41	41	50	50
550	45	47	40	40	59	58	51	53
525	55	55	47	47	73	73	60	50
500	60	65	50	53	77	80	65	65
475	63	68	55	57	89	89	69	71
450	73	75	60	65	93	96	72	91
425	83	86	70	73	98	100	80	89
400	93	95	83	88	105	108	80	90
375	93	98	95	102	112	117	103	110
350	110	116	109	115	122	127	112	131

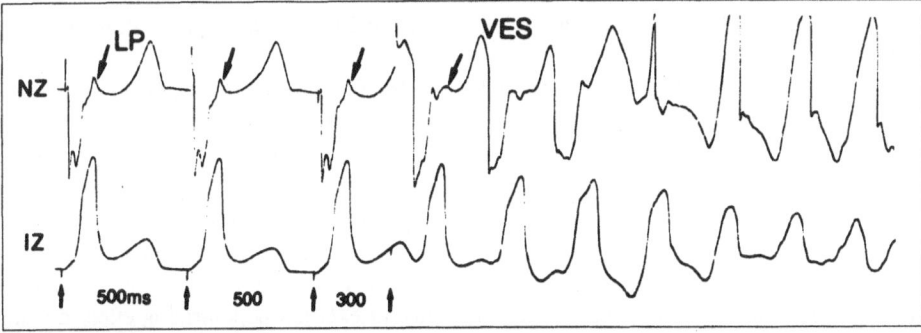

Fig. 3. At programmed stimulation (basic cycle length 500 ms, coupling interval 300 ms) a ventricular tachycardia is induced. The initial action (VES) is preceded by a late potential (↙ LP).

39

Late potentials and intrinsic deflections can be further delayed by premature stimulation. If appropriate prematurity is chosen a tachycardia can be induced.

In Fig. 3 a late potential is shown, which follows the QRS complexes of the normal zone. After premature ventricular stimulation, the delays of the late potential and the intrinsic deflection increase and a ventricular tachycardia begins. The first action of the tachycardia is preceded by a late potential.

Discussion

In contrast to clinical studies we did not use a signal averager, a signal filter or a high gain amplifier to record late potentials. Our experimental set up enables us to record "beat to beat" from the epicardium at low amplification (5 to 10 x) and to preserve the DC content of the signals.

The results demonstrate a good correlation between late potentials and intrinsic deflections. If the ischemic myocardium is activated with progressive delay after LAD occlusion, the intervals between the QRS complexes and the late potentials increase more and more. If 2 : 1 block of the wave of activation into the ischemic zone occurs, the late potentials also appear in a 2 : 1 sequence. If a conduction delay into the ischemic region is created by premature stimulation late potentials and intrinsic deflections are equally delayed.

Our results suggest, that late potentials, recorded in the normal zone are due to electrotonic current flow between the ischemic zone and the normal zone. The current flow is caused by differences in resting membrane potentials, action potential durations and activation times of normal and ischemic myocardium. The current flows across the border zone in regional ischemia and exerts depolarizing effects on the normal zone (8).

Several mechanisms can be distinguished by which flow of current could initiate ectopic activity: Electrotonic current might lower the resting membrane potential to threshold if it flows late enough and if the repolarisation process in the normal myocardium is completed. If current flows during repolarisation only an "electrotonic hump" (a late potential) is seen.

Other mechanisms by which electrotonic current can be arrhythmogenic might be the induction of oscillatory after potentials in partly depolarized fibers, the enhancement of normal phase 4 depolarisation in Purkinje fibers or "reflection", a special kind of reentry in which back and forth transmission of the reentrant impulse takes place along a single pathway (9).

Late potentials recorded by other authors look different from ours (4, 9, 10). Differences in the recording techniques used might be the reason. Filters used in this field of electrocardiography favour some portions of the signal and reject others and can transform a smooth sinusoid into a sharp polyphasic signal.

Our results demonstrate a definite correlation between late potentials and delayed intrinsic deflections in acute regional ischemia. The delayed activation of ischemic myocardium influences the electrogram recorded from the normal zone. Late potentials are due to current flow from the ischemic zone. This current exerts a depolarizing effect on the neighbouring normal myocardium. If the current is sufficient in amplitude and flows late enough in diastole it can disturb the cardiac rhythm.

References

1. Scherlag BJ, Berbari EJ: Glossary. In: Hombach V and Hilger HH (eds), Signal averaging technique in clinical cardiology. Stuttgart–New York, FK Schattauer Verlag 1981; 387–92.
2. Boineau JP, Cox JL: Slow ventricular activation in acute myocardial infarction. Circulation 1973; 48: 702–13.
3. Durrer D, Dam van RTh, Freud GE, Janse MJ: Re-entry and ventricular arrhythmias in local ischemia and infarction of the intact dog heart. Proc K Ned Akad Wet, Biol Med 1971; 74: 321–34.
4. El-Sherif N, Scherlag BJ, Lazarra R, Hope RR: Re-entrant ventricular arrhythmias in the late myocardial infarction period. Circulation 1977; 55: 686–702.
5. Naumann d'Alnoncourt C, Eingartner C, Zierhut W, Lüderitz B: Spätpotential und verzögerte intrinsische Deflektion bei akuter regionaler Ischämie des Herzens. Z Kardiol 1983; 72: 381–84.
6. Fontaine G, Frank R, Gallais-Hamonno F, Allali J, Phan-Thuc H, Grosgogeat Y: Electrocardiographie des potentiels tardifs du syndrome de post-excitation. Arch Mal Coeur 1978; 71: 854–64.
7. Josephson ME, Simson MB, Harken AH, Horowitz LN, Falcone RA: The incidence and clinical significance of epicardial late potentials in patients with recurrent sustained ventricular tachycardia and coronary artery disease. Circulation 1982; 66: 1199–1204.
8. Janse MJ, Capelle v FJL, Morsink H, Kleber AG, Schopman WF, Cardinal R, Naumann d'Alnoncourt C, Durrer D: Flow of "injury" current and patterns of excitation during early ventricular arrhythmias in acute regional myocardial ischemia in isolated porcine and canine hearts. Evidence of two different arrhythmogenic mechanisms. Circ Res 1980; 47: 151–65.
9. Naumann d'Alnoncourt C, Zierhut W, Lüderitz, B: Pathophysiology of ventricular arrhythmias with special reference to late depolarizations. In: Hombach V and Hilger HH, eds. Signal averaging technique in clinical cardiology. Stuttgart–New York, FK Schattauer Verlag 1981; 153–61.
10. Hombach V, Kebbel U, Höpp HW, Winter VJ, Braun V, Deutsch H, Hirche H, Hilger HH: Fortlaufende Registrierung von Mikropotentialen des menschlichen Herzens. Dtsch med Wschr 1982; 107: 1951–56.

Authors' address:
Dr. Chr. Naumann d'Alnoncourt
Medizinische Klinik
Innere Medizin – Kardiologie
Sigmund-Freud-Str. 25
5300 Bonn-Venusberg

Ageing and Atrial Electrophysiologic Properties in Man

A. Michelucci, L. Padeletti, R. M. Lova, G. A. Fradella, D. Monizzi, A. Giomi, P. Seniori*, G. Berni*, F. Fantini

Summary: In order to assess the influence of age on atrial electrophysiologic properties, we studied 17 normal subjects, whose ages were homogeneously distributed between 17 and 78 years, measuring in each of them effective (ERP) and functional (FRP) refractory periods at 3 sites of the right atrium (high, middle and low in the lateral wall) at the same driven frequency (120/min). Two threshold stimuli of 2 msec duration were applied. Dispersion of refractoriness (D) was measured as the longest minus the shortest refractory period. A significant direct correlation was observed between age and D (of ERP: $r = 0.75$, $p < 0.001$; of FRP: $r = 0.82$, $p < 0.001$). Moreover age showed a significant direct correlation with refractoriness at high right atrium (ERP: $r = 0.66$, $p < 0.01$; FRP: $r = 0.76$, $p < 0.001$) but did not correlate with that at the other two sites. In conclusion we suggest that ageing modifies atrial refractoriness in a non uniform manner inducing a progressive increment of D. The impression is that a slow but continuous process takes place from juvenility to old age. Even if it is not easy to establish the clinical relevance of our data we think that they should be considered in view of the differences in susceptibility to and electrophysiologic manifestations of arrhythmias at various ages.

Introduction

Previous studies on humans concerning the influence of age on atrial electrophysiologic properties (1, 2) were performed measuring refractoriness at only atrial site (parasinusal zone). Recent papers (3–5), however, indicated the possibility of performing a more extensive evaluation of atrial excitability in clinical electrophysiology. Results obtained testing more than one atrial site allowed a better definition of some pathophysiological conditions, such as sinus node dysfunction and atrial tachyarrhythmias. If we consider that a possible implication of these studies concerns the role exerted be ageing on clinical electrophysiologic results, it becomes necessary to perform further evaluation of this problem, adopting the more extensive protocol of the above mentioned studies (3–5).

Material and Methods

The study group consisted of 17 normal subjects (14 males and 3 females) whose ages were homogenously distributed between 17 and 78 years. Complete medical history was obtained and physical examination was performed by at least two of the authors. Analysis of blood, urine and chest roentgenograms did not show abnormalities in any subject. Particular attention was given to exclude latent coronary artery disease. In all subjects

Cardiology Unit, University of Florence; * Arcispedale of S.M. Nuova, Florence, Italy.

43

ECG, response to multistage treadmill stress test, systolic time intervals, echocardiogram, and Holter monitoring were normal. The electrophysiological study was carried out: during an atrial pacing performed for atypical chest pain (8 cases) and before a cardiac catheterization performed to exclude the presence of a gradient between right or left ventricles and pulmonary artery or aorta (9 cases).

All patients had: 1. normal sinus rhythm with sinus rates between 60 and 100/min in all recorded resting electrograms; and 2. absence of documented atrial dysrhythmias. The subjects were observed for a period of 12 to 30 months (mean 18 months). Periodic controls confirmed normal cardiac conditions. Blood pressure was normal in all subjects. The subjects were studied in the resting, nonsedated and postabsorptive state after informed consent had been obtained. None of them was receiving cardioactive drugs.

Two electrodes, number 6F USCI quadripolar and number 6F USCI tripolar, were inserted percutaneously via a right antecubital vein and the right femoral vein respectively. The distal pair of electrodes of the quadripolar catheter were used to stimulate the atrium and the proximal pair of electrodes to record a right atrial electrogram (A). The tripolar catheter was positioned across the tricuspid valve and was used to record the His bundle electrogram (HBE). The A, HBE and four surface electrocardiographic leads (I, II, III and V_1) were simultaneously displayed on a Hewlett-Packard eight channel oscilloscope and were recorded on a Elema-Schonander Mingograph 62–6 channel ink-jet at a paper speed of 100 mm/sec. Overdrive and premature programmed atrial stimulation were performed using an electrically isolated battery-powered Medtronics 5325 stimulator. The pulse width was 2 msec and the amplitude was adjusted to twice diastolic threshold. The stimulating electrodes were first positioned at the high right atrium (HRA) near its junction with the superior vena cava to determine corrected sinus node recovery time and total sinoatrial conduction time as previously indicated (6, 7). Atrial extrastimuli were applied at 10 msec decrements after eight beats of atrial pacing at a rate of 120 beats/min until atrial refractoriness was determined. The stimulating poles were then fluoroscopically repositioned, the threshold was reevaluated and atrial stimulation performed at two additional right atrial sites in the lateral wall at least 1 cm distant from the HRA: mid-lateral (MRA) and low-lateral (LRA) right atrium. Atrial functional refractory period (FRP) was the shortest coupling interval recorded on the atrial electrogram. Atrial effective refractory period (ERP) was the longest interval between the stimulus artefact (atrial pacing) and the extrastimulus failing to propagate. Dispersion of atrial refractoriness (D) was determined from the range of refractory periods measured in each subject at the three atrial sites as the longest minus the shortest refractory period. Values are expressed in milliseconds and as mean ± 1 standard deviation. Correlation coefficients for the relationship between age and atrial refractoriness or D were derived using standard linear regression methods.

Results

Sinus cycle length ranged from 700 to 980 msec (mean 828 ± 111 msec). Atrioventricular conduction, corrected sinus node recovery time and total sinoatrial conduction time proved to be normal in each subject. Mean A-H and H-V intervals were respectively 105 ± 10 msec and 44 ± 3 msec. Mean corrected sinus recovery time was 244 ± 55

msec. Mean calculated sinoatrial conduction time was 143 ± 32 msec. Single values of age, of atrial refractoriness (at the three atrial sites) and of D are reported in table 1.

ERP ranged at HRA form 240 to 310 msec (mean 272 ± 20 msec), at MRA from 230 to 290 msec (mean 252 ± 16 msec), at LRA from 200 to 290 msec (mean 256 ± 14 msec).

FRP ranged at HRA from 260 to 330 msec (mean 297 ± 23 msec), at MRA from 250 to 300 msec (mean 275 ± 16 msec), at LRA from 250 to 300 msec (mean 279 ± 14 msec).

D of ERP and of FRP ranged respectively from 10 to 70 msec (mean 42 ± 17 msec) and from 10 to 75 msec (mean 38 ± 19 msec).

A significant direct correlation (Fig. 1) was observed between age and D (of ERP: $r = 0.75$, $p < 0.001$; of FRP: $r = 0.82$, $p < 0.001$). Moreover age showed a significant direct correlation (Fig. 2) with refractoriness at HRA (ERP: $r = 0.66$, $p < 0.01$; FRP: $r = 0.76$, $p < 0.001$) but did not correlate with that at MRA and LRA.

Discussion

Previous studies (3–5) showed that length of refractoriness varies physiologically along the atrial myocardium and that some pathophysiological conditions can induce an abnor-

Table 1. Values of age, of atrial refractoriness (at the three atrial sites) and of D in each subject.

Pt. n°	Sex	Age	EPR				FRP			
			HRA	MRA	LRA	D	HRA	MRA	LRA	D
1	M	17	260	250	260	10	280	270	270	10
2	M	25	250	240	230	20	270	250	250	20
3	M	31	240	240	220	20	270	250	250	20
4	M	37	240	290	230	60	260	300	260	40
5	M	40	250	250	280	30	270	260	285	25
6	M	41	260	230	210	50	270	270	250	20
7	M	44	290	260	280	30	300	280	290	20
8	F	46	300	265	250	50	320	280	270	50
9	M	50	280	250	290	40	320	300	300	20
10	M	53	270	270	240	30	300	280	270	30
11	M	54	270	230	220	50	300	250	250	50
12	F	57	290	260	235	55	300	290	250	50
13	F	60	290	240	270	50	330	270	290	60
14	M	63	290	260	250	40	310	300	260	50
15	M	65	270	260	230	40	295	270	260	35
16	M	73	270	230	200	70	325	285	250	75
17	M	78	310	260	240	70	330	270	260	70
$\bar{x}$		49	272	252	243	42	297	275	265	38
SD		16	20	16	25	17	23	16	16	19

D = dispersion of atrial refractoriness; ERP = efective refractory period; FRP = functional refractory period; HRA = high right atrium; LRA = low right atrium; MRA = middle right atrium.

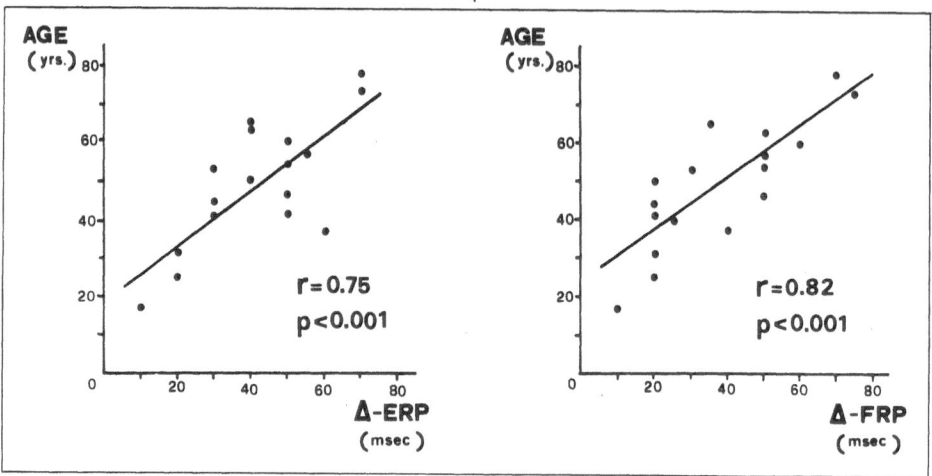

Fig. 1. Age plotted against dispersion of effective (D-ERP) and functional (D-FRP) refractoriness.

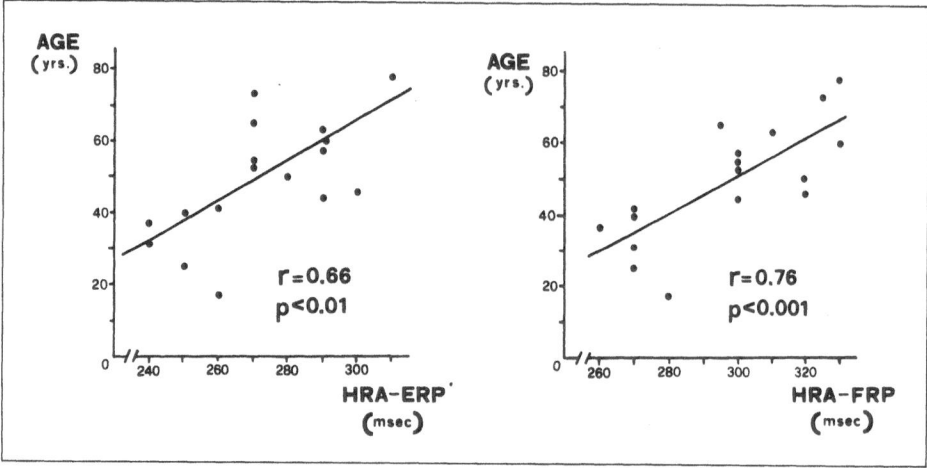

Fig. 2. Age plotted against effective (ERP) and functional (FRP) refractoriness at high right atrium (HRA).

mal increase of the observed differences (a less homogeneous recovery of atrial excitability). Our results indicate that also ageing in itself was able to influence the behaviour of atrial refractoriness. In fact, a significant direct correlation was observed between age and D.

Moreover if we consider separately the three tested atrial sites, only refractoriness at HRA (parasinusal zone) showed a significant correlation with age. A progressive increase of refractoriness from juvenility to old age was observed at this site.

The lack of correlation between age and refractoriness at MRA and LRA (older subjects showed values of refractoriness superimposable to those of younger ones at these sites) did not contradict previous studies (1, 2) as they utilized only the parasinusal zone in order to evaluate the influence of age. On this basis it cannot be simply affirmed, as previously done (1, 2), that ageing induces a lengthening of atrial refractoriness. The impression is that a non homogeneous process takes place from juvenility to old age. Therefore, it can be suggested that ageing modifies atrial refractoriness in a non uniform manner, inducing a progressive increment of D.

Our findings can be interpreted considering that ageing induces structural changes of myocardial tissue (8, 9). Catecholamines (10) and vagal stimulation (11, 12) have been demonstrated to influence the length of refractory periods. Structural changes could make their influence less uniform upon the atrial myocardium, so accounting for the progressive increment of D observed from juvenility to old age. In this regard, it should be remembered that senile hearts are less sensitive to catecholamines (13) and vagal stimulation (14) and that structural changes in themselves have been shown to play a role in inducing inequality of refractoriness and conduction (15). In evaluating our results, however, it should be considered that we controlled the cycle length variable by pacing our subjects at the same driven cycle length. There is evidence that atrial pacing induces a release of autonomic mediators in cardiac tissue (16, 17). This may have made our results more evident.

Even if it is not easy to establish the clinical significance of our data, they should be taken into account when considering the differences in susceptibility to arrhythmias and electrophysiologic manifestations of arrhythmias at various ages. Atrial arrhythmias have many predisposing factors (5, 18, 19) and ageing inducing a progressive increse of D could be one of them.

Finally, we would emphasize that our data should also be taken into account when performing clinical electrophysiologic diagnosis and research.

References

1. Du Brow IW, Fisher EA, Amat-y-Leon F, Denes P, Wu D, Rosen K, Hastreiter AR. Comparison of cardiac refractory periods in children and adults. Circulation 1975; 51: 485–491.
2. Padeletti L, Michelucci A, Franchi F, Fradella GA: Sinoatrial function in old age. Acta Cardiologica 1982; 37: 11–21.
3. Luck JC, Engel TR: Dispersion of atrial refractoriness in patients with sinus node dysfunction. Circulation 1979; 60: 404–412.
4. Franchi F, Michelucci A, Padeletti L: Distribution of right atrial refractoriness in clinical conditions with intermittent atrial tachyarrhythmias: effect of acute administration of verapamil. In: Zanchetti A and Krikler DM, eds. Calcium antagonism in cardiovascular therapy. Amsterdam: Excerpta Medica, 1981: 342–345.
5. Michelucci A, Padeletti L, Fradella GA. Atrial refractoriness and spontaneous or induced atrial fibrillation. Acta Cardiol 1982; 37: 333–344.
6. Strauss HC, Saroff AL, Bigger JT jr, Giardina EGV: Premature atrial stimulation as a key to the understanding of sinoatrial conduction time in man. Presentation of data and critical review of the literature. Circulation 1973; 47: 86–93.
7. Narula OS, Samet P, Javier RP. Significance of the sinus node recovery time. Circulation 1972; 45: 140–158.
8. Davies MJ, Pomerance A: Quantitative study of ageing changes in the human sinoatrial node and internodal tracts. Brit Heart J 1972; 34: 150–152.
9. Guarnieri T, Filburn CR, Zitnik G, Roth GS, Lakatta EG: Contractile and biochemical correlates of Beta-adrenergic stimulation of the aged heart. Am J Physiol 1980; 239: 501–508.

10. Siebens AA, Hoffman BF, Enson Y, Farrell JE, Brooks C McC: Effects of L-epinephrine or L-norepinephrine on cardiac excitability. Am J Physiol 1953; 175: 1–7.
11. Alessi R, Nusynowitz M, Abildskov JA, Moe GK: Nonuniform distribution of vagal effects on the atrial refractory period. Am J Physiol 1958; 194(2): 406–410.
12. Zipes DP, Mihalick Mj, Robbins GT: Effects of selective vagal and stellate ganglion stimulation on atrial refractoriness. Cardiovascular Research 1974; 8: 647–655.
13. Yin FC, Spurgeon HA, Raizes GS, Green HL, Weisfeldt ML, Shock NW: Age associated decrease in chronotropic response to isoproterenol. Circulation 1976; 53–54 (suppl II): 167.
14. Frolkis VV, Bezrukov VV, Shevchuk VG: Hemodynamics and its regulation in old age. Exp Gerontol 1975; 10: 251–271.
15. Demoulin JC, Kulbertus HE: Pathological correlates of atrial arrhythmias. In: Kulbertus, MTP, ed. Reentrant arrhythmias. Mechanisms and treatment. MPT Lancaster, 1977: 99–113.
16. Furchgott RF, De Gubareff T, Grossman A: Release of autonomic mediators in cardiac tissue by suprathreshold stimulation. Science 1959; 129: 328–329.
17. Vincenzi FF, West TC: Release of autonomic mediators in cardiac tissue by direct subthreshold electrical stimulation. J Pharmacol Exptl Therap 1963; 141: 185–194.
18. James TN, Hershey EA: Experimental studies on the pathogenesis of atrial arrhythmias in myocardial infarction. Am Heart J 1962; 63: 196–211.
19. Allessi MA, Bonke FIM, Schopman FJG: Circus movement in rabbit atrial muscle as a mechanism of tachycardia. II The role of non-uniform recovery of excitability in the occurrence of unidirectional block, as studied with multiple microelectrodes. Circ Res 1976; 39: 168–177.

Authors' address:
Dr. Antonio Michelucci
Via Bronzino 163
I-50100 Firenze
Italy

Effectiveness of A-C Bypass Operation for Improvement of Sinus Bradycardia for Patients with Right Coronary Disease and Preoperative Pacing

K. Katsumoto, T. Niibori, K. Takeuchi

Summary: We found various types of right coronary lesion on coronary angiograms in patients who complained of sinus bradycardia and angina pectoris and suspected a blood stream disturbance to the sinus node artery. We experienced improvement of bradycardia after A-C bypass surgery on those patients and also noted in the case of several patients to whom pacemaking was preoperatively indicated, this became unnecessary after A-C bypass. Nineteen patients were entered into study. Four patients were preoperatively indicated for pacemaking due to sinus bradycardia. In one patient to whom a permanent pacemaker was implanted preoperatively for 2 years, all the pacemaker systems were removed during A-C bypass surgery. Inferior infarction was found in 65% of the patients. Permanent pacemakers were implanted in two patients. Preoperative evaluation of conduction system in sinus bradycardic patients revealed AH-time to be 93 ± 21 ms, HV-time 37 ± 8 ms, SNRT 1297 ± 283 ms, ARP 407 ± 99 ms. But there were no statistical differences compared to non-bradycardic patients except HV-time ($p < 0.05$). Total occlusion of the right coronary artery and subsequent disturbance of blood supply for sinoatrial node were noted in 21% of the patients. Sclerotic changes of the sinus node artery were noted in 58% of the patients. Coronary artery spasm was observed in two patients on cineangiogram. RR-interval was found to have improved after A-C bypass from 1.273 ± 0.226 sec to 0.770 ± 0.135 sec. A-C bypass surgery was useful for patients with sinus bradycardia associated with sinus node artery disease and pacemakers were not always needed after A-C bypass surgery

We found various types of right coronary lesions on coronary angiograms in patients who complained of sinus bradycardia and angina pectoris, and suspected a blood stream disturbance to the sinus node artery. We experienced improvement of bradycardia after aorto-coronary bypass surgery on those patients and also noted that in the case of several patients to whom pacemaking was preoperatively indicated, this became unnecessary after A-C bypass surgery. This study was anticipated to delineate the relationship between sinus bradycardia and angiographic findings of the right coronary artery and also physiological examinations of preoperative conduction systems.

Methods

Coronary cineangiography was performed by the Judkin's method with film speeds of 50 frames/sec, utilizing a Thosiba image intensifier. Out of 90 patients 19, who complained of sinus bradycardia with RR-intervals of more than 1.11 sec were entered into study. RR-intervals were calculated from 12 leads EKG charts which were obtained after patients had walked 150 meters to the clinical laboratory. Sinus node artery (coronary angiography), conduction system (His bundle study), sinus node recovery time (SNRT) and RR-interval histogram (Holter recording) were studied. Histograms were obtained using a ICR-Holter cardiography system and compared pre and post operatively.

Electrophysiologic study was performed with premedication of 15 mg of pentazocin and 10 mg of diazepam injected intramuscularly, and SNRT was recorded subsequent to 60 sec of atrial overdrive pacing. Coronary angiography was safely performed for one patient under temporary pacing of the right atrium

His bundle electrogram was recorded utilizing a Toshiba polygraph with biophysiological amplifier and ink jet recorder. A battery powered Medtronic 5880A pacemaker or a Med Data high rate atrial pacemaker was used for evaluation of SNRT and right atrial refractory period (ARP). Four patients needed cardiac pacing before surgery due to slow sinus rhythm.

Results

Nineteen patients were shown in Table 1, who complained of sinus bradycardia with RR-interval of 1.11 sec or more. Of these, 16 cases were male and 3 female. The mean age was 55 ± 8. Old myocardial infarction was seen in 13 patients (68%). Two patients showed exercise induced angina associated with ST elevation and positive cold pressor test. A screw-in pacemaker electrode was attached to 4 patients on their right ventricular anterior wall during A-C bypass surgery. We implanted pacemakers in two patients, one during A-C bypass and the other 14 days after surgery. We tried to put 3 electrodes to the right atrium of the first patient, but we could not pace due to high stimulation threshold of the right atrium and so we changed to VVI mode of pacing. The second patient presented complete right bundle branch block (CRBBB) and so VVI mode was adopted. Programmable pacemakers were used for these two patients and 187 milliseconds of hysteresis were applied with a basic pacing rate of 70 BPM, so therefore pacemaker rhythm was not frequently seen in these 2 patients. Preoperative intermittent CRBBB was converted to normal QRS configuration until 6 months after A-C bypass in another patient (case (10)) who had an old inferior infarction, but this patient has returned to CRBBB thereafter.

Preoperative PR-intervals and RR-intervals were 0.18 ± 0.02 and 1.28 ± 0.22 sec respectively. RR-intervals were found to have improved one month after A-C bypass to 0.770 ± 0.135 sec. On the other hand, RR-interval of consecutive 25 patients who did not present sinus bradycardia preoperatively was also found to have improved one month after A-C bypass to 0.719 ± 0.069 sec. But the rate of shortening was greater in the bradycardic patients 37.6% versus 18.8% ($P < 0.001$) (Table 2). Preoperative evaluation of conduction system for bradycardic patients revealed AH-time to be 93 ± 21 ms, HV-time 37 ± 8 ms, SNRT 1297 ± 283 ms, ARP was 407 ± 99 ms, on the other hand non-bradycardic patients revealed AH-time to be 97 ± 24 ms, HV-time to be 47 ± 15 ms, SNRT to be 1156 ± 266 sec, ARP was 413 ± 78 ms. There were no statistical differences between the two groups except HV-time ($p < 0.05$) according to student's t-test on paired data (Table 3).

Right coronary lesion

Total occlusion or diffuse small caliber of the right coronary artery and subsequent disturbance of blood supply for sinoatrial node were noted in 21% of the patients. Sclerotic

Patient No.	Age (years)	Sex	Preoperative ECG Findings PR (sec)	RR (sec)	Old MI Location	Bundle Branch Block	Preoperative pacing (Days)	1 Month Post Ope RR-intervals (sec)	Electrode Position	Generator Implantation
1	58	M	0.20	1.935	(–)	–	4	0.857	RV	During A-C Bypass
2	53	M	0.20	1.222	high posterior	CRBBB	2	0.882	RV	14 days after A-C Bypass
3	54	M	0.20	1.714	inferior	–	9	0.967	RV	–
4	60	M	0.20	1.200	inferior	–	–	0.508	RV	–
5	63	M	0.18	1.276	anterior	–	–	0.681	–	–
6	67	M	0.20	1.250	inferior	–	–	0.952	–	–
7	42	F	0.16	1.250	(–)	–	–	0.800	–	–
8	63	F	0.18	1.200	inferior	–	–	0.698	–	–
9	48	M	0.16	1.200	(–)	–	–	0.800	–	–
10	47	M	0.16	1.428	inferior	intermittent CRBBB	–	0.723	–	–
11	55	F	0.18	1.176	(–)	–	–	0.789	–	–
12	51	M	0.18	1.132	(–)	–	–	0.706	–	–
13	65	M	0.20	pacing	anterior & inferior	–	750	0.705	Removed	Removed
14	49	M	0.14	1.111	inferior	CRBBB	–	0.638	–	–
15	41	M	0.18	1.091	(–)	–	–	0.667	–	–
16	49	M	0.18	1.154	subendocardial	–	–	0.895	–	–
17	53	M	0.16	1.154	inferior	–	–	1.000	–	–
18	68	M	0.16	1.276	subendocardial	–	–	Died	–	–
19	58	M	0.14	1.250	high posterior	incomplete RBBB	–	0.600	–	–
$\overline{m} \pm SD$	55 ± 8	85% M	0.18 ± 0.02	1.278 ± 0.216				0.770 ± 0.135		

Legend = Old MI = Old myocardial infarction
RV = Right ventricle (anterior wall)
M = Male, F = Female
CRBBB = Complete Right Bundle Branch Block

51

Table 2. Preoperative and Postoperative RR-Intervals and Its Shortening after A-C Bypass.

Group	Preoperative RR-intervals* (sec)	1 M. Postoperative RR-intervals** (sec)	% RR-interval shortening* $\left(\dfrac{\text{Pre}-\text{Post}}{\text{Pre}}\%\right)$
Sinus Bradycardic Group (n = 19)	1.278 ± 0.216 (n = 18)***	0.770 ± 0.135 (n = 18)	37.6 ± 12.0% (n = 17)****
Non-bradycardic Group (n = 25)	0.895 ± 0.120 (n = 25)	0.719 ± 0.069 (n = 25)	18.8 ± 9.6% (n = 25)

Student's t-test on paired data
    * $P < 0.001$
   ** Not significant
  *** case 13 excluded
**** case 18 excluded

Table 3. Preoperative Comparison of Sinus Bradycardic Group and Non-Bradycardic Gruoup.

Group	Cardiac Index (L/min/M²)	His Bundle Elecrogram AH-Time* (ms)	HV-Time**** (ms)	Atrial Overdrive Pacing SNRT* (ms)	C-SNRT* (ms)	ARP* (ms)
Sinus Bradycardic Group	3.16 ± 0.74*** n = 16	93 ± 21** n = 11	37 ± 8** n = 11	1297 ± 283** n = 11	352 ± 239** n = 11	407 ± 99** n = 11
Non-bradycardic group	3.34 ± 0.80 n = 17	97 ± 24 n = 17	47 ± 15 n = 17	1156 ± 266 n = 17	319 ± 217 n = 17	413 ± 78 N = 17

    * Not significant (Student's t-test on paired data)
   ** Case 1 ~ 6, 9 and 10 were not studied
  *** Case 3, 9, 10 were not studied
**** $P < 0.05$
Legend = SNRT   = Sinus node recovery time
          C-SNRT = Corrected SNRT
          ARP   = Atrial refractory period
          ms   = milli seconds

change of the sinus node artery (SNA) was noted in 58% of the patients. Almost complete occlusion or diffuse small caliber of the proximal portion of the right coronary artery was found in cases 1, 3, 4, 14 (Fig. 1). In case 3, complete occlusion of the proximal right coronary artery was found, but there was only a conus branch visualized, from which collaterals went along the anterior wall of the right ventricle towards the apex, but SNA was not continuous from the right coronary artery. Pacemaker was indicated for this patient 9 days preoperatively due to persistent sinus bradycardia of 38 beats per minute, but during

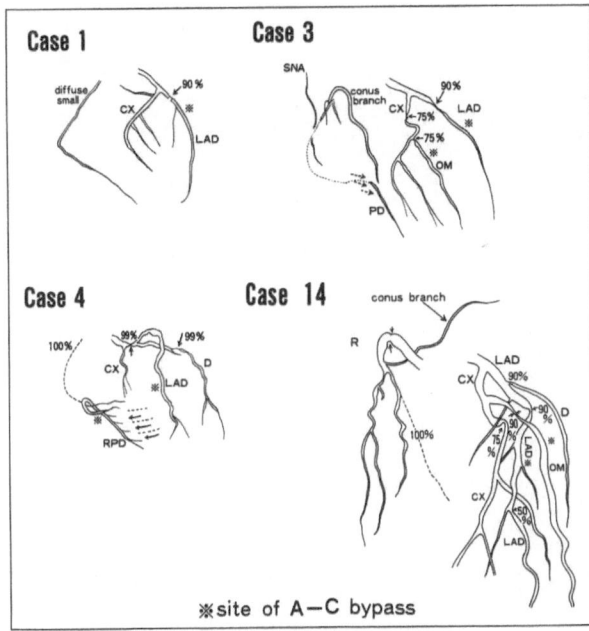

Fig. 1. Complete stenosis or diffuse small caliber of the proximal portion of the right coronary artery.

A-C bypass we put only a permanent epicardial electrode on the right ventricular wall, and this patient is still doing well after 3 years now, without implantation of a permanent pacemaker.

Stenosis of SNA at its origin from the major coronary artery was found in cases 2, 6, 7, 8, 9, 10, 11, 14, 16, 17. In cases 5 and 19, SNA was supplied from the circumflex coronary artery and found a stenosis at its junction.

Coronary spasm

Four patients were associated with either Prinzmetal's angina or coronary spasm. Two patients (Case 15, 18) complained of effort angina with ST-elevation on ECG and one of these patients who showed, during cold pressor test, total spastic occlusion of the right coronary artery just distal to an organic stenosis, died due to right atrial perforation after A-C bypass (Case 18). Other 3 patients (8, 15, 16) survived the operation and both sinus bradycardia and angina disappeared. Spasm of the left anterior descending coronary artery was seen in one patient who responded to sublingual nitroglycerin (Case 16).

RR-interval histogram and a case of pacemaker removal

A RR-interval histogram was compared in case 1 using Holter monitor pre and postoperatively (Fig. 2). Upper column shows histogram before A-C bypass and lower column shows one month after A-C bypass. From midnight to 2 a.m. before surgery, RR-interval was prolonged to about 1.6–1.7 sec, and this was shortened to 0.8 sec after bypass.

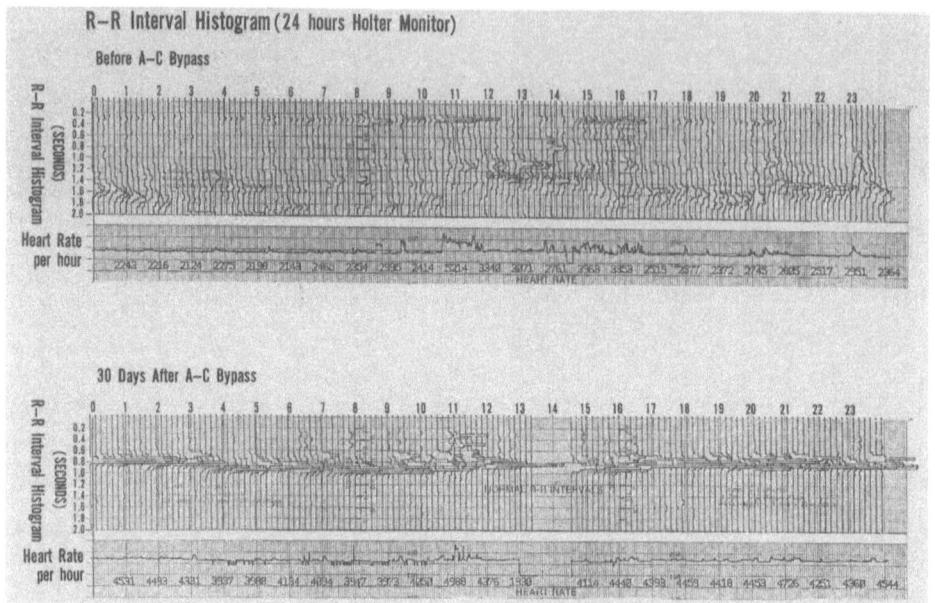

Fig. 2. A RR-interval histogram was compared in case 1 using Holter monitor pre and post operatively. Upper column shows histogram before bypass and lower column shows one month after A-C bypass.

A 65 year old man (case 13) was affected by anterior and inferior infarction 2 years ago and complete A-V block was continued for more than 2 weeks and so a permanent pacemaker was implanted transvenously. Thereafter, complete A-V block improved but sinus bradycardia remained. Preoperative RR-intervals were evaluated in this patient with a Holter monitor applied with chest wall stimulation before A-C bypass, and maximal RR-interval was peaked at 1.20 sec. It seemed likely that for this patient sinus bradycardia could be improved and a pacemaker would not be necessary for him after A-C bypass, so the electrode and generator were removed during A-C bypass. The electrode was safely extracted at the end of cardiopulmonary bypass. Sinus bradycardia was not seen in this patient after A-C bypass on RR-interval histogram (Fig. 3), and he is doing well after one year.

Discussion

There are a number of reports that decrease of blood supply to the sinoatrial node is a causative factor of S-A block or sinus bradycardia at the onset of acute myocardial infarction (2, 3, 4).

Simonsen (5) reported sinus node dysfunction in 128 patients and ischaemic heart disease was most frequently seen and diagnosed in 56% of all patients with sick sinus syndrome and 42% of patients with sinus bradycardia.

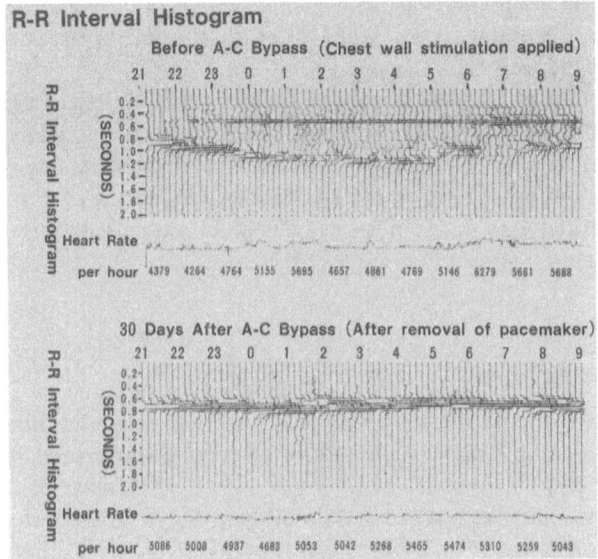

R-R Interval Histogram

Before A-C Bypass (Chest wall stimulation applied)

Fig. 3. Preoperative RR-intervals were evaluated with a Holter monitor applied with chest wall stimulation. After A-C bypass, his pacemaker was removed and sinus bradycardia was not seen in this patient.

Parameswaran (6) reported the difference between patients with sinus bradycardia and those with bradycardia-tachycardia syndrome. And 5 out of 7 patients with bradycardia-tachycardia syndrome required permanent pacing, whereas none of the 13 patients with sinus bradycardia alone required permanent pacing, though one patient had continued to have sinus bradycardia during repeated follow-up examination. It is possible to make sinus bradycardia or S-A block experimentally in a dog with ligation of blood supply to S-A node, and when a multiple blood supply to the sinus node was observed, it was necessary to occlude all major arteries to make slowing of the sinus rate (7). One reason for the improvement of sinus bradycardia after A-C bypass is seemed to be due to the improvement of blood supply to the S-A node and also it is considered that, as indicated in the coronary angiogram of the case 3, blood supply to SNA would be stealed (8) preoperatively from the conus branch which had a role of collateral blood supply to the obstructed right coronary artery, and the coronary flow distribution was balanced by A-C bypass, resulting in recovered S-A node function.

From coronary angiograms of case 1 and case 2, the right coronary artery of case 1 was diffuse small and SNA in case 2 was obstructed at its junction to the right coronary artery and so the effect of A-C bypass was not anticipated, however there was yet improvement of sinus bradycardia, and it seems likely therefore that the increase of collateral blood supply from the atrial branch of circumflex coronary artery was brought fouth after A-C bypass. From 80 unselected coronary artery diseases, Engel et al (9) has found 21% of angiographic disease of, or significant obstruction proximal to, the SNA and they concluded that there was no correlation between coronary disease particularly that of sinus node and sick sinus syndrome from the study of sinus node recovery time, and that 5 patients with SSS exhibited no angiographic evidence of SNA involvement. On the other hand, Jordan et al. (10) found sinoatrial conduction time (Strauss Method) for 10 patients with severe stenosis (75%) proximal to the origin of the sinus node artery (SNA)

55

to be significantly longer than other groups of 17 patients with insignificant proximal stenosis, but they could not find statistical differences either in the atrial refractory period, or in the sinus rate between those groups.

Narula (10) studied A-V conduction in 75 patients with sick sinus syndrome (mean age 73 years), and demonstrated that sinus bradycardia including sinoatrial block and tachycardia-bradycardia syndrome was often (67%) associated with A-V conduction abnormalities. It was unfortunate that we did not examined the His bundle electrogram of 8 patients, ie: from case 1 to case 6 and case 9, 10, however, out of 11 patients only two (18%) showed slight prolongation of HV-time (50 msec, each).

Conclusion

1. RR-intervals were found to have improved after A-C bypass surgery in both sinus bradycardic group and non-bradycardic group but its rate of shortening was greater in bradycardic group (37.6 ± 12.0%)
2. Sclerotic changes of sinus node artery were noted in 58% of the patients. Total occlusion of the proximal right coronary artery and subsequent disturbance of blood supply for sino-atrial node were noted in 21% of the patients.
3. Angiographically demonstrated coronary artery spasms were noted in 3 patients among 19 sinus bradycardic patients.
4. Preoperative evaluation of conduction system in sinus bradycardic patients revealed AH-time to be 93 ± 21 ms, HV-time 37 ± 8 ms and there were no statistical differences compared to non-bradycardic group except HV-time which was rather longer in non-bradycardic group ($p < 0.05$).
5. A case of pacemaker explantation after A-C bypass was reported, to whom a permanent pacemaker had been implanted until A-C bypass.

References

1. Anderson K, Ho SY, Anderson RH: Location and vascular supply of sinus node in human heart. Brit Heart J 1979; 41: 28-32.
2. Haden RF, Langsjoen H, Rapaport M, McNerney JJ: The significance of sinus bradycardia in acute myocardial infarction. Dis Chest 1963; 44: 168-173.
3. Lippestad C Th, Marton PF: Sinus arrest in proximal right coronary artery occlusion. Am. Heart J 1967; 74: 551-556.
4. Simonsen E, Nielsen BL, Nielsen JS: Sinus node dysfunction in acute myocardial infarction. Acta Med Scand 1980; 208: 463-466.
5. Simonsen E, Nielsen JS, Nielsen BL: Sinus node dysfunction in 128 patients. Acta Med Scand 1980; 208: 343-348.
6. Parameswaran R, Ohe T, Goldberg H: Sinus node dysfunction in acute myocardial infarction. Brit Heart J 1976; 38: 93-96.
7. Billette J, Elharrar V, Porlier G, Nadeau RA: Sinus slowing produced by experimental ischemia of the sinus node in dogs. Am J Cardiol 1973; 31: 331-335.
8. Becker LC: Conditions for vasodilator-induced coronary steal in experimental myocardial ischemia. Circulation 1978; 57: 1103-1110.
9. Engel TR, Meister SG, Feitosa GS, Fischer HA, Frankl WS: Appraisal of sinus node artery disease. Circulation 1975; 52: 286-291.

10. Jordan J, Yamaguchi I, Mandel WJ: Characteristics of sinoatrial conduction in patients with coronary artery disease. Circulation 1977; 55: 569-574.
11. Narula OS: Atrioventricular conduction defects in patient with sinus bradycardia. Circulation 1971; 44: 1096–1110.

Authors'address:
K. Katsumoto, M.D.
Saitama National Hospital
2-1 Suwa Wako City
Saitama P./Japan

The Human Sinus Node Electrogram on the Overdrive Suppression Test and Estimated Sinoatrial Conduction Time Measurements

I. Yamaguchi, T. Togo, H. Suzuki, T. Kurusu, K. Iida, T. Sekiguchi,
Y. Sugishita, I. Ito

Summary: Sinus node electrograms (SNEs) on atrial overdrive suppression test (AOD) and estimated sinoatrial conduction time (SACT) measurements were recorded. Typical SNE (TSNE), characterized by low-frequency, anatomically localized pre-P wave potentials (Reiffel et al.) were obtained in 12 of 18 patients (pts) with normal sinus node function (group I) and 15 of 26 pts with sick sinus syndrome (SSS) (group II). In 9 of 15 SSS pts but only 2 or 12 in group I "atypical" SNEs (ASNE) with inverted waves at the beginning of P wave were recorded on SNE recordings of the first sinus recovery beat by overdrive atrial pacing (OAP) for either AOD or SACT measurements, or both. On the basis of ASNE following OAP, the 26 SSS pts fell into 3 subgroups: TSNE with the same configuration as recorded before OAP was observed without ASNE throughout the study in 6 pts (IIA). ASNE was observed without TSNE throughout the study in 11 pts (IIB). TSNE before OAP and ASNE following OAP were recorded in 9 pts (IIC). Corrected sinus node recovery time in IIB was significantly longer than in either IIA or IIC ($P < 0.0005$). Estimated SACT (Narula's method) for either A, B or C was significantly ($P < 0.0005$) longer than in group I. There was no significant difference in either estimated SACT or directly measured SACT between IIA and IIC. A significant correlation existed between estimated SACT and directly measured SACT in group I ($r = 0.88$) and IIA ($r = 0.75$) ($P < 0.01$) but not in IIC ($r = 0.48$). ASNE may result from a pacemaker shift.

The human sinus node electrogram (SNE) recording has been used as the method for evaluating human sinus node function (1–3). However, there is no report regarding assessment of the significance of impossibility of SNE recording or morphological alterations in SNE. The purpose of this study is to evaluate the significance of the sequence of the sinus node electrogram on the overdrive suppression test and estimated sinoatrial conduction time measurements in the sick sinus syndrome.

Patient population and methods

The patient population included 18 patients with normal sinus node function, ages 19–64 (group I) and 26 patients with sick sinus syndrome, ages 30–66 (group II). In this study, bipolar SNEs were obtained in the manner of Reiffel et al (2). We used 6 quadripolar catheters with 1 cm interelectrode distances. SNE recording obtained from the distal two poles of the catheter was displayed on a multichannel oscilloscope at low-pass filter frequencies of 0.1–50 Hz and high-gain amplification of 50–100 μV/cm. High right atrial electrogram, His bundle electrogram, surface leads I, aV_F and V_1 were as well as SNE recorded on a photographic oscilloscopic recorder at a paper speed of 100 and 150 mm/sec on atrial overdrive suppression test and estimated sinoatrial conduction time measurement by Narula's method ($SACT_N$).

Results

Typical sinus node electrograms (TSNEs) were obtained in 12 to 18 patients (67%) with normal sinus node function and in 15 of 26 patients (58%) with SSS. In 9 of 15 SSS patients but only 2 of 12 in group I "atypical" SNE (ASNE) with an inverted wave at the beginning of P wave was recorded on SNE recordings of the first sinus recovery beat by overdrive atrial pacing for either atrial overdrive suppression test or SACT measurements, or both. In 2 patients of group I, TSNE was restored within 10 spontaneous beats, meanwhile in 9 patients of IIC TSNE was not found before 30 spontaneous sinus beats following sudden termination of overdrive atrial pacing. On the basis of ASNE appearance before and following overdrive atrial pacing, 26 SSS patients fell into 3 subgroups; TSNE with the same configuration as recorded before overdrive atrial pacing was observed without ASNE throughout the study in 6 patients (IIA), ASNE was observed without TSNE throughout the study in 11 patients (IIB), and TSNE before and ASNE following overdrive atrial pacing were recorded in 9 patients (IIC).

Corrected sinus node recovery time in IIB was significantly longer than in either IIA or IIC ($P < 0.0005$ in either) (Figure 1). There was no significant difference in directly measured SACT between IIA and IIC (Figure 2). $SACT_N$ for either IIA, IIB or IIC was significantly longer than in group I ($P < 0.005$ in either) (Figure 3).

A significant correlation existed between $SACT_N$ and $SACT_C$ in group I ($r = 0.88$) and IIA ($r = 0.75$, $P < 0.01$), but not in IIC ($r = 0.48$).

Fig. 1. Relationship between the sequence of sinus node electrogram for SCRTC measurement and SNRTC in group II.

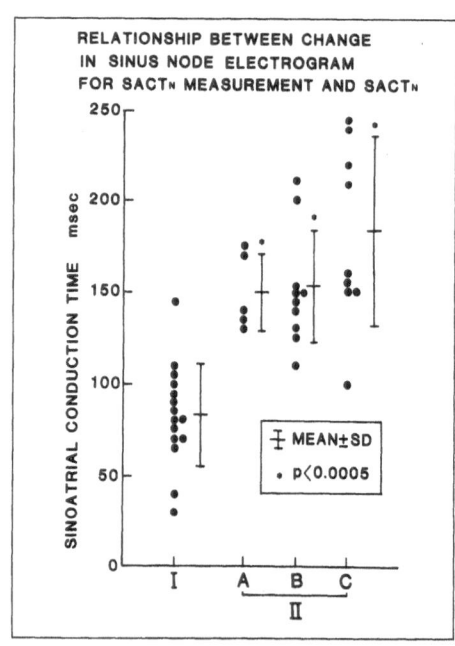

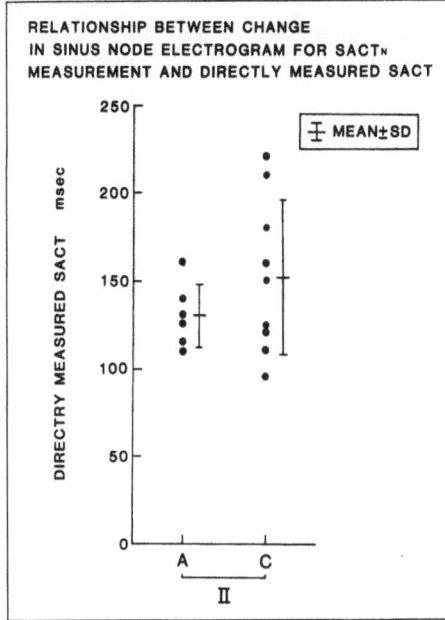

Fig. 3. Relationship between the sequence of sinus node electrogram for SACT$_N$ measurement and SACT$_N$.

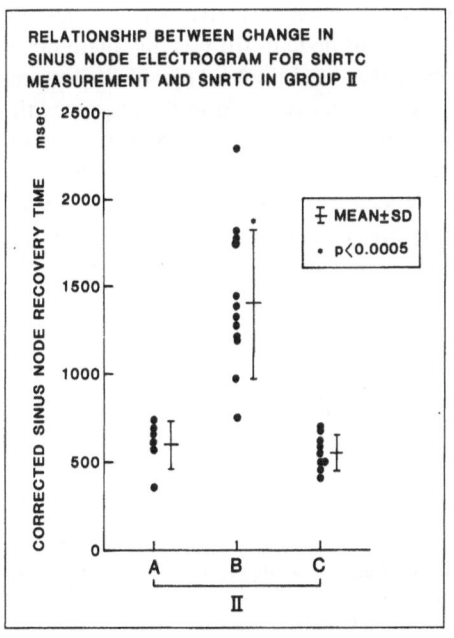

Fig. 2. Relationship between the sequence of sinus node electrogram for SACT$_N$ measurement and directly measured SACT.

Fig. 4

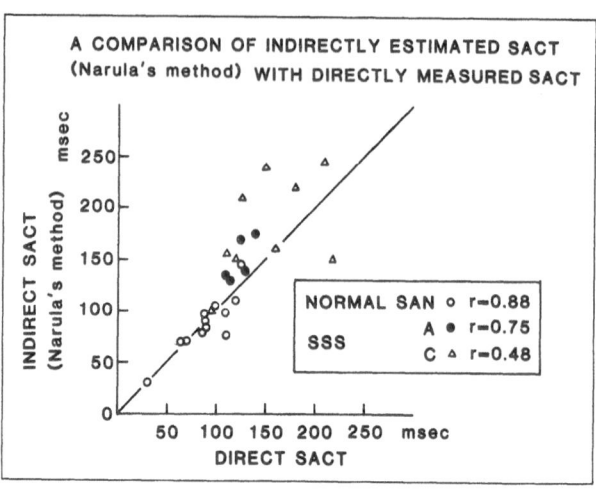

A COMPARISON OF INDIRECTLY ESTIMATED SACT
(Narula's method) WITH DIRECTLY MEASURED SACT

NORMAL SAN o r=0.88
A • r=0.75
SSS
C △ r=0.48

Discussion

In 2 patients of group I and in 20 patients of group II we observed ASNE on SNE recordings of the first sinus recovery beat by atrial overdrive pacing. TSNE was restored within 10 spontaneous beats following sudden termination of overdrive atrial pacing in group I. TSNE could not be obtained throughout the study in 11 patients of group II (IIB), but could be obtained in 9 patients of group II (IIC) though it was restored after at least 30 spontaneous beats following sudden termination of overdrive atrial pacing. These observations may suggest that pacemaker shifts occurred following overdrive atrial pacing in 2 patients of group I and 9 IIC patients, and that the sinus node in IIB was not anatomically localized in the catheter tip position in which TSNE could not be recorded. Restorations from ASNE to TSNE may suggest that TSNEs do not result from the change of the catheter tip position. Discrepancy between directly measured SACT and SACT$_N$ may result from a pacemaker shift of the first recovery beat used for estimated SACT. P waves before overdrive atrial pacing are morphologically identical with those of the first recovery beats in surface ECG leads even in IIC. Therefore, we must be careful when the estimated SACT in SSS is measured and evaluated.

References

1. Hariman RJ, Krongrad E, Boxer RA, Weiss MB, Steeg CN, Hoffman, BF: Method for recording electrical activity of the sinoatrial node and automatic atrial foci during cardiac catheterization in human subjects. Am J Cardiol 1980; 453 775–781.
2. Reiffel JA, Gang E, Gliklich J, Weiss MB, Davis JC, Patton JN, Bigger JT: The human sinus node electrogram. A transvenous catheter technique and a comparison of directly measured and indirectly estimated sinoatrial conduction time in adults. Circulation 1980; 62: 1324–1334.

3. Gomes JAC, Kang PS, El-Sherif N: The sinus node electrogram in patients with and without sick sinus syndrome. Techniques and correlation between directly measured and indirectly estimated sinoatrial conduction time. Circulation 1982; 66: 864–873.

Authors' address:
Dr. Iwao Yamaguchi
University of Tsukuba
School of Medicine
1-1-1 Tennodai, Sakura-Mura
Niihari-Gun, Ibaraki 305
Japan

A Study on Atrial Potential – Characteristics and its Relation to ECG

M. Murase, T. Ishihara, M. Kawamura, Y. Iyomasa

Summary: Seventy-three measurements of the atrial potential in 64 cases were recorded and studied at the time of physiological pacemaker implantation. The amplitude of the atrial potential in patients with Sick Sinus Syndrome (SSS) was significantly lower than in those with Atrio-Ventricular Block (AVB) (by PSA, 2.2 ± 1.3 mV vs. 3.9 ± 1.1 mV, $p < 0.001$; by endocardial electrogram, 2.7 ± 1.5 mV vs. 4.6 ± 1.7 mV, $p < 0.001$). The slew rate was slightly, but not significantly, faster in AVB than in SSS. The amplitude of the atrial potential recorded with bipolar lead was not significantly different from that with unipolar lead (by PSA 2.6 ± 1.5 mV vs. 2.3 ± 1.6 mV; by electrogram, 3.3 ± 1.4 mV vs. 2.8 ± 1.5 mV, NS). In the cases in which P-wave failed to appear after various procedures, the retrograde atrial potential was markedly low ($p < 0.001$). The atrial potential correlated relatively well with the total of P-wave voltages of lead I, II and III of the body surface ECG ($Y = 0.24 \pm 0.039$ X, $r = 0.446$, $p < 0.01$). This can be used in predicting the endocardial atrial potential preoperatively.

I. Introduction

During recent years, the usefulness of physiological pacing has been recognized (1, 2) and has been increasingly used clinically (3, 4). Nevertheless, the atrial potential is lower electrically than the ventricular potential (5), and, though atrial sensing is important, there are still problems to be resolved.

In sick sinus syndrome (SSS) the atrium is primarily affected. In atrio-ventricular block (AVB), the main lesion is in the atrio-ventricular conduction tissue and the atrium is almost free from the disease. These conditions may cause changes in the amplitude of the endoatrial electrogram.

In view of this, we have carried out a study of the atrial potentials measured at the time of pacemaker implantation in relation to physiological pacing.

II. Material and methods

We used sixty-four cases for the basis of this study; the patients population breaks down as follows: 42 had SSS, 19 had AVB, and 3 had both SSS and AVB. In cases of SSS, bipolar J-shaped electrodes (Medtronic*) 6990, 6990U, 4502) were used for AAI pacing. The surface area of the tip of these electrodes was 11 mm², and the ring area was 48 mm². The unipolar leads of the Medtronic 6991U type (electrode tip surface area of 11 mm²) were used in AVB and AVB + SSS, for physiological pacings (VAT in 6 cases, VDD in 7, and DDD in 9).

---

*) Medtronic Inc. Minneapolis, Minnesota.

The amplitude of atrial endocardial potential and electrogram was checked in all patients at the time of implantation of pacemakers.

Measurements were taken 73 times – 53 times in SSS and 20 times in AVB – because of reinsertion of the electrodes due to dislodgement, infections, etc. In each case the amplitude of the atrial potential was measured with the pacing system analyzer (PSA) of Medtronic*) model 5309 or 5311. While amplitude measurements and recording endocardial electrograms with an unipolar lead, a plate electrode (Medtronic*) 5803A, surface area 4.0 cm²), placed in the pacemaker pocket, served as a reference lead.

In 27 recent consecutive recordings (SSS: 17, AVB: 10), the amplitude and the slew rate of the atrial potential were analyzed. Electrogram recordings were made under the following conditions; the input impedance was approximately one megaohm and the band pass was $10 \sim 1000$ Hz.

Amplitudes were determined as the maximum positive-to-negative excursion of the signal with the most rapid dV/dt, and averaged over five beats. The slew rate or dV/dt was recorded at a sweep speed of 500 millimeters per second. It was determined as the mean dV/dt of the fastest changing limb of endocardial electrograms. Data were compared using Student's T-test. A probability level greater than 95% was chosen for significance.

III. Results

The atrial amplitude in SSS measured by PSA was 2.2 ± 1.3 mV (mean ± SD) and 3.9 ± 1.1 mV in AVB. There was a statistically significant difference ($p < 0.001$). The peak to peak amplitude of endocardial electrogram is SSS (2.7 ± 1.5 mV) was significantly lower than in AVB (4.6 ± 1.7 mV). The slew rates of the atrial electrogram in AVB were slightly, but not significantly, faster than those in SSS. These data were obtained from unipolar recordings in AVB, and from bipolar recordings in SSS (Table 1, Fig. 1). Therefore, we also measured unipolar potentials in some of the cases of SSS at the time

Table 1. Abbreviations; AVB: atrioventricular block, NS: not significant, PSA: pacemaker system analyzer, SD: standard deviation, SSS: sick sinus syndrome.

Atrial Potential (SSS and AVB) mean ± SD			
	SSS (bipolar)	AVB (unipolar)	p
PSA	Amplitude (mV) 2.2±1.3 (n = 45) (range 0.3–5.4)	3.9±1.1 (n = 20) (range 1.7–6.0)	p < 0.001
Endocardial Electrogram	Amplitude (mV) 2.7±1.5 (n= 17) (range 0.6–6.3)	4.6±1.7 (n = 10) (range 1.4–8.0	p < 0,001
	Slew Rate (v/s) 0.83±0.64 (n = 17) (range 0.21–2.1)	1.99±1.44 (n = 10) (range 0.52–5.67)	NS

of insertion of bipolar electrodes. As shown in Table 2, when measured by PSA, the amplitude of unipolar lead was 2.3 ± 1.6 mV, and that of bipolar lead was 2.6 ± 1.5 mV. By endocardial electrogram, those were 2.8 ± 1.5 mV and 3.3 ± 1.4 mV respectively. These data were obtained from the same patients and bipolar amplitudes were somewhat higher than unipolar amplitudes, although the difference between them was not significant (Table 2). In the recent cases of SSS, measurements with unipolar electrodes, as in the cases of AVB, were possible, and they also showed that the potentials were significantly lower ($p < 0.001$) in those with SSS (2.4 ± 1.4 mV by PSA, 2.8 ± 1.4 mV by endocardial electrogram) when compared with the cases of AVB (3.9 ± 1.1 mV by PSA, 4.6 ± 1.7 mV: by endocardial electrogram). But the slew rate showed no significant difference, though a rather faster slew rate was observed in AVB.

When combined, these results showed that the atrial potential of the patients with SSS was generally lower than that of the patients with AVB.

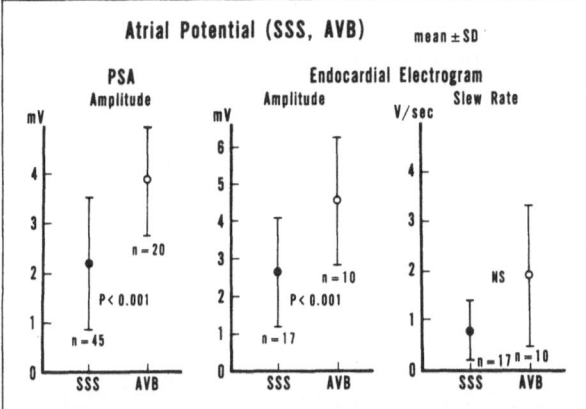

Fig. 1. Comparison of atrial potential in SSS and AVB. Amplitude in AVB was significantly higher than in SSS by both PSA and endocardial electrogram. Slew rate was not significant but faster in AVB.

Table 2. Abbreviations; see Table 1.

Atrial Potential (unipolar and bipolar) mean ± SD

	Unipolar	Bipolar	
PSA (n = 17)	Amplitude (mV) 2.3 ± 1.6 (range 0.6–5.8)	2.6 ± 1.5 (range 1.2–5.4)	NS
Endocardial Electrogram (n = 11)	Amplitude (mV) 2.8 ± 1.5 (range 0.6–5.7)	3.3 ± 1.4 (range 0.9–6.3)	NS
	Slew Rate (v/s) 1.09 ± 1.05 (range 0.02–2.78)	1.05 ± 0.70 (range 0.21–2.1)	NS

67

In eight cases of SSS, only atrio-ventricular junctional rhythm was observed and a sinus P-wave did not appear even after intravenous injection of atropin sulfate or by other means. Retrograde atrial potential were confirmed by simultaneous recording of the intra-atrial electrogram and the amplitude of measured retrograde atrial potentials was 0.6 ± 0.4 mV by PSA, and 0.8 ± 0.1 mV by endocardial electrogram analysis. These were significantly lower than antegrade atrial potentials (Fig. 2).

In cases in which both recordings of the retrograde and antegrade potential were possible, the retrograde potential was lower than the antegrade potential.

We also studied the standard electrocardiogram of body surface leads in these patients.

We measured the voltage of the P-wave in the standard limb leads I, II and III of ECGs recorded before pacemaker implantation. In the total of P-wave voltages in leads I, II and III of the surface ECG, there was a significant difference between the patients with SSS and those with AVB (0.30 ± 0.11 mV vs. 0.46 ± 0.12 mV: $p < 0.001$) (Table 3). Compared with the control group with no heart disease (0.35 ± 0.10 mV), the total of P-wave

Fig. 2. Amplitude of the atrial potentials in the patients with only retrograde P-wave at operation was remarkably lower than that in the others. Slew rate was not significant.

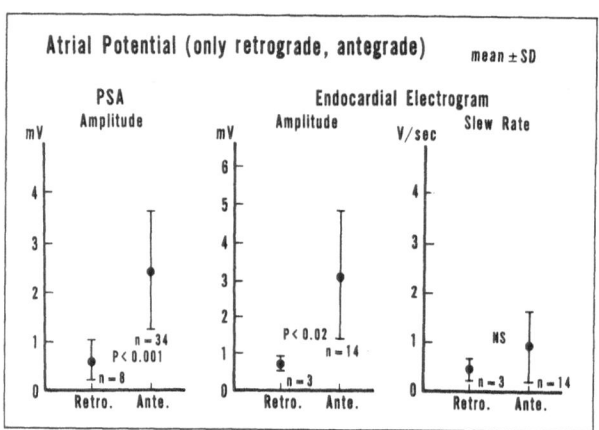

Table 3. Abbreviations; AVB: atrioventricular block, pt. No: patient number, SD: standard deviation, SSS: sick sinus syndrome.

P-Voltage (total of lead I, II and III) mean ± SD

	SSS	AVB	Control
Pt. No.	n = 42	n = 19	n = 44
Voltage	0.30 ± 0.11 mV	0.46 ± 0.12 mV	0.35 ± 0.10 mV
Range	0.06–0.58	0.22–0.70	0.15–0.55
p		$p < 0.001$ $p < 0.001$	
		$p < 0.05$	

voltages was significantly lower in SSS, and higher in AVB. We compared the cases of physiological pacing to find any correlation between the atrial potential and the total of P-wave voltages of lead I, II and III of the preoperative standard ECG and it was found that the total of P-wave voltages of lead I, II and III had a relatively good correlation with the atrial potential at $Y = 0.24 + 0.039X$, $r = 0.446$, $p < 0.01$ (Fig. 3).

IV. Discussion

During recent years, with the advances in atrial electrodes and improvements in generators, physiological pacing has come into use. However, as the atrial potential is lower than the ventricular potential, the atrial sensing still has many problems to be resolved. As the atrial potential is low, and in order to increase the sensitivity for the atrial sensing, as well as to prevent oversensing due to myopotentials, we have used "J" bipolar electrodes in SSS patients. However, physiological pacemakers such as DDD, VDD, have unipolar lead systems. It has become necessary for us to use unipolar electrodes in patients with AVB or AVB + SSS.

Several reports about the intra-atrial electrogram have been published (6, 7, 8), but a comparative study of the atrial potential between SSS and AVB has not been reported.

According to the study of all cases, the amplitude of the atrial potential in SSS was significantly lower than in AVB. However, in SSS, the value was obtained from bipolar lead, and in AVB from unipolar lead.

In some cases of SSS, measurements with both unipolar leads and bipolar leads were taken, and the results, as shown in Table 2, showed no remarkable difference. In the past,

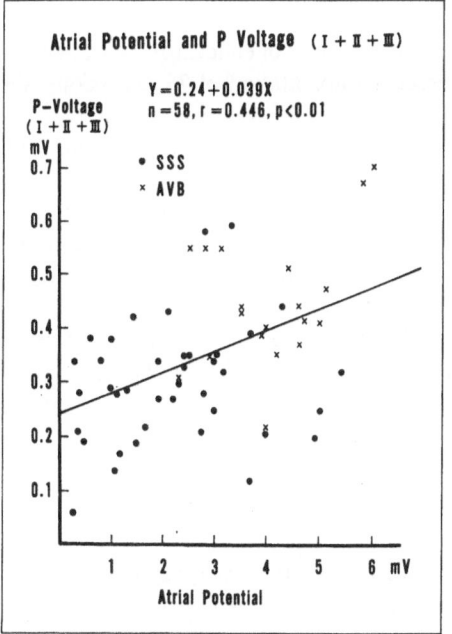

Fig. 3. Amplitude of the atrial potential correlated relatively well with the total of P-wave voltages of lead I, II and III.

ventricular potential in ventricular pacing had been considered to be higher when measured with a unipolar electrode, however, according to a recent report even the ventricular potential showed no remarkable difference between measurements with unipolar and bipolar electrodes (9). The same results were found in atrial potential (10).

Considering only amplitudes with unipolar lead the mean of the amplitudes in SSS (PSA: 2.4 ± 1.4 mV n = 21, Endocardial Electrogram: 2.8 ± 1.4 mV n = 14) was significantly lower than that in AVB (PSA: 3.9 ± 1.1 mV n = 20, Endocardial Electrogram: 4.6 ± 1.7 mV n = 10; $p < 0.001$, $p < 0.01$ respectively).

From these, it was reasonable to assume that the atrial potentials of the patients with SSS were generally lower than those of the patients with AVB.

When antegrade P-waves failed to appear at the time of pacemaker implantation, a large dose of atropin sulfate was given intravenously in addition to other inductive procedures, but there were cases in which these procedures did not result in the appearance of P-wave. In these cases, we found that the retrograde atrial potentials were remarkably and significantly ($p < 0.001$) low. It was presumed in these patients that the pathologic changes of the atrium were more severe and broader with less electrical force than other patients.

Analysis of the P-wave voltages of the standard leads I, II and III of the surface ECG showed that the total of P-wave voltages was high in AVB, low in SSS, and moderate in the control group with no heart disease. These results were the same as the results obtained from the intra-atrial potential analysis. As shown in Fig. 3, the atrial potentials correlated highly with P-wave voltages of the body surface ECG, therefore, this should be used in predicting the atrial potential so as to select the best suitable and safest pacing mode and pacemaker type for a particular patient.

V. Conclusion

Physiological pacing was used in 64 cases. Based on the study of endocardial atrial potentials which were measured at the time of pacemaker implantation of 73 occassions, the following conclusions were reached.

1. Atrial potentials of the patients with SSS were lower than those of the patients with AVB.
2. In some patients, P-waves failed to appear after various procedures for induction of this wave. The retrograde atrial potentials in these patients were markedly low, probably showing high degrees of pathologic changes in the atrium. Generally, the retrograde atrial potentials were lower than the antegrade atrial potentials.
3. The atrial potentials correlated relatively well with the total of P-wave voltages of leads I, II, III of the body surface ECG. This can be used in predicting the endocardial atrial potential preoperatively, which will serve as an aid in the selection of a suitable pacemaker.

References

1. Sutton R, Perrins J, Citron P: Physiological cardiac pacing. Pace 1980; 3: 207–219.
2. Stone JM, Bhaka RD, Lutgen J: Dual chamber sequential pacing management of sinus node dysfunction: Advantages over single-chamber pacing. Am Heart J 1982; 104: 1319–1327.

3. Sutton R, Citron P: Electrophysiological and haemodynamic basis for application of new pacemaker technology in sick sinus syndrome and atrioventricular block. Br Heart J 1979; 41: 600–612.
4. Curtis JJ, Madigan NP, Whiting RB, Mueller KJ, Pezzella AT, Walls JT, Heineman FM: Clinical experience with permanent atrioventricular sequential pacing. Ann Thorac Surg 1981; 32: 179–185.
5. Murase M, et al: Atrial pacing, evaluation of leads, threshold, and p voltage (In Japanese). Artif Organs 1981; 10: 115–118.
6. Parsonnet V, Myers G, Kresh YM: Characteristics of intracardiac electrograms II: atrial endocardial electrograms. Pace 1980; 3: 406–417.
7. Kruse I, Rydén L, Ydse B: A new lead for transvenous atrial pacing and sensing. Pace 1980; 3: 395–404.
8. Murase M, Abe T, Washizu T, Tanaka M, Kawamura M, Takeuchi E, Kakihara R, Iyomasa Y, Ishihara T, Miyata T, Ohmiya T, Tamaki S: A study of atrial endocardial signals (In Japanese). Artif Organs 1982; 11: 1005–1008.
9. Breivik K, Engedal H, Ohm O: Electrophysiological properties of a new permanent endocardial lead for uni- and bipolar pacing. Pace 1982; 5: 268–274.
10. Griffin JC: Sensing characteristics of the right atrial appendage electrode. Pace 1983; 6: 22–24.

Authors' address:
M. Murase, M.D.
1st Dept. of Surgery
Nagoya University
Showa-ku,
Tsurumai-Cho 65
Nagoya 466/Japan

Blood Volume Changes and Sinus Node Function

V. Hossmann, U. Alt, E. Dundalek, R. Griebenow, F. Saborowski

Summary: In twenty-three patients (38–82 yrs, mean age 62.2 yrs) with a history of light-headedness or syncope sinus node recovery time (SNRT) was measured following atrial stimulation of 85 and 145/min, whereby pulmonary arterial pressure (PAP) and systemic intraarterial pressure (SAP) were continuously recorded, cardiac output (CO) measured by thermodilution and venous blood withdrawn for radioenzymatic determination of plasma norepinephrine (PNE) and epinephrine (PE) after 15 min of rest and at the end of each stimulation period, lasting 3 min. The hemodynamic and electrophysiological measurements were repeated in the same way during volume load (VL) by tilting up the legs and volume depletion (VD) induced by a) venous occlusion of the legs and b) by i.v. injection of 20 mg frusemide. During VL mPAP increased significantly by 2 mmHg from 10.9 ± 0.8 to 12.9 ± 0.9 mmHg at sinus rhythm, SNRT from 1313 ± 58 msec to 1348 ± 57 msec at 85/min, and from 1149 ± 65 msec to 1232 ± 58 msec at 145/min, max. cSNRT from 337 ± 38 msec to 433 ± 37 msec. VD induced by venodilation due to frusemide significantly reduced SNRT to 1056 ± 58 msec at 85/min, 1034 ± 52 msec at 145/min ($P < 0.01$). CO decreased significantly from 6.0 ± 0.5 l/min to 4.9 l/min at 85/min and from 5.2 l/min to 4.3 l/min at 145/min ($p < 0.01$), and peripheral vascular resistance significantly increased, as did PNE: from 0.35 ± 0.07 ng/ml to 0.55 ± 0.09 ng/ml ($p < 0.05$). Baroreceptor mediated adaptation of the autonomic nervous system to volume depletion is evidently responsible for the reduction of SNRT.

Introduction

Sinus node recovery time varies widely inter- and intraindividually, due to a complex of intrinsic electrophysiological properties and extrinsic factors (1–3). Among the extrinsic factors the most important is probably the autonomic nervous system, which modifies sinus node function to a large extent and which has been examined extensively in clinical studies, namely by comparing sinus node function prior to and after autonomic blockade (4–6). Another extrinsic factor which may influence sinus node function is the blood volume.

The aim of this study was to examine whether blood volume shifts influence sinus node function and to what extent the sympathetic nervous system participates in this regulatory process.

Patients and Methods

Twenty-three patients (38–82 yrs, mean age 62.2 yrs, 14 males, 9 females) with a previous history of light-headedness or syncope were included into the study. All medication was discontinued at least 7 days prior to the investigation. Each patient gave his written informed consent.

The study was performed in a cardiac catheterization laboratory with the patient in a nonsedated, postabsorptive state.

Two catheters were placed into the femoral vein by Seldinger technique. Under fluoroscopic control one dipolar stimulation catheter (5 F, USCI) was positioned at the junction

73

of the superior vena cava and the high right atrium for atrial stimulation (AS). The other, a Swan-Ganz thermodilution catheter was placed into the pulmonary artery for continuous recording of the pulmonary artery pressure (PAP) and measurement of cardiac output (CO) by thermodilution using an Edwards cardiac output computer.

A micro-Seldinger catheter (Seldicath, intra) was inserted into the right femoral artery and connected with a Statham 23 Db transducer for continuous recording of the systemic arterial pressure (SAP). Finally an indwelling catheter was inserted into a left antecubital vein for blood sampling. Standard ECG was continuously monitored on a 6 channel polygraph (Cardirex 62, Siemens-Elema, Stockholm) at varying paper speed.

After a stabilization period of 15 min the following control recordings were performed: PAP, SAP, ECG, and CO. 10 ml of blood were withdrawn from the antecubital vein, filled in chilled EDTA-containing tubes, placed on ice and centrifuged at 2000 g and + 4 °C for 10 min within 30 min.

The plasma obtained was stored at −20 °C for subsequent measurement of plasma epinephrine (PE) and plasma norepinephrine (PNE) by using a modified radioenzymatic assay according to Da Prada and Zürcher (1976) and Peuler and Johnson (1977; 7, 8).

Sinus node recovery time (SNRT) was measured following atrial pacing with rectangular stimuli of 2 msec duration and twice diastolic threshold at 85 and 145/min with an USM 30 (Biotronic, Berlin). The respective stimulation period lasted 3 min. While SAP and PAP were continuously recorded, CO was measured twice during the third minute of stimulation and blood for determination of plasma catecholamines was withdrawn immediately before the end of stimulation.

SNRT was recorded as the interval to the return of spontaneous atrial activity after abrupt termination of atrial pacing. Corrected sinus node recovery time (cSNRT) was measured as SNRT minus the mean of 8 prepaced basic cycle lengths.

Thereafter, the legs were tilted up to about 60–70 ° and following a subsequent stabilization period of 10 min the same measurements during volume load (VL) were performed as described above: hemodynamic measurements, determination of PNE and PE, during sinus rhythm and AS of 85 and 145/min, as well as SNRT following AS.

Volume depletion (VD) was obtained in two ways:
a) by venous occlusion (VO) with a pneumatic cuff placed around the proximal third of the thighs and being inflated to 80 mmHg
b) by intravenous injection of 20 mg frusemide.

The hemodynamic and electrophysiological studies were performed after a stabilization period of 10 min after VO and 5 min after i.v. injection of frusemide.

Pulmonary vascular resistance was calculated from the ratio mean PAP/CO, pulmonary arteriolar resistance as (mean PAP − diastolic PAP)/CO, peripheral vascular resistance as mean SAP/CO.

Statistical comparisons were performed by paired and unpaired t-tests using two-tailed probabilities throughout the analysis. Values are expressed as mean ± SEM.

Results

The blood volume changes, as described here, induced different hemodynamic and electrophysiological alterations of sinus function at rest, and during atrial stimulation of 85 and 145/min. During atrial stimulation of 145/min these changes were dependent upon the AV-conduction. In 12 of 23 patients rapid atrial pacing resulted in intermittent AV-block of 2 : 1 or of Wenckebach type, irrespective of the blood volume changes. In these patients e.g. the reduction in systolic blood pressure and in cardiac output was less pronounced, than in the patients group with normal AV-conduction. The differences of the mean values of the whole patient group, therefore, are less marked.

1. Pulmonary artery pressure

Volume load by tilting up the legs induced a significant increase in mean pulmonary artery pressure (mPAP) of 2 mmHg during sinus rhythm (10.9 ± 0.8 vs. 12.9 ± 0.9 mmHg; p < 0.05), as well as during AS of 85/min (10.9 ± 0.8 vs. 12.5 ± 0.8 mmHg: p < 0.05), while at 145/min this increase was no more detectable (Fig. 1). On the other hand reduction of mPAP due to volume depletion by venous occlusion of the legs, as well as injection of frusemide became only apparent during atrial stimulation of 85/min (10.9 ± 0.8 vs. 9.3 ± 0.6 mmHg during VO; p < 0.05) and 145/min (13.4 ± 1.2 vs. 11.2 ± 0.9 mmHg; p < 0.05), whereby mPAP decreased by 1.6–2.2 mmHg, when compared with AS of the same frequency during the control period.

Interesting to note, that the failing decrease in mPAP during VL and sinus rhythm was accompanied by a significant increase in pulmonary vascular resistance, while pulmonary arteriolar resistance was not influenced by either change of blood volume during sinus rhythm and during AS of 85/min.

2. Cardiac output

Cardiac output significantly increased by 11.7% from 5.3 ± 0.4 l/min during sinus rhythm of 61.3 ± 2.6 beats/min to 6.0 ± 0.5 l/min during AS of 85/min (p < 0.05; Fig. 2). AS of 145/min only slightly decreased CO (5.2 l/min). The same changes were observed during volume load. Volume depletion, however, induced a significant reduction

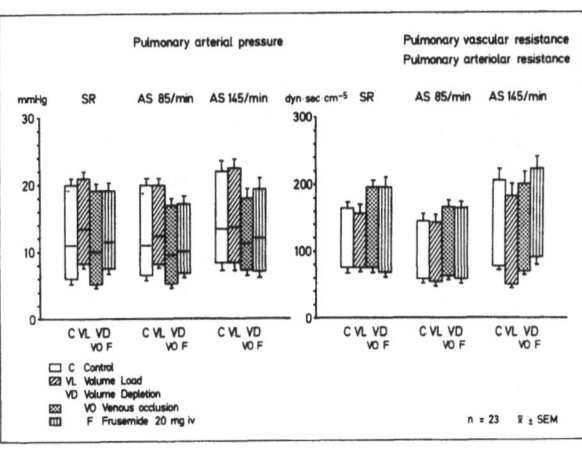

Fig. 1. Pulmonary arterial pressure (left), pulmonary vascular resistance (right above) and pulmonary aterіolar resistance (right below) under normal steady-state condition (C), during volume load (VL) and volume depletion (VD) induced by venous occlusion (VO) and i.v. injection of frusemide 20 mg (F) at rest and during atrial stimulation (AS) of 85 and 145/min.

in CO during AS of 85/min (5.2 ± 0.4 l/min during VO; 4.9 l/min after frusemide; $p < 0.01$) and 145/min (4.5 ± 0.4 l/min during VO; 4.3 ± 0.4 l/min after F; $p < 0.01$). After frusemide CO was already reduced at sinus rhythm (4.8 ± 0.4 l/min).

3. Systemic arterial blood pressure

The changes in systemic arterial blood pressure and peripheral vascular resistance are listed on Table 1. The most interesting findings are a significant reduction in arterial

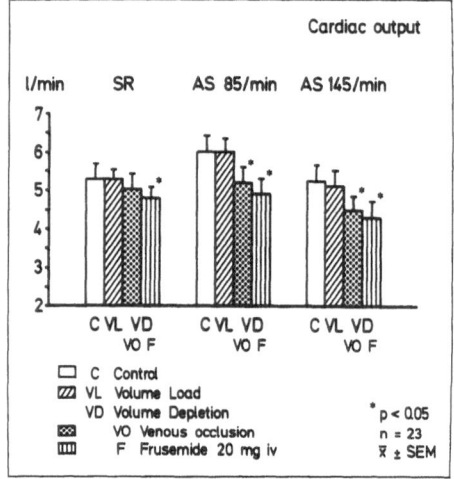

Fig. 2. Cardiac output (CO), measured by thermodilution under steady-state condition (C), during volume load (VL) and volume depletion (VD) induced by venous occlusion (VO) and i.v. injection of frusemide 20 mg (F) at rest and during atrial stimulation (AS) of 85 and 145/min.

Table 1.

		Blood pressure (mmHg)		Peripheral vascular resistance
		Systolic	Diastolic	(dyn. sec. cm$^{-5)}$
Control	Sinus rhythm	140.9 ± 4.8	77.1 ± 3.2	1561 ± 170
	AS 85/min	143.7 ± 5.2	82.6 ± 3.4	1648 ± 128
	AS 145/min	143.8 ± 6.0	89.7 ± 3.3	1776 ± 165
Volume load	Sinus rhythm	145.4 ± 5.0	82.8 ± 3.3	1597 ± 111
	AS 85/min	149.3 ± 4.5	87.0 ± 3.5	1530 ± 111
	AS 145/min	147.1 ± 4.8	92.2 ± 3.4	1896 ± 180
Volume depletion	Sinus rhythm	140.8 ± 5.6	80.0 ± 3.5	1630 ± 171
(VO)	AS 85/min	138.7 ± 4.9	85.1 ± 3.1	1733 ± 150
	AS 145/min	132.8 ± 5.2	87.1 ± 2.6	1894 ± 163
Volume depletion	Sinus rhythm	148.8 ± 4.7	82.6 ± 2.1	1958 ± 154
(Frusemide)	AS 85/min	146.5 ± 4.6	85.5 ± 2.4	1933 ± 175
	AS 145/min	144.7 ± 5.2	91.5 ± 4.2	2238 ± 258

blood pressure only in the volume depleted state, a moderate increase in blood pressure during volume load at SR as well as during AS of 85 and 145/min and a significant increase in systemic vascular resistance during AS of 85 and 145/min during volume depletion.

4. Catecholamines

Plasma norepinephrine was in the normal range during sinus rhythm in normal steady-state, as well as during VL and VD (Fig. 3). However, a significant increase in PNE was obtained during AS of 85 and 145/min in the course of volume depletion by i.v. injection of frusemide. PNE increased from 0.35 ± 0.07 ng/ml during sinus rhythm to 0.55 ± 0.09 ng/ml during AS of 145/min. This increase in PNE was reflected by the significant increase in peripheral vascular resistance as shown in Table 1. Plasma epinephrine on the other hand varied widely and seemed not to be influenced by the different blood volume changes.

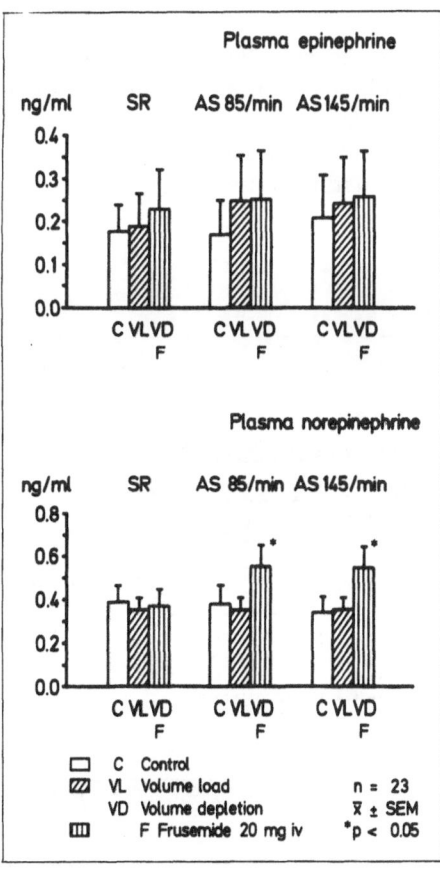

Fig. 3. Plasma epinephrine and plasma norepinephrine under steady-state condition (C), during volume load (VL) and volume depletion (VD) induced by i.v. injection of frusemide 20 mg (F) at rest and during atrial stimulation (AS) of 85 and 145/min.

In 4 of the 23 patients SNRT was $\geq$ 1500 msec and cSNRT $\geq$ 450 msec. The alteration of SNRT due to volume changes was similar. Therefore, the groups were not separated. SNRT was 1313 ± 58 msec following AS of 85/min and 1149 ± 65 msec following AS of 145/min. The correspondent cSNRT was 337 ± 38 msec resp. 173 ± 37 msec. During volume load SNRT increased to 1348 ± 57 msec (85/min) and 1232 ± 58 msec (145/min). The increase of cSNRT was similar being 433 ± 37 msec at AS 85/min and 318 ± 33 msec at 145/min. Volume depletion by venous occlusion did not influence SNRT significantly when compared with the control measurements: 1250 ± 66 msec at 85/min and 1094 ± 64 msec at 145/min, cSNRT: 315 ± 42 msec at 85/min and 212 ± 37 msec at 145/min.

Volume depletion induced by venodilation after i.v. injection of frusemide, however, had a marked effect on both SNRT and intrinsic heart rate. SNRT decreased to 1056 ± 58 msec at 85/min, 1034 ± 52 msec at 145/min; cSNRT to 160 ± 37 msec at 85/min and 139 ± 39 msec at 145/min. The intrinsic heart rate at the same time increased from 61.3 ± 2.8 to 67.0 ± 3.3 beats/min ($p < 0.01$; Fig. 4).

Discussion

The results of this study indicate that blood volume changes influence sinus node function in a different way. Although there was a small increase in SNRT due to volume load, this increase, however, did not attain statistical significance. This observation coincides with that obtained by Yamaguchi et al. 1982 (9), who did not show significant changes of the corrected SNRT in normal controls during autonomic blockade, where

Fig. 4. Sinus node recovery time (SNRT) after atrial stimulation (AS) of 85 and 145/min under normal steady-state condition (control), during volume load and volume depletion induced by venous occlusion and i.v. injection of frusemide 20 mg.

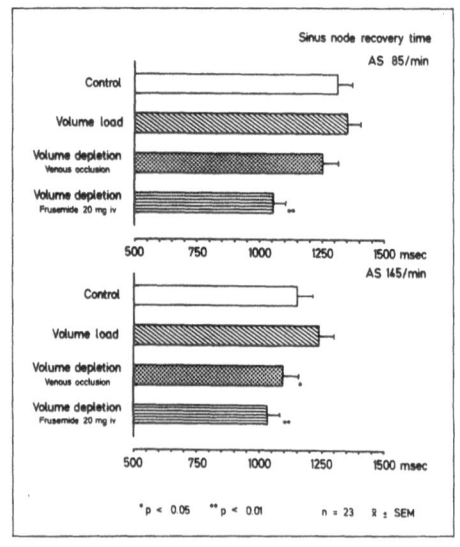

volume load was obtained by infusion of low molecular weight dextran, thereby increasing right atrial pressure by about 4 mmHg. Yamaguchi et al. (9) found an increase in cSNRT and intrinsic heart rate only in patients with intrinsic sinus node dysfunction.

Of the 4 patients in our series with increased cSNRT under normal steady state conditions only two showed an increase in SNRT and cSNRT during volume load.

Volume depletion due to venodilation following i.v. injection of frusemide was accompanied by a significant reduction in SNRT and cSNRT. The hemodynamic changes were much more pronounced as during volume load especially during atrial stimulation. The reduction in cardiac output resulted in an increase in peripheral vascular resistance, which in turn was evidently due to an increase in sympathetic tone, since PNE increased significantly by more than 60%, when compared with the basal value. It is therefore most likely, that the shortening of SNRT, cSNRT and spontaneous heart rate was due to an activation of sympathetic tone.

Mean plasma norepinephrine was 0.35 ± 0.07 ng/ml during the first measurement after a resting period of 15 min following the placement of the different catheters. This value is in the normal range, when compared with PNE concentration in recumbent healthy age-matched controls after a similar resting period following placement of a venous cannula. Therefore, it can be concluded, that emotional stress, due to the catheterization procedure is only of minor importance in influencing the results of invasive measurements of sinus node function. Only 5 of the 23 patients showed an elevation of PNE at the first measurement of more than 0.5 ng/ml but not more than 0.7 ng/ml, whereby after the first stimulation procedure PNE returned to normal values, too. This result supports the observation made by Jewell et al. 1980 (10) who measured urinary catecholamines and systolic time intervals before, during and after the catheterization procedure and who were not able to detect an increased sympathetic activation during the catheterization.

The results obtained so far may have practical implications. Dehydrated patients, especially those being chronically treated with diuretics, may demonstrate false-negative results, when sinus node function is measured. Strict bedrest of only 48 hrs may induce a decrease in blood volume of about 500 ml, which, too, may seriously disturb a correct measurement of SNRT. Whether hypervolemic states such as in congestive heart failure increase SNRT may be doubted since the well – known increase of sympathetic tone will overcome the possibly volume dependent increase in SNRT.

References

1. Thormann J, Schlepper M: Zur Reproduzierbarkeit der Sinusknotenerholungszeit in Abhängigkeit von Tageszeit und "Overdrive"-Testfrequenz. Z Kardiol 1980; 69: 542–550.
2. Tonkin AM, Tornos P, Heddle WF, Rapp H: Variability of the normal sinus node recovery time. Aust N Z J Med 1978; 8: 571.
3. Jordan JL, Yamaguchi I, Mandel WJ: Studies on the mechanism of sinus node dysfunction in the sick sinus syndrome. Circulation 1978; 57: 217–223.
4. Alboni P, Malcarne C, Pedroni P, Masoni A, Narula OS: Electrophysiology of normal sinus node with and without autonomic blockade. Circulation 1982; 65: 1236–1242.
5. Desai JM, Scheinman MM, Strauss HC, Massie B, O'Young J: Electrophysiologic effects of combined autonomic blockade in patients with sinus node disease. Circulation 1981; 63: 953–960.
6. Kang PS, Gomes JAC, El-Sherif N: Differential effects of functional autonomic blockade on the variables of sinus nodal automaticity in sick sinus syndrome. Am J Cardiol 1982; 49: 273–282.

7. Da Prada M, Zürcher G: Simultaneous radioenzymatic determination of plasma and tissue adrenaline, noradrenaline and dopamine within the fentomole range. Life Sci 1976; 19: 1161–1174.
8. Peuler JD, Johnson GA: Simultaneous single isotope radioenzymatic assay of plasma norepinephrine, epinephrine and dopamine. Life Sci 1977; 21: 625–636.
9. Yamaguchi I, Togo T, Sekiguchi T, Ito I: The effects on sinus node function of increases in right atrial pressure. In: Cardiac pacing. Electrophysiological and pacemaker technology, Ed. Feruglio GA, pp. 51–54. Piccin Medical Books Padova (Italy) 1982.
10. Jewell GM, Magorien RD, Schaal SF, Leier CV: Autonomic tone of patients during an electrophysiological catheterization. Am Heart J 1980; 99: 51–57.

Authors address:
PD Dr. V. Hossmann
Lehrstuhl Innere Medizin II
Ostmerheimer Str. 200
5000 Köln 91

Loss of Sinus Activity after Long-Term Permanent VVI Pacing

S. Feldman, H. N. Neufeld

Summary: In 183 out of 763 patients (24%) without sinus node dysfunction belonging to the atrio-ventricular conduction defect group, a spontaneous loss of sinus activity was detected after a 2–3 year follow-up period, following permanent VVI pacemaker implantation. Atrial fibrillation and/or atrial fibrillo-flutter may precede this final stage of loss of sinus activity.

These findings could be a result of the natural history of the disease, with the involvement of the sinus node in the organic process i.e. fibrosis of the conduction tissue.

This evolution may jeopardize the effect and the usefulness of the dual chamber mode of pacing in the long-term follow-up, by the appearance of atrial electro-mechanical dissociation.

Introduction

For many years VVI has been the preferred mode of pacing, replacing the first VOO system.

With the development of the double chamber pulse generators, the behaviour of the sinus activity became an important electrophysiologic and hemodynamic factor (1). We became interested in the evolution of the sinus activity after pacing.

Material and methods

Knowing that the disease of the sinus node is an inherent characteristic of the Sick Sinus Syndrome (Sinus Insufficiency Snydrome) (2, 3) we selected our material only from the atrio-ventricular conduction defect group, with normal sinus node activity during the implant and a high degree of pacemaker dependency during the long-term follow-up.

Out of 1,067 patients with permanent VVI pacemaker, 763 were selected (70%). Of them 62% were male and 38% female. The mean age was 68 years.

The etiology of the disease was fibrosis of the conduction system in 72%, ischemic heart disease in 23%, and miscellaneous in 5%.

The ECG pattern showed narrow QRS in 321 patients (42%) and different patterns of multifascicular block (mostly 1º AVB + CRBBB + left anterior fascicular block, or 1º AVB + CLBBB) in 442 (58%).

No sinus node dysfunction was documented; the corrected sinus recovery time was normal in all the patients, as well as the sino-atrial conduction time (by Narula's method) when measurement was feasible. Carotid body hypersensitivity was not present. All the patients had VVI unipolar pacemaker, 80% of them programmable. Follow-up over a 5 year period was performed by routine clinical examination and ECG. However patients in whom loss of P wave was detected, underwent chest X-ray fluoroscopy, and the permanent pulse generator was temporarily programmed at a slow rate, usually at 30 spikes per minute. During replacement of non-programmable pacemakers, the ECG was recorded with an external programmable pulse generator at a progressive slow rate down to 30 spikes per minute.

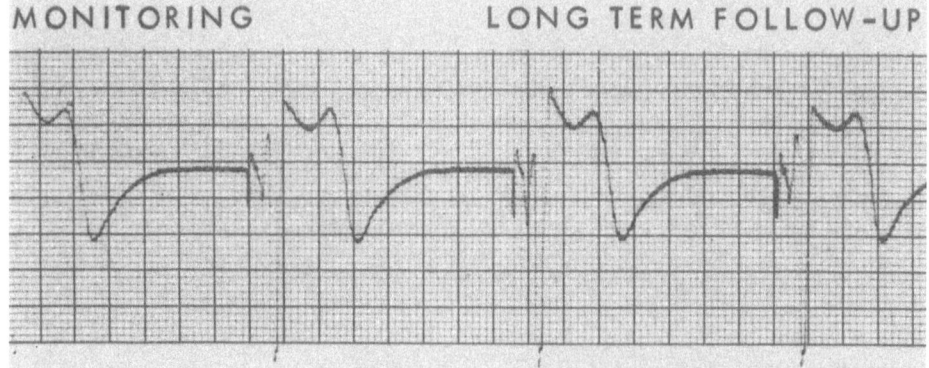

Fig. 1. Case 1 – Ventricular pacing at 30 spikes per minute without signs of sinus node activity.

Fig. 2. Case 2 – Routine ECG shows 1° degree AVB, CRBBB and left anterior scicular block.

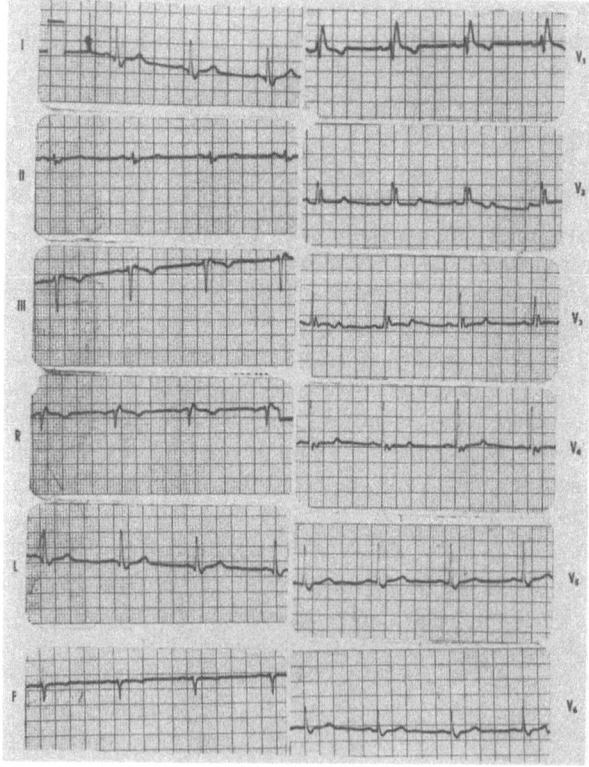

The chest wall stimulation test (4) was not used due to the high degree of pacemaker dependency in our cases.

Our patients were usually free of drug treatment, particularly digitalis, beta-blockers, verapamil and amiodarone.

Results

From 2 to 3 years after commencement of follow-up, it was seen that the P wave disappeared in 183 patients (24%), despite the absence of the clinical "pacemaker syndrome". Occasionally the disappearance of the P waves was preceded by the appearance of atrial fibrillo-flutter.

Case 1: A 68 year old male patient was admitted because of syncope. The clinical examination, echocardiography and hemodynamic investigations were compatible with the diagnosis of idiopathic subaortic stenosis. The ECG showed: P mitrale, left ventricular hypertrophy and strain. A CAVB was detected intermittently by ECG monitoring. No sinus node dysfunction was found. After a follow-up of 26 months the P waves disappeared (Fig. 1) after a short period of atrial fibrillo-flutter.

Case 2: A 73 year old male patient was admitted because of Adams-Stokes attacks. A multifascicular block (1º AVB + CRBBB + Left Anterior Fascicular Block) (Fig. 2) of unknown etiology was found. The sinus node was normal. The A · H was 90 ms and the

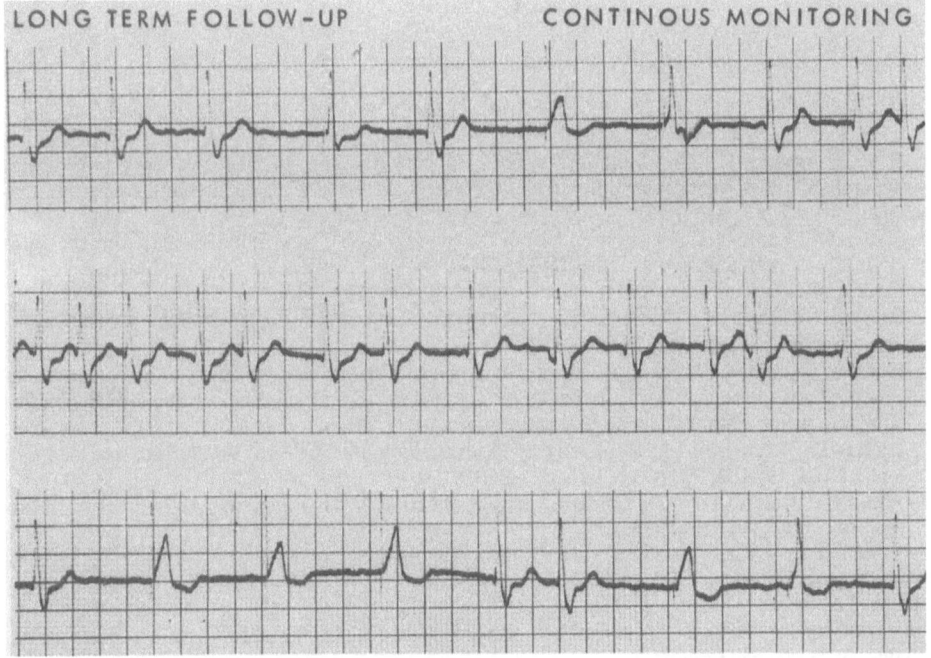

Fig. 3. Case 2 – After a 3 year follow-up an intractable atrial fibrillation appeared and remained unchanged.

H · V 100 ms. After a long-term follow-up, close to 3 years after the permanent pacemaker implant, an intractable atrial fibrillation appeared and remained unchanged without the reappearence of P waves (Fig. 3).

Discussion

The possible reasons for loss of sinus activity are:

1. *Overdrive suppression of the sinus function.* During programmed pacing at 30 spikes per minute, a normal sinus node will take over. Our method avoids overdrive suppression by a progressive slowing of the pacemaker's rate.
2. *Asynchronized atrio-ventricular activity* during VVI pacing with loss of atrial compliance and contraction during the long-term follow-up. However this seems improbable due to the fact that the clinical pacemaker syndrome was absent in our patients and retrograde conduction was a rare finding.
3. *Natural history and spontaneous evolution* of the atrio-ventricular conduction disturbances, with involvement of the sinus node in the organic process i.e. fibrosis of the conduction tissue (5).

This seems to us to be the only feasible reason for the loss of sinus activity and atrial contraction. This unexpected evolution of the sinus node function may jeopardize the effect and the usefulness of the dual chamber mode of pacing (6, 7).

In fact, a clinical trial is currently being carried out in our hospital involving 12 patients with loss of sinus node function who underwent temporary DVI during pacemaker replacement under ECG monitoring and fluoroscopy control. Neither reappearance of the P waves nor atrial activity were detected.

References

1. Kruse I, Arnman K, Conradson TB, Ryden L: A comparison of the acute and long term hemodynamic effects of ventricular inhibited and atrial synchronous ventricular inhibited pacing. Circulation 1982; 65: 846–855.
2. Feldman S, Yahini JH, Krakover R, Kishon Y, Neufeld HN: Sinus insufficiency syndrome. Clinical results of permanent ventricular pacing. El Torax 1981; 27: 19–21.
3. Ferrer I: The sick sinus syndrome. Circulation 1973; 47: 635–641.
4. Staessen J, Ector H, De Geese H: The underlying heart rhythm in patients with an artificial cardiac pacemaker. Pace 1982; 5 (6): 801–807.
5. Feldman S, Yahini JH, Palant A, Shem-Tov A, Neufeld HN: Natural history of atrio-ventricular conduction disturbances in 115 patients. In: Cardiac Pacing. Proceedings of the VIth International Symposium. Ed Y Watanabe. Excerpta Medica 1977; 89–92.
6. Dreifus LS, Michelson EL, Kaplinsky E: Brady-arrhythmias. Clinical significance and management. JACC 1983; 1: 327–338.
7. Parsonnet V, Bernstein AD: Cardiac pacing in the 1980's. Treatment and techniques in transition. JACC 1983; 1: 339–354.

Authors' address:
Shlomo Feldman,
Heart Institute
Chaim Sheba Medical Center,
Tel Hashomer
Israel

Long-Term Follow-Up of Paced Patients with Sick Sinus Syndrome

S. Sasaki, A. Takeuchi, M. Ohzeki, H. Kishida, T. Nishimoto, S. Kakimoto, H. Fukumoto

Summary: Seventy-eight patients with sick sinus syndrome underwent pacemaker implantation during the period from September 1970 to December 1981. The pacing methods employed were atrial pacing (AP) in 36 (including 2 cases of sequential atrioventricular pacing) and ventricular pacing (VP) in 42 patients. The study was made to compare AP with VP with respect to cardiac output, symptoms and incidence of thromboembolism, and to evaluate the long-term results of all paced patients.

Cardiac index (CI) in AP was greater than 3.0 l/min/m² at rest in 60% of the patients. In the remaining 40% in whom CI at rest was less than 3.0 l/min/m², the increase in CI after exercise was more than 3.0 l/min/m². In VP patients, on the contrary, CI at rest and the increase in CI after exercise were lower than those in AP patients. Symptoms present before pacemaker implantation disappeared in 82% of AP and 62% of VP patients. Thromboembolic episodes were observed in none of AP, while the incidence of this complication was 35% in VP and it was fatal in 50% of those patients. Thromboembolism in VP was irrespective of the type of arrhythmia (bradycardia or bradytachycardia) or history of atrial fibrillation prior to the study. Prophylactic anticoagulant therapy for VP patients reduced the incidence of thromboembolism to 7%.

Atrial pacing is a more physiological approach in the treatment of sick sinus syndrome. In addition, AP appears to be of particular value in avoiding the incidence of thromboembolic complications. Prophylactic anticoagulant therapy is necessary and useful especially in the patients with VP.

Recently, there has been a growing tendency to use cardiac pacemakers in the treatment of sick sinus syndrome. The results of permanent pacing for this condition, however, are not uniformly excellent, and it may be due in part to improper selection of pacing mode. The present study was designed to review our experience with permanent atrial and ventricular pacing for sick sinus syndrome with special reference to the long-term results.

Patients and Methods

Seventy-eigth patients with sick sinus syndrome underwent pacemaker implantation during the period from September 1970 to December 1981. This is equivalent to 35% of all 223 patients who have been treated with cardiac pacemakers at our institute. All patients were characterized by any one of the ECG criteria of sick sinus syndrome. The major indications for pacing were symptoms of cerebral ischemia such as syncope and dizziness, prolonged sinus or escaped pause ($\geq$ 4 sec) after rapid atrial pacing, and bradytachyarrhythmias refractory to medical treatment.

For the study, patients were divided into two groups. Forty-one patients with Rubenstein's (1) groups I and II bradycardias formed group B, and 37 patients with his group III bradycardia-tachycardia syndrome were classified as group BT.

Atrioventricular conduction was tested by His bundle electrogram and rapid atrial pacing in 52 of the 78 patients to determine the feasibility of atrial pacing (AP).

Consequently, AP was employed in 34, sequential atrioventricular pacing (SAVP) in 2 and ventricular pacing (VP) in the remaining 42 patients. As the number of patients with SAVP was small, they were included in AP patients in this study.

Epicardial electrodes were used in 57 patients (73%): 31 AP, 1 SAVP and 25 VP patients. Subxiphoid approach was our preference in implanting epicardial electrodes.

The study was made to compare AP with VP with respect to cardiac output, symptoms, complications, and to evaluate the long-term results. Student's test was used for statistical comparison.

Results

Cardiac output

At the time of initial implantation, cardiac output at the same rate (70 ppm) was higher in AP than in VP with a mean increase of 26%. At the chronic stage, cardiac index was measured in 15 patients with AP and 37 with VP at rest and after exercise. In 9 of the 15 AP patients, the resting cardiac index was greater than 3.0 l/min/m², and the increase after exercise was more than 3.0 l/min/m² even in the patients whose cardiac indices were less than 3.0 l/min/m² at rest. In 26 of the 37 VP patients, on the contrary, the resting cardiac index was less than 3.0 l/min/m², and the increase after exercise remained less than 3.0 l/min/m² in all 37 but one patient.

Symptoms

At the time of study, 32 patients were being paced atrially and 46 were ventricularly paced (4 crossovers from AP to VP). Symptomatic relief was observed in the majority of the patients without regard to pacing mode. The symptoms present before implantation disappeared in 55 patients (70%). However, the symptom-free rate was much higher in AP with a rate of 81% compared to 63% in VP patients. This rate was greater in descending order of AP for group B, VP for group B, AP for group BT and VP for group BT. The difference between AP for group B and VP for group BT was statistically significant (p < 0.01) (Table 1).

Complications

Three AP patients had a rise in stimulation threshold, and in all the pacing mode was switched to VP. Infection at the site of the pulse generator pocket occurred in one AP patient and necessitated switching to VP. Thromboembolic episodes were observed in 17 patients (20 occasions) for an incidence of 22%. Sixteen of the 17 patients were being paced by VP when thromboembolism occurred. Thus, the incidence in this patient group was 35%. In the remaining one patient, the complication developed during temporary interruption of pacing. Thromboembolism in VP patients occurred irrespective of the type of arrhythmia (B or BT) or history of atrial fibrillation prior to the study (Table 2).

Anticoagulant therapy for VP patients

Since 1976 warfarin sodium has been used in 14 VP patients. Of the 14 patients, 7 had no history of thromboembolism and the therapy was prophylactic. In the other 7, however, it was initiated after having thromboembolic episodes for preventing the recurrence. In the 14 patients, thromboembolism occurred in only one case, for an incidence

Table 1. Symptoms after pacemaker implantation for sick sinus syndrome.

	No Symptom	Dizziness	Palpitation	Chest Pain	Edema
VP (46)	29 (63.0%)	6	5	2	4
B 20	B 15 (75.0%)	B 1	B 2	B 1	B 1
BT 26	BT 14 (53.8%)	BT 5	BT 3	BT 1	BT 3
AP or SAVP 32	26 (81.3%)	1	3	1	1
B 21	B 19 (90.5%)	B 0	B 1	B 1	B 0
BT 11	BT 7 (63.6%)	BT 1	BT 2	BT 0	BT 1

AP: atrial pacing; B: bradycardia group; BT: brady-tachycardia group; SAVP: sequential atrioventricular pacing; VP: ventricular pacing.

Table 2. Thromboembolism during ventricular pacing for sick sinus syndrome.

16 patients (19 times) ·········· 34.8%

B	8/20	40.0%	] N.S.
BT	8/26	30.8%	
af	7/23	30.4%	] N.S.
Non af	9/23	39.1%	

af: atrial fibrillation; B: bradycardia group; BT: brady-tachycardia group.

of 7.1%. On the contrary, in 4 patients in whom anticoagulant therapy was not attempted in spite of a history of thromboembolism, a recurrence was seen in 3 patients (75%). Thromboembolism-free actuarial curves for VP patients with and without anticoagulant therapy showed 92% and 69%, respectively, of patients thromboembolism-free at the end of one year. The difference was statistically significant ($p < 0.01$) (Fig. 1).

Late results
There were 15 deaths. Of the 15 deaths, 8 were due to systemic thromboembolism (Table 3).
Actuarial survival curves for pacemaker patients showed no difference of survival rate between A-V block and sick sinus syndrome through all whole follow-up years. This was in contrast of the actuarial curves constructed at the end of 1978: the survival was significantly better for A-V block through the initial four years after pacemaker implantation (Fig. 2).

Fig. 1. Thromboembolism-free curves in patients with ventricular pacing for sick sinus syndrome. Thromboembolism-free rate is significantly higher in patients with anticoagulant therapy than in those without the therapy at the end of one year follow-up.

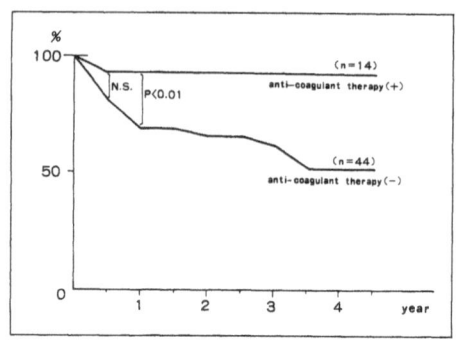

Table 3. Cause of deaths during pacing for sick sinus syndrome.

Thromboembolism	8 (VP)
Neoplasm	2
Senility	2
Aplastic anemia	1 $\left.\begin{matrix} \text{VP} : 1 \\ \text{AP} : 1 \end{matrix}\right)$
Unknown (sudden)	2
Total	15

AP: atrial pacing; VP: ventricular pacing.

Fig. 2. Actuarial survival curves in patients with permanent pacemakers. Actuarial survival curves constructed in 1978 show a significantly lower survival rate in sick sinus syndrome than in A-V block during the first 4 years after implantation (upper pannel). There is disappearance of this difference in 1981 (lower pannel).

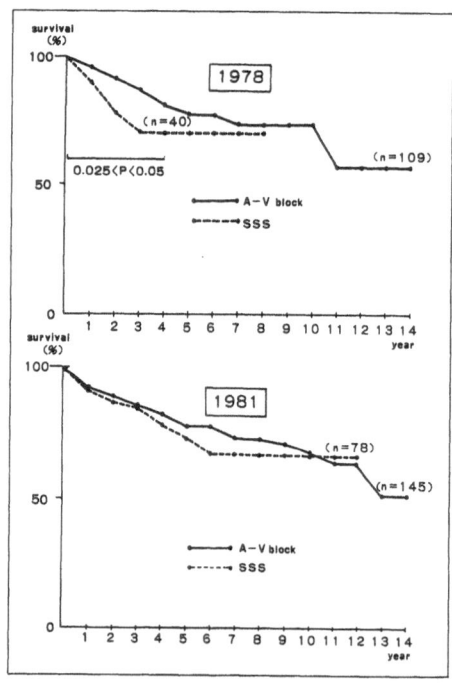

Discussion

Pacemaker implantation in patients with sick sinus syndrome has been increasing during recent years. At the end of 1981, 35% of the patients treated with cardiac pacemakers at our institute had sick sinus syndrome.

Atrial pacing has been our preference in the treatment of sick sinus syndrome. This approach seems to be logical for obtaining better hemodynamics by preserving the normal sequence of atrioventricular contraction (2, 3). However, atrial pacing can not be applied in the presence of atrioventricular conduction disturbance or chronic atrial fibrillation. For the former, when "physiological pacing" is desirable, the use of atrioventricular sequential pacing should be considered. In addition to hemodynamic superiority, atrioventricular sequential pacing is useful in controlling ectopic rhythm and re-entry tachyarrhythmia (4).

We have been using epicardial electrodes in most of the patients, though successful endocardial pacing using J-shaped electrodes has been reported (5). The subxiphoid approach has been used almost exclusively without mortality and morbidity. The oldest patient who underwent this procedure was 86 years old at the time of surgery.

Symptoms present before pacemaker implantation disappeared in AP patients with a higher rate than in VP patients, although the difference was not significant. The lowest improvement was obtained in VP for group BT. This fact suggests that the use of a pacemaker alone is able to prevent tachyarrhythmia only in a small part of the patients (1).

It is well known that the risk of thromboembolism is considerably high in patients with sick sinus syndrome and it is particularly evident in patients with bradycardia-tachycardia syndrome (1, 6). A high incidence of thromboembolism in patients with pacemakers also has been reported (7). It should be stressed that, in this series, this complication occurred only in VP patients except one, and 8 of the 16 patients with VP eventually died, and that the incidence was independent of the type of arrhythmia. Although there was no significant difference in the incidence of thromboembolism between patients with and without history of atrial fibrillation, it may be difficult to document transient one.

After recognizing the prevalence of thromboembolism in VP patients, we have treated this group with warfarin sodium whenever possible. The results confirmed the importance of anticoagulant therapy which has been advocated previously (7).

In 1978, actuarial survival curves for paced patients demonstrated a significantly lower rate in sick sinus syndrome than in A-V block during the first four years after implantation. However, the curves constructed in 1981 showed no significant difference between them. The facts are attributed to recent more frequent use of "physiological pacing" in sick sinus syndrome and anticoagulant therapy in VP patients.

References

1. Rubenstein JJ, Schulman CL, Yurchak PM, DeSantis RW: Clinical spectrum of the sick sinus syndrome. Circulation 1972; 46: 5–13.
2. Samet P, Castillo C, Bernstein WH: Hemodynamic sequelae of atrial, ventricular, and sequential atrioventricular pacing in cardiac patients. Am Heart J 1966; 72: 725–729.
3. Kosowsky BD, Scherlag BJ, Damato AN: Re-evaluation of the atrial contribution to ventricular function. Am J Cardiol 1968; 21: 518–524.

4. Fields J, Berkovits BV, Matloff JM: Surgical experience with temporary and permanent A-V sequential demand pacing. J Thorac Cardiovasc Surg 1973; 66: 865–877.
5. Smyth NPD, Citron P, Keshishian JM, Garcia JM, Kelly LC: Permanent pervenous atrial sensing and pacing with a new J-shaped lead. J Thorac Cardiovasc Surg 1976; 72: 565–570.
6. Fairfax AJ, Lambert CD, Leatham A: Systemic embolism in chronic sinoatrial disorder. New Eng J Med 1976; 295: 190–192.
7. Radford DJ, Julian DG: Sick sinus syndrome: Experience of a cardiac pacemaker clinic. Brit Med J 1974; 24: 504–507.

Authors' address:
S. Sasaki, M.D.
Dept. of Thoracic Surgery
Osaka Medical College
2–7 Daigaku-cho
Takatsuki-shi 569
Japan

Termination of Pacing in Patients with Sick Sinus Syndrome and Implanted Pacemakers who Developed Chronic Atrial Fibrillation

S. Amikam, M. Yahalom, E. Riss

Summary: A significant number of patients (pts) with sick sinus syndrome (SSS) treated with implanted ventricular pacemakers (PM), develop consequently chronic atrial fibrillation (AF) which terminates their clinical syndrome. In these pts, termination of permanent pacing (PP) may be considered. Among a group of 100 pts with SSS, treated with implanted PMs, 27 pts (27%) developed chronic AF following implantation. Of this group, long-term PP was terminated in 10 pts. In 2 pts pacing was ceased unexpectedly as a result of PM or electrode malfunction. In 8 pts it was terminated intentionally as batteries exhausted and were not replaced. All 10 pts were asymptomatic when pacing was discontinued and have been followed closely since; their ages ranged from 53 to 80 years (mean 70) and the duration of PP before termination ranged between 12 to 76 months (mean 46). Follow-up period since termination of pacing ranged from 12 to 40 months (mean 30). In 5 pts PP had to be reinstituted (by replacing the PM): 3 became asymptomatic due to AF with slow ventricular rate and 2 had symptomatic recurrences of sinus of junctional bradycardia. The other 5 pts remained well and asymptomatic without PP. In conclusion, in some paced SSS pts who developed chronic AF, termination of PP is possible as AF is stable and the ventricular rate is adequate but in some, slow ventricular rate or unstable AF indicates the continuation of pacing.

Introduction

At the Montreal meeting we presented a study on the natural history of patients with sick sinus syndrome treated with permanent pacemakers (1). We identified a sub-set of patients with so-called "transient form" of the sick sinus syndrome who converted to stable chronic atrial fibrillation following pacemaker implantation. In this group, the establishment of atrial fibrillation had been shown to terminated in some the clinical syndrome (2). We than suggested that in this subset of patients termination of permanent pacing may be considered. Since than we have continued to follow this group and additional SSS pts and the follow-up results show that among our first 100 pts with SSS treated with pacemakers, 27 pts (27%) developed chronic atrial fibrillation during a period of few days to several years after the implantation. Among this group of 27 pts who converted to chronic atrial fibrillation, in 10 pts, permanent pacing was discontinued. This study summarizes the follow-up results of these 10 patients since the termination of pacing.

Material and methods

This group of 10 pts included 4 males and 6 females. Their age ranged from 53 to 80 years (mean 70) and pacing was terminated after a period that ranged from 12 to 76 months following implantation (mean 46 months). The initial indication for pacing was Bradycardia-Tachycardia in 6 patients and bradyarrhythmias in 4 pts. The termination of pacing occured under two different circumstances. 1. When pacing was unexpectedly interrupted as a result of electrode or pulse-generator malfunction and despite of it the patient remained completely asymptomatic. This occured in 2 of our cases. 2. When the termination of pacing was preplanned and carried out on our initiative. In 8 cases we decided not to replace the unit when the batteries exhausted. In these cases, termination of pacing was affected only after a protacted and close follow-up period at the pacemaker clinic. The follow-up program included repeated Holter monitoring examinations that showed that the patients were in stable atrial fibrillation and did not need pacemaker support. We continued this close follow-up after the termination of pacing: patients were seen at the clinic twice a month during the first two months following pacing interruption and once monthly thereafter. Except for one case in which pacing was interrupted for pouch infection, we did not remove the pacemaker system after the termination of pacing. The exhausted pulse-generators and the electrodes were not remove and remained in place. This enabled us to reinstitute pacing easily should it become necessary.

Results

Out of the 10 patients, 5 remained asymptomatic and are still without pacemaker support during a period of 24 to 40 months (mean 30) since the discontinuation of pacing. In the other 5 patients, permanent pacing had to be reinstituted during a period of 4 to 12 months (mean 7) following pacing interruption, as they became symptomatic due to bradycardia. In 3 patients despite stable atrial fibrillation the ventricular rate was slow and induced symptoms of low cardiac output like dizziness or fatigue. In one patient syncope due to sudden return of nodal bradycardia following 12 months of stable atrial fibrillation and 4 months without pacing support. Another patient became symptomatic as sinus bradycardia returned after 26 months of stable atrial fibrillation and 16 months without pacing. In 4 of these 5 pts, pacing was resummed by replacing the pulse-generator and only in one patient a new pacing system had to be reimplanted.

Discussion

It is generally understood that whenever permanent pacing is established it will have to be continued throughout the patient's life. However, in a few selected cases, it might be possible to terminate pacing without causing any harm to the patient. This can happen under the following circumstances: 1. When the dysrrhythmia resulted from drugs that have been withdrawn. 2. When the dysrrhythmia resulted from acute or sub-acute disease or intervention from which the patient recovered as in acute myocardial infarction, Cardiac surgery, Thyrotoxicosis etc. 3. When stable atrial fibrillation terminated the clinical syndrome of sick sinus syndrome. 4. When the original indication for pacing ultimately proved erroneous (and this might indeed happen). If one of these situations is met, the decision to stop permanent pacing has to be very carefully weighed and further checked by closed long-term follow-up prior to termination to prove that pacing is indeed unnecessary. The follow-up is much more important after pacing is discontinued. When the follow-up is expected not to be adequate or the patient might be lost to follow-up or transfers to another place, discontinuation of pacing should not be planned. In our group of 10 patients half became symptomatic and required the reinstitution of pacing.

Crelinsten et al. in 1979 (3) were first to describe a group of 20 patients in whom permanent pacing was discontinued. Sixteen of these patients suffered from atrioventricular conduction disturbances and 4 patients form sick sinus syndrome. All were asymptomatic at the time of pacing interruption. Seventeen of this group remained asymptomatic during a mean non-paced period of 1.7 years, 2 patients required reinstitution of pacing and one patient died. They concluded that certain sub-groups of patients may tolerate well the termination of pacing. Most of their patients belonged to the AV block group, and only 4 to the sick sinus syndrome. Among this latter group, in only one patient resumption of pacing was required. We in 1980 (4) described a mixed group of 12 patients in whom permanent pacing was discontinued; 6 patients of this group are also included in the present survey. At the time we presented the results, only in 2 of the 12 patients, reinstitution of pacing due to recurrence of symptoms, was required. However, after a longer follow-up period, in 5 additional patients of our first group, pacing had to be reinstituted. Three of them had atrioventricular disease and 2 belonged to the sick sinus syndrome group. After having this bad experience with termination of pacing in patients with atrioventricular conduction defects, we are now considering interruption of pacing only in sick sinus syndrome patients who converted to chronic atrial fibrillation.

In patients with rate-programmable units, decreasing the rate of the pacemaker to its lower rate may be helpful in taking the decision to terminate permanent pacing. In some of the new pacemakers available now or those that would be available in the future, a mini-Holter is included which can tell by telemetry if the pacemaker was used for pacing and for what percentage of the time, or if it is only used in sensing and did not pace at all. Improvement in this regard of pacemaker memory and telemetry technology would ensure the physician that the pacemaker was not used and that pacing is unnecessary. Some of the patients are psychologically dependant on the functioning of the pacemaker. Even if it was found that the pacemaker is superfluous on medical grounds, they remain psychologycally pacemaker-dependant, and there in no choice in these patients but to continue permanent pacing for ever.

In conclusion, some patients with sick sinus syndrome who converted to chronic atrial fibrillation, remain asymptomatic despite termination of long-term treatment with implanted pacemaker. Close follow-up program is mandatory when pacing is discontinued, as symptoms due to bradycardia may reoccur in some patients and restitution of pacing is required.

References

1. Amikam S, Riss E: The Natural history of sick sinus syndrome following permanent pacemaker implantation. Pace 1979; 2: 262 (Abstract).
2. Vera Z, Mason DT, Awan NA, Miller RR, JanzenD, Tonkon MJ, Vismara LA: Improvement of symptoms in patients with sick sinus syndrome by spontaneous development of stable atrial fibrillation. Br Heart J 1977; 30: 160–164.
3. Crelinsten GL, Morin J, Gagne P, Meere C, Noble E: Termination of Cardiac Pacing. In: Meere C, Proceedings of the VIth Symposium on Cardiac Pacing, Montreal 1979, Chap. 18–6.

4. Amikam S, Yahalom M, Riss E: Experience in patients in whom permanent pacing was discontinued. Pace, 1980; 3: 361 (Abstract)

Authors' address:
S. Amikam, M.D.
Rambam Medical Center,
Dept. of Cardiology,
Haifa, 34601, Israel

Electrophysiologic Effects of Reduced Oxygen Supply on the Transmembrane Potential and Membrane Current Systems of the Rabbit Atrioventricular Node

T. Katoh, M. Nishimura, Y. Tsuji, S. Hiromasa, Y. Watanabe

Summary: Effects of ischemia on atrioventricular (AV) conduction were studied in 11 isolated, perfused rabbit hearts by reducing the coronary flow from 17 to 8.5 ml/min. Within 10 minutes, all the hearts showed a 2° AV block, with significant prolongation of intraatrial (16%), intra-AV nodal (223%) and His-Purkinje (23%) conduction times before the 2° AV block developed. Effects of hypoxia were studied in 7 spontaneously beating small (0.2 × 0.2 × 0.1 mm) AV nodal preparations. When pO_2 of the perfusate was reduced from 550 to 30 mmHg, the preparations showed a slowing of firing from 122 to 112/min and a reduction of the maximal diastolic potential (from -67 to -63 mV) as well as the maximal rate of depolarization (from 17 to 14 V/sec). Action potential duration was unchanged. When pO_2 was further reduced to 19 mmHg, all preparations ceased their firing (n = 5). This was accompanied by hyperpolarization and an increased resting tension even in a Ca^{++} free medium containing 5 mM EGTA, suggesting increased intracellular Ca^{++} concentration possibly by Ca^{++} release from mitochondria and/or sarcoplasmic reticulum. Voltage clamp experiments (n = 5) by double microelectrode techniques revealed that hypoxia reduced the slow inward current by 28% and outward K^+ current tail minimally, although the background current flowed outwardly by 3–5 nA. These results suggest that hypoxia depresses AV nodal conduction by reducing the slow inward current and increasing intracellular resistance, and depresses automaticity by reducing the slow inward current and shifting the background current outwardly.

It is well known that ischemic heart disease, especially acute myocardial infarction, is often accompanied by atrioventricular (abbreviated as AV in the subsequent text) block and the lack of adequate AV nodal escape mechanism. However, the mechanisms by which ischemia depresses conduction and automaticity in the AV node have not been fully elucidated mainly because reproduction of clinically encountered "ischemia" is extremely difficult in in-vitro experiments and application of voltage clamp method to an in-vivo AV node is impossible. In the present study, we used isolated, perfused rabbit hearts to study AV conduction times under ischemia. Small rabbit AV nodal preparations were used to record transmembrane potentials and ionic currents under hypoxia as an in-vitro model of ischemia.

Material and Methods

Rabbits weighing 1.5–2.0 kg were anesthetized by an intravenous injection of pentobarbital sodium (35 mg/kg). The chest was opened and the heart quickly isolated. Perfusion of the coronary arteries was immediately started, through a glass cannula inserted into the ascending aorta, at a constant flow rate of 17 ml/min using a microtube pump. The heart was driven at a constant rate by a bipolar silver electrode attached near the sinoatrial node. Using His bundle electrogram, we measured the intraatrial, AV nodal and His-Purkinje conduction times. After a period of control recording, the coronary flow rate was reduced to one-half the control to see the effects of ischemia on AV conduction times.

To study the effects of hypoxia on AV nodal action potentials and membrane current systems, small AV nodal preparations were used. The central portion of the AV node was dissected to make a strand of 0.2 mm in width and 1.0 mm in length, which was then ligated at several sites by silk fibers to electrically isolate one section from another. The final dimension of the preparation thus obtained was approximately $0.2 \times 0.2 \times 0.1$ mm. Transmembrane potentials were recorded by a glass microelectrode and ionic currents by voltage clamp using double microelectrode techniques. Normoxic and hypoxic perfusions were obtained by saturating the perfusate with either 100% oxygen or 100% nitrogen. Their oxygen pressures were measured as 500–550 and 18–30 mmHg, respectively. Composition of the modified Tyrode solution was as follows: NaCl 136.9, KCl 4.0, $CaCl_2$ 1.8, $MgCl_2$ 1.0, NaH_2PO_4 0.33 and Na_2HPO_4 2.24, in mM, and its pH was adjusted to 7.4.

Results

1. Effects of ischemia on AV conduction

In 11 isolated, perfused rabbit hearts, effects of a reduction of coronary flow to one-half the control level were studied. The total AV conduction time was prolonged from 87.1 ± 5.6 to 170.2 ± 45.3 msec ($P < 0.001$). The AV nodal conduction time showed the greatest increase, with a change from 33.3 ± 4.8 to 107.7 ± 44.4 msec ($P < 0.001$). The intraatrial and His-Purkinje conduction times were also prolonged, but to lesser extents, from 19.4 ± 2.9 to 22.4 ± 3.6 msec ($P < 0.01$) and from 34.3 ± 4.1 to 40.1 ± 4.3 msec ($P < 0.01$), respectively. Within ten minutes of ischemia, a second degree AV nodal block was observed in all hearts, progressing from the Wenckebach type of conduction to a 2:1 block. This finding suggests that the AV nodal conduction is most sensitive to ischemia in the specialized conducting system.

2. Effects of hypoxia on spontaneous action potentials of the AV node

In all seven experiments in which a mild hypoxia ($pO_2 = 30$ mmHg) was produced, the AV node showed a reduction in the spontaneous firing frequency. Figure 1 shows a typical experiment. Under the hypoxic perfusion, the spontaneous cycle length was prolonged from 492 to 538 msec mainly due to a reduction of the rate of diastolic depolarization from 60.4 to 38.6 mV/sec. The maximal diastolic potential and the maximal rate of depolarization were also decreased from -67 to -63 mV and 17 to 14 V/sec, respectively. On the other hand, the overshoot and the action potential duration remained unchanged.

A more severely hypoxic perfusion ($pO_2 = 19$ mmHg) showed a stronger negative chronotropic effect, finally leading to a cessation of spontaneous firing (n = 5). Figure 2 shows a low speed recording in such an experiment. Shortly after the hypoxic perfusion was started, the maximal diastolic potential and the spontaneous firing frequency were decreased as in Figure 1. Cessation of spontaneous action potentials was followed by subthreshold

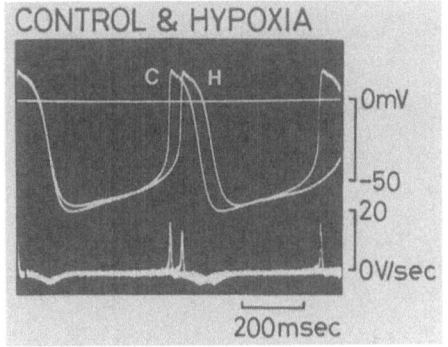

CONTROL & HYPOXIA

C H

0mV

-50

20

0V/sec

200msec

Fig. 1. Effects of mild hypoxia (pO_2 = 30 mmHg) on the spontaneous action potential of the rabbit AV node. The upper tracing shows the transmembrane potential and the lower, its first derivative, or the maximal rate of depolarization.
C denotes the action potential during control perfusion, and H denotes that during hypoxic perfusion.

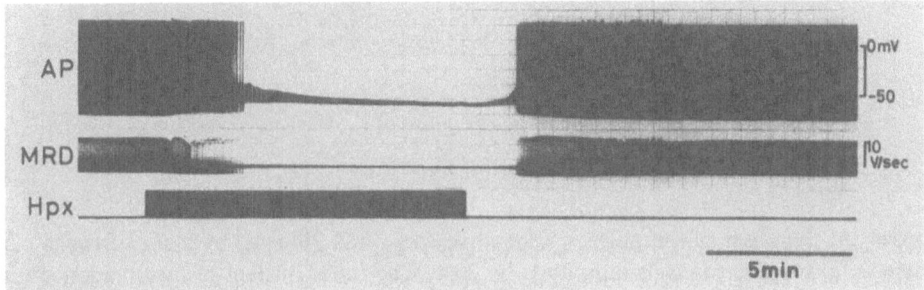

AP

0mV

-50

MRD

10 V/sec

Hpx

5min

Fig. 2. Effects of severe hypoxia (pO_2 = 19 mmHg) on the spontaneous action potential of the rabbit AV node. AP = action potential, MRD = maximal rate of depolarization, Hpx = the duration of the hypoxic perfusion. Note that the tracings were recorded at a low speed.

oscillatory potentials with a gradual decrease in their amplitude and by a subsequent hyperpolarization. This hyperpolarization was observed even in a Ca^{++} free medium containing 5 mM EGTA, and was accompanied by an increase in the resting tension. After returning to the control oxygenation, oscillatory potentials reappeared with a gradually increasing amplitude, leading to the resumption of spontaneous firing.

When 10 mM glucose was added to the perfusate during a prolonged hypoxic perfusion in five other experiments (not shown), spontaneous firing was always restored despite the maintenance of hypoxic perfusion, suggesting that the effects of hypoxia on the AV node could be reversed by glucose.

3. Effects of hypoxia on membrane current systems of the AV node

In order to inactivate the fast Na^+ current, the membrane potential was clamped at -40 mV. Then, either depolarizing or hyperpolarizing pulses of different amplitudes were applied. Figure 3 shows superimposed current tracings obtained during the control and hypoxic perfusions. In the upper panel, the membrane was depolarized to -15 mV for 500

Fig. 3. Effects of mild hypoxia ($pO_2 = 30$ mmHg) on the membrane current systems of the rabbit AV node.

The upper and lower panels show current tracings obtained on depolarization to -15 mV and on hyperpolarization to -75 mV, respectively, from the holding potential of -40 mV. C denotes the current during control perfusion, and H denotes that during hypoxic perfusion.

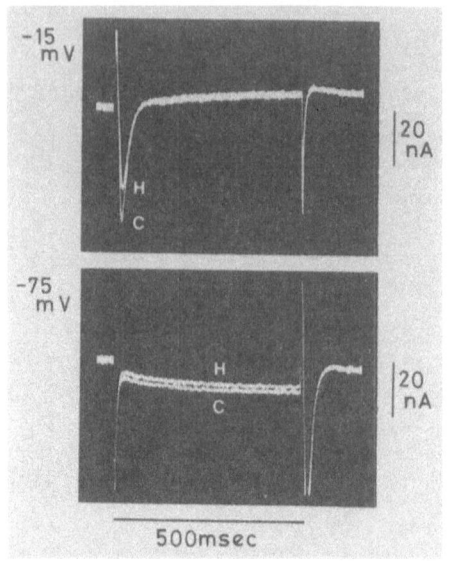

msec. At the onset of the pulse, a capacitive surge was followed by a slow inward current. Hypoxia decreased its amplitude by 23%. The time constant of inactivation of the slow inward current was measured as 14 and 13 msec under the control and hypoxic perfusions, respectively, suggesting that hypoxia did not change the kinetics of inactivation of the slow inward current. The steady-state outward current was minimally increased, probably reflecting an outward shift of the holding current under hypoxia. However, the tail of the outward current observed on repolarization to the holding potential appeared unaffected or slightly decreased. In the lower panel, the membrane was hyperpolarized to -75 mV from the holding potential, again for 500 msec. The background inward current recorded at the onset of the pulse as the magnitude of the current jump was decreased under hypoxia, but the hyperpolarization-activated inward current was not at all affected by hypoxia.

Discussion

Two major electrophysiologic functions of the AV node are to conduct atrial impulses to the ventricles and to act as a subsidiary pacemaker when atrial impulses fail to control the ventricles at an adequate rate (1, 2). Although both of these functions were shown to be impaired by a reduction of oxygen supply, their mechanisms are not necessarily the same.

As is well known clinically and has been shown in the present experiments, the AV node was most sensitive to a reduction of the coronary flow in the specialized conducting system. Such a depression of AV nodal conduction appeared to be caused mainly by a reduction of the slow inward current, which is responsible for the upstroke phase of the AV nodal action potential (3–5). However, when discussing the mechanisms for impulse conduction, one should also consider passive electrical properties of the membrane. Although we did not specifically study the effects of hypoxia on passive electrical properties in the current experiments, our finding that the membrane was hyperpolarized with a concomitant increase in the resting tension suggests that the intracellular Ca^{++} concentration was increased by hypoxia. The intracellular Ca^{++} concentration is said to regulate the potassium conductance (6–7), and an increase in this concentration is expected to increase the intracellular resistance (8) and further aggravate the AV nodal conduction.

The ionic mechanisms responsible for the pacemaker activity of the AV node include deactivation of the outward K^+ current, activation of the slow inward current and the presence of a background inward current in the potential range of the slow diastolic depolarization (5). Our study has confirmed that hypoxia exerts a negative chronotropic effect on the AV node by decreasing the rate of diastolic depolarization, which, in turn, was caused by a reduction of the slow inward current and an outward shift of the background current. The latter phenomenon, which might result from an increase in the time-independent outward K^+ current possibly activated by a high intracellular Ca^{++} concentration, probably caused the subsequent hyperpolarization after the cessation of the automatic activities. However, it is noteworthy that hypoxia-induced depression of automaticity was antagonized by an addition of glucose. This observation can be explained that ATP synthesis in the electron transport system impaired by hypoxia can very well be compensated by ATP synthesis through glycolysis occurring in the cytoplasm, although the amount of ATP synthesized by the latter mechanism may be much smaller than that by the former mechanism under normal conditions. This finding suggests that glucose-insulin-potassium infusion therapy during acute myocardial infarction could facilitate the recovery of myocardium from hypoxic or ischemic damages, and improve impaired electrophysiologic functions of the AV node, provided that such a solution could reach the ischemic tissue.

Conclusions

1. The AV node is very sensitive to a reduced oxygen supply, showing a depression of conduction as well as automaticity.
2. These changes are dependent mainly on a reduction of the slow inward current in the presence of a mild hypoxia.
3. An increase in the background outward current contributes to membrane hyperpolarization in the presence of a more severe hypoxia, further aggravating conduction and automaticity in the AV node.
4. Such effects of hypoxia on the AV node can be antagonized by glucose.

References

1. Watanabe Y, Dreifus LS: Factors controlling impulse transmission with special reference to A-V conduction. Am Heart J 1975; 89: 790–803.
2. Watanabe Y, Dreifus LS: Sites of impulse formation within the atrioventricular junction of the rabbit. Circ Res 1968; 22: 717–727.
3. Kokubun S, Nishimura M, Noma A, Irisawa H: The spontaneous action potential of rabbit atrioventricular node cells. Jpn J Physiol 1980; 30: 529–540.

4. Noma A, Irisawa H, Kokubun S, Kotake H, Nishimura M, Watanabe Y: Slow current systems in the A-V node of the rabbit heart. Nature 1980; 285: 228–229.
5. Kokubun S, Nishimura M, Noma A, Irisawa H: Membrane currents in the rabbit atrioventricular node cell. Pflügers Arch 1982; 393: 15–22.
6. Meech RW, Standen NB: Potassium activation in Helix aspersa neurons under voltage clamp: A component mediated by calcium influx. J Physiol (London) 1975; 249: 211–239.
7. Isenberg G: Cardiac Purkinje fibers. $[Ca^{2+}]_i$ controls the potassium permeability via the conductance components g_{K1} and g_{K2}. Pflügers Arch 1977; 371: 77–85.
8. DeMello WC: Effect of intracellular injection of calcium and strontium on cell communication in heart. J Physiol (London) 1975; 250: 231–245.

Authors' address:
Dr. Takakazu Katoh
Cardiovascular Institute
Fujita Gakuen University
Toyoake, Aichi 470–11
Japan

Catheter Biopsy Assessed Cardiomyopathic and Post-myocarditic Changes in Cases with Atrioventricular or Intraventricular Conduction Disturbance

Motonari Hasumi, Morie Sekiguchi, Shinichiro Morimoto, Machiko Take,
Michiaki Hiroe, Satoshi Ohnishi, Hiroshi Kasanuki, Koshichiro Hirosawa

Summary: To determine the cause of A-V block or intraventricular conduction disturbance (IVCD) at the clinical level is usually difficult. Our experience with endomyocardial biopsy which exceeds 1300 cases has revealed that biopsy is useful in diagnosing and assessing myocardial disease. A serial biopsy study in 10 cases with acute viral myocarditis has enabled us to define the histopathological criteria of postmyocarditic change (PMC). Eighty-eight cases with A-V block and 51 cases with IVCD underwent biopsy in order to better understand the nature and incidence of myocardial change. Those cases where the ECG abnormalities were the most pertinent to the clinical findings were selected for this study. Accordingly, 91 of 139 cases were idiopathic. Diagnosis of cardiac sarcoidosis in 2 cases and of cardiac amyloidosis in 1 case were made with the biopsy. Twenty-three of 91 idiopathic cases (25%) showed significant myocardial pathology. In 38 of 91 idiopathic cases (42%), PMC was detected. His-bundle electrogram revealed that in cases with A-V block, H-V prolongation was correlated with the significant pathology. Most of the cases were not classified into either dilated or hypertrophic cardiomyopathy but were classified according to our proposed term: "Arrhythmia-conduction disturbance type of cardiomyopathy". A long-term follow up of up to 13 years in 87 cases among the 139 cases revealed that the apparent heart muscle diseases such as sarcoidosis, amyloidosis, dilated cardiomyopathy (DCM) and hypertrophic cardiomyopathy (HCM) were more prone to have short prognosis. It is concluded that in those cases where the A-V block or IVCD exists and when pacemaker implantation is considered, biopsy is useful in making diagnosis and also in recognizing the nature of the disease and its severity.

Introduction

In most of the cases with A-V block and/or intraventricular conduction disturbance (IVCD), the etiology is unclear and it is usually said that the pathology is "localized degeneration" and/or "fibrosis" of the conduction system (1, 2, 3). But in cases of myocardial diseases such as acute myocarditis or cardiac sarcoidosis, we have realized that such electrocardiographic abnormalities are due to the myocardial disease in which the conduction system is involved (4, 5).

To determine the cause of A-V block or IVCD at the clinical level, endomyocardial biopsy (biopsy) was applied and histopathological assessment was made through our experience with more than 1300 cases (6, 7).

Materials and methods

Among the patients who underwent biopsy over a 15 year period from 1968 to 1982, except for cases with congenital or valvular heart diseases, 139 cases with A-V block or IVCD which was one of the most pertinent clinical findings were studied (Table 1). In

101

those cases, routine cardiac examinations such as chest roentgenography, echocardiography, cardiac catheterization including ventriculography were performed. The biopsy was performed employing Konno-Sakakibara's bioptome and the specimen was taken from the right ventricle in most of the cases (6). In 2 cases, the biopsy was taken from the left ventricle. Because of the high frequency of non-specific histopathological findings in biopsied specimens, we used our own criteria of histopathological assessment (7). Each finding which consisted of 23 parameters were graded into four categories, and the final assessment in hypertrophy, degeneration, interstitial fibrosis and disarrangement of the muscle bundles was made (7). If at least one of the above four parameters exceeded grade 2 and the sum of the grade of these exceeded a score of 4, it would qualify the cases as a significant pathology which might be the cause of conduction disturbance (Table 2). The incidence of significant pathology was analized.

Table 1. Clinical Diagnosis of Patients with A–V block or IVCD.

			Low grade A–V B.	High grade A–V B.	LBBB	RBBB	Bifas-cicular	Other IVCD
DCM	(n = 18)	13%	2	7	2	3	1	3
HCM	(n = 7)	5%	2		1		3	1
Myocarditis	(n = 11)	8%		10			1	
Myocardial D.	(n = 8)	6%		3		1	3	1
IHD	(n = 2)	1%		2				
Others	(n = 2)	1%					1	1
Idiopathic	(n = 91)	66%	13	49	8	10	7	4
Total	(n = 139)	100%	17	71	11	14	16	10

Low grade A–V B.: I°, II° Wenckelbach type. High grade A–V B.; II° Mobitz type, Advanced, complete A–V block; LBBB: Left bundle branch block (complete, incomplete); RBBB: Right bundle branch block (complete, incomplete); Bifascular: bifascular block; IVCD: Intraventricular conduction disturbance; DCM: Dilated cardiomyopathy; HCM: Hypertrophic cardiomyopathy; Myocardial D.: Specific myocardial disease (except Myocarditis); IHD: Ischemic heart disease.

Table 2. Endomyocardial Biopsy Assessment of A–V Conduction Disturbance.

A. Parameters	B. Criteria for Significant Pathology
1. Hypertrophy	1. At least one of A_{2-4} should exceed grade 2
2. Degeneration	2. Sum of A_{1-4} should exceed a score of 4
3. Interstitial fibrosis	
4. Disarrangement	

Grading

–	+	++	+++
0	1	2	3

A serial biopsy study in 10 cases with acute myocarditis of viral origin enabled us to define the histopathological criteria of postmyocarditic change (PMC) (4, 8). At the convalescent stage of myocarditis, biopsy findings showed disarrangement, scarcity of myofibrils, fragmentation of the muscle bundles, abnormal branching, proliferation of large mononuclear cells, and interstitial fibrosis. Accordingly, the incidence of PMC was studied.

The left ventriculography was evaluated with the use of Kasser's method (9) and the ejection fraction was calculated. His bundle electrograms (HBE) were recorded with the use of Sherlag's method (10), and the results were compared with the biopsy findings. Those cases which were finally diagnosed to be idiopathic in nature, were further analyzed in order to determine the etiology of the disease, both clinically and histopathologically. In cases where the long term follow-up of up to 13 years (mean 4.5 ± 3.9 years) could be made (87 cases), the clinical features were compared with the biopsied findings. The electrocardiographic diagnosis was made with the use of a new coding system by Robles de Medina (11).

Results

Among the 1300 cases which have been biopsied in the 15 year period, 139 cases were matched according to our selection criteria for this study. Table 1 illustrates the breakdown of the cases. It was recognized that the cases which were classified as idiopathic were most frequent (91 cases; 66%). 18 cases (13%) were diagnosed as dilated cardiomyopathy (DCM), that showed an ejection fraction of less than 50% with an increase in left ventricular diastolic volume. 7 cases (5%) were diagnosed as hypertrophic cardiomyopathy (HCM). Myocarditis was seen in 11 cases (8%). The diagnoses were made according to our criteria for clinical diagnosis and all cases were presumed to be of viral origin (12). There were 8 cases (6%) which were diagnosed as specific myocardial diseases; sarcoidosis in 5 cases, amyloidosis in 1 case, polymyositis in 1 case, and congenital myopathy in 1 case. Among them, 2 cases of sarcoidosis and 1 case of amyloidosis were confirmed by the biopsy as a sole diagnostic element. Ischemic heart disease was found in 2 cases with the aid of coronary arteriography. The rest of the cases were diagnosed as having mitral valve prolapse and left ventricular tumor.

Hypertension was associated with 16 out of the 91 idiopathic cases (18%). Familial occurrence defined according to our criteria (13) was confirmed or highly suspected in 18 cases (20%). It was also noted that in 22 of the 91 idiopathic cases (24%), ECG abnormalities were found in patients of less than 15 years of age. History revealed the presence of "flu" symptoms in 21 cases (23%). The symptoms consisted of high fever, arthralgia, myalgia and symptoms of upper respiratory infection and were found within 10 days prior to the occurrence of the cardiac manifestations. It was also noted that the presence of a past history of diphtheria was found in 7 cases (8%).

To determine the nature of the 91 cases which we classified into the idiopathic group, we evaluated the biopsy findings. Fig. 1 shows incidence of PMC and significant pathology in 91 idiopathic cases compared to 18 DCM cases. The incidence of PMC was 38 of the 91 cases (42%) in the idiopathic group, while it was found in 6 of the 18 cases (33%) in the DCM group. There was no significant difference between the idiopathic and DCM groups.

The incidence of significant pathology in this study was 23 of 91 cases (25%) in the idiopathic group and 9 of 18 cases (50%) in the DCM group. There were no apparent differences in the incidence of significant pathology between DCM and each of the idiopathic conduction disturbance group except for the low grade A-V block group. The reason why we have compared the 2 groups is that the DCM is a characteristic type of cardiomyopathy and often showed PMC or significant pathology in our previous study (8).

Next we studied the comparison between His bundle electrogram and biopsy findings (Fig. 2-A). In all the A-V block cases studied, 31 of 56 cases showed normal H-V interval, and 25 cases showed prolonged H-V interval. The incidence of significant pathology was 48% and apparently higher in H-V prolonged cases than in H-V normal cases

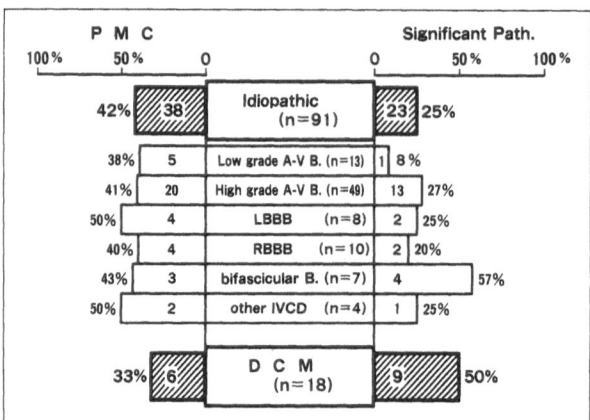

Fig. 1. Left hand side shows the incidence of postmyocarditic change (PMC).
Right hand side shows the incidence of significant pathology. Each incidence was compared with the incidence of the DCM group. There were no significant differences in the incidence of PMC between the idiopathic and the DCM groups. In the incidence of significant pathology, there were no apparent differences between the 2 groups, except for the low grade A-V block (P < 0.025).
PMC: postmyocarditic change, Path: Pathology,
DCM: dilated cardiomyopathy

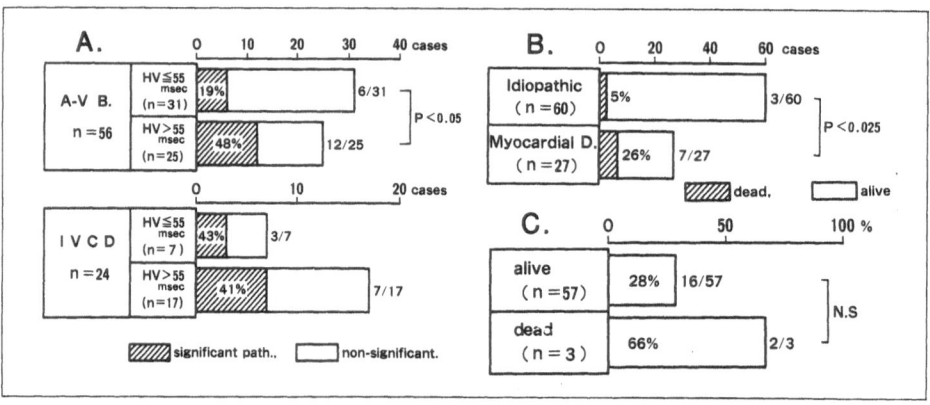

Fig. 2: A: Comparison between HBE and biopsy findings. See text for explanation.
B: Long-term follow up of patients with A-V and/or IVCD. See text for explanation.
C: Comparison of the incidence with significant pathology between alive and dead cases in the idiopathic group. See text for explanation.
        B: block, IVCD: intraventricular conduction disturbance,
        D: disease

which was 19%. However in IVCD, the incidence of significant pathology was high having no correlation with H-V interval.

Mean ejection fraction of the left ventricle in the idiopathic group was 64.9 ± 6.6% in cases with A-V block, and 63.9 ± 9.2% in cases with IVCD, showing fairly good contraction force.

A long-term follow-up of up to 13 years in 87 cases revealed that there were 3 deaths out of 60 cases (5%) in the idiopathic group and 7 deaths out of 27 cases (26%) in myocardial disease group (Fig. 2-B). There was a significant difference between the 2 groups (P < 0.025). In 3 fatal cases in the idiopathic group, 2 (67%) showed a significant pathology, while in 57 non-fatal cases in the idiopathic group, 16 cases (28%) showed significant pathology. There was no apparent difference between fatal and nonfatal groups because of the small number of fatal cases (Fig. 2-C).

Case presentation

Case 1: A 41 year old female with "flu" symptoms and PMC (Fig. 3).
This patient had a history of "flu" symptoms which consisted of productive cough and symptoms of upper respiratory infection 6 days before complete A-V block was detected. ECG showed III° A-V block. She experienced syncopal attacks. LVEF showed 57% and

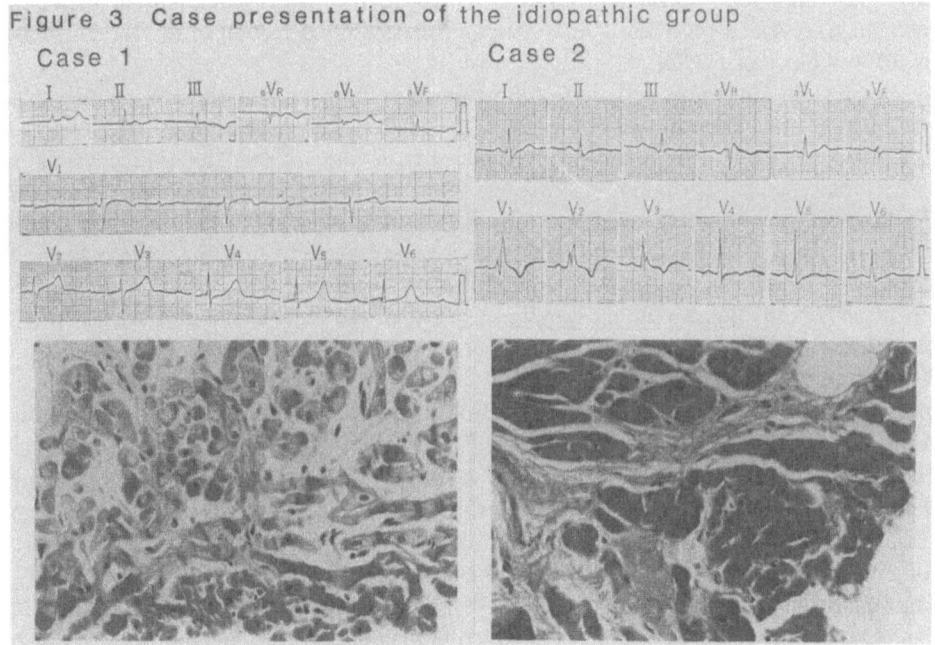

Figure 3 Case presentation of the idiopathic group
Case 1   Case 2

Fig. 3. Case 1: A 41 year old female with "flu" symptoms. ECG shows complete A-V block and the biopsy shows postmyocarditic change.
Case 2: A 53 year old male with a familial occurrence. ECG shows CRBBB and the biopsy shows significant pathology.

105

left ventricular volume was normal. There was no significant stenosis in the coronary angiogram. In HBE, intrahissian block was seen. The biopsy findings shows PMC.

Case 2: A 53 year old male with familial occurrence of complete right bundle branch block (Fig. 3).

Biopsy from the right ventricle shows fragmentation (+) and disarrangement (+) of muscle bundles, hypertrophy of myocytes (+) and interstitial fibrosis (++). According to our experience, this kind of pathology can be differentiated from the postmyocarditic change and diagnosed as showing "significant pathology". In this case, left ventricular ejection fraction was 75% and there was no significant coronary artery stenosis. HBE showed normal A-H and H-V interval.

Discussion

In cases with A-V block and/or IVCD, analysis of the endomyocardial biopsy findings revealed that there existed a certain number of cases where the biopsy was of final diagnostic value in which sarcoidosis or amyloidosis were demonstrated (5, 6, 7). So it should be stressed that the biopsy is an important diagnostic tool in cases with conduction disturbance.

Our experience of performing serial myocardial biopsy in 10 cases with acute myocarditis of viral origin enabled us to define the histopathological criteria of postmyocarditic change (PMC). Utilizing this experience, we have analyzed the cases which were classified into the idiopathic group and PMC was found in 42% of the cases. Among them, 13 cases (42%) revealed preceding "flu" symptoms before the detection of ECG abnormalities of A-V block or IVCD.

In our previous study (14), long-term follow-up of acute myocarditis where the diagnosis was accomplished with the aid of the biopsy revealed that there were cases with residual A-V block or IVCD. It is therefore presumed that in some of the idiopathic cases as in case 1, the origin of conduction disturbance was a residual phenomenon of myocarditis. Furthermore, we reported that there were a certain number of cases where the LVEF was lower than 50% after they suffered from myocarditis and were able to be diagnosed as DCM (15). In cases which we classified into DCM in this study, PMC was also frequently observed and also the flu symptoms preceded the onset of the disease. In 4 of 18 cases (22%) which were classified into DCM, we presumed that the origin of conduction disturbance was an after effect of myocarditis.

In our present study, the incidence of significant pathology was 25% in the idiopathic group (Fig. 1). And HBE revealed that significant pathology in A-V block had some influence upon H-V prolongation. In IVCD cases, the incidence of significant pathology was high having no correlation with H-V prolongation (Fig. 2-A). We considered that in IVCD, the significant pathology influenced the intraventricular conduction time. So we concluded that significant pathology might be the cause of conduction disturbance.

The significant pathology that we have observed in cases in the idiopathic group were too diseased to consider as a result of conduction disturbance and therefore we think that the disease is occurring primarily in the ventricle and involved the conduction system of the heart. This concept can be applied to the existence of cardiomyopathy in which the A-V block or IVCD is the main clinical feature, as those cases revealed no apparent dilatation of the left ventricle and also revealed no apparent thickening of the ventricular wall. It can be classified into our classification system of non-hypertrophic, non-dilated, arrhythmia · conduction disturbance type of cardiomyopathy. We finally put the 23 cases (25%) of idiopathic group into this classification system.

A long-term follow-up of 86 cases among the 139 cases studied revealed 3 deaths among the 60 idiopathic cases (5%) and 7 deaths among the 27 cases with myocardial diseases (26%) (Fig. 2-B). This indicates that the apparent heart muscle diseases such as amyloidosis, sarcoidosis, DCM and HCM are more prone to have short prognosis. And in idiopathic cases, the incidence of significant pathology was 28% of 57 non-fatal cases and 66% of 3 fatal cases (NS). The number of cases was small so further study is needed (Fig. 2-C).

It is to be stressed here that in those cases where the A-V block or IVCD exists and when pacemaker implantation is considered, the study employing endomyocardial biopsy is very informative in making the diagnosis and also useful for the recognition of the prognosis of the patients. It may also be useful for the selection of the mode of pacemaker implantation such as endocardial or epicardial pacing and selection of the leads.

It has to be mentioned finally that the incidence of detecting myocardial diseases or significant pathology in cases with conduction disturbance in our study is rather high. The reason may be due to our selection in which the biopsies were performed in those cases where the myocardial disease was suspected.

Acknowledgement

English correction by Mr. Michael Johnson is appreciated.
This study was supported by a Research Grant for Intractable Diseases from the Japanese Ministry of Health and Welfare.

References

1. Lev M: Anatomic basis for atrioventricular block. Am J Med 1964; 34: 742–748.
2. Dhingra RC, Khan A, Pouget JM, Rosen KM: Lenegre's disease in a young adult. Am Heart J 1974; 88: 487–492.
3. Davies MJ, Anclerson RH, Becker AE: The conduction system of the heart. London: Butterworths, 1983: 228–300.
4. Sekiguchi M, Hiroe M, Take M, Hirosawa K: Clinical and histopathological profile of sarcoidosis of the heart and acute idiopathic myocarditis. Concepts through a study employing endomyocardial biopsy. II. Myocarditis. Jpn Circul J 1980; 44: 264–273.
5. Sekiguchi M, Numao Y, Imai M, Furuie T, Mikami R: Clinical and histopathological profile of sarcoidosis of the heart and acute idiopathic myocarditis. Concepts through a study employing endomyocardial biopsy. I. Sarcoidosis. Jpn Circul J 1980; 44: 249–263.
6. Konno S, Sakakibara S: Intracardiac heart biopsy. Dis Chest 1963; 44: 345–350.
7. Sekiguchi M, Hiroe M, Ogasawara S, Nishikawa T: Practical aspects of endomyocardial biopsy. Ann Acad Med Singapore 1981; 10 (4) suppl: 115–128.
8. Take M: A clinicopathological study on a case of idiopathic cardiomyopathy and arrhythmia and conduction disturbance employing endomyocardial biopsy. J Tokyo Wom Med Coll 1982; 52: 1417–1442 (In Japanese with English abstract).
9. Kasser IS, Kennedy JW: Measurement of left ventricular volumes in man by single-plane cineangiocardiography. Invest Radiol 1969; 4: 83.

10. Scherlag BJ, Lav SH, Helfant RH, Berkowitz WD, Stein E, Damato AN: Catheter technique for recording His-bundle activity in man. Circulation 1969; 39: 13–18.
11. Robles de Medina EO: A new coding system for electrocardiography. Amsterdam: Excerpta Medica, 1972.
12. Take M, Sekiguchi M, Hiroe M, Hirosawa K: Early clinical profile of cases with histopathologically proven acute idiopathic myocarditis and proposal for diagnostic criteria. Jpn Circul J 1981; 45: 1415–1420.
13. Sekiguchi M, Hasegawa A, Ando A: A proposal for analyzing the familial occurrence of cardiomyopathy in the clinical situation. In: Sekiguchi M, Olsen EGJ, eds. Cardiomyopathy. Clinical, pathological and theoretical aspects. Tokyo, Baltimore: Univ Tokyo Press and Univ Park Press, 1980: 445–453.
14. Take M, Sekiguchi M, Hiroe M, Hirosawa K: Long-term follow up of electrocardiographic findings in patients with acute myocarditis proven by endomyocardial biopsy. Jpn Circul J 1982; 46: 1227–1234.
15. Hasumi M, Sekiguchi M, Morimoto S, Hiroe M, Take M, Hirosawa K: Ventriculographic findings at the convalescent stage in eleven cases with acute myocarditis. Jpn Circul J 1983; 47: (in press).

Authors' address:
Dr. Motonari Hasumi
The Heart Institute of Japan,
Tokyo Women's Medical College
10 Kawada-cho
Shinjuku-ku
Tokyo 162 / Japan

Atrial Contribution in VVI Pacing

Yutaka Yamamoto, Jiro Sugai

Summary: Frequency of at random atrio-ventricular (A-V) sequence in VVI pacing was studied by using a simulated model and by applying 24-hour Holter ECGs for 12 paced patients with complete A-V block. A ratio of the number of QRS complexes preceded by P waves to the total number of QRS complexes (atrial contribution rate, ACR) was calculated. ACR was also calculated as a ratio of T-R interval to P-P interval when atrial rate was fixed. Under ventricular pacing at rate of 70/min and T-R interval of 500 msec, ACR was 46%, 62%, 74%, 79%, 87% and 94% at atrial rate of 59/min, 78/min, 88/min, 97/min, 107/min and 117/min, respectively. On the exercise model, ACR was calculated as 61% to 81%. In the paced patients, maximal ACR of the day ranged from 47% to 93% with a mean of 72 ± 14%, minimal ACR ranged from 24% to 50% with a mean of 39 ± 8%, and mean ACR of the day ranged from 40% to 63% with a mean of 51 ± 7%. Higher ACR was seen in the daytime. Thus, at random A-V sequence occurs at substantial rates, especially during exercise. Nevertheless, atrial contribution should not be overemphasized in the majority of cases, as it is not a major factor in keeping cardiac output equal to hemodynamic demands.

A considerable number of studies have been conducted demonstrating improved hemodynamics with atrial or atrio-ventricular (A-V) sequential pacing, as compared to fixed rate ventricular pacing (1–18). In some of these studies (3–6), the hemodynamics of atrial or A-V sequential pacing were compared to ventricular pacing with P waves during ventricular systole. However, in patients with complete A-V block, treated by VVI pacing, some of the atrial contractions must occur coincidentally during ventricular diastole. The purpose of the present study is to clarify how often this at random AV sequence does occur in VVI pacing.

Methods

1. Simulation study

Simulated QRS-T signals and atrial signals were entered into ECG monitoring systems their own rates. Ventricular rates and T-R interval (an interval between the end of T wave and the beginning of the QRS complex) were fixed at 70/min and 500 msec, respectively. Two minutes recordings were taken at atrial rates of 60/min, 80/min, 90/min, 100/min, 110/min and 120/min.

As a simulation of exercise, the atrial rates were changed during the recording as follows; the study was started at an atrial rate of 75/min, which was increased to 85/min in 30 seconds, then to 90/min in the next 30 seconds. It was maintained at 90/min for 3 minutes, and it was then decreased to 75 min for 1 minute. Other modes of exercise simulation were performed by atrial rate changes of 75–90–100–75/min, 75–100–110–75/min, and 75–110–120–75/min within the time schedule as mentioned above.

A ratio of the number of QRS complexes preceded by P waves to the total number of QRS complexes (atrial contribution rate, ACR) was calculated in each study. When the atrial rate was fixed, ACR was also calculated as a ratio of T-R interval to P-P interval (theoretical ACR).

2. Clinical study

Twenty-four hours' Holter ECGs were taken in 12 ambulatory patients with complete A-V block, who were completely dependent on fixed rate ventricular pacing. Their age ranged from 52 to 85 years, with a mean of 72 ± 8 (SD) years. The average pacing rate was 72 ± 2 beats/min, and the average T-R interval was 398 ± 17 msec. When the Holter ECGS were reviewed, one minute records were made hourly and the ACR was calculated.

Results

1. ACR in the simulated model

Actual and theoretical ACR at different atrial rates are shown in Table I. Both ACR were nearly identical and were higher at higher atrial rates. ACR was as low as 46% at an atrial rate of 59/min, but this increased to more than 90% when the atrial rate was increased to 117/min.

The simulated exercise study, with atrial rate changes, showed ACR ranging from 61% to 81% (Table 1). Exericse of higher levels, with higher atrial response, was associated with higher ACR.

Table 1. ACR in VVI pacing

Atrial rate	ACR
59/min	46 (49)%
78	62 (65)
88	74 (73)
97	79 (81)
107	87 (89)
117	94 (94)
75– 90–75/min	61
75–100–75	67
75–110–75	77
75–120–75	81

* theoretical ACR in ( )

$$ACR = \frac{QRS\ preceded\ by\ P}{Total\ QRS}$$

$$= \frac{T\text{–R interval}}{P\text{– interval}}$$

2. ACR in the paced patients

Maximal, minimal, and mean ACR during 24 hours in the 12 patients were 72 ± 14%, 39 ± 8% and 51 ± 7%, respectively (Table 2). Maximal ACR of cases A, B, and C were higher than 90%. Half of the patients showed on average an ACR of more than 50%. Diurnal change of ACR is shown in Fig. 1. ACR was around 45% between 1 a.m. and 5 a.m., then began to increase until reaching the peak value of 61% at 9 a.m. It then decreased gradually to 45% at midnight.

ACR of cases B, E, and L are shown in Fig. 2. Case B is a 68 year-old active housewife, whose sinus node responded well to her daily activity resulting in a wide range of atrial rate changes. ACR, while awake, maintained a level of 60 to 70%. Above all, ACR at 7 a.m., at 9 a.m., and at 3 p.m. were as high as 84%, 92%, and 79%, respectively. To the contrary, case L is a 85 year-old inactive lady, whose ACR remained at a lower level of 33 to 47%, possibly due to her inactivity and/or associated sinus node dysfunction.

Discussion

The present study was aimed at clarifying the frequency of at random A-V sequence in VVI pacing. The study, using both simulated models and real paced patients, demonstrated that atrial contractions occurred during ventricular diastole at substantial rates, especially during exercise. Whether all of these A-V sequences are hemodynamically effective for ventricular filling, is another subject. Uncertainty still exists regarding the proper A-V interval. Leinbach et al. (17) and Chamberlain et al. (16) found that the optimal A-V in-

Table 2. ACR during 24 hours

Patient	Age	Sex	Pacing rate xp (beats/min)	T–R interval (msec)	ACR (%) max	min	mean	SD
A	84	M	70	400	93	39	52	12
B	68	F	68	440	92	48	63	11
C	72	M	70	400	90	33	48	11
D	68	M	74	400	77	37	48	10
E	78	F	73	400	73	53	61	5
F	67	M	72	400	73	50	60	5
G	70	M	74	400	70	40	53	8
H	52	M	74	360	69	33	48	10
I	73	F	71	400	61	44	52	5
J	70	M	71	380	60	33	48	8
K	76	F	73	400	55	24	44	7
L	85	F	73	400	47	33	40	4
mean	72		72	398	72	39	51	
SD	8		2	17	14	8	7	

SD: Standard deviation

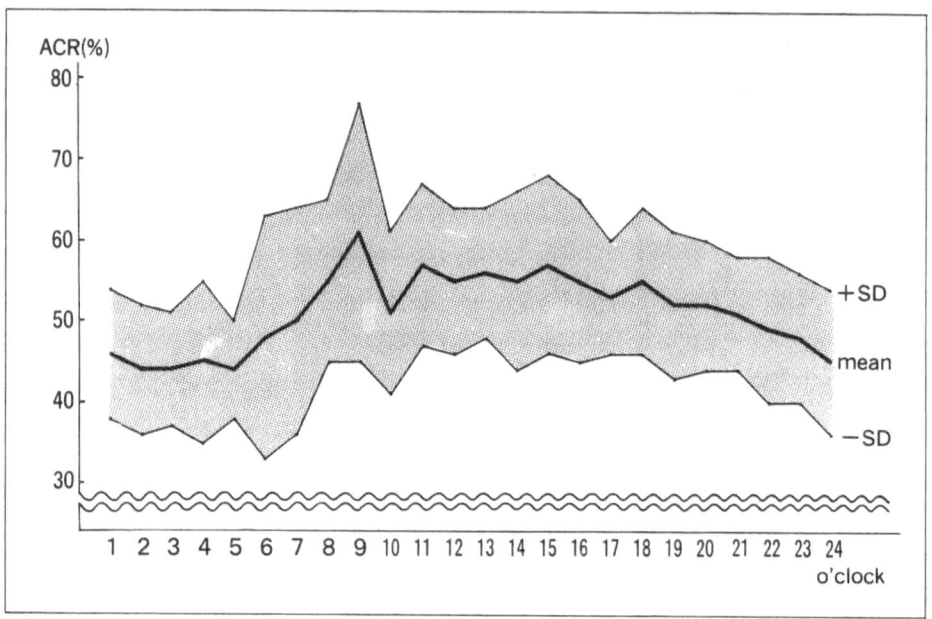

Fig. 1. Diurnal change of atrial contribution rate (ACR) in 12 paced patients with complete heart block. Average ACR of the 12 patients is 61% at 9 a.m. and average ACR while awake ranges from 50 to 55%.

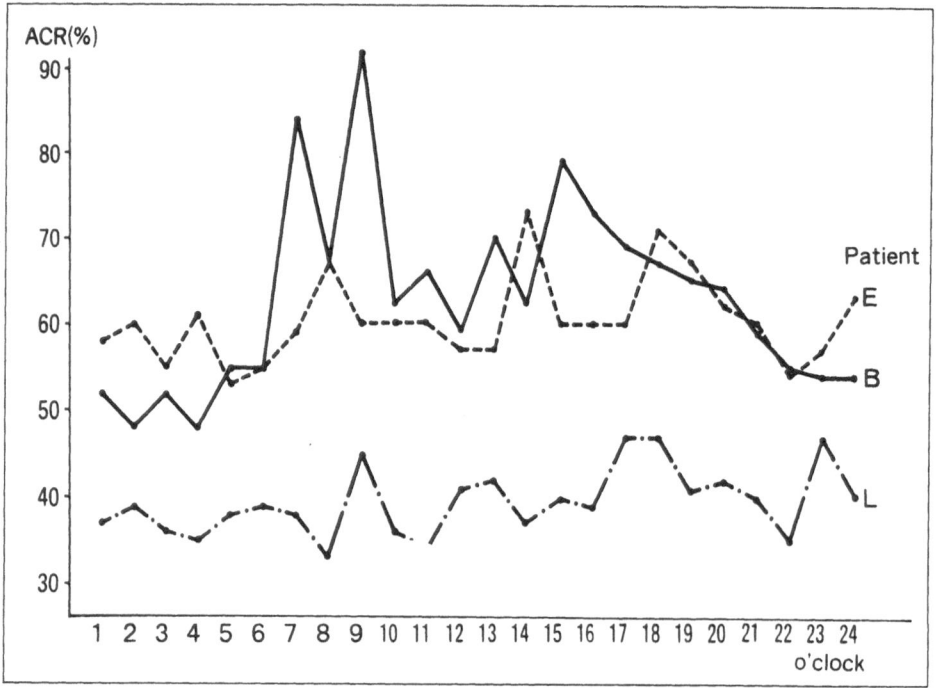

Fig. 2. Diurnal change of atrial contribution rate (ACR) in case B, E and L. Case B and E show relatively higher ACR and case C shows low ACR through 24 hours.

terval was 150 msec in patients with chronic, complete A-V block and 100 msec or less in patients with heart block complicating acute myocardial infarction. Hartzler et al. (14) studied A-V sequential pacing after cardiac surgery and demonstrated that the optimal A-V interval ranged from 150 to 250 msec in adults. Benchimol et al. (7) reported an increase in ejection time, isometric contraction time, systemic arterial systolic pressure, dp/dt of arterial pressure, and tension-time index at a P-R interval of 1 to 300 msec, as compared with figures obtained during a time when atrial systole occurs during ventricular systole. The same authors (10) also demonstrated a higher peak arterial flow velocity at a P-R interval of 1 to 200 msec. Bashour et al. (13) measured systolic time intervals, and they demonstrated that a P-R interval of 180 to 200 msec was associated with a maximal left ventricular ejection time, a minimal pre-ejection period, and an optimal stroke volume. In their data, some degree of contribution of atrial contractions is evidenced even at a P-R interval of less than 180 msec or more than 200 msec. ACR is much modified by the atrial rate as is shown in the present study, but it is also influenced by the T-R interval (Fig. 3). As the average T-R interval in the patients paced at a ventricular rate of 72 ± 2/min was found to be 400 msec, this figure must be applied to Fig. 3, which shows an ACR of 50% at an atrial rate of 75/min and 80% at 120/min. If the range of P-R intervals effective for ventricular filling is narrower than the T-R interval, we can apply this range to Fig. 3 instead of the T-R interval. Assuming that this range of P-R intervals is 350 msec, ACR is calculated as 70% at an atrial rate of 120/min and 44% at 75/min. These figures are greater than was previously thought.

This study also suggests that a comparison between A-V sequential and VVI pacing should be done, considering that at random A-V sequence in VVI pacing occurs more frequently during exercise. Nevertheless, atrial contribution should not be overemphasized in the majority of cases in whom the heart may function at a wide range of work loads with an increment of stroke volume, though the A-V sequence may be of some significance under certain circumstances such as the decompensated heart. It is well known that one of the major factors in increasing cardiac output is ventricular rate, and our effort

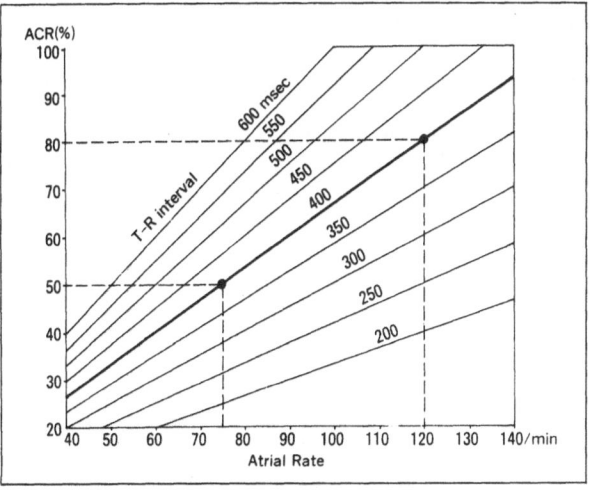

Fig. 3. Interrelation of atrial contribution rate (ACR), atrial rate and T-R interval. When T-R interval is 400 msec, ACR is 80% at atrial rate of 120/min and 50% at 75/min.

should be directed to the developement of pacemakers that provide an automatic adjustment of the pacing rate according to the hemodynamic needs.

References

1. Nathan DA, Samet P, Center S et al: Long-term correction of complete heart block. Clinical and physiologic studies of a new type of implantable synchronous pacer. Progr Cardiovasc Dis 1964; 6: 538.
2. Judge RD, Wilson WS, Siegal JH: Hemodynamic studies in patients with implanted cardiac pacemakers. New England J Med 1964; 270: 1391.
3. Samet P, Bernstein W, Levine S: Significance of the atrial contribution of ventricular filling. Am J Cardiol 1965; 15: 195–202.
4. Samet P, Bernstein WH, Nathan DA et al: Atrial contribution to cardiac output in complete heart block. Am J Cardiol 1965; 16: 1–10.
5. Samet P, Castillo C, Bernstein WH: Hemodynamic consequences of sequential atrioventricular pacing. Am J Cardiol 1968; 21: 207–212.
6. Befeler B, Hildner FJ, Javier RP et al: Cardiovascular dynamics during coronary sinus, right atrial, and right ventricular pacing. Am Heart J 1971; 81: 372–380.
7. Benchimol A, Duenas A, Ligget MS et al: Contribution of atrial systole to the cardiac function at a fixed and at a variable ventricular rate. Am J Cardiol 1965; 16: 11–21.
8. Benchimol A, Ellis JG, Dimond EG: Hemodynamic consequences of atrial and ventricular pacing in patients with normal and abnormal hearts. Am J Med 1965; 39: 911–922.
9. Benchimol A, Ligget MS: Cardiac hemodynamics during stimulation of the right atrium, right ventricle, and left ventricle in normal and abnormal hearts. Circulation 1966; 33: 933–944.
10. Benchimol A: Significance of the contribution of atrial systole to cardiac function in man. Am J Cardiol 1969; 23: 568–571.
11. Carleton RA, Passovoy M, Graettinger JS: The importance of the contribution and timing of left atrial systole. Clin Sci 1966; 30: 151–159.
12. Kosowsky BD, Dcherlag BJ, Damato AN: Re-evaluation of the atrial contribution to ventricular function. Am J Cardiol 1968; 21: 518–524.
13. Bashour TT, Naughton JP, Cheng TO: Systolic time intervals in patients with artificial pacemakers. Am J Cardiol 1973; 32: 290.
14. Hartzler GO, Maloney JD, Curtid JJ et al: Hemodynamic benefits of atrioventricular sequential pacing after cardiac surgery. Am J Cardiol 1977; 40: 232–236.
15. Greenberg B, Chatterjee K, Parmley WW et al: The influence of left ventricular filling presure on atrial contribution to cardiac output. Am Heart J 1979; 98: 742–751.
16. Chamberlain DA, Leinbach RC, Vassaux CE et al: Sequential atrioventricular pacing in heart block complicating acute myocardial infarction. New England J Med 1970; 282: 577–582.
17. Leinbach RC, Chamberlein DA, Kastor JA et al: A comparison of the hemodynamic effects of ventricular and sequential A-V pacing in patients with heart block. Am Heart J 1969; 78: 502–508.
18. Kappenberger L, Gloor HO, Babotai I et al: Hemodynamic effects of atrial synchronization in acute and long-term ventricular pacing. Pace 1982; 5: 639–645.

Authors' address:
Yutaka Yamamoto, M.D.
663-31, Odzenji,
Asao-ku, Kawasaki-shi
215 Japan

Stability of AV Conduction in Patients with Implanted Atrial Pacemakers

D. L. Hayes, S. Furman

Summary: Single chamber atrial pacing is effective in the management of sinus node dysfunction, subject to the uncertainty of longterm atrioventricular conduction. Despite the accepted observation that many patients with sinus node dysfunction also have atrioventricular conduction disease, data does not exist on the development of atrioventricular block in those patients with permanent single chamber atrial pacing. Of 70 patients who received single chamber atrial pacing from 1967 to 1982 (mean duration of pacing was 33 months) only 2 patients (2.9%) developed atrioventricular block which occurred after 14 months in one patient and after 23 months of successful atrial pacing in the other. Of the 70 patients, 37 had assessment of AV conduction by incremental atrial pacing at the time of implant and 20 patients underwent atrial pacing on the basis of surface electrocardiogram and clinical judgment. Electrophysiologic studies were conducted only in those patients being paced for control of supraventricular arrhythmias. Only 5 of the 70 patients required conversion to ventricular pacing for technical difficulties; three of these conversions occurred in the early 1970's before the advent of atrial tined or J leads, one was for irreparable lead fracture, and only one occurred in a patient with a newer design atrial lead. In conclusion, progression to AV block in patients with permanent atrial pacing is uncommon, that formal electrophysiologic studies are necessary mainly in patients with supraventricular arrhythmias and that in the majority of patients, AV conduction can be assessed at the time of implant. Continued improvement in atrial leads should make atrial pacing even more successful.

Implanted single chamber atrial pacing is an accepted mode for pacing those patients with sinus node dysfunction (without atrial fibrillation or flutter) including sinus bradycardia, sinus arrest, supraventricular tachycardia, etc. (1, 2). An argument against single chamber atrial pacing is the possibility of later development of atrioventricular block which would expose the patient to failure of ventricular response and would necessitate conversion to ventricular or dual chamber pacing (3). Because of this uncertainty, some have avoided single chamber atrial pacing in favor of ventricular or dual chamber pacing. Many of the patients with intact antegrade conduction also have retrograde (ventriculo-atrial) conduction and permanent single chamber ventricular pacing (VVI) may leave them as symptomatic as the intrinsic node dysfunction. An issue in regard to permanent single chamber atrial pacing is which pre-implant studies, if any, are necessary prior to committing a patient to long-term atrial pacing. To determine the natural history of patients with implanted single chamber atrial pacing, we reviewed our fifteen-year experience.

Methods and materials

From 1967 to 1982, 70 patients underwent implantation of single chamber atrial pacing at Montefiore Hospital and Medical Center. In this population there were 40 males and

Table 1. Leads Utilized in Atrial Position.

Lead	# of Patients
Coronary Sinus (Cordis)	18
6990 (Medtronic)	1
6990u (Medtronic)	16
6991 (Medtronic)	9
6991u (Medtronic)	1
Continuous Lead (Cordis)	5
483-01 (Intermedics)	4
Epicardial-Atrial (Cordis)	4
6961 (Medtronic)	2
6907 (Medtronic)	2
6901 (Medtronic)	1
IVE (Biotronik)	2
Miscellaneous	5

30 females with mean age of 64 years (range of 26 to 82 years). The underlying rhythm disturbances necessitating permanent pacing were: sick sinus syndrome (without atrial flutter or fibrillation) in 4 patients; sinus bradycardia in 26 patients; sinus arrest in 28 patients; supraventricular or re-entrant tachycardias in 12 patients. Follow-up has been carried out for a mean of 30 months (range from 1 month to greater than 10 years). Mean thresholds at the time of initial implants were: 0.1 ms, 5.27 mA: 2.44 V; 0.2 ms, 4.09 mA: 1.43 V; 0.5 ms, 2.28 mA: 0.98 V; 1.0 ms, 1.44 mA: 0.81 V; and 2.0 ms, 1.00 mA: 0.75 V. The mean P wave amplitude was 5 mV, mean slew rate was 1.9 mV/ms and mean impedance was 477 ohms. A variety of leads were utilized and are listed in Table 1. A number of ventricular leads were used in the atrial position. Four patients were paced epicardially and of the 66 patients paced intravenously, 42 were paced from the right atrial appendage and 24 from the coronary sinus. Data from atrial leads which were initially part of dual chamber pacing systems is not included.

The decision to commit a patient to implanted single chamber atrial pacing was made in one of three ways:

1. a previous electrophysiologic study;
2. incremental pacing at the time of implant to determine the status of AV conduction;
3. clinically by electrocardiogram and history.

Of the 70 patients, 13 had formal electrophysiologic studies of whom 12 had supraventricular or re-entrant tachycardias which required electrophysiologic evaluation for definition of the rhythm disturbance. The remaining patient was a 26-year-old man with syncope and documented sinus arrest who was studied to rule out an inducible tachycardia which had not been documented during long-term electrocardiographic monitoring, but which might be a factor in the syncope.

Thirty-six patients had intraoperative evaluation of AV conduction including incremental atrial pacing and recording of PR interval as well as the rate at which Wenckebach conduction of AV block occurred. In some patients a sinus node recovery time was recorded and in a few patients a simple His bundle recording was obtained. The remaining 21 patients were paced on the basis of their clinical presentation, history and surface electrocardiogram, as well as electrocardiographic recording during carotid sinus massage.

Results

During the follow-up period, 5 patients have been lost to follow-up and 10 patients have died. None of the deaths were considered to be pacemaker related.

Two of the 70 patients developed atrioventricular conduction disease during the follow-up period. One patient was a 78-year-old female who was initially paced for sick sinus syndrome. After 14 months of successful atrial pacing, intermittent complete heart block was found during a follow-up visit. She subsequently underwent permanent ventricular pacing (VVI) and continues to do well. The second patient was a 74-year-old man who had had syncope and documented sinus arrest without AV block on carotid sinus massage. Thirty months later he had another syncopal episode. Electrocardiogram showed alternating bundle branch block and carotid sinus massage revealed complete AV block. He underwent ventricular pacing. The development of AV block occurred early after implant in both patients. The 95% cumulative survival for development of AV block was reached during the third year after implant and has not deteriorated (Table 2).

Five patients have required conversion to ventricular pacing because of technical difficulties; none has developed AV conduction disease during follow-up. Of the patients requiring conversion to VVI pacing for technical reasons, 3 occurred prior to 1976, i.e. before the availability of newer tined atrial or J leads. A fourth patient sustained a lead fracture after 80 months of successful pacing from the coronary sinus. At the time of revision to ventricular pacing, a secure position in the right atrial appendage where thresholds were acceptable could not be found. The remaining patient, a 26-year-old male with sinus arrest, developed high pacing threshold and failure to capture in the very early post-implant period without radiographic evidence of displacement. He opted for conversion to VVI pacing and is known to have retained AV conduction one year following implant, though he is now followed elsewhere.

Table 2. Cumulative Survival for Conversion to Atrioventricular Block.

Mos	# PTS	AV B	Deceased	LTF	PTL Ex	RVC	Annual surv	Cum surv %
0– 12	70	0	5	2	13	3	100	100
13– 24	47	1	1	0	7	1	98	98
25– 36	37	1	1	2	7	0	97	95
37– 48	26	0	0	1	4	0	100	95
49– 60	21	0	2	0	6	0	100	95
61– 72	13	0	1	0	4	0	100	95
73– 84	8	0	0	0	3	0	100	95
85– 96	4	0	0	0	0	0	100	95
97–108	4	0	0	0	2	0	100	95
109–120	2	0	0	0	1	0	100	95
121–126	1	0	0	0	1	0	100	95
Total	70	2	10	5	48	5	–	95

AV B	= Conversion to AV block
LTF	= Lost to follow-up
PTL Ex	= Partly exposed
RVC	= Conversion to right ventricular pacing for technical reasons

Discussion

Despite the increasing use of implanted pacing for sinus node dysfunction, permanent single chamber atrial pacing is utilized infrequently in comparison for ventricular pacing. Three reasons have been advocated for the limitations of atrial pacing (3):
1. atrial electrode instability compared to ventricular electrodes;
2. P wave sensing of less reliability than QRS sensing and
3. the uncertainty of distal conduction system disease developing in patients with sinus node dysfunction.

Recent advances in implant technique, pulse generator sensing circuitry and atrial electrodes, have minimized the first two concerns (4, 5, 6). The major unanswered question is whether or not a significant number of patients with sinus node dysfunction will deteriorate and develop clinically significant AV conduction disease. Our experience with 70 patients with implanted single chamber atrial pacing with follow-up for greater than 5 years in 10 patients and greater than 10 years in 2 patients reveals an incidence of only 2.9% (2 of 70) developing clinically significant AV conduction disturbance. Although several authors have reported on the frequency of AV conduction disease in patients with sinus node dysfunction or sinus bradycardia, there is no documentation of the incidence of symptomatic atrioventricular conduction disease developing in patients with sinus node dysfunction (7, 8, 9, 10). Several series of long-term atrial pacing have been reported, but none deal with the incidence of developing distal conduction disease (3, 4, 5, 11, 12, 13, 14).

Of the 2 patients demonstrating AV conduction abnormality, one was a 78-year-old female initially paced for sick sinus syndrome and the other was a 74-year-old male initially paced for sinus arrest and syncope. Both had intraoperative assessment of AV conduction and one was asymptomatic at the time the AV conduction disturbance was discovered. Not only have the patients been paced safely, but also atrial pacing has allowed retention of the normal AV sequence and has avoided the "pacemaker syndrome", i.e. symptomatic retrograde ventriculo-atrial conduction (15, 16, 17, 18). Syncope has been relieved in all except the 74-year-old who developed AV block; of the 12 patients with supraventricular or re-entrant tachycardias, all have had a marked reduction in tachycardia episodes or have had satisfactory specific antitachycardia management by the implanted pacemaker.

Formal electrophysiologic studies are necessary only in those patients with documented or suspected supraventricular or re-entrant tachycardias for definition of the tachycardia mechanism and determination of whether pacing or pharmaceutical managment is appropriate (19). In the patients with sinus node dysfunction, intraoperative assessment of AV conduction is adequate to insure safe permanent atrial pacing.

Intraopertive techniques consisted of incremental atrial pacing beginning at a rate of 60 (or the lowest rate at which the sinus mechanism could be surpassed) and then at rates of 80, 100, 120, 140 and higher in some cases depending on AV nodal response. The electrocardiogram was displayed on a physiologic recorder*) and hard copy of the electrocardiogram made. The tracings were analyzed for prolongation of P–R interval at various

---

* Electronics-For-Medicine, Pleasantville, NY

pacing rates, rates at which Wenckebach conduction occurs, and any development of higher degrees of AV block. The value of His bundle recordings in patients with sinus node dysfunction has been disputed and is not currently part of the assessment at the time of implant (20). Similarly, in those patients with sinus node disease in whom implantable pacing has been selected, the value of sinus node function tests is of questionable value and this measurement is no longer performed in our institution during evaluation for atrial pacing (21). Although 20 patients received implanted atrial pacing on the basis of clinical presentation, history, and surface electrocardiogram and although none have developed AV conduction disease, the majority of these patients received their initial implant during the early part of the study. In the current state of practice almost all patients receiving implanted atrial pacing have intraoperative assessment of AV conduction. The procedure as described above is performed with the atrial lead after it is in place and adds little time to the implant procedure. Of the 5 (7%) patients who had technical difficulties and required conversion to ventricular pacing, it is noteworthy that 3 of these conversions occurred prior to the availability of the newer tined or atrial J leads.

Permanent atrial pacing has been found to be as reliable as ventricular pacing of the same era. Once instituted, a low 2.9% incidence of the development of AB block occurred and this threat should not, therefore, be considered a substantial problem in properly selected patients. The quality of patient benefit has been as great as in ventricular pacing for some, and greater for those with retained AV conduction.

References

1. Mond H: The bradyarrhythmias: current indications for permanent pacing (Part II). Pace 1981; 4: 538–547.
2. Hayward R: Who do we pace? Br J Hosp Med 1981; 466–473.
3. Joseph SP, White J: Long-term atrial pacing for sinus node disease without output-terminal programmable pacemakers. J Thorac Cardiovasc Surg 1979; 78: 292–297.
4. Kleinert M, Bock M, Wilhelmi F: Clinical use of a new transvenous atrial lead. Am J Cardiol 1977; 40: 237–42.
5. Geddes JS, Webb SW, Clements IP: Clinical experience with transvenous atrial pacing. Br Heart J 1978; 40: 589–595.
6. Zucker IR, Parsonnet V, Gilbert L: A method of permanent transvenous implantation of an atrial electrode. Am Heart J 1973; 85: 195.
7. Rosen KM, Loeb HS, Sinno MZ, Rahimtoola SH, Gunnar RM: Cardiac conduction in patients with symptomatic sinus node disease. Circulation 1971; 43: 836–844.
8. Narula OS: Atrioventricular conduction defects in patients with sinus bradycardia. Circulation 1971; 44: 1096–1110.
9. Rubenstein JJ, Schulman CL, Yurchak PM: The clinical spectrum of the sick sinus syndrome. Circulation 1972; 46: 5–13.
10. Edhag O: Associated conduction disturbances in patients with symptomatic sinus node disease. Acta Med Scand 1981; 210: 263–270.
11. Smyth N, Citron P, Keshishian J, Garcia J, Kelly L: Permanent pervenous atrial sensing and pacing with a new J shaped lead. J Thorac Cardiovasc Surg 1976; 72: 565
12. Moss AJ, Rivers RJ, Jr: Atrial pacing from the coronary vein. Ten-year experience in 50 patients with implanted pervenous pacemakers. Circulation 1978; 57: 103–106.
13. Kramer DH, Moss AJ: Permanent pervenous atrial pacing from the coronary vein. Circulation 1970; 42: 427.
14. Van Hemel NM, Van Riempst Ales, Bakema H, Swenne CA: Longterm follow-up after pacemaker implantation in sick sinus syndrome. Pace 1981; 4: 8–13.

15. El Gamal Mih, Van Gelder LM: Chronic ventricular pacing with ventriculo-atrial conduction versus atrial pacing in three patients with symptomatic sinus bradycardia. Pace 1981; 4: 100–105.
16. Wirtzfeld A, Himmler FCH, Paaeur HW, Klein G: Atrial and ventricular pacing in patients with sick sinus syndrome. In C Meere (ed) Proceedings VIth World Symposium On Cardiac Pacing, Montreal, Pacesymp 1979, Ch 15–5.
17. Ogawa S, Dreifus LS, Shenoy PN, Brockman SK, Berkovits BV: Hemodynamic consequences of atrioventricular and ventriculo-atrial pacing. Pace 1978; 1: 8–15.
18. Johnson AD, Laiken SL, Engler RL: Hemodynamic compromise associated with ventriculo-atrial conduction following transvenous pacemaker placement. Am J Med 1978; 65: 75–79.
19. Fisher JD: Role of electrophysiologic testing in the diagnosis and treatment of patients with known and suspected bradycardias and tachycardias. Prog Cardiovasc Dis 1981; 24: 25–90.
20. Gould L, Ramana Reddy CV, Brevetti GC, Cifarelli F, Maghazeh P, Shin CS: His bundle electrograms in 51 patients requiring permanent transvenous pacemakers. J Thorac Cardiovasc Surg 1977; 74: 28–36.
21. Breithadt G, Seipel L: Comparative study of two methods of estimating sinoatrial conduction time in man. Am J Cardiol 1978; 42: 965–972.

Authors' address:
David L. Hayes, M.D.
Mayo Clinic
Rochester, Minnesota 55905
USA

Atrio-Ventricular and Ventriculo-Atrial Conduction in Patients with Symptomatic Sinus Node Dysfunction

R. van Mechelen, F. Hagemeijer

Summary: Van Mechelen, R. et al.: Atrio-ventricular and ventriculo-atrial conduction in patients with symptomatic sinus node dysfunction. In 26 patients (pts) with symptomatic sinus node dysfunction (SND) electrophysiological studies were performed before pacemaker implantation. Patients were divided into two groups: Group I pts (18) with intact antegrade AV conduction (AVNW $\geq$ 130/min); Group II pts (8) with impaired antegrade AV conduction (AVNW < 130/min).
VA conduction was present in 20/26 pts (77%) of the total patient population. In 17/18 pts (94%) of Group I and in 3/8 pts (37%) of Group II VA conduction could be demonstrated (p < 0.01). In regard to a pacemaker syndrome, VVI pacing is therefore not the optimal pacemaker therapy in SND patients with VA conduction. However, the presently available alternatives (AAI, DVI, DDD pacemakers) have their imperfections too.

Introduction

Some patients with symptomatic sinus node dysfunction are not suitable candidates for permanent ventricular demand pacing (1–6). In these patients retrograde conduction to the atria during ventricular pacing results in atrial contraction against closed mitral and tricuspid valves. The symptoms of this so called "pacemaker syndrome" are in some patients so disabling that their demand unit has to be explanted (6).

Three years ago we started to perform electrophysiological studies (EPS) in these patients to demonstrate the presence or absence of retrograde conduction during ventricular pacing. In addition sino-atrial, AV nodal and infranodal conduction were evaluated, in order to select the most appropriate permanent pacing mode.

Methods

The decision to implant a pacemaker in patients with sinus node dysfunction was based upon symptoms of dizziness, dyspnea and/or syncope in relation with sinus bradycardia, sinus arrest, or sinoatrial block, documented by telemetry or by holter monitoring. Patients on drug therapy that might impair sino-atrial function were not included in this study.

Electrophysiological studies (EPS)

Following informed consent, EPS were performed in patients who met the selection criteria. The patients received no medication prior to the study. Catheters were placed for both stimulation and recording of intracardiac electrograms at the right ventricular (RV) apex, tricuspid valve ring, and high right atrium (HRA). Patterns of AV and VA conduction, refractory periods, were determined using the extrastimulus technique during pacing from the HRA and RV apex at several basic cycle lengths of pacing (7). Incremental ventricular pacing was initiated at a rate 10–15% faster than the spontaneous sinus rate or AV junctional rate, up to a rate at which second degree VA block occurred. Pacing rate was increased in steps of 10 beats/min; each pacing period lasted one minute. Criteria for the acceptance of 1 : 1 VA conduction were the following:

1. atrial activation sequence from the low right atrium to the high right atrium;
2. identical ventricular and atrial cycle lengths at the ventricular paced rate;
3. constant VA conduction time at one and the same pacing rate.

Incremental atrial pacing was performed up to a rate at which second degree AV block occurred. A normal response to atrial pacing at incremental rates was defined as the development of AV nodal Wenckebach at a heart rate of least 130 beats/min (7). The development of second degree AV block at heart rates below 130/min suggested impaired AV conduction. Patients were divided into two categories: Group I patients with intact antegrade AV conduction; Group II patients with impaired antegrade AV conduction.

An estimate of cardiac automaticity was obtained by pacing the atrium at approximately 120/min for a minimum of 30 seconds. Upon cessation of pacing, the interval from the last pacing impulse to the first sinus node recovery beat was measured (SNRT). The corrected sinus node recovery time (CSNRT) was calculated by subtracting the basic sinus rhythm cycle length form the sinus node recovery time. If asystole persisted for 5 seconds without escape rhythm, atrial pacing was resumed.

Autonomic tone was assessed by carotid sinus stimulation and the intravenous administration of atropine, starting with 0.5 mg up to a maximum dose of 2 mg. A normal response to atropine was defined as an increase of sinus rate to greater than 90/min, and an increase over the spontaneous rate of 20–50%.

Results

The clinical and electrocardiographic data are listed in Table 1. Table 2 and 3 show the results of EPS. Sinus node recovery time ranged from 1400–5500 msec in Group I, and from 1100–6400 msec in Group II. Corrected sinus node recovery time ranged from 250–600 msec in Group I, and from 250–1100 msec in Group II. These differences were not statistically significant. The response to atropine was blunted in 9 patients of Group I, and in 4 patients of Group II. VA conduction was present in 20/26 or 77% of the total patient population. The incidence of VA conduction in patients of Group I was 17/18 (94%); the incidence of VA conduction of Group II patients was 3/8 (37%). The difference between the two groups was a statistically significant difference associated with a p-value of < 0.01 (8). Therefore this difference might be of clinical importance. The rate up to which VA conduction remained intact during incremental ventricular pacing varied considerably in both groups, and was not related to the atrial rate up to which 1 : 1 AV conduction was present. However, in the majority of patients in both groups antegrade AV conduction remained intact up to higher rates during incremental atrial pacing, than retrograde conduction did during incremental ventricular pacing.

Table 1.

Clinical and Electrocardiographic	Data
Patients	26
Male/Female	10/16
Sinus bradycardia	14
Sinusarrest/sino-atrial block	10
Tachy-brady syndrome	2
ECG Heart rate (bpm)	16–150
PR interval (s.)	0.14–0.22
QRS duration (s.)	0.08–0.140
QRS morphology	
RBBB	3
RBBB + LAHB	1
LAHB	2
LBBB	1

Table 2. Electrophysiological data. Abbreviations: VERP = ventricular effective refractory period; 2° VA block = the rate up to which second degree VA block occurred; VACT = VA conduction time, VA interval was measured from the ventricular stimulus artifact to the onset of atrial depolarization at the HRA electrogram.

	Group I	Group II	
Patients	18	8	
AH interval (ms)	80–130	80–180	
HV interval (ms)	40–60	40–60	
VERP (ms)	200–320	190–300	
VA conduction	17/18	3/8	$(p < 0.01)$
2° VA block (bpm)	60–160	90–120	
VACT (ms)	130–420	150–220	
2° AV block ≥ 2° VA block	15/17	2/3	
2° AV block < 2° VA block	2/17	1/3	

Table 3. Electrophysiological data of Patients with impaired AAVC. Abbreviations: AVJR = AV junctional rhythm; SR = sinus rhythm; AVB II = second degree AVnodal block; AVC = the rate up to which antegrade conduction remained intact during incremental atrial pacing; VAC = the rate up to which retrograde conduction remained intact during incremental ventricular pacing; VACT = VA conduction time.

PTS. of group II HR and Rhythm during study (bpm)		AVC (bpm)	VAC (bpm)	VACT (ms)
1. AVJR	50	110	120	150
2. AVJR	45	70	–	–
3. SR	40	100	–	–
4. SR, AVB II	40	60	–	–
5. SR, AVB II	30	50	–	–
6. SR	60	120	90	150
7. SR	55	110	–	–
8. SR	80	120	110	220

Initially, we implanted AAI pacemakers in patients of group I; later (1982), when the AV universal (DDD) units became commercially available, we also implanted several DDD units (Fig. 1). In patients of Group II we implanted DVI units when VA conduction was present during EPS, and VVI units when VA conduction was absent during EPS. We also implanted a DDD unit in two patients of Group II. Follow-up ranges from three months to three years (mean follow-up 22 months). In none of 14 patients with AAI units 2/3 degree AV block developed; 3 AAI units were reprogrammed to AAT mode because of false inhibition, probably by sensing of myopotentials as was documented by holter recordings. In patients with VA conduction in whom a DDD unit was implanted, programmable parameters (AV delay period, refractory period of the atrial channel) had to be adjusted to prevent pacemaker mediated tachycardia. One patient with a DVI unit developed chronic atrial fibrillation despite antiarrhythmic therapy and elective cardioversion 8 months after pacemaker implantation. The course of the 4 patients with VVI units was uneventful.

Discussion

Patients with symptomatic sinus node dysfunction, in particular patients with intact antegrade AV conduction will frequently evidence VA conduction during ventricular pacing.

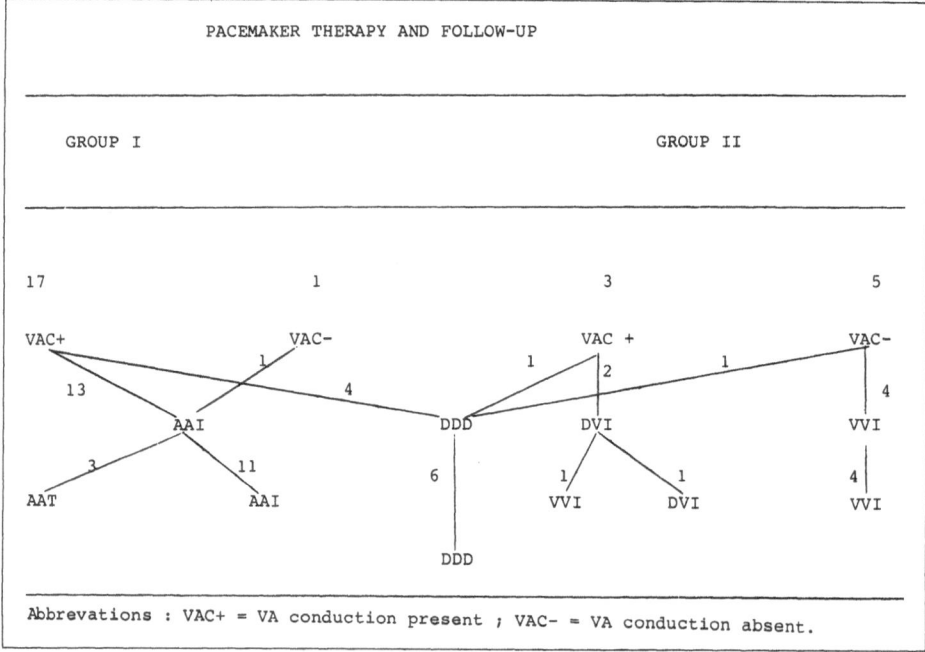

Fig. 1. Pacemaker therapy and follow-up. Abbreviations: VAC+ = VA conduction present; VAC- = VA conduction absent.

These patients may develop a pacemaker syndrome after implantation of a ventricular demand (VVI) pacemaker. Therefore, permanent ventricular demand pacing is not the optimal therapeutic approach (9).

However, the presently available alternatives have their imperfections too. When second or third degree AV block develops in a patient with a AAI unit, pacemaker reintervention is necessary. DVI pacing has several imperfections:

1. dual chamber pacing without atrial sensing might induce atrial fibrillation (10);

2. many of the available units have an AV delay which is too short to respect normal antegrade AV conduction, and artificial ventricular pacing occurs despite intact antegrade AV conduction at the programmed DVI pacing rate. With DDD pacemakers we also encountered the problem of artificial ventricular despite intact antegrade AV conduction. Besides, there was the problem of pacemaker mediated tachycardia. Fortunately, we could adjust programmed parameters (AV delay period, refractory period of the atrial channel) of the DDD units (Cordis 233D) we applied, to prevent pacemaker mediated tachycardia.

Additional refinements of presently available DDD and DVI pulse generators will be necessary to avoid artificial ventricular pacing despite intact antegrade AV conduction and to solve the problem of pacemaker mediated tachycardia.

References

1. Wirtzfeld A, Himmler FCH, Prauer HW et al: Atrial and ventricular pacing in patients with the sick sinus syndrome. In C. Meere (Ed): Proceedings of the VIth World Symposium on Cardiac Pacing, Montreal, Pacesymp, 1979, Chap. 15–5.
2. Ogawa S, Dreifus LS, Shenoy PA et al: Hemodynamic consequences of atrio-ventricular and ventriculo-atrial pacing. Pace, 1978; 1: 8.
3. Johnson AD, Laiken SL, and Enhler RL: Hemodynamic compromise associated with ventriculo-atrial conduction following transvenous pacemaker placement. Am J Med 1978; 65: 75.
4. Alicandri C, Fonad FM, Tarazi RC et al: Three cases of hypotension and syncope with ventricular pacing: Possible role of atrial reflexes. Am J Cardiol 1978; 42: 137.
5. Amikam S, and Riss E: Untoward hemodynamic consequences of permanent ventricular pacing associated with ventriculo-atrial conduction. In C Meere (Ed): Proceedings of the VIth World Symposium on Cardiac Pacing, Montreal, Pacesymp, 1979, Chap. 15–6.
6. El Gamel MIH, and Van Gelder LM: Chronic ventricular pacing with ventriculo-atrial conduction versus atrial pacing in three patients with symptomatic sinus bradycardia. Pace 1981; 1: 100.
7. Rosen KM, Loeb HS, Ziad Sinno et al: Cardiac conduction in patients with symptomatic sinus node disease. Circulation, 1971; 43: 836.
8. Armitage P: Statistical Methods in Medical Research. (Second printing), Blackwell Sci Publ, Oxford, 1973.
9. Van Mechelen R, Hagemeijer F, De Boer H, Schelling A: Atrio-ventricular and ventriculo-atrial conduction in patients with symptomatic sinus node dysfunction. Pace 1983; 6: 13–21.
10. Furman S, and Cooper JA: Atrial fibrillation during AV sequential pacing. Pace 1982; 5: 133–135.

Authors' address:
Rob van Mechelen, M.D.
Department of Cardiology
Sint Franciscus Gasthuis
Kleiweg 500
3045 PM Rotterdam The Netherlands

Deleterious Clinical and haemodynamic Effects of V-A Retroconduction in Symptomatic Sinus Brady-arrhythmias (S.S.B.) Treated with V. V. I. Pacing: their Regression with A. A. I. Pacing

G. Curzi, A. Purcaro, E. Molini, C. Viola, U. Berrettini, V. Di Luzio*)

Summary: Fifty-six pts. with "isolated" Symptomatic Sinus Brady-arrhythmias (S.S.B.) treated by V.V.I. p., showed 1:1 V-A retroconduction. They were followed for a mean period of 51 monts (12–122 m.). Twentynine pts. (52%) showed a progressive deterioration of cardiac function and c. heart failure. A high incidence of a. fibrillation (46%), thromboembolic complications (12.5%) and of syncopal episodes was also observed. Total survival was 80%, and 50% of deaths occurred within 2 years from PM implantation. Of the whole group 18 pts., who were not in A. F. were studied by L. and R. heart catheterization before and after 5 m' of temporary A.A.I. pacing was instituted to a p. rate sufficient to inhibit the V.V.I. apparatus. Mean aortic pressure showed an increase(m.) of 20%, C. Index increased from a mean 2.6 (range 2.2–3.1) to 3.5 (3.2–4.0), mean P. wedge p. decreased from a mean of 17.8 mmHg (12–24) to 12 mmHg (9–14), R.A.P. from 13.7 (8–18) to 5.5 mmHg (3–7). These changes were all statistically significant. No statistically significant variations were seen for P.A.P., RVEDP and LVEDP. Permanent A.A.I. pacing was therefore instituted in all 18 pts.– After a mean follow-up period of 2 yrs. survival is 100%, all pts. are still asymptomatic and no complications have occurred. The clinical-haemodynamic deleterious effects due to V-A retroconduction (in pts. with S.S.B. and V.V.I. pms) are reversible using the A.A.I. mode of pacing which should be regarded as the treatment of choice for these conditions.

Patients with "isolated" symptomatic sinus brady-arrhythmias (S.S.B.) are usually treated by permanent cardiac pacing. In most of these patients antegrade as well as retrograde conduction is not impaired and permanent ventricular pacing may cause several clinical-haemodynamic problems even if an underlying myocardial disease is not present.

Haemodynamic problems are not limited to those caused by ventricular asynchrony (1–3) or by the loss of atrial contribution to ventricular filling, but they involve mostly the effects of persistent V-A retroconduction, a phenomenon which has been recognized to cause acute haemodynamic changes simulating mitral and tricuspid incompentence (8–10) and the long-term clinical significance of which is still unknown.

The purpose of this study has been:

– To evaluate the long-term clinical-haemodynamic effects of V-A retroconduction in patients with "isolated" S.S.B. treated by V.V.I. pacing.

– To assess if, in the same subjects, the potential deleterious effects of this phenomenon on survival, clinical and haemodynamic status are reversible using the A.A.I. mode of pacing.

– To compare the long-term result of V.V.I. and A.A.I. pacing in patients with the above mentioned sinus node dysfunction.

---

*) Ospedale cardiologico "Lancisi", Ancona, Italy

Patients and methods

Of a total 86 patients with "isolated" S.S.B. (episodic or persistent s. bradycardia, with or without periods of s. arrest or s-a block, and in the absence of an underlying manifest myocardial disease) treated by transvenous V.V.I. permanent pacing since 1971 at the "Lancisi Hospital"-Ancona (Italy), 56 showed spontaneous and persistent V-A retroconduction during a routine follow-up mean period of 6 years (6 months–12 years). Of these 56 patients (Group A) 31 were males and 25 females, aged between 39 and 78 years (mean 65 yrs). They were followed for a mean period of 51 months (12–122 m.) and seen at the PM clinic at intervals of 3 or 6 months. Historical assessment of symptoms, clinical examination, ECG and P.M. testing together with chest X-rays were performed at each programmed interval either in this group (group A) or in the group of 30 V.V.I. treated pts. who did not show V-A retroconduction (group B).

Eighteen pts. of group A (who had an underlying sinus rhythm) underwent an acute haemodynamic study by left and right heart catheterization, to assess the relative haemodynamic effects of V.V.I. pacing with V-A retroconduction and those of atrial pacing. Right atrial, right ventricular, pulmonary arterial, simultaneous pulmonary wedge and left ventricular pressures, as well as aortic pressures were firstly recorded at the end of 5 m' periods of stable ventricular pacing (at a mean p. rate 72 beats/m'), together with 3 consecutive thermodilution estimations of cardiac output. 5 m' after temporary atrial pacing was instituted at a pacing rate just sufficient to inhibit the V.V.I. apparatus (mean p. rate 74 beats/m'), repeat measurements were done.

Since acute haemodynamic studies showed significant improvements in cardiac performance in all 18 pts. studied, A.A.I. permanent pacing was instituted in all. The mean follow-up period of this group (group A_1) from the new P.M. implant is of approximately 2 years (12–36 months).

Fig. 1. See text.

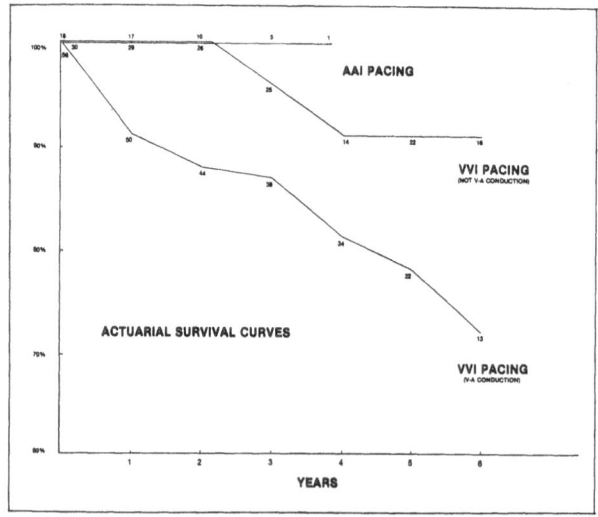

Results

Mortality

The actuarial survival curves of the 3 groups of patients (A, B and A_1) are illustrated in Fig. 1 –
The mortality rate was consistent in the 56 V.V.I. treated pts. with V-A retroconduction (group A). This attained to 20% at 51 months, with 50% of deaths occurring within the first 2 years. Deaths were due to ictus cerebri in 4 pts, c. heart failure in other 4 pts, while in 3 instances they were presumably due to ventricular fibrillation (sudden).
Mortality was significantly lower in group B (10% at 51 months). All pts. who had V.V.I. pacing changed to the A.A.I. mode (group A_1) are still alive after a mean follow-up period of 2 years.

Clinical observations

All 56 pts. of group A showed a progressive deterioration of the cardiac function and symptoms and signs of c. heart failure were present in 29 of them (52%), which could not welle managed by the treatment with digitalis and diuretics. The vast majority of pts. presented with new symptoms which were absent or less severe from those prior to the V.V.I. pacemaker implantation.
The commonest complaints were dyspnoea, fatigue and fainting sensations, while the main physical sign in all pts. were regular giant "cannon waves" in the jugular veins which were observed only during V-A retroconduction. In many pts. a pulsating liver was also felt, simulating the clinical signs of severe tricuspid regurgitation.
As illustrated in tables I (a-b-c) a high incidence of complications was observed in group A:
– *Atrial fibrillation* occurred in 26 pts. (46%) of this group and only in 1 pt. of group B
– *Thromboembolic complications* occurred in 7 pts. of group A (12.5%) and in only 1 pt. of group B.
– *Syncopal episodes,* not due to P.M. malfunction, were recorded only in 4 pts. of group A.

In contrast, no complications were observed in pts. of group A_1 after a mean follow-up period of 2 years (A.A.I. paced group).

Table 1. The incidence of various complications in the 3 Groups of pts. – The V.V.I. treated pts. with V-A retroconduction (Group A) showed a very high incidence of c. heart failure and a. fibrillation, while no complications were seen in the A.A.I. paced group (Group A_1).

Complications	Group A (V-A retro- conduction)	Group B	Group A_1 (A. pacing)
A. Fibrillation	46 %	2%	0%
Thromboembolic e.	12.5%	2%	0%
Syncope	9 %	0%	0%
C. Heart Failure	52 %	0%	0%

Cardiac Index: All 18 pts. with V.V.I. pacing and V-A retroconduction had a low c. index in resting basal conditions. Mean value attained 2.6 (range 2.1–3.1). This was significantly lower (p 0.001) than that found in the same pts. prior to V.V.I. pacemaker implantation and lower than that measured in 15 V.V.I. paced pts. of group B (without V-A retroconduction) which could be considered normal (3.2–3.7, mean 3.4).

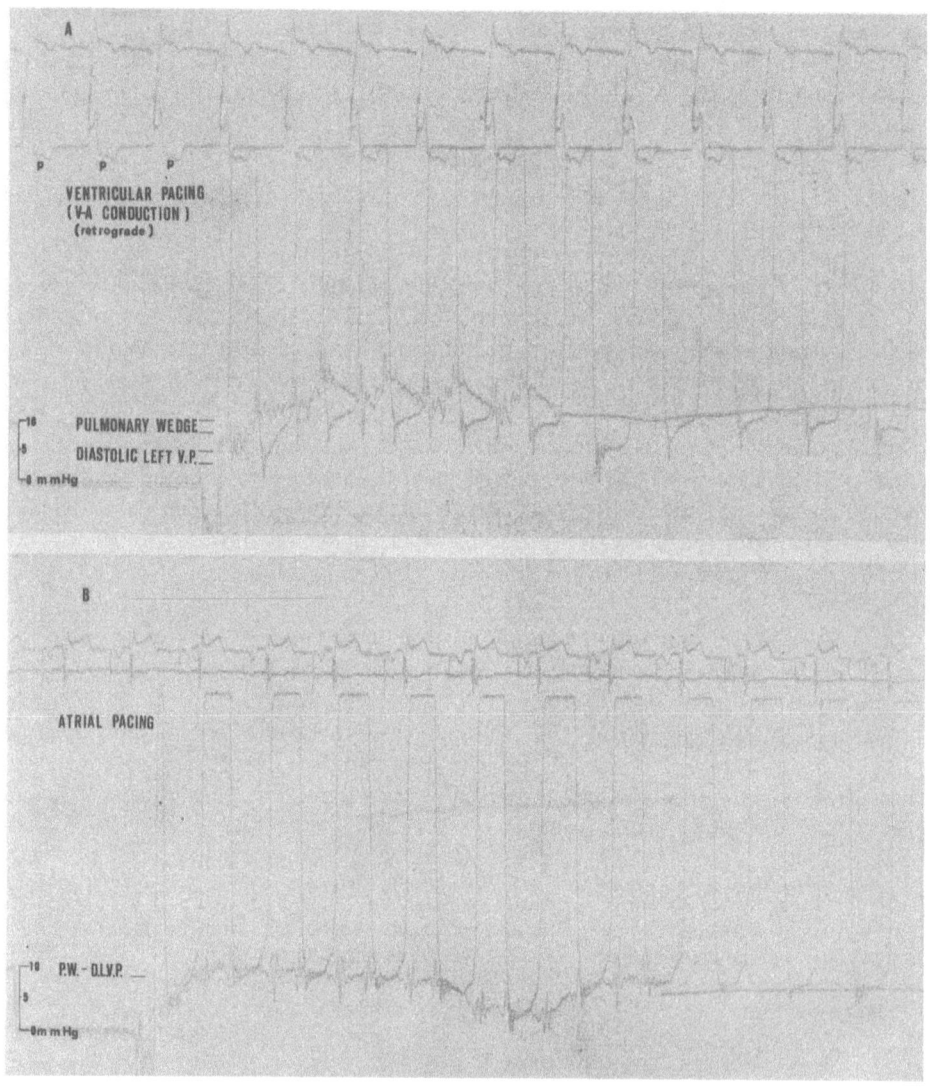

Fig. 2. Simultaneous recording of P.W.P. and LVDP during V. pacing and V-A retroconduction, and during A. pacing. There is an elevation of the mean P.W.P. during retroconduction due to repetitive "cannon waves" in the left atrium and the pulmonary venous system. There is also the persistence of a pressure gradient between P.W.P. and LVDP which simulate the haemodynamic pattern of mitral stenosis and incompetence.

During atrial pacing c. index in group A increased significantly (p 0.001) to a mean value of 3.7 (range 3.2–4.0). No significant variations in c. index were found during a. pacing in patients of group B.

Pulmonary wedge (P.W.) and right atrial pressures (R.A.P.)

Both mean P.W.P. and R.A.P. at rest were increased during V.V.I. pacing with V-A retroconduction. Mean P.W.P. was 17.8 mmHg (range 13–24 mmHg) while mean R.A.P. was 13.7 mmHg (range 6–18 mmHg). Atrial pacing led these pressures to decrease significantly to the mean values of 12 mmHg (range 9–14) and 5.5 mmHg (range 3–7) respectively.

R.V.E.D.P. and L.V.E.D.P.

During V.V.I. pacing and V-A retroconduction mean RVEDP and LVEDP were 6 ± 2 and 10 ± 3 mmHg respectively. During atrial pacing we observed occasional increases in both RVEDP and LVEDP but these were not statistically significant.

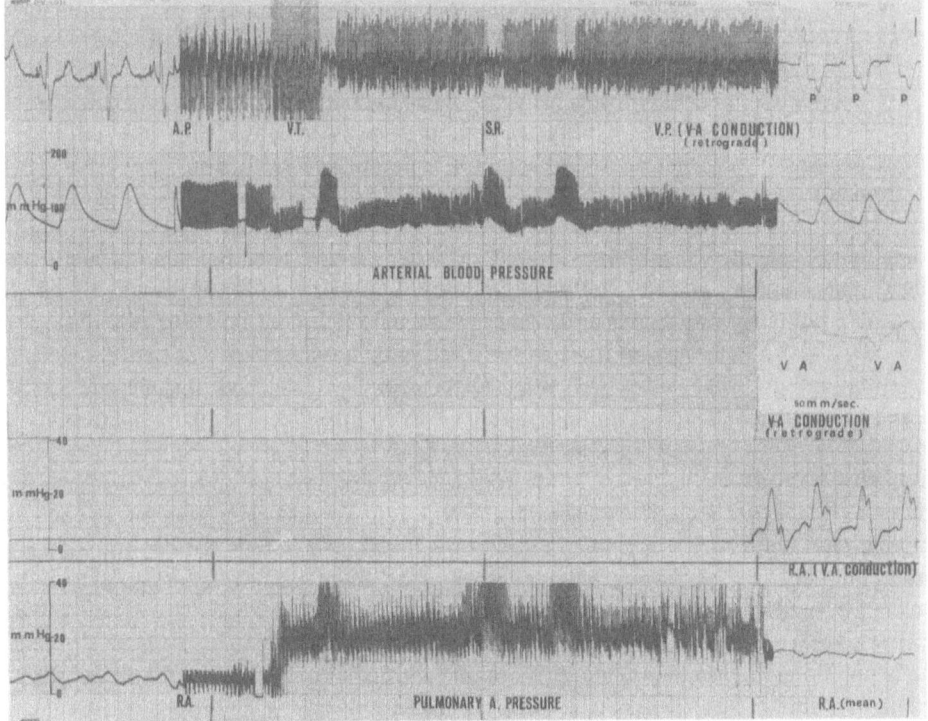

Fig. 3. Variations of the Pulmonary a., Right atrial (R.A.) and Aortic pressures during A. pacing (A.P.), ventricular tachycardia (V.T.), Ventricular pacing with V-A retroconduction (V.P.) and sinus rhythm (S.R.). During V-A retroconduction there is a marked decrease of Aortic pressure and a relevant increase of the mean R.A. pressure with systolic "cannon waves".

131

During V.V.I. pacing and V-A retroconduction mean values of aortic p. were within normal limits in all pts. studied. Mean aortic systolic p. was 122 mmHg (range 105–136); mean diastolic p. was 78 mmHg (range 74–90 mmHg). During atrial pacing we observed a mean increase of mean aortic p. of 20% (range 14–26%), which passed from 88 mmHg to 105 mmHg, mainly due to an increase of systolic values (+ 28%). No significant variations of P.A.P. were seen in the same pts. changing from V.V.I. and V-A retroconduction to the A.A.I. mode of pacing. Mean values of mean P.A.P. changed from 20 to 18.4 mmHg.

Discussion

In patients with S.S.B. and intact ventriculo-atrial conduction permanent ventricular pacing (V.V.I. p.), in our experience, leads very often to a condition of stable ventriculo-atrial retroconduction. This means retrograde stimulation of the atria immediately following ventricular activation.

As known, this phenomenon induces haemodynamic disturbances as a result of regular repetitive contractions of the atria always against closed A-V valves, which produce systolic "cannon waves" in both the atria and their corresponding inflow veins. As a consequence there is a permanent elevation of the mean right atrial and pulmonary wedge pressures, a reduction of cardiac output and a decrease of aortic pressure.

As was reported by others (8, 10), haemodynamic changes of V-A retroconduction simulate haemodynamic effects of mitral valve and tricuspid incompetence; obviously they are more deleterious when an additional myocardial disease is present.

It is widely accepted that the long-term prognosis of patients with S.S.B. and pacemakers depends on the patients age, presence or absence of heart failure and the underlying cardiac pathology, since deaths related to P.M. system failure have become unusual in recent years. Among our V.V.I. treated patients, those with V-A retroconduction have shown a mortality rate significantly higher than those who did not have this phenomenon. Of the whole group, at the time of P.M. implantation, none showed the signs of heart failure nor other cardiac pathology, apart from their sinus node disfunction. By these observations, therefore, it would seem that V-A retroconduction "per se" can influence survival in V.V.I. treated pts. for "isolated" S.S.B. –

We have also shown that, even in subjects who do not have an underlying myocardial disease, the long-term clinical significance of V-A retroconduction is relevant. Patients in fact become frequently symptomatic during the apparently normal cardiac pacing, even more than before P.M. implantation, because of fatigue, dyspnoea, reduction of exercise tolerance, fainting sensations and, although much less frequently, they experience syncopal episodes.

It is our opinion that these clinical manifestations, similar to those referred as "Pacemaker syndrome" (11–12), are due to the characteristic haemodynamic effects of V-A retroconduction which, at times, can even induce syncope because of a crytical drop of the cardiac output and of the arterial blood pressure. Apart from the symptoms of congestive heart failure (cardiomegaly, dyspnoea on mild or moderate exertion, distension of the jugular veins and congestion of the liver) which were present in 52% of the pts., of particular importance is also the high incidence of serious complications, which has been observed only in the group of V.V.I. paced pts. with V-A retroconduction.

Atrial fibrillation was the commonest and occurred in 46% of the cases. This was probably due to the persistent haemodynamic changes secondary to retroconduction, similar to those of mitral valve disease and tricuspid incompetence. Thromboembolic complications occurred in 12.5% of the pts., and all pts. who had these episodes were in atrial fibrillation.

Syncopal episodes occurred in 9% of pts. independently from P.M. malfunction. These pts. showed the lowest c. index and aortic pressures when studied haemodynamically.

Alicandri et al. (13) have suggested a vasodilating reflex mediated by atrial vagal receptors to explain the critical hypotension in these pts., induced by sudden right atrial distension (caused by the prominent cannon waves). The reflex would cause a paradoxic reduction of total peripheral resistances and syncope. We think that this mechanism, even if proved, does not operate in all circumstances. Two of our pts., who were followed by Holter monitoring, had syncope during a long standing ventricular rhythm with V-A retroduction.

Eighteen V.V.I. treated pts. with V-A retroconduction, who were symptomatic because of dyspnoea, fatigue and fainting sensations, showed a significant improvement of their haemodynamic status when they were atrially paced. In these pts., following permanent A.A.I. pacemaker implantation, no complications have been observed after a mean follow-up period of 2 years. All of them are still alive and practically symptoms-free.

These observations show that the clinical-haemodynamic deleterious effects of V-A retroconduction in V.V.I. treated pts. for S.S.B. are reversible by using A.A.I. mode of pacing. A.A.I. pacing must be regarded as the treatment of choice for pts. with S.S.B. without A-V conduction disorders.

References

1. Samet P, Castillo C and Bernstein WH: "Haemodynamic consequences of atrial and ventricular pacing in subjects with normal hearts". Am J Cardiol 18; 522–525 (1966).
2. Samet P, Bernstein WH, and Levine S: "Significance of the atrial contribution to ventricular filling" Am J Cardiol vol 15, 195–199 (1965).
3. Benchimol A, Ellis JG, and Dimond E: "Hemodynamic consequences of atrial and ventricular pacing in patients with normal and abnormal hearts" Am J Med, vol 39, 911–918 (1965).
4. Furman S: "Therapeutic uses of atrial pacing" Am Heart J, vol 86, 835–840 (1973).
5. Gilmore JP, Sarnoff SI, Mitchell JH: "Synchronicity of ventricular contractions: observations comparing hemodynamic effects of atrial and ventricular pacing". Br Heart J, vol 25, 299–305 (1963).
6. Samet P, Castillo C, Bernstein WH: "Hemodynamic sequelae of atrial, ventricular, and sequential atrio-ventricular pacing in cardiac patients". Am Heart J, vol 72, 725–729 (1966).
7. Samet P, Bernstein WH, Levine S, and Lopez A: "Atrial contribution to cardiac output in complete heart block". Am J Cardiol, Vol 16, 1–6 (1965).
8. Amikam S, and Riss E: "Untoward hemodynamic consequences of permanent ventricular pacing associated with ventriculo-atrial conduction". VIth World Symp. on Cardiac Pacing Montreal 1979, Abstracts (n. 238).
9. Perrins J, and Sutton R: "Haemodynamic effects of atrial and ventricular pacing in sick sinus syndrome". VIth World Symp on Cardiac Pacing Montreal, 1979, Abstracts (N 232).
10. Berkovits BV: "Hemodynamic consequences of atrio-ventricular and ventriculo-atrial pacing". Pace, vol 1, 8–13 (1978).

11. Haas JM, and Strait GB: "Pacemaker-induced cardiovascular failure: Hemodynamic and angiographic observations". Am J Cardiol, Vol 33, 295–301 (1974).
12. Patel AJ, and Thomsen JH: "A deleterious effect of cardiac pacing in a patient with mitral insufficiency". Acta Med Scand, vol 202, 331–334 (1977).
13. Alicandri C, Fouad FM, Tarazi RC, Castle L, Morant V: "Three cases of hypotension and syncope with ventricular pacing: possible role of atrial reflexes". Am J Cardiol, vol 42, 137–142 (1978).
14. Ihara K, Sato S, Ogitani N, et al: "Evaluation of atrial pacing therapy for sick sinus syndrome. A comparison with ventricular pacing therapy". VIth World Symp on Cardiac Pacing Montreal, 1979, Abstracts (N 263).

Authors' address:
G. Curzi, M.D.
Ospedale Lancisi di Ancona,
Via Candia 90/c,
I-60100 Ancona

Intra-Atrial Recording of Ventriculoatrial Conduction During Pacemakers' Implantation

D. A. Gascon, F. Errazquin, J. Nietò, A. Martinez,
M. Gil-Fournier, L. Castillon

Summary: Ventriculoatrial conduction (VAC) is the causative factor of some cases of the so-called 'pacemaker syndrome' in patients with VVI pacemakers and can induce the 'endless-loop arrhythmias' (ELA), which is the principal drawback against the spreading of VDD or DDD pacemakers.
During the last 30 months the presence of VAC was studied in 215 patients during the PM implantation; 104 (48%) were paced with a VVI unit, 100 (47%) with a dual-chamber system and 11 (5%) with a single leads' VDD device. In the first 56 cases the ventricular pacing was initiated at 80 bpm or 10 bpm higher than the intrinsic rate, maintained during 2 minutes and ended at 130; in the rest of patients the pacing began at 50 bpm and ended at 150 bpm, because of the finding that some patients showed VAC only below 70 bpm. At the end of the study the response of VAC to the intravenous administration of amiodarone (150–300 mg) was tested. The atrial activity was recorded by way of the guide wire of the introducer or the ventricular lead left in the atrium in cases paced with VVI pacers.
There was VAC in 68 patients (31.6%), 27 with high degree AV block and 41 (60.3%) with sick sinus syndrome. The ventriculoatrial interval was lower than 160 ms in 19, between 170–240 ms in 26 and longer than 250 ms in 23. The VAC appears at rates lower than 70 bpm in 16, between 80 and 110 in 13 and at higher rates in 39. A retrograde Wenckebach block appears in 19 and A 2 : 1 VA block in 8. The VAC disappear with amiodarone in 31 patients (45.6%). After excluding the cases with VAI lower than 160 ms rest at risk the 72% of the patients and the 45.5% after excluding the cases with VAC at rates lower than 80 bpm and VAI longer than 160 ms. The presence of retrograde Wenckebach or 2 : 1 VA block decreases the risk to 32.9% and the response to amiodarone left a 17.2% of patients exposed to the risk of ELA.

Since the original description of retrograde conduction by Mines (1) in 1913, its study have not received very much attention until recently (2, 3, 4). It is necessary to distinguish between retrograde conduction, which can be concealed, and ventriculoatrial conduction (VAC) which, by definition (4), requires an effective propagation to the atria. VAC with an 1 : 1 sequence can be a causative factor for the so-called "pacemaker syndrome", since the reversing of the normal atrioventricular relationship implies an atrial contraction against closed atrioventricular valves and the atrial empting into the pulmonary veins with the resultant fall of atrial blood volume when the atrioventricular valves open after the ventricular systole. In our country, Candel et al. (5) found that the presence of VAC was responsible for the symptoms referred by 40 patients (60.6%) with AV block, whereas only a 38.5% of patients without VAC present symptoms.

Actually, VAC is the principal drawback against the spreading of the pacemakers which pace the ventricle triggered by the atrial activity (VDD and DDD), the most physiological pacing modes availables at present. In 1969, Castellanos and Lemberg (6) described the possibility that pacemakers triggered by the atrial sensig can act as an accesory pathway giving rise to the appearance of pacemakers-mediated tachycardias, now named with a very descriptive term: "Endless-loop arrhythmias" (ELA) (7). Because of the difficulties to establish the diagnosis of VAC from a surface ECG, it is necessary to study it by invasive means. Since it is not always possible to perform an electrophysiological study in each patient who needs a pacemaker it is mandatory to discard the presence of VAC before any implantation of a pacemaker with atrial triggered capabilities. This point can be accomplished during the operative implantation and the results of the study gives information about the risk of ELA if the patient shows VAC.

Our involvement in the field of physiological pacing prompted us to began, 30 months ago, a study on the presence of VAC during the surgical implantation of pacemakers with the objetives to determine, in our pacemakers' population, the incidence of VAC, its variation with time, the duration of the ventriculoatrial interval, the characteristics of the retrograde waves and its response to different maneuvers and drugs. The intraoperative nature of the present study did not allow the recording of the His bundle deflection. This implies that only cases with true ventriculoatrial conduction were detected and no one with retrograde conduction.

Material and Methods

All consecutive patients operated on by one of us were selected as the study population to avoid any type of bias introduced by personal interpretation of the study protocol. Evidently, only cases in sinus rhythm were selected. The group comprises 215 patients, 91 of whom were females (42%), age between 10 and 88 years (mean of 60.3; S.D. 13.96 years). The diagnosis were high degree AV block in 117 patients (54.4%), congenital in 4 (3.4%), surgical-induced in 1 (0.9%) and degenerative in the rest, and sick sinus syndrome in 98 (45.6%). Four patients presented, in addition to the sick sinus syndrome (SSS), episodes of reentrant tachycardia. An electrophysiological study was obtained in 164 patients (76.3%), 89 with SSS (90.8%) and 75 with AV block (64.1%). VAC was present in 57 cases (34.7%), 38 (42.7%) in patients with SSS and 19 (25.3%) in patients with AV block. One hundred patients were paced with VVI devices, 100 with dual-chamber pacemakers

Table 1. Types of PMs implanted

Type of pacing	Number of Pacemakers	Total
WI:		104 (48%)
P	49 (23%)	
M	37 (17%)	
NO P	18 (8%)	
VDD1*		11 (5%)
DCH:		100 (47%)
VAT	2 (1%)	
VDD2*	8 (4%)	
DVI**	39 (18%)	
DDD	51 (24%)	

* VDD1 = VDD with single AV lead
  VDD2 = VDD with two leads
** both, committed and uncommitted

and 11 with single-lead VDD pulse generators as shown in table 1. The surgical approach was through the subclavian vein puncture technique in 197 patients (91.6%).

The intracavitary recording was obtained with the aid of a four channel Mingograf recorder, without any parallel load and employing only the filters incorporated to such recorder. For the study of VAC only the 25 and 50 mm/sec speed were used. VAC was considered as present if there was a fixed or cyclic changed relationship between the ventricular impulse and P waves following it; after excluding that it was not due to a random location of a sinus P wave behind the ventricular spike. Almost the study of VAC was made before any other measurement if the patients were candidate to a VVI or a VDD1 (single-lead VDD) pacemaker, leaving the tip of the lead at the atrial level and pacing with the temporary ventricular lead or recording the atrial activity by way of the guide wire of the introducer. Patients who were candidates for dual-chamber pacemakers the study of VAC was obtained after the placement of the atrial lead.

In the first 56 cases, ventricular pacing was initiated at 80 bpm or 10 bpm higher than the intrinsic rate and maintained during 2 minutes, rising it at increments of 10 bpm until the 130 bpm level was reached. Thereafter, the ventricular pacing began at 50 bpm and was rised up to 150 bpm, because of cases with VAC only below a rate of 70 bpm. Once established the presence of VAC and its characteristics the patient received an intravenous injection of amiodarone (150 mg), repeated after 10 minutes if there was not any modification in the pattern of the VAC. We prefer for the study bipolar leads, since they permit the stimulation and intracavitary recording through the same lead. In the last cases of dual chamber pacemaker implantation we used a bipolar lead with "in line" connection (Medtronic SP 2014), systematically, in spite of using unipolar pulse generators. The ventriculoatrial interval (VAI) and the pacing rate at which the VAC disappears or changed to a retrograde Wenkebach phenomenon or to a 2 : 1 or lower VA block were measured. For the analysis the patients were grouped in respect to both measures. For statistical analysis a Hewlett-Packard HP-85 were used with a statistic program developed by us.

Results

At implantation VAC was present in 68 patients (31.6%), 27 (39.7%) with a diagnosis of high degree AV block and 41 (60.3%) with SSS. VAC was absent in the others. Any of the patients who received a VDD pacemaker showed VAC (its presence contraindicates its use in our opinion). The distribution of the cases with VAC according to the diagnosis and to the pacing rate at which it disappears or changes is summarized in table 2. VAC was present at rates below 70 bpm in 16 patients (23.5%), between 80 and 110 bpm in 13 (19%) and at rates higher in 39 (57.4%). In patients with SSS the incidence of VAC was significantly higher than in patients with AV block (p < 0.005). The ventriculoatrial conduction time as reflected by the mean VAI was 226.9 ± 46.1 ms (mean ± SEM), with a range between 120 and 380 ms. The patients were allocated into 3 groups according to the VAI: A. those with VAI lower than 160 ms, formed by 19 patients (27.9%); B. those with VAI between 170 and 240 ms, formed by 26 patients (38.2%); and C. those with VAI higher than 250 ms, integrated by 23 patients (33.8%). The VAI limits were randomly choiced taking into account the future atrial refractory period of dual-chamber pacemakers and the ease of its measurement in the operating room. The mean ± SEM values for each group were 150.5 ± 40.7 ms (120–160) for the group A; 210 ± 33.2 ms

Table 2. Ventriculoatrial conduction

	< 70 bpm	80–110 bpm	any rate*	Total
AVB	12 (17.6%)	10 (14.7%)	5 (7.4%)	27 (39.7%)
SSS**	4 (5.9%)	3 (4.4%)	34(50 %)	41 (60.3%)
Total	16 (23.5%)	13 (19 %)	39 (57.4%)	68

* up to 150 bpm
** VAC was significantly more frequent (p < 0.005)

Table 3. Ventriculoatrial conduction analysis

	< 80 bpm	> 80 bpm	Total
VAC	16 (23.5%)	52 (76.5%)	68 (100 %)
VAI:			
< 160 ms	1 (1.5%)	18 (26.4%)	19 (27.9%)
> 160 ms	15 (22 %)	34 (50 %)	49 (72 %)
Retr. Wenck.	3 (4.4%)	16 (23.5%)*	19 (27.9%)
2 : 1 VA Block	1 (1.5%)	7 (10.2%)	8 (11.8%)
No VAC after			
Amiodarone**	10 (14.7%)	21 (30.9%)	31 (45.6%)†

VAI = Ventriculoatrial Interval
 * 5 patients with intermittent 2 : 1 VA Block
** Most of the patients showed VAI > 160 ms
 † Without previous Retr. Wenck. or 2 : 1 VAB

(170–240) for the group B; and 299.1 ± 34.1 ms (250–380) for the group C. There was not significant difference between groups in respect to age, sex and diagnosis, but there was a trend for patients with AV block to show longer VAI than patients with SSS.

Since the DDD pacemakers availables to us during the period of the study had a maximum rate for atrial pacing of 80 bpm, the patients were divided in two groups according to the presence of VAC at pacing rates lower or higher than 80 bpm (Table 3). The VAC appears below 80 bpm in 16 patients (23.5%) (group I) and at rates higher than 80 bpm (group II) in 52 (76.5%). The VAI was lower than 160 ms in only 1 patient of the group I and in 18 (26.4%) of the group II, and was higher than 160 ms in 15 (22%) and 34 (50%), respectively. During the recording of VAC a retrograde Wenckebach phenomenon appeared in 19 patients (27.9%), 5 of whom showed also intermittent 2 : 1 VA block. In 3 (4.4%) it appeared at rates lower than 70; in 5 (7.4%) at rates between 80 and 110 bpm; and in 11 (16.2%) at rates higher than 120 bpm. A 2 : 1 VA block appeared below 70 bpm in 1 (1.5%); between 80–110 bpm in 4 (5.9%); and at rates higher than 120 bpm in 3 (4.4%). After amiodarone administration VAC disappeared at the rates it was present before or its pattern changed to a retrograde Wenckebach or a 2 : 1 VA block in 31 patients (45.6%), 9 of this group did not show any disturbance of the VA conduction previously. 26 of them showed previously a VAI longer than 160 ms (p < 0.01). There was not any statistical difference in respect to age and sex, but patients with AV block and

VAC with VAI interval longer than 160 ms responded with a significant higher rate to amiodarone (p < 0.05) than patients with SSS or AV block and short VAI. In two patients with VAI interval lower than 160 ms, VA lengthened after amiodarone.

There was a trend for patients with SSS and younger than 55 years to show VAC of short VAI at rates higher than 120 bpm. A disagreement between the incidence of VAC during the electrophysiological study, present in 57 patients (34.7%), and during the operation was observed. In 36 patients VAC was detected at both studies, in 32 only at the implantation and in 21 only during the electrophysiological study. Adding this last cases to the 68 with VAC detected at the implantation, there were a total of 89 patients with VAC in both studies (41.4%). The results were concordant in 36 patients (40.4%) and discordant in 53 patients (59.6%). This disagreement could be explained by a higher dose of sedative and analgesic drugs during the implantation (p < 0.05) and the time difference between both procedures (p < 0.01), since most of them were performed on different days (1 to 13) and at different hours (electrophysiology in the morning and implantation in the afternoon). In the figures 1 and 2 are two examples of the intraoperative recording of VAC.

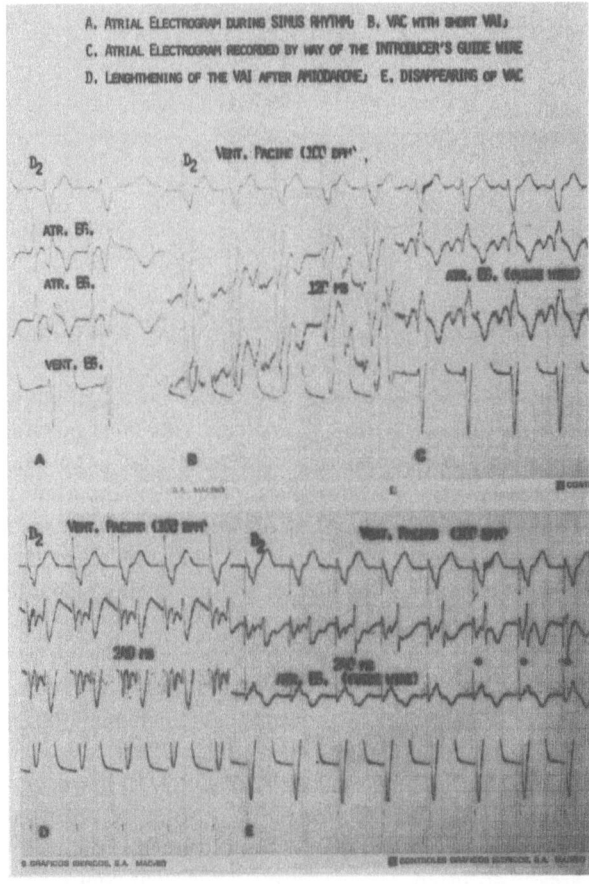

Fig. 1. In A the recording of a surface ECG lead (D2), two atrial electrogram (EG) and the ventricular electrogram sinus rhythm during. In B the presence of VAC with a short VAI demonstrated. In C the atrial EG was recorded by way of the guide wire of the introducer. In D the VAI lengthened after the administration of amiodarone and in E the VAC disappeared after the three last ventricular impulses. (VAC = ventriculoatrial conduction; VAI = ventriculoatrial interval).

Fig. 2. In the upper part of the figure the recording of a retrograde Wenckebach phenomenon at a ventricular pacing rate of 75 bpm, with lengthening of the VAI from 240 ms until 420 ms is shown. In the lower part after administration of amiodarone there is not VAC at ventricular pacing note of 80 bpm. (VAI = ventriculoatrial interval; VAC = ventriculoatrial conduction.)

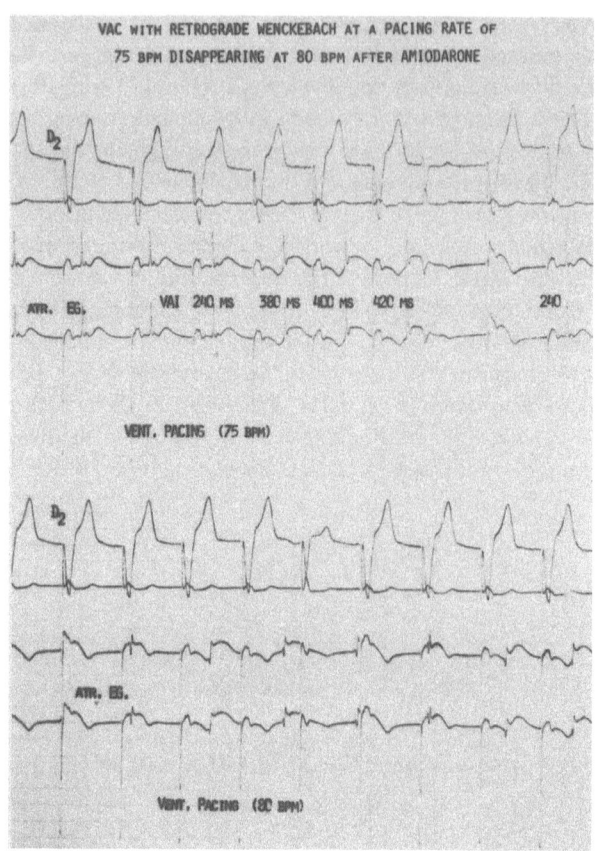

Discussion

Our study can not determine the absolute incidence of VAC because of the impossibility to record the His bundle deflection in the operating room. Concealed VAC is of no clinical significance for the development of endless-loop arrhythmias since there is not conduction to the atrium. Our study can also introduce some bias for the determination of the incidence of VAC due to the bad quality of the recording obtained through the guide wire of the introducer. VAI recorded through the guide wire is 20–60 ms longer than measured with other methods. We don't belive that the lock of parallel load or signal filtering affects the objectives of our study.

VAC was present in the 41.4% of the patients if the cases only detected at the electrophysiological study, and 31.6% if only the cases with VAC at operation are considered. The risk of VAC is higher in patients with normal or near normal AV conduction (60.3% for SSS vs 39.7% for AV block). In our group of patients we consider as risk factors for the development of endless-loop arrhythmias the presence of VAC with VAI longer than 160 ms the presence of pacing rates higher than 80 bpm, the absence of retrograde Wenckebach or 2 : 1 VA block and no response to drugs. In clinical practice the factors that contribute to its appearance are the occurrence of premature ventricular contractions and the fall of the intrinsic rate below the minimum rate of the pacemaker or the rise of the patients rate above the programed maximal rate with the appearance of the pseudo-Wenckebach phenomenon. If there is not fatigue of the pathways, the VAC is maintained at high rates, and the endless-loop arrhythymia will perpetuate itself.

From our point of view it is important to assess the effects of drugs on the VAC, since some patients with short VAI can show a lengthening of this interval in response to different drugs, as it was the case with amiodarone in two of our patients. Actually, we think that VDD pacemakers are more exposed to endless-loop arrhythmias since there is no possibility for pacing the atrium. This could reduce the incidence of VAC, principally with rates of at least 80 bpm. We also consider as dangerous the use of low minimum rates or long AV intervals, and also a low maximal atrial track rate. In accordance with these ideas we prefer DDD,M pacemakers to VDD,M and the devices with programable atrial refractory period and DDD function at any rate as the Sequicor II from Cordis or the probability of lengthening the atrial refractory period after sensing of a premature ventricular contraction as the Versatrax II from Medtronic or the 674 from Siemens. The next step will be a pacemaker which automatically changes the atrial refractory period dependent on the presence of VAC. This requires a pacemaker with discrimination facilities between P waves of sinus origin and those conducted from the ventricular impulse.

Analysing our population with VAC at risk for developing endless-loop arrhythmias, the incidence of VAC with VAI lower than 160 ms decreases the risk to 72% (Fig. 3). In regard to patients with VAC and VAI longer than 160 ms but only at rates below 80 bpm the resultant figure is 45.5%. After excluding all cases with retrograde Wenckebach or 2 : 1 VA block the population at risk is 32.9%. Since amiodarone interfere with VAC in certain patients the theoretical population at risk is 17.2% in this group of patients. We concluded that, in spite of the results of the electrophysiological study, the presence of VAC must be studied during all the implantations of DDD-pacemakers because the risk of endless-loop arrhythmia is high and can be disminished with a proper selection of the pulse generator to be implanted.

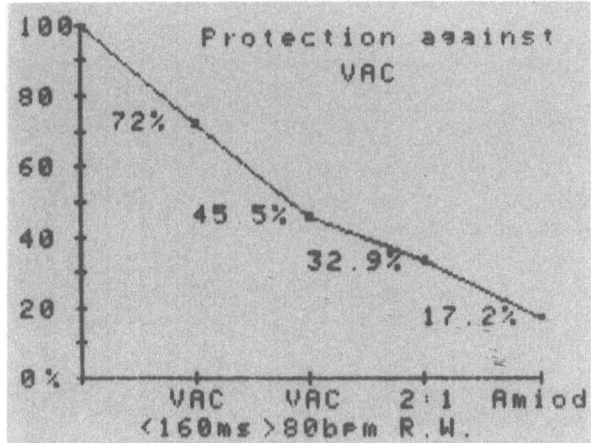

Fig. 3. Correlation between risk of ELA and VAC.

References

1. Mines GR: "On dynamic equilibrium in the heart". Arch J Physiol 1913; 46: 349 (quoted in reference 7).
2. Schuilenburg RM: "Patterns of VA conduction in the human heart in the presence of normal and abnormal AV conduction". In HJJ Wellens, KI Lie and MJ Janse (Eds): "The conduction system of the heart. Structure, function and clinical implications". Philadelphia: Lea and Febiger, 1976: 485
3. Gupta PK and Waft JL: "Retrograde ventriculoatrial conduction in complete heart block". Am Heart J 1970; 30: 408
4. Akhtar M: "Retrograde conduction in man". Pace 1981; 4: 548
5. Candel M: "La activación ventricular retrógrada en la estimulación ventricular". 1982, personal communication.
6. Castellanos A and Lemberg L: "Electrophysiology of pacing and cardioversion". New York: Appleton Century Crofts, 1969: 54
7. Furman, S: "Arrhythmias of dual chamber pacemakers". Pace 1982, 5: 469

Authors' address:
Damian A. Gascon, M.D.
Residencia Sanit.
Virgen del Rocio
Avda Reina Mercedes 19C, 5 4
Sevilla/Spain

A Comparative Analysis of the Effect of Glucagon and Atropine in the Sinus and Atrio Ventricular Nodes

P. I. Altieri, J. M. Toro, H. Banch, L. del Valle, Mary Torres

Summary: The drug management of sick sinus syndrome (SSS.) at the present time is not optimal. Due to this we decided to investigate the effect of Atropine (A) and Glucagon (G) in this syndrome. The effect of Glucagon and A in the sinus (SN) and atrioventricular node (AVN) was compared in 11 patients (pts.), 5 with sick sinus syndrome and 6 with normal sinus node function (N) G shortened the sino-atrial recovery time (SART) in N. by 16.6% (1046 ± 112 to 856 ± 61 msec) $P < 0.025$ and by 23% in SSS (1408 ± 16 to 1058 msec + 110) $P < 0.025$ A shortened the SART in N by 19.5% (1046 ± 112 to 832 msec + 77) $P < 0.025$ and by 26.7% in SSS (1335 ± 193 to 945 msec ± 182) $P < 0.10$. G increased AVN conduction in N by 12% (165 to 141.6 msec ± 34) $P < 0.010$ and A by 19% (178 ± 27 to 142 msec ± 21) $P < 0.0025$. The effects in SSS was similar. G increased the heart rate (HR) by 17% in N and 26% in SSS (NS). A increased the HR by 26% in N and SSS. In conclusion G and A have similar effects of shortening the SART and increasing AVN conduction, although pts with SSS are more sensitive to both drugs than N. The effect of G lasted up to 5 minutes while A up to 10 minutes. These electrophysiologic findings show that drugs can be used for the temporary management of patients with SSS.

The syndrome of sick sinus is under investigation due to the fact that its pathogenesis is not completely understood and the present therapy is not optimal. Several investigators have reported the usefulness of digitalis preparations and atropine in the management of some of the arrhythmias seen in the syndrome (1, 2). On basis of the above observations we decided to study the electrophysiologic changes by glucagon and compare them to atropine and in this way find out if they can be potentially used to manage patients with sick sinus syndrome.

Methods and Materials

Ten patients with history of sinus bradycardia, syncope or related symptoms such as episodic light headeness were studied without premedication in the post absortive state. The mean age was 60 years. Five were found with sick sinus syndrome (SSS) and five were considered normal. None of the patients received cardioactive medications during the week prior to the study. Atrial pacing was performed with a catheter advanced from the right basilic vein and positioned at the lateral wall of the right atrium. Rectangular stimuli 2 msec in duration and 1.5 diastolic threshold were delivered from a Medtronic Programmable stimulator model 5325. Sino atrial recovery times (SART) were recorded after abrupt termination of rapid atrial pacing at rates from 100 to 160 beats per minutes. SART was measured from the last paced P wave to the next spontaneous P wave or junctional beat. His bundle electrograms were recorded in all patients from a catheter inserted percutaneously into the femoral vein and placed across the triücuspid valve. Three standard leads were simultaneously recorded along with and atrial electrogram. A-H interval and H-V interval was recorded. The A-H interval was used as atrioventricular node conduction. After basal recordings each patient received 5 mgs of glucagon intravenously. Recordings of heart rate, SART, A-H and H-V intervals were done every minute for 20 minutes. Thirty minutes after the last recording, one mg of atropine was injected intravenously. Recordings of the same intervals were done every minute for twenty minutes.

The results obtained were expressed as means and standard error of the mean. A statistical comparison was done using the student T test for paired observations. The glucagon and atropine results were compared between them.

Results

Glucagon shortened the SART in normals by 16.6% (1046 ± 112 msec to 856 ± 6 msec) $P < 0.025$ and by 23% in patients with SSS (1048 ± 167 msec to 1058 ± 110 msec) $P < 0.025$ (Fig. 1). Atropine shortened the SART in normals by 19.5% (1046 ± 112 msec to 832 ± 77 msec) $P < 0.025$ and by 26.7% in SSS (1335 ± 193 msec to 945 ± 182 msec) $P < 0.10$ (Fig. 1).

Glucagon increased the atrioventricular conduction in normals by 12% (165 ± 15 msec to 141 ± 36 msec) $P < 0.010$ and atropine by 19% (178 ± 27 msec to 142 ± 21 msec) $P < .025$ (Fig. 2).

A similar change was seen in patients with SSS (13% by glucagon and 18% by atropine).

Glucagon increased the heart rate by 17% in normal and 26% in SSS Atropine increased the heart rate by 26% in normals and in the SSS.

It was noticed that the effect of glucagon disappeared at 5 minutes while atropine lasted up to 10 minutes and that the sinus node of the SSS group is more sensitive than the ones of normals.

Fig. 1. Compares the shortening of the sinus node recovery time by glucagon and atropine.

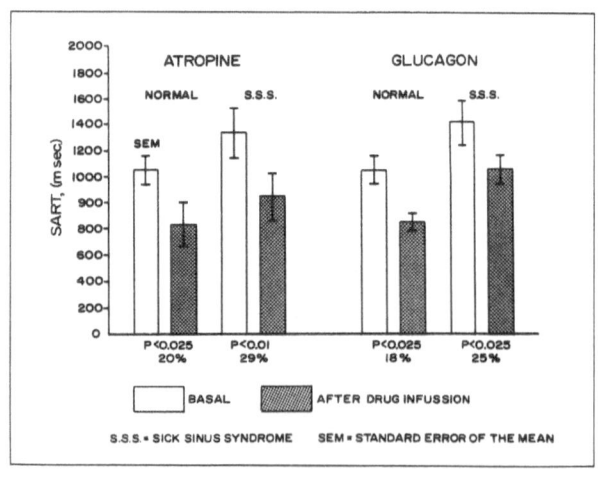

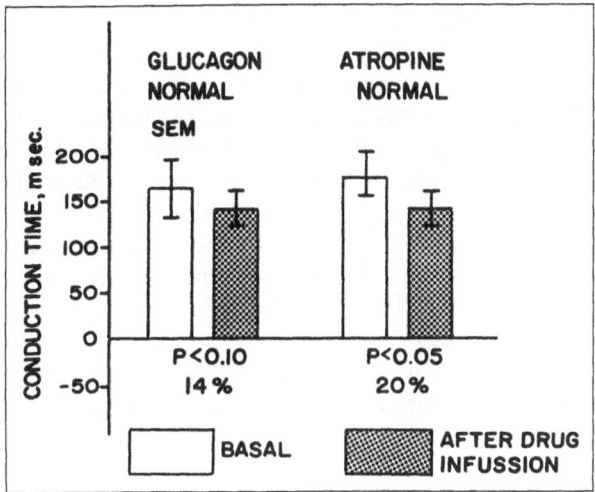

Fig. 2. Compares the atrioventricular conduction time changes between atropine and glucagon.

Discussion

The sick sinus syndrome describes patients having sinus node dysfunction. Usually they present with sinus bradycardia, arrhythmias or sinus node arrest (1). Also it has been shown that these patients usually have left ventricular dysfunction due to coronary disease or the aging process (3). Due to the fact that survival is not related to the implantation of a pacemakers but to the underlying heart disease (4), several investigators have been looking for the management of this syndrome with drugs, rather than with a pacemaker.

Engel and Schaal (2) reported the usefulness of digitalis preparations in the management of this syndrome. They reported the normalization of the SART in some patients both by oubain and atropine. Engel also reported the improvement of sino-atrial function by hydralazine (5).

Glucagon is a hormone produced by the pancreas which has been shown to be very important in the homeostasis of glucose, certain amino acids and perhaps of free fatty acids. Several investigator have been interested in the cardiac effects of this hormone. Burton (6) and coworkers is showed that glucagon did not significantly affect the heart rate, cardiac index, left ventricular end-diastolic pressure or mean brachial artery pressure enter at rest or during mild supine leg exercise. Lucchesi (7) showed a positive inotropic and chronotropic response in the isolated dog papillary muscle which was not abolished by beta-receptor blockade. He showed that the possible mechanism of action was an increase in the intracellular concentration of cyclic 3' 5' AMP.

Steiner (8) and coworkers found that glucagon increased the speed of A-V conduction without increasing ventricular automaticitiy. Lucchesi (9) had the same observation and he suggested that glucagon possesses and advantage over the catecholamines due to this property.

Due to the characteristics of improving left ventricular function with an improvement of atrioventricular conduction, we thought pertinent to study the effect of glucagon in sinus node function. We were surprised to find out a dramatic improvement in sinus node function with normalization in many patients. The effect was similar to atropine with the advantage of not increasing automaticity and improving the left ventricular function.

This dual effect is an advantage, because most of the patients with sick sinus syndrome one old patients already having left ventricular dysfunction. Another advantage is that glucagon can be given as a constant infusion (1 mg/minute) and in this way the effect in the sinus an atrioventricular nodes and in the myocardium can be prolonged until the patient can be stabilized. Also they will benefit of an increase in heart rate.

In our opinion glucagon can be used in patients with sick sinus syndrome and left ventricular dysfunction, because of its dual effect in the sinus node and atrioventricular nodes with the benefical effect of improving the left ventricular function.

Another possible use of glucagon is in an acute inferior myocardial infarction with transient sinus and atrioventricular node dysfunction. A constant infusion of glucagon may improve sinus node function and atrioventricular conduction and in this way avoid the insertion of a temporary pacemaker.

In conclusion we have shown that glucagon improves the sinus and atrioventricular node function. This effect may help patients with chronic or acute sinus and atrioventricular node dysfunction.

References

1. Ferrer MI: The sick sinus syndrome. Circulation 1973; 47: 635.
2. Engel TR, Schaal SF: Digitalis in the sick sinus syndrome: The effect of Digitalis on sinoatrial automaticity and atrioventricular conduction. Circulation 1973; 48: 1202–1207.
3. Moss AJ, Davis RJ: Brady-Tachy syndrome. Progress cardiovasc Dis 1974; 16: 439–454.
4. Simon AB, Zloto AN: Symptomatic sinus node disease: Natural history after permanent ventricular pacing. Pace 1979; 2: 305–314.
5. Engel T, Leddy C, González A, Meister S, Frankl WS: Electrophysiologic effect of hydrazaline on sinoatrial function in patients with sick sinus syndrome. Amer J Cardiol 1978; 41: 763–769.
6. Burton G, McCallister BD, Fryerl: Effect of glucagon on resting and exercise hemodynamics in patients with coronary disease. Br Heart J 1972; 34: 924–929.
7. Lucchesi BR: Cardia actions of glucagon. Circulation Res 1968; 22: 777–787.
8. Steiner C, Wit AC, Damato A: Effects of glucagon on atrioventricular conduction and ventricular automaticity in dogs. Circulation 1969; 24: 167–177.
9. Lucchesi BR, Stutz DR, Winfield RA: Glucagon. Circulation Res 1969; 25: 183–190.

Authors' address:
Pablo I. Altieri, M.D.
Department of Medicine
Medical Science Campus
University of Puerto Rico
San Juan, Puerto Rico

Conducting System Assessed by his Bundle Electrograms from the Permanent Atrial Electrode at Implantation

D. B. O'Keeffe, J. S. Geddes

Summary: His bundle electrograms were recorded from conventional J-shaped atrial electrodes in twelve consecutive patients, at pacemaker implantation for sinus node disorder. Five patients with impairment of atrioventricular conduction, received atrioventricular (DVI) pacemakers. His bundle recording by this method is simple and reliable, avoids the discomfort of the conventional technique, and represents a new application for the well established atrial "J" electrode.

Introduction

A substantial proportion of patients with sino-atrial disease also show disturbance of atrioventricular conduction (1, 3) and the presence or absence of such disturbance may determine the need for ventricular pacing in a particular patient. The presence of such conducting system disease may not be obvious from the surface electrocardiogram but may nevertheless exist in as many as 60% (1) of these patients and may progress to complete heart block (2, 3). When physiological pacing is indicated and conducting system disease is identified, it has been recommended that electrodes should be placed in both atrium and ventricle (2).

Measurement of intracardiac conduction times from the His electrogram allows diagnosis of conducting system disease not otherwise apparent, and may be used to guide the choice of pacing mode. We envisaged that it might be possible to acquire His bundle electrograms by manipulation of the permanent atrial electrode introduced by the subclavian or cephalic vein, before implantation in the right atrium, using standard recording equipment.

This report concerns 12 consecutive cases of permanent pacemaker implantation involving the use of atrial electrodes in which it was possible to obtain good quality His bundle electrograms from the permanent atrial electrode placed against the septal leaflet of the tricuspid valve. These electrograms were obtained easily, with no discomfort to the patient and with minimal extension of pacemaker implantation time. This information affected the choice of pacemaker system in 5 of the 12 patients.

Methods

Patients

Eight male and four female patients (ages 34 to 83 years) who were considered for atrial pacing because of sinus bradycardia, were investigated. All of the 12 required treatment with betablockers and/or anti-arrhythmic drugs because of angina or co-existant tachycardias. Eight patients had coronary artery disease, two had valvular heart disease and two had no evidence of structural heart disease.

A Medtronic 6990U bipolar tined atrial J electrode with an interelectrode distance of 15 mm was used (Fig. 1). Atrial and, when required, ventricular electrodes were inserted through the left cephalic vein or by direct puncture of the subclavian vein.

Standard equipment was employed for recording intracardiac electrograms.

Technique of His Bundle Electrogram Acquisition

The atrial J electrode was first advanced, with the stylet fully inserted, to the right ventricular outflow tract (Fig. 2A). The stylet was then partially withdrawn so as to restore some, but not all, of the J shape to the distal portion of the electrode. The electrode was then given a counter clockwise twist to press the tip against the septum, and withdrawn so that the bipole rested against the septal leaflet of the tricuspid valve (Fig. 2B). Intracardiac electrograms were taken from this position, with minor adjustment to obtain an optimal His bundle electrogram. The electrode was then further withdrawn, rotated clockwise and the stylet withdrawn to allow the tip to rest in the right atrial appendage (Fig. 2C), for permanent atrial pacing.

Results

In all 12 patients a satisfactory His bundle electrogram (Fig. 3) was obtained without difficulty and within 5 minutes of electrode insertion. There was evidence of impairment of

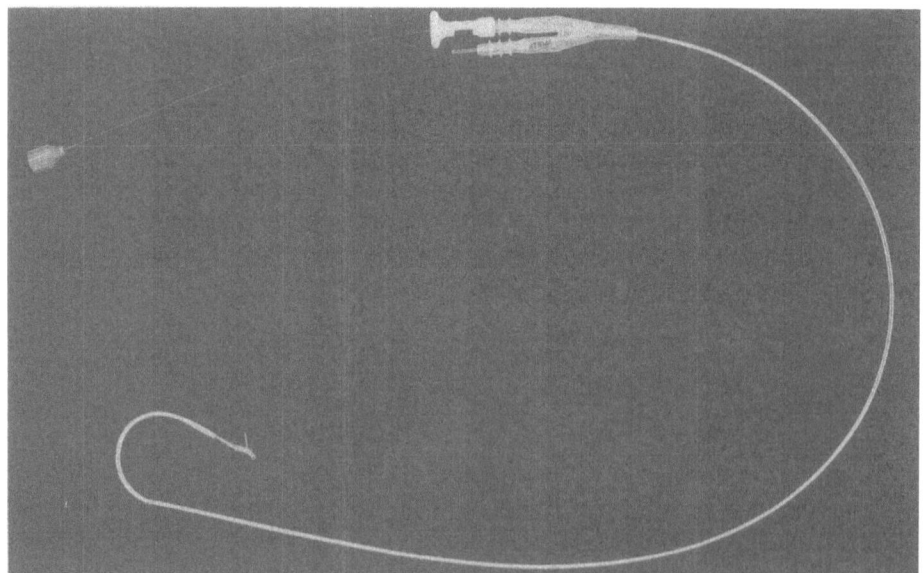

Fig. 1. A Medtronic 6990U atrial tined "J" endocardial electrode, of the type used in this study. The interelectrode distance is 15 mm.

148

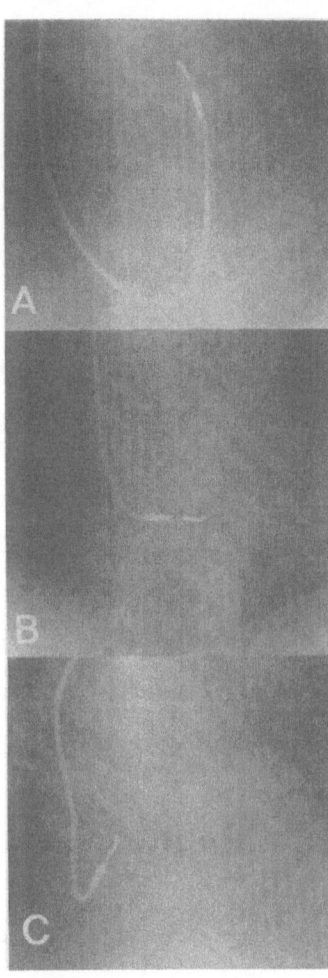

Fig. 2. A Initial position of pacing catheter in the right ventricular outflow tract with stylet fully inserted.
B Catheter withdrawn to the tricuspid valve for His bundle recording.
C Catheter placed in the right atrial appendage for Permanent pacing.

atrioventricular conduction in 5 of the 12 patients, as judged by the criteria of Hecht and Kossman (5) (that is to say the A-H time was greater than 130 ms, or the H-V time was greater than 55 ms), or the rate at which atrioventricular Wenckebach block occurred during atrial pacing was less than 100 beats/minute.

In 1 patient the A-H time was prolonged and in 4 patients the H-V time was prolonged despite a normal P-R interval. In one other patient the rate at which atrioventricular Wenckebach block occurred was 100 beats/minute.

In 4 of the 12 patients there was evidence of atrioventricular conducting system disease on the surface E.C.G. This took the form of abnormal axis in 2 cases, abnormal axis and right bundle branch block in 1 case and prolonged P-R interval in a fourth case. These findings on surface ECG were present in only 2 of the patients with abnormal intracardiac conducting times, and in the other 2 patients were present in spite of normal intracardiac conduction times. The surface ECG was therefore neither a sensitive not a specific predictor of intracardiac conduction time abnormalities in this study.

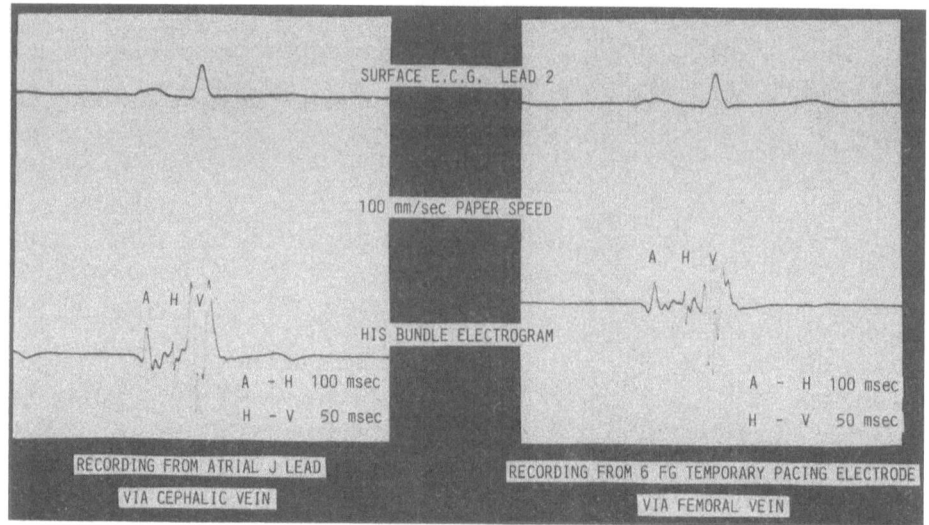

Fig. 3. Simultaneous recordings of surface electrocardiographic lead II, and the His bundle endocardial electrogram obtained by the orthodox recording technique using the femoral approach (right hand record), and on the left hand recording, the His electrogram obtained from a permanent atrial "J" electrode as described in the text.

Similar records were obtained by both techniques giving the same measurements (AH time 100 msecs and HV time 50 msecs).

The 6 patients without evidence of conducting system disease had the atrial electrode implanted and attached to an atrial demand unit (AAIM pacing). In the remaining 6 with such evidence, the atrial bipolar electrode was implanted, and in 5 an additional ventricular electrode was also implanted. DVI pacing was employed in 3 cases, and AAI in the remainder.

No complications either at implantation or on follow-up, have been encountered in this group of patients over a mean follow-up period of 7.7 months.

Discussion

Measurement of intracardiac conducting times has been advocated as a means of assessing the atrioventricular conduction system in sino-atrial disease (1, 2, 3, 4) as a guide to the appropriate mode of pacing. The results of this study show that a His bundle electrogram can be easily, conveniently and reliably obtained from a conventional permanent atrial electrode at the time of pacemaker implantation. The disadvantages of femoral vein catheterisation for His bundle recording (6), in addition to the usual procedure of permanent pacemaker implantation, are avoided.

Simple atrial pacing is often adequate for the control of symptomatic sinus bradycardia. Mild abnormalities of atrioventricular conduction at the time of pacemaker implantation may, however, be the precursors of higher grades of block (1, 3). In the presence of such abnormalities, serious consideration is given to DVI pacing. Further information relating

to the possibility that disturbance of atrioventricular conduction may develop later, even in patients with normal conduction at the time of pacemaker implantation, is required.
The ease and convenience with which intracardiac conduction times can be measured from the permanent atrial electrode leads us to recommend that this procedure should be performed when detailed analysis of atrioventricular conduction is required during pacemaker implantation.

References

1. Narula OS: Atrioventricular conduction defects in patients with sinus bradycardia. Circulation 1971; XLIV: 1096–1110.
2. Sutton R and Citron P: Electrophysiological and haemodynamic basis of application of new pacemaker technology in sick sinus syndrome and atrioventricular block. Br Heart J 1979; 41: 600–612.
3. Rosen KM, Loeb HS, Ziad Sinno M, Rahimtoola SH and Gunnar RM: Cardiac conduction in patients with symptomatic sinus node disease. Circulation 1971 XLIII; 836–844.
4. Puech P: Atrioventricular block: The value of intracardiac recordings. In: Krikler DM and Goodwin JF (Eds): Cardiac arrhythmias: The modern electrophysiological approach. W. B. Saunders Co. Ltd. London, Philadelphia, Toronto 1975; p 81.
5. Hecht HH and Kossman CE: Atrioventricular and intraventricular conduction. AM J of Cardiology 1973; 31: 232.
6. Curry PVL: Fundamentals of arrhythmias: Modern methods of investigation. In: Krikler DM and Goodwin JF (Eds): Cardiac arrhythmias: The modern electrophysiological approach. W. B. Saunders Co. Ltd., London, Philadelphia, Toronto 1975; p 39.

Author's address:
D. B. O'Keeffe
Senior Registrar
Cardiology Department
Belfast City Hospital
Lisburn Road
Belfast, BT9 7AB
Northern Ireland

Functional Sinoatrial Node Disorders: An Association with Dual Atrioventricular Node Pathways

S. Saksena, Katherine Liptak

Summary: Six symptomatic patients (2 males, 4 females, aged 15–43, mean 32 ± 12 years) with un-explained paroxysmal supraventricular tachycardia (SVT) or sinus bradycardia were evaluated. Pre-senting symptoms were palpitations (3 patients) and/or near syncope/syncope (5 patients). Non-invasive and invasive cardiac studies including programmed electrical stimulation (PES) were per-formed before and after autonomic blockade. Postural induction and termination of SVT was seen in 3 patients, inappropriate sinus bradycardia with escape junctional rhythm in 3 patients and spontan-eous atypical type I second degree AV block in 1 patient.

During PES, patients with sinus bradycardia demonstrated prolongation of corrected sinus node re-covery time (2 patients) and sinoatrial conduction time (2 patients) which corrected after atropine. In 3 patients with SVT, postural induction and termination was noted. SVT could not be induced us-ing PES in any patient, but could be induced by atropine and terminated with propranolol. Atrial activation during SVT suggested a right atrial origin in all 3 patients. Patients with bradyarrhythmias and tachyarrhythmias showed discontinuous A1–A2/H1–H2 and A1–A2/A2–H2 curves.

We conclude: 1. Functional disorders in the sinoatrial node region may result in symptomatic bra-dyarrhythmias and tachyarrhythmias. 2. Reflex changes in autonomic tone may mediate the onset and termination of these arrhythmias. 3. There may be an association between longitudinal dissocia-tion of AV nodal conduction and functional sinoatrial arrhythmias.

Introduction

Autonomic influences often play a significant role in supraventricular arrhythmias. Sinus node dysfunction may be due either to intrinsic abnormalities in sinus node function or to extrinsic factors like disorders of autonomic tone (1). Paroxysmal reentrant supraven-tricular tachycardia (PSVT) can be terminated by physical manoeuvres enhancing vagal tone (2). Recently we reported induction and termination of an automatic right atrial ta-chycardia presumably mediated by changes in autonomic tone (3). PSVT is most com-monly due to reentry with the atrioventricular node and, much less commonly, the sino-atrial node. Longitudinal dissociation of conduction within these structures may be the underlying mechanism (4, 5). In this report we describe six patients with functional sino-atrial arrhythmias (bradyarrhythmias and tachyarrhythmias) with coexistent longitudinal dissociation of atrioventricular nodal conduction.

Methods

Symptomatic patients with unexplained paroxysmal sinus bradycardia or supraventricu-lar tachycardia were evaluated. Electrocardiographic documentation of the arrhythmia and its correlation with symptoms was determined using noninvasive techniques.

a) Noninvasive Studies

A resting ECG was obtained in all patients. Postural ECG changes were recorded. All patients underwent a continuous 24-hour ambulatory ECG recording. A symptom limited treadmill exercise test was performed using a modified Bruce protocol.

b) Electrophysiologic Studies

Patients underwent baseline electrophysiologic studies in the nonsedated postabsorptive state. Informed consent was obtained. All cardioactive drug therapy was discontinued for a period of at least five drug half lives prior to the study. Standard venous and arterial catheterization techniques were utilized. A Berkovits-Castellanos hexapolar electrode catheter was used for atrial and ventricular pacing. A tetrapolar electrode catheter was used to record His Bundle electrograms. Additional tetrapolar electrode catheters were used to record other intracardiac electrograms. Recording sites include high, mid and low lateral right atrium, proximal and distal coronary sinus and the right ventricular apex. Three surface ECG leads (1, AVF and V1) were recorded simultaneously "with" intracardiac electrograms. Arterial blood pressure was monitored using an indwelling femoral arterial cannula. A multichannel display recorder (Electronics for Medicine VR-12, White Plains, N.Y.) was used to display electrograms. Hard copy recordings were obtained at paper speeds of 100–250 mm/sec. Programmed electrical stimulation (PES) was performed using a custom-made programmed stimulator (Bloom Associated, Ltd. Narberth, Pa) which delivered rectangular pulses of 1 msec duration at twice diastolic threshold.
The PES protocol used in this study included:

1. Single premature atrial extrastimuli during sinus and high right atrial drive rhythms at two or more cycle lengths (usually 700 and 500 ms).
2. Rapid atrial pacing with incremental rates until the Wenckebach phenomenon was observed.
3. Two premature atrial extrastimuli during atrial drive rhythm.
4. High rate atrial pacing up to rates of 800/min for induction of sustained atrial flutter/ fibrillation.
5. Single premature ventricular extrastimuli in sinus rhythm and during two ventricular drive rhythms.
6. Rapid ventricular pacing at cycle lengths of 400–250 ms or ventricular refractoriness, whichever was longer.

Extrastimuli were introduced late in diastole in the spontaneous or paced rhythm. Coupling intervals of the extrastimuli were reduced in 10–20 ms decrements until refractoriness was reached. Additional extrastimuli were introduced at coupling intervals 50 ms greater than the refractory period and the interval was gradually reduced. If initial stimulation sites (high right atrium, right ventricular apex) were unsuccessful in arrhythmia induction, alternative atrial sites (low right atrium, coronary sinus) were used and the PES protocol repeated.

154

c) Autonomic Testing:

Autonomic reflexes were tested using physical and pharmacologic manoeuvres. Physical manoeuvres included carotid sinus massage and changes in posture. Pharmacologic manoeuvres included administration of atropine (0.04 mg/kg) and propranolol (0.1 mg/kg) intravenously after baseline stimulation studies were completed.

d) Study Parameters:

The parameters analysed in this study were:
1. Standard ECG intervals (RR, PR, QRS, QTc).
2. Intracardiac conduction intervals (PA, AH and HV).
3. Sinus node function studies. This included sinoatrial conduction time (according to the method of Strauss and Bigger), corrected sinus node recovery time (1) and measurement of intrinsic heart rate when possible.
4. Atrial and ventricular refractory periods.
5. Electrophysiologic properties of the atrioventricular node. A1–A2/A2–H2 and A1–A2/H1–H2 conduction curves were constructed. A discontinuous curve was defined as one in which both conduction parameters (A2–H2 and H1–H2) increased by 50 msec or more for a 10–20 msec decrement in the A1A2 interval.
6. Spontaneous arrhythmias during electrophysiologic study.
7. Arrhythmia induction during PES.
8. Response to provocative autonomic testing.

Results:

1. Clinical Characteristics

Six patients, 4 females and 2 males, with paroxysmal sinus bradycardia or supraventricular tachycardia, age range 16–45 (mean 32 ± 12) years were studied. Five patients had no significant heart disease and one patient had mitral valve prolapse. The presenting symptoms were palpitations in three patients and near syncope or syncope in five patients. Three patients had both symptoms. The duration of symptoms ranged from 3 to 192 (mean 58 ± 72) months. Symptoms were typically nonexertional occurring at the time of change of posture in 3 patients.

2. Electrocardiographic Manifestations:

Inappropriate sinus bradycardia with an escape junctional rhythm was noted in three patients. Two patients had escape junctional rhythms on termination of SVT. All 5 patients had symptoms of near syncope/syncope.
Spontaneous alternating long and short PR intervals were noted in 2 patients. Intermittent atypical Wenckebach AV conduction was noted in one of these patients. The PR in-

terval was normal in 4 patients. There was no abnormality noted in the QRS or QTc intervals in any patient.

Three patients demonstrated paroxysmal SVT. During SVT, P wave morphology was upright in the inferior leads with small morphologic changes from sinus rhythm. The rate of SVT varied from 110–140/minute.

3. Conduction Intervals:

Intracardiac conduction intervals were within normal limits in all patients. P-A interval ranged from 25 to 40 (mean 33 ± 7) ms, A-H interval from 55 to 125 (mean 79 ± 45) ms and HV from 35 to 45 (mean 40 ± 4) ms.

4. Sinus Node Function:

Sinoatrial conduction time ranged from 170–510 (mean 288 ± 137) ms before autonomic blockage. It was markedly prolonged in one patient (510 ms) and mildly prolonged (300 ms) in another patient with sinus bradycardia. It could not be measured after autonomic blockade due to induction of SVT.

Corrected sinus node recovery time (SNRT) ranged from 350–1040 (mean 516 ± 319) ms. Two patients with sinus bradycardia showed significant prolongation of SNRT which normalized after autonomic blockade. Intrinsic heart rate could be measured in 2 patients and was normal in both patients. Figure 1A shows corrected sinus node recovery time in the control state and after atropine in three patients with sinus bradycardia. Note the prolonged recovery time in the control state in two patients normalizing after atropine.

5. Atrial and Ventricular Refractory Periods

The effective and functional refractory periods of the right atrium and ventricle were normal in all patients.

6. Electrophysiologic Properties of the Atrioventricular Node

Discontinuous A1–A2/A2–H2 and A1–A2/H1–H2 curves were observed in all patients. The effective refractory periods of the fast conduction pathways ranged from 420–600 (mean 504 ± 74) ms and of the slow conduction pathway from 320–470 (mean 385 ± 63) ms. The atrial pacing cycle length inducing second degree atrioventricular nodal block ranged from 400–600 (mean 467 ± 82) ms. Atypical second degree AV block during atrial pacing was observed in 4 patients. This was due to intermittent failure of conduction in the longitudinally dissociated AV nodal pathways. Figure 1 B shows atrial pacing in patient D.S. at the time of vagal reaction. Two distinct PR intervals are noted at the same pacing cycle length. Figure 1 C shows discontinuous AV nodal conduction curves in another patient with supraventricular tachycardia. Ventriculoatrial block du-

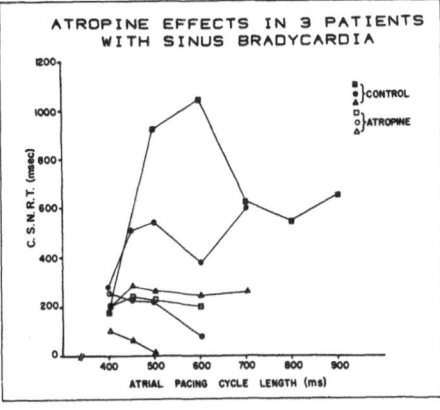

Fig. 1. Sinus and AV Nodal Conduction in Patients with Sinus Bradycardia

A: Corrected sinus node recovery time before and after atropine in 3 patients with sinus bradycardia. Note prolonged time in the control state in 2 patients which normalized after atropine.

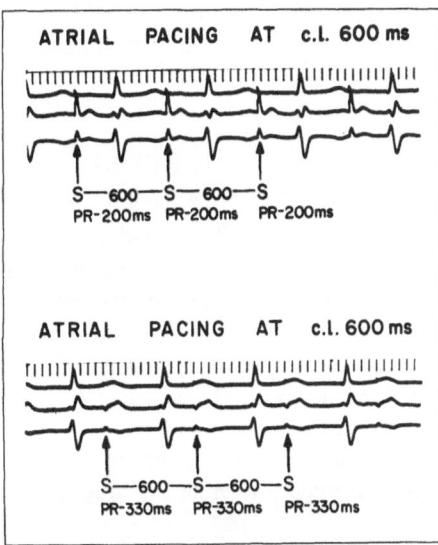

B: Atrial pacing at 600 ms in patient D.S. showing two distinct PR intervals.

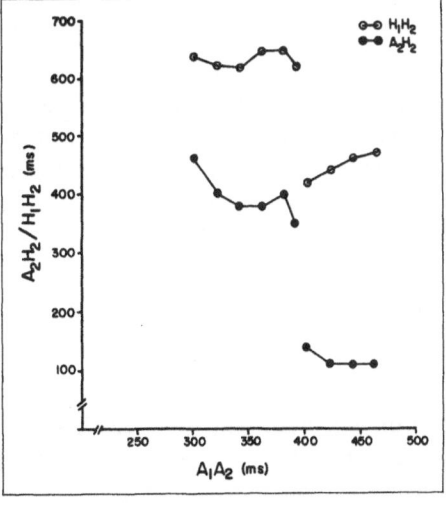

C: Discontinuous A1–A2/H1–H2 and A1–A2/A2–H2 curves in another patient.

157

ring programmed ventricular stimulation was observed in 5 patients in whom it could be measured.

7. Spontaneous Arrhythmias during EPS

One patient had a spontaneous vagal reaction with constitutional symptoms, intermittent sinus arrest and alternating long and short PR intervals. Two patients had spontaneous paroxysms of nonsustained SVT at rest.

8. Arrhythmia Induction with Programmed Electrical Stimulation

Electrical stimulation did not induce or terminate sustained or nonsustained SVT in any patient. Isolated sinus nodal or AV nodal echo beats were also not observed in any patient.

9. Effects of Physical and Pharmacologic Manoeuvres

Carotid sinus hypersensitivity was not present in any patient. SVT was induced by assumption of the upright posture and terminated in the supine position in 3 patients. Figure 2A illustrates postural induction and termination of SVT in one such patient. During the arrhythmia, upright P waves with a long RP and short PR interval were observed in each patient. During SVT, atrial mapping revealed a right atrial tachycardia origin and a "warm up" phenomenon was noted (Figure 2B). Atropine induced incessant SVT in all three patients with transient type 1 second degree AV nodal block in one patient (Figure 3A). In the remaining 3 patients, normal sinus acceleration was noted. Propranolol terminated the arrhythmia in two of these 3 patients who could tolerate the drug (Figure 3B).

10. Management:

Oral propantheline controlled symptoms in one patient with sinus bradycardia and reduced the severity of symptoms in another. One patient did not improve and required permanent demand pacemaker implantation. Propranolol controlled symptoms in two of three patients with SVT. One patient was intolerant of propranolol and responded to digoxin. Quinidine was also effective in one patient to whom it was administered.

Discussion:

The influence of the autonomic nervous system on S-A node and A-V node has been established (6). Symptomatic sinoatrial bradyarrhythmias due to abnormal autonomic tone have been reported in patients with the sick sinus syndrome (1). Similarly, symp-

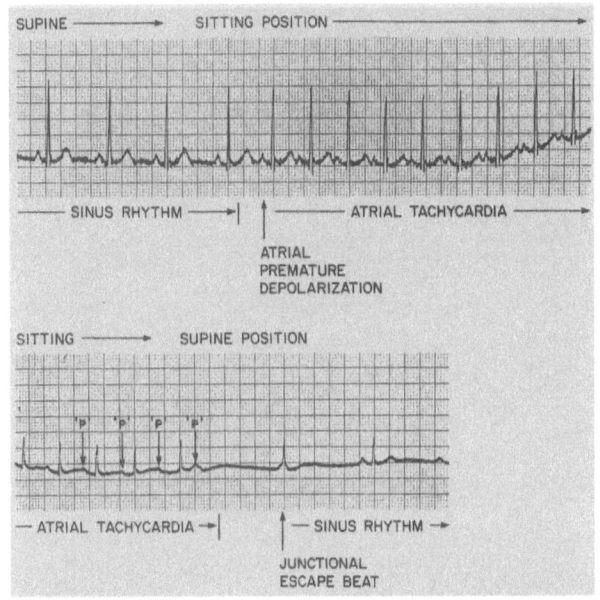

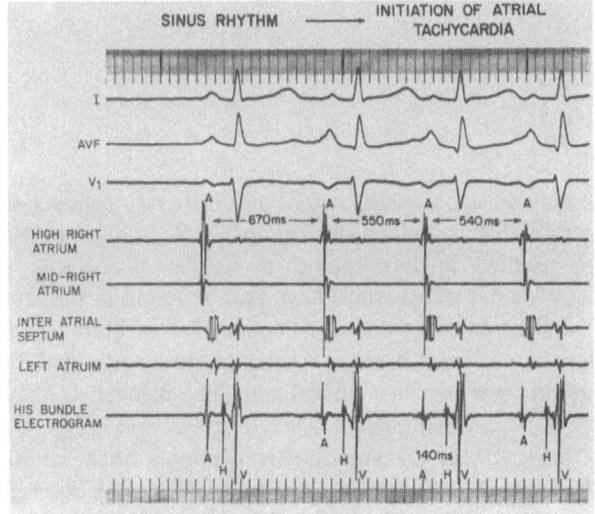

Fig. 2. A: Postural induction and termination of supraventricular tachycardia in patient M.F. Note nonconducted P-wave prior to termination.

B: Intracardiac recordings during spontaneous SVT in patient M.F. showing right atrial origin of SVT and gradual "warm up" of tachycardia. (Figure reproduced with permission of C.V. Mosby Co., Ltd, St. Louis, Missouri.)

toms have been reported in patients with functional type I second degree A-V nodal block, though the overall prognosis of this disorder is generally benign (7, 8).

Longitudinal dissociation of A-V nodal conduction is believed to be the commonest mechanism underlying reentrant SVT (9). It is unclear if this dissociation has a functional and/or anatomic basis. The electrophysiologic properties of the dissociated pathways change after parasympathetic blockade with atropine (10). Atropine shortens the refrac-

Fig. 3. Effect of Autonomic Block on SVT in Patient M.F. A: Atropine acceleration of SVT with type I second degree AV nodal block (see text).

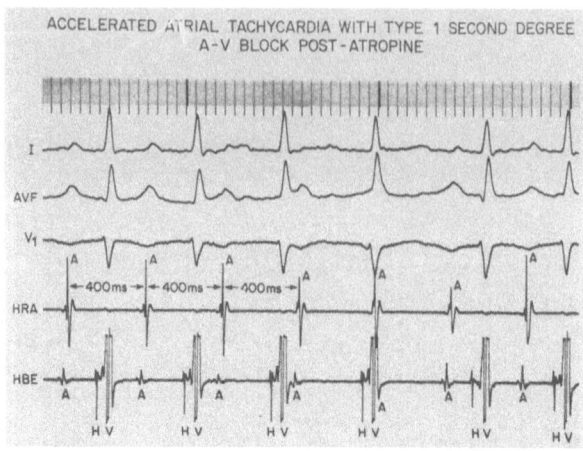

B: Propranolol termination of SVT (see text). (Figure reproduced with permission of C.V. Mosby Co., Ltd., St. Louis, Missouri.)

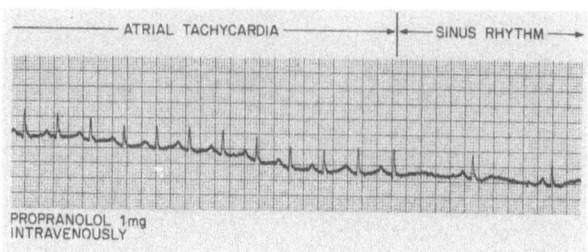

tory periods of the pathways and may mask or unmask latent dissociation of conduction. Acute ischemia has been associated with longitudinal dissociation of A-V nodal conduction (11). Resolution of ischemia resulted in disappearance of manifest dissociation of conduction. Reentrant S-A and A-V nodal tachycardias have been reported in the same patient implying simultaneous longitudinal dissociation of conduction in both regions (12). While these data could imply a functional basis or component in longitudinal dissociation of A-V nodal conduction in some patients, clinical and pathologic reports have suggested an anatomic basis in other patients with dual AV nodal pathways (13, 14).

Our observations would confirm the occurrence of symptomatic functional sinoatrial bradyarrhythmias in patients without structural heart disease. In addition, we observed symptomatic automatic supraventricular tachyarrhythmias originating in the right atrium reflexly induced and terminated by changing autonomic tone probably mediated through the baroreceptor reflex. While postural induction and termination of reentrant PSVT and atrial flutter have been described, similar observations for an autonomic atrial tachycardia have been recently reported (3).

The surprising observation of longitudinal dissociation of atrioventricular nodal conduction in each case deserves comment. This phenomenon has been reported as an incidental observation in patients without supraventricular arrhythmias (15, 16). Estimates of its frequency range from 10–35%. The frequency may be higher in children who also may have more vagotonic influences. The presence of this finding in all our patients is, significant. The changes observed in refractory periods with autonomic blockade and the frequent overlap in conduction curves for the slow and fast pathways could imply a dynamic process like autonomic tone modulating dissociation of conduction. Autonomic imbalance could therefore explain sinoatrial arrhythmias and overt ECG manifestations of longitudinal dissociation of AV nodal conduction.

The implications of our observations is that abnormal autonomic tone could be involved in the induction of automatic atrial arrhythmias and influence dissociation of conduction in the atrio-ventricular node. These data would suggest that investigation of functional sinus node disorders should be accompanied by an evaluation of A-V conduction. Such information may provide greater insight into the mechanisms of conduction and arrhythmogenesis in these structures.

References

1. Jordan JL, Yamaguchi I, Mandel WJ: Studies on the mechanism of sinus node dysfunction in the sick sinus syndrome. Circulation 1978; 57: 217.
2. Waxman MB, Bonet JF, Finley JP, Wald RW: Effects of respiration and posture on paroxysmal supraventricular tachycardia: Circulation 1980; 62: 1011.
3. Saksena S, Siegel P, Rathyen W: Electrophysiologic mechanisms in postural supraventricular tachycardia. Am Ht J 1983; 106: 151.
4. Goldreyer BN, Bigger JT Jr: Site of reentry in paroxysmal supraventricular tachycardia in man. Circulation. 1971; 43: 15.
5. Narula OS: Sinus node reentry. A mechanism for supraventricular tachycardia. Circulation 1975; 35: 492.
6. Strauss HC, Prystowsky EN, Scheinman MM: Sino-atrial and atrial electrogenesis. Progress in Cardiovasc Dis 1977; 19: 385.
7. Young D, Eisenberg R, Fish B, Fisher JD: Wenckebach atrioventricular Block (Mobitz Type I) in children and adolescents: Am J Cardiol 1977; 40: 393.
8. Strasberg B, Amat-y-Leon F, Dhingra RC, Palileo E, Swiryn S, Bauernfiend R, Wyndham C, Rosen KM: Natural history of chronic second-degree atrioventricular nodal block. Circulation 1981; 63: 1043.
9. Josephson ME: Paroxysmal supraventricular tachycardia. An electrophysiologic approach. Am J Cardiol 1978; 41: 1123.
10. Wu D, Denes P, Bauernfiend R, Dhingra RC, Wyndham C, Rosen KM: Effects of atropine in the induction and maintenance of atrioventricular nodal reentrant tachycardia. Circulation 1979; 59: 779.
11. Sclarovsky S, Strasberg B, Lewin R, Agnoli J: Dissociation of the atrioventricular node acute inferior wall myocardial infarction. 2. Longitudinal dissociation (Dual atrioventricular nodal pathways). Chest 1978; 73: 638.
12. Paulay KL, Ruskin JN, Damato AN: Sinus and atrioventricular nodal reentrant tachycardia in the same patient. Am J Cardiol 1975; 36: 810.
13. Bharati S, Bauernfiend R, Schienman M, Massie B, Cheitlin M, Denes P, Wu D, Lev M, Rosen KM: Congenital abnormalities of the conduction system in two patients with tachyarrhythmias. Circulation 1979; 59: 593.
14. Sung RJ, Waxman HL, Saksena S, Juma Z: Sequence of retrograde atrial activation in patients with dual atrioventricular nodal pathways. Circulation 1981; 64: 1059.
15. Denes P, Wu D, Dhingra RC, Amat-y-Leon F, Wyndham C, Rosen RM: Dual atrioventricular nodal pathways, a common electrophysiological response. Br Heart J 1975; 37: 1069.

16. Casta A, Wolff GS, Mehta AV, Tamer D, Garcia OL, Pickoff AS, Ferrer PL, Sung RJ, Gelband H: Dual atrioventricular nodal pathways: A benign finding in arrhythmia free children with heart disease. Am J Cardiol 1980; 46: 1013.

Authors' address:
Sanjeev Saksena, M.D.
Cardiac Electrophysiology
Newark Beth Israel Medical Center
201 Lyons Avenue
Newark, N.J. 07112 (USA)

Early Clinical Experience with a DDD Pacemaker

P. H. Belott, St. S. Sands

Summary: Fifty-six patients with a Universal AV [DDD] pacemaker have been followed a minimum of three months with thorough rhythm analysis to assess appropriate pacemaker function. A total of fifty-three patients demonstrated evidence of VA conduction. Of all patients programmed to the DDD mode, three required programming to the DVI mode because of symptomatic sustained pacemaker mediated tachycardia (PMT). Thirty-five patients chronically programmed to the DDD mode demonstrated asymptomatic self-limited runs of PMT. These episodes consistently related to ventricular ectopic activity. The pacemaker demonstrated appropriate function as designed. Although most PMTs are asymptomatic and self-limited their prevalence and association with ventricular ectopy suggests the importance of post ventricular atrial refractory period programmability, post premature ventricular contraction atrial refractory period extension and post premature ventricular contraction DDD operation.

Now that atrial lead stability is achievable (1) and dual lead implantation techniques (2) are firmly established, dual chamber pacing is possible in a wide range of patients. The ideal approach would appear to be one which preserves atrial ventricular relationships at all times and offers rate responsiveness, for optimal hemodynamics (3) and effective arrhythmia control. Such a device is the Universal AV (4) [DDD] (5) pacemaker which incorporates the beneficial features of the AV sequential [DVI] and P wave synchronized [VDD] pacing systems. This pacemaker has complex operation and function. One must be concerned with refractoriness in both atrium and ventricle, appropriate AV delay, safe tracking windows and be cognizant of potential VA conduction with resultant pacemaker mediated tachycardia (6). Primitive concerns over appropriate sense and capture in one chamber expand to those of pacemaker induced arrthythmias, self inhibition and spurious reprogramming. One must have a thorough understanding of pacemaker atrial and ventricular refractory period and the concepts of blanking and crosstalk and appropriate responses to high atrial rates.

How a particular peacemaker deals with ectopic ventricular activity is extremely important. Early clinical experience with a DDD pacemaker is reported demonstrating the importance of these operating features for proper programming and analysis of appropriate function (7).

Methods

All patients were considered as candidates for DDD pacing except those with chronic atrial fibrillation or atrial paralysis. The patients received Medtronic*) Versatrax Model 7000 AV Universal pacemaker. The device has six programmable modes DDD, DVI,

---

*   Medtronic, Inc., Minneapolis, MN

VVI, DAT, DOO, VOO. The atrial refractory period starts with an atrial paced or sensed event and continues for 155 milliseconds after a ventricular event. The device protects against premature ventricular contraction ventriculo-atrial activation by disabling the atrial ventricular timer for 340 milliseconds following a PVC. The upper rate characteristics exemplify a Wenkebach type response. To avoid the problem of cross-talk or self inhibition the device exhibits "ventricular safety pacing"*). That is, if a signal is detected by the ventricular amplifier during the first 110 milliseconds of the AV interval following an atrial paced event, a ventricular stimulus is emitted at the end of the 110 millisecond period.

All patients received a Medtronic*) unipolar 6957 J screw in polyurethane atrial electrode and a Medtronic*) 6971 ring tip tined ventricular polyurethane electrode.

At the time of implant, standard threshold and sensing measurements were taken in both chambers. Patients were also screened for ventriculo-atrial conduction by pacing the right ventricle at rates 80, 90 and 100 BPM while simultaneously recording the right atrial endocardial electrogram on an E for M**) AR 12 recorder.

Post operative follow-up included early in-patient telemetry monitoring and subsequent outpatient pacemaker clinic evaluations at one week, one month and three months. Each patient underwent ambulatory monitoring acutely and at three months. Clinic evaluation included analysis for appropriate sensing and capture in both chambers, screening for myoinhibtion, testing for rate responsiveness and appropriate upper rate characteristics (8).

Results

Fifty-six patients have been followed a minimum of three months with thorough rhythm analysis. Thirty-two patients had primary AV block and twenty-four had sick sinus syndrome. Initially forty-two patients were programmed to the DDD mode, twenty-four with AV block and eighteen with sick sinus syndrome. Fourteen patients were initially programmed to the DVI mode, eight with AV block and six with sick sinus syndrome. After three months, thirty-five patients were still programmed to the DDD mode, twenty-three with AV block and twelve with sick sinus syndrome, while twenty-one were in DVI mode, nine with AV block and twelve with sick sinus syndrome (Table 1). Seven patients were programmed from DDD to DVI modes. Of these patients, three required reprogramming because of symptomatic sustained pacemaker mediated tachycardia (9); while four patients were reprogrammed because of poor rate responsiveness or profound bradycardia (Table 2).

Ventriculo-atrial conduction analysis (Table 3) demonstrated that nineteen patients, seven with AV block and twelve with sick sinus syndrome, had demonstrated VA conduction at time of implant. Post operative VA conduction manifesting as pacemaker mediated tachycardia was observed in thirty-four patients, twenty-two with AV block and twelve with sick sinus syndrome. A total of fifty-three patients demonstrated evidence of

---

* Medtronic, Inc., Minneapolis, MN
** Electronics for Medicine, Orange, CA

Table 1.

PACEMAKER PROGRAMMED				
MODE ANALYSIS				
INITIAL				
AVB	SSS		MODE	
24	18	42	DDD	75%
8	6	14	DVI	25%
3 MONTHS				
23	12	35	DDD	63%
9	12	21	DVI	37%

Table 2.

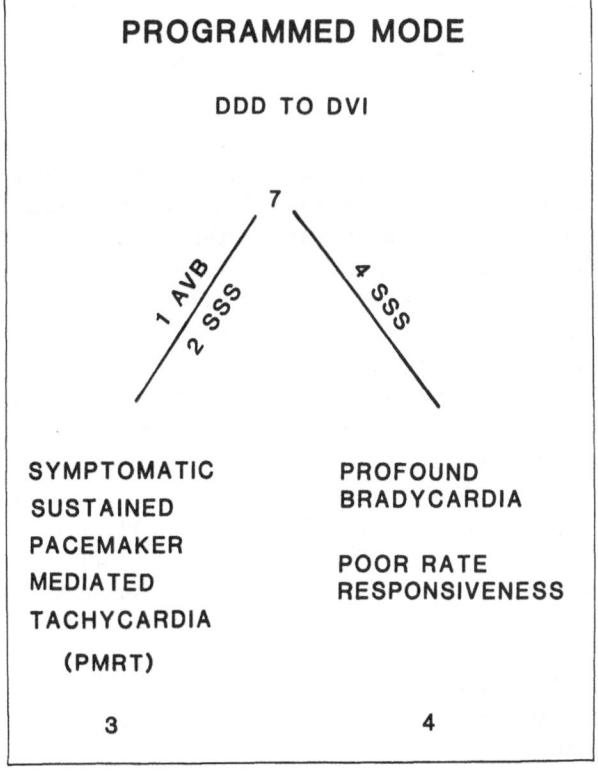

PROGRAMMED MODE

DDD TO DVI

SYMPTOMATIC SUSTAINED PACEMAKER MEDIATED TACHYCARDIA (PMRT)

PROFOUND BRADYCARDIA

POOR RATE RESPONSIVENESS

Table 3.

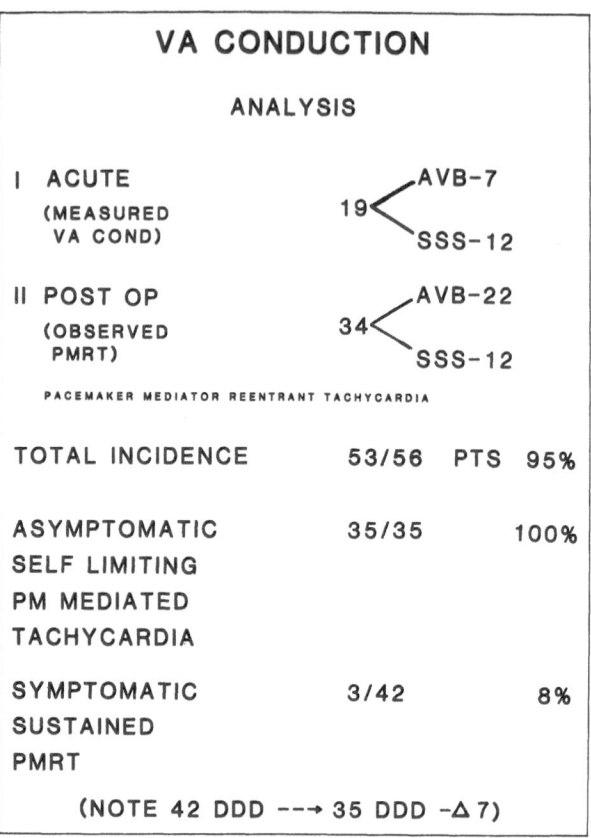

VA CONDUCTION

ANALYSIS

I ACUTE
(MEASURED
VA COND)
19 < AVB−7
SSS−12

II POST OP
(OBSERVED
PMRT)
34 < AVB−22
SSS−12

PACEMAKER MEDIATOR REENTRANT TACHYCARDIA

TOTAL INCIDENCE	53/56 PTS	95%
ASYMPTOMATIC SELF LIMITING PM MEDIATED TACHYCARDIA	35/35	100%
SYMPTOMATIC SUSTAINED PMRT	3/42	8%

(NOTE 42 DDD −−→ 35 DDD −Δ7)

VA conduction. All thirty-five patients chronically programmed to the DDD mode demonstrated asymptomatic, brief, selflimited bursts of pacemaker mediated tachycardia.
Rhythm analysis consistently demonstrated appropriate atrial synchronous and AV sequential operation with Wenckebach upper rate characteristics. A common rhythm pattern was observed with all pacemaker mediated tachycardias. This pattern is demonstrated by analysis of actual representative rhythm strips. In Fig. 1 there is normal sinus rhythm until the appearance of a PVC (forth complex on the ECG) which initiates an atrial refractory period, the A–V disable period, and the upper rate interval. At the end of the atrial refractory period but before the completion of the 340 milliseconds disable period, a retrograde event is sensed which restarts the atrial refractory period. With no further intrinsic activity, the lower rate (V–V internal) counter expires, delivering a ventricular stimulus. This is followed by a retrograde p-wave which is sensed and which triggers a ventricular stimulus at the end of the A–V interval. The patient then spontaneously reverts to sinus rhythm. The reason that only a ventricular stimulus was delivered in the fifth complex is that although the V–A interval had expired, the atrial amplifier was refractory, precluding the delivery of an atrial stimulus. The patient in Figure 2 is in sinus rhythm until interrupted by a PVC that conducts retrogradely to the atrium. As in the preceding example, no further intrinsic activity occurs, and the pacemaker delivers a ventricular stimulus at the end of the lower rate (V–V) interval (no atrial stimulus is de-

166

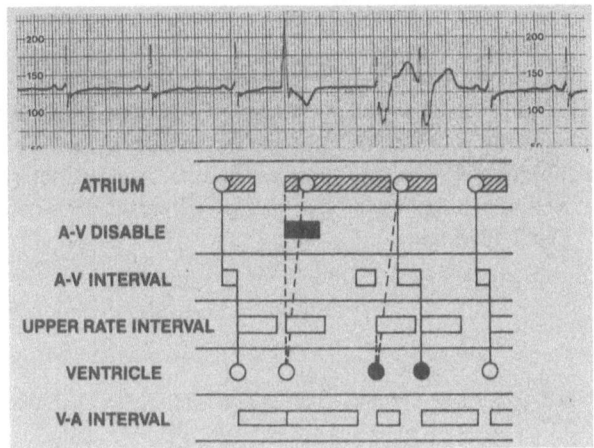

Fig. 1. Rhythm analysis of a self-limited pacemaker mediated tachycardia reentrant loop.

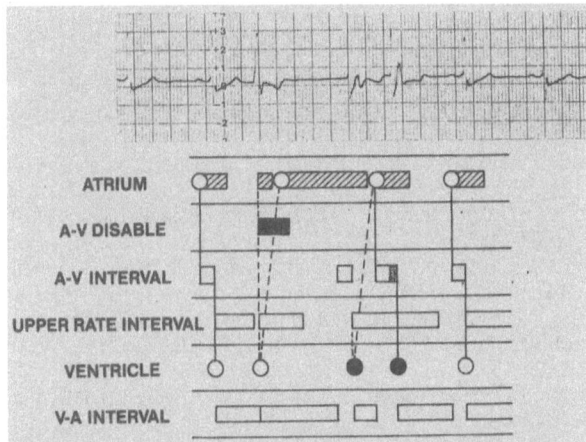

Fig. 2. Rhythm analysis of a self-limited pacemaker mediated tachycardia reentrant loop with operation at the upper rate limit.

livered because the atrial amplifier is refractory). Following this ventricular event is a retrograde p-wave which is sensed by the pacemaker. The ventricular stimulus, however, which is normally delivered at the end of the A–V interval is delayed until the end of the upper rate interval. Normal sinus rhythm then returns.

These brief pacemaker-mediated events were clinically insignificant asymptomatic and self-limited without hemodynamic compromise. Their occurrence stresses the importance of careful post implant follow-up including thorough ambulatory holter monitoring. Retrograde conduction can be expected in most patients including those with third degree AV block.

Conclusions

This first generation Universal AV pacemaker has been very instrumental in leading the way to more effective dual chamber Universal AV pacing. The device demonstrated safe and appropriate function as designed. This early experience has demonstrated the extremely common occurrence of VA conduction and resultant pacemaker mediated tachycardia. Most pacemaker mediated tachycardias were asymptomatic and self limited; while sustained tachycardia was unusual. The observed prevalence of VA conduction and resultant pacemaker mediated tachycardia has demonstrated the importance of post ventriculo-atrial refractory programmability. The association of pacemaker mediated tachycardia with PVCs reinforces the need for an extended post PVC atrial refractory period and the preservation of post PVC DDD operation.

References

1. Messenger John C, Castellanet Mark J, Stephenson Nancy L: New Permanent Endocardial Atrial J Lead: Implantation Techniques and Clinical Performance. Pace 5(S) Sept–Oct 1982: 767–772.
2. Belott Peter H: Retaining Guidewire, Introducer Technique for Unlimited Access to the Central Circulation: A Review. Clinical Progress in Pacing and Electrophysiology Vol 1, No 1, 1983: 59–69.
3. Shapland JE, MacCarter D, Tockman B, Knudson M: Physiologic Benefits of Rate Responsiveness. Pace Vol. 6 March-April Part II 1983; 329–332.
4. Funke HD: Cardiac Pacing with Universal DDD Pulse Generator. In: Barold SS, Mugica J, eds. Third Decade of Cardiac Pacing. Mount Kisco, New York: Futura Publishing Company, 1982: 191.
5. Parsonnet V, Furman S, Smyth NPD: A Revised Code for Pacemaker Identifications. Pace Vol 4, 1981: 400.
6. Dulk Karel Den, Lindemans Fred W, Bar Frits W, Wellens Hein JJ: Pacemaker Related Tachycardias. Pace Vol 5, July–Aug 1982: 476–485.
7. Barold S Serge, Ong Ling S, Falkoff Michael D, Heinle Robert: Programmable Pacemakers: Clinical Indications, Complications and Future Directions. In: Barold SS, Mugica J, eds. Third Decade of Cardiac Pacing. Mount Kisco, New York: Futura Publishing Company, 1982: 27.
8. Hauser Robert G: The Electrocardiography of AV Universal DDD Pacemakers. Pace Vol 6, March–April Part II, 1983: 399–409.
9. Furman Seymour, Fisher John D: Endless Loop Tachycardia in an AV Universal (DDD) Pacemaker. Pace Vol 5, July–Aug 1982: 486–489.

Authors' address:
Peter H. Belott, M.D.
1625 East Main Street
El Cajon, CA. 92021
USA

Comparison of Left Ventricular Myocardial Blood Flow During Atrial and Ventricular Pacing

A. Nakamura, Z. S. Zheng, S. Nakaji, I. Hashimoto

Summary: In order to compare left ventricular myocardial blood flow (MBF) during atrial pacing (AP) and ventricular pacing (VP), this experimental study was performed. Twenty house rabbits, weighing 2.5 to 4.0 kg (3.3 ± 0.4) were used. After sinus arrest (SA) was produced, the measurements of regional MBF (hydrogen gas clearance method), cardiac output and the pressure of LV and AO were undertaken. Regional MBF was measured at the area of apex, circumflex (CX) coronary artery, left anterior descending (LAD) artery and interventricular septum, using wire-type platinum electrodes.
As a result, cardiac output was higher by 54.3% during atrial pacing as compared with VP (p < 0.001). Regional MBF at the area of LAD, septum and apex during VP was significantly reduced as compared with AP (p < 0.05) except CX area. However, there was no significant difference between the MBF of AP and SA, VP and SA. The distribution of MBF between 4 areas during SA, AP and VP was uniform, and MBF of CX area was larger than that of septum during AP and VP (p < 0.05). But, there were no significant differences among the another area.
In conclusion, the results from this present investigation indicate an important role of atrial contraction and ventricular normal depolarization in the left cardiac function. Also, it demonstrates that atrial pacing results in an increase in myocardial flow and cardiac output than ventricular pacing.

Ventricular pacing in the treatment of bradyarrhythmia has been strikingly successful. However, it is prevailing opinion that this mode has a hemodynamic disadvantage which is induced by the asynchrony between atrial and ventricular contraction.

On the other hand, atrial pacing is beneficial hemodynamically, due to the booster pump action of atrium and normal ventricular depolarization, as compared with ventricular pacing. In fact, the excellent cardiac performance has been evaluated by many investigators.

In this study, regional myocardial blood flow of left ventricle during SA, AP and VP was compared.

Methods

Studies were carried out in 20 house rabbits weighing 2.5 to 4.0 kg and anesthetized with sodium pentobarbital (35 to 40 mg/kg) into peritoneal cavity. After tracheostomy, a bilateral thoracotomy was performed under controlled respiration maintained with pancuronium bromide (0.3 mg/kg) intravenously.

An electromagnetic flowprobe was applied around the ascending aorta. Teflon catheters were inserted into the aorta and left ventricle for the recordings of pressure. Myocardial blood flow was determined with hydrogen gas clearance method (Aukland's technique) (1). The platinum electrodes were placed on the myocardial middle layer at 4 areas, apex, CX region, LAD region and IVS. The indifferent electrode was implanted into the subcutaneous tissue. Hydrogen gas was introduced from the lateral orifice of the tracheal cannula for 3 to 5 minutes, and the gas concentration was mantained at 10% of respiratory volume. Hydrogen gas clearance curve was obtained, using the blood flowmeter (Unique Medical Co. UH meter) and analyzed with the data processer.

After the above operation was prepared, sinus arrest was produced by applying a few drops of formalin at sinus node.

1. Five minutes after sinus arrest, cardiac output, aortic pressure, left ventricular pressure and myocardial blood flow were measured.
2. In next study, the right atrium was stimulated at a rate equal to resting state prior to sinus arrest. After 5 minutes, when stable state was given, the same parameters were studied.
3. Then, the right ventricle was paced at a rate equal to atrial pacing. Also, the same measurements were undertaken.

Results

During AP and SA, cardiac output increased significantly as compared with VP (AP : VP $p < 0.001$, SA : VP $p < 0.01$), but there was no significant difference between AP and SA (Fig. 1).

Left ventricular pressure is shown in Table 1. Left ventricular enddiastolic pressure (LVEDP) was unchanged during SA, AP and VP.

Fig. 1. Cardiac output in the conditions of SA, AP and VP.

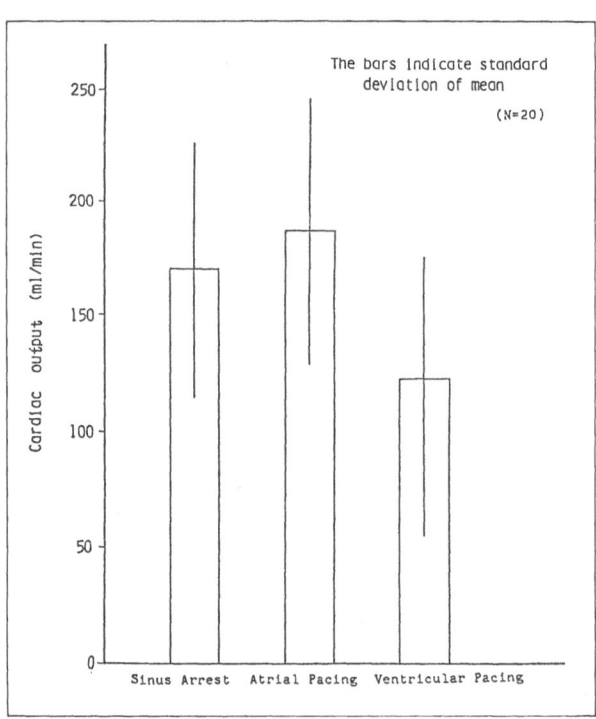

Table 1. Pressure of the aorta and the left ventricle in the conditions of SA, AP and VP.

Rabbit No.	Sinus Arrest		Atrial Pacing		Ventricular Pacing	
	Ao	LV	Ao	LV	Ao	LV
1	86/70 (78)	88/ 5 (45)	80/64 (70)	84/ 4 (38)	80/66 (70)	84/ 4 (39)
2	84/71 (74)	124/ 0 (60)	68/56 (62)	106/ 2 (48)	72/59 (63)	126/ 0 (40)
3	66/50 (58)	106/12 (46)	51/40 (43)	96/10 (35)	62/48 (56)	106/ 8 (44)
4	39/28 (34)	56/ 0 (18)	37/26 (29)	44/ 0 (17)	46/34 (38)	56/ 0 (20)
5	86/65 (70)	104/ 3 (39)	66/51 (64)	90/ 0 (43)	76/58 (65)	98/ 3 (42)
6	77/59 (67)	77/ 6 (34)	67/57 (62)	64/ 6 (32)	54/46 (52)	50/ 6 (28)
7	75/56 (63)	90/ 4 (34)	64/54 (62)	76/ 6 (40)	48/42 (45)	58/ 6 (28)
8	68/50 (58)	88/ 2 (34)	68/56 (64)	80/ 2 (50)	48/40 (44)	58/ 6 (30)
9	70/46 (60)	88/ 4 (48)	48/36 (44)	70/ 6 (34)	35/26 (32)	53/ 5 (26)
10	61/44 (54)	80/16 (38)	62/50 (55)	88/16 (50)	54/44 (46)	72/17 (40
11	68/44 (58)	80/ 6 (72)	68/53 (61)	84/ 0 (54)	62/47 (58)	77/ 0 (39)
12	68/60 (66)	77/ 4 (32)	72/57 (63)	81/ 4 (37)	72/58 (61)	80/ 4 (34)
13	40/26 (34)	64/10 (40)	44/36 (42)	66/14 (44)	28/20 (22)	40/12 (22)
14	66/56 (64)	73/ 6 (40)	74/58 (64)	88/ 2 (33)	48/40 (43)	62/ 6 (32)
15	86/62 (74)	95/ 2 (50)	86/66 (75)	96/ 3 (50)	76/67 (68)	84/ 2 (41)
16	50/37 (42)	74/ 8 (28)	58/41 (47)	87/ 6 (43)	56/42 (48)	84/ 9 (38)
17	63/50 (57)	70/ 4 (59)	43/34 (36)	50/ 7 (32)	43/34 (36)	46/ 8 (30)
18	64/54 (56)	70/ 4 (44)	44/38 (39)	44/12 (33)	31/21 (23)	34/ 8 (16)
19	78/60 (74)	90/ 6 (40)	94/77 (83)	104/ 3 (64)	55/42 (46)	81/ 1 (34)
20	66/50 (56)	76/ 4 (34)	74/58 (67)	86/ 2 (46)	58/46 (50)	65/ 5 (33)
Mean	68.1/51.9	83.5/5.3	63.9/49.9	79.2/5.3	55.7/44.0	70.8/5.5
± SD	(59.9 ± 12.0)	(41.8 ± 11.8)	(57.1 ± 14.4)	(41.2 ± 10.0)	(48.3 ± 13.4)	(32.8 ± 7.6)

Ao: syst./diast. (mean) mmHg, LV: syst./EDP (mean) mmHg

Aortic pressure was used as mean value. Mean arterial pressure was significantly higher during AP than VP ($p < 0.05$).

Regional MBF is shown in Fig. 2. Regional MBF at the area of LAD, septum and apex during VP was significantly reduced as compared with AP ($p < 0.05$) except CX area. However, there was no significant difference between MBF of AP and SA, VP and SA.

The distribution of MBF between 4 areas during SA, AP and VP was uniform, and MBF of CX area was larger than that of septum during AP and VP ($p < 0.05$). But, there were no significant differences among another area.

Discussion

The fact that AP dominates to VP on the standpoint of cardiac output is well known. In our studies, also, cardiac output was higher by 54.3% during AP as compared with VP ($p < 0.001$).

Cardiac output is regulated by stroke volume and heart rate. Pre-load, after-load, contractility of the myocardium and compliance of the ventricle were mentioned as factors to influence upon the stroke volume. Pre-load is influenced by atrial contraction, circula-

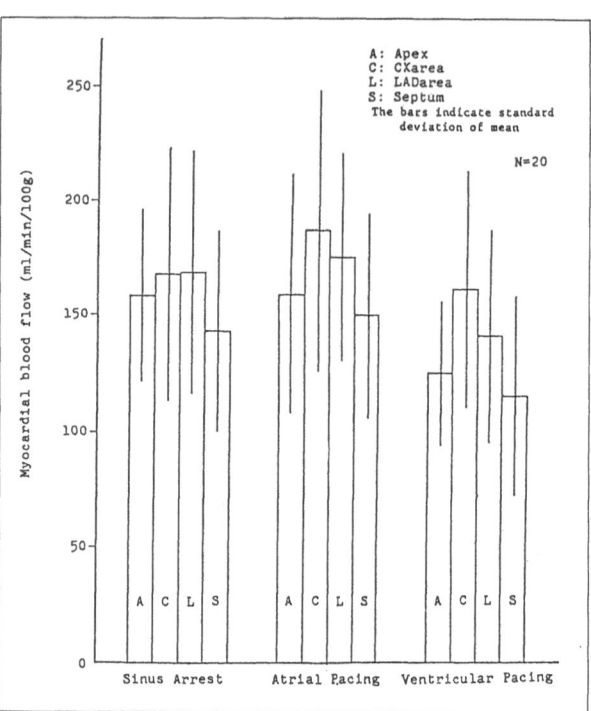

Fig. 2. Regional myocardial blood flow of 4 areas in the conditions of SA, AP and VP.

tory blood volume, venous return, intrathoracic pressure, intrapericardial pressure and posture. Afterload is controlled by stroke volume and peripheral vascular resistance. Contractility is controlled by preload, afterload, increased heart rate, catecholamine, ischemia and acidosis. Thus, cardiac output is regulated by complex interaction of many factors as mentioned above.

In this studies, cardiac output was evaluated by the difference of stroke volume, because the pacing rate of AP and VP was kept uniform throughout the experiments.

In AP with normal conduction, inflow blood volume increased into the ventricle by the effective atrial contraction. So, it was considered that LVEDV increased. As summarized in Table 1, there were no significant difference of LVEDP during AP and VP. This phenomenon was explained as the dependence upon ventricular compliance. Therefore, the atrium had the function as a booster pump of ventricle and contributed to effective closure of atrioventricular valve. Either increased LVEDV and increased initial length of myocardial fiber were conducted to increase stroke volume.

On the other hand, during VP the booster pump effect was lost because of a synchronized atrial and ventricular contraction, more over, VP had the disadvantage concerning with abnormal ventricular depolarization. They produced the loss of cooperating ventricular contraction, and consequently reduced cardiac output and coronary flow due to a lack of squeezing effect of myocardium.

From the reason mentioned above, we considered that different cardiac output between AP and VP was based on the results of different stroke volume.

172

Concerning with cardiac output during SA, there was no significant difference as compared with AP, but cardiac output during SA increased significantly by 130% compared with VP, in spite of lower heart rate during SA.

These results were induced by the different conduction mode. In SA, ventricular conduction was kept in normal fashion followed to junctional rhythm. But, VP had a mode considered as a kind of ventricular extrasystole. This fact was understood in the same during AP and VP. However, in AP heart rate should also be taken into consideration. Since our study was performed in acute phase of 5 to 10 minutes later producing SA, it was considered that heart maintained the function to regulate EDV. We suspected that prolongation of diastolic phase resulted in increase of stroke volume by means of increasing ventricular filling. Thus, it was explained that the decreased heart rate might influence slightly upon cardiac output.

On the other hand, in chronic phase cardiomegaly will occur, because these control mechanisms will be lost gradually relating to decreased ventricular contractility, in spite of increased ventricular filling.

The factors conributing to the variation in regional MBF could be attributed to the differences in contraction, anatomic composition and coronary vascular reaction. If a comparison were made of MBF of 4 areas during SA, AP and VP, the value of MBF decreased in the next order: AP > SA > VP. We believed that the cause of these differences can possibly be explained in part by hemodynamic factors. Since the coronary circulation was under hemodynamic, metabolic and neurogenic regulation, the decrease of MBF during VP was most likely related to

1. A fall in aortic diastolic pressure
2. A rise in transmural pressure
3. A decrease in afterload and wall tension which resulted in decrease in myocardial oxygen consumption (2, 3).

But, when greater cardiac output is required, the myocardial oxygen consumption rises because of increase of inotropic state and initial tension during VP. However, the high transmural pressure will result in a decrease in MBF.

Due to these mechanism MBF will not be increased and the ischemia will occur even when there is increase in cardiac output, a rise in aortic pressure, and MBF of 4 areas will decrease at the same ratio to one another.

Conclusions

The results from present investigation indicate an important role for the atrial contraction and ventricular normal conduction in the left cardiac function. It also demonstrates that AP can result in an increase in MBF, cardiac output and other parameters of ventricular function other than VP.

References

1. Aukland K, Bower BF, Berliner RW: Measurement of local blood flow with hydrogen gas. Circ Res 1964; 14: 164–187.

2. Downey JM, Kirk ES: Distribution of coronary blood flow across the canine heart wall during systole. Circ Res 1974; 34: 251–257.
3. Baird RJ, Manktelow RT, Shah PA, Ameli FM: Intramyocardial pressure. A study of its regional variation and its relationship to intraventricular pressure. J Thorac Cardiovasc Surg 1970; 59: 810–823.

Authors' address:
Dr. A. Nakamura
Dept. of Surgery
Kyoto Pref. University of Medicine
Kawaramachi Hirokoji, Kamikyo-ku
Kyoto 602/Japan

Influence of Atrio-Ventricular Contraction Interval on Hemodynamics

J. J. Curtis, J. T. Walls, Theresa M. Boley, N. P. Madigan, G. C. Flaker, J. C. Reid

Summary: This study was designed to determine if changes in the delay between atrial contraction and ventricular contraction would affect hemodynamics in patients following open heart surgery. Temporary pacing wires were placed on the right atrium and right ventricle of consecutive patients undergoing open heart surgery. Duplicate thermodilution cardiac outputs (CO), left atrial pressure (LA), mean arterial pressure (MAP), and stroke volume index (SVI) were determined during atrial (A) pacing, ventricular (V) pacing, A-V sequential pacing at A-V intervals of 50, 100, 125, 150, 175 and 200 milliseconds (msecs) concluding with repeat A pacing. If the CO with A pacing at the end of the study varied more than 10% from that at the beginning of the study, it was concluded that observations in the interim might be due to factors other than the A-V contraction interval. Data from these "unstable" patients were excluded. Fifty-three patients met the study design criteria and the data from these studies was analyzed by response surface analysis and Wilcoxon matched pairs signed ranks test, with $p < 0.05$ being considered significant. There was a significant curvilinear relationship between A-V interval and CO. A-V sequential pacing with an A-V interval of 50 msecs increased the CO significantly over that observed with V pacing, with further significant increases at 100 and 150 msecs. LA dropped significantly from 19 to 16 mmHg when changing the A-V interval from 50 to 150 msecs. MAP increased significantly at an A-V interval of 50 msecs over V pacing, with a further significant increase at an A-V interval of 150 msecs. Average CO at 200 msecs was significantly lower than that seen at 125 and 150 msecs, though there were noteworthy individual patient exceptions. SVI increased significantly with each 50 msecs lengthening of the A-V interval to an A-V interval of 100 msecs. The timing of A-V synchrony is important to achieve optimal hemodynamics following open heart surgery.

During the past decade there was emerged tremendous interest in cardiac pacing modalities which maintain atrio-ventricular synchrony. There is excellent documentation that atrial contraction should precede ventricular contraction for optimal hemodynamics (1–17). However, with noteworthy exceptions, little attention has been given to the importance of the atrio-ventricular contraction interval. The purpose of our study was to determine the effects of varying atrio-ventricular contraction intervals on hemodynamics in patients following open heart surgery.

Materials and Methods

Temporary pacing wires were placed on the right atrium and right ventricle of patients undergoing open heart surgery. During the postoperative period, when hemodynamics were stable, mean left atrial and systemic pressures and duplicate thermodilution cardiac outputs were determined during atrial pacing, ventricular pacing, A-V (atrio-ventricular) sequential pacing at A-V intervals of 50, 100, 125, 150, 175 and 200 msecs, concluding with repeat atrial pacing. Those patients who could not be consistently A-V sequentially paced at longer A-V intervals because of competitively shorter PR intervals were taken as

175

far in the protocol as possible before concluding with repeat atrial pacing. All pacing was at 100 beats per minute and a 3-minute equilibration period was allowed at each new pacing modality. Each patient served as his own control, in that, if the cardiac output with atrial pacing at the end of the study varied more than 10% from that at the beginning of study, it was concluded that observations in the interim might not be due to the A-V contraction interval but to other factors. Data from these patients were excluded from statistical analysis. Data meeting the specifications of the internal control were analyzed using the Wilcoxon Matched Pairs Signed Ranks test and Response Surface Analysis.

The patient population consisted of 53 patients who met the protocol design criteria. There were 37 males and 16 females. Age ranged from 36–78 years with a median age of 55.5 years. The ejection fraction of these patients ranged from 24–83% with a median of 57.7%. Thirty-nine patients had undergone isolated coronary artery bypass grafting, 6 patients combined coronary artery bypass grafting with a valvular procedure and 8 patients had undergone isolated valve replacement.

Results

The results of this study are compiled in Table 1 where average hemodynamic values are listed on all 53 patients studied. The hemodynamic parameters with atrial pacing at the beginning of the study and at the end of the pacing protocol are quite similar indicating that patients were "hemodynamically stable" during the pacing protocol. This allows one to conclude that the varying hemodynamics observed are indeed due to the pacing modality and A-V contraction interval being tested, rather than to other factors.

The now well recognized adverse effect of ventricular pacing on hemodynamics when compared to atrial pacing at the same rate was, once again, well documented. Left atrial pressure rose from 15 mmHg to 19 mmHg when changing from atrial to ventricular pacing. Also, mean arterial pressure fell from 87 mmHg to 80 mmHg and the average cardiac output fell from 6.08 ml/min to 4.74 ml/min. This was due predominantly to a change in stroke volume with the stroke volume index falling from 30.9 ml/beat/min to 24.3 ml/beat/min with total loss of the atrial contribution to ventricular filling. With restoration of A-V synchrony, albeit with a short A-V contraction interval of only 50 msecs, mean arterial pressure, cardiac output and stroke volume index all improved (Table 1). As the A-V contraction interval was fractionally lengthened to 150 msecs by protocol, all hemodynamic parameters improved, whereupon, further lengthening of the A-V contraction interval to 200 msecs resulted in deterioration of hemodynamics (see Table 1).

Forty of the 53 patients (75%) demonstrated maximal cardiac output with an A-V contraction interval of between 125 and 175 msecs. However, there was great individual variation and the A-V interval which would produce maximal cardiac output could not be anticipated. Four patients had maximal cardiac output produced at an A-V interval of 50 msecs and 6 patients had maximal cardiac output produced at an A-V interval of 100 msecs (10 of 53 patients or 18.9%). Three patients (5.7%) had maximal cardiac output produced with an A-V interval of 200 msecs. However, only 31 of the 53 patients (58.5%) could be paced at an A-V interval of 200 msecs as A-V capture could not be maintained at 200 msecs. Therefore, of the 31 patients who could be paced at an A–V interval of 200 msecs, 9.8% had maximal cardiac output with an A-V contraction interval of 200 msecs.

When the cardiac output at varying A-V interval was examined by Response Surface Analysis, a highly significant ($p < 0.0001$) curvilinear relationship was confirmed.

The magnitude of change in the hemodynamic parameters with 50 msecs incremental changes in the A-V contraction interval is summarized in Table 2. Average percent change for all patients is listed. Comparison of the average data obtained with each of the contraction intervals was analyzed by the Wilcoxon Matched Pairs Signed Ranks test with a p value less than 0.05 being considered significant. The asterisks' in Table 2 designate a significant difference when comparing the average values at the two A-V contraction intervals tested. Left atrial pressure did not change significantly when going from ventricular to A-V sequential pacing at 50 msecs. However, a significant decrease in left atrial pressure occurred with lengthening the A-V interval from 50–100 msecs. By in-

Table 1. Effect of Pacing Modality on Hemodynamics.

Pacing Mode	LA	MAP	CO	SVI
Atrial	15	87	6.08	30.9
Ventricular	19	80	4.74	24.3
AVS-50 msecs	19	84	5.28	27.1
AVS-100 msecs	18	86	5.55	29.2
AVS-125 msecs	17	85	5.96	30.6
AVS-150 msecs	16	87	6.01	31.0
AVS-175 msecs	16	85	5.86	30.4
AVS-200 msecs	17	87	5.67	29.4
Atrial	15	88	5.85	30.2

See text for description.

AVS = Atrioventricular Sequential, CO = Cardiac Output (l/min); LA = Left Atrial Pressure (mmHg); MAP = Mean Arterial Pressure (mmHg); msecs = Milliseconds; SVI = Stroke Volume Index (ml/beat/m²).

Table 2. Percent Change in Hemodynamic Parameters With Varying Atrioventricular Contraction Intervals.

	V-AVS 50 msecs	AVS 50–100 msecs	AVS 100–150 msecs	AVS 150–200 msecs
LA	0	−5.3*	−11*	+6.3
MAP	+5.0*	+2.4*	+1.2	0
CO	+11.4*	+5.1*	+8.3*	−5.7*
SVI	+11.5*	+7.7*	+6.2	−5.2

See text for description.

AVS = Atrioventricular Sequential; CO = Cardiac Output; LA = Left Atrial Pressure; MAP = Mean Arterial Pressure; msecs = Milliseconds; SVI = Stroke Volume Index, V = Ventricular; * = $p < 0.05$.

creasing the A-V interval to 150 msecs, another significant decline in left atrial pressure of 11% was observed. By changing the A-V interval from 150 msecs to 200 msecs the left atrial pressure rose 6.3%, though, this was not statistically significant. Mean arterial pressure rose significantly when changing from ventricular pacing to A-V sequential pacing at 50 msecs with an additional significant increase being observed when lengthening the A-V interval to 100 msecs. Further lengthening of the A-V sequential interval to 150 and 200 msecs did not significantly change the mean arterial pressure. As can be seen from Table 2, cardiac output changed significantly with each 50 msecs increment in A-V interval. A positive hemodynamic effect was observed with lengthening the A-V interval to 150 msecs, whereupon, further prolongation of the A-V interval to 200 msecs resulted in an adverse hemodynamic effect.

A statistically significant difference in all hemodynamic parameters was observed when changing the A-V interval from 50 msecs to 150 msecs. Left atrial pressure fell from 19 to 16 mmHg (15.8%), mean arterial pressure increased from 84 to 87 mmHg (3.6%), cardiac output increased from 5.28 to 6.01 l/min (13.8%) and stroke volume index increased from 27.1 to 31.0 ml/beat/m² (14.3%).

Conclusions

Small changes in the time delay between atrial and ventricular contraction significantly alter hemodynamics in patients following open heart surgery. Not only is it important for atrial contraction to precede ventricular contraction but the timing of A-V synchrony is important to achieve optimal hemodynamics.

References

1. Little RC: Effect of atrial systole on ventricular pressure and closure of the AV valves. Am J Physiol 1951; 166: 289–295.
2. Linden RJ, Mitchell JH: Relation between left ventricular diastolic pressure and myocardial segment length and observations on the contribution of atrial systole. Circ Res 1960; 8: 1092–1099.
3. Gilmore JP, Sarnoff SJ, Mitchell JH, Linden RJ: Synchronicity of ventricular contraction: Observations comparing haemodynamic effects of atrial and ventricular pacing. Brit Heart J 1963; 25: 299–307.
4. Skinner NS, Mitchell JH, Wallace AG, Sarnoff SJ: Hemodynamic effects of altering the timing of atrial systole. Am J Physiol 1963; 205: 499–503.
5. Carleton RA, Passovoy M, Graettinger JS: The importance of the contribution and timing of left atrial systole. Clin Sci 1966; 30: 151–159.
6. Samet P, Castillo C, Bernstein WH: Hemodynamic sequelae of atrial, ventricular, and sequential atrioventricular pacing in cardiac patients. Am Heart J 1966; 72: 727–729.
7. Chamberlain DA, Leinbach RC, Vassaux CE, Kastor JA, DeSanctis RW, Sanders CA: Sequential atrioventricular pacing in heart block complicating acute myocardial infarction. New Eng J Med 1970; 282: 577–582.
8. Daggett WM, Bianco JA, Powell WJ, Austen WG: Relative contributions of the atrial systole-ventricular systole interval and of patterns of ventricular activation to ventricular function during electrical pacing of the dog heart. Circulation Res 1970; 27: 69–79.
9. Curtis JJ, Maloney JD, Barnhorst DA, Pluth JR, Hartzler GO, Wallace RB: A critical look at temporary ventricular pacing following cardiac surgery. Surgery 1977; 82: 888–893.
10. Hartzler GO, Maloney JD, Curtis JJ, Barhorst DA: Hemodynamic benefits of atrioventricular sequential pacing after cardiac surgery. Am J of Cardiol 1977; 40: 232–236.

11. Ogawa S, Dreifus LS, Shenoy PN, Brockman SK, Berkovits BV: Hemodynamic consequences of atrioventricular and ventriculoatrial pacing. Pace 1978; 1: 8–15.
12. Curtis JJ, Madigan NP, Whiting RB, Mueller KJ, Pezzella AT, Walls JT, Heinemann FM: Clinical experience with permanent atrioventricular sequential pacing. Ann of Thorac Surg 1981; 32: 179–187.
13. Curtis JJ, Walls JT, Madigan NP, Boley T, Reid J: Effect of varying atrioventricular contraction intervals on cardiac output in man. Surgical Forum 1982; 33: 285–287.
14. Kruse I, Arnman K, Conradson TB, Ryden L: A comparison of the acute and long-term hemodynamic effects of ventricular inhibited and atrial synchronous ventricular inhibited pacing. Circulation 1982; 65: 846–855.
15. David D, Michelson EL, Naito M, Chen CC, Schaffenburg M, Dreifus LS: Diastolic "locking" of the mitral valve: The importance of atrial systole and intraventricular volume. Circulation 1983; 67: 640–645.
16. Naito M, Dreifus LS, David D, Michelson EL, Mardelli J, Kmetzo JJ: Reevaluation of the role of atrial systole to cardiac hemodynamics: Evidence for pulmonary venous regurgitation during abnormal atrioventricular sequencing. American Heart Journal 1983; 105: 295–302.
17. Sutton R, Morley C, Chan SL, Perrins J: Physiological benefits of atrial synchrony in paced patients. Pace 1983; 6: 327–328.

Authors' address:
Prof. Dr. J. Curtis
University of Missouri
Medical Center
1 Hospital Drive
Columbia, Missouri 65212
USA

The Effect of Pacing Mode on External Work and Myocardial Oxygen Consumption

Yukihiro Koretsune, Kazuhisa Kodama, Shinsuke Nanto, Kiyomu Ishikawa, Koichi Taniura, Masayoshi Mishima, Michitoshi Inoue, Hiroshi Abe

Summary: The clinical significance of atrial kick and synchronicity of ventricular contraction when the impulse is normally propagated were evaluated by comparing the effects of atrial and ventricular pacing with the effects of A-V sequential pacing on hemodynamics, coronary circulation, and energy efficiency. Twenty-one patients with sinus bradycardia undergoing cardiac catheterization were studied. Aortic pressure, pulmonary arterial end-diastolic pressure, and cardiac output were recorded during each pacing which were performed at 60–70 per minute. Coronary sinus flow was recorded by the continuous thermodilution technique. Energy efficiency was calculated as left ventricular pressure-volume area divided by myocardial oxygen consumption. Comparing A-V sequential with ventricular pacing to evaluate the atrial kick, pulmonary arterial end-diastolic pressure did not significantly change, but mean aortic pressure and cardiac output increased in A-V sequential pacing. Coronary sinus flow and myocardial oxygen consumption didn't noticeably change. Comparing A-V sequential with atrial pacing to evaluate the synchronicity of ventricular contraction, cardiac output increased and myocardial oxygen consumption decreased significantly in atrial pacing. Energy efficiency is highest in atrial, second highest in A-V sequential, and lowest in ventricular pacing. We conclude that the atrial kick has beneficial effect on hemodynamics and the synchronicity of ventricular contraction has a saving effect on myocardial oxygen consumption.

Permanent, implanted cardiac pacemakers have been used clinically since 1959. As is common with new developments, the initial usage was restricted. In this instance, implanted cardiac pacemakers were intended primarily for ventricular stimulation in cases of complete atrioventricular block with Adams-Stokes seizures. These early pacing systems maintained a constant, regular cardiac rhythm by stimulating the ventricle asynchronously at a fixed rate.

As a fuller understanding of cardiac pacing was realized, usage expanded to include management of symptomatic bradyarrhythmias, tachyarrhythmias, and restoration of optimal hemodynamics. As a result, the operational types of artificial pacemakers evolved so that there now exists an armamentarium of atrial and ventricular pacemaker systems, each appropriate to certain pathological situations within a broad range of cardiac diseases.

It is well known that the atrial pacemaker has a beneficial effect on hemodynamics compared with a ventricular pacemaker because of the atrial kick and the ventricular synchronicity. In recent years, bradyarrhythmias combined with ischemic heart disease, in which the increase in myocardial oxygen consumption should be avoided, are many. Little is known, however, about the effects of ventricular pacing and other physiological pacing on coronary circulation and energy efficiency.

The aims of this study are to clarify the clinical significance of the atrial kick and the ventricular synchronicity respectively, from the viewpoint of energy efficiency and myocardial oxygen consumption as well as hemodynamics by comparing atrial and ventricular pacing with A-V sequential pacing.

Materials and Methods

Twenty-one patients with severe bradycardia, who were undergoing diagnostic cardiac catheterization, were studied. All of the patients signed informed consent forms before cardiac catheterization, and all agreed to have coronary sinus flow measurements performed. There were 13 men and eight women, aged 17 to 75. PQ intervals of these patients ranged from 160 to 280 msec (Table 1). Swan-Ganz catheter, ventricular pacing, and atrial pacing catheters were introduced through the right femoral vein. After systemic heparinization, pressure transducer with single lumen (Gaeltec Co. Ltd.) was inserted through the right femoral artery. Wilton-Webster thermodilution catheter with two electrodes was introduced through the left basilic vein into the coronary sinus for sampling and the measurement of coronary sinus flow. If we can use Webster catheter for coronary sinus pacing, atrial pacing catheter is not needed. After cardiac catheterization, atrial pacing, ventricular pacing, and A-V sequential pacing were carried out at random for three minutes at five minutes intervals. To analyze each parameter on physiological heart rate, each pacing was performed at 60–70 per minute and the pacing rate was fixed in each patient. When we performed DVI, A-V delay was settled at 150 msec. Hemodynamic parameters, aortic pressure, pulmonary arterial pressure, and cardiac output were recorded before pacing and every one minute to three minutes at each pacing mode. Coronary sinus blood flow measurements and paired samplings from coronary sinus and aorta were performed before and at the end of each pacing. Then, we performed left ventriculography at a 30° right anterior oblique projection in each pacing mode with simultaneous recording of left ventricular pressure in five patients.

Table 1. Subjects of this study

	Name	Age & Sex	Clinical Diagnosis	PQ Interval
1.	A.W.	54 M	I° AV Block	0.26"
2.	T.Y.	73 F	S S S	0.18"
3.	Y.M.	60 M	E A, S S S	0.16"
4.	K.T.	55 F	S S S	0.22"
5.	H.K.	20 M	S S S	0.16"
6.	M.I.	17 F	S S S	0.16"
7.	F.Y.	63 M	Hypertensive Heart	0.16"
8.	H.O.	58 F	II° AV Block	0.16"
9.	T.K.	61 F	S S S	0.18"
10.	S.O.	58 M	I° AV Block	0.26"
11.	F.S.	41 M	Chest Pain Syndrome	0.16"
12.	F.G.	56 M	S S S	0.16"
13.	F.I.	56 F	E A, S S S	0.17"
14.	M.K.	24 M	I° AV Block	0.28"
15.	S.T.	75 F	S S S	0.17"
16.	M.Y.	52 F	S S S	0.18"
17.	S.S.	64 M	S S S	0.16'
18.	T.T.	45 M	S S S	0.21"
19.	M.A.	27 M	S S S	0.16"
20.	Y.Y.	63 M	S S S	0.18"
21.	R.S.	46 M	S S S	0.20"

Myocardial oxygen consumption (MVO$_2$) and lactate uptake (LU) were calculated as follows:

$$M\dot{V}O_2 \ (ml/min) = 1.34 \times Hb \times (SaO_2\text{-}ScO_2) \times CSF/10^4$$

$$LU \ (mg/min) = (La\text{-}Lc) \times CSF/10^2$$

where Hb is hemoglobin; SaO$_2$ is O$_2$ saturation in aortic blood; ScO$_2$ is O$_2$ saturation in coronary sinus blood; La is lactate level in aortic blood; Lc is lactate level in coronary sinus blood.

The mean ± SD was determined for each variable. Data was compared by utilizing paired t-test. Probability with a value of less than 0.05 was accepted as significant.

Results

A-V sequential pacing vs ventricular pacing:

To evaluate the clinical significance of atrial kick, we compared A-V sequential with ventricular pacing (Fig. 1). Pulmonary arterial end-diastolic pressure did not significantly change (DVI vs VVI; 9.5 ± 3.1 vs 10.4 ± 3.1 mmHg, mean ± SD), but mean aortic pressure and cardiac output increased clearly in A-V sequential pacing (mean AoP; 107 ± 16 vs 101 ± 16 mmHg, CO; 4.6 ± 1.0 vs 4.1 ± 0.9 l/min). Coronary sinus flow, myocardial oxygen consumption, and lactate uptake didn't noticeably change.

These results suggest that the atrial kick has beneficial effect on hemodynamics without remarkable increase in myocardial oxygen consumption.

A-V sequential pacing vs atrial pacing:

Comparing A-V sequential with atrial pacing to evaluate the synchronicity of ventricular contraction (Fig. 2), pulmonary arterial end-diastolic pressure and mean aortic pressure did not significantly change, but cardiac output increased in atrial pacing (DVI vs AAI; 4.6 ± 1.0 vs 4.9 ± 1.0 l/min). On the other hand, coronary sinus flow and myocardial

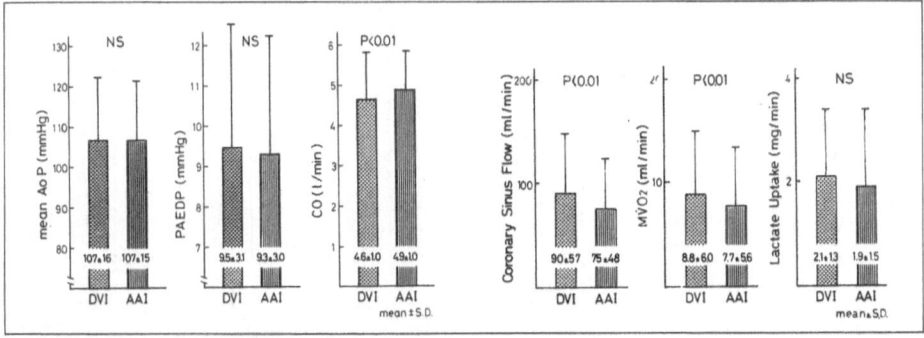

Fig. 1. A-V sequential pacing vs ventricular pacing

oxygen consumption were lower in atrial pacing (CSF; 90 ± 57 vs 75 ± 48 ml/min, MVO_2; 8.8 ± 6.0 vs 7.7 ± 5.6 ml/min, DVI vs AAI, respectively).

These results strongly suggest that the ventricular synchronicity has a beneficial effect on hemodynamics and a saving effect on myocardial oxygen consumption.

Energy efficiency of each pacing mode:

In recent years, pacemaker implantations for elderly patients associated with ischemic heart disease have increased. In these patients, it is very important to find out how much external work can be achieved with restricted coronary blood flow. So, we evaluated the energy efficiency of each pacing mode.

As the indicia of external work, we selected the left ventricular pressure-volume area. Left ventriculography at a 30° right anterior oblique projection were performed of each pacing mode with 20 ml of 76% Urografin. Simultaneously, left ventricular pressure was recorded with pressure transducer. Then, left ventricular pressure-volume relationships were analyzed and inner areas were calculated with a planimeter. We evaluated the energy efficiency of left ventricular pressure volume area divided by myocardial oxygen consumption (Fig. 3).

Atrial pacing, which has both the atrial kick and the synchronicity of ventricular contraction, was found to be the best. A-V sequential pacing, which has only the atrial kick without ventricular synchronicity was ranked second. Ventricular pacing, which has neither of them, was found to be the least effective (AAI vs DVI vs VVI; 8.5 ± 3.1 vs 6.5 ± 2.3 vs 4.4 ± 2.4 unit).

Discussion

Several investigators, by recording intraventricular pressures and cardiac output, have studied the differences in the effects of atrial and ventricular pacing on cardiac function.

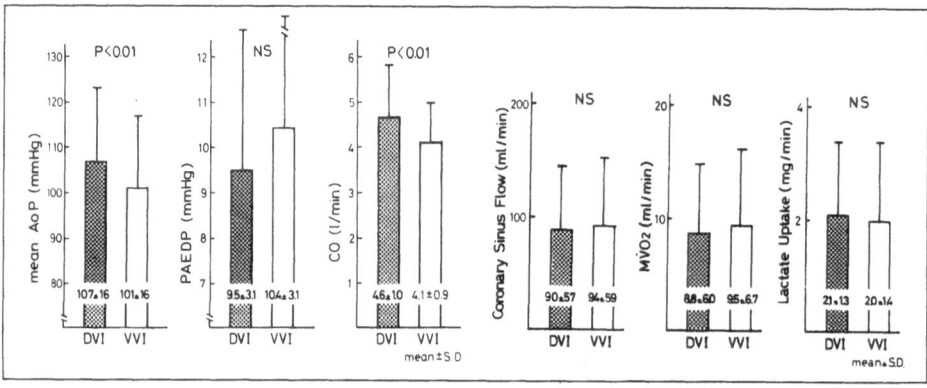

Fig. 2. A-V sequential pacing vs atrial pacing

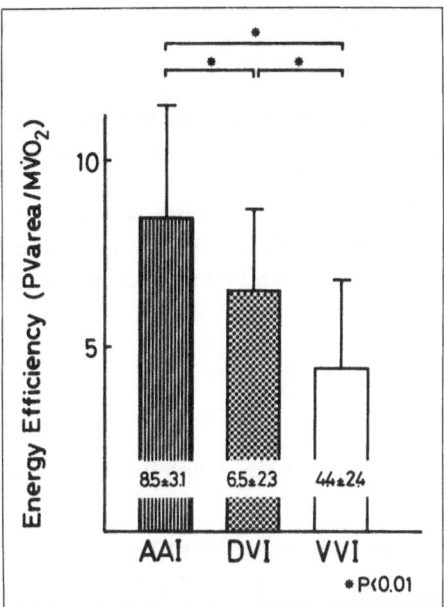

Fig. 3. Energy efficiency of three pacing modes

The differences have been explained by a less synchronous ventricular contraction or lack of atrial kick.

We examined these factors, respectively, and tried further examination on hemodynamics and left ventricular external works of these pacing modes by pressure-volume relationship.

Eber et al. said that the ventricular asynchronicity by the stimulation of ventricle has been observed associated with prolongation of systolic expansion of the ventricular cavity being localized to the site of ventricular stimulation in the ventricular premature beat or ventricular tachycardia.

Our observations suggest, however, that the ventricular asynchronous contraction by the stimulation of right ventricular apex does not obviously affect the ventricular pressure-volume relationship. On the other hand, comparing ventricular pacing with A-V sequential pacing, the atrial kick increases the cardiac output, left ventricular end-diastolic volume, and left ventricular systolic pressure. These results suggest that the atrial kick has a beneficial effect on hemodynamics, but the ventricular synchronous contraction does not provide as much of a beneficial effect.

Comparing atrial pacing with A-V sequential pacing, however, myocardial oxygen consumption is significantly lower in atrial pacing, and this means the ventricular synchronous contraction has a saving effect on myocardial oxygen consumption.

Conclusion

1. The clinical significance of atrial kick and synchronicity of ventricular contraction were evaluated from the viewpoint of hemodynamics, coronary circulation, and energy efficiency.

185

2. Comparing DVI with VVI to evaluate the atrial kick, mean aortic pressure and cardiac output increased in DVI. Coronary sinus flow myocardial oxygen consumption did not noticeably change.
3. Comparing DVI with AAI to evaluate the synchronicity of ventricular contraction, cardiac output increased and myocardial oxygen consumption decreased significantly in AAI.
4. Energy efficiency is the highest in AAI, second highest in DVI, and lowest in VVI.
5. These results lead us to conclude that the atrial kick has a beneficial effect on hemodynamics and the synchronicity of ventricular contraction has a saving effect on myocardial oxygen consumption.

References

1. Sowton E: Hemodynamic studies in patients with artificial pacemakers. British Heart J 1964; 26: 737.
2. Gilmore JP, Sarnoff SJ, Mitchell JH, Linden RJ: Synchronicity of ventricular contraction: observations comparing hemodynamic effects of atrial and ventricular pacing. British Heart J 1963; 25: 299.
3. Samet P, Castillo C, Bernstein WH: Hemodynamic sequelae of atrial, ventricular, and sequential atrioventricular pacing in cardiac patients. Am Heart J 1966; 72(6): 725.
4. Benchimol A, Liggett MS: Cardiac hemodynamics during stimulation of the right atrium, right ventricle, and left ventricle in normal and abnormal hearts. Circulation 1966; 33: 933.
5. Friesen WG, Woodson RD, Ames AW, Herr RH, Starr A, Kassebaum DG: A hemodynamic comparison of atrial and ventricular pacing in postoperative cardiac surgical patients. J Thorac Cardiovasc Surgery 1971; 55: 271.
6. Samet P, Bernstein WH, Levine S, Lopez A: Hemodynamic effects of tachycardias produced by atrial and ventricular pacing. Am J of Medicine 1965; 39: 905.
7. Eber LM, Berkovits BV, Matloff JM, Gorlin R, Cooke JM: Dynamic characterization of premature ventricular beats and ventricular tachycardias. Am J of Cardiol 1974; 33: 378.

Authors' address:
Dr. Y. Koretsune
Osaka Police Hospital
10–31 Kitayama-cho Tennoji-ku
Osaka-Shi 543
Japan

Left Ventricular Pump Function after Long-Term Treatment with Ventricular Pacing compared to Atrial Synchronous Pacing

S. K. Pehrsson, H. Åström

Summary: The effect of VVI and VAT pacing on the left ventricular pump function was determined by cardiac catheterization after long-term treatment in 9 patients with high degree heart block. Measurements were made in supine at rest, with the patients legs elevated, during steady state work and the procedure was ended with a period of stepwise increase in load of $10 \ W \times 1 \ min^{-1}$ until exhaustion (W_{max}). Function curves were constructed by plotting stroke work index (SWI) and left ventricular power index (LVPI) against left ventricular end-diastolic pressure (LVEDP).

Cardiac output (CO) increased with VAT vs VVI pacing at rest by 22% (5.5 vs 4.5 l/min, $p < 0.01$). An increased stroke volume constituted the difference (75 vs 63 ml, $p < 0.05$). The ventricular rate being the same. At W_{max} CO increased with VAT vs VVI by 40% (10.2 vs 7.3 l/min, $p < 0.01$). Atrial rate (AR), systolic aortic pressure (SP) and systemic vascular resistance (SVR) was reduced during exercise with VAT vs VVI pacing. The function curves with SWI vs LVEDP demonstrated a shift to the right with a significant decrease in SWI during exercise with VAT vs VVI, whereas LVPI vs LVEDP showed a shift to the left with a significant increase in LVPI at W_{max} with VAT vs VVI.

The changes in function curves, as the reduction in AR, SP and SVR appear to be constituted by a decrease in sympathetic activity with the VAT vs VVI.

The present study demonstrates that hemodynamic advantages with VAT pacing are still obtainable after several years of prior VVI pacing.

Cardiac catheterization was performed in order to evaluate the influence of long-term treatment with VVI and of VAT pacing on cardiac performance in patients with symptomatic high degree AV-block.

Patients

The study comprised six men and three women, mean age 60 years (range 39–72). They had been treated with VVI pacing for on average 4.2 (range 1–8) years prior to the first of two investigations, which was performed just before the change to VAT pacing. The investigative procedure was repeated 4.4 (range 2–8) months after VAT pacing was begun. The switch to VAT pacing mode was made in all cases because of complaints of impaired physical fitness.

Methods

The cardiac function was assessed by cardiac catheterization using a Swan-Ganz thermo-dilution catheter positioned in the pulmonary artery. Another catheter was placed in the left ventricle in seven of the nine patients, and in the aortic root in the other two, who had aortic valve prothesis. In these two patients the pulmonary capillary venous pressure was used as a measure of the left ventricular end-diastolic pressure.

Measurements were made with the patients in the supine position 1. at rest 2. with the legs elevated 15 cm from the table, 3. during steady-state work and 4. after a period of stepwise increase in work load ($10 \text{ W} \times 1 \text{ min}^{-1}$) until symptoms ($W_{max}$). Cardiac output was measured with thermodilution technique and at rest and during steady state work also with the Fick method. The correlation between simultaneous measurements of cardiac output with the thermodilution technique and the Fick method calculated from 32 determinations had a correlation coefficient $r = 0.82$.

Left ventricular function curves were constructed by plotting stroke work index (SWI) and left ventricular power index (LVPI) against left ventricular end-diastolic pressure (LVEDP). SWI and LVPI were calculated according to the formulas $SWI = (LVSP-LVEDP) \times SV \times C \times BSA^{-1}$ (J/beat/m² BSA) and $LVPI = SWI \times HR \times \frac{1}{60}$ (W/m² BSA) where BSA = body surface area (m²), HR = heart rate (beats/min), LVSP = left ventricular systolic pressure (mmHg), LVEDP = left ventricular end-diastolic pressure (mmHg), SV = stroke volume (ml), C = constant = 1.33×10^{-4}.

Relative heart volume (ml/m² BSA) was measured on chest x-ray in the erect position (1).

Results

Physical working capacity (W_{max}) during catheterization in the supine position was 12 per cent greater with VAT than with VVI pacing ($p < 0.05$). The relative heart volume was

Fig. 1. Relation between the atrial rate (AR) at rest during VVI pacing and the increase in cardiac output ($\varDelta \dot{Q}$) during exercise following a change from VVI to VAT pacing.

$$\varDelta \dot{Q} = \frac{\dot{Q}_{VAT} - \dot{Q}_{VVI}}{\dot{Q}_{VVI}} \times 100$$

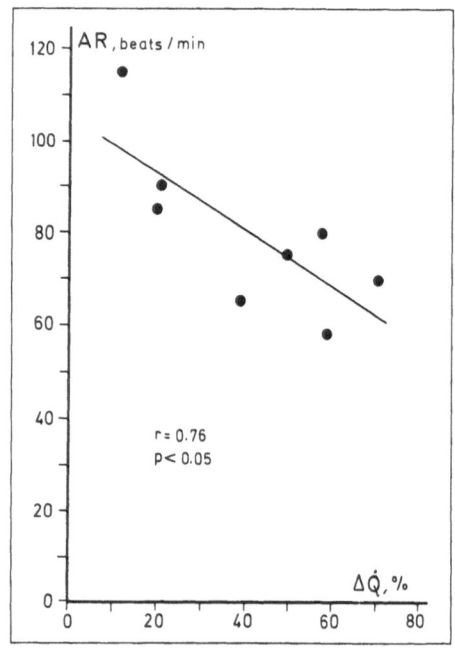

Table 1. Hemodynamic data in 9 patients with VVI vs VAT pacing.

	At rest			Legs elevated			Steady state exercise			Maximum work load		
	VVI	VAT	(p)	VVI	VAT	(p)	VVI	VAT	(p)	VVI	VAT	(p)
Work load (W)							43 ±10	43 ±10	(NS)	75 ±33	84 ±34	(<0.05)
Atrial rate (beats/min)	79 ±17	74 ±14	(NS)	81 ±15	73 ±15	(<0.05) ±12	124 ±12	109 ±15	(<0.01)	145 ±15	133 ±18	(<0.05)
Ventricular rate (beats/min)	72 ±3	74 ±14	(NS)	71 ±4	73 ±15	(NS)	73 ±4	108 ±15	(<0.001)	71 ±3	130 ±15	(<0.001)
Cardiac output (l/min)	4.5 ±1.5	5.5 ±1.6	(<0.01)	5.4 ±1.4	5.8 ±1.8	(NS)	6.1 ±2.0	8.3 ±1.9	(<0.001)	7.2 ±1.0	10.2 ±2.5	(<0.01)
Stroke volume (ml)	63 ±21	75 ±18	(<0.05)	75 ±20	78 ±18	(NS)	87 ±29	79 ±25	(NS)	100 ±13	77 ±21	(<0.01)
Arterio-venous oxygen difference (ml/min)	55 ±8	47 ±6	(0.01)				128 ±18	106 ±4	(<0.001)			
Oxygen uptake (ml/min)	238 ±40	253 ±58	(NS)				779 ±195	881 ±177	(<0.02)			
Left ventricular systolic pressure (mm Hg)	140 ±21	146 ±19	(NS)	157 ±25	159 ±15	(NS)	191 ±21	172 ±17	(<0.02)	200 ±13	190 ±12	(<0.01)
Left ventricular end-diastolic pressure (mm Hg)	12 ±3.3	11 ±2.7	(NS)	15 ±2.5	18 ±4.6	(NS)	28 ±4.3	28 ±8.6	(NS)	35 ±2.8	33 ±9.2	(NS)
Mean right atrial pressure (mm Hg)	7 ±1.1	5 ±1.7	(<0.01)	9 ±1.5	8 ±1.3	(<0.01)	15 ±2.5	12 ±3.6	(NS)	15 ±2.7	14 ±3.1	(NS)
Pulmonary artery systolic pressure (mm Hg)	25 ±5	26 ±7	(NS)	31 ±6	30 ±6	(NS)	52 ±7	49 ±7	(NS)	53 ±10	57 ±10	(NS) ±11
Stroke work index (J/beat m² BSA)	0.73 ±0.30	0.73 ±0.13	(NS)	1.00 ±0.50	0.80 ±0.16	(NS)	1.27 ±0.48	0.92 ±0.21	(<0.05)	1.28 ±0.18	1.05 ±0.28	(<0.05)
Left ventricular power index (W/m² BSA)	0.86 ±0.30	0.91 ±0.27	(NS)	1.2 ±0.57	1.0 ±0.36	(NS)	1.49 ±0.62	1.58 ±0.54	(NS)	1.52 ±0.18	2.18 ±0.74	(<0.05)
Systolic vascular resistance (dynes-sec-cm⁻⁵)	3300 ±697	2520 ±498	(<0.001)							1480 ±508	1000 ±474	(<0.001)

reduced from 476 to 430 ml/m² BSA (p < 0.001). Hemodynamic mean values are presented in Table 1. Cardiac output at rest was higher with VAT than with VVI pacing (5.5 v. 4.5 l/min, p < 0.01), and increase of 22 per cent. As the ventricular rate at rest was the same with both modes of pacing, an increased stroke volume was responsible for the difference in cardiac output (75 v. 63 ml, p < 0.05). The increase in stroke volume at rest probably reflected the contribution of a properly timed atrial systole. The arteriovenous oxygen difference was lower with VAT versus VVI pacing (47 vs 55 ml/l, p < 0.01).

During exercise cardiac output rose with both types of pacing. With VVI the rise was attributable to an increase in stroke volume and with VAT to an increase in heart rate. The increase in cardiac output during exercise was significantly larger with VAT than with VVI, at W_{max} the difference was 40 per cent. The arteriovenous oxygen difference decreased during submaximal steady state work from 128 ml/l with VVI to 106 ml/l with VAT pacing (p < 0.001).

Left ventricular end-diastolic pressure was not affected by the change from VVI to VAT pacing, either at rest or during exercise. Systolic aortic pressure and systemic vascular resistance were significantly lower during work with VAT vs VVI pacing. The atrial rate during exercise likewise was significantly lower with AT.

The resting atrial rate with VVI pacing showed good inverse correlation (r = 0.76, p < 0.05) to the improvement in cardiac output during exercise after the change to VAT pacing (Fig. 1).

The left ventricular function curve, SWI plotted as a function of LVEDP showed during exercise a shift to the right after the change to VAT pacing (Fig. 3). The curve with LVPI as a function of LVEDP, on the other hand, showed a significantly higher LVPI at W_{max} during VAT than during VVI pacing, as a result of the heart rate increase (Fig. 2).

Fig. 2. Mean left ventricular function curves for patients on VVI pacing (full line) and after change to VAT pacing (broken line). The lower part illustrates the relationship between left ventricular end-diastolic pressure (LVEDP) and stroke work index (SWI) and the upper part the relationship between LVEDP and left ventricular power index (LVPI). (The data represent in each curve from left to right 1) rest, 2) legs up, 3) steady state exercise and 4) W_{max}.)

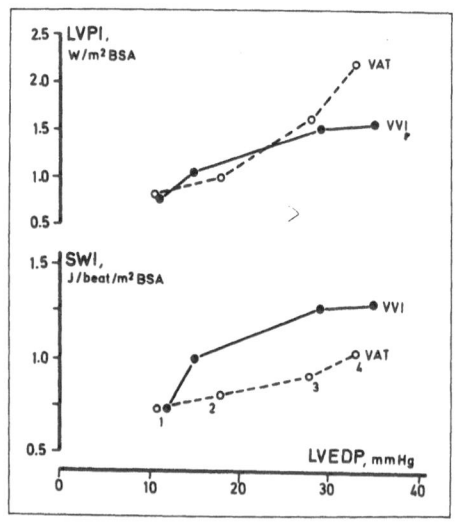

190

Discussion

The short-term improvement in hemodynamic performance at rest achieved with properly timed atrial systole has been well documented (2–6). In these studies the cardiac output at rest rose 10 to 25 per cent when A-V synchrony was restored. It has been suggested that in many cases the acute deleterious effects of loss of atrial contraction are only temporary and can be relatively rapidly overcome by adaptational mechanisms (7). Other authors, however, found that improvement after a change from VVI to VAT mode persisted both at rest and during exercise at reevaluation three months later (5, 6).

Proposals for curves to describe left ventricular function were based on experimental animal studies (8), in which ventricular stroke work was recorded over a range of atrial or ventricular end-diastolic pressures. A "familiy" of such curves was considered to reflect a spectrum of contractile states, with the relative position of a given curve providing a description of ventricular contractility. The path of the curve represents a Frank-Starling effect, with complex interaction between preload, afterload and contractility. Displacement of such a curve upward (= to the left) or downward (= to the right) signifies, respectively, positive and negative inotropic effects, i.e. augmentation or depression of contractility.

The changes in the left ventricular function curves in the present study may thus be interpreted as an increase in contractility during VVI pacing, possibly due in turn to a higher sympathetic activity, as indicated by the higher atrial rate during exercise with VVI compared with VAT pacing. However, despite the reduction in stroke work with VAT versus VVI pacing the ability to increase heart rate with VAT resulted in an increased power – heart work/min; i.e. LVPI.

The study demonstrated that hemodynamic advantages with VAT pacing are still obtainable after several years of VVI pacing. The improvement after transition to VAT was evidenced by improved physical working capacity and increased cardiac output. The atrial rate at rest during VVI pacing showed a good inverse correlation ($r = 0.76$, $p < 0.05$) with the increment in cardiac output during steady state exercise after the change to VAT pacing. The mechanism might be that patients with a higher atrial rate than pacing rate at rest are in fact underpaced and thus have to compensate their relatively low pacing rate by an increased stroke volume in an attempt to adjust cardiac output to their metabolic demands. Such a compensatory increase in stroke volume is probably mediated by an increased sympathetic activity that is higher at any load in these patients compared to those with an atrial rate at rest similar to their pacing rate. What these patients with a high atrial rate then gain in heart rate after a change to VAT pacing they lose in stroke volume, resulting in only a slight or moderate increase in cardiac output. Patients with an atrial rate at rest similar to their pacing rate may, on the other hand, indicate that they are well adapted to that rate and may therefore exploit the advantages of VAT pacing without any marked lose in stroke volume during exercise.

However, even though the correlation is significant the atrial rate is not good enough as a predictor of cardiac output improvement because of the scatter (Fig. 1).

In conclusion the present study demonstrates that hemodynamic advantages with VAT pacing are still obtainable after seval years of prior VVI pacing. The implication thereof is that in connection with replacement of the pulse generator in patients with VVI pacing and in sinus rhythm, change to VAT should always be considered if physical working performance is reduced because of circulatory limitations.

References

1. Jonsell S: A method for the determination of the heart size by teleroentgenography (A Heart Volume Index). Acta Radiol 1939; 20: 325–48.
2. Center S, Nathan DA, Wu C-Y, Samet P, Keller W: The implantable synchronous pacer in the treatment of complete heart block. J Thorac Cardiovasc Surg 1963; 46: 744–54.
3. Karlöf I: Haemodynamic effect of atrial triggered versus fixed rate pacing at rest and during exercise in complete heart block. Acta Med Scand 1975; 197: 195–206.
4. Ogawa S, Dreifus LS, Shenoy PN, Brockman SK, Berkovits VB: Hemodynamic consequences of atrioventricular and ventriculoatrial pacing. Pace 1978; 1: 8–15.
5. Kappenberger L, Gloor HO, Babotai J, Stenbrunn W, Turina M: Hemodynamic effects of atrial synchronization in acute and long-term ventricular pacing. Pace 1982; 5: 639–45.
6. Kruse I, Arnman K, Conradson T-B, Rydén L: A comparison of the acute and long-term hemodynamic effects of ventricular inhibited and atrial synchronous ventricular inhibited pacing. Circula tion 1982; 65: 846–55.
7. Sowton E, Thorburn C, Roy P: Haemodynamic changes during cardiac pacing. Proceedings of the IVth International Symposium on Cardiac Pacing. Van Gorcum Assen, 1973.
8. Sarnoff SJ, Berglund E: Ventricular function. Starling's law of the heart studied by means of simultaneous right and left ventricular function curves in the dog. Circulation 1954; 9: 706–18.

Authors' address:
Dr. K. Pehrsson
Division of Cardiology
Department of Medicine
Thoracic Clinics
Karolinska Hospital
Stockholm/Sweden

Underestimation of Stroke Volume (SVI) and Cardiac Index (CI) by TM-Echocardiography during Ventricular Pacing

B. Maisch, K. Kochsiek

Summary: Left ventricular function can be assessed precisely by TM-echocardiography. During ventricular pacing, however, abnormal septal motion is observed regularly. To determine if stroke volume (SVI) and cardiac index (CI) can be assessed correctly by echocardiography during ventricular pacing, both indices were measured by thermodilution and simultaneous echocardiography in ten patients during ventricular and atrial pacing. From TM-echocardiography volume measurements were computed according to Teichholz et al. During ventricular pacing the cardiac index was reduced by $13.8 \pm 11.8\%$, the stroke volume index by $15 \pm 13.2\%$ as measured by thermodilution. The correlations between thermodilution and echocardiography were $r = 0.87$ for SVI and $r = 0.92$ for the CI, respectively, during spontaneous sinus rhythm. By atrial pacing with 100 and 120 bpm the correlation coefficients were still $r = 0.84$ and $r = 0.85$ for SVI and CI, respectively. During ventricular pacing echocardiography regularly underestimated the SVI by $26.8 + 14\%$ and the CI by $20.6 \pm 14.1\%$, thus giving less stronger correlations ($r = 0.83$). This was primarily due to an underestimation of the endsystolic left ventriculard diameter. Consequently, left ventricular fraction of shortening and computed ejection fraction were also grossly underestimated. A correction factor of 1.27 for SVI and 1.21 for CI during ventricular pacing is suggested to correct the respective TM-echocardiographically computed indices.

Introduction

One and two dimensional echocardiography provide a precise and reproducible method for the assessment of left ventricular function. In a number of cases abnormal septal motion is observed e.g. after cardiac surgery (1, 2), pericardial effusion (3, 4, 5), right ventricular overload (6, 7), Wolff-Parkinson-White syndrome (8, 9, 10, 11), and left bundle branch block (12). It can be observed regularly in patients with VVI-pacemakers, since ventricular pacing causes an early excitation of the apex. Consequently, abnormal septal motion occurs. In these patients the enddiastolic and endsystolic diameters do not necessarily represent the true performance of the entire left ventricle (2, 11).

It was therefore the purpose of this study to answer the following questions:

1. Can abnormal septal motion be observed regularly during ventricular pacing?
2. Does abnormal septal motion cause underestimation of stroke volume and cardiac index when assessed by TM-echocardiography?
3. Is it feasible to correct the proposed underestimation by a correction factor?

Patients and Methods

The study included 10 patients (7 coronary artery disease with minor stenosis and without infarction, 1 dilated cardiomyopathy , 2 normal coronary arteries and ventricular volumes) who underwent routine heart catheterisation. In all patients the cardiac index

193

was measured by thermodilution at sponteneous rate, and at 100 and 120 bpm during atrial and ventricular stimulation by a stimulation catheter. (Retrograde conduction was observed in 3 of the 10 patients.) Simultaneously TM-echocardiography was performed from the 3rd or 4th intercostal space on an Irex II (Kontron) or on a Varian 3400 DPDM (Sonotron). Three measurements were evaluated by thermodilution. The echocardiographic measurements (enddiastolic and endsystolic diameters) were measured according to the recommendations of the American Society for Echocardiography (leading edge) by two independent observers. Three measurements of one diameter were taken, the mean was calculated and used only when the interobserver variability was less than 10%. Volume estimations from TM-echocardiography were made using the formula proposed by Teichholz et al. 1976 (13): [V = (LVID)³ × 7 : (2,4 + LVID); V = Volume, LVID = left ventricular inner diameter]. They were compared with the corresponding data obtained by thermodilution. Linear regression analysis was performed to compare data obtained by thermodilution or by echocardiography.

Fig. 1. During ventricular pacing the cardiac index (CI) and the stroke volume index (SVI) are significantly reduced when compared to atrial pacing (CI: $p < 0.001$, SVI: $p < 0.001$).

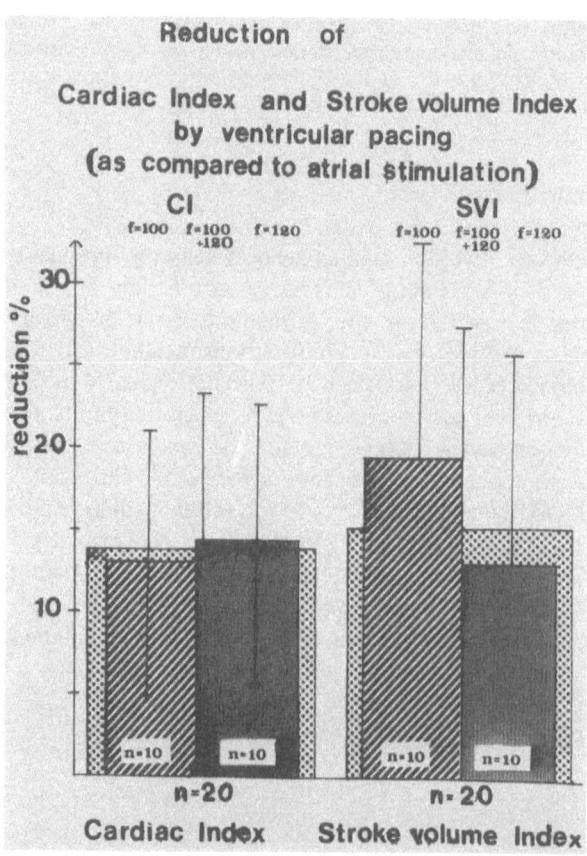

194

Results

Abnormal septal motion is observed in ventricular pacing regularly. During ventricular pacing the cardiac and the stroke volume indices were diminished. At 100 bpm the reduction of the CI was $13.6 \pm 10.9\%$, at 120 bpm $14.1 \pm 12.1\%$. Since the difference at both rates was insignificant data were combined. They added up to a reduction of $13.8 \pm 11.8\%$ for the cardiac index. Similarly the stroke volume index was reduced by $19.1 \pm 12.1\%$ at 100 bpm and by 13.5 ± 12.1 at 120 bpm. The reduction of the SVI for both rates was $15.8 \pm 13.9\%$, when ventricular pacing was compared to atrial stimulation (Fig. 1).

There was a good correlation between the cardiac indices measured by thermodilution and echocardiography (Fig. 2 left side; $y = 1.12 x + 0.19$; $r = 0.92$) and the computed stroke volume indices (Fig. 2 right side; $y = 0.72 x + 9.82$, $r = 0.87$) at spontaneous rate. When CI and SVI during atrial pacing were compared to the same indices during ventricular stimulation, the correlations were less strong for ventricular pacing: At 100 bpm the correlations of CI and SVI during atrial pacing were comparable to those at spontaneous rate (CI: $r = 0.91$; SVI: $r = 0.89$), but worse, when measured during ventricular pacing (CI: $r = 0.73$; SVI: $r = 0.72$, Fig. 3a). At 120 bpm correlations between the CI and SVI assessed by thermodilution and echocardiography during atrial pacing were also excellent (CI: $y = 1.13 x + 0.4$; $r = 0.91$; SVI: $y = 1.13 x + 0.23$; $r = 0.92$), whereas during ventricular pacing a shift of the curve to the left was observed and correlations were worse (CI: $y = 0.81 x - 0.17$; $r = 0.83$; SVI: $y = 0.81 x - 1.4$; $r = 0.83$; Fig. 3b).

In an overall assessment of the percent underestimation of stroke volume and cardiac indices by TM-echocardiography the SVI was underestimated by $26.8 \pm 14.0\%$ and the CI by $20.6 \pm 14.1\%$. Although the standard deviation of this underestimation is fairly large a correction factor of 1.27 for SVI and of 1.21 for CI computations during ventricular pacing may be helpful, since it is evident, that in patients with abnormal septal motion the fraction of shortening or the ejection fraction assessed or computed by TM-echocardiography is too low. It can be normalized only by employing the respective cor-

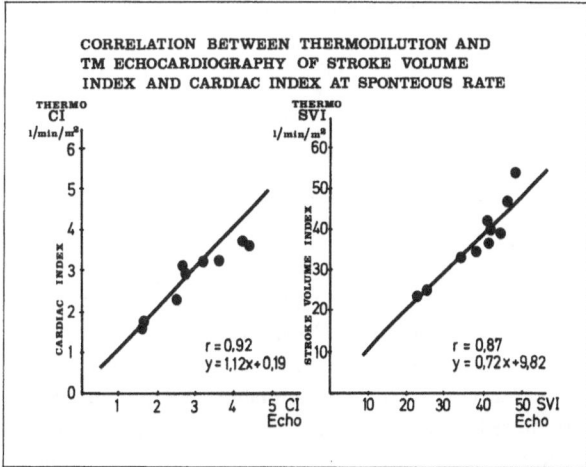

Fig. 2. There is a good correlation between the different methods of assessing stroke volume and cardiac indices.

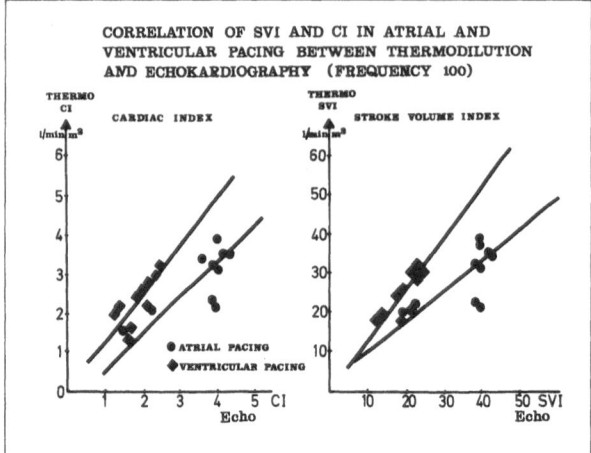

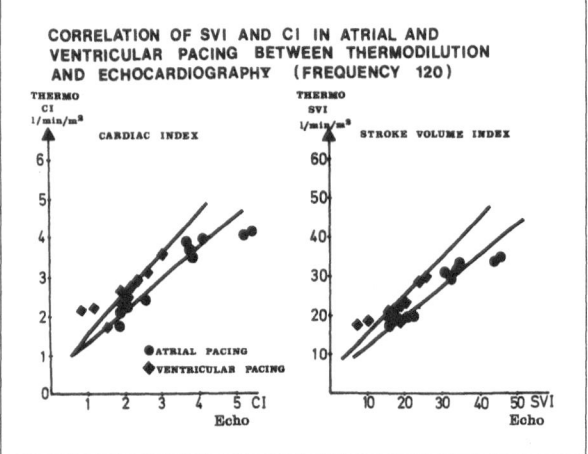

Fig. 3.a/b By ventricular pacing the regression curves of the cardiac and stroke volume indices are shifted to the left indicating the underestimation of both parameters by TM-echocardiography by frequencies of 100 bpm (a) and 120 bpm (b).

rection factors. It is obvious that the underestimations of both indices by TM-echocardiography are due to a falsely measured endsystolic left ventricular diameter.

Discussion

Abnormal septal motion is the cause of problems in the determination of volumes and diameters as assessed by TM-echocardiography (2, 11, 13). It has therefore been proposed that changes in left atrial dimension could be helpful in the determination of the true fraction of shortening or ejection fraction (2, 5, 11) in these patients, since abnormal septal motion can be due to several causes e.g. pericardial effusion (3, 4), right ventricular overload (6, 7), Wolff-Parkinson-White syndrome (9, 12). This possibility is not feasible when volume and cardiac indices are computed. Thus an estimate of the proper correction, that should be made, was attempted in patients who underwent ventricular and atrial pacing. It could be demonstrated that a factor for SVI and CI can be computed, which helps to correct the underestimation caused by abnormal septal motion in patients with a ventricular pacemaker.

References

1. Burggraf GW, Craige E: Echocardiographic studies of left ventricular wall motion and dimensions after valvular heart surgery. Am J Cardiol 1975; 35: 473–480.
2. Maisch B, Kochsiek K: Beziehung zwischen linksatrialer Amplitudenänderung und linksventrikulärer Verkürzungsfraktion im TM-Echokardiogramm. Z Kardiol 1981; 70: 347 (Abstract).
3. Cosio FG, Martinez JP, Serrano CM, de la Calzada C, Alcaine CC: Abnormal septal motion in cardiac tamponade with pulsus paradoxus – Echocardiographic and hemodynamic observations. Chest 1977; 71: 787–789.
4. D'Cruz IA, Cohen HC, Prabhu R, Glick G: Diagnosis of cardiac tamponade by echocardiography – Changes in mitral valve motion and ventricular dimensions, with special reference to paradoxical pulse. Circulation 1975; 52: 460–465.
5. Maisch B: Echokardiographische Diagnostik der Herzinsuffizienz. Der Kassenarzt 1982; 22: 2546–2569.
6. Hagan AD, Francis GS, Sahn DJ, Karliner JS, Friedman WF, O'Rourke RA: Ultrasound evaluation of systolic anterior septal motion in patients with and without right ventricular volume overload. Circulation 1974; 50: 248–254.
7. Weyman AE, Wann S, Feigenbaum H, Dillon JC: Mechanism of abnormal septal motion in patients with right ventricular volume overload: A cross-sectional echocardiographic study. Circulation 1976; 54: 179–186.
8. Chandra MS, Kerber RE, Brown DD, Funk DC: Echocardiography in Wolff-Parkinson-White syndrome. Circulation 1976; 53: 943–946.
9. Hishida H, Sotobata I, Koike Y, Okumura M, Mizuno Y: Echocardiographic patterns of ventricular contraction in the Wolff-Parkinson-White syndrome. Circulation 1976; 54: 567–570.
10. Ticzon AR, Damato AN, Caracta AR, Russo G, Foster JR, Lau SH: Interventricular septal motion during preexcitation and normal conduction in Wolff-Parkinson-White syndrome. Am J Cardiol 1976; 37: 840–847.
11. Maisch B, Kochsiek K: Assessment of left ventricular function by changes in left atrial dimension (submitted).
12. Abbasi AS, Eber LM, McAlpin RN, Kattus AA: Paradoxical motion of interventricular septum in left bundle branch block. Circulation 1974; 49: 423–427.
13. Teichholz LE, Kreulen T, Herman MV, Gorlin R: Problems in echocardiographic volume determinations: Echocardiographic-angiographic correlations in the presence or absence of asynergy. Amer J Cardiol 1976; 37: 7–11.

Authors' address:
Dr. B. Maisch
University Hospital of Internal Medicine
Josef-Schneider-Str. 2
D-8700 Würzburg
Federal Republic of Germany

Study of the Left Ventricular Performance During Sequential and Ventricular Pacing by Quantitative Two Dimensional Echocardiography

J. Creplet, A. Sartieaux, P. Bohyn, F. Achkar, J. Sacre, J. L. Adda, I. Azancot, D. De Mey*

Summary: The purpose of our work is to evaluate the response of the left ventricular end-diastolic volume (EDV), stroke volume (SV), ejection fraction (EF), and blood pressure (BP), to sequential (S), and ventricular (V) pacing. Five patients, two women and three men, aged 74 ± 3 (mean ± 1 SD) years, were studied by quantitative two dimensional echocardiography (Q2DE) during S and V at 80, 100 and 120 beats/min. EDV, SV, and EF were calculated using Simpson's Rule on a four chamber view. Samples of 3 to 10 (mean 5) volumes were obtained at each rate for the two pacing modes. The results at 80–100–120/min are for EDV: 95–95–78 ml in S ($p = 0.01$), 76–75–70 ml in V (NS). For SV: 58–58–44 ml in S ($p = 0.05$), and 46–43–38 ml in V (NS). EDV is higher in S at 80 ($p = 0.02$), and 100/min ($p = 0.05$); SV is higher in S at each frequency ($p = 0.02$). EF is unaffected by frequency and pacing mode. BP is unchanged with frequency, buth higher in S at 80 and 120/min. We conclude that Q2DE is a promising tool to study the hemodynamic effects of pacing. In patients with normal or subnormal EF, the hemodynamic advantages of sequential pacing are better filling and better SV of the LV, without change of EF.

Introduction

The hemodynamic effects of different pacing modes have been studied by several techniques: catheterization (1, 2), radionuclide ventriculography (3), and systolic time intervals (4). M mode echocardiography has been used to assess the effects of atrial pacing on the left ventricle (5). Quantitative two-dimensional echocardiography is a promising technique for the non-invasive evaluation of left ventricular volume and ejection fraction (6). It has been applied in the study of left ventricular function during arrhythmias in the dog (7). Nevertheless, at this time, quantitative two-dimensional echocardiography has not been used to appreciate the hemodynamic effects of pacing. This can be partly attributed to difficulties in the practical utilisation of the method: lack of accepted standards for endocardium recognition, systematic underestimation of the left ventricular volume, and tedious, time-consuming analysis of the signal. In a program having as its first purpose an evaluation of the validity of quantitative two-dimensional echocardiography, we tested the sensitivity of this technique to changes in left ventricular volume and ejection fraction. These changes were induced by accelerating the heart rate in ventricular and A-V sequential pacing modes.

---

* With the technical assistance of I. Deboeck.

Methods

Study group: Five patients, two women and three men, aged 70 to 77 years (mean 74) were selected for the study on the basis of the following criteria: the implantation of a programmable dual-chamber pacemaker for greater than one week, the absence of clinical signs of ischemic heart disease and heart failure, and the possibility of recording a high quality echocardiogram in the four chamber view. Indication for pacing was sinus node disease in three cases; carotid sinus syncope and bradycardia, trifascicular block and syncope in the two others.

Cardiac pacing: two series of pacing were performed at 80–100–120 beats/min, one in ventricular (VVI), and the other in sequential (DVI, A-V 150 msec) mode, without any preferential order. The duration of the stimulation at each frequency was fixed at two minutes. A delay of ten minutes separated the two modes, to allow for the recovery of the basal conditions. The echocardiogram and the blood pressure were registered during the second minute of each step.

Two-dimensional echocardiography: Real-time two-dimensional echocardiography was performed with a wide-angle rotary mechanical sector scan (ATL Mark 5). Care was taken to place the patient in an optimal position, in order to obtain a satisfactory apical 4 chamber view. The orientation of the exploratory plane was adjusted to visualise the longest mitral-apical length, the largest mitral annulus diameter, and the maximal amplitude of movement of the mitral valve.

Analysis of the data: the echocardiograms were recorded on a VHS videorecorder, Panasonic NV 8200. The best sequences were registered from this record to a video-disc, Sony SVM 1010. The video-disc allows a frame by frame, backward and forward analysis of a signal of 10 sec duration, and gives an optimal fixed image.

The end-diastolic and end-systolic endocardium of the ventricle in a 4 chamber view was outlined on a transparent sheet. End-diastole (ED) was taken at the largest cavity area,

Fig. 1. Example of digitized end-diastolic and end-systolic endocardium of the left ventricle in 4 chambers view. Left: sequential mode – Right: ventricular mode. Frequency: 80/min. The numbers refer to an analysis of the regional function not taken into consideration for this study. Scale ½.

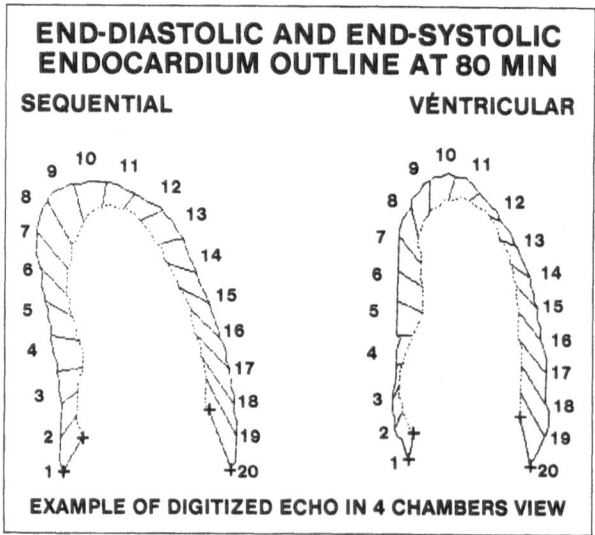

END-DIASTOLIC AND END-SYSTOLIC ENDOCARDIUM OUTLINE AT 80 MIN

SEQUENTIAL   VÉNTRICULAR

EXAMPLE OF DIGITIZED ECHO IN 4 CHAMBERS VIEW

just before the closure of the mitral valves; end-systole (ES) at the smallest area on the descending part of the T wave. After introduction of the scale, the ED and ES contours were traced on a HP 9874A digitizer, interfaced with a HP 9845B calculator with 64 K octets of central memory. The left ventricular volumes were calculated using Simpson's integration rule, reconstructing the ventricular geometry by 30 circular slices, perpendicular to the long axis. Fig. 1 shows an example of digitized 4 chamber view. Samples of 3 to 10 (mean 5) values were obtained at each step, and their mean retained as the measured value.

Statistical analysis: To study the effect of frequency in the same pacing mode, we used a two way analysis of variance, associated with Duncan's method to compare the means (8). The significance of the difference between the two pacing modes was examined by a paired t-test.

Table 1. End-diastolic and end-systolic volumes (ml).

EDV						ESV					
80		100		120		80		100		120	
S	V	S	V	S	V	S	V	S	V	S	V
73	53	68	56	53	49	24	19	24	18	17	16
101	74	100	62	79	74	23	19	26	21	26	23
95	66	98	69	85	68	46	27	45	34	39	35
89	82	98	92	76	78	43	37	35	40	40	41
116	104	110	97	96	81	49	47	54	49	48	46
M 95	76	95	75	78	70	37	30	37	32	34	32
p 0.02		0.05				0.05					

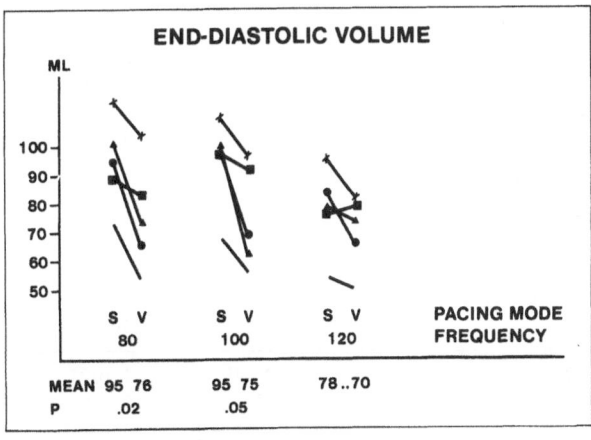

Fig. 2. Comparison of end-diastolic volumes during sequential (S) and ventricular (V) pacing at 80, 100, 120/min. . . . refers to the analysis of variance in studying the effects of frequency; p refers to the effects of pacing mode.

Results

EDV and ESV are presented in Table 1. EDV in the sequential mode diminishs from 95 ml at 80 and 100/min, to 78 ml at 120/min (p = 0.01).

In the ventricular mode, there is no significant reduction of EDV with frequency: 76 ml at 80/min, 75 ml at 100/min, and 70 ml at 120/min.

EDV is higher in the sequential mode at 80/min (p = 0.02), and at 100/min (p = 0.05). ESV is not affected by the frequency in either pacing mode. ESV is slightly higher in the sequential mode at 80/min (p = 0.05). EF remains unaffected by the frequency and pacing modes: 61% in either mode at 80/min, 62% in the sequential, and 58% in the ventricular mode at 100/min and 57 and 55% at 120/min, respectively. SV (Fig. 3) follows the evolution of EDV (Fig. 2): reduction from 58 ml at 80 and 100/min, to 44 ml at 120/min in the sequential mode (p = 0.05); slight reduction, insignificant, from 46 ml at 80/min to

Fig. 3. Comparison of stroke volumes during sequential (S) and ventricular (V) pacing at 80, 100, 120/min. ... refers to the analysis of variance on the effects of frequency; p refers to the effects of pacing mode.

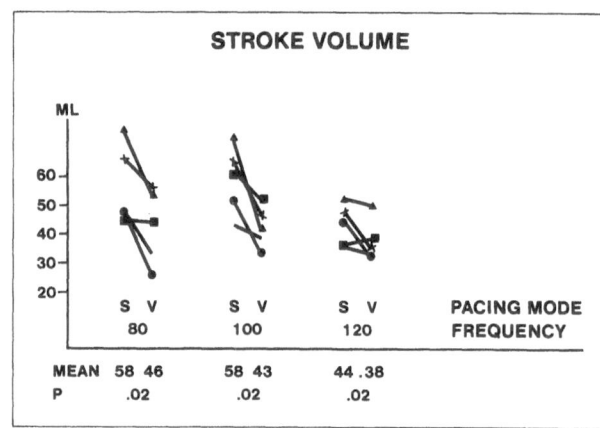

Table 2. Blood pressure (mm Hg).

80		100		120	
S	V	S	V	S	V
134/81	127/80	140/84	124/83	128/91	117/84
99	96	103	97	103	95
130/80	116/74	128/88	126/80	127/92	107/80
97	92	101	95	104	89
125/72	121/72	121/76	122/77	125/81	97/74
90	88	91	92	96	82
105/74	100/64	107/76	112/76	111/76	97/76
88	76	86	88	88	83
150/86	117/92	147/95	127/88	139/98	131/89
107	103	112	101	112	103
M 129/79	116/76	127/86	122/81	126/88	110/81
96	90	99	95	101	90

43 ml at 100/min, and 38 ml at 120/min in the ventricular mode. SV remains significantly higher in the sequential mode (p = 0.02) at each frequency.
Systolic and mean blood pressure (Table 2) are unaffected by the frequency, but slightly higher in the sequential mode at 80 min (p = 0.05), and 120/min (p = 0.05).

Discussion

The accuracy of volume determination by two-dimensional echocardiography has been appreciated most often by comparison with angiography and radionuclide ventriculography (9, 10, 11). In vitro studies on models (12) and beating hearts (13) were also performed. Another important aspect to be considered in validating a quantitative method is its sensitivity to the changes induced by acute or chronic interventions. In this study, we used ventricular and sequential pacing at 80, 100, and 120/min to assess the response of EDV, ESV, SV, and EF, measured by Simpson's rule on 4 chamber views.
This method is based upon the geometric assumption that sections perpendicular to the long axis are circular.
The object of the study being to observe changes in the same patient, the effects of errors on this assumption can be neglected.
Table 3 resumes the conclusions of this study. They are in agreement with the results obtained by other methods. The reduction of EDV at a high rate, with little change in EF, has been observed with radionuclide ventriculography (3) and M mode echocardiography (5). Hung (3) also demonstrated the reduction of stroke volume. Nevertheless, the studied frequency was higher (160/min). Toss (14) and Benchimol (15) observed the constancy of heart output with frequency, thus implying a reduction of stroke volume. The hemodynamic advantages of the sequential pacing mode have been demonstrated on the blood pressure and the cardiac output (2). The higher EDV and SV, and the unchanged EF, are confirmed by isotopic studies (3). Due to the little number of selected patients, these results can only be considered as preliminary. The determinants and clinical significance of better filling and better stroke volume with sequential pacing remain to be defined.
Nevertheless, these results demonstrate that quantitative two dimensional echocardiography can be a useful tool to assess some hemodynamic effects of different pacing

Table 3. Conclusions.

Variable	Effects of frequency from 80 to 120/min		Effects of pacing mode from S to V		
	S	V	80	100	120
EDV	−18**	=	−27**	−18*	=
SV	−24**	=	−31**	−14**	−8**
EF	=	=	=	=	=
BP	=	=	↘*	↘*	

Changes are expressed in %.

modes. Unfortunately, the tedious and time-consuming treatment of the data, in the actuel state of the art, precludes and extensive use of this method. Much is expected of automatic processing of two-dimensional echocardiograms in the near future to resolve this problem (16).

References

1. Kappenberger L, Gloor HO, Babotai I, Steinbrunn W, Turina M: Hemodynamic effects of atrial synchronization in acute and longterm ventricular pacing. Pace 1982; 5: 639–645.
2. Fananapazir L, Srinivas V, Bennett DH: Comparison of resting hemodynamic indices and exercise performance during atrial synchronized and asynchronous ventricular pacing. Pace 1983; 6: 202–209.
3. Hung J, Kelly DT, Hutton BF, Uther JB, Baird DK: Influence of heart rate and atrial transport on left ventricular volume and function: relation to hemodynamic changes produced by supraventricular arrhythmia. Am J Cardiol 1981; 48: 632–638.
4. Whiting RB, Madigan NP, Heinemann FM, Curtis JJ, Reid J: Atrioventricular sequential pacing: comparison with ventricular pacing using systolic time intervals. Pace 1983; 6: 242–246.
5. De Maria AN, Neumann A, Schubart PJ, Lee G, Mason DT: Systematic correlation of cardiac chamber size and ventricular performance determined with echocardiography during alterations in heart rate in normal persons. Am J Cardiol 1979; 44: 447–451.
6. Henry WL: Evaluation of ventricular function using two-dimensional echocardiography. Am J Cardiol 1982; 49: 1319–1323.
7. Uchiyama T, Corday E, Meerbaum S, Lang TW, Gueret P, Povzhitkov M, Peter T: Characterization of left ventricular mechanical function during arrhythmias with two dimensional echocardiography. I Premature ventricular contractions. Am J Cardiol 1981; 48: 679–689.
8. Duncan DB: A Bayesian approach to multiple comparisons. Technometrics 1965; 7: 171–222.
9. Folland ED, Parisi AF, Moynihan PF, Jones DR, Feldman LL, Tow DE: Assessment of left ventricular ejection fraction and volumes by realtime, two-dimensional echocardiography. A comparison of cineangiographic and radionuclide techniques. Circulation 1979; 60: 760–766.
10. Schiller NB, Acquatella H, Prots TA, Drew D, Goerke J, Ringertz H, Silverman WH, Brundage B, Botvinick EH, Boswell R, Carlsson E, Parmley WW: Left ventricular volume from paired biplane two-dimensional echocardiography. Circulation 1979; 60: 547–555.
11. Starling MR, Crawford MH, Sorensen SG, Levi B, Richards KL, O'Rourke RA: Comparative accuracy of apical biplane cross-sectional echocardiography and gated equilibrium radionuclide angiography for estimating left ventricular sizef and performance. Circulation 1981; 63: 1075–1084.
12. Erbel R, Krebs W, Henn G, Schweizer P, Richter HA, Meyer J, Effert S: Comparison of single-plane and biplane volume determination by two-dimensional echocardiography. Asymmetric model heart. Eur Heart J 1982; 3: 469–480.
13. Weiss JL, Eaton LW, Kallman CH, Maugham WL: Accuracy of volume determination by two-dimensional echocardiography: defining requirements under controlled conditions in the ejecting canine left ventricle. Circulation 1983; 67: 889–895.
14. Ross J, Linhart JW, Braunwald E. Effect of changing heart rate in man by electrical stimulation of the right atrim. Circulation 1965; 32: 549–558.
15. Benchimol A, Liggett MS. Cardiac hemodynamics during stimulation of the right atrium, right ventricle and left ventricle in normal and abnormal hearts. Circulation 1966; 33: 933–944.
16. Garcia E, Gueret P, Bennett M, Corday E, Zwehl W, Meerbaum S, Corday S, Swan HJC, Berman D: Real time computerization of two-dimensional echocardiography. Am Heart J 1981; 101: 783–792.

Authors' address:
Dr. J. Creplet
I Bracops Hospital, Av. Dr. Huet 79
1070 Brüssel, Belgium

Mitral Valve Function and Cardiac Dimensions During Ventricular (VVI) and Sequential Atrio-Ventricular (DVI) Pacing. Echocardiographic Study

G. Gershony, B. Goldman, E. Noble, C. Pollick

Summary: We studied 16 patients with implanted multiprogrammable DVI pacemakers, utilizing M-mode and two dimensional (2D) echocardiography, during DVI and VVI pacing.
Left ventricular dimensions in both systole and diastole were significantly larger during DVI pacing compared to VVI ($p < 0.001$). Conversely left atrial (LA) dimensions were significantly smaller during DVI pacing compared to VVI ($p < 0.001$). The duration of "effective" mitral valve opening (MVO) was significantly longer during DVI pacing ($p < 0.001$). All patients demonstrated septal dyssynergy during right ventricular pacing, regardless of the mode. Atrial competition was a frequent finding during DVI pacing and this correlated with an ineffective atrial kick demonstrated echocardiographically.

Introduction

DVI permanent pacemakers have been implanted in Europe and North America since the late 1970's. The proponents of this type of pacing have stressed the importance of maintaining atrio-ventricular (A–V) synchrony to optimize cardiac hemodynamics (1, 2). With the advent of more stable atrial electrodes it is probable that a larger proportion of atrial leads are effectively capturing the atria. Nevertheless it is often difficult to tell from the 12-lead ECG whether or not an atrial pacer stimulus is actually depolarizing the atria. Furthermore electrical atrial depolarization may not be associated with effective mechanical atrial systole.

The effectiveness of atrial systole can be easily ascertained echocardiographically. Anterior mitral valve leaflet motion can identify the presence of an atrial kick by the presence of an "a" wave (3).

Previous hemodynamic studies of A–V sequential pacers have been done mainly in the acute situation and many of the results have been inconclusive. We chose echocardiography to compare DVI to VVI pacing because it is a totally non invasive method of assessing left ventricular function and cardiac dimensions, is especially useful for analyzing intracardiac structures such as the mitral valve and is particularly well suited to performing serial studies on ambulatory patients with permanently implanted pacemakers.

Methods

Patient Selection: 16 patients with multiprogrammable dual chamber pacemakers implanted at Toronto General Hospital were selected according to the following criteria. (a) Indication for pacing – complete heart block (CHB) or sinus node dysfunction. (b) No known valvular or myocardial dysfunction. (c) Absence of atrial fibrillation or underlying left bundle branch block (LBBB), because of its independent effect on LV wall motion.

Patients selected had either committed DVI pacemakers (Intermedics-Cyberlith, Paceset-ter-Programmalith) or DDD pacemakers (Medtronic-Versatrax, Cordis-Sequicor) pro-grammed to DVI mode.

Protocol

Each patient was programmed to rates of 70 and 90 bpm in DVI and VVI mode respec-tively. In each patient the pacemaker was programmed to a rate of 30 bpm to determine their underlying rhythm.

During each pacemaker program the patient was allowed to achieve a steady state for ap-proximately 20 minutes.

12-lead ECG

Each patient had a 12-lead ECG performed in DVI mode at a rate of 70 bpm.

Echocardiography

M-mode and 2-D echocardiograms were performed using a commercially available real-time, wide angle (90°) phased array sector scanner and a 2.5 or 3.5 MHz transducer (Hewlett Packard 77020A). Standard echocardiographic examinations were performed with the patient in the supine and/or left decubitus positions. A simultaneous ECG in the optimal lead demonstrating atrial depolarization was recorded during the study.

Echocardiographic Measurements

1. *Mitral Valve Function*
Each M-mode echocardiogram was analyzed for: (a) The presence and pattern of the "a" wave. (b) The duration of effective MVO ie. the time (secs) from the "D" point to the point of "effective" closure.
Effective closure was defined as the "C" point or the coaptation or near coaptation (with-in 2 mm) point of the mitral valve in mid diastole associated with the pattern of persis-tent mitral valve coaptation or near coaptation for the remainder of diastole (figure 1).

2. *Cardiac Dimensions*
Each echocardiogram was analyzed for: (a) Maximal LA dimension, (b) left ventricular end-systolic (LVES) dimension, (c) left ventricular end-diastolic (LVED) dimension.
Each measurement was carried out during three separate cardiac cycles and the average value was then used.
The simultaneous 2-D echocardiogram was used to ascertain that all M-mode studies were carried out in the standard planes.

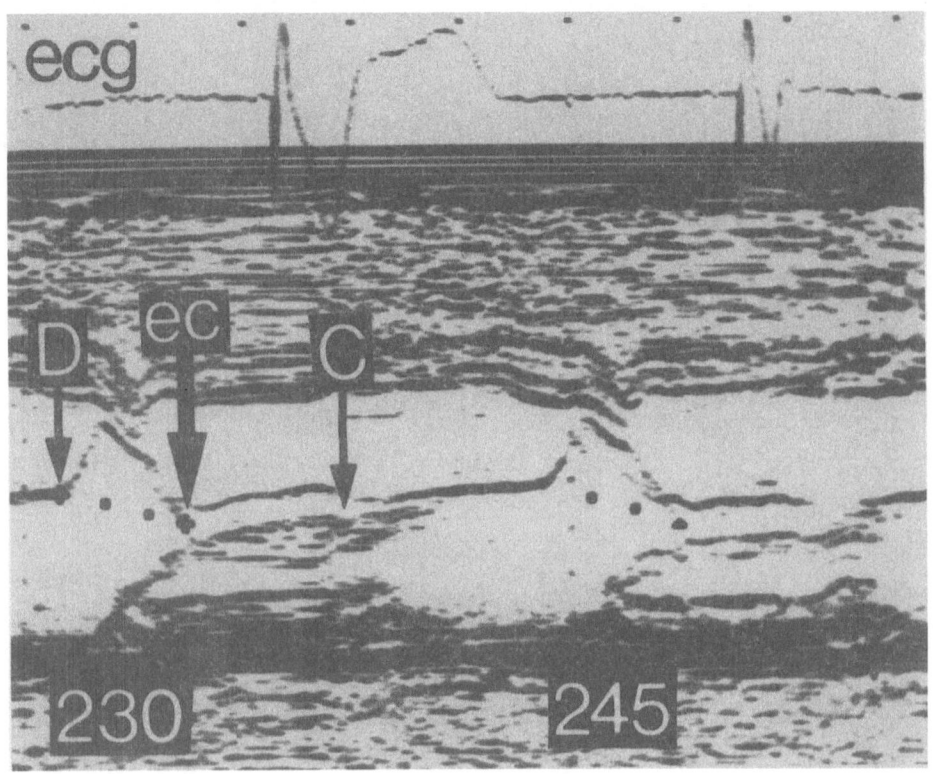

Fig. 1. (a) M-mode echo at the level of the mitral valve during VVI pacing at a rate of 70 bpm. The duration of "effective" mitral valve opening (MVO) is measured from the "D" point to the "EC" (effective closure) point (large arrow). Note that the mitral valve is effectively closed after the "EC" point (C point (small arrow) refers to the "true" closure point). The mitral valve closes prematurely prior to the QRS complex (ECG).

Table 1

	DVI	VVI	p-value	DVI	VVI	p-value
HR (bpm)	70	70		90	90	
LA (cm)	3.6 ±0.5	3.9 ±0.6	0.001	3.5 ±0.5	3.9 ±0.5	0.001
LVED (cm)	5.0 ±0.7	4.4 ±0.7	0.001	4.8 ±0.7	4.4 ±0.08	0.001
LVES (cm)	3.9 ±0.8	3.5 ±0.8	0.001	3.7 ±0.9	3.5 ±0.9	0.01
EMVO (sec)	0.45±0.08	0.31±0.09	0.001	0.32±0.07	0.27±0.05	0.01

EMVO – Effective Mitral Valve Opening
HR   – Heart Rate
LA   – Left Atrium
LVED – Left Ventricular End Diastolic
LVES – Left Ventricular End Systolic

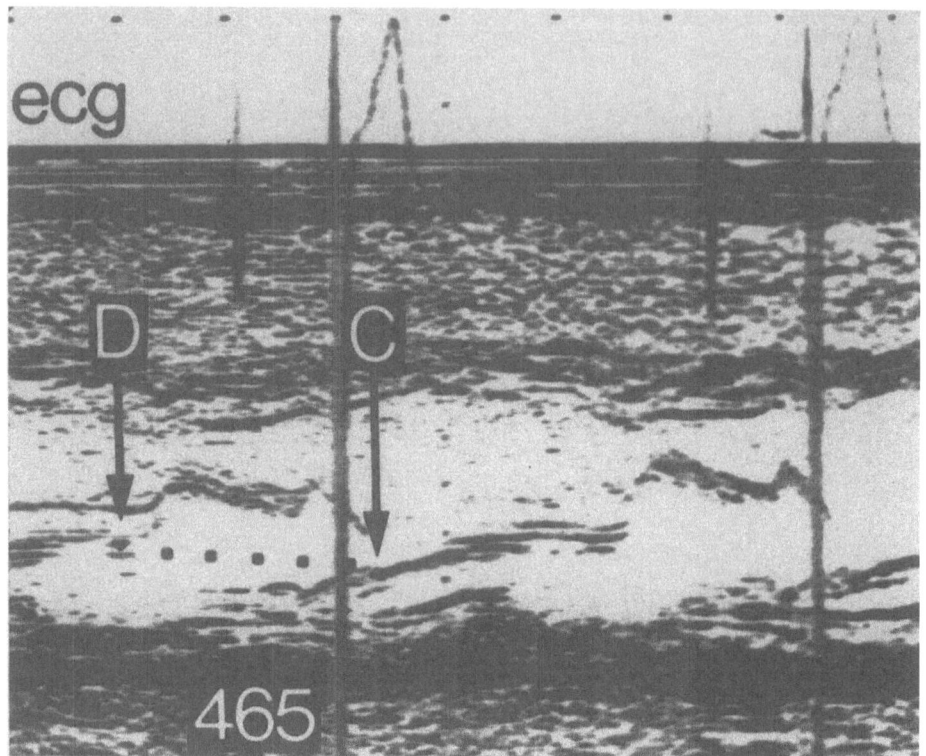

Fig. 1. (b) M-mode echo at the level of the mitral valve during DVI pacing at a rate of 70 bpm in the same patient. Note the significantly longer duration of effective mitral valve opening (465 vs. 230 ms).

3. *Regional Wall Motion*
Studies with sufficient detail of endocardial motion throughout the cardiac cycle were assessed qualitatively from the 2D echocardiogram.

Statistical Analysis: This was performed using the paired t-test.

Results

1. *Mitral Valve Function*
(a) The duration of "effective" MVO was significantly longer during DVI pacing at the heart rates tested ($p < 0.001$ for 70 bpm and $p < 0.01$ for 90 bpm) (Table 1).
The mitral valve echocardiogram demonstrated a pattern of "premature closure" during VVI pacing (figure 1).
(b) Atrial competition was a common finding during DVI pacing. Two patients had over 50% of their cardiac cycles complicated by atrial competition.
M-mode echocardiography shows that there are two distinct types of atrial competition (figure 2). Both result in ineffective atrial systole and resultant shortening of the "effective" MVO duration.

208

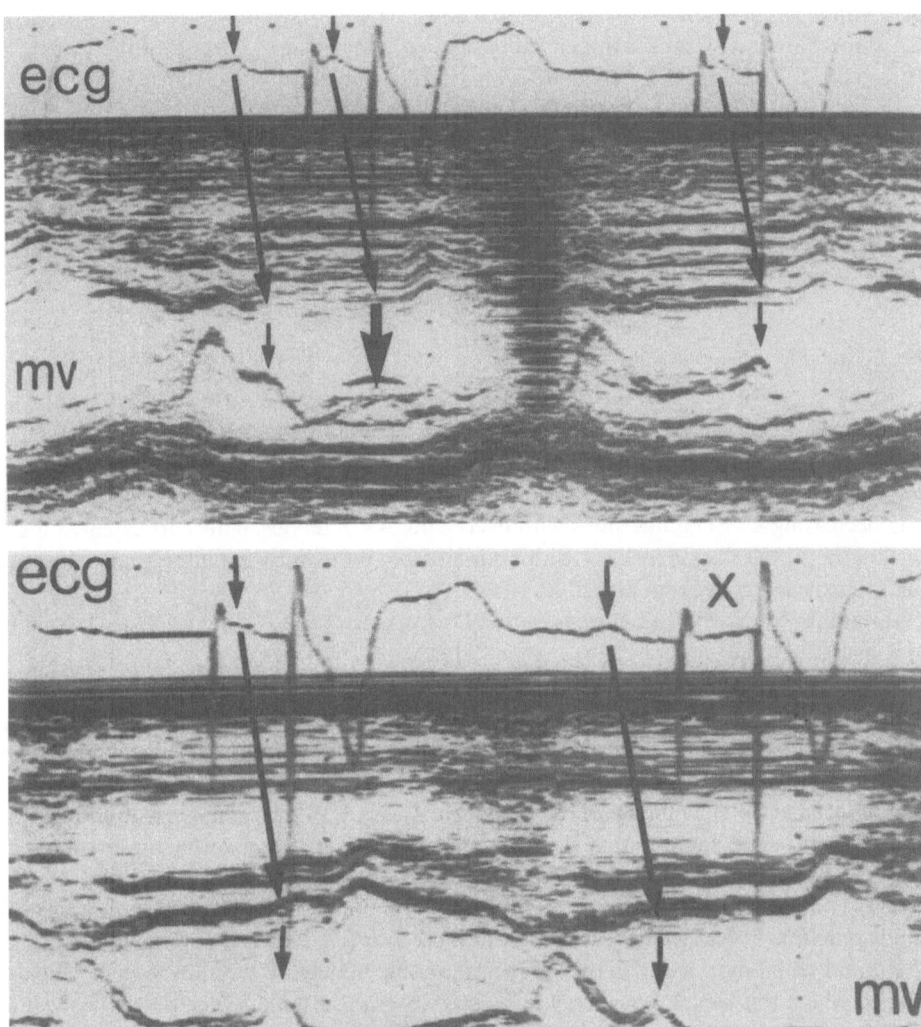

Fig. 2. (a) M-mode echo at the level of the mitral valve during DVI pacing. The ECG is at the top (ECG). There are two cardiac cycles. In the first cycle the top arrows refer to the sinus node "p" wave and the pacemaker "p" wave respectively. Note that the sinus "p" wave is associated with an early blunted "a" kick followed by premature closure of the mitral valve. This is Type I atrial competition during DVI pacing.

The second cardiac cycle shows "normal" DVI function.

(b) M-mode echo at the level of the mitr al valve during DVI pacing. There are two cardiac cycles, the second cycle shows Type II atrial competition. Note the second arrow at the top, which shows a sinus node "p" wave followed by the atrial pacemaker spike. There is no pacemaker "p" wave (X). The duration of mitral valve opening is much shorter in the second cardiac cycle. The first cardiac cycle shows "normal" DVI function.

2. *Cardiac Dimensions*

LA dimensions were significantly smaller during DVI pacing regardless of the heart rate (p < 0.001). LVED and LVES dimensions were significantly larger during DVI pacing (p < 0.001 and p < 0.01 respectively) (Table 1).

3. *Wall Motion*

All patients demonstrated varying degrees of septal dyssynergy during RV pacing regardless of the mode of pacing. Ten patients assessed during sinus rhythm showed normalization of septal motion.

Discussion

Naito et al described the typical mitral valve motion and alterations of LVED and LA end-systolic dimensions with varying A–V and V–A intervals utilizing M-mode and 2-D echocardiography in dogs. They found a definite trend towards increasing LA dimensions and decreasing LVED dimensions with decreasing AV intervals. This correlated with deterioration in the hemodynamics with an increasing pulmonary capillary wedge pressure and decreasing cardiac output (4).

Our findings comparing dimensions during DVI pacing to those during VVI pacing are in agreement with the work of Naito et al.

The fact that ventricular dimensions are larger during DVI pacing and LA dimensions are smaller suggest that during A–V sequential pacing there is better ventricular filling and atrial emptying and therefore the potential for improved cardiac performance based on the Starling mechanism (5).

The associated finding of longer MVO duration during DVI pacing appears to fit with the above findings and suggests that the improved ventricular filling during atrial systole in DVI pacing keeps the mitral valve effectively open for a longer period of diastole.

Reeves et al described abnormal patterns of septal motion during RV pacing utilizing M-mode echo (6). These findings are similar to those found in patients with LBBB (7).

We found septal dyssynergy to be a universal finding in patients with RV pacing. The degree to which this septal dyssynergy influences cardiac output and hemodynamics is unknown at present. However it is possible to speculate that in some patients particularly those with non-compliant ventricles, symptoms of low output post pacemaker implantation i.e. "the pacemaker syndrome" may occasionally be a result of this phenomenon.

The lack of atrial sensing during DVI pacing results in atrial competition in patients with an intact sinus node. We found this to be a particularly common problem during DVI pacing. Echocardiographically we have described two types of atrial competition. Both result in significant shortening of the duration of "effective" MVO. Atrial competition may also lead to arrhythmias such as atrial fibrillation which are particularly deleterious in patients with aortic stenosis or I.H.S.S.

Conclusion

Atrio-ventricular pacing improves ventricular filling and therefore cardiac performance by allowing active atrial emptying with longer effective mitral valve opening.

The lack of atrial sensing during DVI pacing leads to frequent atrial competition with potentially unfavourable hemodynamic consequences secondary to ineffective atrial contraction. This problem can be mitigated by the use of pacemakers with atrial sensing (eg. DDD pacing). Finally RV pacing is universally associated with septal dyssynergy with uncertain consequences. It therefore seems prudent that when pacing is indicated in patients with intact A–V nodes that normal conduction pathways to the ventricles should be preserved.

References

1. Samet P, Costello C, Bernstein WH: Hemodynamic sequelae of atrial, ventricular and sequential atrio-ventricular pacing in cardiac patients. Am Heart J, 1966; 72: 725–729.
2. Ogawa S, Dreifus LS, Shenoy PN, Brockman SK, Berkovits BV: Hemodynamic consequences of atrioventricular and ventriculo-atrial pacing. Pace 1978; 1: 8–15.
3. Feigenbaum H: Echocardiography. Philadelphia: Lea & Febiger, 1981; 76.
4. Naito M, Dreifus LS, Mardelli TJ, Chen CC, David D, Michelson EL, Marcy V, Morganroth J: Echocardiographic features of atrioventricular and ventriculo-atrial conduction. Am J Cardiol 1980; 46: 625–633.
5. Starling EH: Linacre Lecture of the Law of the Heart (1915) London, Longmans Green and Co. Ltd, 1918.
6. Reeves WC: Echocardiographic evaluation of intracardiac pacing catheters: M-mode and 2-D Studies. Circulation 1978; 58: 1049–1056.
7. Dillon JC, Chang S, Feigenbaum H: Echocardiographic manifestations of LBBB. Circulation 1974; 49: 876–880.

Authors' address:
G. Gershony, M.D.
Toronto Western Hospital
Department of Medicine
399 Bathurst Street
Toronto, Canada M5T 2S8

Comprehensive Evaluation of Ventricular Function During Physiological Pacing

P. Liu, R. J. Burns, R. D. Weisel, L. Mickleborough, B. S. Goldman, P. R. McLaughlin

Summary: To assess the effects of the various modes of physiological pacing on left ventricular volume and hemodynamics, we studied 12 pts (age 52 ± 4 yrs) who had intramyocardial tantalum markers implanted at the time of coronary bypass surgery. Left ventricular (LV) end-diastolic volume (EDV) and ejection fraction (EF) were determined from cinefluoroscopic tantalum marker ventriculograms, validated with contrast angiography.

Thermodilution cardiac output (CO) and LV systolic pressure (LVSP) were recorded at rest and after 2 min of pacing, in atrial (AP), ventricular (VP), and A-V sequential (AVP) modes with varying A-V intervals (AVI) and pacing rates (HR). Results were as follows:

Mode	AVI (sec)	CO (L/min)			EDV (ml)		
HR (bpm)		90	110	130	90	110	130
AP		7.6*	7.6*	7.6*	117	108	102
AVP	.10	7.2	7.9	7.5	116	115	110
	.14	7.5*	7.7*	8.0*	119	112	103
	.18	8.1	7.7	7.9	119	111	106
VP		6.4*	6.1*	6.1*	117	112	108

* $p < 0.05$ between VP and AVP or AP

LVSP decreased with VP, as compared to AP and AVP ($p < 0.05$). EF did not differ amongst the different modes and rates of pacing.

Conclusion: 1. Compared to AP and AVP, VP produced adverse effects on LV hemodynamics with decreases in CO and LVSP; 2. CO decreased during VP, but EDV and EF did not change significantly, implying that the decrease in CO was due to asynchronous ventricular contraction with possible mitral regurgitation; 3. There were no significant differences in LV volume and hemodynamics between AP and AVP at various AVI; 4. These data support the functional benefits of physiological pacing.

"Physiological pacing", in the context of preserving the atrio-ventricular synchrony, has recently received a great deal of attention due to the presumed hemodynamic benefits of the preservation of A-V synchrony, and the present availability of a wide variety of "physiological pacemakers". This mode of pacing has been recommended for an increasing number of clinical situations (1, 2), including complete heart block (3), post myocardial infarction (4), post-operative cardiovascular surgery (5, 6), aortic stenosis (7, 8), ischemic heart disease, and congestive heart failure, etc. Unfortunately very few comprehensive documentation exists today to critically evaluate the actual physiological benefits offered by this type of pacing.

We have thus undertaken to compare systematically the left ventricular hemodynamics and function during atrial, ventricular and A-V sequential modes of pacing in the same group of patients. First, we examined these variables during ventricular pacing and compared them with that during "physiological" modes of atrial and A-V sequential pacing. Then we compared within the physiological modes of atrial pacing and A-V sequential pacing, the effects on hemodynamics by varying the heart rate and A-V interval.

In order to assess left ventricular volumes accurately without repeated contrast angiograms, we studied a group of patients with implanted tantalum markers at the time of coronary bypass surgery. This method was originally developed and validated by Ingels et al. (9, 10) at Stanford University, and subsequently applied clinically by McLaughlin (11). Analysis of motion of each marker will allow the calculation of ventricular volumes and ejection fraction during each pacing parameter.

Patients

Twelve patients were selected for the study. Patients must meet the following eligibility criteria prior to entry into the study:
1. Uncomplicated course post bypass surgery;
2. Totally asymptomatic post-op clinical status, and off all cardiac medications;
3. Relatively normal ventricular function as judged clinically and by tantalum markers;
4. Absence of valvular disease or cardiomyopathy.

Method

Tantalum Marker Insertion

All patients underwent coronary bypass surgery with saphenous vein grafts, using standard hypothermia and hyperkalemic cardioplegic techniques. Prior to sternal closure, 9 small tantalum coils (1.5 mm × 0.8 mm) were inserted into mid-left ventricular myocardium along the anterior and posterior aspects of ventricular septum using a special applicator. The markers thus would outline the left ventricular cavity when projected in a 30° RAO position (Fig. 1).

Pacing Protocol

Approximately 8–12 weeks post-op, patients with markers who fitted the eligibility criteria returned to the catheterization laboratory for pacing studies. At the time of catheterization, a Swan-Ganz thermodilution catheter was positioned in the pulmonary artery, with cardiac output measured by an automated computer in triplicate and averaged. A left ventricular pigtail catheter was also introduced to measure LVEDP and LV systolic pressure. Temporary bipolar pacing electrodes were passed via the femoral vein, and were positioned in the vicinity of right ventricular apex and right atrial appendage respectively. The pacing catheters were then connected to an external A-V demand sequential

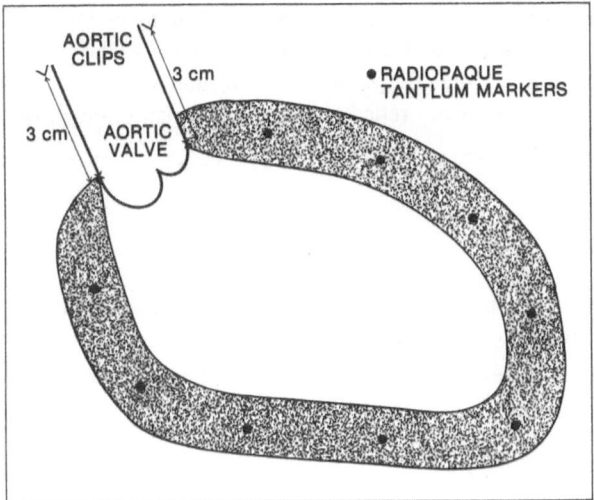

Fig. 1. Midmyocardial tantalum markers positioned to outline the left ventricle in an RAO 30° view.

pulse generator. Tantalum marker cinefluorograms were recorded in an RAO 30° position at 60 frames/second for 3 consecutive cardiac cycles.

Patient then had recordings of cardiacd output, LVEDP, LV systolic pressure and tantalum cinefluorograms at rest, and after 2 minutes of pacing in atrial, ventricular and A-V sequential pacing modes, at pacing rates of 90, 110 and 130/min. During A-V sequential pacing, A-V interval was systematically varied at 0.10, 0.14, and 0.18 seconds, as allowed by patient's native A-V interval.

Tantalum marker cinefluorograms were then validated at the end of procedure with contrast angiography using Kennedy-Dodge's single plane area-length method for LV volume determination. End-diastolic and end-systolic frames were then identified, and the corrected marker cinefluorograms then allowed the calculation of end-diastolic volume (EDV), end-systolic volume (ESV) and ejection fraction.

Results

Patients

There was a total of 12 patients, 11 males and 1 female, with a mean age of 52 ± 4 years. All patients demonstrated normal left ventricular function with normal wall motion and patent bypass grafts at the time of the study. There was an average of 2.67 grafts constructed in this group of patients.

Cardiac Output

Thermodilution cardiac output at the various pacing parameters were displayed in figure 2. Cardiac output during ventricular pacing was significantly lower than atrial or A-V sequential pacing at all pacing rates (p < 0.05). However, there was no significant differ-

215

ence found in cardiac output amongst atrial and A-V sequential pacing at various A-V intervals, even though for each individual patient, there definitely existed a "best" A-V interval to optimize the cardiac output. Cardiac output did not continue to increase with increasing heart rate in each pacing mode, likely reflecting an already maximum cardiac output for a given physiological demand.

End-Diastolic Volume

End-diastolic volumes at various pacing parameters are displayed in Table 1. EDV did not differ significantly in the variuos modes in each of the pacing rates. However, with increasing heart rate in each pacing mode, likely reflecting an already maximum cardiac output for a given physiological demand.

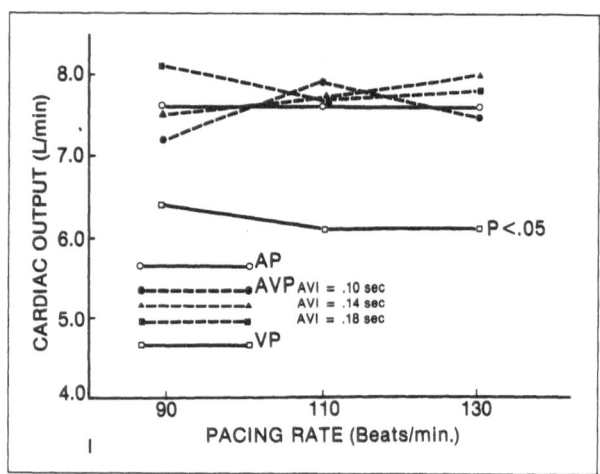

Fig. 2. Thermodilution cardiac output at various rates and modes of pacing. (AP = Atrial Pacing; AVP = A-V Sequential Pacing; AVI = A-V Interval; VP = Ventricular Pacing).

Table 1. End-diastolic volume* (ml) at various modes and rates of pacing.

Heart rate (bpm)		90	110	130
Mode	AVI (sec)			
Atrial		117±31	108±22	102±21
A–V sequential	.100	116±23	115±21	110±19
	.140	118±26	112±23	103±17
	.180	118±28	111±23	106±23
Ventricular		117±34	112±21	108±20
Control (NSR)		(118±25)		

* Data listed as: Mean±S.D.; AVI = Atrio-Ventricular Interval; NSR = Normal Sinus Rhythm.

Left Ventricular Systolic Pressure

LV systolic pressures were plotted in Figure 3. The systolic pressure, as in cardiac output, fell significantly during ventricular pacing at all rates. However there was again no significant difference amongst the physiological modes of pacing, i.e. atrial and A-V sequential modes. None of the patients however was symptomatic during ventricular pacing.

Ejection Fraction

Ejection fraction as calculated from tantalum marker end-diastolic and end-systolic frames were tabulated in Table 2. No significant difference in ejection fraction existed amongst the different modes of pacing or A-V interval. Despite decrease in EDV with increasing rates of pacing, ejection fraction did not rise significantly as might be expected.

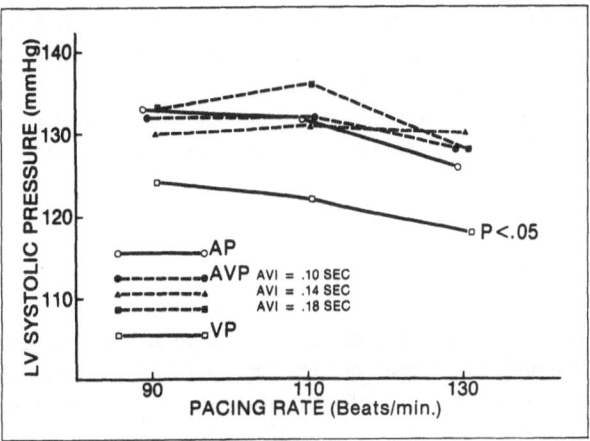

Fig. 3. Left ventricular systolic pressure at various rates and modes of pacing (Abbreviations as in Fig. 2).

Table 2. Ejection fraction* (%) at various modes and rates of pacing.

Heart rate (bpm)		90	110	130
Mode	AVI (sec)			
Atrial		63± 9	60± 8	62±11
A–V sequential	.100	65± 7	60± 9	61± 7
	.140	64± 7	59± 7	59± 8
	.180	62± 7	62±12	59± 8
Ventricular		62± 9	62± 7	61± 7
Control (NSR)		(62± 7)		

* Data listed as: Mean±S.D.; AVI = Atrio-Ventricular Interval; NSR = Normal Sinus Rhythm.

Discussion

The concept of "physiological pacing" with the preservation of atrio-ventricular synchrony has been introduced more than a decade ago, but has been slow in gaining acceptance due to the lack of proof of benefit and the complexity of the pacemaker hardware and expense.

Contribution of Atrial Systole

Investigators have long recognized that the contribution of atrial systole is especially relevant in rapid heart rates and "non-compliant" ventricles, where passive diastolic filling is often impaired in the absence of atrial systole (6, 7, 13, 14, 15). In the setting of acute myocardial infarction and heart block, Chamberlain (4) has demonstrated an average increase of cardiac output by A-V sequential pacing, and Kroetz (7) also demonstrated increased stroke volume and increased cardiac index by A-V sequential pacing in aortic stenosis.

Physiological pacing is also important in the setting of post-cardiac surgery to optimize cardiac output. Curtis (5) has demonstrated a decrease of cardiac output up to 42% by ventricular pacing, whereas atrial pacing will increase cardiac output by an average of 13%, and A-V sequential pacing by 19%. Hartzler (6) in an elegant study also demonstrated the physiological benefits of atrial and A-V sequential pacing post-op, especially in patients with aortic valve disease. Hilton et al. (16) from our institution has in addition demonstrated a decrease in ejection fraction and increased lactate production with ventricular pacing, but not atrial pacing, further attesting to the adverse effects of ventricular pacing.

However in the presence of normal cardiac function, controversy reigns over the true atrial contribution. Benchimol (17) demonstrated little hemodynamic advantage of atrial systole in patients with normal hearts. Carlton (13) in addition claimed that in mitral stenosis, atrial contribution is not significant in consequence. On the other hand, Samet (18) has shown clearly the hemodynamic benefits of physiological pacing in normal hearts. From our study it is also clear that even in patients with relatively normal hearts, the atrial contribution is significant and consistently contributes from 13% to 30% of cardiac output at various pacing rates. In addition the systolic pressure decreased significantly with ventricular pacing.

A-V Synchrony

It is interesting to note that during ventricular pacing, cardiac output, hence stroke volume, decreased significantly as compared to atrial and A-V sequential pacing, yet EDV and ejection fraction was not significantly different. One possible explanation is that in addition to atrial contribution to cardiac output, there may have been in fact mitral regurgitation to maintain the ejection fraction and EDV. Mitral regurgitation has been demonstrated to occur by Little (19) and Skinner (20) in improperly timed atrial contraction and during ventricular pacing. Mitral regurgitation was also seen with premature ventricular complexes and excessively long A-V intervals. Mitral regurgitation would explain the fact that total stroke volume (EDV × EF) is not significantly changed, yet the net forward cardiac output has significantly diminished.

Timing of Atrial Systole

Moreover, it has only become known recently that not only is the atrial contribution important, but the timing of it was also important (14, 17, 21, 22). If the A-V interval was too short, no effective atrial boost will take place. However on the other hand, if A-V interval was excessively long, the ventriculo-atrial regurgitation can result (14, 22). Hartzler (6) has demonstrated elegantly that by altering the A-V interval, one may obtain a further increase in cardiac output beyond atrial pacing alone by 18%. Daggett (14) has also emphasized that A-V interval is an important determinant of left ventricular function during cardiac pacing, especially in diseased states. In our patients, by optimizing the A-V interval, one could obtain an improved cardiac output above that in atrial pacing in 9 of 12 patients. There was a trend toward shorter optimum A-V intervals at faster heart rate, however this was again not significant. Taking the group on the whole, optimizing A-V interval did not increase cardiac output. Thus in this group, of patients with relatively normal known left ventricular function, atrial contribution is important, but the timing of which appeared less important in the range of A-V intervals we used.

A corollary of the above observation is that the abnormal ventricular activation in A-V sequential pacing, which is absent in atrial pacing, contributes no important role in the overall hemodynamic status. Thus it appears that ventricular pacing is adverse hemodynamically mainly because of lack of atrial contribution and possible A-V valvular regurgitation due to A-V dyssynchrony, whereas abnormal activation only played a small negligible role, as observed by Samet previously (18).

Cardiac Output at different Rates

It is also of interest to note that during pacing at rates of 90, 110, and 130 per minute, the cardiac output within each variety of pacing did not increase further with increasing heart rates. This likely reflected intact physiological reflex mechanisms, and due to the lack of further physiological demand, the stroke volume fell appropriately for the increasing heart rate to maintain an already somewhat elevated cardiac output. This would have an important implication in the next generation of "physiological pacemakers", i.e. regulation of heart rate according to physiological demands. It can be seen that there is an optimum heart rate for each given level of physiological demand, such as to minimize the rate of pacing, hence to decrease the myocardial oxygen consumption and to conserve battery power. Yet at the same time the heart rate must be adequate so that stroke volume and EDV are not excessive, again raising myocardial oxygen consumption, yet maintaining the same cardiac output.

Conclusion

Thus we conclude from our study that "physiological pacing" by preserving A-V synchrony will significantly improve left ventricular hemodynamics even in relatively normal functioning ventricles. This is chiefly accomplished by the preservation of atrial filling and avoiding possible mitral regurgitation as the result of A-V dyssynchrony. Optimizing A-V interval achieved only a small further benefit attesting to the fact that abnormal ventricular activation did not produce adverse hemodynamic effects. With present technological advances in dual chamber pacing and increasing clinical expertise in the implantation of the J atrial electrodes, physiological pacing is now a clinical reality. The physiological benefits are real and present even in patients with relatively normal ventricular function. Thus this modality of pacing should be offered to all those patients who are likely candidates to benefit from the hemodynamic advantages of this form of physiological pacing.

References

1. Yashar JJ, Kitzes DL, Arif M, Carleton RA, Goldberg M et al: Atrioventricular sequential pacemakers: Indications, complications, and long-term follow-up. Ann Th Surg 1978; 29: 91–98.
2. Fields J, Berkovits BV, Ing EE, Matloff JM: Surgical experience with temporary and permanent A-V sequential demand pacing. J Th & CV Surg 1973; 66: 865–77.
3. Leinbach RC, Chamberlain DA, Kastor JA, Harthorne JW, Sanders CA: A comparison of the hemodynamic effects of ventricular and sequential A-V pacing in patients with heart block. Am Heart J 1969; 78: 502–8.
4. Chamberlain DA, Leinbach RC, Vassaux CE, Kastor JA, DeSanctis RW, Sanders CA: Sequential atrioventricular pacing in heart block complicating acute myocardial infarction. N Eng J Med 1970; 282: 577–82.
5. Curtis JJ, Maloney JD, Barnhorst DA, Pluth JR, Hartzler GO, Wallace RB: A critical look at temporary ventricular pacing following cardiac surgery. Surg 1977; 82: 888–93.
6. Hartzler GO, Maloney JD, Curtis JJ, Barnhorst DA: Hemodynamic benefits of atrioventricular sequential pacing after cardiac surgery. Am J Card 1977; 40: 232–6.
7. Kroetz FW, Leonard JJ, Shaver JA, Leon DF, Lancaster JF, Beamer VL: The effect of atrial contraction on left ventricular performance in valvular aortic stenosis. Circulation 1967; 35: 852–67.
8. Stott DK, Marpole DGF, Bristow JD, Kloster FE, Griswold HE: The role of left atrial transport in aortic and mitral stenosis. Circulation 1970; 1031–41.
9. Ingels NB, Daughters GT, Stinson EB, Alderman EL: Measurement of midwall myocardial dynamics in intact man by radiography of surgically implanted markers. Circulation 1975; 52: 859–67.
10. Ingels NB, Daughters GT, Stinson EB, Alderman EL: Evaluation of methods for quantitating left ventricular segmental wall motion in man using myocardial markers as a standard. Circulation 1980; 61: 966–72.
11. McLaughlin PR, Kleiman JH, Martin RP, Doherty PW et al: The effect of exercise and atrial pacing on left ventricular volume and contractility in patients with innervated and denervated hearts. Circulation 1978; 58: 476–83.
12. Wolf NM, Kreulen TH, Bove AA, McDonough MT, Kessler KM et al: left ventricular function following coronary bypass surgery. Circulation 1978; 58: 63–70.
13. Carleton RA, Passovoy M, Greaettinger JS: The importance of the contribution and timing of left atrial systole. Clin Sci 1966; 30: 151.
14. Daggett WM, Bianco JA, Powell WJ, Austen WG: Relative contributions of the atrial systole-ventricular systole interval and of patterns of ventricular activation to ventricular function during electrical pacing of the dog heart. Circulation Res 1970; 27: 69–70.
15. Nolan SP, Dixon SH, Fisher RD, Morrow AG: The influence of atrial contraction and mitral valve mechanics on ventricular filling, a study of instantaneous mitral valve flow in vivo. Am Heart J 1969; 77: 784–91.
16. Hilton JD, Weisel RD, Baird RJ, Jablonsky G, Pym J et al: The hemodynamic and metabolic response to pacing following aortocoronary bypass. Circulation 1981; 64(II): 48–53.
17. Benchimol A, Ellis JG, Dimond EG: Hemodynamic consequences of atrial and ventricular pacing in patients with normal and abnormal hearts. Am J Med 1965; 39: 911–22.

18. Samet P, Castillo C, Bernstein WH: Hemodynamic consequences of sequential atrioventricular pacing. Am J Card 1968; 21: 207–212.
19. Little RC: Effect of atrial systole on ventricular pressure and closure of the A-V valves. Am J Physiol 1951; 166: 289.
20. Skinner NS, Mitchell JH, Wallace AG, Saronoff SJ: Hemodynamic effects of altering the timing of atrial systole. Am J Physiol 1963; 205: 499–503.
21. Furman S, Reiss HR, Escher DJW. A-V sequential pacing and pacemakers. Chest 1973; 63: 783.
22. Gilmore JP, Sarnoff SJ, Mitchell JH et al: Synchronicity of ventricular contraction: observations comparing hemodynamic effects of atrial and ventricular pacing. Br Heart J 1963; 25: 299.

Authors' address:
Dr. Peter Liu
Cardiovascular Unit
Toronto General Hospital
Toronto, Ontario M5G 1L7
Canada

Cardiac Adaptation to Dynamic Exercise in Pacemaker Implanted Patients

Jun Matsumura, Masuaki Fujiyama, Yohichiro Furuta, Akihiro Tanabe, Hideo Ikeda, Hironori Toshima

Summary: To clarify the mechanism of cardiac adaptations to dynamic exercise excluding chronotropic effect, supine bicycle ergometer exercise with 2-dimensional echocardiogram was performed in 27 pacemaker implanted patients (PMI-pts), whose heart rate were constant during exercise, and six healthy subjects (control: C). Simultaneously, cuff-blood pressure (BP) and serum catecholamine were measured. Patients were divided into two groups by exercise capacity in the sitting bicycle ergometer. Group I (G-I) consisted of 15 patients with relatively good physical work capacity (maximal load: 80 watt $\leqslant$ in male, 60 watt $\leqslant$ in female) and group II (G-II) of 12 patients with depressed physical work capacity (maximal load: 60 watt $\geqslant$ in male, 40 watt $\geqslant$ in female). The resting left ventricular function was impaired in group II. During the initial stage of exercise, left ventricular end-diastolic dimension (EDD) and percent fractional shortening (%FS) in group I increased significantly greater than those in the other two groups, and left ventricular end-systolic dimension (ESD) in group I decreased greater than that in the other groups (G-I $\geqslant$ G-II > C). Increase of systolic BP, posterior wall velocity and systolic BP/ESD ratio in group I and controls were greater than those in group II (G-I = C > G-II). At the last stage of exercise, increases of ESD and systolic BP/ESD ratio in group I were lower than those in controls. Plasma norepinephrine levels in PMI-pts were significantly higher than in controls at rest and during exercise (G-II $\geqslant$ G-I > C). Thus, group I adapts to exercise mainly due to the Frank-Starling mechanism, and to a lesser degree due to an augmentation of contractility corresponding to an increase of circulatory catecholamines. On the other hand, group II can not adapt sufficiently to exercise because of near limitation of preload-reserve and contractility-reserve at rest, in spite of a remarkable activation of sympathetic nervous system.

It has been known that the increase in stroke volume during the dynamic exercise is partly due to an increase in end-diastolic volume and secondly due to a reduction in end-systolic volume (1, 2). The increase in end-diastolic volume is the role played by the Frank-Starling mechanism, and the reduction in end-systolic volume can be related to increased contractility, mediated by beta adrenergic stimulation (3, 4). However, these changes of volume are usually over- or under-estimated because of the concomitant tachycardia in exercise (5, 6).

Only by observing subjects under the constant heart rate during exercise, it is possible to obtain precise information concerning cardiac adaptations (7). In this study, we investigated the relationship between changes of left ventricular function and of serum catecholamines in patients with pacemaker implantation whose heart rates were kept constant during exercise.

Patients and Methods

Subjects were 27 patients (10 men and 11 women) with complete heart block and an endocardial VVI mode pacemaker system implanted in the right ventricular apex, with a pacing rate of 70 beats per minute. The patients were divided into two groups by their exercise capacity in the preceeding sitting bicycle ergometer stress test.

All of them showed the constant heart rate at rest and during exercise. Group I consisted of 15 patients (7 menand 8 women) with relatively good physical work capacity, whose maximal load were exceeded 80 watts among the men and 60 watts among the women (mean 76 ± 17 watts). Group II consisted of 12 patients (9 men and 3 women) with depressed physical work capacity, whose maximal load were less than 60 watts among the men and 40 watts among the women (mean 47 ± 12 watts). Left ventricular performance was measured by the multi-stage supine bicycle ergometer stress test in 27 patients and 6 (5 men and one woman) healthy persons (control group). The test started at 20 watt and increased 20 watt every 3 minutes until cardiac or other limiting symptoms occurred. Simultaneously, left ventricular echocardiogram, cuff-blood pressure and serum catecholamine were determined at rest and every 3 minutes during exercise. The echocardiograms were recorded at the mitral chordae level, with the sound beam direction determined by 2-dimensional echocardiogram. All echocardiographic measurements were obtained by the averaging at least 3 consecutive beats. From the echocardiographic measurements described above, percent fractional shortening and cardiac output were calculated as follows:

$$\%FS = \frac{EDD-ESD}{EDD} \times 100, \ COP = \{(EDD)^3 - (ESD)^3\} \times HR$$

Serum catecholamines was measured in peripheral venous blood by the trihydroxy indole method with high performance liquid chromatography.

The data were expressed as mean ± SD and statistical evaluation was made using Student's t-test for un-paired data with $p < 0.05$ considered significant.

Results

Resting cardiac parameters (Table 1)

Data were obtained at rest in the three groups. End-diastolic dimension and end-systolic dimension were larger in group II than in the other two groups. Percent fractional shortening and posterior wall velocity in group II were smaller than in the other groups. Age did not differ in these three groups.

Table 1. Resting cardiac parameters and maximal load by sitting bicycle ergometer.

	ESD (mm)	EDD (mm)	% FS (%)	PWV (mm/sec)	age	Max. load (watt)
Group I (n = 15)	32.6 ± 7.3	47.6 ± 6.6	32.7 ± 7.2	49.1 ± 6.9	58.3 ± 7.0	76 ± 17
Group II (n = 12)	43.2 ± 10.3[*§]	55.5 ± 9.1[*§]	22.8 ± 9.2[*§]	39.5 ± 11.9[*§]	57.0 ± 8.9	47 ± 12[*]
Control (n=6)	28.3 ± 2.6	46.0 ± 2.7	38.5 ± 3.0	50.7 ± 7.2	60.7 ± 8.9	

Abbreviations: EDD = end-diastolic dimension, ESD = end-systolic dimension, %FS = percent fractional shortening, PWV = posterior wall velocity.
Values are mean ± SD. * $p < 0.05$ Group I vs Group II. §$p < 0.05$ Group II vs Control.

Changes of cardiac parameters during exercise (1) (Fig. 1)

Patients in group I showed a significantly greater increase in end-diastolic dimension than that in group II and controls at all stage (at 9 minutes, group I: 4.9 ± 1.7, group II: 2.5 ± 1.7, control: – 1.0 ± 1.7 mm). The decrease in end-systolic dimension in group I was significantly greater than that in the other groups at the first three minutes (group I: – 2.5 ± 1.2, group II: – 1.3 ± 1.7, control: – 1.0 ± 1.7 mm). But at 6 and 9 minutes, it did not differ from that in controls (at 9 minutes, group I: – 3.5 ± 1.6, group II: – 1.3 ± 2.2, control: – 3.3 ± 1.5 mm). End-systolic dimension in group II decrease slightly at the initial stage, but no further decrease was observed. The increase in percent fractional shortening in group I was significantly greater than that in group II and controls (at 9 minutes, group I: 11.4 ± 2.7, group II: 6.0 ± 3.5, control: 5.7 ± 5.1%). Cardiac output in group II was significantly lower than in group I and controls (at 9 minutes, group I: 3.3. ± 2.1, group II: 2.4 ± 1.2, control: 3.6 ± 1.6 l/min). The increase in posterior wall velocity in group II was lower than that in the other groups (at 9 minutes, group I: 24.4 ± 5.5, group II: 15.2 ± 4.1, control: 18.7 ± 9.0 mm/sec).

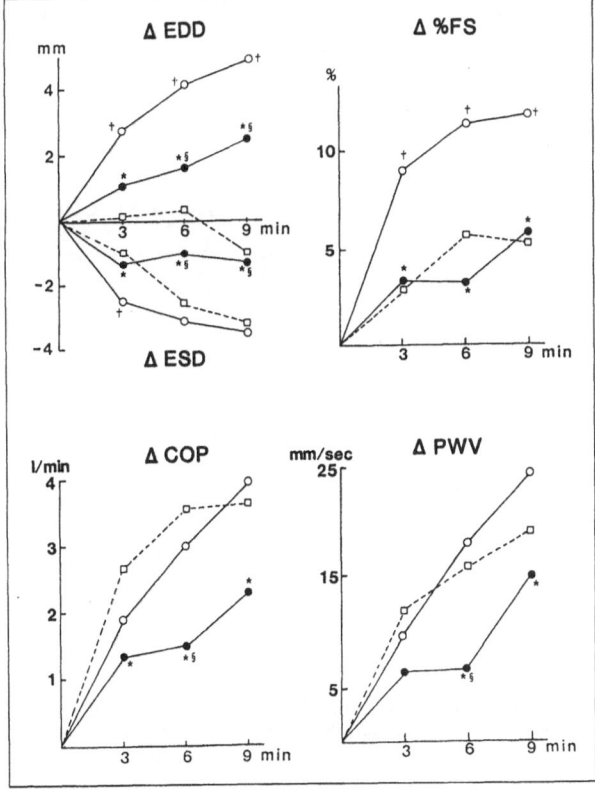

Fig. 1. Changes of cardiac parameters during supine ergometer exercise (1).
*Δ*EDD and *Δ*%FS in group I increase significantly greater than in other groups. *Δ*ESD in group I decreases significantly greater than in other groups at 3 minutes during exercise. Decrease of *Δ*ESD in group II is lower than in other groups at 6 and 9 minutes. Increases of *Δ*COP and *Δ*PWV in group II are lower than in other groups.
Abbreviations: COP = cardiac output, EDD = end-diastolic dimension, ESD = end-systolic dimension, %FS = percent fractional shortening, PWV = posterior wall velocity. Values are mean ± SD.
○——○ group I, ●——● group II, □-----□ control. *p < 0.05 group I vs group II. † p < 0.05 group I vs control. § p < 0.05 group II vs control.

Changes of cardiac parameters during exercise (2) (Fig. 2)

The increase in systolic blood pressure in group I did not differ from that in controls at 3 and 6 minutes (at 6 minutes, group I: 33.4 ± 12.4, control: 34.4 ± 14.4 mmHg), but was lower than that in controls at 9 minutes (group I: 38.7 ± 9.3, control 59.5 ± 20 mmHg). The increase in systolic blood pressure in group II was smaller than that in controls at 6 and 9 minutes (at 9 minutes, group II: 26.7 ± 18 mmHg).

Systolic blood pressure/end-systolic dimension ratio (SBP/ESD), which is an index of the left ventricular contractility at rest (8), increased equally in group I and controls. However, an increase of this ratio in group II was significantly lower than in the other groups at all stages (at 9 minutes, group I: 1.8 ± 0.2, group II: 0.6 ± 0.4, control: 2.3 ± 1.2 mmHg/mm). Mean blood pressure/cardiac output ratio, which is a parameter of peripheral resistance, decreased equally in group I and controls. The decrease of this ratio in group II was significantly lower than in the other two groups at all stages (at 3 minutes, group I: – 3.6 ± 2.6, group II: – 0.9 ± 1.7, control: – 4.4 ± 3.0 mmHg/l).

Changes of serum catecholamines (Table 2)

Group II showed significantly higher serum norepinephrine levels at rest. The rate of increase of norepinephrine during exercise was greater in group II than in the other groups. The response of norepinephrine in group I was similar to that of controls, however a statistical difference was observed at 9 minutes of exercise. Epinephrine also increased during exercise but the changes of epineprhine did not differ in each group.

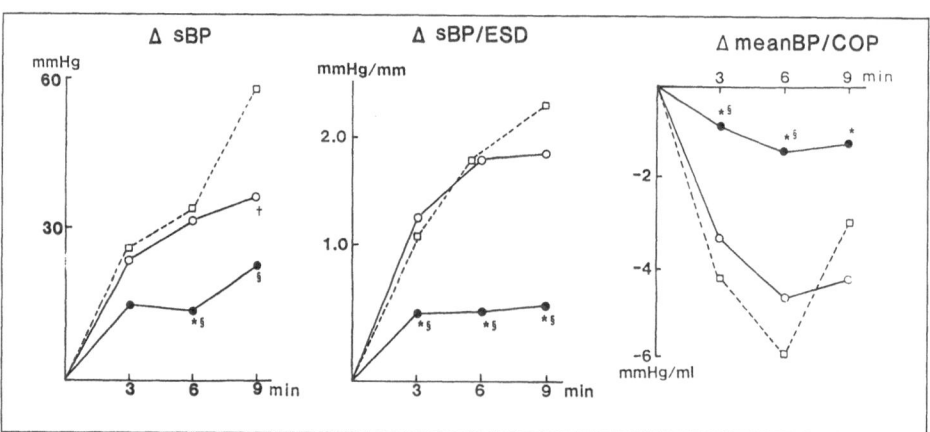

Fig. 2. Changes of cardiac parameters during supine ergometer exercise (2).
Increases of ⊿sBP and ⊿sBP/ESD in group II are lower than in other groups. Decrease of ⊿mean BP/COP in group II is lower than in other groups.
Abbreviations: meanBP/COP = mean blood pressure-cardiac output ratio, sBP = systolic blood pressure, sBP/ESD = systolic blood pressure-end-systolic dimension ratio. Values are mean ± SD.
○——○ group I, ●——● group II, □-----□ control. * p < 0.05 group I vs group II. † p < 0.05 group I vs control. § p < 0.05 group II vs control.

Table 2. Changes of serum catecholamine at rest and during supine ergometer exercise

		during exercise			
	Rest	at 3 min.	at 6 min.	at 9 min.	at 3 min after exercise
Group I NE (ng/ml)	0.14±0.07	0.30±0.14	0.43±0.17	0.64±0.17[†]	0.34±0.14
E (ng/ml)	0.03±0.02	0.03±0.02	0.06±0.06	0.09±0.05	0.04±0.03
Group II NE	0.43±0.30[*§]	0.72±0.53[*§]	1.43±1.20[*§]	2.71±1.35[*§]	1.07±1.40
E	0.03±0.02	0.04±0.03	0.05±0.05	0.05±0.04	0.07±0.06
Control NE	0.15±0.06	0.21±0.08	0.30±0.07	0.47±0.04	0.29±0.09
E	0.03±0.02	0.05±0.03	0.06±0.04	0.08±0.05	0.04±0.02

Abbreviations: E = epinephrine, NE = norepinephrine.
Values are mean ± SD.
*$p < 0.05$ Group I vs Group II.
†$p < 0.05$ Group I vs Control.
§$p < 0.05$ Group II vs Control.

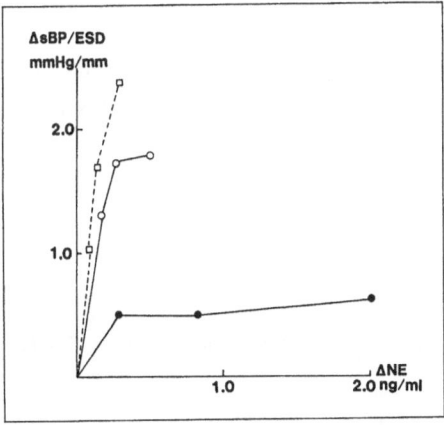

Fig. 3. Relationship between changes of sBP/ESD and changes of norepinephrine.
At first 3 minutes, it is clear in group I that sBP/ESD increases greatly corresponding to increasing of NE. At last 9 minutes, increase of sBP/ESD in group I is lower than in control, furthermore there is a few changes in group II in spite of remarkable increase of NE.
Abbreviations: NE = norepinephrine, sBP/ESD = systolic blood pressure-end-systolic dimension ratio.
○——○ group I, ●——● group II, □-----□ control.

Relationship between changes of systolic blood pressure/end-systolic dimension ratio and changes of norepinephrine (Fig. 3)

At the initial three minutes in group I, systolic blood pressure/end-systolic dimension ratio increased markedly, coinciding with an increse of norepinephrine. However, at 9 minutes there was not further augmentation in this ratio, despite the further increase of norepinephrine. This ratio in group II increased slighly only at the initial stage of exercise, but remained unchanged thereafter, in spite of a remarkable increase of norepinephrine. Similar results were obtained regarding the relation of norepinephrine and end-systolic dimension or posterior wall velocity.

Discussion

Crawford et al. (9) and Horwitz et al. (10) reported that end-diastolic dimension in normal persons decreased or remained unchanged during exercise. But in patients with the constant heart rate, a remarkable increase in end-diastolic dimension were observed, and cardiac output in these patients were similar to that in controls. Thus, these results suggest that the left ventricular adaptation to dynamic exercise in patients with constant heart rate are mainly due to the Frank-Starling mechanism based on an increase of the venous return.

Secondly, we observed decrease in end-systolic dimension and increase in systolic blood pressure/end-systolic dimension ratio and posterior wall velocity corresponding to a remarkable increase of serum norepinephrine.

Thus, the left ventricular adaptation to exercise are secondarily due to an augmentation of contractility with an increase of sympathetic neural activity. On the other hand, in patients with depressed physical work capacity, the left ventricular function is impaired at the lower level of exercise despite maximal contributions of the compensatory mechanisms because their resting ventricular function had already reached its limit (11, 12). These compensatory mechanisms, augmentations of preload and contractility, could be accurately evaluated in patients with the constant heart rate during exercise (13, 14). Therefore, we concluded the following:

Patients with good physical work capacity adapt to moderate exercise mainly due to the Frank-Starling mechanism, and secondarily due to an augmentation of contractility mediated by sympathetic neural activation. Patients with depressed physical work capacity can not adapt sufficiently to dynamic exercise because their cardiac function is impaired even at rest, and preload and contractility are not allowed to compensate for exercise.

References

1. Rushmer RF, Smith O and Franklin D: Mechanisms of cardiac control in exercise. Cir Res 1959; 7: 602.
2. Braunwald E, Coldblatt A, Harrison DC and Mason DT: Studies on cardiac dimensions in tact, unanesthetized man: III. Effects of muscular exercise. Circ Res 1963; 13: 460.
3. Goldstein DS: Plasma norepinephrine as indication of sympathetic neural activity in clinical cardiology. Am J Cardiol 1981; 48: 1147.
4. Levy NM and Blattberg B: The effect of the pattern of cardiac sympathetic activity on myocardial contractile force and norepinephrine overflow in the dog heart. Circ Res 1976; 39: 341.
5. Quinones MA, Gaasch WH and Alexander JK: Influence of acute changes in preload, afterload, contractile state and heart rate on ejection and isovolumic indices of myocardial contractility in man. Circulation, 1976; 53: 293.
6. Sonnenblick EH, Braunwald E, Williams JF and Glick G: Effects and exercise on myocardial force-velocity relations in intact unanesthetized man: Relative roles of changes in heart rate, sympathetic activity and ventricular dimensions. J Clin Invest 1965; 44: 2051.
7. Takamoto T, Iesaka Y, Niwa A, Miyahara Y, Taniguchi K and Takeuchi J: Echocardiographic evaluation of left ventricular performance during fixed heart rate isometric exercise. J Cardiography 1980; 10: 1133.
8. Fujiyama M, Furuta Y, Ikeda H, Uemura S, Itaya M, Takahashi H, Toshima H and Utsu F: Experimental and clinical study of peak left ventricular systolic blood pressure/left ventricular end-systolic volume (LVSP/LVESVI) ratio as an index of left ventricular function. J Cardiography 1980; 10: 831.

9. Crawford MH, White DH and Amon KW: Echocardiographic evaluation of left ventricular size and performance during handgrip and supine and upright bicycle exercise. Circulation, 1979; 59: 1138.
10. Horwitz LD, Atkins JM and Leshin SJ: Role of the Frank-Starling mechanism in exercise. Circ Res 1972; 31: 868.
11. Francis GS, Goldsmith SR, Ziesche SM and Cohn JN: Response of plasma norepinephrine and epinephrine to dynamic exercise in patients with congestive heart failure. Am J Cardiol 1982; 49: 1152.
12. Chidsey CA, Harrison DC and Braunwald E: Augmentation of the plasma norepinephrine response to exercise in patients with congestive heart failure. New Engl J Med 1962; 267: 650.
13. Matsumura J, Fujiyama M, Furuta Y, Tanabe A, Itaya M, Takahashi H, Koga Y, Ikeda H and Toshima H: Left ventricular performance during dynamic exercise in patients with constant heart rate. J Cardiography, 1983; 13: 149.
14. Segal N, Hudson WA, Harris P and Bishop JM: Circulatory effects of electrically induced changes in ventricular rate at rest and during exercise in complete heart block. J Clin Invest 1964; 43: 1541.

Authors' address:
Dr. Jun Matsumura
3rd. Dept. of Int. Medicine
Kurume University School of Medicine
67 Asahi-Machi
Kurume 830
Japan

Doppler Ultrasound Measurement of Cardiac Output in Patients with Physiologic Dual Chamber Pacemakers

V. C. Dicola*, W. J. Stewart, J. W. Harthorne, A. E. Weyman

Summary: Dual chamber pacemakers have recently come into widespread use. They offer practical advantages in restoring atrio-ventricular synchrony and in allowing rate variability in response to physiologic stresses. Doppler ultrasound allows non-invasive assessment of cardiac output in man. We used this technique to determine the changes in resting cardiac output in patients with DDD pacemakers when the mode of pacing was varied from VVI to DDD at fixed heart rates.

Doppler ultrasound measurement of cardiac output was first validated with thermodilution measurements in 12 patients recovering from coronary bypass surgery (R = 0.83). Then twenty-seven patients with DDD pacemakers were assessed at rest with the heart rate fixed and the mode of pacing varied from VVI to DDD. There was a significant increase in cardiac output from 4.2 ± 0.4 (mean $\pm$ SEM) liters per minute in the VVI mode to 5.0 ± 0.4 in the DDD mode ($p < 0.001$). The degree of improvement in cardiac output was independent of ventricular function. The percentage increase in cardiac output averaged $16 \pm 3\%$ in those 12 patients with left ventricular ejection fraction greater than 40% and $27 \pm 8\%$ in those 15 patients with LVEF less than 40% ($p = NS$).

Substantially greater improvements in cardiac output occurred however, in those patients with evidence of the pacemaker syndrome or intact ventriculo-atrial conduction. In these 9 patients, there was a mean improvement of $39 \pm 10\%$ in cardiac output between VVI and DDD as opposed to an average increase of only $14\% \pm 3\%$ in the 18 patients without VA conduction ($p < 0.02$). The patients with poor left ventricular function and VA conduction showed the most marked improvements. Thus, Doppler ultrasound can be used to quantitate the improvement in cardiac output which occurs in patients at rest with DDD pacing versus VVI pacing. This improvement is independent of the level of left ventricular function but is substantially higher when there is evidence of VA conduction or the pacemaker syndrome.

Introduction

The hemodynamic advantages of proper atrioventricular synchrony were appreciated long before the availability of AV sequential pacing systems (1, 2). Advances in the miniaturization of sophisticated electronic circuitry and the development of stable and reliable atrial electrode systems however, have made such pacemaker systems generally available. Unfortunately, the physiologic benefit derived from these more sophisticated, complex, and costly devices has been difficult to quantitate in a systematic manner without the use of invasive monitoring.

Doppler ultrasound is a relatively new technique that can be used to measure blood flow in the heart and great vessels (3, 4) and offers a non-invasive and easily repeatable method of assessing cardiac output in a wide range of patients (5, 6, 7). The purpose of this

* Albert S. Hyman Research Fellow in Cardiac Pacing, North American Society of Pacing and Electrophysiology

study was to determine: 1. whether Doppler assessment of cardiac output can be used successfully in pacemaker patients; 2. what changes in hemodynamics occur with changes from ventricular demand (VVI) mode to dual-chamber (DDD) mode; and 3. whether intact ventriculo-atrial conduction or left ventricular function can be used to predict which patients are most favorably affected by DDD pacing.

Methods

Patient Population: The study population consisted of 27 patients who had physiologic (DDD) dual-chamber pacemakers. There were 22 males and 5 females. The mean age was 66 years (range 28 to 85 years). The indication for pacing was high grade conduction system disease or complete AV block in 22 patients and sick sinus syndrome in 5 patients. There were a variety of associated cardiac disorders present including 14 patients with overt coronary artery disease, 8 of whom were status post coronary bypass surgery. Five patients had complete heart block following valvular surgery. Four patients had hypertensive heart disease and nine patients had a history of congestive heart failure. Nine patients had either ventriculo-atrial conduction documented at the time of pacemaker implantation (6 patients) or had previously been unable to tolerate ventricular pacing (6 patients) because of symptoms consistent with the pacemaker syndrome (8).

Left ventricular function was assessed by radionuclide ventriculography. In fifteen of the twenty-seven patients, left ventricular systolic function was depressed with an ejection fraction (LVEF) of 40% or less. All Doppler studies were made within three weeks of insertion of or revision to a DDD pacing system.

Doppler echocardiographic methods: All non-invasive assessments of cardiac output were made with the patients supine and in a resting state. In the first 17 patients, ultrasound measurements were made with an automated Doppler instrument (Ultracom, Lawrence Medical Systems, Redmond, Washington). Using this instrument, the internal diameter of the ascending aorta (D) was measured using an A-mode echo to derive an aortic diameter to calculate cross-sectional area. Then a single-crystal continuous wave Doppler probe was applied to the suprasternal notch to measure maximum flow velocity in the ascending aorta. Transducer direction was guided by the audio feedback of the Doppler shift and the visual feedback of a computer-derived velocity integral. This represents an automated integral of the systolic portion of the smoothed maximum frequency shift and is proportional to stroke volume. Cardiac output is the product of cross-sectional area times mean velocity, which is calculated from the velocity integral divided by the cycle length (see Figure 1). In this group, patients with aortic valve prostheses were excluded.

Experience with measurement of cardiac output using this technique had been gained previously by measurement of cardiac output in post-coronary artery bypass graft (CABG) patients. The acoustic window in that population is more difficult to optimize due to problems relating to patient position and recent surgery. Nonetheless, the comparison between thermodilution and Doppler cardiac output yielded a good correlation (r = 0.83) (Fig. 2).

In the second group of 10 patients, cardiac output was measured in the pulmonary artery using an instrument which combines two-dimensional echo with range-gated Doppler (MK 500 Advanced Technology Laboratories, Bellevue, Washington). No patient had intrinsic disease of the pulmonic valve. The cross-sectional area was derived by measuring

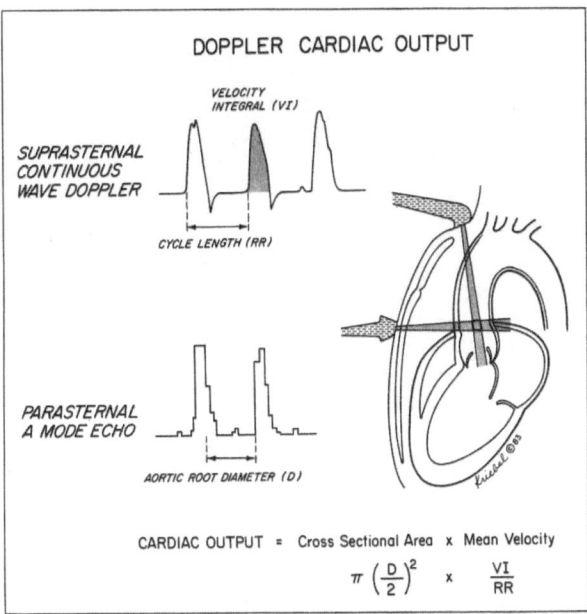

Fig. 1. Doppler ultrasound determination of cross sectional area and mean flow velocity. Cardiac output is the product of these measurements.

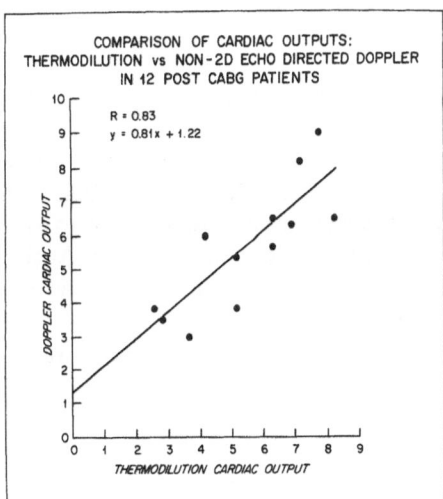

Fig. 2. Comparison of thermodilution and doppler ultrasound determinations of cardiac output in post coronary artery bypass graft (CABG) patients.

the systolic diameter of the pulmonic valve annulus from a parasternal two-dimensional echo image (see Fig. 3). The Doppler signal was optimized using the audio signal and the spectral velocity display. Only cycles with a narrow frequency band width indicating undisturbed flow were used, avoiding phases in VVI pacing mode where independent atrial activity provided fortuitously appropriate atrio-ventricular synchrony. The velocity inte-

233

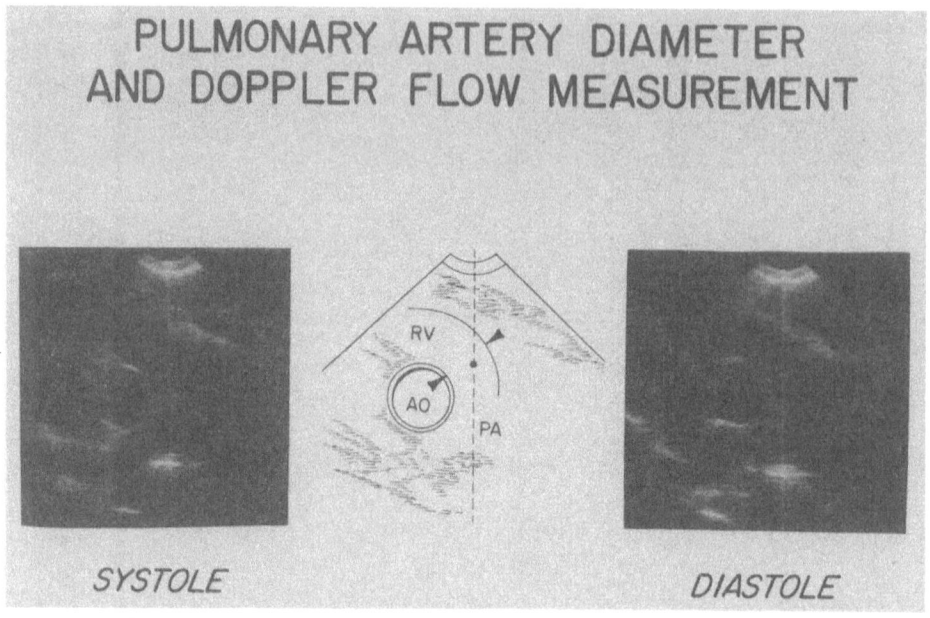

Fig. 3. Two dimensional echocardiogram of pulmonary artery with Doppler cursor superimposed. Arrows denote the pulmonic valve annulus. AO = aorta, PA = pulmonary artery, RV = right ventricle.

gral and cycle length were measured from the video spectral velocity using a computer graphics analysis system (Easyvue II, Microsonics, Inc., Indianapolis, Indiana).

Experimental Protocol: In each of four or more phases, the pacemaker was programmed either to DDD mode or to ventricular demand (VVI) mode, in a random order unknown to the echocardiographer. In each instance the heart rate was held constant just above the sinus rate. Rhythms were confirmed by surface electrocardiographic recording. After a period of equilibration of 3 minutes in each pacing mode, three or more Doppler recordings were made over a 5 to 15 minute period and averaged.

Statistical methods: The student's "t" test was utilized for statistical analysis. All values are given as mean + standard error of the mean.

Results

Improved cardiac output with DDD pacing. The mean cardiac output for all patients in VVI mode was 4.2 ± 0.4 liters/min. The mean cardiac output during DDD pacing was 5.0 ± 0.4 liters/min. The difference between these values was significant at the $p < 0.001$ level (see Fig. 4).

In 22 of 27 patients, cardiac output was consistently better in DDD mode compared to VVI mode. In the entire group maintenance of continuous atrioventricular synchrony with DDD pacing provides a mean improvement of 22% in cardiac output compared to ventricular demand (VVI) pacing.

234

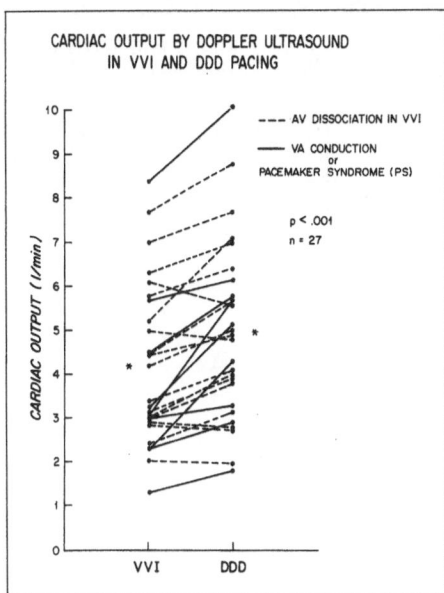

Fig. 4. Comparison of cardiac output in VVI and DDD pacing in all pacemaker patients studied.

Intact V-A conduction. In the 9 patients with ventriculo-atrial conduction and/or the "pacemaker syndrome", the cardiac output in DDD pacing was 39.1 ± 10.1 greater than the VVI level. In the 18 patients without V-A conduction, the increment in cardiac output was 13.7 ± 3.3. The difference between these groups was significant ($p < 0.02$) as shown in Fig. 5. Indeed 3 of the 9 patients had greater than 50% increments in cardiac output when switched from VVI to DDD mode.

Impaired LV function. In the 12 patients in whom left ventricular ejection fraction was greater than 40%, the mean improvement in cardiac output from VVI to DDD pacing was $16.4 \pm 3.3\%$ (mean $\pm$ SEM). In the 15 patients with LVEF less than 40%, the mean improvement was $26.8 \pm 7.7\%$. The difference in the mean improvement between these groups was not statistically significant as shown in Figure 6. The improvement in cardiac output with DDD pacing therefore, appears to be independent of the level of left ventricular performance.

Discussion

The observation that atrial contraction provides a significant increment of ventricular filling and forward flow was made over 70 years ago (9). Several mechanisms have been elucidated to account for this augmentation. Properly-timed atrial systole maintains a low mean atrial pressure thus facilitating venous return; it coordinates atrioventricular valve closure and abolishes AV valve regurgitation; finally, it augments ventricular filling significantly and increases ventricular contractile force via the Starling principle (10–15).

In patients with disorders of atrio-ventricular conduction or impulse generation, therapeutic options in the choice of a pacemaker have been expanded by the development of reliable atrial leads (16, 17) and the miniaturization of increasingly sophisticated elec-

Fig. 5. The percentage change in cardiac output with DDD when patients are segregated according to radionuclide left ventricular ejection fraction.

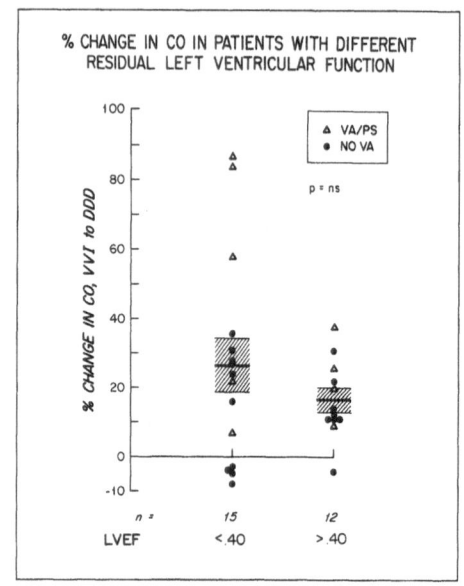

Fig. 6. The percentage change in cardiac output with DDD when patients are segregated according to the presence or absence of either VA conduction or the pacemaker syndrome.

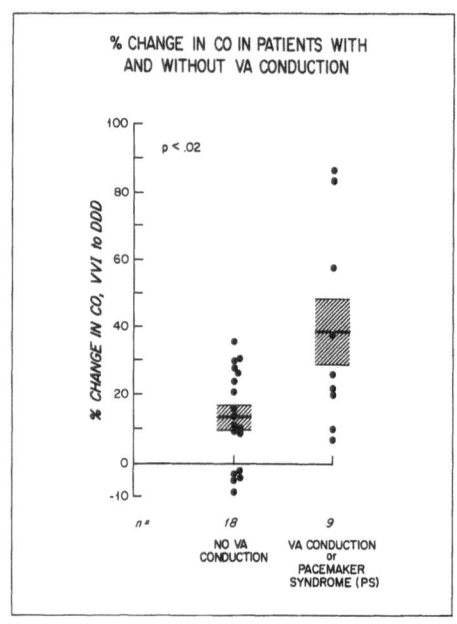

tronics (18). Some guidelines for selection of an appropriate pacemaker have been published (19). However, estimates of the need and indications for dual chamber devices range from less than 10% to 85% of all patients (20–22). Thus, in individual cases, choice of a pacing system is often based on subjective clinical assessment rather than objective data. Equally important, the adjustment of programmable parameters has been largely arbitrary and dependent on the patient's subjective sense of well-being. Serial measurement of cardiac output by Doppler echocardiography offers an objective means for non-invasively assessing the results of dual chamber pacing and for quantitating its effects both acutely and chronically.

The 23% average increment in cardiac output at rest demonstrated by the present study is similar to values found by others with invasive techniques (13, 23, 24). In addition, it is comparable to what has been shown under controlled conditions in an experimental animal model (12).

Kruse et al. performed invasive catheter studies at rest and during upright bicycle exercise to determine work capacity and cardiac output during both VVI and VDD pacing (25). The increment in cardiac output afforded by VDD compared to VVI was significant at rest. During exercise the increase was of a larger magnitude despite a substantial compensatory increase in stroke volume with VVI pacing.

The second objective of the present study was to delineate which patients would have the greatest improvement in cardiac output with DDD. We demonstrated that the presence of ventriculo-atrial conduction or the pacemaker syndrome clearly identified those patients who would have the most substantial improvements with DDD. This is in agreement with studies by Ogawa et al. who concluded that maintenance of a physiologic AV interval is the critical determinant of overall cardiac performance during pacing (26). DDD pacing systems should be considered for all patients in whom ventriculo-atrial conduction has been documented.

The degree of improvement we observed was not related to the degree of impairment of left ventricular function as has previously been suggested (27–29). Similar improvements in cardiac output occurred in patients with both normal and depressed left ventricular function. Thus left ventricular dysfunction should not be the sole criteria by which a patient is considered for a more sophisticated pacing system. It should be noted however, that our patient groups were relatively small and a more clearly defined effect of ventricular function might become apparent with a larger sample size.

The greatest improvements in cardiac output occurred in those patients who had both impaired left ventricular function and VA conduction. This is consistent with previous studies showing that the atrial contribution to cardiac output is proportionately greater in patients with left ventricular dysfunction (27–29). Thus in these patients, ventriculo-atrial conduction would be most deleterious because they are dependent on the booster pump function of the atria.

The measurement of cardiac output using Doppler has been previously reported by various authors. Most of these determinations have been in the ascending aorta (6, 7), although flow through the mitral valve (30) and pulmonary artery (31) have also been measured successfully. Comparing Doppler cardiac output with other techniques has yielded correlation coefficients ranging from 0.78 to 0.96 (7, 30, 31).

Several assumptions are necessary with this technique. In this study, we were most interested in changes in each patient's cardiac output. This should be accurately reflected by the Doppler velocity integral alone (32, 33) so that errors in the cross-sectional area values are of less importance.

The unique advantage of this technique is that it is non-invasive and can be repeated easily with minimal patient discomfort. Using this technique, we demonstrated a clearcut improvement in cardiac output with DDD pacing versus VVI using a simple, widely applicable technique. The improvement in cardiac output was greatest in patients with ventriculo-atrial conduction or the pacemaker syndrome but occurred at all levels of ventricular function. The technique of Doppler ultrasound should be of value in the initial evaluation as well as during follow-up of patients with DDD pacemakers.

References

1. Folkman MJ, Watkins EJ: An artificial conduction system for the management of experimental complete heart block. Surg Forum 1958; 8: 331–334.
2. Nathan DA, Samet P, Center S, Wu CY: Long term correction of complete heart block. Clinical and physiologic studies of a new type of implantable synchronous pacer. Prog Cardiovas Dis 1964; 6: 538–565.
3. Light LH: Non-injurious ultrasonic technique for observing flow in the human aorta. Nature 1969; 224: 1119–1121.
4. Hatle L, Angleson B: Doppler ultrasound in cardiology, physical principles and applications. Lea and Febiger, Philadelphia, 238 pp, 1982.
5. Brubakk AO, Gisvold SE: Pulsed Doppler ultrasound for measuring blood flow in the human aorta. In Hatle L and Angleson B, op cit, pp 185–193.
6. Mackay RS: Non-invasive cardiac output measurement. Microvasc Res 1972; 4: 438–452.
7. Magnin PA, Stewart JA, Myers S, VonRamm O, Kisslo JA: Combined Doppler and phased-array echocardiographic estimation of cardiac output. Circ 1981; 63: 388–392.
8. Mitsui T, Mizuno A, Hasegawa T, Kobayashi H, Hori M, Suma K, Laigusa M: Atrial rate as an indicator for optimal pacing rate and the pacemaking syndrome. Ann Cardiol Angeiol 1971; 20: 371–379.
9. Gesell, RA: Auricular systole and its relation to ventricular output. Am J Physiol 1911; 29: 32–63.
10. Little, RC: Effect of atrial systole on ventricular pressure and closure of the AV valves. Am J Physiol 1951; 166: 289–295.
11. Skinner NS, Mitchell JH, Wallace AG, Sarnoff SJ: Hemodynamic effects of altering the timing of atrial systole. Am J Physiol 1963; 205: 499–503.
12. Gilmore JP, Sarnoff SJ, Mitchell JH, Linden RJ: Synchronicity of ventricular contraction: Observation comparing hemodynamic effects of atrial and ventricular pacing. Brit Heart J 1963; 25: 299–307.
13. Samet P, Castillo C, Bernstein WH: Hemodynamic consequences of sequential atrioventricular pacing. Subjects with normal hearts. Am J Cardiol 1968; 21: 207–212.
14. Benchimol A, Duenas A, Liggett NS, Dimond EG: Contribution of atrial systole to the cardiac function at a fixed and at a variable ventricular rate. Am J Cardiol 1965; 16: 11–21.
15. Braunwald E, Frahm CJ: Studies on Starling's law of the heart. IV. Observations of the hemodynamic functions of the left atrium in man. Circ 1961; 24: 633–642.
16. Smyth, NPD, Citron P, Keshishian JM, Garcia JM, Kelly LC: Permanent pervenous atrial sensing and pacing with a new J-shaped lead. J Thorac Cardiovasc Surg 1976; 72: 565–570.
17. Kleinert M, Block M, Wilhemi F: Clinical use of a new transvenous atrial lead. Am J Cardiol 1977; 40: 237–242.
18. Schaldach M, Furman S (Eds): Advances in pacemaker technology. Page 55–75. Springer-Verlag, New York, Heidelberg, Berlin, 554 pp, 1975.
19. Parsonnet V, Bernstein AD: Treatment and techniques in transition. J Am Coll Cardiol 1983; 1: 339–354.
20. Cohen SI, Frank HA: Preservation of active atrial transport: An important clinical consideration in cardiac pacing. Chest 1982; 81: 51–4.
21. Sutton R, Perrins J, Citron P: Physiologic cardiac pacing. Pace 1980; 3: 207–219.
22. Goldman B, Curtiss JJ, Madigan NP, Whiting RB, Mueller KJ, Pezzalla AT: Discussion: Clinical experience with permanent atrioventricular sequential pacing. Ann Thorac Surg 1981; 32: 179–187.
23. Hartzler GO, Maloney JD, Curtis JJ, Barnhorst DA: Hemodynamic benefits of atrioventricular sequential pacing after cardiac surgery: Am J Cardiol 1977; 40: 232–235.

24. Leinbach RC, Chamberlain DA, Kastor JA, Harthorne JW, Sanders CA: A comparison of the hemodynamic effects of ventricular and sequential AV pacing in patients with heart block. Am Heart J 1969; 78: 502–508.

25. Kruse I, Arnman K, Conradson TB, Ryden L: A comparison of the acute and long-term hemodynamic effects of ventricular inhibited and atrial synchronous ventricular inhibited pacing. Circulation 1982; 65: 846–855.

26. Ogawa S, Dreifus LS, Shenoig PN, Brockman SK, Berkovits BV: Hemodynamic consequences of atrioventricular and ventriculo atrial pacing. Pace 1978; 1: 8–15.

27. Rahimtoola SH, Ehsani A, Sinno MZ, Loeb HS, Rosen KM, Gunnar RM: Left atrial transport function in myocardial infarction. Am J Med 1975; 59: 686–694.

28. Chamberlain DA, Leinbach RC, Vassaux CE, Kastor JA, DeSanctis RW, Sanders CA: Sequential atrioventricular pacing in heart block complicating acute myocardial infarction. NEJM 1970; 282: 577–582.

29. Benchimol A, Ellis JG, Dimond EG: Hemodynamic consequences of atrial and ventricular pacing in patients with normal and abnormal hearts. Effect of exercise at a fixed atrial and ventricular rate. Am J Med 1965; 39: 911–922.

30. Fischer DC, Sahn DJ, Friedman MJ, Larson D, Valdes-Cruz LM, Horowitz S, Goldberg SJ, Allen HD: The mitral valve orifice method for noninvasive two-dimensional echo Doppler determination of cardiac output. Circ 1983; 67: 872–877.

31. Sanders SP, Yeager S, Williams RG: Measurement of systemic and pulmonary blood flow and QP/QS ratio using Doppler and two-dimensional echocardiography. Am J Card 1983; 51: 952–956.

32. Steingart RM, Meller J, Barovick J, Patterson R, Herman MV, Teichholz LE: Pulsed Doppler echocardiographic measurement of beat-to-beat changes in stroke volume in dogs. Circ 1980; 62: 542–548.

33. Colocousis JS, Huntsman LL, Curreri PW: Estimation of stroke volume changes by ultrasonic Doppler. Circ 1977; 56: 914–917.

Authors' address:
J. Warren Harthorne, M.D.
Massachusetts General Hospital
Boston, MA 02114

Influence of Pacing Mode and Parameter of Left Ventricular Function (LVF) Measured by Tc-Nucleidventriculography (Tc-N)

G. Unger, Ch. Bialonczyk, K. Frohner, H. Leonhartsberger, H. Köhn, F. Meisl, A. Mostbeck, K. Steinbach

Summary: In 10 patients the effect of VVI- and DDD-pacing was evaluated by means of Tc-N. No difference in global ejection fraction (EF) and regional wall motion was seen with both pacing modes. During DDD-pacing peak empting rate (PER) showed a significant increase, peak filling rate (PFR) a significant decrease, in comparison to VVI-pacing. PFR and PER were of the same range, in patients with and without retrograde conduction during VVI-pacing. We conclude that PER and PFR are useful parameters to differentiate the effects of different pacing modes on hemodynamics.

Introduction

The treatment of bradycardias as a cause of heart failure and/or Adams-Stokes attack with permanent cardiac stimulation is a well established method. In recent years an increasing number of different PM-systems has become available which allow to adapt the stimulation method to the underlying arrhythmia. In theory, AV-sequential pacing, as physiological pacing mode, seems to be the treatment of choice, especially in patients with an impairment of left ventricular function (1). It has not yet been established whether AV-sequential pacing is the treatment of choice for all patients, when considering the aspect of increasing cardiac output (2, 3). The significance of difference invasive and non-invasive methods for the measurements of left ventricular function is currently under investigation. The present study was undertaken to evaluate the influence of VVI- and DDD-pacing on the behaviour of global EF, regional wall motion, PER and PFR.

Patients and Methods

10 patients (3 females, 7 males), age 53–86 years (mean age 70.6 y), formed the study group. In 9 patients, the underlying heart disease was CHD, in 1 patient dilative CMP (Table 1). The patients were paced at the same rate (60–80 stimuli/min) in VVI- and DDD-mode. The AV-interval in DDD-pacing was between 150 and 200 msec. In 4 patients retrograde VA-conduction was detected.

Equilibrium gated blood pool Radionucleidventriculography with 20mCI 99 mTc in vitro labelled red cells was performed at rest during AV-sequential pacing. Then the PM was switched to VVI-mode and after 10 minutes the second study was started. Heart rhythm was monitored continuously.

Data were collected in a 32×32 matrix with analogue and digital zoom (amplification 2–2.8), the cardiac cycle divided into 32 frames. After temporal and spatial low pass filtering (4) the study was interpolated into a 64×64 matrix.

Utilizing the first Fourier sine and cosine coefficients amplitude and phase images and by using the latter, the standard deviation of the phase histograms of the left ventricle was calculated.

According to these parametric scans regional wall motion abnormalities were classified as hypo-, a- and dyskinetic.

The left ventricular region of interest is a compromise between a second derivative edge detection algorithm, amplitude image and the minimum of the septum. For assessment of global and regional EF we used on the one hand a program by Maddox et al. (5) and on the other hand our own program, which divides the left ventricle into 10 equiangular regions from its center of gravity. PFR and PER were calculated by substituting the original by a five harmonic Fourier curve.

Results

Global EF during DDD-pacing showed no significant change in comparison to VVI-pacing (DDD-pacing 41.6 ± 17.0%, VVI-pacing 43.1 ± 17.1%). There was no difference between patients with and without retrograde VA-conduction during VVI-pacing (Table 1), (Fig. 1).

All 10 patients had regional wall motion abnormalities (2 patients hypokinetic segments, 3 patients akinetic segments, 5 patients dyskinetic segments with paradox volumes). The degree of wall motion abnormality was not influenced by the pacing mode.

The mean value of the maximum PER increased from 2.25 ± 0.8 EDV/sec in VVI-pacing to 2.49 ± 0.92 EDV/sec in DDD-pacing. Also there was no difference between patients with and without retrograde VA-conduction (Fig. 2).

Table 1. Demographic data of patients, pacing mode, underlying heart disease and pre-pacing ECG (RC = retrograde conduction).

Name	Age	Sex	PM	Month since impl.	Diagnosis	Pre-pacing ECG	R.C.
E.J.	53	m	DVI	11	dilat. CMP	Sinusbradycardia + A-V bl. II°	no
P.M.	73	m	DDD	4	CHD	A-V block II° + III°	yes
B.L.	72	m	DVI	9	CHD	A-V block II°	no
S.M.	77	f	DDD	15	CHD	trifasc. block	no
SCH.F.	64	m	DDD	4	CHD	A-V block II°	no
E.L.	72	f	DDD	2	CHD	trifasc. block	yes
F.K.	74	f	DDD	1	CHD	Sinusbradycardia intermitt. LBBB	yes
S.F.	86	m	DDD	9	CHD	trifasc. block	yes
P.A.	72	m	DDD	12	CHD	LBBB + A-V bl. II°	no
B.F.	63	m	DDD	7	CHD	A-V block II°	no

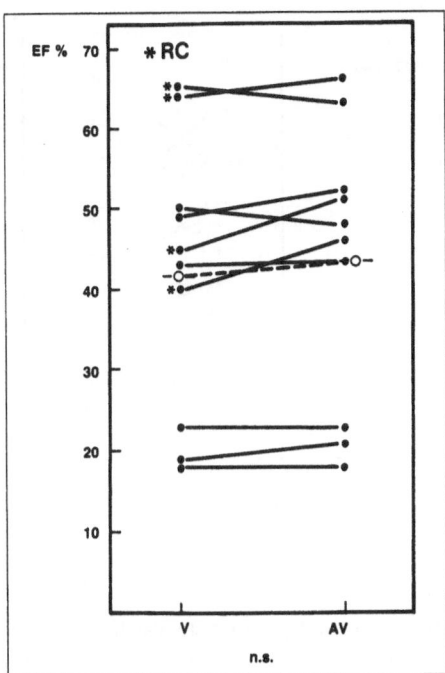

Fig. 1. Global ejection fraction during VVI- and AV-sequential pacing.

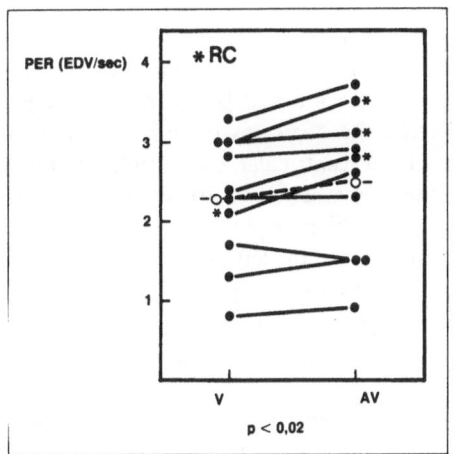

Fig. 2. Peak ejection rate during VVI- and AV-sequential pacing.

Maximum PFR decreased from 2.13 ± 0.82 EDV/sec during VVI-pacing to 1.63 ± 0.92 EDV/sec during DDD-pacing. Again no influence of retrograde VA-conduction was detected (Fig. 3).

243

Fig. 3. Peak filling rate during VVI- and AV-sequential pacing.

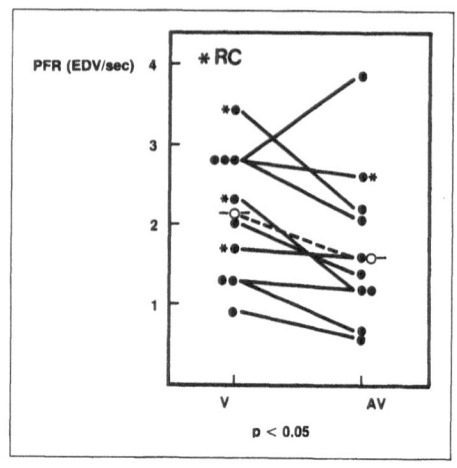

Discussion

The influence of atrial contraction on diastolic filling of the left ventricle was first observed by W. Harvey (6), 1628, and was determined in animal experiments by Mitchell (7, 8) and Linden (9). Linden demonstrated that the effect on fiber-length increase caused by the atrial contraction, depends on the pressure/volume curve of the left ventricle and on the preload. The present study corroborates the above investigation and demonstrates a significant increase of PER during DDD-pacing in comparison to VVI-pacing, whereas global EF remained unchanged.

Recent reports by Kemper and Pollak (10), Manzini (11), Adam and Bitter (12) described PFR during rest and exercise as a sensitive parameter of impairment of diastolic function in patients with CHD, even if the systolic parameters are still in the normal range. According to our results, one could speculate that the decreases of PFR during AV-sequential pacing is in relation to the increased left ventricular enddiastolic volume, caused by active atrial contraction. In this case the increased left ventricular enddiastolic volume could lead to higher wall tension especially of the segments with impaired function. As a result, PFR expresses the impaired compliance of the left ventricular wall.

The study demonstrates the positive effect of DDD-pacing in comparison to VVI-pacing on systolic and a possibly negative effect on diastolic function. Possibly this finding can be explained by allodromic conduction of the electrical activation from the right to the left ventricle.

When considering that for the time being no established method exists to predict the ideal pacing mode for any particular patient, parameters like PER, which can be calculated easily by using non-invasive methods, are of practical value. Studies are under way to evaluate the behaviour of PFR in patients with normal global and regional wall motion. For practical purposes it is important that DDD- and VVI-pacing can be differentiated by this parameter during rest. Exercise tests, especially in an elderly population, are difficult to perform because of technical reasons (low working capacity).

No difference between PER and PFR was observed in patients with and without retrograde conduction during VVI-pacing. No final decision can be reached, as yet, whether in this small patient group, VA-conduction has a negative effect on hemodynamics, or whether an influence can not be detected by using this method.

References

1. Sutton R, Perrins J, Citron P: Physiological cardiac pacing. Pace 1980; 3: 207–219.
2. Greenberg B, Chatterjee K, Parmley WW, Werner JA, Holly AN: The influence of left ventricular filling pressure on atrial contribution to cardiac output. Am Heart J 1979; 98: 742–751.
3. Reiter MJ, Hindman MC. Hemodynamic effects of acute atrioventricular sequential pacing in patients with left ventricular dysfunction. Am J Cardiol 1982; 49: 687–692.
4. Mostbeck A, Köhn H, Bialonczyk CH: Das Low-pass-Filter als bildverbesserndes Verfahren in der Radionuklidventrikulographie. Acta Med Austriaca 1983; 10: 40–44.
5. Maddox DE, Wynne J, Uren R, Parker JA, Idoine J, Siegel LC, Neill JM, Cohn PF, Homan BL: Regional ejection fraction: A quantitative radionuclide index of regional left ventricular performance. Circ 1979; 59: 1001–1009.
6. Harvey W: Movement of the heart and blood in animals. An anatomical essay. KJ Blackwell, Oxford Scientific Publications; 1957: 34.
7. Mitchell JH, Gilmore JP, Sarnoff SJ: The transport function of the atrium: Factors influencing the relation between mean left atrial pressure and left ventricular enddiastolic pressure. Am J Cardiol 1962: 237–247.
8. Mitchell JH, Gupta DN, Payne RM: Influence of atrial systole on effective ventricular stroke volume. Circ 1965; XVII: 11–18.
9. Linden RJ, Mitchell JH: Relation between left ventricular diastolic pressure and myocardial segment length and observations on the contribution of atrial systole. Circ 1960; VIII: 1092–1099.
10. Polak JF, Kemper AJ, Bianco JA, Parisi AF, Tow DE: Resting early peak diastolic filling rate: A sensitive index of myocardial dysfunction in patients with coronary artery disease. J Nucl Med 1982; 23: 471–478.
11. Mancini GBJ, Slutsky RA, Norris SL, Bhargava V, Ashburn WL, Higgins CB: Radionuclide analysis of peak filling rate, filling fraction and time to peak filling rate. Am J Card 1983; 51: 43–51.
12. Adam WE, Bitter F: Advances in heart imaging. Med Radionuclide Imaging 1980: 195–215.

Supported in part by "Jubiläumsfond der Österreichischen Nationalbank; Projekt Nr. 1983" and Hochschuljubiläumsstiftung der Stadt Wien.

Authors' address:
Dr. G. Unger
Wilhelminenspital
III. Medical and Cardiac Dept.
Montleartstr. 32
A-1160 Wien/Österreich

Effect of Right Ventricular Pacing Rate on the Asynchronous Contraction of the Ventricles Studied by a Phase Analysis of Multigated RN Angiocardiogram

Keiji Ueda, Hiroshi Tabuchi, Hajime Murata, Hideo Yamada,
Shinichro Ohkawa, Makoto Sakai, Satoru Matsushita, Masaya Sugiura

Summary: The effect of the rate of right ventricular, endocardial pacing on the asynchronous contraction of the ventricles was studied by the phase analysis of the regional volume curves of the right and left ventricles on multigated, equilibrium RN angiocardiogram in ten adult control subjects (mean age, 38.0 years) and eight aged patients (mean age, 77.8 years) receiving ventricular demand pacemaker.

In paced aged patients, the average value of the phase delay of the left ventricle from the right ventricle was increased in five patients; an average of the delay was 8.4 msec for pacing rate of 50 bpm, 24.4 msec for 90 bpm, and 33.8 msec for 110 bpm. No change was noted on the electrocardiogram or on a body surface map when the pacing rate was increased from 50 bpm to 90 or 110 bpm. An augmented asynchronism of ventricular contraction may reflect pacing-induced left ventricular dysfunction in aged patients.

Recent advances in the data processing of heart imaging, especially that using the phase of the basic frequency of Fourier analysis (1), allows precise recognition and analysis of uncoordinated myocardial motion. Asynchronous contraction accompanying bundle branch block (2) has been analysed with the help of the phase scan.

We studied the extent of asynchronous contraction of the right and left ventricles in aged cases with right ventricular endocardial pacemaker and the effect of pacing rate on the asynchronism of the regional contraction of the ventricles.

Material and Method

The study group consisted of ten control subjects (control group, mean age: 38.0 years) showing normal electrocardiogram and no apparent cardiovascular disorders, and eight patients (paced group, mean age: 77.8 years) with implanted endocardial, multiprogrammable right ventricular pacemaker (VVI). The paced patients included six patients with complete A-V block and two patients with sinus brady-arrhythmia (sick sinus syndrome). The transvenous lead was placed in the apical portion of the right ventricle in all patients studied. In four patients, electrocardiograms showed QRS complex of left bundle block pattern and in another four patients, RS pattern of the QRS complex in precordial leads from V_1 through V_6. No paced patient had congestive heart failure or hypertension at time of the study.

A multigated, equilibrium radionuclide (RN) angiocardiogram was obtained in modified LAO position with the injection of 20 mc of technetium-99m red blood cells in both groups. In the paced group, pacing rate was increased by 20 bpm and equilibrium RN angiocardiogram was repeated: in three patients pacing rate was increased by 20 bpm from

50 bpm to 110 bpm, in four patients from 50 bpm t0 90 bpm, and in one patient from 70 bpm to 110 bpm. Precordial lead electrocardiogram (V_5 or V_6) and blood pressure were monitored during the study.

Data obtained with a parallel hole collimeter were processed with a computer and the quantitative phase at each pixel of the both ventricles was calculated by the Fourier transform at fundamental frequency (1). Then mean phase values of the right and left ventricle were obtained using a phase histogram. Regional phase values of the small ROIs located at the apex of the right ventricle and near the free walls of the both ventricles (lateral portion of the right and left ventricles) were also obtained.

The phase image was depicted as a functional colour image representing 15 msec difference in the phase per one colour as reported elsewhere (3).

A body surface map was recorded in four patients with a pacing rate of 70 bpm and 110 bpm. The details of the method of recording and the analysis were reported elsewhere (4).

Results

1. Comparison of the phase image of regional volume curve.

In the control group, contraction of the right and left ventricles was observed almost simultaneously with slight delay in the outflow tract of the right ventricle. The difference between the phase images between the two ventricles was 12.5 ± 10.8 (m $\pm$ SD) msec.

In paced patients, the contraction was first observed in the apical portion of the right ventricle where the tip of the lead was placed and regional contraction spread to the rest of the right ventricle and to the left ventricle (Fig. 1). The time delay of the initiation of the

Fig. 1. Phase image of regional contraction in Case 2. Delay of the contraction of the left ventricle is evident when pacing rate was increased from 50 bpm to 70 or 90 bpm.

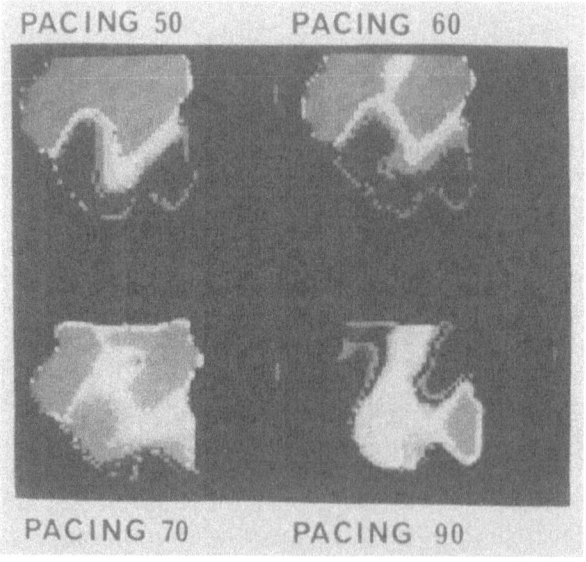

PACING 50   PACING 60

PACING 70   PACING 90

contraction between the apex and lateral portion of the right ventricle, and between the apex of the right ventricle and the lateral portion of the left ventricle were 42.38 ± 22.06 msec and 58.38 ± 23.39 msec, respectively (Table 1).

2. Effect of the increase in pacing rate on asynchronous contraction of the ventricles.

As pacing rate was increased from 50 bpm (from 70 bpm in one patient) to 90 bpm (four patients) or to 110 bpm (four patients), the time delay in the contraction of the right and left ventricle, defined as the difference between the mean values of the phase histogram of both ventricles, was increased in six patients, and decreased slightly in two patients (Fig. 2).

Mean values of the phase delay of the left ventricle from the right ventricle were: 8.43 ± 27.8 msec with pacing rate of 50 bpm (seven patients), 16.43 ± 15.67 msec with

Table 1. Clinical spectrum and phase difference at pacing rate of 70 bpm.

Case	Age (years)	Sex	Arrhythmia	ECG	Phase difference (rate 70 bpm) (msec)		
					RV_A–RV_L	RV_A–LV_{OL}	RV_L–LV_L
1. S.M.	74	M	C–AVB	LBBB pattern	60	103	43
2. H.I.	79	F	C–AVB	LBBB pattern	21	40	19.
3. S.G.	75	F	C–AVB	LBBB pattern	21	40	19
4. S.Sa	80	M	C–AVB	RS pattern	20	40	20
5. S.Su.	69	F	C–AVB	RS pattern	58	56	−2
6. F.N.	88	F	C–AVB	LBBB pattern	38	68	30
7. C.S.	76	M	SSS	RS pattern	41	41	0
8. Y.O.	81	M	SSS	RS pattern	80	79	−1
mean	77.75				42.38	58.38	16.0
± SD	± 5.65				± 22.06	± 23.39	± 16.16

Abbreviations: C–AVB = complete atrioventricular block, F = female; LV_L = lateral portion of the left ventricle; M = male; RV_A = apical portion of the right ventricle; RV_L = lateral portion of the right ventricle; SSS = sick sinus syndrome.

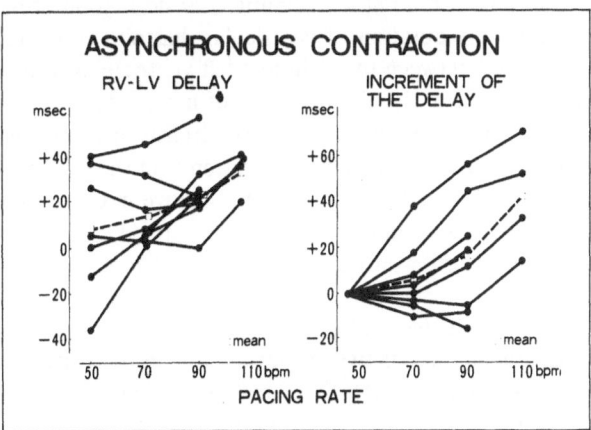

ASYNCHRONOUS CONTRACTION

Fig. 2. Phase delay between the right and left ventricle at various pacing rates.

70 bpm (eight patients), 24.38 ± 15.99 msec with 90 bpm (eight patients), and 33.75 ± 9.47 msec for 110 bpm (four patients) (Table 2). They tended to increase as the pacing rate was increased.

3. Effect of the increase in pacing rate on electrocardiogram and precordial mapping.

On precordial lead electrocardiogram and body surface map, no appreciable change in QRS complex, ST segment, and T wave was observed with the increase in the pacing rate.

Discussion

The temporal sequence of regional contraction in both ventricles, depicted by the phase image of RN angiocardiography, usually follows the spread of the excitation wave-front over the right and left ventricular myocardium when the endocardium of the right ventricular apex is stimulated. A phase difference of an average of 42 msec between the right ventricular apex and the lateral portion of the right ventricle may be mainly due to the time required for the excitation wave-front to reach the right bundle branch through local muscular conduction. The excitation of the left ventricle shows a delay of 58 msec, as an average, mainly due to the time required for the excitation wave-front to reach the left side of the interventricular septum. It has been noted that the QRS complex of the 12-lead electrocardiogram, especially those of precordial leads, during right ventricular pacing may be influenced by the location of the tip of the lead in the right ventricle. However, the precise mechanism by which the difference of the spread of excitation wave is reflected in various patterns of the QRS complex on the electrocardiogram could not be accurately analysed in the present study with LAO RN angiocardiogram.

An increase in the time delay of the phase between the right and left ventricular contraction, observed in the majority of cases when the pacing rate was increased to 90 bpm or 110 bpm, is of interest. Although the precise mechanism of this finding could not be confirmed in the present study, several possibilities may be involved. These include: 1. the limitation of the comparison of phase parameters in Fourier transform for cases with markedly different heart rate, 2. the change in the spread of excitation induced by an increase in heart rate, and 3. manifestation of hemodynamic derangement induced by pacing tachycardia.

It has been recognized that the parameters of the phase in Fourier transformation of regional of volume curve is influenced by the duration of ventricular diastole. However, when the regional contraction is compared between the right and left ventricle, of which the duration of diastole did not differ significantly, the influence of heart rate may not contribute to the result of comparison of phase parameter of Fourier transformation. The possibility that pacing tachycardia may modify the spread of excitation over the right and left ventricle appears to be unlikely, because usually no appreciable change in QRS complex on 12-lead electrocardiogram is observed when the pacing rate is altered, and in the present study, the body surface map failed to show any alteration of the pattern of ventricular excitation.

Pacing tachycardia increases minute oxygen demand of the myocardium and may induce myocardial ischemia in cases with significant obstructive lesions in the coronary arteries, resulting in disturbance of left ventricular function (5). Since regional function curve of RN angiocardiogram actually represents regional ejection fraction, pacing-induced myocardial ischemia in aged patients may impede regional ejection fraction which may be reflected in the change of the phase of Fourier transformation. Ischemic ST-T changes during pacing tachycardia could not be detected in the present study, probably due to the presence of L-BBB pattern of QRS complex and secondary ST-T changes accompaning right ventricular pacing.

Angina pectoris was clinically recognized in one patient (case No. 3) and significant stenosis of three main branches of the coronary artery was found at the autopsy in one patient (case No. 8). Among other patients, histories of hypertension were noted in three cases (case's No's 2, 4, 6), mitral regurgitation in one patient (case No. 8), and aortic regurgitation in one patient (case No. 7). Left ventricular dysfunction may be induced by pacing tachycardia in aged patients with ischemic heart disease and/or left ventricular hypertrophy, and this may contribute to the increase in delay of the phase of the left ventricle.

References

1. Adam WE, Tarkowska A, Bitter F, Stauch M, Geffers H: Equilibrium (Gated) Radionuclide Ventriculography. Cardiovasc Radiol 1979; 2: 161–173.
2. Swiryn S, Pavel D, Byrom E: Sequential regional phase mapping of radionuclide gated biventriculograms in patients with left bundle branch block. Am Heart J 1981; 102: 1000–1010.
3. Toyama H, Murata H, Iio M, Takaoka S: The temporal Fourier analysis of the cardiac multigated by the first pass and the equilibrium method. J Medical Imaging 1981; 1: 81–88.
4. Yamada K, Toyama J, Wada M, Sugiyama S, Sugenoya J, Toyoshima H, Mizuno Y, Satohata I, Kobayashi T, Okajima HM: Body surface isopotential mapping in Wolff-Parkinson-White syndrome: Noninvasive method to determine the localization of the accessory atrioventricular pathway. Am Heart J 1975; 90: 721–734.
5. Graber JD, Conti CR, Lappe DL, Ross RS: Effect of pacing-induced tachycardia and myocardial ischemia on ventricular pressure-velocity relationships in man. Circulation 1972; 46: 74–83.

Authors' address:
Dr. Keiji Ueda
Department of Medicine and Department of Nuclear Medicine
and Radiological Science
Tokyo Metropolitan Geriatric Hospital
35-2 Sakaecho, Itabashi-ku, Tokyo 173, Japan

Rate Responsive Pacing Using the TX Pacemaker

A. F. Rickards, R. M. Donaldson

Summary: We have evaluated clinically a rate-responsive pacemaker which uses the evoked QT principle as indicator of physiological demand. This pacemaker is microprocessor-based and fully programmable noninvasibly through radiofrequency coupling to an external microcomputer.

To date this system has been implanted in 15 patients. With this QT sensing pacemaker the rate response to exercise was smooth and progressive, and gradually returned the basic paced rate after termination of activity. Physiological rate responsive pacing resulted in significant improvement in exercise tolerance and a 40% increase in cardiac output when compared to fixed-rate pacing in 8 patients.

This initial experience confirms the possibility of obtaining a physiological response to exercise using a pacing system dependent only on a unipolar electrode which is independent of the problems of atrial activity and sensing. Rate responsive pacing might prove to be a useful alternative to atrial synchronous systems, particularly advantageous in those patients whose sinoatrial function is abnormal or who suffer from atrial arrhythmias.

Introduction

The alteration of cardiac output in relation to metabolic needs is a fundamental property of the intact cardiovascular system. Although pacemakers capable of adjusting heart rate according to changes in atrial activity were introduced more than 19 years ago (1), the majority of patients receiving pacemakers for the treatment of bradycardia do not have 'physiological' control of cardiac hemodynamics. Whilst the normal atrium must still remain the ideal input to a physiological pacing system, there remain major problems in the technology of atrial sensing and in differentiating between normal and retrograde atrial activation or pathological and physiological tachycardias. Patients with abnormal sinus function are potentially limited if the atrium is used as physiological marker.

We have recently described a rate responsive pacemaker which uses the QT principle as an indicator of physiological demand (2) independent of the requirement to synchronise with atrial activity. In this study we report our clinical experience with this pacing system.

Patients

To date (April, 1983) 15 QT pacemakers have been implanted in patients with complete, established heart block; 12 of the 15 patients had either abnormal sinus node function or atrial fibrillation.

253

The Pacemaker

The design of the rate responsive (TX) pacemaker* using the QT principle as well as the initial evaluation of the paced evoked response has been reported by us (2–4).

Algorithms simulating normal physiological response alter the paced rate in response to relative changes in the sensed stimulus to T wave interval; these pacing algorithms can also be modified noninvasibly. Following delivery of a stimulus the pacemaker is refractory for 200 ms, then anables a T wave sensing window (around 350 ms) which terminates the refractory period and enables QRS sensing. The subsequent stimulus escape interval is then set as a function of the proceeding stimulus-T time. A decrease in this interval causes a rate increase and viceversa. The sensitivity (slope) or the system to the stimulus-T changes (from 0.5 to 5 beats $min^{-1}ms^{-1}$) and the slow exponential drift (null) back to the basic rate (from 35 to 125 beats $min^{-1}hour^{-1}$) were programmed noninvasibly soon after implantation and tailored individually to produce steady rate increases (with a maximal rate of change set at 30 beats min^{-2}) to reach the pre-set upper rate value up to 145 beats/min over a 6 to 12 minute period, and then gradually decrease to the basic pacing rate. The T wave sensitivity can be modified according to the amplitude of the evoked T wave.

Assessment study

Changes in treadmill exercise tolerance and cardiac output were evaluated in 8 patients.

1. *Exercise testing.* For each of the 8 patients, the effects of ventricular inhibited, fixed rate pacing (VVI) at 70 beats/minute and of rate-responsive pacing (with a maximal rate set at 125 beats/min) were comparatively assessed on two separate occasions by measurements of treadmill exercise tolerance following the Bruce protocol. Studies were performed on average 2 weeks after pacemaker implant and the patients were unaware of the particular pacing mode evaluated. All exercise was reported in terms of METS (METS = O_2 uptake ml $min^{-1} \times kg^{-1}/3.5$).
2. *Cardiac output* was measured in triplicate both at rest and on peak exercise with both modes of pacing by the thermodilution technique (CVI model 600, Edwards Lab Model 9510A) following the insertion of a Swan Ganz flow directed triple lumen catheter (CVI model 600-017 Edwards Lab model No. 93A 131 7F) positioned in the pulmonary artery.
3. *Statistical analysis.* The difference in the means and Student's t-test was applied to evaluate changes in cardiac output with both forms of pacing.

Results

The initial experience reported was obtained over a 6 month follow-up period. In one patient with cardiomyopathy and low amplitude (1 mV) T waves, transient loss of T wave

---

* Vitatron Medical BV, The Netherlands.

sensing occurred from 2 to 5 days after the acute electrode implant. There were no other sensing or pacing problems at this early follow-up stage.

1. *Exercise stress testing*

Fig. 1 illustrates the smooth and progressive ventricular rate adaptation during treadmill exercise testing. This progressive decrease in the paced cycle length is seen in the continuous ECG recording during exercise shown in Fig. 2. A gradual rate decline ensued from the 8 minute period of exercise (Fig. 1) coinciding with peak exercise workload, and enabling the patient to maintain fast rates for the duration of the exercise.

Exercise tolerance in METS at fixed rate (70 beats/min) and at the maximally achieved rate response to the stimulus-T shortening (125 beats/min) is shown in the Table. Maximal exercise capacity at the rate 70 beats/min was 5.56 ± 1.35 (SD) METS whilst at the paced rate 125 beats/min the peak exercise achieved was 8.0 ± 1.22 METS ($p < 0.005$).

2. *Cardiac output*

The changes in cardiac output on exercise paralleled the increased exercise tolerance (Table). Resting cardiac output was mean: 5.83 ± 1.43 l/min at fixed paced rates of 70 beats/min and on peak exercise this increased to 9.99 ± 1.43 l/min ($p < 0.001$). With rate responsive pacing resting cardiac output was similar (5.62 ± 1.35 l/min) at mean paced rates of 66 beats/min and increased with maximal exercise to 14.02 ± 3.14 l/min. The difference between resting and exercise cardiac output with rate responsive pacing was highly significant ($p < 0.001$). The difference between maximal cardiac output with

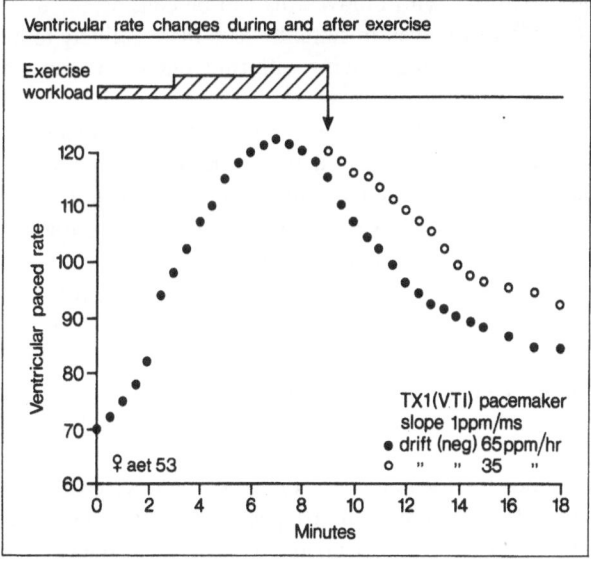

Fig. 1. Rate responsive pacing during treadmill exercise testing, showing smooth and progressive ventricular rate increase and decrease (see text for details).

Fig. 2. Continuous ECG recording during the treadmill exercise test, showing a gradual decrease in the paced cycle length as exercise workload progresses.

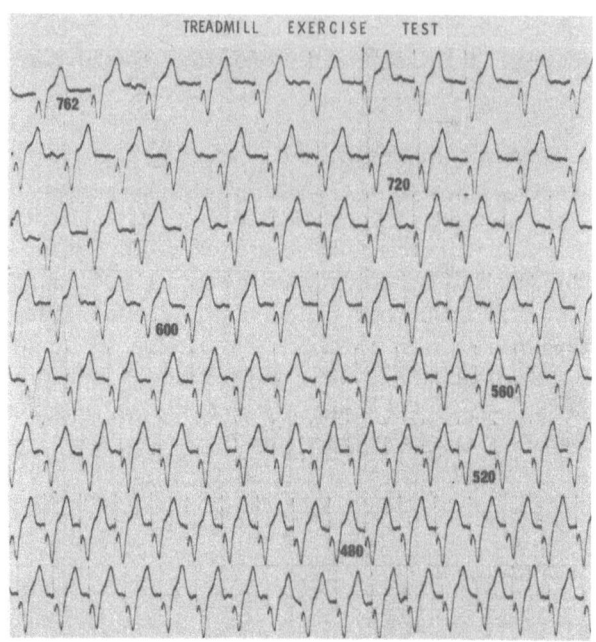

fixed rate pacing and rate responsive pacing was also significant ($p < 0.001$) in the 8 cases.

Discussion

Approximately 25% of all patients presenting with bradycardia can be considered suitable for atrial synchronous pacing (5). However, even in suitable cases there is likely to be a decrease in the effectiveness of atrial synchronous pacing with time due to progressive sino-atrial disease.

When single chamber ventricular pacing is being employed, or when sinoatrial function is abnormal, alternate methods of sensing the physiological demands need to be employed, which can be effective in producing a physiological rate response to exercise. Two rate responsive approaches have been explored. The first uses an orthogonal atrial electrogram detector, which senses average atrial rate and the change in atrial rate as indicative of metabolic demands; this information is then used to control the ventricular rate (6). The second approach to rate responsiveness has been to use indicators of physiological demand which are independent of the atrial electrogram. In addition to the evoked QT, changes in pH (7), central venous O_2 content (8) and respiratory rate (9), have been evaluated as indicators of increased metabolic demands for the development of physiological pacing systems.

Advantages of the TX pacemaker include the use of a conventional unipolar electrode for pacing and sensing, the independence of the system from atrial activity and atrial sensing problems and the absence pacemaker-induced reentrant arrhythmias. Because the QT in-

Table 1. Changes in maximal workload (in mets) and cardiac output in 8 patients during pacing at VVI (70 bpm) and with TX pacing with a maximal rate set at 125 beats/min.

Patient No.	Maximal workload (mets)		Cardiac output (l min^{-1})			
			Fixed rate pacing (70 bpm)		Rate responsive pacing	
	Fixed rate pacing (70 bpm)	Rate responsive pacing (mx 125 bpm)	Rest	Exercise	Rest (mean rate: (66 bpm)	Exercise (mx 125 bpm)
1	6	8.5	5.2	7.2	5	14.4
2	4.5	9	6	8.5	5.5	12.6
3	4	8	6.3	8.6	5.8	11.4
4	7	9.5	7	13	7.2	16.3
5	5	7	4.4	9.3	4.6	13
6	4	6	3.8	7.8	3.6	9.2
7	7	7	5.64	11	5.48	14.8
8	7	9	8.3	14.5	7.8	20.5
Mean ± SD	5.56 ± 1.35	8 ± 1.22	5.83 ± 1.43	9.99 ± 2.61	5.62 ± 1.35	14.02 ± 3.14

terval varies between individuals and may be affected by a variety of drugs, physiological limitations have to be considered. The use of a slow drift back and sensing of QT interval change rather than QT interval itself largely avoids these problems.

As in the studies reported by Knudson (6) and MacCarter (10) we found an almost linear relationship between exercise tolerance and the peak heart rates achieved on exercise (Table). The mean exercise tolerance increased from 5.56 ± 1.35 METS (with fixed rate pacing at 70 beats/min) to 8.0 ± 1.22 (at rate-responsive paced rates to a maximum of 125 beats/min). Furthermore, the improved exercise tolerance was mimicked by a 40% increase in the mean exercise cardiac output from 9.99 ± 2.61 l/min (at 70 beats/min) to 14.02 ± 3.14 (at rates of 125 beats/min) (p < 0.001).

This initial experience confirms the possibility of obtaining a physiological response to exercise using a pacing system dependent only on a conventional endocardial electrode which independent of problems of atrial activity and sensing. The development of a single chamber rate responsive pacemaker should be seen as a step in the development of potential dual chamber devices. Rate responsive pacing might prove to be a useful alternative to atrial synchronous systems, particularly advantageous in those patients whose sinoatrial function is abnormal or who suffer from atrial arrhythmias.

References

1. Samet P, Castillo C, Bernstein WH: Hemodynamic sequelae of atrial ventricular and sequential atrioventricular pacing in cardiac patients. Am Heart J 1966; 72: 725–729.
2. Rickards AF, Norman J: Relation between QT interval and heart rate. New design of physiologically adaptive cardiac pacemaker. Br Heart J 1981; 45: 56–61.
3. Donaldson RM, Fox K, Rickards AF: Initial experience with a physiological, rate responsive pacemaker. Br Med J 1983; 286: 667–671.

4. Rickards AF, Donaldson RM: The use of the QT to determine pacing rate. Early clinical experience. Pace 1983; 6: (2) 346–354.
5. Rickards AF, Donaldson RM: Rate responsive pacing. Clin Progr Pacing & Electrophysiol 1983; 1: 12–19.
6. Knudson MB, Amundson DC, Mosharrafa M: In: Barold S, Mugica J, eds. The Third Decade of Cardiac Pacing. Futura Publishing Co, New York, 1982; 249.
7. Camilli L, Alcidi L, Risani R: Results, problems and perspectives in the autoregulating pacemaker (Abs). Pace 1982; 3: 365.
8. Wirtzfeld A, Goedel-Meinen L, Block T et al: Central venous oxygen saturation for the control of automatic rate responsive pacing. Pace 1982; 5: 829–835.
9. Rossi P, Pliccui G, Canducci G et al: Cardiac pacemaker with stimulation rate controlled by breathing frequency. Proceedings 5th International Seminar "La Nuova Frontiera Delle Aritmie", Trento, Italy. 1982 (In press).
10. MacCarter D, Santini A, Goicoles A et al: Improved exercise tolerance and arrhythmia protection with a new dual chambered rate responsive pacing system (Abs). Circulation 1982; 66 II: 218.

Authors' address:
Anthony F. Rickards, FRCP, FACC
National Heart Hospital
Westmoreland
London W1
England

A Pacemaker which Automatically Increases its Rate with Physical Activity

D. P. Humen, K. Anderson, D. Brumwell, S. Huntley, G. J. Klein

Summary: Although atrial synchronous pacemakers (VAT, VDD) are being used successfully to give some patients a physiologic heart rate increase with exercise, there are others who cannot benefit from these devices because of sinus node dysfunction. We constructed a novel pacemaker with an internal transducer which senses the quantity of physical activity and a special circuit which translates that quantity into a pacing rate. We initially tested the device in 5 normal subjects who wore the pacemaker on the chest surface while an ambulatory monitor recorded both the patient's ECG and the stimulation rate of the pacemaker. The recordings demonstrated an excellent correspondence between two rates. The device was then implanted in two patients with sinus node dysfunction who subsequently demonstrated a physiological rate response with exercise and improved exercise tolerance.

Dual-chamber pacing may provide benefits to the patient through enhancement of ventricular filling by atrial systole and by allowing physiological rate increases by atrial tracking. The relative contributions of the latter 2 mechanisms have been the focus of debate (1, 2). Although Samet (3) demonstrated a 25% increase in resting cardiac output with DVI pacing as compared to VVI pacing, Sowton (4) was not able to demonstrate an increase in exercise tolerance when switching from VVI to DVI pacing. Kruse (5) demonstrated nearly an 80% increase in exercise tolerance with a VDD device – a device which gives atrial assist AND rate responsiveness. In the latter report, the benefits of atrial systole were less important than rate responsiveness in patients with congential A-V block. These patients did not have a limited cardiac performance despite A-V block because of their ability to increase heart rate with exercise. This does not demean the importance of atrial systole in the compromised heart but rather points to rate responsiveness as a crucial component in achieving maximal cardiac output.

It is clear that appropriate rate responsiveness with a VDD or DDD device requires normal sinus node function and absence of atrial fibrillation and other atrial arrhythmias. However, it has been reported that approximately 30% or more of all pacemaker patients may exhibit these contraindications (6). The latter underscores the need for a rate-responsive pacemaker which is triggered by a parameter other than atrial rate. Many parameters have been tried including Ph (7), respiratory rate (8, 9), ventricular repolarization (10) and oxygen saturation (2). We felt that physical activity was an important variable and have chosen it as the parameter determining heart rate. Ours is an activity-sensing, rate-responsive pacemaker and has the benefits of simplicity and universal applicability regardless of atrial disease.

Description of the Pacemaker

The sensor we have developed for this purpose is bonded to the inner surface of the pacemaker enclosure for portection from mechanical and chemical abuse. The sensor not only detects activity from local muscle motion but also is sensitive enough to detect muscle activity propagated from the extremities. Ambulation results in typical electrical signals emanating from the sensor. Other activities (somersaulting, rope climbing, for example) show similar waveforms. Important to note is that, as the degree of activity increases, so do both the strength AND occurrence of the sensor signals. These parameters (strength and occurrence) are used to tailor the heart rate response to individual patients.

The pacemaker can be noninvasively programmed to ignore low level signals (Fig. 1a). Only those signals above a programmed level are entered as "counts". In this way, only filtered "counts" eminate from the circuit and indicate that activity is being undertaken. More activity produces more "counts". The counts are multiplied by a preselected gain (or sensivitiy) to give the continuously varying pacing rate. Only very low strength counts are ignored so that "occurrence" of sensor electrical activity has a greater impact than "strength". For this reason the origin of the activity, be it the extremities or thorax, makes little difference. The system treats all activity equally.

There are 10 sensitivities (Fig. 1b), any one of which can be noninvasively programmed. The pacemaker is designed to modulate the rate between a programmable lower rate (of which the minimum is 55 bpm) and an upper rate (of which the maximum if 120 bpm), the specific rate dependent upon the activity level and the sensitivity setting. Lower rates of 60, 70, 80 or 90 bpm are programmable as well as an upper rate of 100 bpm. The pacemaker has a fast attack, slow decay response in an attempt to simulate normal phys-

Fig. 1. Pacemaker Function
a) Circuitry schematic of the activity-sensing pacemaker.
b) Ten programmable rate sensitivities.
c) Time restraints of attack and decay.

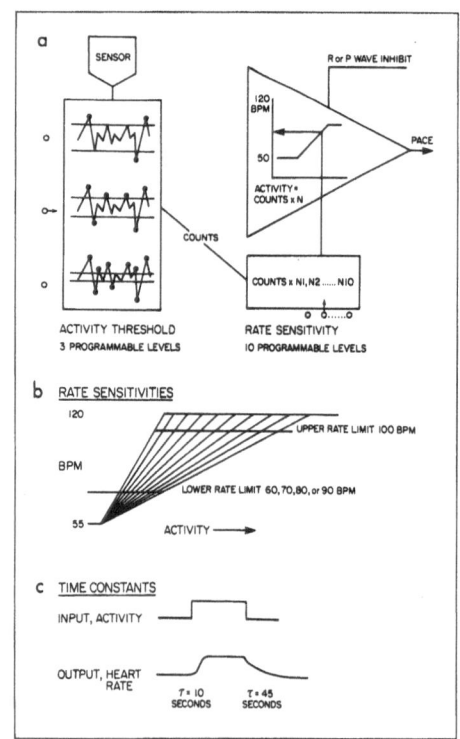

iology (Fig. 1c). An example of such a hypothetical activity would be to quickly stand up, walk around and then quickly sit down. Note the heart rate increase is purposely faster than the decay. For a slowly increasing or slowly decreasing activity the heart rate will not lag behind the activity. This approximates the response of the normal heart.

Evaluation of Normal Subjects

The efficacy of the device was then tested in normal subjects. Of primary importance was how well the pacing rate approximated a normal person's intrinsic rate. False increases or decreases in pacing rate were especially looked for. For that purpose, we securely taped the devices to the chest of five normal subjects. The pacing output was fed into channel 1 of an ambulatory monitor while channel 2 recorded the subject's intrinsic heart rate. The subjects were told to perform their normal daily routine. The spontaneous heart rates of the patients were then compared to the pacing output rate.

Results

Following evaluation of the Holter monitor recordings (Fig. 2) it became clear that the pacing rate follows the intrinsic rate remarkably well. When the intrinsic rate rises or falls so does the pacing rate. A couple of incidents are noted where a rise in the intrin-

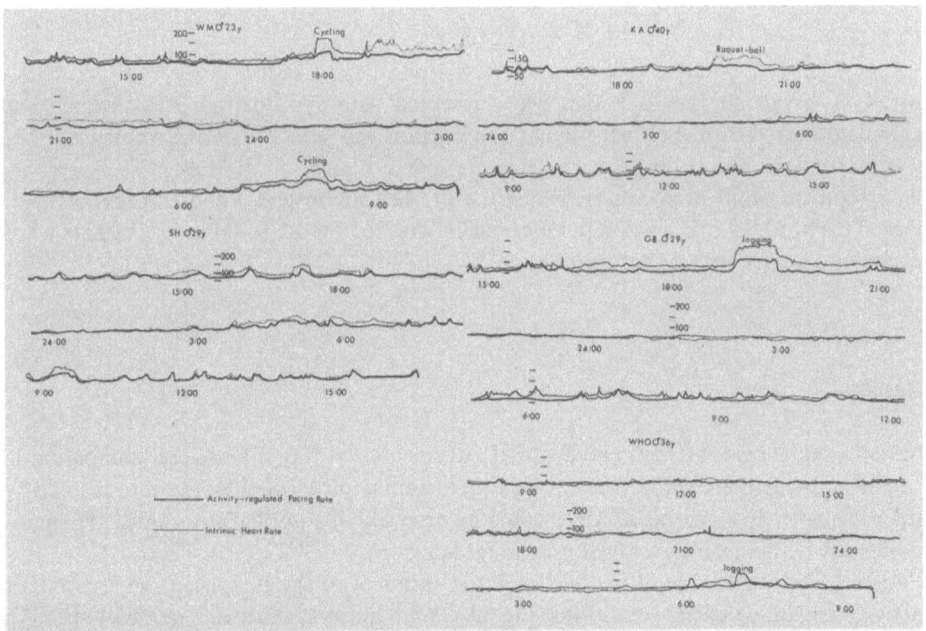

Fig. 2. Holter Monitor Heart Rate Histograms. The rate of pacing impulses closely follow the intrinsic heart rates.

sic rate is not accompanied by a rise in pacing rate. The log reveals that this event was not associated with physical activity.

There is one instance where the pacing rate exceeds the intrinsic rate. This occurred in subject WHO during deep sleep. The difference noted in heart rates recorded was only slight.

When the subjects underwent strenuous exercise the intrinsic rates rose to 150 bpm and often to 180 but the paced rate remains limited to 120 bpm. The pacemaker was specifically designed to regulate from 55 to 120 bpm since the literature (11) suggests further increases above 120 bpm are not accompanied by further significant increases in cardiac output.

Patient Implants

Having gained confidence in this device's ability to simulate a healthy sinus node, units were implanted in two patients.

Case One

Mr. M.H. is a 44 year old man who presented with sinoatrial node dysfunction accompanied by syncope which was induced by Amiodarone required for control of malignant ventricular arrhythmias. Because atrioventricular conduction was found to be normal, an atrial lead was inserted for AAI pacing.

Case Two

Mr. G.T. is an 80 year old man who presented with syncopal spells associated with complete heart block. Left ventricular dysfunction was also present. A ventricular lead was inserted for VVI pacing.

Naughton treadmill protocols (13) were used to test the response and efficacy of the device. This protocol offers a gradual increase in workload more suitable for patients whose exercise tolerance may be compromised.

Results

Several weeks post-implant patient M.H. was exercised (Fig. 3a). When comparing his response to age-matched normals following a similar protocol (12), the rate response of the pacemaker is very near to what would be expected of a normal sinus node. The paced patient by design reaches a lower maximum however.

Patient G.T. was exercised in the Naughton protocol in the nonpaced, VVI paced and activity-regulating paced conditions (Fig. 3b). With an idioventricular rate of 40 bpm, he barely started the protocol when the exercise was discontinued because of fatigue and dyspnea at 3/4 MET. Fixed rate VVI pacing at 70 bpm permitted 1 1/2 MET's and the

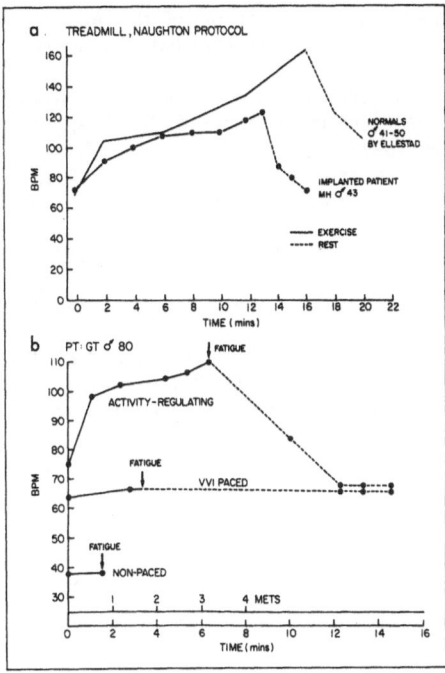

Fig. 3. Patient Treadmill Data
a) Rate response of M.H. as compared to normals.
b) Enhanced exercise tolerance in patient G.T.

activity regulating mode with a peak pacing rate of 120 bpm permitted exercise to 3 MET's.

It is clear that, although fixed rate VVI pacing doubles his exercise tolerance, activity sensing rate-responsive pacing doubles it further.

Summary

We have developed a rate-responsive, activity-sensing pacemaker which produces a physiologic pacing rate response. With this feature the potential exists for increased exercise tolerance and a more active lifestyle than could be attained with a nonregulating pacemaker.

References

1. Goldreyer BN: Physiologic Pacing: The Role of A-V Synchrony. Pace, 1982; 5: 613.
2. Wirtzfeld A, Goedel-Meinen L, Bock T, Heinze R, Liss H, and Munteanu J: Central Venous Oxygen Saturation for the Control of Automatic Rate Responsive Pacing. Pace 1982; 5: 829.
3. Samet P, Bernstein WH, and Levine S: Significance of the Atrial Contribution to Ventricular Filling. Am J Cardiol 1965; 15: 195.
4. Sowton B, Thorburn C, and Roy P: Hemodynamic Changes During Cardiac Pacing. In: Proceedings of the IVth International Symposium On Cardiac Pacing, Thalen HS, editor, Assen Von Gorcum, 1973, p 24.

5. Kruse I, Arnman K, Conradson T, and Ryden L: A Comparison of the Acute and Long-Term Hemodynamic Effects of Ventricular-Inhibited Pacing. Circulation, May 1982; 65(5): 846–855.
6. Sutton R, Perrins J, and Citron P: Physiological Cardiac Pacing. VIth World Symposium on Cardiac Pacing, Montreal, 1979. Cardiac Pacing – State of the Arts, 1979: Proceedings. Montreal, Quebec: Pacesymp 1979, pp 16–17.
7. Camilli L, Alcidi L, and Papeschi G: A New Pacemaker Autoregulating the Rate of Pacing in Relation of Metabolic Needs. Cardiac Pacing. Proceedings of the Vth International Symposium. Excerpta Medica, Amsterdam, 1977: p 414.
8. Funke HD: Ein Herzschrittmacher mit belastungsabhängiger Frequenzregulation. Bio-Med Technik, 1975; 20: 225.
9. Krasner J, Voukydis P, and Nardella P: A Physiologically Controlled Cardiac Pacemaker. JAAMS, Nov/Dec 1966; 1(3): 476–485.
10. Rickards A, and Norman J: Relation Between QT Interval and Heart Rate. New Design of Physiologically Adaptive Cardiac Pacemaker. Br Heart J, Jan 1981; 45(1): 56–61.
11. Escher DW: In: Heart Disease: A Textbook of Cardiovascular Disease. Braunwald E, editor, WB Saunders, 1980, p 756.
12. Ellestad M: Stress Testing, Principles and Practice, FA Davis, pub 1975.
13. In: Exercise and the Heart, FA Davis, pub, 1978, p 176.

Authors' address:
Dr. D. P. Humen
Cardiac Investigation Unit
University Hospital
Box 5339, Station A
London, Ontario
Canada N6A-SA 5

Automatic Atrial-Guided Adjustment of Ventricular Pacing Rate in Complete AV Block

S. Sermasi, M. Marzaloni, L. Rusconi, M. Pauletti*, C. Contini*,
G. E. Antonioli

Summary: The clinical feasibility of achieving permanent, atrial guided pacing via a transvenous single catheter with double electrodes has previously been proposed by the AA and recently adopted. A morphological modification of the atrial sensor has subsequently been reported by other AA and applied to a ventricular pacing system that automatically responds to variations in the atrial rate without AV synchrony. The validity of such a device, the RS4/SRT system, has been evaluated in 8 patients with advanced AV block, normal sinus function and acceptable ventricular performance. 3 to 22 month follow-up studies (373 ± 166 days) with the RS4 demonstrated the following:
- Choerent rate response of the system according to device specifications at rest (pharmacological tests).
- Greater exercise tolerance (ergometric tests) with RS4 in the RS mode vs. VVI mode.
- Ripetitive adjustment of ventricular pacing rate as response to variations in sinus rate (Dynamic 24-hour ECG monitoring).
- Greater subjective well-being of patients during normal activities with the RS mode compared to VVI one.

The results obtained show that the RS4/SRT system constitutes a valid progress compared to the traditional VVI pacing.

The increase of heart rate is one of the first mechanisms which occurs to elevate cardiac output during increased patients activity. One of the limits of ventricular pacing in complete AV block is the absence of automatic adjustment of the pacing rate in relation to necessary patients demands.

In cases of advanced AV block with intact sinus function, at present time, an atrial-guided system represents the most effective solution for pacing.

Our group demonstrated the possibility of recording atrial signals of sufficient amplitude and frequency for pacemaker sensing circuitry, without contacting the endocardial wall using a coaxial transvenous catheter with a ring electrode (unipolar) for sensing in the atrium and an electrode for ventricular pacing (1–5).

From these preliminary studies we developed a simplified system for permanent atrial-synchronized pacing which demonstrated a satisfactory working in repeated tests (6).

In 1981 CPI presented a rate responsive pacing system, called RS4, utilizing a single transvenous catheter (the SRT lead) for both atrial sensing and ventricular pacing: the atrial ring was subdivided in two orthogonal semi-rings (bipolar) for discriminating the floating atrial signal with the elimination of the far field ventricular electrogram component (7). The RS4 system does not result in consistent 1 : 1 AV synchrony, but variations

---

* CNR Institute of Clinical Physiology – Pisa, Italy. Cardiology Dept. Ospedale Infermi – Rimini, Italy.

in ventricular rate are induced as result of sensed variations in the atrial rate, in a randomized AV synchronous fashion.

The ventricular response to a change in the atrial rate appears withing a few seconds and tends to complete itself within 30 seconds. The ventricular pacing rate varies between 63–65 ppm and 115 ppm in relation to the atrial rate.

Preliminary clinical evaluations demonstrates the advantages of such system and the possibility to resolve some problems related to traditional ventricular pacing in the treatment of patients with advanced AV block, normal sinus function and acceptable ventricular performance (8–12).

This study reports an experience of eight RS4/SRT implanted and their follow-up.

Materials, methods and results

RS4 units were implanted in eight patient (Tab. 1). In all cases catheter entry was via cephalic vein. Aside from rigidity of the tip-tines which impaired maneuverability of the catheter, no particular difficulties in the introduction and positioning were encountered. The medium to hig position in the atrium always guaranteed an optimal sensing of the atrial signal (Fig. 1). The P-wave recorded by an Electronic for Medicine VR 12 photographic recorder, measured in each case within one respiratory cycle, demonstrated an average amplitude of 3.85 ± 1.43 mV.

Correct working of the pacing system in the Rate Responsive (RS) mode was verified in each patient by pharmacological tests. In Fig. 2 is shown an example of intravenous infu-

Table 1. RS paced patients (Pts).

Pts	Age	Sex	Indications	Date of implantation
PV	76	M	3rd degree AV block	12. 2. 1981
MR	74	M	2nd degree AV block Mobiz II + 3rd degree AV block (intermittent)	11. 6. 1981
GU	61	M	Trifascicular block (1st degree AV block + RBBB + LAH) + 2nd degree AV block Mobiz II (intermittent)	10. 8. 1981
SA	70	M	3rd degree AV block	6. 10. 1981
MA	70	M	3rd degree AV block	1. 12. 1981
PG	72	M	2nd degree AV block Mobiz II + 3rd degree AV block (intermittent)	22. 4. 1982
DDM	44	F	3rd degree AV block	15. 6. 1982
MM	71	F	3rd degree AV block	3. 9. 1982

Fig. 1. See text.

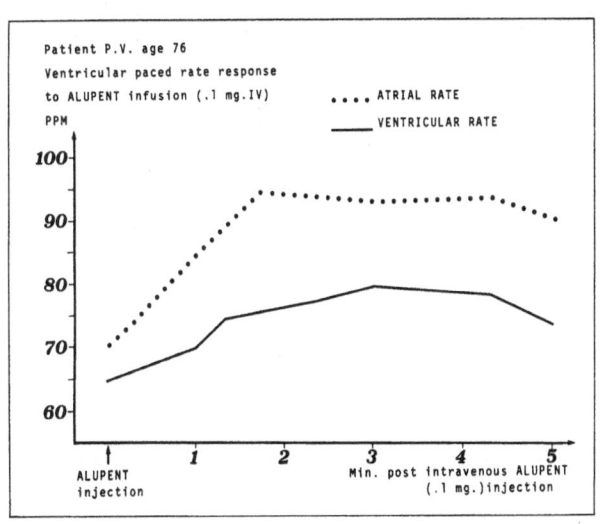

Fig. 2. See text.

sion of Alupent able to produce an increase of atrial rate with subsequent automatic increase in paced ventricular response and the following algorithm-induced rate decay.

On the fourth week post-implant, a patient stress test was performed on a cycle ergometer (Del Mar-Avionics ExerStress Analyzer 3100) with the pulse generator converted to VVI mode.

A similar study was repeated one week later in the RS mode.

The results of the stress (Tab. 2). demonstrated in 7 cases a greater work capacity (expressed as total work done) in RS mode.

One patient was not evaluable for the presence of constant sinus rhythm.

The average follow-up has been 373 ± 166 days; i.e. from a minimum of 3 to a maximum of 22 month.

Two patients (PV and SA) died respectively 314 and 174 days after implant for causes not related to the pacemaker. In one patient (DDM) the correct working of the RS mode was documented but frequent and prolonged pauses due to myopotential inhibitions were documented too. 237 days after implant the pacemaker was explanted and a traditional programmable VVI replaced, switched to VOO because myopotential inhibitions were still present.

Follow-up studies performed via dynamic 24-hour ECG monitoring demonstrated in all cases proper adherence of the RS4 system to its rate response design specifications. An example of automatic changes in the RS4 paced rate according to patient activity is shown in Fig. 3. By testing for several seconds only the phases immediately following a detected algorithm-induced increase, the average paced ventricular rate in relation to the sinus rate (real-time Holter recording), was quite high: $87.1 \pm 3.4\%$. The latest follow-up subjectively evaluated patient tolerance to non-synchronous, rate responsive pacing.

For several days, the patients were not informed they were being paced in the VVI mode. At check-up time, all reported reduced physical capacity to perform their activities. These subjective comments ceased with reconversion to the RS mode of pacing.

Table 2. Exercise Stress Testing: RS vs VVI pacing (Bruce protocol).

Pts	Age	KgMt (VVI)	KgMt (RS)	%	VR max (VVI)	VR max (RS)
PV	76	22.2	35.5	59.4	72	96
MR	74	19.4	28.8	48.4	72	92
GU	61	21.8	30.0	27.3	72	86
SA	70	33.6	48.0	42.9	72	80
MA	70	18.0	24.4	37.8	72	96
PG	72	21.6	32.4	33.3	72	98
MM	71	12.6	16.2	22.2	72	88

KgMt = Total work load $\times 10^2$
VR max = Maximum ventricular paced rate in ppm

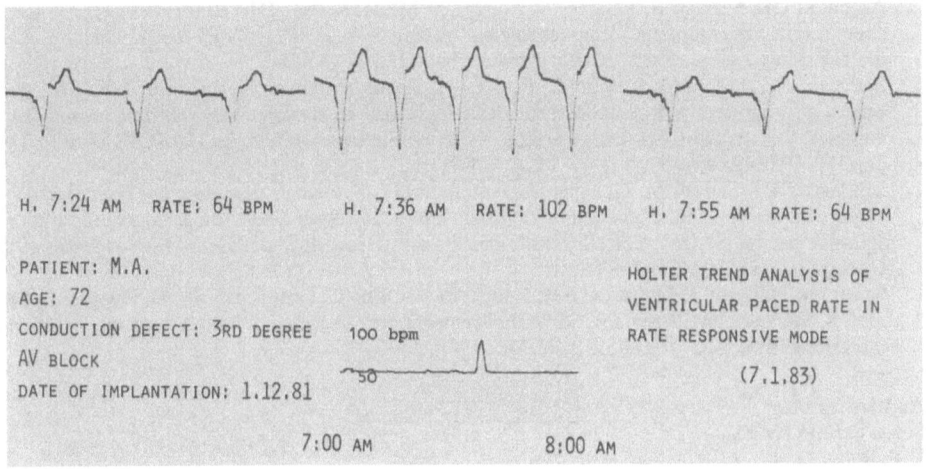

H. 7:24 AM   RATE: 64 BPM   H. 7:36 AM   RATE: 102 BPM   H. 7:55 AM   RATE: 64 BPM

PATIENT: M.A.   HOLTER TREND ANALYSIS OF
AGE: 72   VENTRICULAR PACED RATE IN
CONDUCTION DEFECT: 3RD DEGREE   100 bpm   RATE RESPONSIVE MODE
AV BLOCK   (7.1.83)
DATE OF IMPLANTATION: 1.12.81

                                7:00 AM   8:00 AM

Fig. 3. See text.

Comment

The results obtained show the RS4/SRT system constitutes a valid progress compared to the traditional VVI pacing. It is well understood that optimized cardiac pacing will be attained once a pulse generator is developed which not only is atrial-guided, yet respects the atrioventricular sequence of the normal heart; on the other hand the developement of an automatic, rate adjustable pulse generator in response to the patient's daily life activity is certainly an achievement in pacemaker therapy.

References

1. Antonioli, GE, Grassi G, Baggioni GF, Andreuccetti, D, Paone F, Marzaloni M: "A simple P-sensing, ventricular stimulating lead driving a VAT generator". In C Meere (Ed), Proceedings of the 6th World Symp on Cardiac Pacing. Pacesymp Montreal, Canada 1979; chap 34–9.
2. Antonioli GE, Grassi G, Baggioni GF, Andreuccetti D, Papone F, Marzaloni M: "A simple new method for atrial triggered pacemaker". G Ital Cardiol, 1980; 10: 679.
3. Antonioli GE, Grassi G, Baggioni GF, Marzaloni M, Andreuccetti D, Sermasi S: "VAT and VDT system using a single bipolar catheter". 1st Asian-Pacific Symp. on Cardiac Pacing. Jerusalem 1980 Pace, 1980; 3: 362 (Abstr).
4. Antonioli GE, Grassi G: "Stimolatore atrio-comandato e ventricolo-sincrono con catetere unico a doppio elettrodo". Pacemaker in Italia 1980; 9: 3.
5. Antonioli GE, Grassi G, Marzaloni M, Rusconi L, Sermasi S: "Catetere unico per stimolazione atrio-guidata. Rassegna critica". Cardiostimolazione, 1983; 1: 74.
6. Antonioli GE, Grassi G, Marzaloni M, Sermasi S: "A new implantable VDT pacemaker using a single catheter with a doble electrode". 2nd European Symp. on Cardiac Pacing. Florence 1981 Pace, 1981; 4: A-80 (Abstr).
7. Goldreyer BN, Olive AL, Leslie J, Cannom DS, Wyman MG: "A new orthogonal lead for P synchronous pacing". Pace, 1981; 4: 638.
8. MacCarter DJ, Alliegro A, Hector H, Rollies L, Dubert A, Antonioli GE, Sermasi S, Mugica J, Letouzey JP, Santini M: Frequenzadaptierte Schrittmachertherapie beim Menschen unter verschiedenen Belastungsbedingungen". Herz-Medizin, 1981; 3: 145.

9. Antonioli GE, Sermasi S, Pesaresi A, Marzaloni M, MacCarter DJ: "Improved exercise tolerance in man via automatic" 'rate responsive' pacing. A case history". IX World Congr of Cardiology, Moscow June 1982; 20–26: Abstract book II, pag 13 n°43.
10. Sermasi S, Marzaloni M, Rusconi L, Pesaresi A, Pasini W, Albani A, Antonioli GE: "Adeguamento atrio-guidato non sincronizzato della frequenza di stimolazione ventricolare nel BAV completo". Atti XIII Congr Naz Cardiol ANMCO, Firenze 3–6 Giugno 1982 OIC Press, c 277, pag 389, 1982 (Abstr).
11. MacCarter DJ, Santini M, Goicolea A, Antonioli GE, Sermasi S, Knudson M, Goldreyer BN: "Improved exercise tolerance and arrhythmia protection with a new dual chambered rate responsive pacing system". 55th Scientific Session Am Heart Ass, Dallas 15–18 November 1982 Circulation, 1982; 66.3 II-219 (Abstr).
12. Santini M, Alliegro A, Di Mascolo R, Rocchi M, Messina G, Dini P, Ialongo D, Rusconi L, Sermasi S, Marzaloni M, Antonioli GE: "Il pacemaker atrio-regolato. Un nuovo approccio alla stimolazione fisiologica". Cardiostimolazione 1983; 1: 37.

Authors' address:
Sergio Sermasi, M.D.
V. le Boito, 26
47049 Viserba di Rimini (Italy)

Mixed Venous Oxygen Saturation for Rate Control of an Implantable Pacing System

A. Wirtzfeld, K. Stangl, R. Heinze, Th. Bock, H. D. Liess, E. Alt

Summary: One of the main disadvantages of most pacing systems available today is their inability to increase stimulating rate with exercise. This paper describes the concept of an autoregulating pacing system the rate of which is determined by changes in mixed venous oxygen content. For the realisation of this concept an optical sensor mounted on the pacing lead has been developed which allows continuous monitoring of the oxygen saturation in the right ventricular cavity. The advantages of this parameter over other physiologic hemodynamic or metabolic variables are discussed.

There is no denying the fact that for most patients cardiac pacing is unable to truly normalize or at least optimize circulatory performance since there are a number of defects inherent in this mode of treatment as it is usually applied today (1). This is especially reflected by the hemodynamic situation of the paced heart in patients with myocardial impairment; the symptoms of failure are often heardly improved by pacing (2, 3), and most individuals remain markedly limited in their working capacity (4, 5). The underlying cardiac disease as well as pacing itself must be made responsible for this undesirable situation.

The major defect in contemporary pacemakers is their inability to increase pacing rate with changing physiological requirements. This serious disadvantage of most pacing systems has not been redressed with the introduction of so called "physiologic pacing" (6). A number of studies have shown that the exercise capacity can markedly be augmented by rate-responsive pacing systems (7–11) and that reinstitution of AV synchrony alone without an increase in pacing rate does not appreciably improve cardiac performance during exercise (12). The significance of AV synchrony appears especially unimportant in patients with cardiac failure as with progressively higher left ventricular filling pressures the atrial contribution to ventricular filling becomes progressively less (6). Furthermore, it is known from the work by Karlöf et al. (8) on patients with atrial-triggered pacemakers (VAT) that for the improvement in cardiac output during exercise an increase in heart rate is much more important than the restoration of AV synchrony. With the exception of VAT-(VDD)-units, however, pacing rate is fixed and it must be assumed that the rate at which the unit is set will not be optimal for the patient most of the time (1). A truly physiologic pacemaker, therefore, should be able to autoregulate its pacing rate even in the absence of normal atrial activity.

The development of a pacemaker responsive to increasing metabolic demands by increasing pacing rate is dependent upon the input or sensing system which "informs" the pacemaker that an altered metabolic state requiring a higher rate exists. Various biological parameters such as blood pH (13, 14), respiratory rate (15–17), central body temperature (18, 19) or QT-interval of the intracardiac electrogram (20, 21) have been proposed as input signals for such a pacemaker. As we have pointed out, however, we believe that mixed venous oxygen saturation (S_{O_2}) would be a more suitable parameter for pacemaker rate control (22).

Behaviour of S_{O_2} during exercise

By raising oxygen consumption, any increase in physical activity requires an increase in the oxygen transporting capacity of the circulation which is accomplished by two factors: an increase in cardiac output and an enhancement of oxygen extraction from arterial blood. This latter change leads to an increase in arterio-venous oxygen difference (AVD-O_2) which is the consequence of a drop in mixed venous oxygen saturation as arterial saturation remains unchanged (23).

As more oxygen is extracted from arterial blood by the working muscles, S_{O_2} falls immediately from the beginning of exercise and reaches a new plateau within a period of about 1 minute (Fig. 1). The extent of the drop in S_{O_2} is dependent on the level of exercise and on cardiac output. The product of cardiac output and arterio-venous oxygen difference is the amount of oxygen used by the body ($\dot{V}O_2 = CO \cdot AVD-O_2$). If cardiac output cannot adequately be increased the fall in S_{O_2} will be more pronounced and the maximum oxygen uptake, i.e. the aerobic power will be reduced. In patients with decompensated heart failure mixed venous S_{O_2} will be reduced even at rest.

Any therapeutic intervention which improves hemodynamics in the sense of augmenting cardiac output will immediately lead to a rise in mixed venous S_{O_2}. In patients with pacemakers, therefore, any improvement in cardiac performance seen with various pacing modalities will be reflected by a higher mixed venous S_{O_2}. As we have demonstrated during exercise tests performed on ten patients with implanted programmable VDD units, mixed venous S_{O_2} was about 7 vol% higher on VDD- as compared to VVI (70/min) pacing (Fig. 2). This quite appreciable difference, the fast response of S_{O_2} and its dependency

Fig. 1. Drop of mixed venous oxygen saturation measured in the right ventricular cavity with our S_{O_2} sensor during a 25 Watts exercise test.

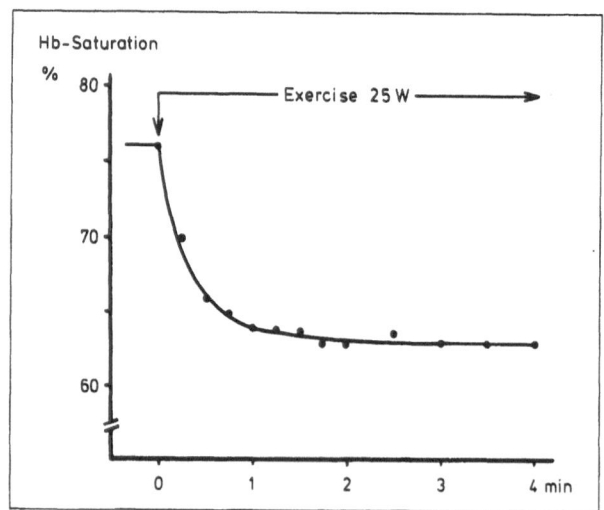

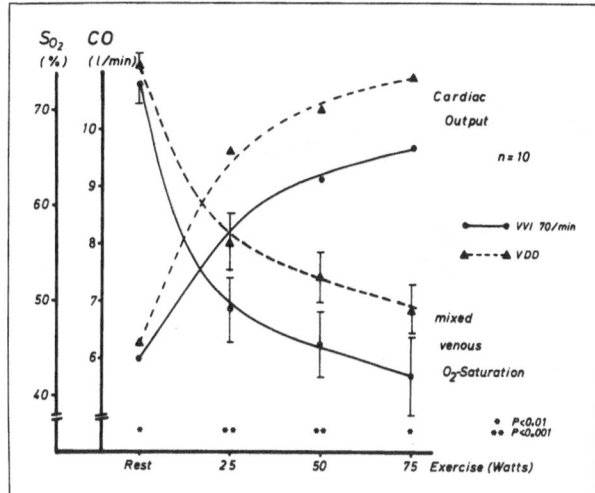

Fig. 2. Cardiac output and mixed venous oxygen saturation at rest and during an exercise test performed on 10 patients at VVI- and VDD-pacing.

on the level of exercise should make this parameter the ideal input signal for an autoregulation rate-responsive pacing system.

Optical sensor for monitoring mixed venous S_{O_2}

The sensor developed at our institution (24) is incorporated within the pacing lead at some distance from the stimulating tip so that the oxygen saturation in the right ventricular cavity can be monitored (Fig. 3 and 4). S_{O_2} is measured opto-electronically by means of the well-known principle of hemoreflectorimetry. The optical head consists of the light emitting (LED) and light receiving (phototransistor) part of the system. Light of a wave length of 660 nm is emitted by the LED, reflected by the red blood cells and received by the phototransistor (Fig. 5). The voltage coming from the S_{O_2}-sensor lies around 2.5 Volts. Its dependency on the oxygen saturation of the blood is also shown on Fig. 5. Coating of the surface of the sensor by fibrin causes a downward displacement of this relationship but does not alter the characteristic of the curve.

When used in vivo, the signal received from the S_{O_2}-sensor shows characteristic fluctuations with each cardiac cycle (Fig. 6a). These are probably due to artefacts produced by the movements of the sensor. By using the intracardiac electrogram detected by the pacing electrode for triggering the sensor, in other words by restricting the measurement to enddiastole exclusively, a very stable S_{O_2}-signal can be obtained (Fig. 6b). In the case of a stimulating pacemaker, the pacing spike, of course, would trigger the S_{O_2}-sensor. The time required for the LED to flash up is less than 1 ms. Thus the current consumption of the entire S_{O_2}-measuring system can be kept very low (3–4 uA).

Our experience so far has shown that with the S_{O_2}-sensor working in the triggered mode, a reliable reproduction of mixed venous S_{O_2} can be obtained. As an example, in Fig. 7 the course of S_{O_2} during an exercise test performed on a patient with normal hemodynamics and normal rate increase on exercise is demonstrated. There is a marked fall in oxygen

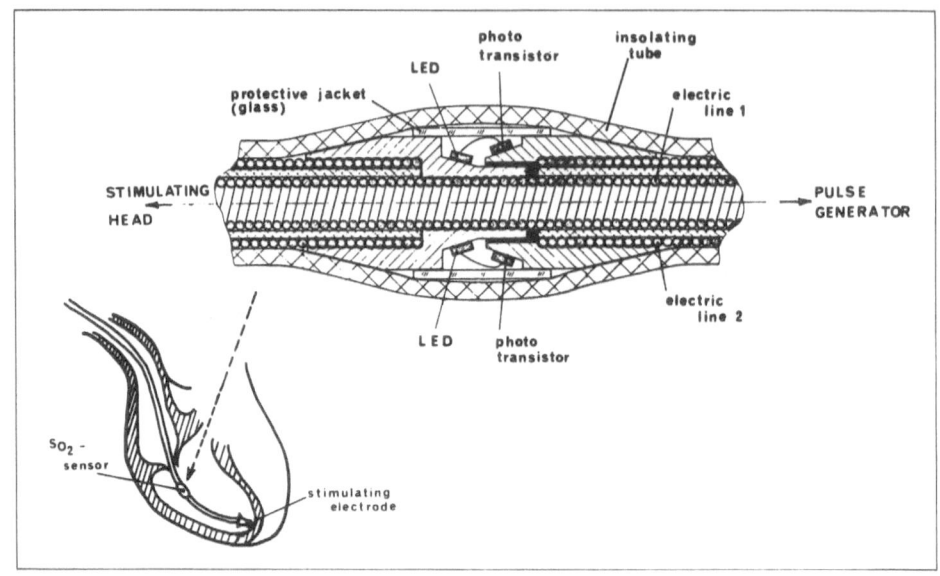

Fig. 3. Cross-section through the S_{O_2}-sensor.

Fig. 4. Laboratory model of the S_{O_2} electrode used for our studies

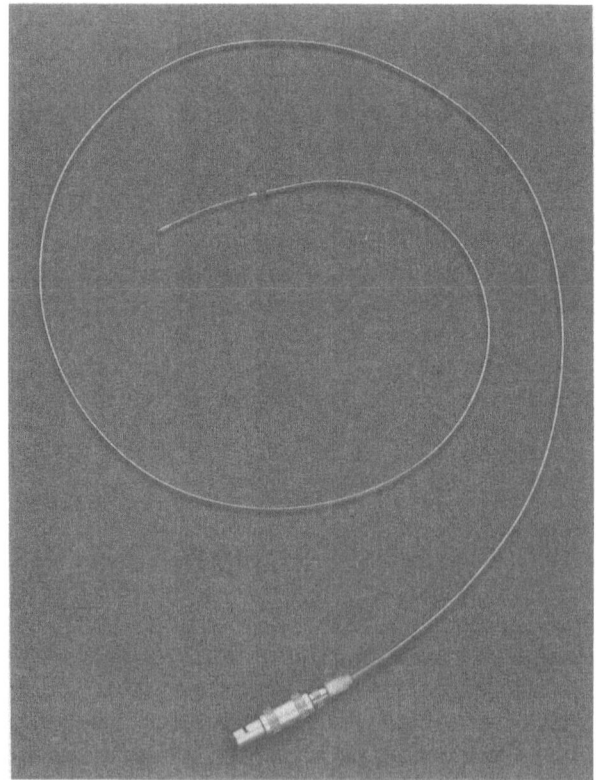

274

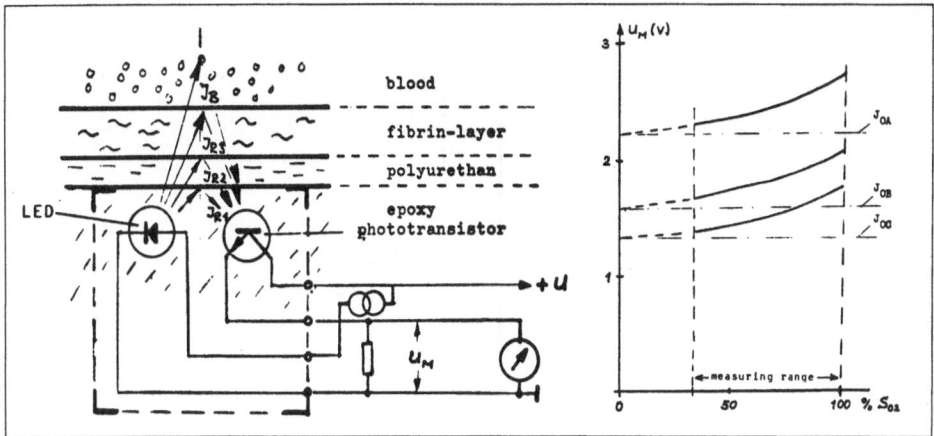

Fig. 5. Mode of operation of the active S_{O_2}-sensor
Left: principle of measurement. Total intensity of reflected light reaching the phototransistor: $J_G = J_B + J_O$ when J_B = light reflected on red blood cells; J_O = light reflected by different material layers and their interfaces; $J_O = J_{R1} + J_{R2} + J_{R3}$
Right: Voltage measured at the phototransistor as a function of hemoglobin oxygen saturation and its dependence on fibrin layers surrounding the S_{O_2}-sensor. A = clear surface; B = fibrin layer 0.6 mm; C = fibrin layer 1.0 mm

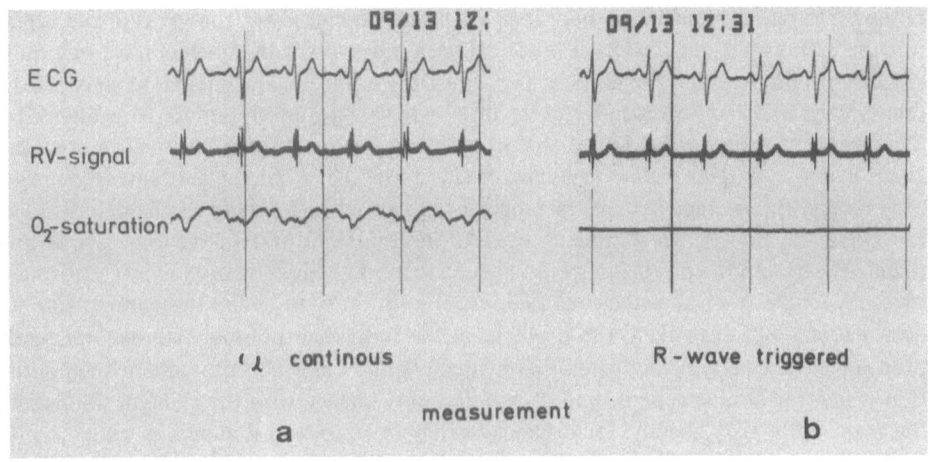

Fig. 6. Signal received from the S_{O_2}-sensor.

saturation starting right from the beginning of the test and a clear relationship between the degree of exercise and the decrease of S_{O_2}. On each level of exercise a new plateau is reached within a period of about 60 sec. After the test is finished, there is a rapid return of the S_{O_2} towards the pre-exercise resting value.

275

Fig. 7. Mixed venous oxygen saturation recorded during an exercise test.

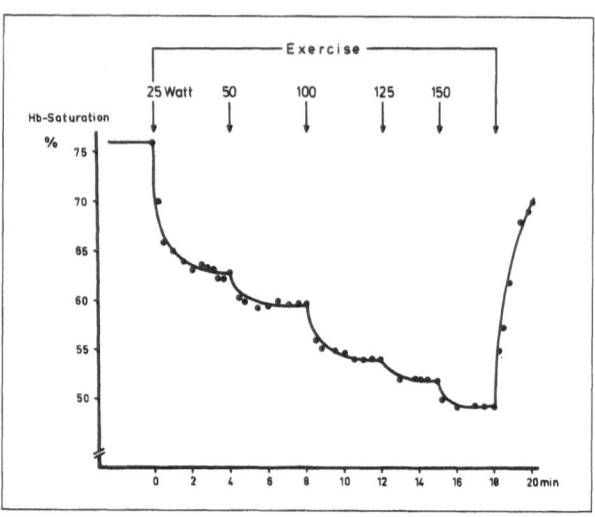

Advantages of a S_{O_2}-regulated pacing system

There are a number of advantages of S_{O_2} as input signal for an autoregulating pacemaker which would make this parameter superior to other physiological parameters that could be used for rate-responsive pacing (Tab. 1). Besides their slower change with the beginning or with any change in the level of exercise, these other parameters have one quite significant disadvantage in common: they must use a fixed characteristic, namely a fixed relationship between pacing rate and the physiological parameter used for is regulation!

This means that one will never be able to optimize the hemodynamic situation in all patients as due to different rate-output curves (25) a rate that would be adequate in one case may be bad for another patient. In practice that would mean that the characteristics of rate versus the physiologic parameter used for its regulation would have to be a programmable feature and the physician would have to determine individually (invasively or noninvasively?) the most advantageous rate response in order to define the optimal rate for each patient. But even then, the problem of the individual optimal rate has not really been solved since any hemodynamic assessment would only reflect the momentary situation which might change any time. It will certainly change with the aging of the patient but it may also vary acutely, for instance during an episode of ischemia in patients with coronary heart disease. Therefore it seems unlikely that a frequency-regulated pacing system using a fixed characteristic between rate and a physiologic parameter would be acceptable for a significant proportion of our pacemaker patients.

Mixed venous S_{O_2}, on the other hand, is the only parameter which does not require a fixed relationship to pacing rate. Irrespective of the individual values for mixed venous S_{O_2} (which may vary quite considerably indeed among various patients, expecially during exercise!) the highest S_{O_2} value achieved with the lowest pacing rate will always be the "optimal" rate at this particular instant. Mixed venous S_{O_2} can therefore be used for the realization of a fully automatic physiological pacemaker with a closed feedback loop regulation of pacing rate. The idea of this concept is a pacemaker which at any given mo-

Table 1. Comparison of the various parameters proposed for rate responsive pacing.

Parameter	Advantages	Disadvantages	open questions
pH	– reflects actual work load	– no direct relationship to CO – takes relatively long to return to resting level after discontinuing exercise – must use a fixed characteristic (i.e. rate vs ph)	– long term reliability of the sensor?
Respiration Rate	– easy to measure – reacts relatively fast	– special extracardiac sensor required – can be influenced voluntarily – must use a fixed characteristic (i.e. respiratory vs heart rate)	
central blood temperature	– easy to measure	– changes are slow and do not occur with low work loads – may rise due to fever – must use a fixed characteristic (i.e. rate vs temperature)	
QT interval	– easy to measure – no special sensor required – reacts relatively fast	– only works if the unit is actually pacing – causes rate increase for only short periods ("nulling") – is influenced by drugs and may change independently of exercise (e.g. during an episode of ischemia) – must use a fixed characteristic (i.e. rate vs QT interval)	– long term behaviour of QT interval? – reliability of T wave sensing in myocardial disease?
mixed venous O_2 saturation	– fast response to exercise – exclusively determined by CO and O_2 demand – no evaluation of hemodynamic response required – only parameter suitable for a closed feedback loop system for optimizing pacing rate – could also select other pacing parameters (e.g. mode, AV interval etc.)	– difficult to measure	– long term reliability of the sensor?

ment paces at the lowest rate achieving the highest S_{O_2}. This means that at rest the pacing rate may well be below 70/min and that during exercise unnecessary high rates are avoided. Thus the pacemaker will always pace at the optimal frequency whatever the patient's rate output curve or state of activity may be. Since there is no fixed relationship between S_{O_2} and pacing rate, the system will function in patients with a reduced mixed venous S_{O_2} at rest, such as patients with decompensated heart failure or chronic pulmonary insufficiency, just as well. Such a pacemaker could be implanted without the need for preoperative (or postoperative) evaluation of the individual rate/S_{O_2}-response, and any change in this relationship occurring with further progression in myocardial impairment would automatically be taken care of.

Conclusion and future perspectives

Summarizing the advantages of mixed venous S_{O_2} for the control of a rate-responsive pacemaker, it can be stated that
- S_{O_2} starts to decline immediately from the beginning of exercise,
- the changes of S_{O_2} are exclusively determined by cardiac output and peripheral O_2 demand and
- S_{O_2} is the only parameter suitable for the realization of a closed feedback loop regulating pacing rate.

The principle of S_{O_2}-regulation may be used for any type of pacemaker including AAI- and DVI-units. It actually could finally make a truely physiologic pacemaker of the DDD units which are available today. Such a pacemaker could be the system of choice for the great majority of our patients in which VDD pacing is not suitable because of the lack of a reliable atrial signal (patients with Sick Sinus Syndrome, binodal disease, intermittent or permanent atrial fibrillation, patients with retrograde ventriculoatrial conduction initiating circus movement tachycardias).

At this time we are studying the long-time behaviour of the S_{O_2}-sensor and are working on the elaboration of the best algorithm for control of the system.

References

1. Morse D: What's wrong with pacing? Pace 1982; 5: 455.
2. Davidson DM, Braak CA, Preston TA and Judge RD: Effect on long-term survival, congestive heart failure, and subsequent myocardial infarction and stroke. Ann Intern Med 1972; 77: 345.
3. Dolder E, Halter J and Nager F: Schrittmacherimplantation bei bradykarder Herzinsuffizienz. Dtsch med Wschr 1975; 100: 2070.
4. Segel N, Hudson WA, Harris P and Bishop JM: The circulatory effects of electrically induced changes in ventricular rate at rest and during exercise. J Clin Invest 1964; 43: 1541.
5. Eimer HH and Witte J: Zur Leistungsbreite bei Patienten mit festfrequentem Herzschrittmacher unter Berücksichtigung von Hämodynamik, arteriovenöser Sauerstoffdifferenz und Lungenfunktion. Z Kardiol 1974; 63: 1099.
6. Goldreyer B: Physiologic pacing: the role of AV synchrony. Pace 1982; 5: 612.
7. Westermann KW: Hämodynamische Untersuchungen bei Schrittmacherträgern während AV-Block, starrfrequenter und vorhofgesteuerter Stimulation. Intensivmedizin 1972; 9: 360.
8. Karlöf I: Haemodynamic effect of atrial triggered versus fixed rate pacing at rest and during exercise in complete heart block. Acta med Scand 1975; 197: 195.
9. Wirtzfeld A, Himmler FC and Blömer H: Klinische Gesichtspunkte der Schrittmachertherapie bei bradykarden Herzrhythmusstörungen. Verh Dtsch Ges Kreislaufforsch 1981; 47: 98.
10. Kruse I, Arnman K, Conradson TB, and Ryden L: A comparison of the acute and long-term hemodynamic effects of ventricular inhibited and atrial synchronous ventricular inhibited pacing. Circulation 1982; 65: 846.
11. Shapland JE, McCarter D, Tockman B and Knudson M: Physiologic benefits of rate responsiveness. Pace 1983; 6: 329.

12. Sowton E, Thorburn C and Roy P: Haemodynamic changes during cardiac pacing. In: Thalen H J Th (Ed): Cardiac Pacing. Van Gorcum, Assen 1973.
13. Cammilli L, Alcidi L and Papeschi G: A new pacemaker autoregulating the rate of pacing in relation to metabolic needs. In: Watanabe, Y (Ed): Cardiac Pacing, Excerpta Medica, Amsterdam 1977.
14. Cammilli L, Alcidi L, Shapland E and Obino S: Results, problems and perspectives with the autoregulating pacemaker. Pace 1983; 6: 488.
15. Funke HD: Ein Herzschrittmacher mit belastungsabhängiger Frequenzregulation. Biomed. Technik 1975; 20: 225.
16. Ionescu VL: An „on demand pacemaker" responsive to respiration rate. Pace 1980; 3: 375.
17. Rossi P, Plicchi G, Canducci G, Rognoni G and Aina F: Respiratory rate as a determinant of optimal pacing rate. Pace 1983; 6: 502.
18. Weisswange A, Csapo G and Perach W: Frequenzsteuerung von Schrittmachern durch Bluttemperatur. Verh Dtsch Ges Kreislaufforsch 1978; 44: 152.
19. Griffin JC, Jutzky KR, Claude JP and Knutti JW: Central body temperature as a guide to optimal heart rate. Pace 1983; 6: 498.
20. Rickards AF and Norman J: Relation between QT interval and heart rate. New design of physiologically adaptive cardiac pacemaker. Brit Hert J 1981; 45: 56.
21. Rickards AF, Donaldson RM and Thalen HJTh: The use of QT interval of determine pacing rate: early clinical experience. Pace 1983; 6: 346.
22. Wirtzfeld A, Goedel-Meinen L, Bock TH, Heinze R, Liess HD and Munteanu J: Central venous oxygen saturation for the control of automatic rate-responsive pacing. Pace 1982; 5: 829.
23. Holmgren A and Linderholm H: Oxygen and carbon dioxyde tensions of arterial blood during heavy and exhaustive exercise. Acta Physiol Scand 1958; 44: 203.
24. Wirtzfeld A, Heinze R, Liess HD, Stangl K and Alt E: An active optical sensor for monitoring mixed venous oxygen saturation for an implantable rate-regulating pacing system. Pace 1983; 6: 494.
25. Sowton E: Haemodynamic studies in patients with artificial pacemakers. Brit Heart J 1964; 26: 737.

Authors' address:
Prof. Dr. A. Wirtzfeld
I. Med. Klinik rechts der Isar
der Technischen Universität
Ismaninger Str. 22
8000 München 80

Output Programmable Pulse Generator Adjustment: Pulse Duration or Amplitude

E. Astrinsky, S. Furman

Summary: Altering pacemaker output compensates for threshold rise and maintains a "safety factor" for chronic pacing. A common practice for "safety" is to double the threshold pulse duration at constant output voltage. It is the charge (mean current × pulse duration), which produces cardiac contraction at a given pulse duration. The "safety factor" depends on the ratio of output charge, which increases with both pulse duration and output voltage, to threshold charge, which increases with pulse duration only. The effect of doubling output voltage versus doubling pulse duration was determined with the Medtronic 5985 output programmable pulse generator (OPPG) connected to chronic leads of 26 to 88 months longevity, during pulse generator replacement in 7 patients. Voltage and current waveforms were acquired as the OPPG reduced pulse duration in its "auto-threshold" mode for both 2.7 and 5 volts. Similar measurements were taken at threshold for pulse duration ranging from 0.1 to 2 ms using a calibrated external pacing system analyzer. The charge per pulse was calculated from the current waveforms stored by a digital oscilloscope using its computing capability. From plots of charge vs pulse duration for threshold, 2.7 and 5 volt generator output, "safety factors" were determined. The pulse duration at which the 2.7 volt output curve intersects the threshold curve was termed threshold pulse duration. Doubling output voltage at threshold pulse duration always resulted in a larger "safety factor" by at least 20%, than doubling threshold pulse duration at 2.7 volts. Pulse duration programming is useful at shorter pulse duration and voltage programming at all pulse durations.

Alteration of the output (amplitude or pulse duration) of implanted output programmable pulse generators is readily achieved non-invasively by programming, facilitating the management of post-implant transient threshold rise (1). Programming also makes possible the reduction in output to conserve battery capacity and increase the implant's longevity. This is particularly important when dual chamber stimulating devices are used as the current drain may be so high that even lithium battery powered pacemaker's longevity is reduced to that of single chamber mercury battery powered pacemakers.

Threshold

The threshold of cardiac stimulation is the least cathodal electrical stimulus which, when delivered in diastole after the absolute, relative refractory and the hypersensitive periods, is able to maintain consistent capture of the heart. The per pulse values of current in milliamperes (mA), voltage (V), charge in microcoulombs (μC) and energy in microjoules (μJ) have all been used to quantify threshold (2, 3, 4, 5).

Voltage is an indirect measure of threshold as the actual voltage drop across responsive myocardium producing cardiac excitation cannot be separated from the voltage drop across the lead resistance and the nonlinear drop across the electrode-tissue interface. Energy per pulse is also an unsuitable parameter for quantifying threshold as it involves multiplication of the voltage by the current and pulse duration.

281

We have chosen charge per pulse as the measure of threshold stimulus as well as the measure of pulse generator output.

$$Q(t) = \int_0^T i(t) \cdot dt \qquad [1]$$

$$= \bar{I} \cdot T \qquad [2]$$

where $Q(t)$ is the charge per pulse at time t, $i(t)$ is the instantaneous current at time t, $\bar{I}$ is the mean current during the impulse, and T is the pulse duration.

It has been shown that the threshold at a given pulse duration depends primarily on the applied charge (6) which is relatively independent of stimulator output impedance for square wave pulses (7). Charge per pulse has also been chosen as it relates directly to the amount of electricity removed from the pacemaker battery each time a stimulus is delivered. Battery capacity is rated in units of charge i.e. milliampere hours. Because the current, in the series circuit formed by the pulse generator, lead, electrode and heart, is the same no matter where it is measured in the circuit, charge can be measured anywhere in the circuit.

Safety factor

Output cannot be reduced arbitrarily. The output must be left at a high enough level to maintain an adequate safety factor between output and threshold and accommodate threshold variation which occurs during normal daily activities such as sleeping, eating, exercise and the effect of medication (8). Safety factor or suprathreshold safety margin has been described increasingly in the literature (9, 10, 11).

At a given pulse duration:

$$\text{Safety Factor}$$

$$= \frac{\text{Pulse Generator Output} - \text{Threshold Value}}{\text{Threshold Value}} \qquad [3]$$

$$= \frac{\text{Output Charge} - \text{Threshold Charge}}{\text{Threshold Charge}} \qquad [4]$$

The effect on safety factor of varying output by varying pulse amplitude is different from that resulting from changing pulse duration. This is due to the shape of the charge strength duration curve which rises nearly linearly with increasing pulse duration (12) as well as the complex interaction of the pacemaker with the electrode-heart combination (13) whose impedance is a function of both amplitude and pulse duration. A series of measurements were undertaken to find the safety factor resulting from varying pacemaker output amplitude or pulse duration.

Materials and methods

All measurements were taken during pulse generator replacement on seven patients, having chronic stable leads of 26 to 88 months implant duration (Table 1). Each patient was in a resting, post absorptive stable state under local anesthesia. Chronic leads were used

Table 1. Data on leads used

Subject	Manufacturer	Lead model	AGE (mos.)
DB	Medtronic	6961	49
SH	Medtronic	6907	88
MD	Biotronik	IE65-I	48
BD	Biotronik	PE60-I-2	36
BN	Biotronik	PE60-I-2	26
MF	Cordis*	4113	44
MM	Cordis	CL	62

* Cordis Corp., Miami, Florida

to avoid short term fluctuations in threshold which occur with acute lead implants (14). In each case the lead was connected to the negative output of a Biotronik* ERA 3SDH external pacemaker modified for constant voltage output. A stainless steel retractor with a 30 cm² surface area in the pacemaker pocket served as the indifferent electrode connected to the positive output of the pulse generator through a series 10 ohm resistor. Using a Nicolet** 4094 Digital Oscilloscope, output voltage and current (voltage drop across the 10 ohm resistor) waveforms were acquired at a 2 MHz sampling rate at 12 bits precision, and displayed on the oscilloscope screen.

Threshold was determined at pulse durations of 0.1 to 2.0 ms by reducing the pulse generator's output to the lowest value which maintained capture. This method gives lower values for threshold than that found by increasing amplitude from subthreshold values due to the Wedensky (15) or hysteresis effect (16). Measurements also have better repeatability (17). Voltage and current waveforms at threshold were saved on the digital oscilloscope and stored on floppy disks for later analysis.

The external pulse generator was then replaced in the circuit by a Medtronic*** 5985 programmable pulse generator. Using the programmer in the "auto-threshold mode" output pulse duration was decreased automatically in 0.1 ms steps every six impulses from 1.7 ms until capture was lost. This was done for output programmed to 5 volts (Full) and 2.7 volts (Half). Voltage and current waveforms for each value of pulse duration for both output voltages were acquired and stored on the floppy disk.

Using the Nicolet 4094's waveform analysis and computing capability the area under the current waveform was found and the charge per pulse calculated for each of the stored current waveforms.

From graphs (Figure 1) of charge per pulse vs pulse duration for charge at threshold (the charge strength duration curve), charge at Full output and charge at Half output, the safety factor for doubling voltage was compared with that for doubling pulse duration. Note that programming from Half to Full output approximately doubles the mean output voltage even though the output is rated at 2.7 and 5 volts.

 * Biotronik Sales Inc., Lake Oswego, Oregon
 ** Nicolet Instrument Corp., Madison, Wisconsin
*** Medtronic, Inc., Minneapolis, Minnesota

Figure 1. Illustration of method of estimating charge safety factor. $Q_{P.G. (Full)}$ and $Q_{P.G. (Half)}$ are curves of charge output vs pulse duration for the pulse generator programmed to 5.0 and 2.7 volts respectively. The threshold point occurs at a pulse duration, t, where $Q_{P.G. (Half)}$ intersects the charge strength duration line, Q_{TH}. The safety factor from doubling voltage at t is A'/A, and that from doubling pulse duration to 2 t, is B'/B.

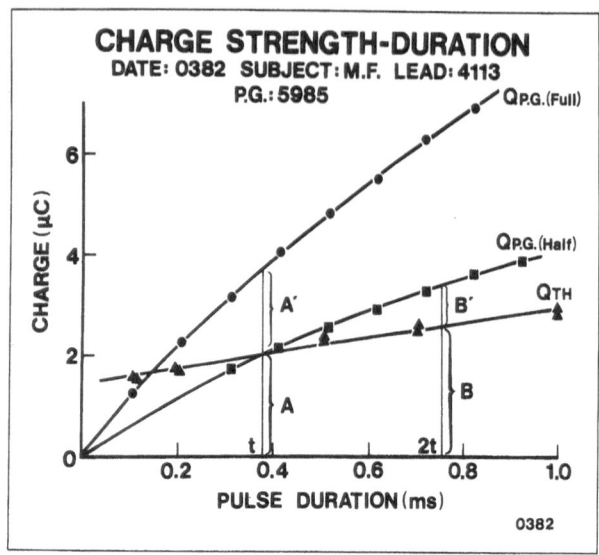

Using the formula:

Relative increase in safety factor

$$= \frac{\text{Safety factor from doubling voltage} - \text{safety factor from doubling pulse duration}}{\text{Safety factor from doubling pulse duration}} \qquad [5]$$

the relative increase was calculated for each subject.

Discussion

From Table 2 it can be seen that doubling voltage usually results in increasing the charge output by between 90 and 100% giving safety factors equal to these values. The exception in the case of BN was due to an abnormally low mean impedance of less than 300 ohms over the range of pulse durations and output voltages used. This low impedance was probably a consequence of insulation failure at the electrode. A similar case involving this electrode has been described (18) showing the bared electrode and resulting large surface area. The low impedance results in loading of the pulse generator's output and a drop in output voltage. Doubling the pulse duration from threshold at 2.7 volts never doubles the safety factor. This is readily explained by considering the interaction of the pulse generator with the heart-electrode combination.

Figure 1 shows three curves. First the charge strength duration line, Q_{TH}, then the pulse generator output curve at 2.7 volts $Q_{P.G. (Half)}$ and third the pulse generator output curve at 5 volts, $Q_{P.G. (Full)}$. Q_{TH} depends on the excitability of the heart, the proximity of the electrode to stimulatable tissue and properties of the electrode such as area, material, etc. The slope of the Q_{Th}-pulse duration line is given by the current rheobase (12) (the lowest value of current which will capture the heart no matter how long the pulse duration). This means that the line will be steep if the rheobase is elevated.

The $Q_{P.G. (Half)}$ curve has a position and slope on the charge-pulse duration plane determined by the mean equivalent impedance. The mean equivalent impedance depends on

Table 2. Charge values and safety factors for doubling pulse duration or voltage

Subj.	Pulse dura-tion	Charge per pulse			Safety factors		Relative increase in S.F.
		Threshold	"Half" output	"Full" output	Double PD	Double voltage	
	ms	μC	μC	μC			%
DB	0.08	0.52		1.06	0.68	1.04	53
	0.16	0.57	0.96				
SH	0.10	0.62		1.18	0.65	0.90	38
	0.20	0.71	1.17				
MD	0.13	1.02		2.00	0.79	0.96	21
	0.26	1.12	2.00				
BD	0.17	1.20		2.40	0.54	1.00	85
	0.34	1.40	2.15				
BN	0.23	2.55		4.66	0.60	0.83	38
	0.46	2.84	4.55				
MF	0.38	2.01		3.78	0.33	0.88	167
	0.76	2.59	3.44				
MM	0.52	2.20		4.40	0.47	1.00	113
	1.04	2.51	3.70				

Full = 5.0 volts PD = pulse duration
Half = 2.7 volts SF = safety factor

Table 3. Charge values and pulse durations for maintaining safety factor

Subject	Safety factor AT PD = t ms & "Full" output	Pulse duration		Charge values		Relative charge increase	Relative PD increase
		t	tSF	PD = t output "Full"	PD = tSF output "Half"		
		ms	ms	μC	μC	%	%
DB	1.04	0.08		1.1			
			0.22		1.6	45	175
MD	0.96	0.13		2.0			
			0.32		2.3	15	146
BD	1.00	0.17		2.4			
			0.63		3.5	46	271
BN	0.83	0.23		4.7			
			0.60		5.6	19	161

Full = 5.0 volts t = pulse duration at which threshold equals „Half" output
Half = 2.7 volts tSF = pulse duration at „Half" output at which safety factors is the same as
PD = pulse duration   that at a pulse duration of t and „Full" output

Figure 2. Effect of maintaining the same safety factor at Half output (2.7 volts) by increasing pulse duration as by doubling output amplitude from threshold at Half output.

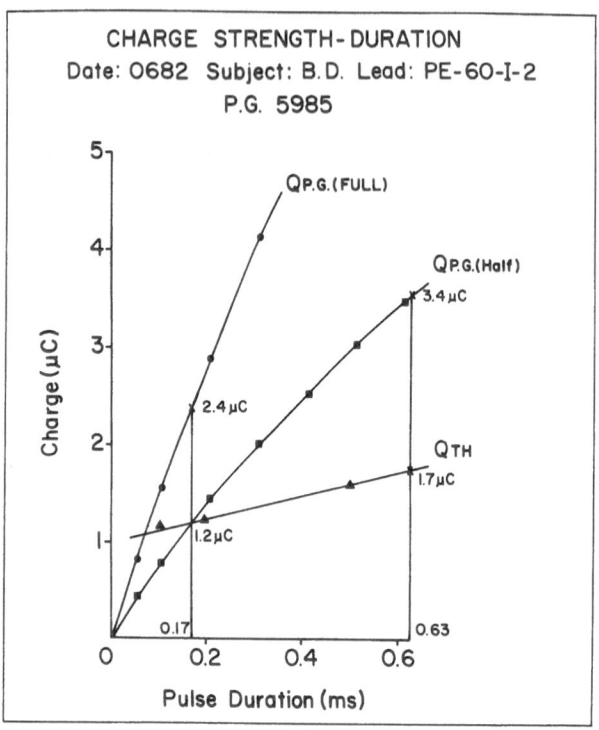

CHARGE STRENGTH-DURATION
Date: O682 Subject: B.D. Lead: PE-6O-I-2
P.G. 5985

electrode and electrolyte parameters (19). The higher the impedance level the flatter the $Q_{P.G. (Half)}$ curve.

A condition can arise where a high impedance lead is used in a patient who has a high current rheobase. Under these circumstances Q_{TH} would not intersect $Q_{P.G. (Half)}$ and the 2.7 volt output could not capture the heart no matter how great the pulse duration. Such conditions do occur in clinical practice. This explains the high relative increase in safety factor for doubling voltage compared with pulse duration for subjects MF and MM. In these cases both rheobase and mean equivalent impedance are relatively high. The low relative increase in safety factor in the case of BN is anomalous due to a high threshold but low mean impedance.

Because the current drain from the pulse generator battery increases with increasing charge per pulse, a study was carried out on the effect of increasing pulse duration at Half output until the charge safety factor reached the same value as found by doubling output voltage (Figure 2) (Table 3). In every case more charge per pulse was used by increasing pulse duration than by doubling voltage. When considering pulse generator longevity, battery current drain may favor keeping voltage low and increasing pulse duration not withstanding the relative increase in charge per pulse. This is because the efficiency of doubling voltage may be low enough to counteract the effect of requiring less charge per pulse to achieve the desired safety factor. The effect of efficiency varies with the design of the pulse generator's output circuit.

Conclusions

From threshold at a low voltage output, doubling voltage always produces a higher charge safety factor than doubling pulse duration at the low output voltage. Doubling voltage normally results in a safety factor of at least 90% unless very large electrode area, low mean impedance leads are used. Except for the activated carbon tip electrodes most modern leads have small surface area and relatively high mean equivalent impedance.

If the safety factor from doubling voltage is to be maintained by increasing pulse duration only, then the charge per pulse delivered to the lead-heart circuit is greater than that delivered by doubling voltage.

The primary concern in cardiac pacing is to maintain capture and hence maintain an adequate safety factor to overcome threshold variation. It is better to double output voltage than pulse duration. Practically, when programming the output of a pulse generator connected to stable chronic leads it is recommended that voltage be left at double threshold for a given pulse duration. If pulse duration programming only is possible then the pulse duration should be left at three times that at which threshold occurred.

Pulse generator longevity, though very important especially in the case of dual chamber pacemakers, should be treated as of secondary importance when compared with maintaining adequate safety factor. More detailed recommendations have recently been published (20).

References

1. Furman S, Pannizzo F: Output programmability and reduction of secondary intervention after pacemaker implantation. J Thorac Cardiovasc Surg 1981; 81: 713–717.
2. Sowton E, Barr I: Physiological changes in threshold. Ann NY Acad Sci 1969; 167: 679–685.
3. Davies JG, Sowton E: Electrical threshold of the human heart, Br Heart J 1966; 28: 231.
4. Hurzeler P, Furman S, Escher DJW: Cardiac pacemaker current threshold versus pulse duration. In HT Silverman, IF Miller, AJ Salkind (eds): Electrochemical bioscience and bioengineering. New Jersey, The Electrochemical Society, 1973, p 124.
5. Furman S, Parker B, Escher DJW, Solomon N: Endocardial threshold of cardiac response as a function of electrode surface area. J Surg Res 1968; 8: 161.
6. Babotai I: Die elektrochemischen Impedanzen und die elektrische Reizschwelle des Herzens bei Stimulation mit Schrittmachern. Doctoral Thesis, Eidgenössische Technische Hochschule Zürich, Diss Nr 1971, 4618.
7. Astrinsky EA, Napoli K, Parker B, Furman S: The electrode-heart impedance at threshold. In W Welkowitz (ed): Bioengineering. Proc 9th Northeast Conference, New York: Pergamon Press, 1981; pp 255–258.
8. Preston TA, Judge RD: Alteration of pacemaker threshold by drug and physiological factors. Ann NY Acad Sci 1969; 167: 686–692.
9. Barold SS, Winner JA: Techniques and significance of threshold measurement for cardiac pacing. Relationship to output circuit of cardiac pacemakers. Chest 1976; 70: 760–766.
10. Vera Z, Klein RC, Mason DT: Recent advances in programmable pacemakers. Am J Med 1979; 66: 473–483.
11. Scoblionko DP, Rolett EL: Short-term threshold behavior of human ventricular pacing electrodes: Noninvasive monitoring with a multiprogrammable pacing system. Pace 1981; 4: 631–637.
12. Irnich W: The chronaxie time and its practical importance. Pace 1980; 3: 292–301.
13. Astrinsky EA, Parker B, Furman S: Development of a graphical method for estimating pacing threshold. In BA Cohen (ed): Frontiers of engineering in health care. IEEE, New York: 1981; pp 274–276.

14. Ohm OJ, Morkrid L, Skagseth E: Temporary pacemaker treatment in open heart surgery: Variation in myocardial threshold, tissue and interface impedances in man. Pace 2: 162, 1979.
15. Sylven JC, Hellerstedt M, Levander-Lindgren M: Pacing threshold interval with decreasing and increasing output. Pace 1982; 5: 646–649.
16 Furman S, Escher DJW: Factors affecting electrical stimulation. In S Furman, DJW Escher (eds): Principles and techniques of cardiac pacing. New York, Harper & Row, 1970, p 53.
17. Bando T, Iwa T, Misaki T, Sakurai T: Development of automatic threshold analyzer. In C Meere (ed): Cardiac pacing. Montreal, Pacesymp, 1979, Chap 28–9.
18. Furman S, Pannizzo F, Campo I: Comparison of active and passive adhering leads for endocardial pacing. Pace 1979; 2: 417–427.
19. Mansfield PB: Myocardial stimulation: The electrochemistry of electrode-tissue coupling. Am J Physiol 1967; 212: 1475–1488.
20. Astrinsky EA, Furman S: Pacemaker output programming for maximum safety and maximum longevity. Clin Prog Pacing Electrophysiol 1983; 1: 51–58

Author's address:
E. Astrinsky, Ph.D.
Montefiore Medical Center
111 East 210th Street
Bronx, N.Y. 10647 USA

External-Type All-Purpose Cardiac Pacemaker

H. Makino*, Y. Saito*, T. Kiryu*, K. Tamura**, M. Yamazoe***

Summary: The external-type all-purpose cardiac pacemaker was designed to prevent fatal arrhythmias from occurring in highly susceptible individuals when they are in coronary or intensive care units and/or hospital environment. This pacemaker system consists of catheter, plate electrode, sense amplifier, microcomputers, and defibrillator controller. Once the transvenous catheter is inserted and positioned in the right ventricle, the all-purpose cardiac pacemaker is able to detect ventricular tachycardia, and to control it with burst pulse pacing. When bradyarrythmia occurs, demand pacing program works. This system can also function only as a demand pacemaker by programming. Ventricular fibrillation is diagnosed by recognizing the decrease of blood pressure. Hypotension continuing for more than 10 sec causes the pacemaker to trigger a pulse which turns-on the transvenous defibrillator.

Introduction:

After cardiac surgery, an external-type cardiac pacemaker is used for temporary pacing or for determining whether permanent-type pacemaker implantation is necessary. Until now, however, the optimal stimulation current or the rate has had to be adjusted manually with difficulty in the control procedures. And this type of pacemaker is only effective for tachycardia or bradycardia. So, a new system was designed to solve these problems by using two microcomputers (1). The system has three functions: Demand pacing, burst pulse pacing (2), and defibrillator control (3).

System:

The basic configuration of the system is presented in Fig. 1. ECG and blood pressure signals are amplified by high-input impedance preamplifier to a level between 1.0 and 1.5 Vp-p. The input signal is A-D converted, and the data is fed to a signal processing computer where the R-wave threshold level and R-R time intervals are calculated. This microcomputer and output control microcomputer are connected through a subchannel adapter. Operator interaction is via a keyboard and color CRT display. Two cardiac stimulators containing D-A converters are also provided for atrial and ventricular stimulation. Defibrillator controller contains two relay circuits and one buzzer for alarm.

---
* Faculty of Engin. and *** School of Med., Niigata Univ., ** Dept. of Med., Yamanashi Medical School, Japan.

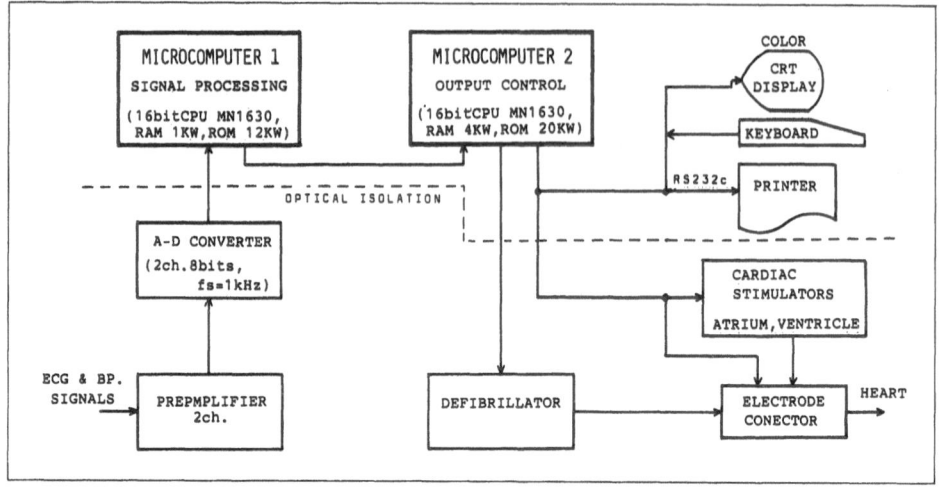

Fig. 1. Hardware configuration
A preamplifier and A–D convertor are constructed using low power OP amplifiers and CMOS ICs. The microprocessors are 16bit CPU MN1630 (PANAFACOM Co., Ltd., Japan). All operation programs are stored in ROM including Basic interpreter, and they can be used immediately by pushing reset switch. The cardiac stimulator and defibrillator are also operated by dry batteries. The two relays and one buzzer are used for defibrillator control, electrode connection, and alarm.

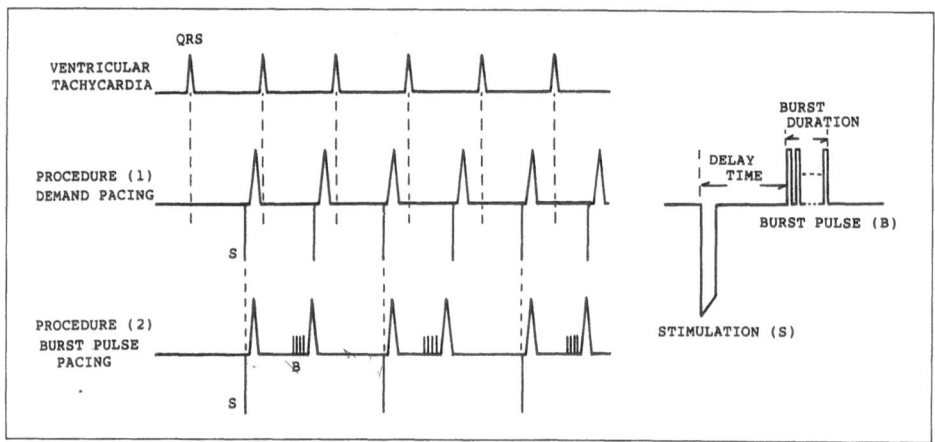

Fig. 2. The schema of the impulse given in "burst pulse" pacing
In procedure (1), high-rate stimulations are added to the heart as timing settlement and threshold measurement. In the procedure (2), to prevent ventricular fibrillation, special attention was paid to the burst pulse pacing. The polarity of the burst pulse is reversed compared with that of the first stimulus, the current is lower than half of the first stimulation, and the energy is dispersed by the way of bursts of rapid ventricular pacing.

Methods:

The operation of this system is divided into three modes, and one of them works according to the ECG and blood pressure condition.

1. Demand pacing mode: The system works as a demand pacemaker. The R-wave and action potential after pacing are monitored by the signal processing computer.
2. Burst pulse pacing mode: Fig. 2 shows the schema of burst pulse pacing. Initially, demand pacing with first stimulus is started with a little higher heart rate than ventricular tachycardia. Shortly after this take-over of rhythm by pacing. The second stimulus, consisting of bursts of rapid ventricular pacing is given with a certain delay of time from the first stimulus, and this time delay is controlled automatically by the output computer (4). Duration, frequency, and voltage of bursts are also controlled. During the experiment, special attention is paid to controlling blood pressure so as not to drop too low because hypotension itself could cause ventricular fibrillation before provocation of this arrhythmia. For this reason, escape function is provided to change the mode to demand pacing.
3. Defibrillation mode: Ventricular fibrillation is diagnosed also by recognizing the decrease of blood pressure. Hypotension continuing for more than 10 sec causes the pacemaker to trigger a pulse which turns on the transvenous defibrillator.

Results:

The results are described under three headings: Demand pacing, burst pacing for tachycardia control, and defibrillation.
1. Demand pacing: Fig. 3-(a) shows the results of demand pacing in a dog (13 kg). In the middle of the figure, demand function is confirmed against arrhythmia.
2. Burst pacing for tachycardia control: Fig. 3-(b) shows the results of burst pacing in a dog (12 kg). Before the control of tachycardia, ten high-rate stimulations are added to the heart as timing settlement. After stimulation, the heart rate decreased to 65% of original rate. Fig. 3-(c) shows the escape function of pacing in case of low blood pressure.
3. Defibrillation: The experiment of defibrillation using a catheter succeeded by the specially designed circuits. Fibrillation was detected by the signal processing computer which checks the blood pressure as well as the ECG (Fig. 3-(d).

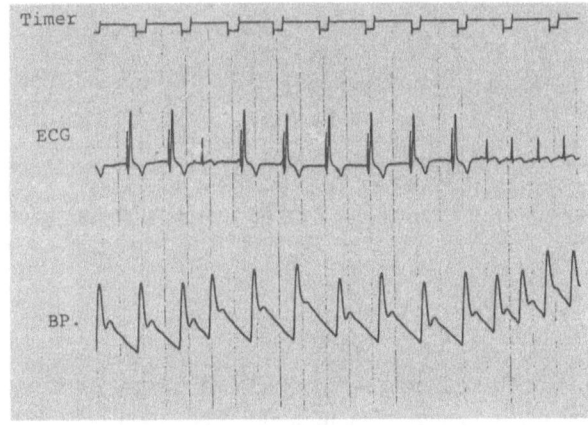

Fig. 3(a). Demand pacing
In the middle of the figure, demand function is confirmed against the arrhythmia. R-wave is detected by it's amplitude and pulse width in the signal processing computer.

Fig. 3(b). Burst pulse pacing

The experimental results of automatic tachycardia control using a mongrel dog. Procedure (1) was demand pacing as a timing settlement. After eight stimulations, procedure (2), burst pulse pacing was begun and the delay time was automatically controlled. At point (A), the delay time was fixed, because tachycardia was controlled four times continuously. Finally, the heart rate dropped to 70 bpm from 107 bpm.

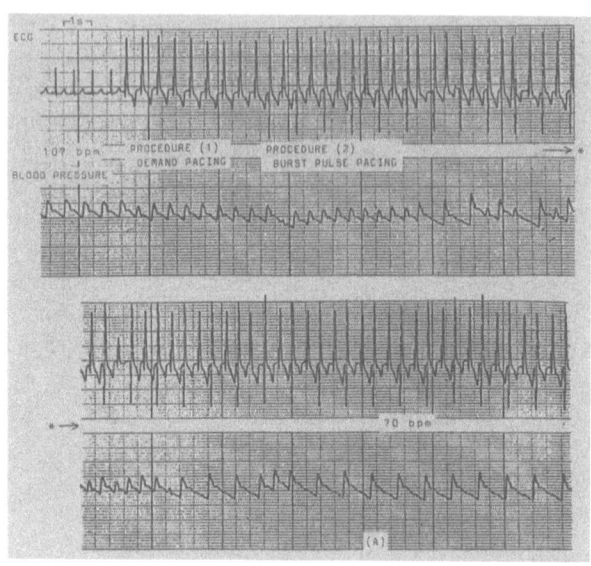

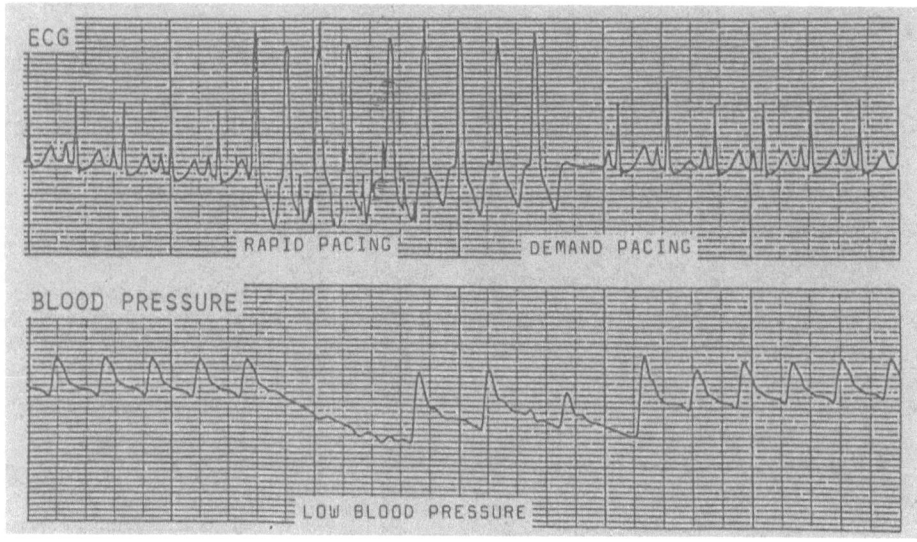

Fig. 3(c). Escape function

During the experiment, special attention was paid to preventing blood pressure from droping so low because hypotension itself could cause ventricular fibrillation. Once low blood pressure is detected by the signal processing computer, stimulation is stopped automatically for a while and the operation mode becomes the demand pacing mode.

Conclusion:

A Microcomputer based all-purpose cardiac pacemaker was developed, and the functions were confirmed in animal experiments. In demand pacing mode, stimulation pulse was

292

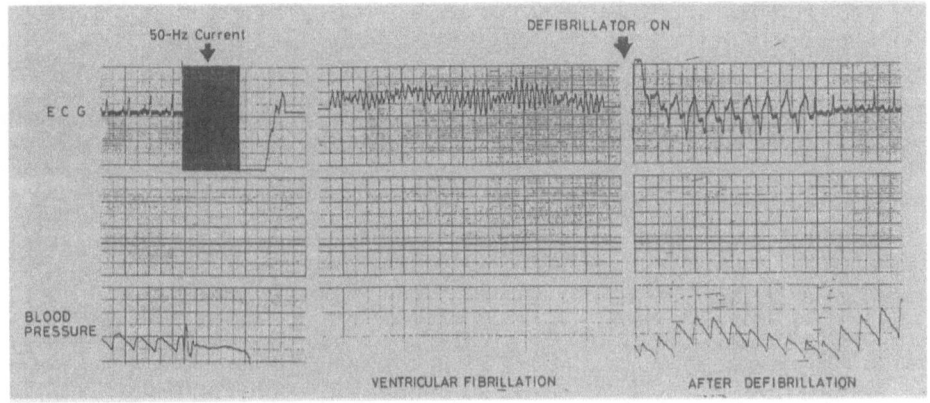

Fig. 3(d). Typical fibrillation-defibrillation sequence

Defibrillation using a catheter electrode succeeded by the specially designed circuits. Fibrillation was detected by the signal processing computer which checks the blood pressure as well as the ECG.

continuously generated and inhibited by R-wave. In burst pacing mode, timing of burst pulse was automatically controlled to find the appropriate stimulation timing, and the heart rate was sensed by the microcomputer using blood pressure signal. Consequently, heart rate was reduced to 68% of the original rate. In defibrillation mode, ventricular fibrillation was diagnosed also by recognizing the decrease of blood pressure, and the pacemaker generated the pulse which turned on the transvenous defibrillator.

This study was supported in part by a grant to Mr. Makino from the Sakkokai foundation.

References:

1. Makino H et al: "A Basic Design for All-Purpose Cardiac Pacemaker", Proc of Conf Japan Soc ME&BE (May, 1982).
2. Tamura K et al: "Termination of Ventricular Tachycardia by Pervenous Burst Pulse Pacemaker", Proc of 6th World Symp on Cardiac Pacing (1979).
3. Yamazoe M et al: "Ventricular Defibrillation through Intracardiac Catheter Electrode and Subcutaneous Plate Electrode of the Anterior Chest Wall", Abstract of 7th World Symp on Cardiac Pacing (1983)
4. Makino, H et al: "An Automatic Tachycardia Control Method for All-Purpose Cardiac Pacemaker ", Proc. of 2nd Symposium of Medical Precision Engineering, Sapporo, Japan (1983, in Japanese)

Author's address:
Hideo Makino
Boimedical Controls
Research Institut of Applied Electricity
Hokkaido University
Sapporo 060, Japan

Clinical Investigation of a Multi-Programmer

B. Dodinot*, L. Kubler*, J. Buffet**, J. F. Meunier**

Summary: Between April and December 1982, 200 programmations were made through an MP in 156 patients treated by 26 various programmable P. M. made by 13 companies.
The MP is made of a micro-computer connected to an interface terminated by 4 different programming heads. 3 accidents:
– 1 electrical shock without consequences, 2 cardiac arrests were observed during the first attempts of programmation. Impossible or difficult programmations occurred in 25% of the cases. They were related to several causes:
– insufficient power of the signals, lack of specificity of the programming heads. Improvements of the circuits, the design of two additional programming heads solved most of the problems. Erroneous programmations occurring in 6% of the cases were related to errors in the programmation of the software. Debugging immediately corrected these potentially dangerous behaviours.
In May 1983, the MP is capable of programming 66 PM made by 13 Companies. Its advantages are: reliability, simplicity, MP replacing or doubling individual programmers, other capabilities such as photoanalysis, mementoes, the suppression of the implanting physicians dependence of the manufacturers. The disadvantages are: the slowness of the system, occasional programming difficulties, the absence of telemetry (these faults should be corrected in the near future), possible legal problems.
The future of the MP depends on the absence or presence of a consensus between pacemaker Companies, the complexity of the future programming system making it extremely difficult for an independent Company to keep it up to date.

In 1978, a French pacemaker (PM) Clinic capable of programming any PM patients implanted in Europe had to possess 6 different programmers. In 1983, 21 programmers must be kept in stock, some of them needing a permanent charge! In 1978, the French Pacing Group organized a meeting with all European companies in order to design a common, unique multi-programmable pacing system. This idea appeared irrealistic for two reasons:
– the existence already of advanced studies by each Company,
– risks of blocking progress by uniformity.
In 1981, the University of Nancy Pacing Group had the idea of designing a system capable of programming through a single computer most, if not all, pacemakers implanted in Europe. In the absence of consensus between PM Companies, the only way of achieving our goal was to find a technical partner willing to accept this new concept and capable of designing such a multi-programmer (MP). A French pacemaker company*) offered to work in close but independent cooperation with our pacemaker Clinic. 3 different steps can be differentiated in the development of the MP:

---

* = Clinique Cardiologique – CHU Nancy-Brabois – Vandoeuvre (France).
** = Cardiofrance, Zone Industrielle des Richardets, 1 bis rue des Aérostiers, 93160 Noisy-le-Grand
*) Cardiofrance: Zone Industrielle des Richardets, 93160 Noisy-le-Grand.

Step 1: Elaboration of the Catalogue of the Programming Codes

In order to achieve this first step, programmable pacemakers and their respective programmers were loaned to the laboratory by the PM Clinic. Programming codes were studied and reproduced. For this purpose, a desktop micro-computer**) associated with a specific interface had been worked out (Fig. 1). A Basic-program (software) took into account all variables (rates, pulse-widths, refractory periods, etc...). The orders given by the computer were transferred to an interface generating the electric signals. These signals were either directly transmitted (cutaneous stimulation programmation) or transformed into magnetic or radiofrequency energies by various transducers (the programming heads).

Step 2: In Vitro Tests

The purpose of these tests were the evaluation of the effectiveness and accuracy of programmation via the MP; each PM had been repetitively programmed in the laboratory.

Step 3: In Vivo Study

This clinical evaluation was performed in our institution in patients treated by implantable programmable PM. The original programmer was always within reach in order to immediately correct possible mis-functions and prevent accidents.

Results

Clinical evaluations of the MP started on April 20, 1982. *Programmation* consisted of one or several transmissions of coded messages in order to modify one or several parameters in the same patient. Clinical evaluation was arbitrarily considered as completed

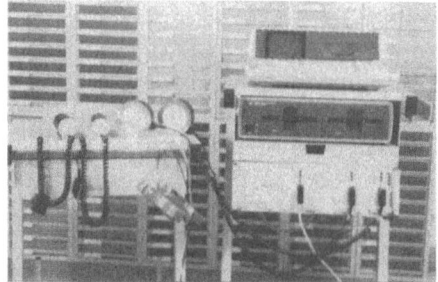

Fig. 1. The multi-programmer in its 1983 version with the 4 programming heads.

**) Hewlett-Packard 85.

when 200 programming sessions were done, in 156 patients. As of 22nd of December 1982, the use of the MP was considered as a standard routine procedure. However, it must be taken in account that:

a) the use of the MP for other purposes than programmation such as oscillogram recordings was not taken into account in this clinical evaluation,

b) permanent improvements and extensions of the MP make the distinction between clinical evaluation and routine use artificial; the principle of the MP has to be a perpetually evolving device.

Out of 200 programmations made in 156 patients 3 accidents were observed:

a) *One electrical leakage* occurred during the very first clinical use of the MP. The magnetic transducer designed for programmation of CORDIS, CPI and ARCO PM induced a painful shock at the level of the plate of the ECP (right leg). This accident was related to a defective insulation of the transducer. Changes of the programming head (increase of the thickness of the insulation, definitively suppressed this type of accident).

b) *Cardiac arrest*

In 2 patients, a cardiac arrest was induced following output programmation below threshold and could not be immediately corrected due to the complexity of the manipulation of the computer. Consequently, the incorporation of a panic button, independent from the computer, was decided. Pressing the button resumes maximum output at a high rate (Fig. 2). This button can be activated at any phase of programma-

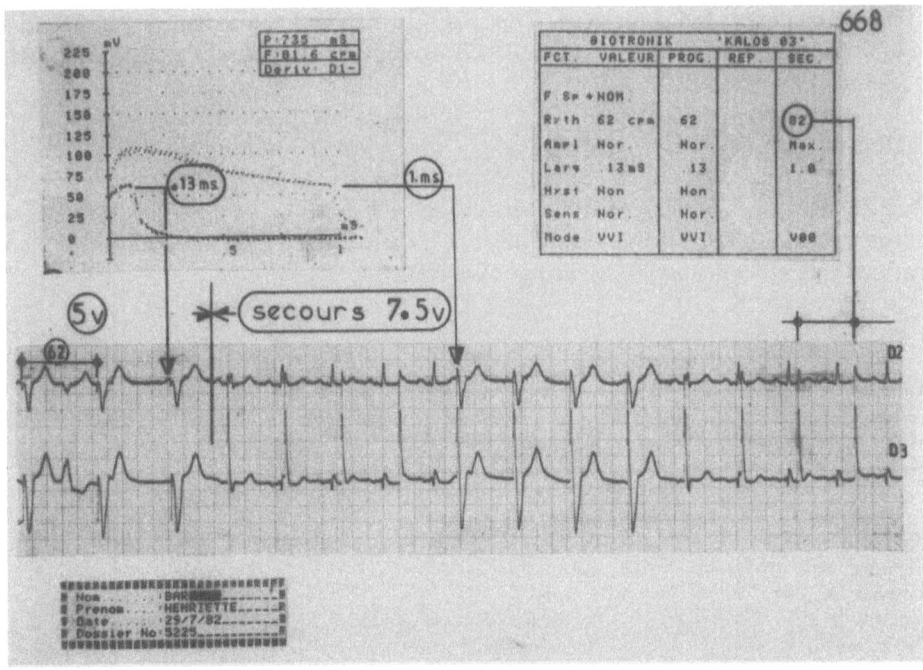

Fig. 2

tion. This safety procedure was designed with all systems with the exception of the Siemens-Elema and Telectronics Optima for technical reasons. It was not necessary with ELA and Cardiofrance systems since magnet application resumes maximum output at a high rate.

I. Modes of Responses to Programmation

Four modes of responses can be differenciated:
- *satisfactory:* immediate effective programmation. This was obtained in 138 cases (69%).
- *difficult:* programmation is effective but following several attempts: 27 cases (13,5%)
- *impossible:* in spite of several attempts of programmation with various positions of the transducers; 23 cases (11,5%)
- *erroneous:* programmation, either immediate or difficult, results in unpredicted results: 12 cases (6%).

II. Comments

The main purpose of this clinical evaluation was to point out and solve the problems. During this evaluation, 31% of the problems of varying importance were faced.
- *Difficult or impossible programmation.* In 25% of the cases, it was impossible or difficult to program, impossibility being not strictly different from difficulty. It is not acceptable for the physician to repetitively send programming messages in order to change one or several parameters. The causes of these difficulties depend on the mode of transmission of the messages. Table 1 lists the various modes of transmission used by each Company 1982.

A) Radiofrequency

Table 2 shows that problems vary depending on each system. The Biotronik system, less advanced and protected than others, being by far the easiest to program. Problems initially faced with other systems (E.M. and P) were related to:

Table 1.

Modes of Transmission		
Radiofrequency	Magnetic	Cutaneous stimulation
Biotronik	ARCO	
ELA Medical	CPI	
Intermedics	Cordis	Cardiofrance
Medtronic	Siemens	
Pacesetter	Telectronics	
Precimed 215	Vitatron	

1. the existence of a safety key, if the PM does not recognize the key, it refuses programmation,
2. insufficient power of the signal. This was corrected by an increase (× 2) of the power transmitted by the transducer,
3. absence of telemetry. This limitation, not yet corrected, was an obvious handicap with ELA and Pacesetter systems. It must be pointed out that in many instances problems faced with the MP were also present with the original programmers. This is the major limitation of radiofrequency transmission systems. The original programmers are not always sufficiently powerful resulting in difficulties when PM are deeply implanted.

B) Magnetic

Table 3 demonstrates that no obvious differences were found during our limited experiences. Problems are related to various causes:
1. *Output power insufficiency.* The redesign of the circuit was decided to increase power of the signals.
2. *Geometry of the transducers.* It is not possible to design a universal magnetic programming head. During clinical evaluation, 2 types of transducers differing as to the magnetic field orientations were used.

The first one incorporating a magnet was specifically designed for systems relying on rapid short bursts of impulses (Siemens, Telectronics Optima); a second one was made for systems using longer pulses of lower frequency (CPI, CORDIS, VITATRON, ARCO). Recently, a 3rd transducer differing form the 2nd one by the number of wire-turns of the solenoid was specifically created to solve the problems faced with the CPI system.

To eliminate all problems, the ideal solution is to use one transducer per system. Practically, a compromise must be found to avoid transforming the MP into a kind of octopus with multi-pole tentacles.

It must be pointed out that, contrary to R.F. systems, it was always possible to program by using the original programmer (when these devices were properly charged!).

Table 2. Radiofrequency.

Biotronik	ELA Medical	Intermedics	Medtronic	Pacesetter	Total		
	0/18	4/8	4/15	7/20	7/10	22/71	(31%)

Table 3. Magnetic.

ARCO	CPI	Cordis	Siemens	Telectronics (Optima)	Vitatron (P 4000)	Total
3/8	4/13	9/39	3/7	1/9	6/13	26/89 (29.2%)

299

C) Cutaneous Stimulation

Programming problems with this system were related to errors in the polarity of the wires; they were quickly and definitively solved.

III. Programmation Errors

To program a rate of 100, output at 10 mA and obtain a rate of 30 and 2 mA output can be catastrophic. We did however have to deal with these abnormal unexpected programmations in 12 instances (6%). These abnormalities were all related to errors in the microcomputer software. They appeared with all modes of transmissions, the abnormality being located in the computer itself. Incomplete in vitro tests, where all possibilities of programmation cannot be tested, explain the late discovery of these abnormalities during clinical evaluation. It must be pointed out that, in one case of code inversion of the sensing levels, the diagnosis was made through telemetry using the original programmer (Pacesetter). Correction of these major malfunctions was immediate and consisted of a software "debugging". The presence of a telemetry seems useful to avoid such mistakes.

IV. Advantages and Disadvantages

In its modified and up to date version, the MP has the following advantages and disadvantages:

A) Advantages

1. *reliability:* the programmation, if not always rapid and easy, is effective and accurate. A printed document is provided.
2. *convenience:* the MP can replace most systems or offer redundancy. We had the opportunity to appreciate its presence for replacing defective or exhausted programmers made by former manufacturers (ARCO, MEDCOR, for instance).
3. *additional capabilities.*
   The computer used with the MP provides a catalogue of each programmable PM with its various functions. Oscillogram recordings can be made through the MP.
4. *independence of the PM Centers.* It is not acceptable to rely one or several companies for the maintenance of programmers. The choice of the PM should not be related to the presence of the programmmer; in the case of the disappearance of a Company, the implanted PM must be still programmable. With an MP, an PM Center can follow patients treated by most programmable PM.

B) Disadvantages

1. *slowness of the system:* this appears to be the major practical clinical problem. It takes several minutes to trigger the machine, select a proper diskett and transducer, send the

messages. This however can be corrected in the future by selecting a more elaborate computer and improving the program of the software.

2. *complexity of the handling.* The daily use of the MP is mandatory to avoid errors. The presence of 4 and soon 5 transducers is a handicap. It is however more simple to get used to a single machine than to several.

3. *limitations.* Up to now, telemetry is not available. Technical problems seem much greater in precisely reproducing telemetry than programmation.

4. *the cost.* The cost of an MP must be compared with the cost of several independent programmers. It must be taken in account that, in France, all programmers are given to physicians, if a minimum of PM are implanted.

5. *Up-dating*

   A new programmation system appears every other month. The MP will never be totally updated in the absence of consensus between Companies. The reproduction of the complex new programmation system by an independent Company appears to become more and more complex.

6. *Legal problems*

   Accidents with the MP have little chance of occurring during precise clinical evaluation. It must be remembered that the presence of an accident related to the absence of the right programmer can be avoided if an MP is at hand. Advantages of the MP are the presence of a panic button, the use of a single programming machine, avoiding training on various systems (which may however prevent programming errors).

Conclusion

Based on this clinical evaluation, it can be concluded:

1. An MP can be designed by a single company without comporting major clinical problems.

2. Following improvements and corrections of several electronic errors, the presently available MP 1982 appears as a reliable, convenient tool which might however be improved to provide a faster programmation and to include telemetry.

The future of this concept is however hypothetic; the complexity of the new programming systems including sophisticated telemetries, electrogram transmission makes updating by an independent Company hardly feasible.

It is however not unrealistic to think that, under the influence of the medical pacing community, a consensus will finally be reached between companies to develop a common programmer replacing these costly electronic odds and ends.

Why not offer, rather than a new custom designed program, the adequate interface and program adapted to a computer designed for programmation and other purposes in a pacemaker clinic?

It is however more probable that commercial considerations and rivalries between companies will slow down such a project than pseudo-technical or legal considerations.

Authors' address:
Dr. B. Dodinot, Clinique Cardiologique
CHU Nancy-Brabois, Vandoeuvre/France

Polyurethane as a Pacemaker Lead Insulator

G. C. Timmis, S. Gordon, D. Westveer, R. O. Martin, K. Stokes

Summary: We have previously shown in canine studies that the surface change regularly observed on both intra- and extravascular segments of explanted leads failed to affect physical or electrical lead integrity within 29 weeks of implant. Neither electron nor infrared spectroscopy has identified a chemical cause for surface changes. More recent studies have exonerated the elution of processing aids as their cause. Environmental stress cracking, a time-limited release of surface stresses (process-induced molecular malorientation) which appears to stop at a plane of zero stress between the polyurethane skin and core, may be responsible. Thus, surface changes at 15 months progressed insignificantly at 31 months in canine studies.

At this institution, we have implanted 254 polyurethane leads of 10 different types from two manufacturers representing a total experience of 348 lead years and a mean ($\pm$ SEM) implant time of $1.37 \pm .06$ years. There have been no insulation failures. Noninvasive impedance telemetry data has not shown a loss of insulation integrity in 101 serially monitored patients over a period of 11 months. This data is concordant with the worldwide experience with 225,000 polyurethane leads among which there have been only 104 known insulation failures (.044%).

In conclusion, surface changes are regularly found on explanted polyurethane leads but do not appear to affect their functional integrity. These changes appear to be more physical than chemical in origin and do not predict lead insulation failure.

Polyurethane as a Pacemaker Lead Insulator

Polyether urethane has been singled out from a family of thermoplastic polymers for clinical use as a lead insulator because it has been shown to be a tough, lubricious elastomer with a high tensile modulus and tear strength. It retains its physical stability at physiologic temperatures and on exposure to physiologic fluids, resists hydrolysis, oxidation, flex fatigue, and has a high dielectric strength and low electric conductivity (1, 2). Additionally, it has been extruded in tubular form of sufficiently small caliber that more than one lead can be passed transvenously for bifocal pacing through a single vessel of average caliber. Although available in a wide range of shore hardness, a specific species, Pellathane® 2363-80A (Upjohn) has had the broadest medical application. Considerable anxiety and controversy has arisen over the significance of polyurethane surface changes on chronic exposure to physiologic environments (3–9). Debate has centered around the nature and depth of surface fissuring (6, 8, 9), its relationship to processing aids, catalyzers, solvents, or colorizers (3, 10), the effect of various sterilization techniques, and polyurethane's absorption of water, inorganic ions, lipids, and proteins allegedly resulting in hydrolysis and oxidation (10). Whatever the cause, surface changes are not unique to polyurethane catheters or pacemaker lead insulators. Similar changes have been observed in the research and development of the artificial heart (11). Thus, questions have arisen regarding the progressive nature of the surface fissuring process, whether or not mechanical stability is affected by surface cracking, and how the "physiologic milieu reacts to these changes" (12). Another key question is whether this process is progressive or self-limited by the ultimate release of "molded-in" stresses.

Environment Stress Cracking. When a thermoplastic material is prepared to function as a lead insulator, after melting it is extruded with force into a cold mold resulting in the "freezing" of surface molecules in conformations which differ from core molecules (13–15). This results in residual intrinsic differential stresses between the skin and the core of polyurethane tubing. These stresses are compounded by the absorption of physiologic fluids which cause polymer swelling to the extent allowed by the tensile strength of molecular entanglements (16). If the latter is exceeded, the swelling force may produce breaks especially at the interface of soft segment (polyether) and hard segment (hydrogen-bonding diisocyanate derivatives) polyurethane linkages (10). Moreover, the composition of this two-phase material differs between the skin (more soft segments) and the core (more hard segments) of polyurethane tubing presumably as a result of surface-free energy and the manufacturing process (17). Thus, surface fissuring and cracking may appear especially with the additional application of extrinsic forces. These cracks will propagate inward toward the core of polyurethane tubing until residual intrinsic stresses have been spent (zero stress boundary). Extrinsic forces include lead flexion and torsion, which may be superimposed on residual tension resulting from expansion-contraction fitting of small bore polyurethane tubing stretched around a relatively wide bore conductor coil. Other points of unusual stress result from stretch forces immediately adjacent to the lead tie-down point. Of 61 leads returned for study, insulation defects have been found in the atrial J-curve of 17 6991U leads and immediately adjacent to the ligature site in another 44 (Medtronic 6990U, 6991U, 6971, and 6972) (3). Since the assembly process for atrial leads has been revised with reduction of stresses in the J-curve, insulation failures at this point have been almost nonexistent. Gentler handling, the learning curve of surgical experience (18), and the employment of a protective sleeve at the lead tie-down point have additionally reduced the failure rate of polyurethane.

Surface changes are not restricted to segments subjected to unusual forces. Thus, our own studies have shown a relatively homogeneous distribution of surface changes in all lead segments (Fig. 1A). Table 1 lists mean scores (Fig. 1B) for cracks and fissures which were uniformly 10 to 20 microns or less in depth (Fig. 1B) and may be equivalent to what others refer to as "surface frosting" (19). We have not been able to assign significant changes in the physical characteristics of polyurethane leads to this phenomenon (infra vide). Although cracks of greater depth have been reported, this does not disqualify the zero stress boundary theory since the superimposition of external forces on intrinsic surface stresses may cause an inward displacement of this boundary. However, one of us (KS) has failed to identify in any segment of four leads explanted from dogs at 31 months, surface changes of greater depth or density than those observed in similar studies at 15 months.

Physical Characteristics of Explanted Polyurethane Leads. We studied seven atrial and seven ventricular polyurethane leads which were forcibly extracted from canine hearts in our laboratory at 26 and 28 weeks, respectively. Physical testing (Table 2) showed that while urethanes are generally resistant to the plasticizing effects of fluids (1, 20) wet strength had decreased at explantation for both lead types and especially the larger atrial leads. There was a 10% reduction in tensile strength in 4 Fr leads and a 33% reduction in 6 Fr leads (2). These changes were unlikely due to physiologic environments since they were also observed in control polyurethane samples soaked in 0.9 normal saline for one week at 37 °C. Although the reduction in tensile strength for atrial leads was greater reflecting their larger cross-sectional area, their break force remained greater than for ven-

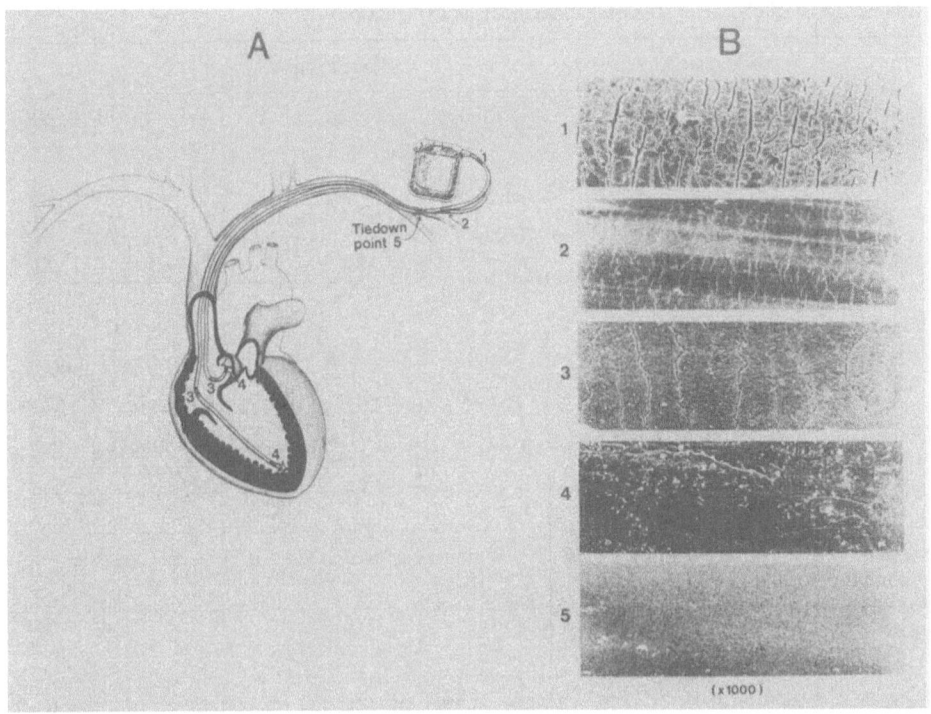

Fig. 1.A. Identification of lead segments studied by scanning electron microscopy and physical testing. **B.** Scoring of surface irregularities detected by scanning electron microscopy (SEM). Lower values identify increasing surface irregularities.

Table 1. Surface change scores determined by scanning electron microscopy (figure 2) according to lead size and sample location (2).

Segment	n	Atrial (6 Fr) mean ± SEM	n	Ventricular (4 Fr) mean ± SEM	p
1	9	2.9 ±.5	7	2.6 ±.4	.626
2	7	3.3 ±.4	8	2.9 ±.4	.457
3	10	2.9 ±.4	8	3.3 ±.4	.390
4	10	3.2 ±.4	8	3.5 ±.4	.545
5	6	2.9 ±.4	6	6.5 ±.4	.579
All	42	2.96±.19	37	3.02±.19	.833

tricular leads. At explant, the elastic modulus of the larger leads increased while that of the smaller leads did not. Similar changes were observed in saline controls. Comparative in vitro physical testing of platinum-cured and conventional silicone rubber tubing showed a superior performance for polyurethane (2). Spearman rho correlations of mean SEM scores and physical testing were not significant (Tab. 3). Surface irregularities of

Table 2. Physical characteristics of lead segments at explanation.

	Tensile strength* (psi)			Elongation* (%)		
Atrial (6 Fr) n	SC 6	IV 6	Controls 12	SC 6	IV 6	Controls 12
	3376 ± 337	3555 ± 289	5147 ± 101	352 ± 51	453 ± 31	280 ± 9
	└─NS─┘ └─$p<.001$─┘ └────── $p<.001$ ──────			└─NS─┘ └─$p<.001$─┘ └────── NS ──────		
Ventricular (4 Fr)n	6	6	12	6	6	12
	9077 ± 1369	8981 ± 1399	$10,055 \pm 924$	1131 ± 103	1149 ± 139	1249 ± 101
	└─NS─┘ └─NS─┘ └────── NS ──────			└─NS─┘ └─NS─┘ └────── NS ──────		

* Strain rate = 20 inches/minutes. SC = subcutaneous (extravascular); IV = intravascular; psi = pounds per square inch (2).

Table 3. Correlation of mean SEM scores by sample location and lead type with ultimate tensile strength (UTS) and elongation. Numbers represent r values (2).

	UTS psi)		Elongation (%)	
n	Atrial 6	Ventricular 6	Atrial 6	Ventricular 6
SEM Score by Location				
subcutaneous	.406	.714	.406	−.600
intravenous	.714	.143	.714	−.086
combined	.600	.371	.600	−.257

explanted leads were not influenced by the method of lead removal (forceful versus surgical extraction), lead size, integrity (i.e., whether or not there were insulation breaks or disconnections from crimp sites, etc.) or as previously indicated, sample location.

The Biochemical Effects of Physiologic Environments on Polyurethane Leads. Changes in polyurethane surface structure have been said to be caused by the absorption of physiologic fluids, lipids, and proteins with resultant hydrolysis and oxidation (10). Thus, biologic enhancement of stress corrosion has been alleged (21). In contrast, previous studies by Stokes et al. employing porcine tallow in vitro (1), and by Boretos et al. (22) with implanted polyurethane specimens in calves for up to 35 weeks showed no lipid absorption. More recently by employing electron spectroscopy for chemical analysis (ESCA) and Auger electron spectroscopy, we have confirmed the apparent absence of lipid adsorption or absorption by explanted polyurethane leads (2). We were also unable to de-

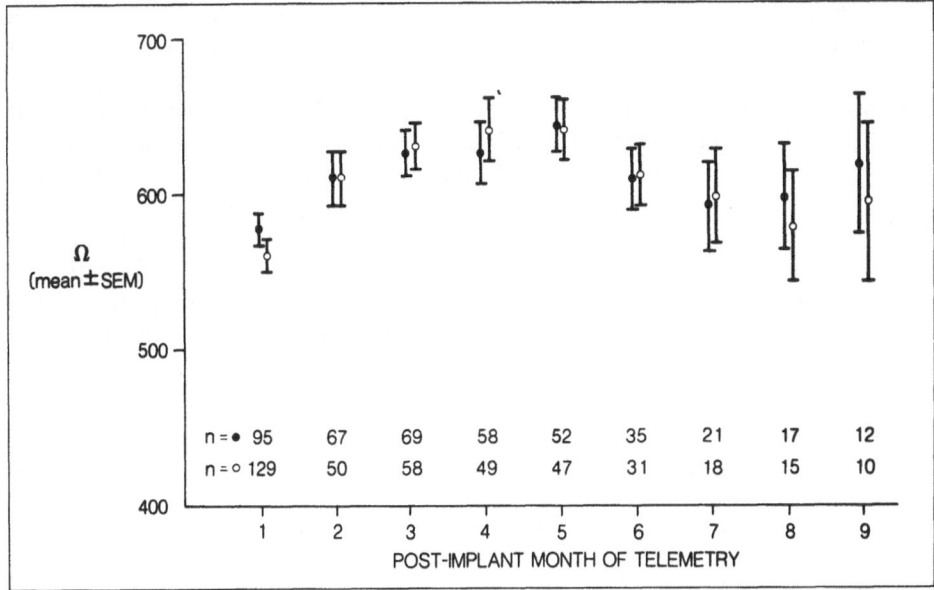

Fig. 2. Noninvasive lead impedance measurements (467) of polyurethane leads obtained by telemetry in 101 patients over a period of 11 months, nine of which are shown. Solid circles represent all data points (mean ± SEM). Open circles represent 378 measurements obtained from the subset of 61 patients in whom at least 4 serial measurements of impedance were made.

monstrate protein absorption. Moreover, scanning microscopy showed no differences between lead segments washed with sodium hydroxide and adjacent control segments (2). If oxidation had contributed to the surface changes, peroxides and aldehydes should have been demonstrable at or near the surface by frustrated multiple internal reflectance which would have shown in increase in carbonyl at 5.75 μ, 8.55 μ and 8.65 μ with a concomitant decrease in aliphatic ether at 9.0 μ. This was not the case. Thus, we are unable to support the existence of the biologically mediated degradative process suggested by others (10, 11).

To explore the possibility that elution of the waxy processing aid for extrusion may cause surface changes (2), an experiment was performed involving two dogs in whom six subcutaneous pockets were surgically created in the flank of each animal. Five standard Pellathane® 2363-80A pellets were placed in the first pocket. Five identical pellets without the processing aid were placed in the second pocket of each animal. Five samples each of Pellathane® compression molded at 360 °F and 420 °F were inserted into the third and fourth pockets of each animal. An equal number of compression molded samples without the processing aid were placed in the fifth and sixth pockets. Scanning electron microscopy of all 60 samples which were explanted after a minimum of three months revealed some degree of surface cracking or fissuring in every specimen ranging from five to ten microns in depth. There was no apparent difference in surface changes which could be related to the presence or absence of the processing aid or to compression mold temperatures. Indeed, those samples molded at 420 °F when examined under cross-polarized light, displayed slightly less surface changes (23).

307

Polyurethane as a Lead Insulator. Polyurethane has been shown to have a high dielectric strength and high volume resistivity which persists after exposure to moisture (20, 24). We found that the combined effects of fissuring and fluid absorption had no apparent effect on the electrical (insulating) performance of polyurethane (2). Thus, the change in canine strength-duration curves over a period of 26 to 28 weeks was comparable to previous reports using silicone rubber insulation (25). Moreover, lead impedance telemetry data has been accumulated in 101 patients who were followed for $3.32 \pm .11$ (mean ±- SEM) months (Fig. 3). There were no changes in this parameter to suggest insulation failure. Only two patients showed a drop in impedance of 10% or more and both continue to pace and sense satisfactorily. Group impedance data was validated by recalculating monthly means in a subset of 61 patients who had at least four serial determinations (Fig. 3).

Clinical Experience. Since their clinical introduction in 1978, insulation failures of polyurethane leads have been relatively few and confined to a single manufacturer. As previously suggested, these insulation failures reflect the combined effects of intrinsic stresses molded in by the manufacturing process and extrinsic stresses of flexion, stretch and torsion. The fact that another manufacturer has had no failures with over 40,000

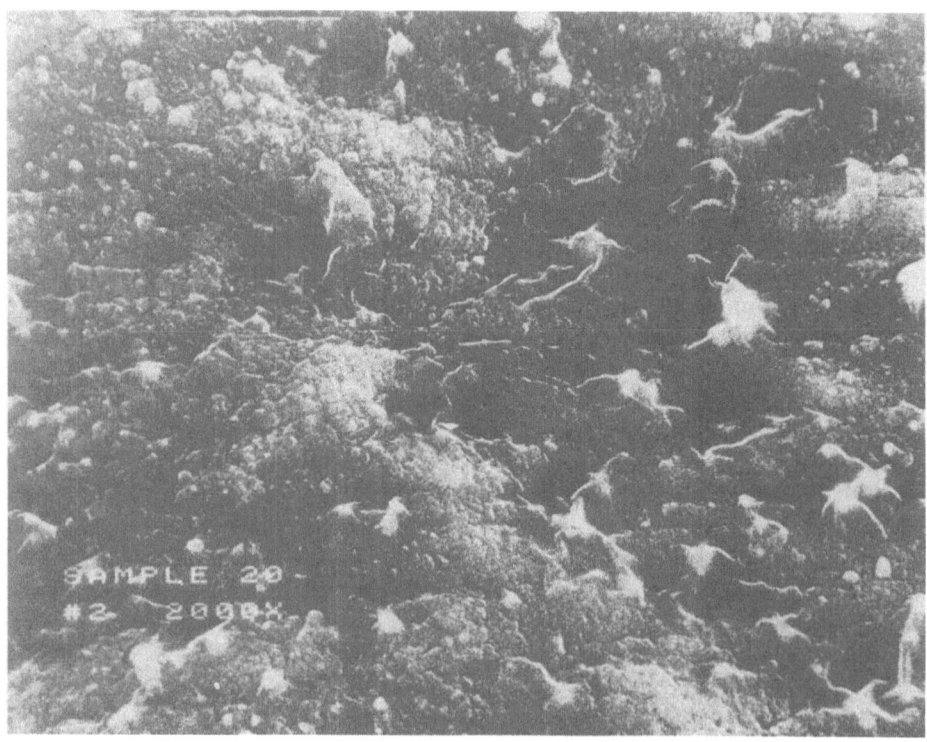

Fig. 3. Scanning electron micrograph of a silicone rubber lead surface removed from patient approximately three months after implant. This is an extravascular segment proximal to the tie-down point.

leads using the same species of polyurethane, underscores the importance of the manufacturing process which since its revision has largely eliminated insulation failures.

As of January 1983, the cumulative worldwide failure rate for 185,000 leads from one manufacturer was 0.16%. This included all types of failure involving crimps, joints, wire, and insulator. Of the 1,200 leads returned for study. 240 displayed areas of surface changes which involved the "skin" only in 136. There were 104 insulation failures (0.056%). The insulation failure rate for all 225,000 polyurethane leads known to have been implanted since January 1977 is less (0.044%). This is no more than for silicone rubber leads. However, in actuarial terms the failure rate for silicone rubber leads may be less because of a longer implant history (12, 26).

A more clinically homogenous experience reported from the University of Frankfurt failed to show any sensing or pacing failure for 1,982 polyurethane electrodes (Medtronic model 6957 and 6959) (27). Similarly, at our own institution we have implanted 254 polyurethane leads (Intermedic model, 490493 (80), 483 (74), 473 (5), 327 (6), Medtronic model 10176 (2), 6991U (1), 6972 (42), 6971 (19), 4951 (7), 4003 (18) representing a total experience of 348 leads and a mean ($\pm$ SEM) implant time of 1.37 ± 0.06 years. There have been no insulation failures.

Conclusions. The diffuse and rather homogeneous surface changes displayed in animal studies and "surface frosting" on polyurethane leads explanted from humans has not been shown to be any more clinically relevant than surface changes on explanted silicone rubber leads (Fig. 3). Insulation failures to date have been found to be largely due to the manufacturing process and surgical technique rather than biologically mediated chemical degradation. Manufacturing revisions, improved manipulative skills and possibly harder polyurethane (28) are anticipated to further enhance our clinical experience so that we can continue to enjoy the advantages of these interesting new leads.

References

1. Stokes K, Cobian K, Lathrop T: Polyurethane insulators, a design approach to small pacing leads. In: Meere C, ed Cardiac pacing. Montreal: Pacesymp, 1979: 28–2.
2. Timmis GC, Westveer DC, Martin R, Gordon S: The significance of surface changes on explanted polyurethane pacemaker leads. Pace (In Press).
3. Stokes K: The polyurethane controversy. Pace 1983; 6: 459–463.
4. Nachnani GH, Lessin LS, Motomiya T, Jensen WN: Scanning electron microscopy of thrombogenesis on vascular catheter surfaces. N Engl J Med 1972; 286: 139–140.
5. Bourassa MG, Cantin M, Sandborn EB, Pederson E: Scanning electron microscopy of surface irregularities and thrombogenesis of polyurethane and polyethylene coronary catheters. Circulation 1976; 53: 992–96.
6. Parins DJ, Black KM, McCoy KD, Horvath NJ: In vivo degradation of a polyurethane. St Paul: Cardiac Pacemakers, Inc, 1981.
7. Stokes K: Polyurethane lead insulation: a study in biostability. Minneapolis: Medtronic News, June 1981.
8. Parins DJ, McCoy KD, Horvath NJ: In vivo degradation of a polyurethane: further evidence. St Paul: Cardiac Pacemakers, Inc, 1981.
9. McArthur WA: Personnal communication. Pacesetter System, Inc, Sylmar, California.
10. Guerin P: Use of synthetic polymers for biomedical application. Pace 1983; 6: 449–453.
11. Coleman DL, Lim D, Kessler T, et al: Calcification of non-textured implantable blood pumps. Am Soc Artif Int Organs 1981; 10: 3.
12. Scheuer-Leeser M, Irnich W, Kreuzer J: Polyurethane leads: facts and controversy. Pace 1983; 6: 454–458.

13. Deanin RD, Hauser DI: Recent developments in environmental stresscrack resistance of plastics. Polym Plast Technol Eng 1981; 17(2): 123–137.
14 Crouthamel DL, Isayev AI, Wang KK: Effect of processing conditions on the residual stress in the injection molding of amorphous polymers. Soc Plast Eng 1982; 28: 295–297.
15. Fujiyama M, Azuma K: Skin/core morphology and tensile impact strength of injection-molded polypropylene. J Appl Pol Sci 1979; 23: 2807–2811.
16. Stokes K: The long-term biostability of polyurethane leads. Stimucoeur 1982; 10(3): 205–212.
17. DeCosta VS, Brier-Russel D, Salzman EW, Merrill EW: ESCA studies of polyurethanes: blood platelet activation in relation to surface composition. Journal of Colloid and Interface Science 1981; 80: 445–52.
18. Byrd CL: Performance of polyurethane leads. Presented at North American Society of Pacing and Electrophysiology, New Orleans, Louisiana, 1983.
19. McArthr W: The polyurethane controversy. Pace 1983; 6: 459–463.
20. Pellethane thermoplastic urethane elastomers. Upjohn Inc, Torrance, California.
21. Emlqvist H: The polyurethane controversy. Pace 1983; 6: 459–463.
22. Boretos JW, Pierce WS, Baier RE, Donachy HJ: Surface and bulk characteristics of a polyether for artificial hearts. J Biomed Mater Res 1975; 9: 327–40.
23. Phillips RE: Unpublished data. Intermedics, Inc. Freeport, Texas.
24. Sluetz J: The polyurethane controversy. Pace 1983; 6: 459–463.
25. Mehra R, McMullen M, Furman S: Time dependence of unipolar cathodal and anodal strength-interval curves. Pace 1980; 3: 526–30.
26. Furman S: The polyurethane controversy. Pace 1983; 6: 459–463.
27. Beyersdorf F: The polyurethane controversy. Pace 1983; 6: 459–463.
28. MacGregor DC: Performance of polyurethane leads. Presented at North American Society of Pacing and Electrophysiology, New Orleans, Louisiana, 1983.

Authors' address:
Dr. G. C. Timmis
William Beaumont Hospital
3601 West Thirteen Mile Road
Royal Oak 48072 Michigan
USA

Immunity Mechanisms Involved in the Degradation of Polyurethane Leads

Comparison between Silicone and Polyurethane

A. Amiel*, G. Lehmann**, G. Touchard***, Ph. Boutaud*, D. Herpin*,
J. Demange*

Summary: The examination by scanning electronic microscopy of polyurethane leads, implanted in rabbits, confirms the biodegradability of the product, and the optical microscopy performed on the blood-vessel and myocardium shows the immunity mechanisms set in action. Three months after implantation, we noticed an important epithelial reaction around the polyurethane lead and particles of the materials embedded in the vein wall. 13 months after implantation a large amount of fibrosis with plastic debris and calcification was present. With silicone and polyethylene there is no degradation of the products 4.5 months after implantation and only a modest tissue reaction without epithelial or pallisadic aspects.

1. Introduction

The use of polyurethane as an insulation for electrodes has brought about significant progress in Cardiac Stimulation, in providing, 1. small diameter leads, the properties of the material (strength, impermeability, etc.,) allowing the use of thinner insulation layers than with usual Silicone and 2. improved slipperiness of the electrode in the vein due to the low coefficient of friction of polyurethane (1, 2, 3, 4, 5). However, several cases of current leakage due to fissures in the polyurethane have been reported, which questions the long term reliability of this material. In the light of studies made (6, 7, 8, 9, 10, 11) and based on our own experience (12) several conclusions were found. In the medium of blood, fissures appear often and fairly rapidly (after several weeks). This degradation could not be reproduced in vitro, in a physiological solution; certain workers conclude that these fissures are due to enzymatic reaction. These fissures are not uniform and appear to congregate at points of stress and, it has not been able to establish the progression of fissures as a function of time. The "Foreign Body" rejection of the polyurethane by the organism is greater than with other biocompatible materials (eg silicone, polyethylene).

We have already reported the results concerning a clinical study involving rabbits (12). We repeat a part of that study in presenting the long term data up to 13 months. The study consists of three parts. 1. Comparison by Scanning Electronic Microscopy (SEM) of the surface of the insulation for Polyurethane, Silicone and Polyethylene. 2. Comparative

---

* Service de Cardiologie B, CHU Poitiers (France)
** Celsa, 86420 Monts-sur-Guesnes (France)
*** Service d'Anatomo-Pathologie, CHU Poitiers (France)

study by Optical Microscopy (O.M.) of the reaction to "Foreign Bodies" of the organism concerned, for the different types of material. 3. Study by SEM and Optical Microscopy of the migration of particles of the material in the organism, in analogy with certain cases reported during chronic haemodyalisis (hepatitis) (13, 14). Only the results of the first two parts of the study are sufficiently advanced to be reproduced here.

2. Methods and Materials

1. The animals

Rabbits (17) were used successfully for this study; these being non-selected offsprings from a rabbit farm.

2. Implant technique

Implantation was performed under anesthetic (Valium IM, on average 20 mg); introduction of the electrode was via the External Jugular, with the ligature at the point of entry; closure made at skin level.

3. The leads

Leads used were completely finished leads, but without electrodes having a length of 15 cm and a diameter as for leads destined for human implants.
– Polyurethane (Type Pellethane 2363 80AE, Up John)
– Silicone (Type Silastic 602-205, Dow Corning)
– Polyethylene (Vygon type 830-20)

4. Sampling

Samples were taken:
– from 3 to 13 months for Polyurethane;
– from 1 to 4.5 months for the Silicone and the Polyethylene.
These were after the animals were sacrificed; except when organs were taken for SEM study.

5. Examinations

The study of the lead surface was made by SEM at the Metallurgical Laboratory of l'Ecole Nationale Supérieure de Mécanique et d'Aéronautique de Poitiers (ENSMA), and examination by SEM and Optical Microscopy of the tissues in the Department of Anatomy-Pathology of Professeur Payen (CHU Poitiers).

The samples for Optical Microscopy were fixed by the standard method (10% Formol and HES staining).

3. Results

1. Study of lead insulation by SEM

With the polyurethane, parallel fissures start to appear 3.5 months after the implantation – At 6.5 months there is only a little evolution; a more serious degradation, with fissures appearing perpendicular to the initial fissures was noticed after 13 months of implantation. With the silicone and the polyethylene there is no degradation 4.5 months after implantation.

2. Study of tissue reaction by Optical Microscopy

Polyurethane

After 3 months an important epithelial reaction was noted around the lead with polynuclear eosinophyles. Some particles of plastic are embedded in the vein wall and are surrounded by multinucleated macrophages (Photo 1).
After 13 months of implantation, the initial epithelial reaction is progressively replaced by fibrosis. In the vein wall (SVC) and in the myocardium (Right Atrium, Right Ventricule) a foreign body reaction developing into fibrosis, with amounts of plastic debris and calcifications, is observed (Photo 2).

Silicone and Polyethylene

After 1 month of implantation, we noted only, for these two materials, a modest reaction without epithelial or palissadic aspects – At 4.5 months, there is a slight fibrosis around the lead in the SVC and in the Right Atrium (Photo 3), but without foreign bodies.

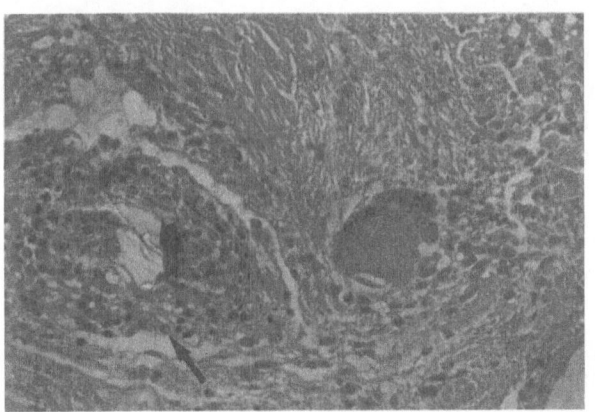

Fig. 1. – x 312 – SVC
Multinucleated macrophages →
Polyurethane ►

Fig. 2. – x 125 – Right Ventricule
Inclusions: →
Calcifications: ▶ ▶

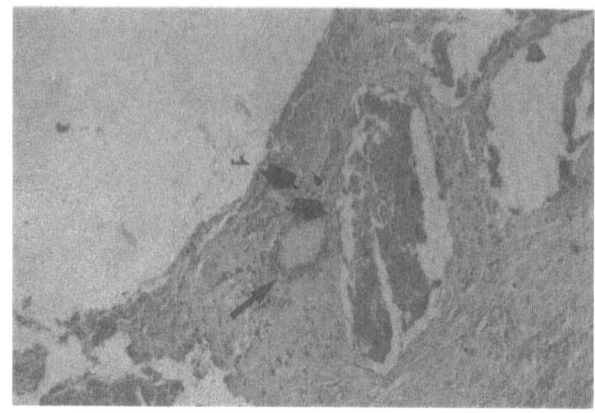

Fig. 3. – x 125 – SVC
Lead ✳

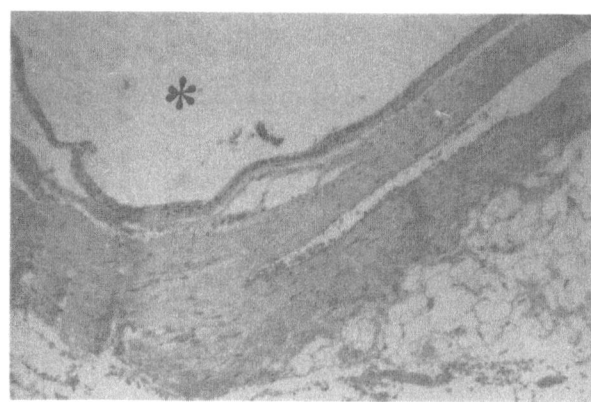

4. Conclusions

Having examined the results, we conclude:

– For the material: Polyurethane rapidly cracks and fissures in an inhomogeneous manner. These areas of degradation are, without doubt, localized in those places where mechanical stress occurs along the length of the lead. These could also be associated with the methods of manufacture (surface defects and structural stresses due to the manufacturing process) (15).

Silicone and Polyethylene are not susceptible to these problems and maintain their integrity during life.

– For the organisms reaction:

Around the lead, Polyurethane provokes a reaction more violent than the other materials.

At a distance (Vein wall, myocardium), foreign particles with inflammatory reaction were found only with the Polyurethane.

314

Silicone and Polyethylene were tolerated best, without foreign particles, no calcification, and without even moderate inflammatory reaction.

The results concerning the third part of the study (examination of the organs) are in the stage of analysis and will be published later. Several cases of "Silicone hepatitis" have been reported in persons subject to chronic haemodialysis caused by particles which detach from the material of the tubes squeezed by the Artificial Kidney pumps. With endocardial leads, the mechanical stresses are much less. However, particles of Polyurethane have been observed in the vessel walls and could be present in organs such as the liver, kidneys, and lungs. Even if the cracks observed with polyurethane are not critical for pacing, it is important to study the possible migration of the product in the organism system and its pathological consequences.

References

1. Irnich W: "Engineering concepts of pacemaker electrodes." Pacemaker technology Ed Springer Verlag Pub 1975.
2. Stokes K, Cobian K, and Co: Polyurethane insulators, a design approach to small pacing leads. Proceeding VI World Symposium on Cardiac Pacing, Pace Symp, 28–2, 1979. – C Meere Ed.
3. Stokes K: Polyurethane lead insulation: a study in biostability, Medtronom 1981: n° 12.
4. Stokes K: Isolant en polyurethane, Medtronom 1981: n° 11.
5. Ploger G, Castet M, Jacquemart JF: Clinical Experience with 300 polyurethane pacing leads, RBM vol 4, n° 5, page 419.
6. Devanathan J, James MS, Shietz E, Keith MS, Young A: In vivo thrombogenicity of implantable Cardiac leads, Biomat, Med Dev, Ant Org, 1980; 814: 369–379.
7. Stokes K: The long term biostability of polyurethane leads. Stimucoeur Medical tome 10 n° 3, 1982: 205–212.
8. Termain Paul: Biostability of urethane cardiac pacing leads, Medtronic Publication Number 4, 1982: April 12.
9. Babotai I: Polyurethane leads – Experimental study in dogs, RBM vol 4, n° 4, page 418.
10. Lieser, Irnich and Kreuzer: Polyurethane leads: Fact and controversy, Pace. March 1983, vol 6, n° 2, part II, pages 404–458.
11. MacArthur WR: Long term Implant effects on three polyurethane leads, Pacesetter Systems Inc 1982 documentation.
12. Amiel A, Roualdes G, Touchard G, Bouchet B, Lehmann G: Biocompatibilité du polyuréthane. A propos d'une étude expérimentale chez le lapin domestique – 15 cas, RBM vol. 4, n° 5, page 417.
13. Leong, ASY, Path C: "Spillation and migration of silicone from blood pump tubing in patients on hemodialysis. The New England Journal of Medecine vol. 306, n° 3, pages 135–141.
14. Bommer P, Eberhard R and Waldhen R: Silicone induced spliaomyolic. The NET of Medecine vol 365, n° 18, pages 1077–1079.
15. Guerin Ph: Use of Synthetic polymers for biomedical application. Pace, Vol. 6, March 83, Part II pp 449–453.

Authors' address:
Dr. A. Amiel
Service de Cardiologie B
CHU Poitiers
France

Comparison of Lead Complications with Polyurethane Tined, Silicone Rubber Tined, and Wedge Tip Ventricular Pacemaker Leads

P. J. Kertes, H. G. Mond, J. K. Vohra, J. G. Sloman, C.-W. Kong, D. Hunt

Summary: A prospective study of lead-related complications was undertaken over a five year period to compare unipolar tined endocardial pacemaker leads with silicone rubber insulation (SR), to those with polyurethane insulation (PU). Overall complications were similar in both groups – 3.6% for the 364 SR leads and 4.2% for the 238 PU leads.

The total series of 602 tined leads (SR + PU) was then compared to a retrospective review of 220 wedge tip silicone rubber ventricular leads. A marked reduction was demonstrated in dislodgements (0.3% vs 7.7%, $P < 0.001$) reoperations (2.0% vs 15.0%, $P < 0.001$) and total complications (3.8% vs 15.5%, $P < 0.001$) with tined leads. We conclude that tined ventricular leads are far superior to wedge tip leads with respect to lead complications. There were no significant differences between the two types of tined leads used in this study.

Lead related complications, in particular dislodgement, were a major problem with early permanent pacing systems (1). In order to improve lead stability, various methods of endocardial fixation were introduced (2) of which one of the earliest and most popular was the wedge tip (WT) lead. A more recent method of passive fixation involved the use of flexible tines near the tip of the lead which were constructed from the same material as the lead insulation. These leads were initially insulated with silicone rubber (SR), but polyurethane (PU) has now been introduced by a number of pacemaker companies. Polyurethane leads are thinner and have a lower friction coefficient in blood than the original designs of SR leads. However, there has been some doubt cast recently on the durability of PU leads (3, 4, 5) but none of these reports are of a clinical series with a substantial number of patients.

We have prospectively studied the lead related complications of 602 consecutively implanted unipolar tined endocardial ventricular pacemaker leads, comparising 364 SR leads and 238 PU leads. We have also compared the complications of the total series of tined leads to an earlier series of 220 unipolar ventricular WT leads.

Methods

Data for the 822 implanted leads in this study were obtained from the pacemaker files of the Cardiology Department which are continuously updated during patient follow-up. Pulse generators were implanted in the sub-clavicular region under local anesthesia, with the lead introduced through the cephalic vein or occasionally by percutaneous puncture of the subclavian vein. All leads studied have been unipolar in type and have included ventricular leads used as part of a dual chamber pacing system (2.7%).

317

At operation, pacing threshold and R-wave amplitudes were measured with a pacing systems analyser (Medtronic 5300*)). Voltage thresholds of less than 1 volt at 0.5 msec pulse duration and sensed R-waves of over 4 mVolts were sought. Pacing at 10 volts was routinely performed to exclude diaphragmatic pacing. With tined leads, gentle traction on the lead was exerted after positioning at the right ventricular apex to ensure that the tines were well anchored beneath or between endocardial trabeculae. The lead was then firmly secured at the venous entry site or to muscle fascia with non-absorbable suture material. Chest radiographs were routinely performed to confirm satisfactory lead positioning.

Wedge tip leads were implanted between June 1975 and February 1978, and were from four manufacturers (Table 1). Tined leads were implanted between November 1977 and October 1982 and were from five manufacturers (Table 1). Polyurethane leads were first implanted in May 1979. The patient populations in all lead groups were well matched with respect to mean age (WT 70 years, SR 73 years, PU 72 years), and sex ratio (males 55% WT, 56% SR, 53% PU). There were no differences between the three groups in indications for pacing, which included high degree atrio-ventricular block in 63 to 67% of patients and sick sinus syndrome in 23 to 30%. Despite a wide range of electrode designs used, there were no major differences between the three groups in voltage and current threshold, R wave measurement and lead resistance at implantation.

Table 1. Lead Manufacturers.

Wedge tip	– Medtronic 6907	114
	Telectronics PY 3802	94
	PY 3804	
	T 176	
	Edwards	10
	Cordis	2
		220
SR tined	– Medtronic 6961	177
	Telectronics 220	123
	Telectronics 227/230/232/233	56
	Cardiac Pacemakers 4130	4
	Pacesetter 841	4
		364
PU tined	– Medtronic 6971	195
	Telectronics 239/240	35
	Intermedics 495	8
		238
	Total –	822

PU = polyurethane
SR = silicone rubber

*) Medtronic, Minneapolis, Minnesota, USA.

Results

Operative Complications

These were encountered in four patients. In one (SR), the tines became permanently entangled in tricuspid valve chordae necessitating insertion of a second lead. Non-fatal air embolism occurred in one patient during positioning of the lead (PU) through a subclavian venous entry site. Two elderly patients (PU) with marked cardiomegaly and a long history of congestive cardiac failure suffered ventricular fibrillation during lead placement in the right ventricle; both were successively resuscitated although one patient died four hours post-operatively from recurrent ventricular fibrillation. This patient also experienced ventricular tachycardia and fibrillation pre-operatively.

Post-Operative Complications

These are summarised in Table 2. A marked reduction in the incidence of dislodgement has been seen with tined compared to WT leads (0.3% vs 7.7%) with no significant differences between PU and SR leads. With tined leads, four perforations of the right ventricle were encountered in three patients, one of which required re-manipulation of the same lead on two occasions. Persistent, troublesome diaphragmatic pacing was seen in one patient (WT) requiring re-positioning of the lead. Two lead conductor fractures were encountered (1 SR 1 WT), both at the point of entry into the external jugular vein. Lead retraction without dislodgement was seen in two patients (SR).

Late high threshold exit block was seen in 16 patients (11 WT, 3 SR, 2 PU) requiring re-operation in 14 (11 WT, 2 SR, 1 PU) and non-invasive re-programming of a pulse generator with high output capability in the other two cases. The longer follow-up period for WT leads (maximum 7.3 years compared to 5 years for tined leads) may partly explain the greater number of late high threshold exit blocks with these leads. Two cases of sensing failure have occurred; one at 3 years post-implantation requiring re-operation (WT) and the other within six months of implantation (PU), corrected by re-programming the sensitivity of the pulse generator.

Total Complications

Both total complications and total re-operations were significant fewer with tined compared to WT leads, with no significant differences between PU and SR tined leads (Table 3). The re-operation rate at one year was also much lower with tined leads, with 17 of 22 wedge tip lead re-operations within the first year due to lead dislodgement.

Discussion

The large experience reported here is in accordance with the findings of previous studies (6–10) demonstrating a marked reduction in the incidence of dislodgement with the use of tined ventricular leads. Although tined leads are rapidly becoming the standard endo-

319

Table 2. Post-operative Complications.

Lead Type	WT	total tined		SR tined	PU tined	
Number	220	602		364	238	
Dislodgement	17 (7.7%)	2 (0.3%)	$P < 0.001$	1	1	N.S.
Retraction	–	2	N.S.	2	1	N.S.
Perforation	2	4	N.S.	3	1	N.S.
Diaphragmatic*) Pacing	2	4	N.S.	2	2	N.S.
High threshold < 1yr exit block	3	5	N.S.	3	2	
total	11	5		3	2	N.S.
Sensing failure	1	1	N.S.	–	1	N.S.
Conductor fracture	1	1	N.S.	1	–	N.S.
Total	34 (15.5%) (22 < 1yr)	19 (3.2%) (all < 1yr)		12 (3.3%)	7 (2.9%)	N.S.

*) Remanipulation only required in one case (WT).

PU = polyurethane
SR = silicone rubber
WT = wedge tip
N.S. = not significant ($P < 0.05$)

Table 3. Total Complications.

Lead Type	WT	total tined		SR tined	PU tined	
Number	220	602		364	238	
Max. follow-up (yrs)	7.3	5		5	3.4	
Post op complications (Table 2)	34 (15.5%)	19 (3.2%)		12 (3.3%)	7 (2.9%)	N.S.
Total complications	34 (15.5%)	23 (3.8%)	$P < 0.001$	13 (3.6%)	10 (4.2%)	N.S.
Total re-operation	33 (15%)	12 (2.0%)	$P < 0.001$	9 (2.5%)	3 (1.3%)	N.S.

PU = polyurethane
SR = silicone rubber
WT = wedge tip
N.S. = not significant ($p > 0.05$)

320

cardial ventricular pacemaker lead used in many pacing centres, wedge tip leads are still being implanted. The results of this study argue strongly in favour of abandoning the use of wedge tip leads altogether.

We have also compared lead complications between SR and PU leads in view of a number of reports (3–5) suggesting a tendency for polyurethane insulation to develop surface cracking in vivo with possible loss of insulation. These reports have been anecodotal (4, 5), and thus challenged (11, 12). While we have not explanted these leads for microscopic examination and testing we have encountered no cases of insulation failure, late high threshold exit block, sensing failure or lead fracture. Thus, our clinical experience with polyurethane over a maximum period of 3 to 4 years has shown this lead insulation material to be safe although the long-term results are still not available.

References

1. Parsonnet V, Bilitch M, Furman S, Fisher JD, Escher DJW, Myers G, Cassady E: Early malfunction of transvenous pacemaker electrodes. A three year study. Circulation 1979; 60: 590–596.
2. Robicsek F, Tarjan P, Harbold NB, Masters TN, Robicsek SA: Self-anchoring endocardial pacemaker leads: Current spectrum of types, advances in design and clinical results. Am Heart J 1981; 102: 775–782.
3. Stimarec Bulletin No. 6, June 30th 1982, Page 1.
4. McArthur, WA: Long-term implant effects of three polyurethane leads in humans. Pacesetter Systems Inc., 1982.
5. Parins DJ, Black KM, McCoy KD and Horvath NJ: In vivo degradation of a polyurethane. Cardiac Pacemakers Inc., 1981.
6. Gordon S, Timmins GC, Ramos RG, Gangadharan V and Hauser J: Improved transvenous pacemaker electrode stability. In: Meere, C. (Ed). Cardiac Pacing. Proceedings of the Sixth World Symposium on Cardiac Pacing. Montreal: Pace-symp, 1979: Chapter 31.3.
7. Painter MW, Harrington OB, Crosby VG, Wolf RY: Implantation of an endocardial lead to prevent early dislodgement. J Thorac Cardiovasc Surg 1979; 77: 249–251.
8. Holmes DR, Gersh BJ, Maloney JD, Merideth J: Follow-up experience with permanent endocardial tined pacemaker electrodes. J Thorac Cardiovasc Surg 1980; 79: 565–569.
9. Mond HG, Sloman JG: The small tined pacemaker lead – absence of displacement. Pace 1980; 3: 171–177.
10. Snow N: Elimination of lead dislodgement by the use of tined transvenous electrodes. Pace 1982; 5: 571–574.
11. Guerrant K: Clinical Engineering Notice, Intermedics Inc, 1982.
12. Termin P: Biostability of urethane cardiac pacing leads. Medtronic Inc. Pacing concept paper No. 4, April, 12, 1982.

Authors' address:
Dr. Paul Kertes
The Royal Melbourne Hospital
Department of Cardiology
c/o Post Office
Melbourne/Australia

A New Polyurethane and Process for Pacer Leads[1]

H. C. Hughes[2], R. D. Bertolet[3], J. T. Kissinger[2], R. R. Brownlee[3]

Summary: Urethane tubing has largely replaced silicone as the insulation of choice on cardiac pacemaker leads. Although urethane has been shown to be biocompatible, there have been reports of insulation defects. This study was on a segmented polyether polyurethane polymer which is applied and bonded directly to the wire. The SPU adds its strength and flexibility to the lead. SPU is heart settable, enabling special configurations (S-A node and J-leads) to be made without significantly affecting the O.D. The modulus of elongation (> 700%), and strength (> 6000 psi) of SPU are superior to silicone (< 500% at 1200 psi) and of urethane (< 400% at 6000 psi). Implants in rats, rabbits, and dogs have shown SPU to be essentially free of blood and tissue reactions. Long-term transvenous atrial and ventricular leads (up to 30 months) have been implanted in dogs without adverse affects and only a 25% decrease in chronic intrinsic P-wave and 20% in R-wave potentials. Threshold strength-duration curves showed changes similar to those reported for other pacemaker leads. Light and scanning photomicrographs show a freedom from cracks, crazing, and internal/external wear defects after over a cumulative 300 months implant experience. Polarized light has failed to show any stress related defects in the SPU coatings.

Introduction

The advent of polyurethane sheathed pacemaker leads, in fact tubes, has resulted in the production of smaller diameter, more supple lead systems. This has permitted the easy introduction of two leads through a single vein for A-V pacing. In addition, their high tissue compatibility has greatly decreased thromboembolic related sequelae. These sheathed leads have been one of the major advances that has made A-V pacing practical. The use of extruded urethane sheaths, however, has not been without complications. Even before their widespread acceptance, there were indications that there may be inherent problems with this type of system. These initial reports indicated that a roughening and cracking appeared on the surface of these leads even after relatively short-term implantation (1). Reports of the loss of lead integrity have continued to surface justifying fears about these urethane leads despite the manufacturer's claims that all is well.

There have been several reasons proposed for these failures. The manufacturer claims that the wire coils are frictionally wearing the polymer out from the inside, especially with J-leads (2). In addition to the actual wearing away from the inside out, insulation defects have occurred at points of tissue contact (3). Another cause of urethane failures is related to the manufacture of the tubing. Changes in the urethane skin occur from accidental "stresses" induced during annealing and/or extruding of the tubing. This is sup-

---

[1]) Supported in part by grants from U.S.P.H.S. (R01 HL13988 and K04 HL00586) and Cardiac Control Systems.
[2]) Department of Comparative Medicine in The Milton S. Hershey Medical Center, The Pennsylvania State University, Hershey, PA (USA).
[3]) Cardiac Control Systems, State College, PA (USA).

ported by the fact that these crazing cracks appear, for the most part, to be superficial (1, 4–6). Some cracks, however, have progressed to the point of disintegration.

Another associated with these urethane sheathed leads is the "creeping" of the polymer away from fixation ligatures. Insulation defects are produced and the pacemaker lead short circuits (4, 5, 7). This is a result of the low modulus of elasticity in the polymer that results in a tendency to creep under pressure. To alleviate this problem, urethane sheathed leads must be secured with a special "suture sleeve".

The purpose of this study was to evaluate a new segmented polyether polyurethane (SPU) coating and process. Similar types of solvent dissolved SPU polymers have been used since the late 1960's (8). Most are presently being used in artificial heart programs since they have been shown to be the strongest, most stable and consistently reliable implantable SPU polymers. SPU's use has been limited, however, because the polymer and the techniques for rapidly and accurately coating wires have not been available.

Materials and Methods

The segmented polyether polyurethane (SPU – CCS/Urethane) used in this study was of the solvent dissolved type. The SPU is dissolved in dimethylacetamide and applied as a 20% (w/v) solution. Prior to use, test samples are evaluated for cytotoxicity (mouse L-929 fibroblast tissue culture). These tests must be negative for cytopathic effects. In addition, samples are examined by infrared spectrographic analysis and compared with standards to assure uniformity.

The dissolved SPU is then coated on quadrafilar MP-35N wire (0.9 mm O.D.) using a cold drawing technique. This process combines the basic techniques used for lacquering with solvent dissolved polymers and the extrusion techniques that have been used for the manufacture of tubing with the thermoplastic urethanes. Rather than making a tube as is now done with other leads, the SPU is coated directly on and to the wire (Fig. 1). Multiple coats are used to build the SPU coat to the desired wall thickness of 0.25 mm. Each coat dissolves into the preceding coat so that "onion skinning" does not occur. High temperatures and pressures are avoided during the entire coextrusion and curing process. Therefore, degradation and stress on the polymer are eliminated during fabrication. Since the polymer is coated on and adhered to the wire, rubbing and frictional wear between the wire and coating cannot occur. The wire and SPU insulation flex as one unit.

Stress-strain analyses were done on 1.4 mm SPU coated leads and compared with conventional urethane tube covered leads of the same diameter and conductor wire. All tests were done in matched pairs. The leads were maintained under constant tension (% elongation) and cycled through minimum and maximum extensions so that life cycle acceleration was extreme (9).

Assessment of biocompatibility was done using procedures similar to the ANSI/ASTM F469–79 standards. Sterile, coated leads were implanted in 15 rabbits, 25 rats, and 65 mongrel dogs. The leads implanted in dogs were of either the ventricular, standard atrial-J, modified atrial-J, or A-V data lead type. All were passed transvenously through the jugular vein and into the heart using asceptic techniques and a fluoroscope. Electrophysiologic measurements, including pacing thresholds and the intrinsic electrograms, were obtained at implantation in the dogs using previously described techniques (10–12). The implants were thereafter examined at regular intervals beginning 2 weeks after implanta-

324

tion and extending to over 2.5 years postimplant. Tissue sections from major organs, with special reference to the heart and vessels, were examined at necropsy and by light microscopy. All leads were examined under light microscopy with representative sections also being examined using scanning electron microscopy and polarized light.

Results

The methods used to coat these pacemaker leads have resulted in highly uniform devices. The leads were coated to a diameter within a 0.05 mm tolerance over the 60 cm length of the lead. Equal uniformity was found from lead to lead. Wall thickness can be varied essentially over an infinite range by varying the concentration of the SPU solution and/or the number of coatings. Coils of different diameters were coated so that it was possible to make leads with different handling characteristics. Finished lead diameters between 1.0–2.5 mm have been made and studied. Since this SPU is heat settable at relatively low temperatures (130 °C), curves and bends were formed in the lead without creating any stress or tension in the polymer coating. It was not necessary to build up extra thicknesses of polymer, nor use stiffer wires, or larger coils in fabricating the bends. Special purpose leads can be fabricated with multiple coils or bends (13). The J-leads had the same wire coil (0.9 mm) and finished (1.4 mm) diameter as the ventricular lead. Leads with a finished outside diameter of < 1.0 mm were also made and passed transvenously in rabbits.

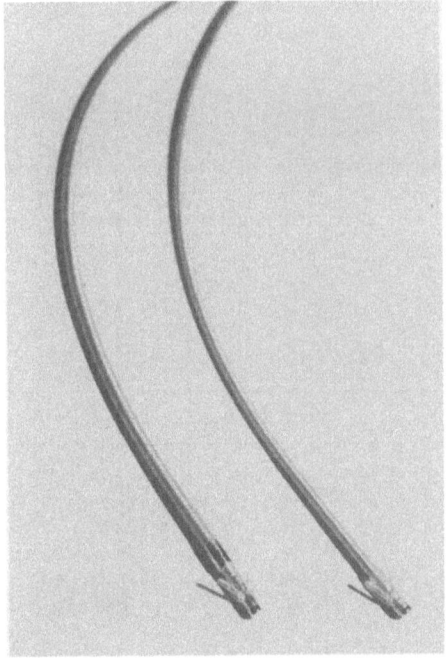

Fig. 1. Finished SPU coated leads. The lead on the left is a coaxial lead (CCS Model BB-102) with a 2.3 mm outside diameter. The lead on the right is a tined unipolar ventricular lead (CCS Model SV-101) with a 1.4 mm diameter.

Because this coating process allows the SPU polymer to penetrate between the wire files, much of the strength and handling characteristics of the SPU are imparted to the wire (Fig. 2, Table 1). The results of the lead stress-strain tests demonstrated that by bonding the SPU to the wire, additional strength and flexibility is added to the wire. The SPU coated leads stress-strain cycled between seven (9% min: 28% max tension) to over 25 times (8% min: 16% max) longer than conventional polyurethane tube sheathed leads.

The tissue reaction to all leads (both SPU test and silicone controls) implanted intramuscularly and subcutaneously, were essentially the same regardless of species. Grossly, there was a thin translucent false capsule surrounding the lead. This tissue would collapse and blend with surrounding tissues when the SPU leads were removed. The silicone leads

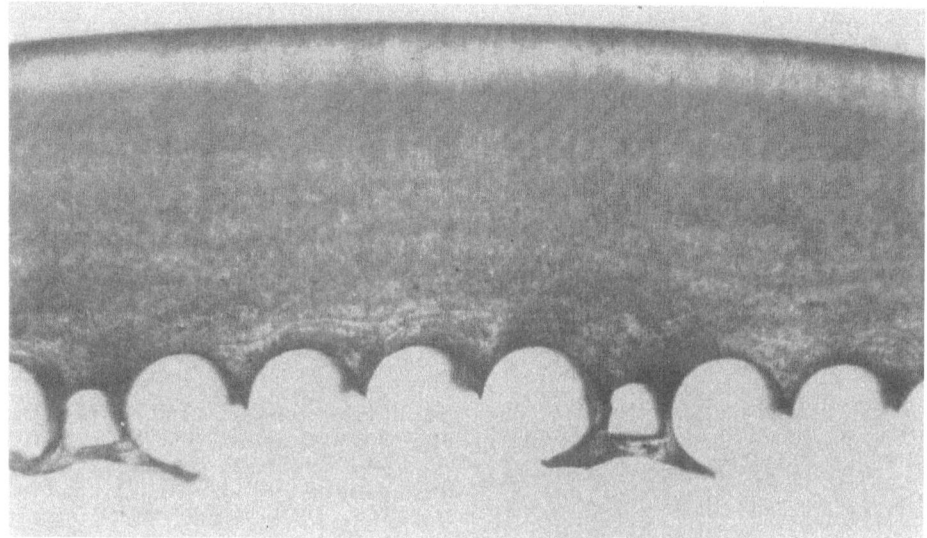

Fig. 2. A longitudinal section of the SPU coating after removal of the quadrafilar wire. The coextrusion process results in polymer penetrating between and bonding to the conductive wires adding the strength and flexibility of the SPU to the wire. (Each individual wire file was 0.13 mm in diameter.)

Table 1. Comparison of Physical Properties between SPU, Silicone, and Urethane.

	SPU	Silicone	Urethane
Tensile Modulus psi ?			
100%	450	160	850
300%	1025		1650
Break	6000	1200	6000
Elongation at break, %	7–800	4–500	3–400
Hardness, Shore A	75	50	80
Specific Grarity	1.1	1.1	1.1

seemed to be slightly adherent to their capsule. Microscopically, only a thin capsule surrounded the leads. Initially, the capsule was only a few cell layers thick and had stabilized at 6–8 cell layers by 8 weeks postimplant. There was no evidence of inflammation, foreign body, or any adverse response to any lead at any time.

In the dogs, the SPU leads were passed transvenously into either the atria or ventricle. All leads handled well and became slippery when wetted with blood or body fluids. At necropsy, there was no evidence of thrombosis or fibrosis along the body of the leads at any time in any animal (Fig. 3). The tined tips of the transvenous leads were firmly attached to the myocardium by a thin fibrous tissue capsule. The pacing threshold requirements for both the atrium and ventricle increased to their maximum levels and the intrinsic deflection of the electrograms were at their minimum between 2–4 weeks postimplant (Tables 2 and 3). These levels returned toward acute levels thereafter, and stabilized by 12 weeks at long-term post postimplantation levels.

All SPU covered leads themselves were completely unaffected by implantation. There was no evidence of pseudoendothelialization, cracking, peeling, delamination, or other internal/external wear defects when the leads were examined grossly, by light microscopy, or by scanning electron microscopy. There has been accumulated over 300 months of implantation experience with the longest being over 2.5 years. There has not been a single lead related adverse effect.

There were no apparent stress-related distortions visible in the SPU leads when examined under polarized light, regardless of whether the leads were examined in their normal straight configuration or severely flexed. Even new conventionally sheathed urethane leads, showed areas of polarized light refraction indicative of extrusion induced stresses.

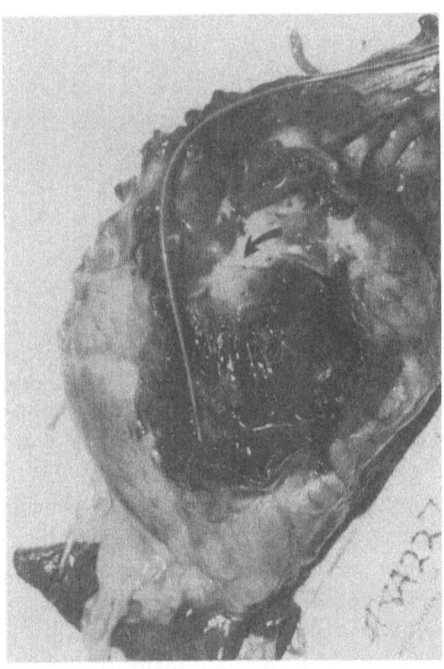

Fig. 3. The heart and vessels of a dog with complete block which had a right ventricular SPU (CCS Model SV-101) lead implanted through the jugular vein for over one year. Only the tip of the lead was fibrosed into the right ventricular apex. The main body of the lead remained free of thrombosis and tissue response along its entire length. (Septal calcification [arrow] was from the induced heart block.)

327

Table 2. Threshold Voltage/Current Requirements and Intrinsic R-wave Potentials for SPU Coated Ventricular Leads.

Weeks	Threshold (Volts/mA)			R-wave Potentials	
	1.0 msec	0.5 msec	0.1 msec	mV	msec
0	0.2±0.2/0.3±0.2*)	0.4±0.2/0.6±0.4	0.8±0.2/1.7±0.4	26±6.7	9.8±4.2
2	1.0±0.3/1.6±0.9	1.4±0.4/2.7±1.2	3.5±1.6/7.9±3.2	23±9.7	9.6±2.3
4	0.8±0.4/1.3±0.8	1.1±0.5/1.8±0.9	2.7±1.4/5.5±2.3	29±8.2	9.2±3.1
12	0.8±0.2/1.1±0.6	1.0±0.3/1.6±0.8	2.4±1.1/4.7±2.5	22±8.7	10±5.6
26	0.8±0.3/1.3±1.0	1.0±0.3/1.9±1.1	2.6±0.9/5.7±2.2	21±7.5	10±3.0

*) Mean ± standard deviation.

Table 3. Threshold Voltage/Current Requirements and Intrinsic R-wave Potentials for the Modified Atrial J-Pacemaker Lead.

Weeks	Threshold (Volts/mA)			R-wave Potentials	
	1.0 msec	0.5 msec	0.1 msec	mV	msec
0	0.5±0.2/0.8±0.7*)	0.7±0.5/1.4±1.2	1.7±1.1/3.9±2.6	7.6±3.4	4.2±1.7
2	2.0±1.1/3.4±3.1	1.9±1.1/4.0±3.3	4.1±2.9/11±9	4.4±1.8	6.5±3.5
4	1.6±0.6/3.1±2.5	2.2±1.3/5.1±4.1	4.7±4.2/10±4.8	6.6±3.5	6.2±2.5
8	1.4±0.5/2.3±1.5	1.8±0.7/3.5±1.9	4.6±2.0/10±4.8	5.7±1.7	4.0±0.8
12	1.4±0.6/2.2±1.4	1.5±0.6/2.8±1.3	3.9±2.1/8.3±4.6	5.7±1.1	4.2±1.1

*) Mean ± standard deviation.

Suture sleeves were not used with any of these SPU leads. Although slight polymer creep was noted under tightly tied fixation sutures, in no case were any insulation defects produced.

Discussion

The term polyurethane and urethane have become generic in their use and are often used to describe a wide variety of polymeric materials of which relatively few are used for biomedical implantation. Most of these polymers are used in the building and textile industries. The most commonly used medical polymer is a thermoplastic polyether polyurethane that is referred to in this paper as urethane. The solvent-dissolved types (SPU) have been used for special application, but much less extensively. Therefore, even though these polymers have distinctly different chemical structural and handling characteristics, they are unfortunately referred to by the same name, polyurethane. This lack of distinction makes differentiation between polyurethane devices difficult.

The process used to form products from the thermoplastic polymers involves relatively high temperatures and pressures which are used to force the non-fluid material through extrusion dyes or injection molds. The solvent-dissolved polymers, on the other hand, are not subjected to these extremes, but their fabrication into devices involves the removal of the solvent by evaporation at relatively low temperatures. The use of these solvent-dissolved SPU polymers have been limited because the lacquer method of application are rather primitive and time consuming. They have consistently, however, been shown to be strong, flexible, biocompatible, and stable for long-term use (8, 14–16).

The leads themselves are made by bonding the SPU to the conductive M-35N wire using a low temperature drawing technique. By using this technique, smooth, uniform, small diameter, yet very strong, pacemaker leads can be made. Because this SPU has a heat set-table, memory-retaining characteristic, it was not necessary to build up extra material or have extra wire at the J-bend of atrial leads in order for the lead to maintain its shape and placement. The result has been the development of atrial leads of the same O.D. as stand-ard ventricular leads (1.4 mm) and special purpose ventricular leads smaller than 1.0 mm and coaxial leads less than 2.3 mm. The stiffness and handling characteristic of each lead can be modified by varying the thickness of the polymer coating over essentially an infinite range. Furthermore, because there is a physical bonding of the SPU to the wire, the strength and elasticity of the polymer is added to that of the wire coils enabling them to flex together smoother and longer than other urethane covered leads.

The stress-strain analysis consistently demonstrated a 7–25 times greater flex life when SPU bonded leads were compared against identical wires covered with urethane tubing. There was no frictional wearing of this SPU polymer from the inside because the polymer and wire are bonded together, therefore, never rubbing against each other. On the other hand, noticeable areas of abrasion and wear were seen in the urethane tubing at areas of maximum flex. In some of these urethane leads, insulation defects were produced prior to wire failure.

By using a multicoating process, each succeeding layer combines with and bonds to the previous layer. This causes any potential surface defects to be sealed by the next coating.

There were no areas of stress created during the manufacture of the SPU polymer leads. The high temperatures and pressure used to make conventional leads are avoided in coat-ing these leads. Even new urethane tubing showed areas of stress-related light defraction patterns when viewed under polarized light. These stress defraction patterns are potential areas for insulation defects to occur. The SPU covered leads have not shown stress-related features or any sign of developing crazing or cracking, either before or after any of the in vivo or in vitro testing.

The results of the animal tests demonstrated the long-term biocompatibility and low thrombogenicity of this SPU polymer. There was never any case of an adverse response to the polymer in any animal. The leads remained thrombus and fibrosis-free along their entire transvenous length (Fig. 3). Muscle and subcutaneous tissue responses were mini-mal. The response of the blood and vascular tissue to SPU was far less than that reported for silicone pacemaker leads (17). The pacing-sensing functions of the SPU leads re-mained at levels comparable to other lead systems (Tables 2 and 3).

In summary, this study has shown that the high modulus of elongation (> 700%), low creep, great strength (> 6000 psi), memory retaining characteristics and great flexibility (> 100 million cycles) make this SPU an ideal insulating material for pacemaker leads as well as many other biomedical applications. Coextruding the lead with the conductive wire results in a highly compliant, stress-free conductive system for pacemakers.

References

1. Parins JF, McCory KD, Horvath WJ: In vivo degradation of a polyurethane: Further evidence. Pace 1982; 5: 302.
2. Welti JJ: Stimarac report of July 1982. Pace 1982; 5: 944.
3. Kruse IM, Mark J, Ryden L: Mechanical wear of pacemaker lead insultation. A cause of loss of pacing. Pace 1980; 3: 159–161.
4. Seligman PL: Polyurethane leads: A more positive view. Stimucour Med 1982; 10: 212–216.
5. Stokes K: The long-term biostability of polyurethane leads. Stimucour Med 1982; 10: 205–212.
6. Godin JF, Welti JJ: Stimarac report of May–June 1982. Pace 1982; 5: 786.
7. Witte AA: Pseudofracture of pacemaker lead due to securing suture: A case report. Pace 1981; 4: 716–718.
8. Boretos JW: Tissue pathology and physical stability of a polyether elastomeric on three-year mplantation. J Biomed Mater Res 1972; 6: 473.
9. Gebhardt VC, Irnich W, Bulles G, Broichhausen J: Multistrand pacemaker leads – a really redundant system. Proc VIth World Symp Cardiac Pacing. 1979. Chapt. 29–4.
10. Furman S, Hurzeler P, DeCaprio V: The ventricular endocardial electrogram and pacemaker sensing. J Thorac Cardiovasc Surg 1977; 73: 258–266.
11. Hughes HC, Brownlee RR, Bertolet RD, Neff PH, Sluetz JE, Tyers GFO: The effects of electrode position on the detection of the transvenous cardiac electrogram. Pace 1980; 3: 651–655.
12. Hughes HC, Tyers GFO: Effect of stimulation site on ventricular threshold in dogs with heart block. Am Heart J 1975; 89: 68–73.
13. Hughes HC, Bertolet RD, Brownlee RR: A new atrial lead with improved stability and optimal P-wave detection. Pace 1983; 6: 726–734.
14. Sparks RE: Chairman's summary: Physical testing of polymers session. Devices and Technology Branch Contractors Meeting Proceedings 1979; 60–62.
15. Shultz JS, Barenberg S, Ciarkowski AA, Lindenauer SM, Penner JA: Evaluation of compatibility of biomaterials. Devices and Technology Branch Contractors Meeting Proceedings 1979; 213–216.
16. Phillips WM, Pierce WS, Rosenberg G, Donachy J: The use of segmented polyurethane in ventricular assist devices and artificial hearts. In: Szycher M, Robinson WJ, eds. Synthetic Biomedical Polymers Concepts and Applications. Westport, CT: Technonic, 1980; 39–51.
17. Fishbein MC, Tan KS, Beazell JW, Schulman JH, Hirose FM, Criley JM: Cardiac pathology of transvenous pacemakers in dogs. Am Heart J 1977; 93: 73–81.

Authors' address:
Howard C. Hughes, V.M.D.
The Miljton S. Hershey Medical Center
500 University Drive
Hershey, PA 17033
USA

Ventricular Lead in Atrial Position

L. Kappenberger, I. Babotai, F. Siclari, L. Egloff, M. Turina

Summary: Longterm function and stability of atrial leads is still a crucial part of dual chamber pacing and sensing. The use of the same type of electrode in the atrium and in the ventricle is an advantage and simplification from technical, surgical and logistic standpoints. We report about the results in 158 consecutive Helifix electrodes in atrial position and 143 Helifix electrodes in ventricular position in the same patients. The 158 patients (85 males, 43 females, mean age 63.5) received a pacemaker system with only atrial sensing (VAT of VDD) in 31%, with atrial pacing and sensing (AAI or DDD) in 44% and with atrial pacing but ventricular sensing only (DVI) in 25%. Electrodes were transvenously inserted via cephalic or subclavian vein. Atrial electrodes were placed underneath the crista terminalis of the lateral right atrium and not in the atrial appendage, the ventricular leads in the right ventricular apex. Atrial threshold at impulse duration of 1.0 ms was 0.85 V (0.37–2.04) and 1.11 mA (0.4–2.0), P-wave was 3.21 mV (1.0–9.5). Ventricular threshold at 1.0 was 0.67 V (0.25–1.70) and 0.89 mA (0.25–2.1), R-wave was 7.9 mV (1.3–20.0). After mean follow-up of 18.2 months overall complication rate was 3%. 3 early displacements (2 within 24 hours and 1 after 3 months). We observed one case of phrenic nerve stimulation. From these results we conclude that an electrode primarily designed for ventricular use is extremely suitable for longterm atrial sensing and stimulation and overall complication is not increased in dual chamber pacing.

The clinical application of atrioventricular pacing has undoubtedly increased over the past few years. Following a first period characterized by technical problems, the clear advantage of sequential pacing has convinced many centers to adapt this technique. One of the major concerns in using dual chamber pacemaker systems was the difficulty in implantation of stable atrial electrodes (1). Today, as for ventricular leads, there is a number of atrial leads to choose for sensing as well as pacing the atrium (2, 3). The problem of a stock of different electrodes for both chambers makes the logistics of a pacemaker clinic more and more complicated. We have earlier reported about the use of the ventricular lead in atrial position (4). With the use of the same electrode for atrial and ventricular pacing as well as sensing, logistics become easier and technical aspects of the operation simpler. We now report about the longterm results of the Helifix electrode in lateral atrial position.

Patients and Method

From August 1979 to November 1982 301 Helifix*) electrodes were implanted in connection to physiologic pacemaker systems. 158 electrodes were placed in the atrium, 143 in the ventricular position. 158 patients, 85 males and 73 females, mean age 63.5 years, with atrial electrodes were followed for an average period of 18.2 months. The total ex-

---

*) Vitatron Medical B.V., Dieren, The Netherlands.

perience reported here covers 2873 patient months. The pacemaker systems used for 143 patients were dual chamber systems with DVI, VAT, VDD, or DDD-mode pacemakers and 15 patients with atrial on demand pacing (AAI).

Pacemaker implantation was performed in over 85% of the cases under local anesthesia. The ventricular electrode was placed first either through cephalic vein approach or by a direct subclavian puncture and introduction with Seldinger technique. The atrial electrode was implanted second using the same venous approach. In all cases, atrial and ventricular electrodes could be introduced from the same side. The electrode for atrial placement was advanced into the lower part of the right atrium. With a preformed bended double stilett (6) it was then turned so that the tip looked upwards and to the lateral wall (Fig. 1). Withdrawing the electrode together with the stilett resulted in hooking of the electrode underneath the crista terminalis in the musculi pectinati (Fig. 2). A clockwise rotation of the electrode helped to screw the tip of the electrode into the musculi pectinati network. After withdrawal of the stilett, the stable position of the electrode was checked by pulling the electrode forwards and backwards.

Threshold measurements were performed with rectangular stimulus at 1.0 ms pulse width. For the ventricular position the mean threshold was 0.67 (0.25–1.7) V and 0.89 (0.25–2.1) mA, respectively. In the atrium with the same type of electrode the mean threshold was 0.85 (0.37–2.04) V and 1.11 (0.4–2.0) mA, respectively. The intracardiac signals were measured on a KO-oscillator over a resistance of 20000 Ohms and recorded on polaroid photos (Fig. 3). The mean amplitude of the R-wave was 7.9 mV (1.3–20) and for the atrial signal 3.21 (1.0–9.5) mV.

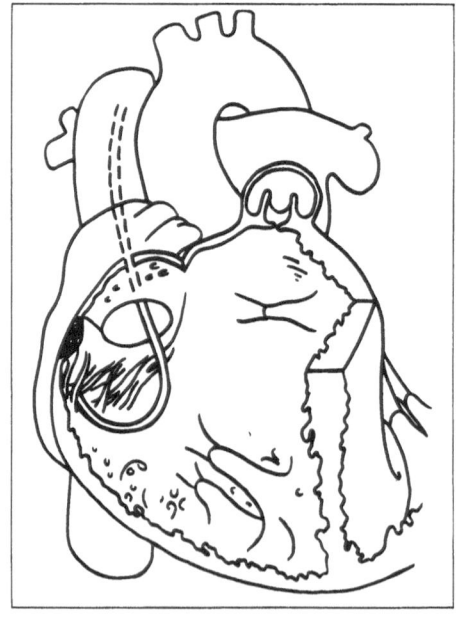

Fig. 1: Artist view of crista terminalis and musculi pectinati of the lateral wall of the right atrium. The electrode is hooked underneath the crista and is passively bended into a U-shape.

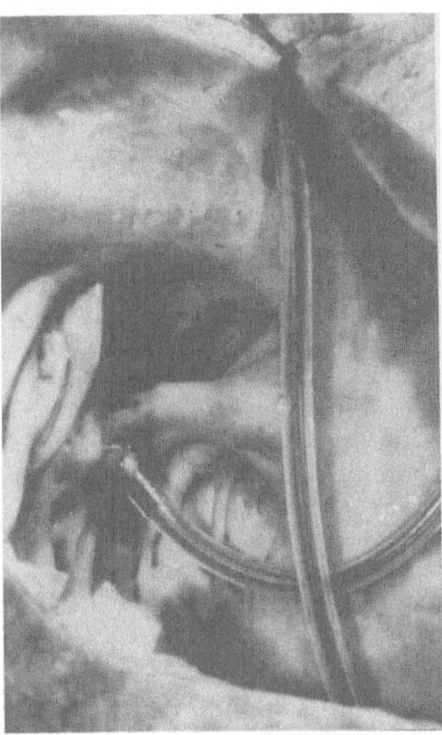

Fig. 2. Autopsy finding 8 months after PM-implantation. The helicoidal tip is wrenched into the musculi pectinati network. The straight wire is the ventricular lead descending from the superior vena cava.

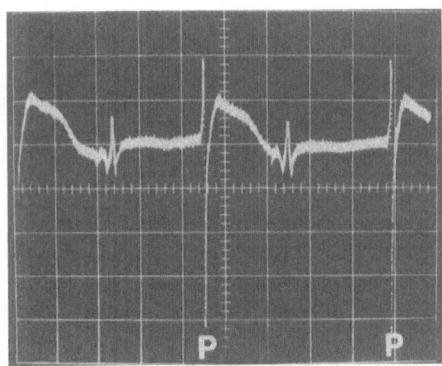

Fig. 3. Intracardiac P-wave signal (P). Horizontal axis 100 msec. per intersection, vertical axis 0.5 mV per division, P-wave amplitude therefore 3.0 mV.

Follow-up

In the above mentioned mean follow-up period of 18.2 months, the overall complication rate, i.e. need for surgical reintervention due to the atrial lead was 3.0%. Three displacements occurred, 2 within the first 24 hours, one 4 months after implant. In one patient, a sensing dysfunction was discovered 2 months after the pacemaker implantation, while in

333

one patient only a phrenic nerve stimulation occurred at the highest output on the atrial lead, which was also present at lower stimulation energies.

Discussion

The use of one type of electrode for ventricular as well as atrial sensing and stimulation for permanent pacing has several advantages. With this study we proved that the position of the Helifix electrode on the lateral wall of the right atrium is stable and efficient for longterm dual chamber pacing (4, 5, 6). The complication rate of the electrode in this position is low and comparable to results of ventricular electrodes in longterm follow-up (7). There is no doubt that alternative electrodes for use in the atrium are bringing as good results as the ones presented here. However, J-shaped leads have a preformed angle that may not be suitable for all atria. With the non-preformed electrode a better and individual adaptation to the size of the atrium is possible. The lateral wall is a suitable position for sensing and/or pacing. Near to the crista terminalis, because of large atrial muscle mass, a good P-wave can be registrated. This technique is equally suitable for patients who have undergone open heart operation with resection of right atrial appendage. So far we were only in one patient unable to find a satisfactory position which proves the versatility of atrial use of ventricular electrodes. The use of the same type of electrode in atrial as well as ventricular position makes logistics easy. There is only one electrode that is used and a discussion about the shape of the required atrial electrode is avoided. By this the stock can be smaller and therefore more economic. In addition with the use of only one type of electrode, the physicians get quicker familiar with the handling of this part of the pacemaker system.

References

1. Lagergren H, Johansson L, Karlöf I, Thornander H: Atrial-triggered pacemaking without thoracotomy: apparatus and results in twenty cases. Acta Chir Scand 1966; 132: 678.
2. Zucker IR, Parsonnet V, Gilbert L: A method of permanent transvenous implantation of an atrial electrode. Amer Heart J 1973; 85: 195.
3. Smyth NPD, Citron P, Keshishian JM, Garcia JM, Kelly LC: Permanent pervenous atrial sensing and pacing with a new J-shaped lead. J thorac cardiovasc Surg 1976; 72: 565.
4. Kappenberger L, Babotai I, Turina M: Modified positioning of Helifix transvenous atrial electrodes. Cardiac Pacing, GA Feruglio (ed), pp 649–651. Piccin Medical Books 1982.
5. Bergdahl L: Helifix, an electrode suitable for transvenous atrial and ventricular implantation. J thorac cardiovasc Surg 1980; 80: 794.
6. Kappenberger L, Münch U, Babotai I, Baumann PC, Steinbrunn W, Turina M: Technik und Langzeitresultate der Schrittmacherbehandlung mit Vorhofelektroden. Schweiz med Wschr 1981; 111: 1706.
7. Babotai I, Meier WE: Erste klinische Erfahrungen mit der neuen intrakardialen Elektrode "Helifix". Schweiz med Wschr 1977; 107: 1592.
8. Levine PA, Brodsky SJ, Seltzer JB: The ventricular tined lead in atrial pacing, an alternative to the preformed J lead. Pace 1983; 6: A-71.

Authors' address:
Dr. Lukas Kappenberger
University Hospital, Dept. of Medicine
Rämistr. 100 CH-8091 Zürich/Schweiz

Atrial Amplitude Mapping to Avoid P Wave Sensing Failure

Takuro Misaki, Takashi Iwa, Tasuhiro Matsunaga

Summary: Physiological pacemaker implantations are increasing in number. However, P wave sensing failure is still a major problem. To determine the best atrial electrode positioning for P wave sensing, the atrial amplitude was measured in 10 dogs, from various epicardial sites, including the endocardium of both appendages. During sinus rhythm, maximum amplitude was obtained from the left atrial free wall. High amplitude was also obtained from the right atrial free wall. However, only low amplitudes were obtained from both appendages. During junctional rhythm, which was obtained by cryosurgery of the sinus node area, patterns of atrial and amplitude mapping changed, but maximum amplitude areas were present on the atrial free walls. Also, atrial amplitude mapping was tried in four clinical cases of WPW-syndrome, during surgery. The maximum amplitude area of the right atrium was located, not on the appendage, but on the free wall, in all cases. These results suggest that J shaped electrode fixation is not adequate to P wave sensing. Even if left a atrial free wall fixation is advisable, this requires a left thoracotomy. Therefore, transvenous fixation to the right free wall should be selected, possibly using a screw-in method.

Introduction:

Following the development in pacemaker technology, physiological pacemaker implantations began increaing in number. However, P wave sensing failure is still a major problem, and the best atrial electrodes positioning for P wave sensing is not get clear. In this paper, atrial and amplitudes were measured from various atrial sites in order to determine the best positioning for P wave sensing.

Methods:

Ten, adult, mongrel dogs weighting from 15 to 20 kg were anesthetized with sodium pentobarbital (30 mg per kilogram of body weight) and ventilated with 40% oxygen through a cuffed endotracheal tube attached to a respirator. Bilateral thoracotomy was performed through the fourth intercostal space. The unipolar peak-to-peak amplitude was obtained from endocardial sites of both the atrial appendages and from 45 different epicardial sites, under quiet respiration. Carbon tip electrodes, with a surface area of 12 sq. mm, were used to pick up electrograms. These electrograms were fed into a specially designed amplifier, duplicating the sensing system of an implantable pacemaker, with a 25 to 150 Hz bandwidth. The output from this amplifier was displayed on an ocilloscope and was recorded on a polygraph. In this way, the atrial amplitude mapping was obtained during sinus rhythm and junctional rhythm with a retrograde conduction. The junctional rhythm was obtained by cryosurgery. A cryolesion was created in the sinus node area by a 120-second exposure to a cryoprobe cooled to −60 °C using expanding nitrous oxide. In addition to amplitude mapping, atrial sequence mapping was obtained at the same time.

A clinical study was performed in four surgical cases of WPW-syndrome. Right atrial amplitude mapping was obtained during sinus rhythm, in order to find the best positioning of electrodes for P wave sensing.

Results:

The results obtained of atrial amplitude mapping in dogs are illustrated in Fig. 1-A. In dog one (upper panel), endocardial amplitude of the right atrial appendage was 4 mV and that of the left atrial appendage was 6 mV. However, the maximum amplitude point (15 mV) was located on the left atrial free wall. Amplitude mapping also demonstrated that the right free wall had a higher amplitude when compared to the right atrial appendage. The same findings were obtained in the other nine dogs. The location of the maximum amplitude points in the 10 dogs, during sinus rhythm, are illustrated in the lower panel of Fig. 1. (All maximum amplitude points are located by asterisks, shown on the left atrial free wall.)

Fig. 1. Atrial amplitude mapping during sinus rhythm in dogs. Upper panel shows amplitude mapping of dog # 1. Lower panel shows the location of the maximum amplitude points of each dog.

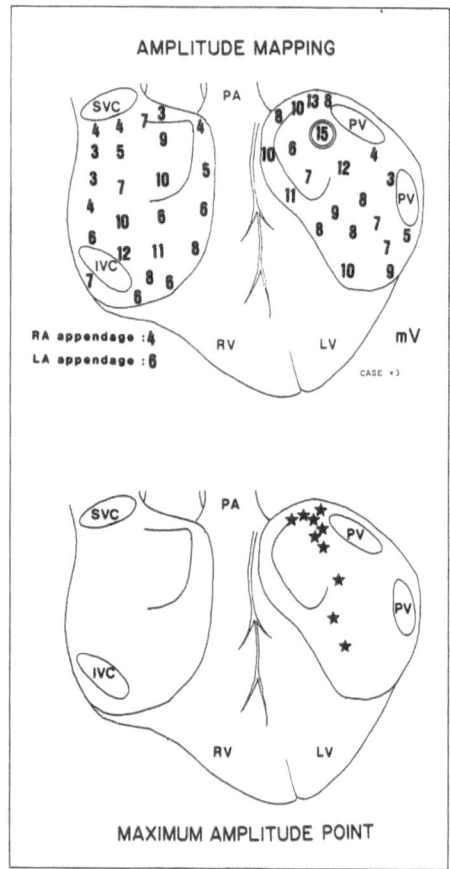

In two out of the 10 dogs, junctional rhythm with retrograde conduction was obtained after cryosurgery. Both amplitude and sequence mapping are illustrated in Fig. 2. The upper panel shows the preoperative, normal sinus rhythm. According to this sequence mapping, location of node area could be easily determined. As illustrated in the lower panel, cryosurgery of this area leads to junctional rhythm with retrograde conduction. Excitation spreads from near the posterior septum. In the same dog, amplitude mapping was obtained pre- and postoperatively. Although atrial amplitude mapping was changed, the maximum area was still present on the left atrial free wall even during junctional rhythm.

In four clinical cases of WPW-syndrome, amplitude mapping was done only on the right side because of difficulty of recording from the left side (Fig. 3). The highest amplitude area was located on the middle right free wall in Case 1, and it was located on the middle free wall near the atrio-ventricular groove in Case 2. In Cases 3 and 4, the highest amplitude areas were located on the lower right free walls near the inferior venae cavae.

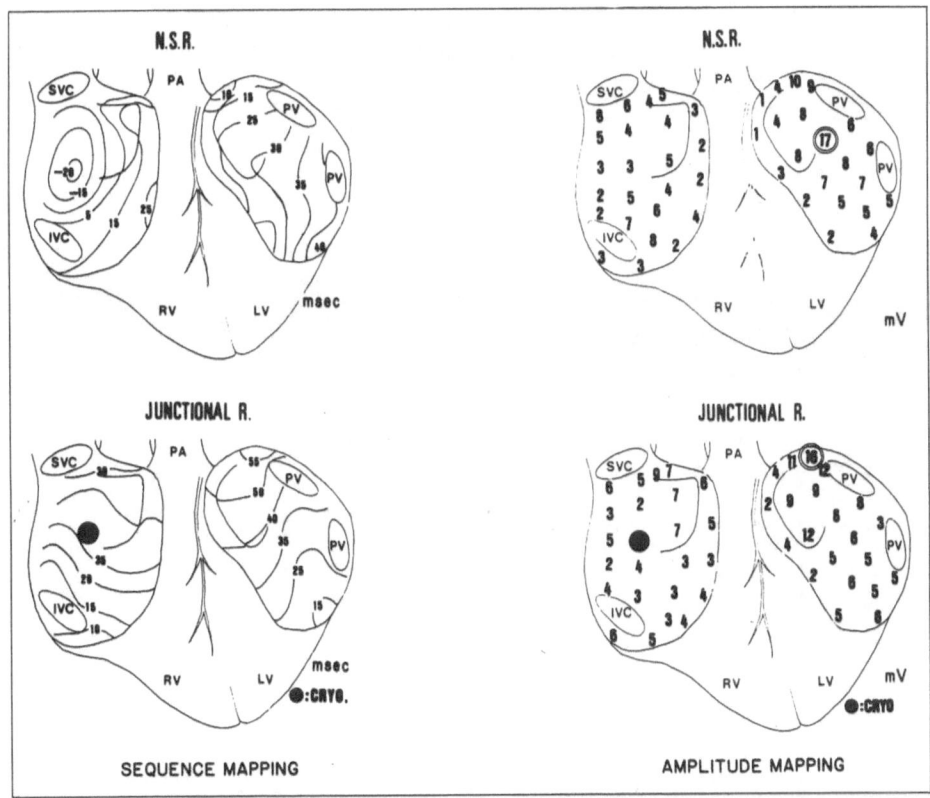

Fig. 2. Atrial sequence and amplitude mapping during sinus rhythm and junctional rhythm which was made possible by cryosurgical method in the dog

Discussion:

Physiological pacemakers are the accpeted mode of management for various arrhythmias because of the many advantages they offer, including atrial kick. However, P wave sensing failure is still a major problem. Several attempts to avoid P wave sensing failure have been made, including the development of an ideal P wave sensing circuit and atrial electrode. In this study, we tried to discover an ideal atrial electrode position for P wave sensing. Transvenous J shaped electrode fixation is now widely used (1) but from our results, the right atrial appendage was not a good positioning place for P wave sensing compared to the free wall. Only low amplitudes were obtained from this area, and this could be a cause of sensing failure, in some cases.

The height of amplitude seems to be decided mainly, by the atrial myocardial volume at the mapping area. The maximum amplitude was obtained from the left atrial free wall. Even when left atrial free wall fixation seemed advisable, it required a left thoracotomy. Moreover, it was discovered that in the case of epicardial fixation, atrial amplitude decreased remarkably during the long-term follow-up period, due to fibrosis around the

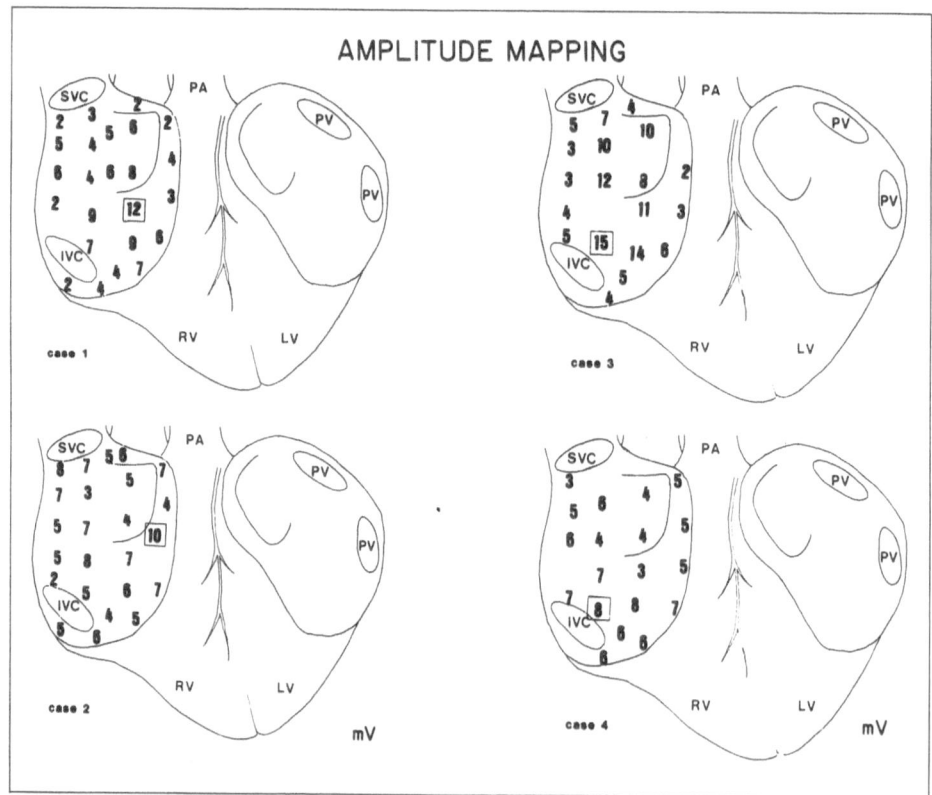

Fig. 3. Atrial amplitude mapping during sinus rhythm in four clinical cases of WPW-syndrome.

electrode (2). Therefore, from a clinical viewpoint, transvenous fixation to the right atrial free wall should be selected, possibly using a screw-in method (3), and a percutaneous atrial puncture intraatrial electrode fixation method (4).

When transvenous approaches are unsuccessful, epicardial atrial amplitude mapping is important, to avoid P wave sensing failure. In a case involving sick sinus syndrome, with a myocardial lesion in addition to a sinus node lesion, amplitude mapping becomes extremely important. Although our experimental study showed that maximum amplitude was achieved on the left atrial free wall during junctional rhythm, in clinical cases, amplitude mapping should be done during sinus rhythm and also during ectopic rhythm.

Conclusion:

1. From these experimental and clinical results, it is suggested that a J shaped atrial electrode, when placed into the right atrial appendage, is not sufficiently adequate for P wave sensing.
2. Even when left free wall fixation is advisable, because of high amplitude, it will require a left thoracotomy. Therefore, from a clinical viewpoint, transvenous fixation to the right free wall should be selected, possibly using a screw-in type method.
3. Atrial amplitude mapping is important to avoid P wave sensing failure in unsuccessful cases of transvenous approach.

References:

1. Smyth NPD, Vasarhelyi L, McNamra W, Kakascik GE: A permanent transvenous atrial electrode catheter. J Thoracic Cardiovasc Surg 1969; 58: 773–782.
2. Nathan D, Center S, Wu C: An implantable synchronous pacemaker for long term term correction of the complete heart block. A, J Cardiol 1963; 11: 362–367.
3. Sutorius DJ: Use of an endocardial corkscrew lead for atrial pacing. In: Meere C, ed. Proceedings of the 6th world symposium on cardiac pacing. Montreal: Pacesymp 1979; Chap 33: 5.
4. Todo K, Kaneko S, Fujiwara T, Sugiki K, Tanaka N, Komastu S: Patient-controlled rapid atrial pacing in long term management of recurrent supraventricular tachycardias. In: Meere C, ed. Proceedings of the 6th World symposium on cardiac pacing. Montreal: Pacesymp 1979; Chap 9: 6.

Authors' address:
T. Misaki, M.D.
Department of Surgery
Kanazawa University School of Medicine
Takaramachi 13–1
Kanazawa 920
Japan

Comparison of Transvenous Atrial Electrodes Employing Active (Helicoidal) and Passive (Tined J-Lead) Fixation in 120 Patients

M. I. H. El Gamal, L. M. van Gelder, J. J. R. M. Bonnier, H. R. Michels

Summary: From November 1977 to February 1983 we implanted transvenous atrial leads in 120 patients for atrial pacing and sensing. The series included 75 helicoidal (Vitatron Helifix) electrodes, and 45 tined J-leads (Intermediccs 483.01/02). The acute and chronic atrial stimulation threshold was acceptable for both types of electrodes with the exception of a single patient in the helicoidal series who developed exit block 9 months after implantation.
Dislodgement occurred in 3 patients (4%) of the helicoidal series, but in only 1 patient (2%) of the J-lead series. Malsensing of spontaneous atrial activity was the most frequently observed complication in the helicoidal series (6 patients = 8%), but did not occur in the J-lead series.
Our results to date with the tined J-leads are superior to those obtained with the helicoidal leads. The series is however smaller and the follow-up is shorter.

A variety of reliable electrodes are presently available for transvenous atrial implantation. Active fixation employing atrial hook (1), cork screw type (2), and helicoidal electrodes (3) has been described. This mode of implantation has a low incidence of electrode dislodgement. Passive fixation initially using J-shaped electrodes hooked in the right atrial appendage had a high incidence of dislodgement (4). The addition of small tines at the distal end significantly reduced the dislodgement rate (5, 6).

The purpose of this study is to evaluate the results obtained with transvenous atrial implantation of helicoidal and tined J-leads in 120 patients.

Material and methods

From November 1977 to February 1983 we implanted transvenous atrial leads in 120 patients. There were 67 males and 53 females. Their ages ranged from 18 to 88 years (mean 60.5 years). Seventy five helicoidal (Vitatron, Helifix) electrodes were implanted between November 1977 and November 1981, and 45 tined J-leads (Intermedics 483.01/0.2) were implanted between January 1981 and February 1983. Twenty-two patients underwent open heart surgery prior to atrial lead implantation, 12 received helicoidal and 10 J-leads. Seventy-two patients received an additional ventricular lead for atrial programmed stimulation. The pulse generators used include 15 AV sequential (DVI), 19 atrial synchronous (VAT, VDD), 38 "universal" (DDD), and 48 atrial demand type (AAI). Lead description:
1. The electrode of the Helifix lead (Fig. 1) consists of platinum iridium (90%–10%) and forms a closed loop. The surface area of the electrode is 12 mm^2. The lead body insulation is silicone rubber.
2. The J-lead (Fig. 2) has a blunt electrode consisting of platinum iridium (90%–10%) with three tines located at the external curve of the J. The surface area of the electrode

Fig. 1. Photograph of the Helifix electrode.

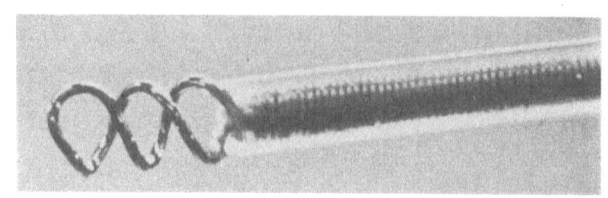

Fig. 2. Photograph of the Intermedics tined J-leads. (Small curve model 483.01, large curve model 483.02.)

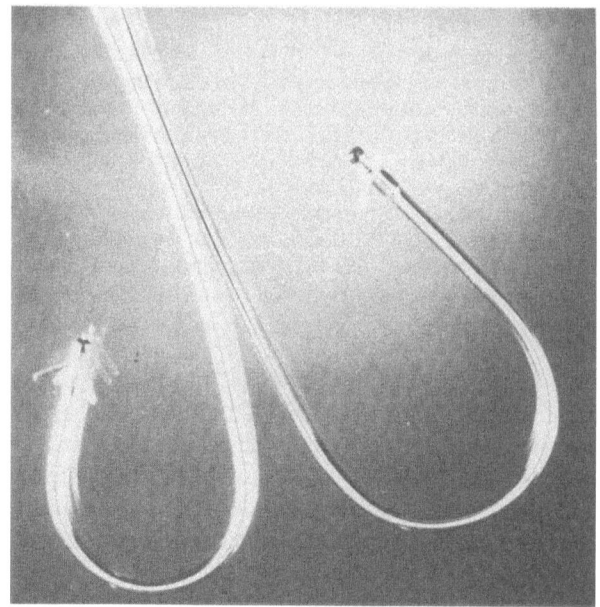

is 11 mm². The insulation of the body is polyurethane. We have used the J-lead with a small curve (483.01) and with a large curve (483.02) depending on the estimated size of the right atrium and right atrial appendage.

Acute stimulation threshold was determined by means of the Medtronic 5300 and 5309 Pacing System Analyzers. P-wave amplitude was measured peak to peak from unipolar intra atrial electrograms recorded on a Gould ES 1000 recorder.

This equipment has a frequency reponse of 0.05–1000 HZ.

Chronic stimulation threshold was assessed by programming the atrial pulse width to a level just above atrial capture. The technical data are summarized in Table 1, follow-up and complications in Table 2.

Follow-up

All patients were clinically examined at the outpatient department one month after discharge and subsequently at 1–3 monthly intervals. Control of pacemaker function was

Table 1. Technical data.

	Helicoidal (N = 75)	Tined J-lead (N = 45)
Electrode surface area (mm²)	12 mm²	11 mm²
Acute stimulation threshold (Volt, 1 ms pulse width)	0.70 (0.4–1.2)	0.78 (0.6–1.3)
Acute stimulation threshold (mA, 1 ms pulse width)	1.35 (0.6–3.0)	1.51 (0.3–3.1)
Chronic stimulation threshold (ms, 5 V output)	0.15 (0.05–0.2)	0.13 (0.05–0.31)
Intra atrial electrogram (mV, peak to peak)	3.12 (1.0–6.0)	3.41 (1.3–7.0)
Number of operators	2	7

Table 2. Follow-up.

	Helicoidal (N = 75)	Tined J-lead (N = 45)
Total follow-up (months)	2542 months (15–63)	521 months (1–26)
Mean follow-up	33.9 months	11.6 months
Dislodgement	3 (4%)	1 (2%)
Malsensing	6	–
Exit block	1	–
Phrenic nerve stimulation	3	1

performed at the same visit. The mean follow-up period for the Helifix series is 33.9 months (total 2542 months), for the J-lead series 11.6 months (total 521 months). Dislodgement of the leads occurred in 3 patients in the Helifix series (4%). Two occurred within 24 hours after implantation and one after 6 months. They were successfully repositioned.

Implantation of the Helifix leads was performed by 2 operators. Seven operators were involved in implantation of the J-leads. Five of the seven operators were beginners. There was only one early dislodgement of a tined J-lead (within 24 hours). Atrial malsensing occurred in 6 patients in the Helifix series but did not occur in the J-lead series. In two patients, the atrial input characteristics of the pulse generator were not optimal for atrial sensing (CPI 505 microlith P). One recovered spontaneously between the 4th and 6th month (atrial electrogram 4.0 mV), the second after replacement of the pulse generator (atrial electrogram 1.5 mV at implantation and 5.5 mV 5 months later). The four patients who continued to exhibit atrial malsensing had atrial electrograms varying between 1.9–3.5 mV mean 2.6 mV. The pulse generators were suitable for atrial demand pacing (Medtronic Spectrax 5985). Exit block occurred in a single patient in the Helifix series 9 months after implantation. A tined J-lead was subsequently implanted, and atrial pacing was restored. The follow-up to date is more than 2 years. Phrenic nerve stimulation occurred in 3 patients in the Helifix group but in only one patient in the J-lead group. Adjustment of the output of the pulse generators solved the problem in 3 patients (2 Helifix, 1 J-lead). A single patient in the Helifix series continued to have mild phrenic nerve stimulation. Reprogramming of the pulse generator was not attempted because of a high stimulation threshold.

There were no cases of perforation of the atrial wall. Twelve patients died during follow-up (9 in the Helifix series and 3 in the J-lead series). The main causes were severe heart failure, and ventricular arrhythmias. There were no deaths related to the pacing system.

Conclusion

Helicoidal and tined J-leads are suitable for transvenous atrial implantation. Our results to date with the tined J-leads show that they are easier to implant and are less likely to dislodge. The absence of atrial malsensing is impressive. The series is however smaller and the follow-up is shorter.

Acknowledgement

We gratefully acknowledge the support of the Foundation for Applied Cardiovascular Research, Eindhoven, The Netherlands.

References

1. Gold, RG: Stimulation electrodes. In: Thalen HJTh, Harthorne JW, eds. To pace or not to pace. The Hague Martinus Nijhoff Medical Division, 1978; 199.
2. Van Hemel NM, El Gamal MIH, Bijkerk P, Bakema H, van Gelder LM: Long term results of endocardial atrial electrodes employing positive fixation. Pace 1981; 4: A77 (Abstr).
3. El Gamal MIH, van Gelder LM: Preliminary experience with the Helifix electrode for transvenous atrial implantation. Pace 1979; 2: 444.
4. Zucker IR, Parsonnet V, Gilbert L: A method of permanent transvenous implantation of an atrial electrode. Am Heart J. 1973; 85: 195.
5. Kleinert M, Bock M, Wilhelmi F: Clinical use of a new transvenous atrial lead. Am J Cardiol 1977; 40: 237.
6. Smyth NPD, Citron P, Keshishian JH, Garcia JM, Kelly LC: Permanent atrial sensing and pacing with a new J-shaped lead. J Thorac Cardiovasc Surg 1976; 72: 565.

Authors' address:
M. I. H. El Gamal
Department of Cardiology
Catharina Hospital
Michelangelolaan 2
5623 EJ Eindhoven
The Netherlands

Improved Electrophysiological Performance Using Porous-Surfaced Electrodes for Atrial Epicardial Pacing

D. C. MacGregor, G. J. Wilson, P. Klement, and R. M. Pilliar

Summary: Porous-surfaced electrodes have been used with success for endocardial pacing, but have not been applied to epicardial pacing in which their performance can be evaluated independent of other active or passive acute fixation means. Moreover, a need clearly exists for an atraumatic lead for atrial pacing from the epicardial surface of the heart. Accordingly, in this study, we compared a porous-surfaced (8–25 μm particle size, 16 μm mean pore size, 36% surface porosity) Elgiloy epicardial electrode (8.8 mm²) with an otherwise identical smooth-surfaced electrode for atrial pacing. Each electrode was mounted on a 9 mm wide silicone rubber pad and peripherally sutured to the anterior epicardial surface of the body of the right atrium. One porous-surfaced and one smooth control electrode were thus implanted in each of nine mongrel dogs. Stimulation thresholds (constant current and constant voltage) at pulse durations from 0.1 to 2.0 ms, sensed peak-to-peak P-wave amplitudes and source impedances were measured acutely and at 1, 2, 3, 4, 8, 12, 16, 20, 24, and 30 weeks thereafter. Analyses of variance on the data for the strength-duration curves at implant showed no significant difference, but by 30 weeks the porous-surfaced electrodes showed superior performance ($p < 0.001$) with thresholds (1.0 ms pulse duration, constant current) of 0.81 ± 0.19 mA (mean-± SD) at 30 weeks versus 1.5 ± 0.87 mA for the smooth controls ($p < 0.05$). Sensing performance for both the porous-surfaced and smooth electrodes was satisfactory, with no significant attenuation in P-wave amplitude from implant (3.9 ± 2.0 mV smooth, 4.4 ± 1.7 mV porous-surfaced) to 30 weeks (4.4 ± 1.3 mV smooth, 5.9 ± 3.4 mV porous-surfaced). There was, however, a significant drop in source impedance ($p < 0.01$) in both groups of electrodes, and at 30 weeks the source impedance of the porous-surfaced electrodes (1.0 ± 0.17 kΩ) was significantly lower ($p < 0.05$) than that of the smooth electrodes (1.4 ± 0.64 kΩ). We conclude that porous-surfaced electrodes provide superior electrophysiological performance and should be particularly useful for atrial epicardial leads in dual chamber pacing.

The development of reliable atrial endocardial pacemaker leads has greatly facilitated the use of dual chamber pacing for the treatment of heart block (1, 2). Despite the popularity of the transvenous approach, there are still situations where the transthoracic approach using epicardial leads is indicated (3). Although satisfactory leads are available for epicardial ventricular pacing (4), epicardial atrial pacing is still a problem because of the thin atrial wall and the low amplitude of the signal associated with atrial depolarization. Previous attempts to sense and pace from the atrium using surface coil (2,5) and "pinch-on" (6) electrodes have met with limited success, although a new small "barbed" electrode (7) has recently shown more promise.

We have previously demonstrated that improved chronic electrophysiological performance can be achieved using a porous-surfaced electrode in the form of an atrial endocardial lead (8, 9). These results can be attributed to electrode fixation by fibrous tissue ingrowth into the surface of the electrode producing a reduction in thickness of the fibrotic capsule plus an enhanced electroactive surface area for reduced polarization and source impedance (10). Because a need clearly exists for an atraumatic lead for atrial pacing from the epicardial surface of the heart, we elected to examine the performance of a porous-surfaced electrode in the context of a permanent atrial epicardial lead.

Materials and Methods

Electrode Fabrication and Characterization

The porous-surfaced electrodes (1.0 mm length, 2.3 mm diameter, 8.8 mm² outer surface area) were fabricated using conventional powder metallurgy techniques which involve bonding 8–25 μm spherical Elgiloy powder particles to each other and to the solid Elgiloy substrate using a high temperature sintering treatment. This process produces a surface region that is approximately 100 μm in thickness and 36% porous with a mean pore size of 16 μm. Conventional smooth-surfaced electrodes of identical outer surface area were used as controls.

Each electrode (9 smooth, 9 porous-surfaced) was incorporated into an atrial epicardial lead comprised of a 9 mm wide silicone rubber pad with four peripherally located suture holes plus a proximal suture groove as illustrated in Fig. 1.

Implant Protocol

Nine mature mongrel dogs, weighing between 18 and 27 kilograms, were given a general anesthetic and subjected to a short right thoracotomy through the fourth intercostal space to expose the anterior surface of the right atrium. Two atrial epicardial leads (1 smooth, 1 porous-surfaced) were sutured to the anterior free wall of the right atrium of each dog equidistant from the base of the appendage, using a continuous 4–0 Tevdek suture as described by Parsonnet (3). A second suture was placed around the proximal suture groove to stabilize the distal portion of the lead, thus ensuring good contact between the electrode and the underlying epicardium. Each lead terminal pin was then connected to a percutaneous access device, positioned subcutaneously in the right flank region, for subsequent electrophysiological measurements as previously described (8). After closing the thoracotomy and taking the initial readings, each dog was recovered and maintained in good health for the duration of the 30 week study.

Fig. 1. The distal portion of the permanent atrial epicardial lead showing the details of its construction. An actual photograph of the lead appears in the right lower corner of the illustration.

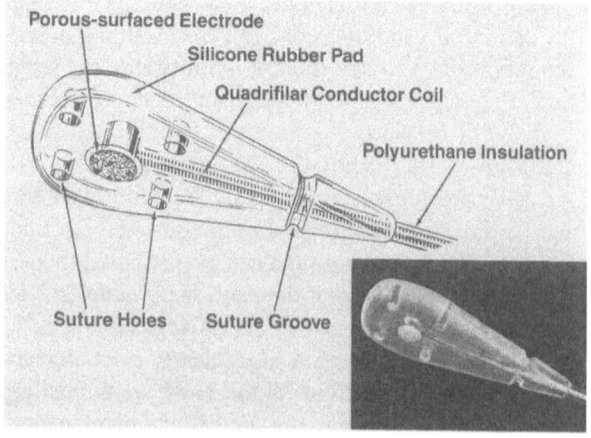

Porous-surfaced Electrode

Silicone Rubber Pad

Quadrifilar Conductor Coil

Polyurethane Insulation

Suture Holes   Suture Groove

Electrophysiological Measurements

With the dog under light general anesthesia, electrophysiological measurements on each lead were made at the time of implant and at 1, 2, 3, 4, 8, 12, 16, 20, 24, and 30 weeks thereafter. Unipolar (cathode) constant current and constant voltage stimulation thresholds were recorded at pulse durations of 0.1, 0.25, 0.5, 0.75, 1.0, 1.5, and 2.0 milliseconds (ms) using a modified Cordis Model 209A Pacer Systems Analyser. Peak-to-peak P-wave amplitudes were displayed on a Tektronix 5441 storage oscilloscope and the source impedance was measured through the use of an external resistance attenuator in parallel with the oscilloscope output terminals.

For each parameter at each time period, the mean value and standard deviation (SD) were calculated for each group of dogs (9 smooth, 9 porous-surfaced). Analyses of variance and Student's t-test for both paired and unpaired data were used to compare the results of the two groups with the level of significance chosen to be $p < 0.05$.

Explant Protocol

After animal sacrifice at 30 weeks, the entire heart with the pacemaker leads in situ was excised and removed from the thoracic cavity. The fibrous tissue capsule overlying the distal portion of each lead was incised and the sutures cut to allow the electrode to be lifted off the anterior wall of the right atrium. After gross inspection of the lead and site of atrial stimulation, the appropriate block of atrial tissue was excised, fixed in 10% buffered formaldehyde, embedded in paraffin, sectioned, and stained with a hematoxylin-phloxine-saffron (HPS) stain. During histological examination, the minimum thickness of the fibrous tissue capsule that developed around each smooth and each porous-surfaced electrode was measured and recorded.

Results

Electrophysiological Measurements

A comparison between the threshold characteristics of smooth versus porous-surfaced atrial epicardial electrodes at implant and explant (30 weeks) is given in Table 1. At the time of implant, under both constant current and constant voltage conditions and a pulse duration of both 0.5 and 1.0 ms, there were no significant differences in stimulation thresholds. In contrast, at 30 weeks, the thresholds achieved with the porous-surfaced electrodes (with the exception of the constant voltage measurements at 0.5 ms which did not quite achieve significance) were significantly lower than the smooth electrodes ($p < 0.05$). Examination of the stimulation thresholds at the chronaxie time demonstrated that the 30 week thresholds for the porous-surfaced electrodes were 50% better than their smooth counterparts under both constant current and constant voltage conditions.

The strength-duration curves for both electrode types at the time of implant under constant current and constant voltage conditions were not significantly different in terms of their appearance (Fig. 2) or on the basis of analyses of variance. In contrast, the strength-duration curves at 30 weeks differed significantly in favor of the porous-surfaced elec-

Table 1. Threshold Characteristics

	Constant Current (mA)					
Pulse duration	0.5 ms		1.0 ms		Chronaxie	
Electrode type	Smooth	Porous	Smooth	Porous	Smooth	Porous
Implant threshold	0.61±0.23	0.53±0.18	0.45±0.18	0.41±0.16	0.74	0.50
p value	NS		NS			
30 week threshold	2.0 ±1.3	1.2 ±0.35	1.5 ±0.87	0.81±0.19	1.5	0.74
p value	<0.05		<0.05			

	Constant Voltage (V)					
Pulse duration	0.5 ms		1.0 ms		Chronaxie	
Electrode type	Smooth	Porous	Smooth	Porous	Smooth	Porous
Implant threshold	0.75±0.18	0.73±0.17	0.62±0.17	0.64±0.15	0.98	1.0
p value	NS		NS			
30 week threshold	2.0 ±1.1	1.4 ±0.57	1.6 ±0.83	1.0 ±0.47	2.3	1.2
p value	NS		<0.05			

All values are mean ±SD (n = 9 per group). Statistical comparisons are made between the smooth and porous groups at the same point in time. NS = not significant.

Fig. 2. Strength-duration stimulation threshold data under constant current and constant voltage conditions for the smooth and the porous-surfaced electrode groups are compared at implant (upper graphs) and at 30 weeks (lower graphs).

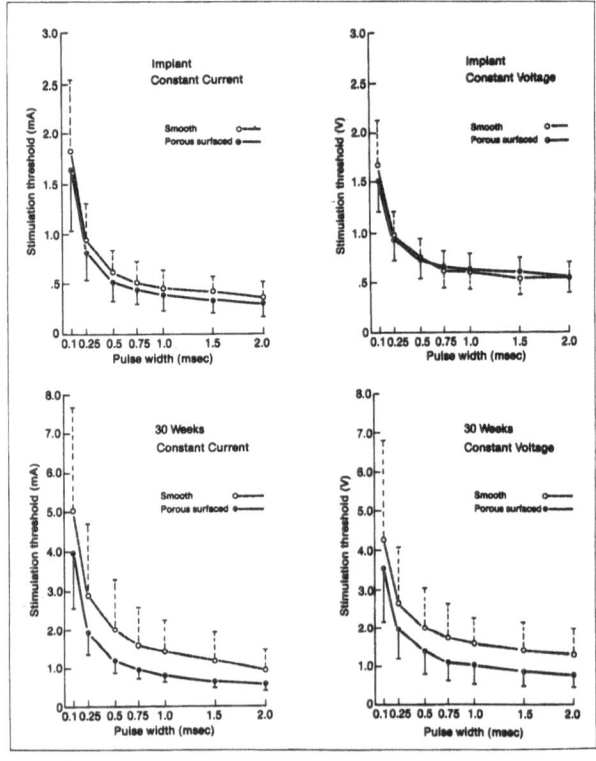

trodes, analyses of variance indicating significance at the 0.001 level under both constant current and constant voltage conditions.

On examining the effects of time on the stimulation threshold, maximum peaking was noted at one week (2.7 ± 1.8 mA and 3.1 ± 2.2. mA for the smooth and porous-surfaced electrodes respectively under constant current conditions, 2.4 ± 1.2 V and 3.1 ± 1.4 V for the smooth and porous-surfaced electrodes respectively under constant voltage conditions, pulse duration 2.0 ms) with rapid resolution thereafter, the improved performance of the porous-surfaced electrodes becoming significant at 12 weeks (p < 0.05).

With respect to the sensing characteristics of the electrodes, a comparison of the peak-to-peak P-wave amplitude and the source impedance of both types of electrode is given in Table 2. At implant, there was no significant difference in either parameter. Although there was no significant difference in the average magnitude of the sensed P-wave, the values for the porous-surfaced electrodes tended to be higher than those for the smooth electrodes with no evidence of signal attenuation between implant and 30 weeks. Source impedance for both groups, although comparable at implant, dropped significantly by 30 weeks (p < 0.01) with the mean value for the porous-surfaced electrodes becoming significantly lower than that for their smooth counterparts (p < 0.05).

Histopathological Findings

On exposing the hearts at autopsy, it was observed that the distal silicone rubber pad onto which the electrode was mounted was completely covered, in all instances, by a thin, semi-transparent fibrous tissue capsule with a smooth, shiny inner lining. After cutting the fixation sutures, the smooth electrodes easily fell away from the epicardial surface of the right atrium, whereas the porous-surfaced electrodes were well attached to the heart by tissue ingrowth into the interstices of the porous surface. Moderate traction resulted in a separation of the tissue bond at the electrode surface such that a small crater remained behind at the site previously occupied by the electrode. In all instances, the electrode site was surrounded by an opaque, pearly white region where the silicone rubber pad was in direct contact with the underlying epicardial surface.

Histological examination of the tissue which surrounded the electrode tips revealed it to be a mature, collagen-rich fibrous connective tissue capsule with spindle-shaped fibrocytes surrounded by an abundant collagen matrix. As illustrated in Fig. 3, the average minimum capsule thickness associated with the porous-surfaced electrodes (140 ± 52 μm) was significantly less than the 222 ± 90 μm thick capsule associated with the smooth electrodes (p < 0.05).

Discussion

This study illustrates the advantage of using porous-surfaced electrodes for permanent pacing from the epicardial surface of the atrium. The improved electrophysiological performance of the porous-surfaced type of electrode is clearly explained by the thinner fibrotic capsule that develops as a result of fibrous tissue ingrowth and stable electrode fixation, plus the increased electrode surface area achieved by the porous structure itself. These findings are consistent with the results of our earlier experiments using endocardial

Table 2. Sensing Characteristics.

Electrode type	P-wave Amplitude (mV)		Source Impedance (kΩ)	
	Smooth	Porous	Smooth	Porous
Implant	3.9 ± 2.0	4.4 ± 1.7	2.5 ± 0.88	2.5 ± 1.3
p value		NS		NS
30 weeks	4.4 ± 1.3	5.9 ± 3.4	1.5 ± 0.64	1.0 ± 0.17
p value		NS		< 0.05

All values are mean ± SD (n = 9 per group). Statistical comparisons are made between the smooth and porous groups at the same point in time. NS = not significant.

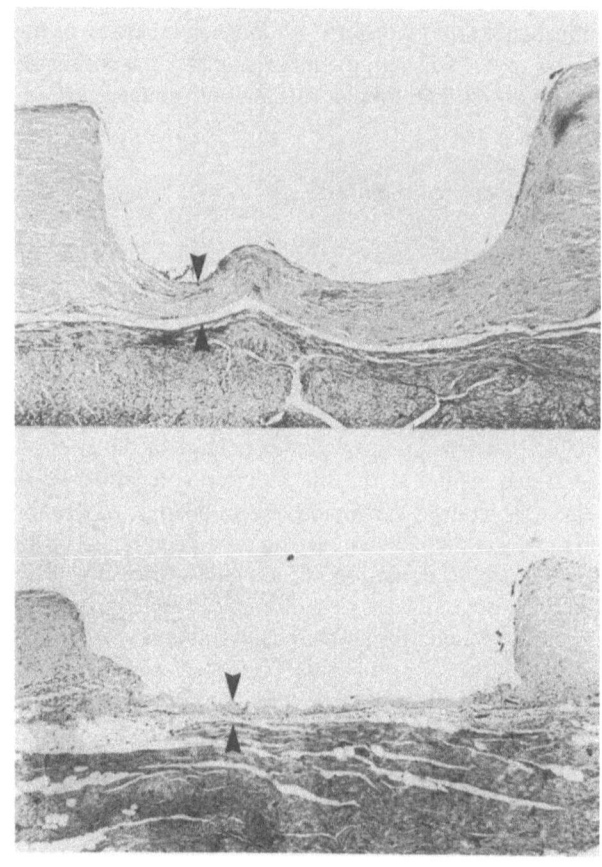

Fig. 3. The typical atrial tissue response to a smooth control electrode (top) is compared (at the same magnification) with the typical tissue response to a porous-surfaced electrode (bottom). Note the marked reduction in the thickness of the fibrous tissue capsule separating the electrode from underlying myocytes (arrows) achieved by using the porous-surfaced structure.

porous-surfaced electrodes in the atrium (8, 9) and ventricle (11). In fact, the 30 week stimulation thresholds achieved in this study do not differ significantly from those obtained from the endocardial surface of the right ventricle using porous-surfaced Elgiloy electrodes of exactly the same size configured as ventricular pervenous leads (0.76 ± 0.19 mA, 1.0 ms pulse duration, constant current) (11).

The relatively high peaking of stimulation thresholds at one week can be explained on the basis of local, reversible tissue trauma at the time of implant as only 5 of the 18 electrodes (3 porous-surfaced, 2 smooth) demonstrated peak thresholds greater than three times the 30 week values. Trauma to the thin-walled atrium can be minimized by not crushing the tissue with surgical instruments, avoiding bleeding near the electrode site, and by using a less traumatic and more tissue compatible suture such as 5–0 polypropylene. A glucocorticosteroid eluting electrode (12), utilizing the porous metal structure, might be particularly applicable in this situation and deserves evaluation.

Despite the fact that Elgiloy was used to fabricate the electrodes used in these experiments, clinical prototypes have been constructed of platinum iridium because of its decreased tendency to corrode when functioning as an anode. The reduced electrode polarization impedance associated with the use of platinum iridium should also provide improved signal energy transmission for both sensing and pacing. This reduced polarization effect could be further enhanced by applying a carbon coating to the porous metal substrate, while retaining the porous architecture for tissue ingrowth and stable electrode fixation.

Although we have described a permanent porous-surfaced epicardial lead for atrial pacing, preliminary studies indicate that similar performance can be expected when it is applied to the ventricle. Because of its small size, this lead would be particularly useful for pediatric epicardial single or dual chamber pacing. A significant improvement over the present design would be a method of attachment, other than by sutures, which would facilitate its implantation through a restricted operative field. By keeping the fixation means remote from the electrode itself, leads of this design should produce less tissue trauma and thus minimize the tissue fibrosis which is the main determinant of electrophysiological performance.

References

1. Smyth NPD, Citron P, Keshishian JM, Garcia JM, Kelley LC: Permanent pervenous atrial sensing and pacing with a new J-shaped lead. J Thorac Cardiovasc Surg 1976; 72: 565–570.
2. Stokes K, Stephenson NL: The implantable cardiac pacing lead – just a simple wire? In: Barold SS, Mugica J, eds. The Third Decade of Cardiac Pacing. New York: Futura, 1982: 365–416.
3. Parsonnet V: Pacemaker Implantation. In: Effler, DB, ed Blades' Surgical Diseases of the Chest. St. Louis: Mosley, 1978: 699–758.
4. Timmis GC, Gordon S, Helland J: Enhanced electrode stability. The endocardial screw. In: Watanabe Y, ed Proceedings of the Vth International Symposium on Cardiac Pacing. Amsterdam: Exerpta Medica, 1977: 516–526.
5. Lajos TZ, Wanka J: Epicardial pacing. Ann Thorac Surg 1978; 25: 64–65.
6. Calvin JW: Permanent atrial pacing: Epicardial approach – "pinch-on" electrodes. Arch Surg 1976; 111: 712–715.
7. Bognolo D, Stokes K, Wiebush W, Vijayanagar R, Eckstein P, Jeffrey D: Experimental and clinical study of a new permanent myocardial atrial sutureless pacing lead. Pace 1983; 6: 113–118.
8. MacGregor DC, Wilson GJ, Lixfeld W, Pilliar RM, Bobyn JD, Silver MD, Smardon S, Miller SL: The porous-surfaced electrode: A new concept in pacemaker lead design. J Thorac Cardiovasc Surg 1979; 78: 281–291.
9. Wilson GJ, MacGregor DC, Bobyn JD, Lixfeld W, Pilliar RM, Miller SL, Silver MD: Tissue response to porous-surfaced electrodes: Basis for a new atrial lead design. In: Meere, ed. Pro-

ceedings of the VIth World Symposium on Cardiac Pacing. Montreal: Pacesymp, 1979: Chap 29–12.

10. MacCarter DJ, Lundberg KM, Corstjens JPM: Porous electrodes: Concept, technology and results. Pace 1983; 6: 427–435.
11. Bobyn JD, Wilson GJ, Mycyk JR, Klement P, Tait GA, Pilliar RM, MacGregor DC: Comparison of a porous-surfaced with a totally porous ventricular endocardial pacing electrode. Pace 1981; 4: 405–416.
12. Timmis GC, Gordon S, Westveer DC, Stewart J, Stokes K, Helland J: A new steroid-eluting low threshold lead. Pace 1983; 6: 31.

Authors' address:
Prof. David C. MacGregor
University of Miami
10421 S.W. 89th Avenue
Miami, Florida 33176
USA

352

Comparative Studies of Ventricular and Atrial Stimulation Thresholds of Carbon-Tip Electrodes

M. P. Kleinert, H. R. Bartsch, K. G. Mühlenpfordt

Summary: The findings can be summarized as follows:
1. At a pulse width of 0.5 ms, the intraoperative atrial voltage thresholds are, on average, 1.7 times higher than in the right ventricle (measured immediately after PMI using the vario-cycle, the factor is 1.56).
2. One to 3 months after PMI, the atrial voltage thresholds have fallen almost to the original values in about 70% of the cases (20 of the 29 patients), while, with the ventricular voltage thresholds, this applies in only 11% of the cases (2 of the 18 patients).
3. Moreover, 6 to 7 months after PMI, the atrial voltage thresholds, at 0.957 V, are below the ventricular values of 1.226 V.
4. One year after PMI, the threshold values are virtually the same, at 1 V, and have apparently become stabilized.
5. The voltage threshold behaviour of carbon-tip electrodes, in particular in the right atrium, is thus incomparably better than that observed to date with all known metal-tip electrodes.

In addition to other objections (1) to permanent atrial pacing was confronted, the atrial voltage thresholds (VTh) of both conventional and screw-in electrodes were described as being 2 to 3 times higher than the voltage thresholds in the right ventricle (2, 3, 4, 5), which would mean that exit blocks could occur at any time. In contrast to this, however, studies on our own patients have shown that voltage thresholds increases were more frequent (3 to 4 times more frequent) in the case of ventricular electrodes.

The question, therefore arose as to what extent to which the use of carbon-tip electrodes, whose extremely favorable voltage threshold behaviour has been described in several recent reports (6, 7, 8, 9, 10, 11), permits an amendment to the above statement.

Studies performed on 99 patients, with the aim of providing an answer to this question, will be discussed in the following pages.

Material and Method

In the case of 20 of the 99 patients (48 female, 51 male, average age 69 ± 11 years), who received carbon-tip electrodes in the period from January 1980 through October 1982, dual-chamber pacemakers were involved. Therefore, for these 20 patients, one electrode was implanted in the atrial and one in the ventricular position (Table 1). In one case, a second carbon-tip electrode had to be implanted contralaterally following an infection caused by the original electrode. With another patient, the carbon-tip electrode was removed from the atrium to the right ventricle following dislocation.

In the case of 6 patients, the carbon-tip electrodes were inserted as second electrodes, following stimulation threshold increases with the metal-tip electrodes that were first implanted – one J-shaped atrial electrode and five screw-in electrodes, one of which was lo-

Table 1. Distribution of carbon-tip electrodes (first as well as second implantation).
RA = right atrium
RV = right ventricle
MPPM = multiprogrammable pacemakers

Pacing Systems		Lead Position		MPPM
		RA	RV	
First Leads	AAI	36		35
	VVI		35	21
	VAT	14	14	
	DDD	6	8	
Second Leads	AAI	1+		
	VVI		2+o	
	VAT		2+	
	DDD	1★	1+	
	Total	58	62	

+ VTh increase
o Lead infection
★ Convertion VVI-to DDD-System

cated in the atrium. Altogether, 120 carbon-tip electrodes, with a surface area of 12 square millimeters were thus implanted.

For all of the patients, the action voltages and the voltage thresholds at 0.25, 0.5 and 1 ms pulse widths were measured intraoperatively. They were recorded on an oscillograph, as were the impedances, at a working voltage of 5 V and a pulse width of 0.5 ms.

Multiprogrammable pulse generators with vario-function were used in 56 patients – 35 in the atrial and 21 in the ventricular position. Thus, in these cases, postoperative, transthoracic measurements of the voltage thresholds were possible. These measurements were taken under the conditions explained above on the same day as implantation, daily during the first 14 days after pacemaker implantation (PMI), 4 weeks later and then at 3-months intervals. The remaining patients were monitored analogously.

The average observation period was 12 months and the maximum observation period was 30 months.

Results

Of the 120 carbon-tip electrodes, 3 – 2 in atrial and 1 in ventricular position – dislodged a few days after implantation. One of the atrial carbon-tip electrodes had to be replaced by a screw-in type, while the second was relocated in the ventricle. The dislocated ventricular electrode was successfully repositioned.

Table 2. Intraoperative electrical characteristics of carbon-tip electrodes measured oscilloscopically. RA = right atrium. RV = right ventricle.

pulse widths		RA n = 45			RV n = 61		
[ms]		U [V]	J [mA]	R [kΩ]	U [V]	J [mA]	R [kΩ]
	min	0.371	0.835	0.350	0.353	0.612	0.420
0.25	m	1.142	2.623	0.444	0.750	1.373	0.556
	max	1.912	5.059	0.612	1.365	3.147	1.094
	min	0.135	0.306	0.380	0.224	0.365	0.426
0.50	m	0.680	1.427	0.488	0.454	0.761	0.621
	max	1.088	2.529	0.627	0.889	1.647	1.121
	min	0.088	0.188	0.416	0.153	0.200	0.507
1.00	m	0.491	0.893	0.561	0.321	0.468	0.713
	max	0.824	1.824	0.741	0.644	1.029	1.379
	min			0.319			0.420
5V/0.50	m			0.486			0.588
	max			0.618			1.022

The electrical characteristics measured intraoperatively in the case of all carbon-tip electrodes are given in Table 2 and Figure 1. This illustrates that the ventricular impedances at 5 V/0.5 ms pulse width exceed the atrial values by 0.100 KΩ.

The correlation between the voltage thresholds for all patients included in the study, and those of the 56 patients with atrial vario-pacemakers, is so close (Table 3), with respect to both the intraoperative, oscilloscopic measurements and the postoperative measurements using the variotechnique (11), that these 56 patients, considered separately to facilitate comparison, can be used as a basis for further discussion.

Thus, on this basis, the voltage threshold values in the right atrium, measured intraoperatively at a mean pulse width of 0.5 ms, exceed those for the right ventricle by a factor of 1.7.

In the postoperative period, as shown in Table 4, a disproportionately high ventricular voltage threshold increase up to 1.508 V (factor 3) occurred until the 11th, 12th and 13th day after PMI. In contrast, the atrial voltage thresholds increased by a factor of only 2.3, namely to 1.739 V (on the 13th day after PMI). The voltage thresholds thus differ merely by a factor of only 1.15. Therefore, there is, on the whole, a close approximation between the atrial and ventricular stimulation threshold/duration curves (Figure 2). Six to 7 months after PMI (in 23 cases), the curves actually cross, as a result of a disproportionate decrease in the atrial voltage thresholds, namely to 0.95 V, compared to the ventricular voltage thresholds of 1.226 V. Twelve to 13 months after PMI, the atrial and ventricular voltage thresholds are virtually the same.

Further observation revealed that additional, although only slight, voltage thresholds decreases were established, at least in the cases involving the atrial electrodes (6 patients). A

Fig. 1. Average acute strength duration curves at 0.5 ms pulse width for voltage thresholds of carbon-tip electrodes in atrial (RA, n = 45) and ventricular position (RV, n = 61) compared with the maximum values on the 11th day (RV) and on the 13th day (RA) after implantation.

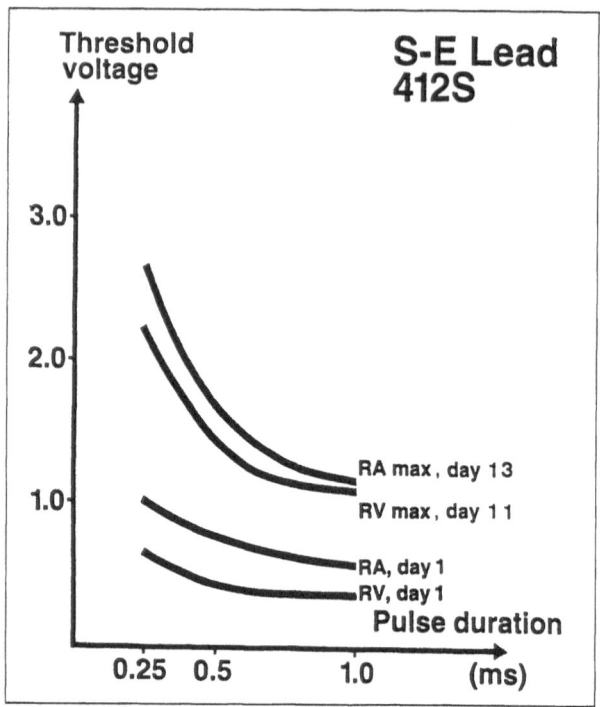

Table 3. Average voltage thresholds of carbon-tip electrodes at 0.5 ms pulse width comparing intraoperative-oscilloscopically measured values to those measured by means of the Vario technique.

method of measurement	RA intraop. osc.		Vario	RV intraop. osc.		Vario
n	45	35	35	61	21	21
pulse widths [ms]	U [V]	U [V]	U [V]	U [V]	U [V]	U [V]
min	0.135	0.335	0.500	0.224	0.224	0.333
0.50　　m	0.680	0.694	0.781	0.454	0.399	0.500
max	1.088	1.088	1.167	0.889	0.588	0.667

similar trend (although in the case of only 3 patients) was indicated for the ventricular electrodes.

Discussion

The voltage threshold behaviour with carbon-tip electrodes observed by others (6, 7, 8, 9) and by ourselves (10, 11) would appear to be extremely remarkable for several reasons.

356

Table 4. Development of atrial and ventricular voltage thresholds measured by means of the Vario technique.

		RA	RV	RA/RV
	t	U [V] (Vario)		quotient
	day of op.	0.781	0.500	1.56
days post op.	11	1.583	1.508	1.05
	12	1.688	1.437	1.18
	13	1.739	1.442	1.21
months post op.	1	1.376	1.266	1.09
	3–4	1.046	1.194	0.88
	6–7	0.957	1.226	0.78
	9–10	0.951	1.121	0.78
	12–13	0.972	1.000	0.97
	15–16	0.917	1.111	0.83
	18–19	0.929	—	—
	21–22	0.945	—	—

First the intraoperative measurements, for both atrial and ventricular positions, showed substantially lower thresholds than in the case of conventional metal-tip electrodes, both flanged and screw-in types. This phenomenon has already been reported by us (10, 11).

Secondly, the atrial voltage thresholds exceeded the ventricular values by the factor of only 1.7 (intraoperative) or 1.56 immediately after operation, measured using the vario-cycle. During further observation after PMI, the factor decreased progressively. On the one hand, the ventricular voltage threshold increase up to the 11th, 12th and 13th day after PMI was much more pronounced than the atrial voltage threshold increase. On the other hand, the later voltage threshold decrease in the right atrial appendage was apparently much more rapid than in the right ventricle. Thus, 4 weeks to 3 months after PMI, the atrial voltage thresholds had fallen almost to their original value in 70% of the cases (20 of the 29 patients). In the case of the ventricular electrodes, this was true only of 11% (2 of the 18 patients).

Expressed in different terms, 3 months after PMI, the atrial voltage thresholds were, overall, only 1.4 times higher than the intraoperative values, while the ventricular values were, in comparison, 2.5 times higher. With respect to the further decreasing tendency of atrial and ventricular voltage thresholds, reference is made to Figure 2.

Following animal experiments, it appears that the favorable voltage threshold behaviour is related to the very thin (less than 0.1 mm) fibrous encapsulation of the electrode tip (9). The thickness of this fibrous tissue, which is not excitable, is, namely, one of the factors responsible for the voltage threshold level. Similarly, the low polarization potentials of

Fig. 2. Development of voltage thresholds of carbon-tip electrodes at 0.5 ms pulse width in atrial (RA, n = 35) and ventricular position (RV, n = 21) during the first 14 days and up to 12 months after PMI.

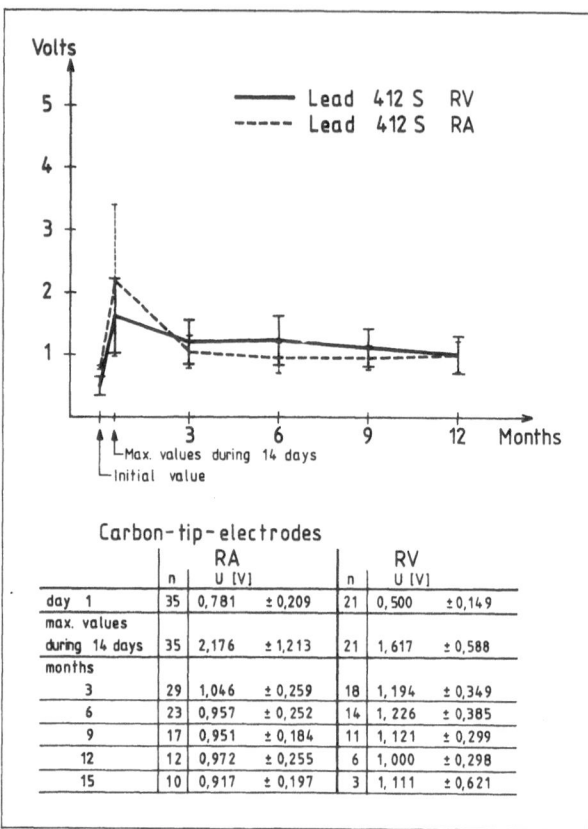

Carbon-tip-electrodes

		RA			RV	
	n	U [V]		n	U [V]	
day 1	35	0,781	± 0,209	21	0,500	± 0,149
max. values during 14 days	35	2,176	± 1,213	21	1,617	± 0,588
months						
3	29	1,046	± 0,259	18	1,194	± 0,349
6	23	0,957	± 0,252	14	1,226	± 0,385
9	17	0,951	± 0,184	11	1,121	± 0,299
12	12	0,972	± 0,255	6	1,000	± 0,298
15	10	0,917	± 0,197	3	1,111	± 0,621

carbon-tip electrodes are significant (7). We do not know to what extent a difference in pressure or lower mechanical load on the electrode tip, depending on the heart cavitiy chosen for implantation, may affect the voltage threshold behaviour. However, such effects are conceivable.

In addition, if one considers the atrial and ventricular values separately, changes in the heart itself would also seem to play a role in the voltage threshold behaviour. Thus, the subdued dynamic stimulation threshold behaviour of the atrium could be related to different thickness of the myocardium in the two heart cavities, or to a conceivable difference in the myocardial metabolism, or perhaps to both these phenomena.

References

1. Witte J, Antonioli GE: Do we have a satisfactory atrial lead? 2nd European Symposium on Cardiac Pacing. Florence, May 1981: 4–6.
2. Smith NPD, Keshishian JM, Basu AP, Bacos JM, Massumi RA, Fletcher RD and Baker NR: Permanent transvenous atrial pacing: An experimental and clinical study. Ann Thorac Surg 1971; 11: 360.
3. Smith NPD, Keshishian JM, Bacos JM, Massumi RA, Fletcher RD and Boivin MR: Permanent pervenous atrial pacing. J Electrocardiol 1971; 4: 299.

4. Smith NPD, and Citron P: Permanent pervenous atrial sensing and pacing. Vth International Symposium on Cardiac Pacing. Tokyo, March 1976: 14–18.
5. Kleinert MP, Bock M and Wilhelmi F: Clinical use of a new transvenous atrial lead. Am J Cardiol 1977; 40: 237.
6. Beck-Jansen P, Schüller H and Winther-Rasmussen S: Vitreous carbon electrodes in endocardial pacing. VIth World Symposium on Cardiac Pacing. Montreal, Oct. 1979: 2–5.
7. Richter GJ, Weidlich E, v. Sturm F, David E, Brandt G, Elmqvist H and Thoren A: Non-polarizable vitreous carbon pacing electrodes in animal experiments. VIth World Symposium on Cardiac Pacing. Montreal, Oct. 1979: 2–5.
8. Beck-Jansen P, Schüller H and Akerström B: Chronical thresholds with carbon-tip endocardial leads. 2nd European Symposium on Cardiac Pacing. Florence, May 1981: 4–6.
9. Richter GJ, Weidlich E, Rao JR, v. Sturm F, Elmqvist H, Akerström B, David E and Brandt G: Chronic threshold of stimulating electrodes: Comparison of activated vitreous carbon with conventional Platin-Iridium electrodes in animal tests. Med Progr Technol 1981; 8: 67.
10. Kleinert MP: New developments of atrial leads. Herz/Kreisl. 1982; 8: 459.
11. Kleinert MP, Bartsch H-R, and Mühlenpfordt K-G: Increased stimulation thresholds: The problem may have been solved. 4th Annual Scientific Session of the North American Society of Pacing and Electrophysiology. New Orleans, March, 1983: 18–19.

Authors' address:
Dr. M. P. Kleinert
Harburg General Hospital
Medical Dept. I.
Eissendorfer Pferdeweg 52
2000 Hamburg 90

359

A New Steroid-Eluting Low Threshold Pacemaker Lead

G. C. Timmis, S. Gordon, D. C. Westveer, J. R. Stewart, K. B. Stokes, J. R. Helland

Summary: Animal studies have shown that dexamethasone sodium phosphate eluting from a silicone core through a porous electrode at focal megadose levels preferentially lowers ventricular thresholds compared with control leads having conventional and porous electrodes. A similar unipolar tined lead with a porous 8 mm² hemispherical electrode attached to a silicone core impregnated with ≤ 1 mg of dexamethasone sodium phosphate was implanted in 18 patients with a special low output generator. Serial thresholds (μJoules) measured at 1.35 volts (0.391 $\pm$ .03 (mean $\pm$ SEM)) at implant, 1582 $\pm$ .07 at one week, and 0.795 $\pm$ 0.07 at 12 weeks) were lower than equivalent values in five control patients with the same generator but with conventional (6971) leads (p $<$ .001). Telemetered R waves were higher throughout the study period than in controls (p $<$ 0.005). These data are in contrast with previous noninvasive tracking studies in this laboratory showing threshold peaking or loss of capture at nominal outputs within 40 days of implant, in 30% of patients with conventional pacing systems emitting voltages two to four times as high. In conclusion, a new corticosteroid-eluting lead has been shown to produce very low and stable thresholds which are significantly better than those seen with conventional leads for up to 12 weeks. Better sensing was also observed over the same period. The mechanism of steroid effect which lasts well beyond the period of elution is unknown but may be anti-inflammatory at the electrode-tissue interface.

A New Steroid-Eluting Low Threshold Pacemaker Lead

Threshold tracking in animals and man have regularly demonstrated an acute rise in stimulation thresholds which begins to level off after three months but continues to increase for several years. The exit block which may ensue reflects the interaction of numerous factors such as electrode composition, surface area, impedance, lead resistivity, voltage, current, and duration of the stimulus (1, 2). Interaction between the lead and the biologic impedance of the heart may result in a nonlinear variation of threshold (3) which is also affected by tissue excitability and the mechanical position of the electrode within the heart. Surgical experience, multiprogrammability and modifications in lead design have overcome many threshold problems (4). Lead resistivity has been reduced (5). Generator and lead impedances have been better matched (1, 2). Changes in the geometry and size of the electrode have increased current density at the delivery site (6). Bandwidths of both generator and lead have been revised to conform with the frequency spectra of intracardiac electrograms (7). Moreover, lead fixation modifications have acutely stabilized the condition of the electrode-tissue interface with an additional salutary effect on thresholds (8, 9). To date there have been no lead designs which utilize the alteration of thresholds by drugs and physiologic factors although corticosteroids have long been known to favorably affect threshold (3, 10). In this report we describe our experience with an innovative pacemaker lead employing corticosteroid elution from a silicone core through a porous electrode.

Methods

The test device (Medtronic model 4003; Figure 1A) is a polyurethane tined lead with a platinum-coated porous titanium 8 mm² hemispherical electrode attached to a silicone rubber core impregnated with dexmethasone sodium phosphate. The content of steroid in the silicone plug, and on the surface of the electrode itself to which the steroid has been absorbed, is approximately 1 mg (0.96 ± 0.20 mg). All components of this lead were tested in vitro (thermal shock, flex testing of conductor coil, resistance between connector pin and electrode, bond pull-strength testing, and crimp pull-strength testing). The differential effects of various eluates (albumin, Heparin, ibuprofen (Motrin) and dexamethasone sodium phosphate) were tested in three dogs each. The lead employed for this purpose was an atrial drug-eluting device (1X041) which is similar to the commercially available Medtronic model 6991U but with an axial 7 mm² platinum electrode and four tines. Stimulation thresholds and R wave amplitude were compared at three weeks to implant values. Corticosteroid elution rates were tested by immersing the electrode of ten leads in agitated pooled human plasma warmed to 37 °C. At given intervals the plasma was decanted and replaced with fresh plasma. The steroid elution rate was measured with a high pressure liquid chromatograph (Varian model 5060 with a Vista UV 50 Variable Wave Length Detector).

Serial steroid lead recordings were then obtained in five dogs of voltage threshold (at the leading edge of a 0.5 msec impulse), pacing resistance (i.e., V/mA calculated from leading edge values), electrographic R wave amplitudes (mV) and source impedance (Kohm).

Fig. 1A. Schematic diagram of the lead tip displaying a silicone rubber core (MCRD) impregnated with approximately 1 mm of dexamethasone sodium phosphate. **B.** Time-concentration curve displaying cumulative steroid elution from the test lead into a 5 cc plasma bath at 37 °C.

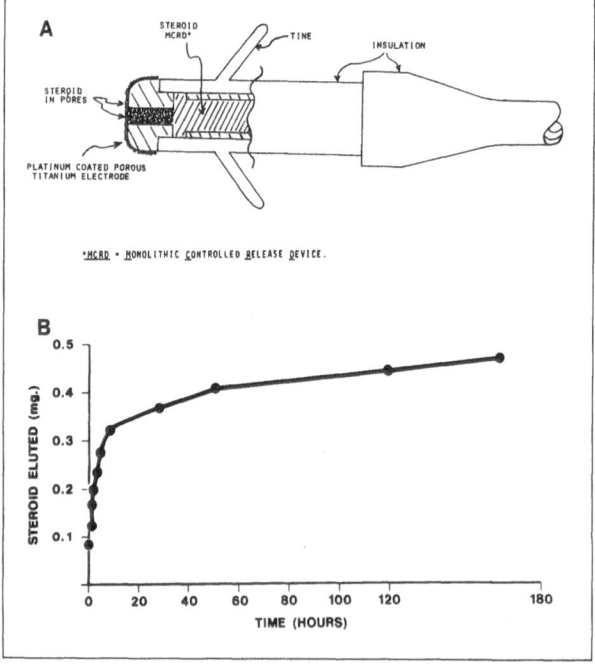

These variables were measured with either a Medtronic model 5300, 5309, or 5309A pacing systems analyzer (PSA). Pulse width thresholds were obtained with a special generator, model 1556. Peak to peak R wave amplitudes were obtained using a Nicolet oscilloscope, model 1090A. Source impedances were obtained with a decade resistance box, by recording the resistance that attenuates the R wave amplitude by 50%. These data were compared to the equivalent values for test leads without steroid (1×397; n = 3) and conventional leads (6971; n = 5).

Twenty-three patients were similarly studied, 18 with the test lead (4003) and five randomly interspersed recipients of a conventional lead (6971). In all but one case, a custom generator enabling a four-fold reduction in output (to 1.35 V) was employed (Spectrax SXT-L, 2443). In a single patient receiving a test lead, a standard generator was employed (Spectrax SXT, 8423). Implant strength-duration thresholds and lead resistance (i.e., V/mA at the leading edge of a 0.5 msec impulse) were calculated using a Medtronic model 5311 PSA. Ventricular electrograms were measured at implant with the 5311 PSA and/or Nicolet model 2090-3B Explorer III digital oscilloscope. Within 24 hours, implant R-wave amplitudes were compared with data telemetered by a Medtronic model 5907C programmer-receiver. Telemetered electrographic signals were calibrated with a four millivolt pulse and displayed on an electrocardiographic (ECG) strip recorder for calculation as follows:

$$R_c = \frac{R_{tf}(mm)}{G_f(mV)} \times \frac{R_m(mV) \times G_a(mm/mV)}{R_{ta}}$$

where R is the ventricular electrogram and G, the ECG gain factor. The subscripts c refer to corrected; m, measured; t, telemetry; a, acute; and f, follow-up. Sequential energy (E) data was calculated employing serial pulses width threshold measurements at 1.35 V (9701C) as follows:

$$E \, (\mu \, \text{Joules}) = \frac{V^2}{R(ohms)} \times t(msec) \times 1000 \, (mV/V)$$

where R is resistance at implant and t, variable pulse-width. Serial peak-to-peak R waves were calculated as indicated above.

Values are expressed as mean ± SEM unless otherwise specified. Lead performance was analyzed by a two-way analysis of variance (ANOVA). All estimates of significance were two-tailed. Human investigations were performed at William Beaumont Hospital with the informed consent of all patients after the procedure, test devices, and ongoing system of patient surveillance had been approved by our Internal Review Board.

Results

In Vitro Testing. Figure 1B depicts steroid elution as an exponential function. Logarithm replotting of data suggested second order kinetics reflecting the effects of diffusing through two media. Thus, steroid on the electrode surface is readily dissolved and elutes rapidly. However, only after moisture penetrates the silicone core does the dexamethasone sodium phosphate diffuse in response to a concentration gradient, eluting at a slower more sustained rate.

Animal Studies. Drug-free leads and leads eluting albumin, heparin, and ibuprofen (silicone core impregnated with 200 mg/cc solution of each substance) displayed threshold increases of 530%, 200%, 140% and 120% respectively. In contrast, the increment with dexamethasone sodium phosphate was only 50%. Pacing impedance fell with each preparation to a degree similar to that observed with the steroid eluting lead (from 1500 ± 650 to 870 ± 180 ohms (mean $\pm$ SD)). The decrease in R wave amplitude over the three week test period was 18% for the steroid lead compared with decreases of 70%, 23%, 33% and 32% respectively for the four different control leads.

Figures 2A–D compare the effects of the ventricular test lead (4003) with the steroid free control (1X397) and conventional (6971) leads. Mean thresholds fell while both groups of controls displayed the rise usually seen with most conventional leads. Resistance fell with all leads, remaining significantly lower with the test lead. Serial R wave amplitudes were the same for the test and conventional leads. They were slightly higher for steroid-free control leads. Serial source impedance was significantly less in the test lead compared with controls.

Histopathologic studies showed no significant differences in tissue reaction around electrodes through which steroid had eluted compared with that of steroid free porous leads. However, the fibrous reaction at the electrode-tissue interface was considerably less with the porous electrodes than with solid electrodes in canines at 12 weeks.

Human Studies. Implant strength-duration curves were significantly less for test leads compared with controls (Figure 3A). Thresholds remained relatively stable over the first 12 weeks in contrast to the rise seen in controls (Figure 3B). Serial R wave amplitudes were higher, increasing throughout the period of observation compared with lower and more stable values in controls (Figure 3C).

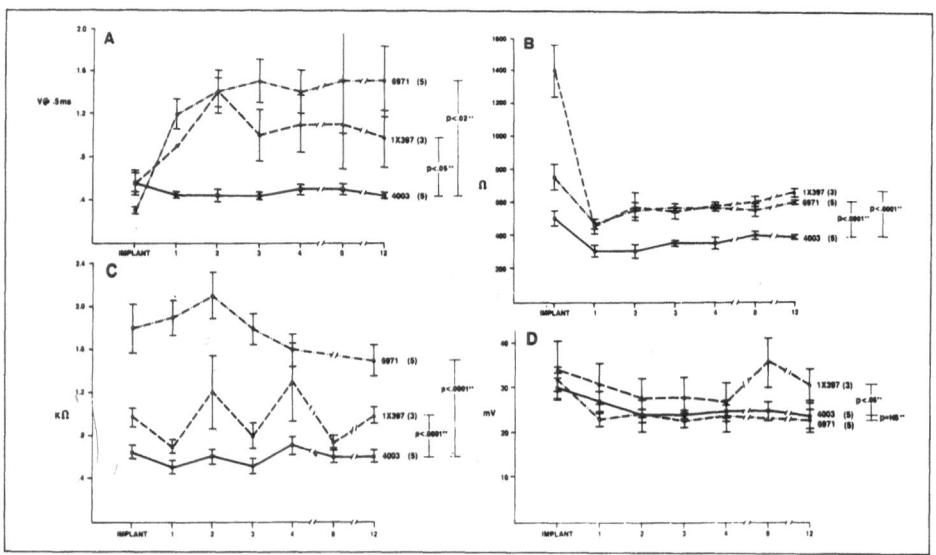

Fig. 2A. Serial effect on stimulation threshold of steroid-eluting test leads (4003) compared with steroid-free porous leads (1X397) and conventional leads with platinum ring electrodes (6971). Comparative effects on lead impedance (actually pacing resistance since current and voltage were measured at the leading edge of a 0.5 msec stimulus) are shown in B, source impedance in C, and R-wave amplitude in D. Significance levels were calculated by the group t-test at twelve weeks.

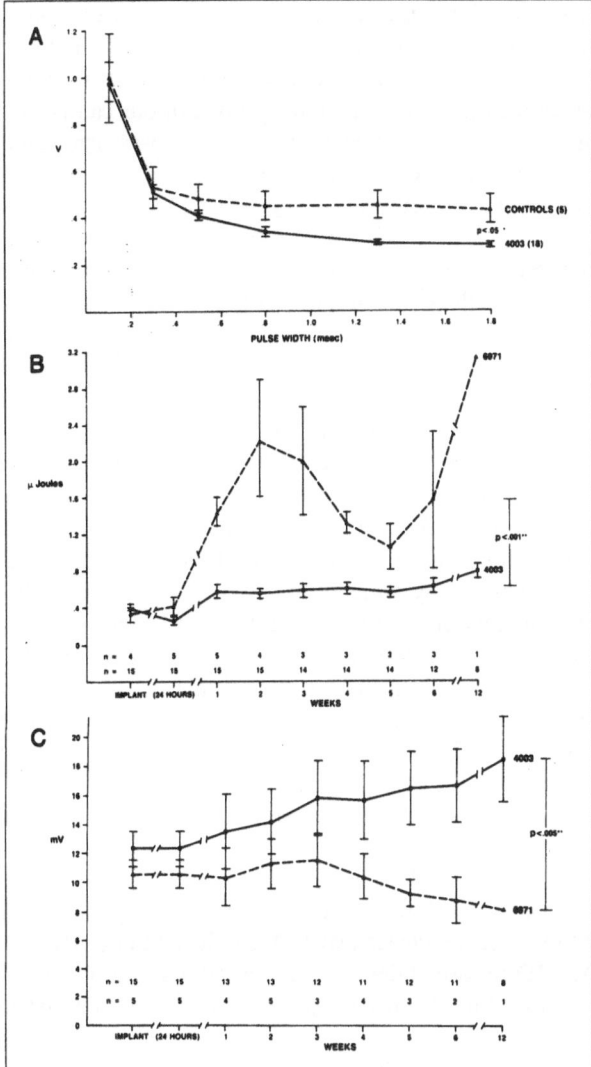

Fig. 3A. Strength-duration curves measured in patients at pacemaker implantation. **B.** Serial thresholds measured non-invasively in patients comparing the effect of the test leads (4003) with that of the conventional leads (6971). See text. **C.** Comparative effect of test leads (4003) and control leads (6971) in patients on serial noninvasively estimated R wave amplitudes. See text.

Discussion

Threshold tracking in our Pacemaker Surveillance Clinic has shown a rise in thresholds sometimes to the point of exit block at nominal outputs (2.7–5.4 V, or 0.5 msec), in 30% of patients with multiprogrammable pacemakers and conventional leads within 40 days of implant (11). A rise in sensing threshold was seen in twelve of these patients (concordant with an increase in pacing threshold in four). Thus, unlike our test lead experience, threshold changes were common within the first several weeks of implantation. However, before assigning the favorable effects of the new lead to the elution of dexamethasone sodium phosphate, several mechanisms must be considered. Although Berman's group claimed that electrode porosity had little effect on thresholds (12), Guarda et

365

al. have shown that intracardiac electrode fixation is remarkably more rapid with porous electrodes than with solid electrodes with less inflammation and fibrosis around the former (13). The thicker fibrous capsule around platinum-iridium electrodes may have an unfavorable effect on thresholds and source impedance. This was shown in our canine studies wherein the threshold increase with the steroid-free porous electrode was significantly less than with the platinum ring electrodes. Nevertheless, there still remained a significant difference between test leads with and without steroid suggesting an additional salutary pharmacologic response.

Too little is known about steroid effects on the heart to explain our findings. It has long been suspected that corticosteroids alter cellular membrane permeability producing significant and sustained threshold changes which abet pacing (3). Thus, a variety of corticosteroids have been used clinically for exit block (3, 10). They may increase the cellular efflux of potassium decreasing the transmembrane gradient of this cation which has been shown to increase excitability (3, 14). However, since the effect of glucocorticoids and minerocorticoids are antagonistic with respect to excitability (3), potassium shifts unlikely mediate the steroid effect seen in our study. Moreover, the electrophysiologic response to glucocorticoids is not particularly striking. Thus, Kriett et al. found that dexamethasone sodium phosphate had minimal effects on rabbit atrial electrophysiological properties (15). Accordingly, the mechanism by which corticosteroids decrease pacing threshold is unclear. Their antiinflammatory effects may account for lower thresholds by decreasing tissue reaction at the electrode site (15). The extremely focal nature of this effect has been demonstrated by the fact that a control electrode within 1 cm from a steroid-eluting electrode in the same ventricle performs like a conventional lead (unpublished data). Our demonstration of a significant difference in strength-duration curves observed in patients at implant is not inconsistent with the anti-inflammatory thesis and may simply reflect the difference between the porous electrode of the test lead and the conventional electrode used in our controls.

Since 1964 it has been known that steroids could diffuse in and out of silicone rubber which in a physiologic environment has been shown to release drugs from implants at a uniform rate in a manner similar to the release device (MCRD) employed in our steroid-eluting test leads (Fig. 1A). The MCRD release of dexamethasone sodium phosphate was probably complete in about two weeks time, further suggesting that late steroid effects may be anti-inflammatory.

Some limitations of our study include the assumptions made in noninvasively serializing our data. Moreover, energy estimates do not ideally measure the excitability of the heart and additionally are impedance-dependant. However, since canine pacing resistances tended to fall over the same period of time in which our human studies were conducted, changes in excitability were probably not obscured. Our sensing data is based on a stable relationship between telemetered electrograms and directly measured R waves throughout the study. We have also assumed that the spatial relationship of electrodes to intrinsic signals was constant throughout or that any variation was the same for both test and control leads. We were unable to assess the polarizing characteristics of the test lead in our human studies because of the confounding effects of the QRS complex superimposed on polarizing signals in the recorded recharge pulse of our telemetered Spectrax SXT-L data. In conclusion, the corticosteroid-eluting lead shows better pacing and sensing performance than similar steroid-free control and conventional leads in animals and man. This appears to be a result of an interaction between the pharmacologic properties of dexamethasone sodium phosphate and the characteristics of the electrode itself. Although steroid elution is spent in about two weeks, the favorable (anti-inflammatory?) effects of the test lead appear to persist in man for about 12 weeks. If clinical studies of longer duration confirm these preliminary results, we may be entering a new era of lead design.

References

1. Thalen HJ, Van Den Berg JW, Van Der Heide JNH, Nieveen J: The artificial cardiac pacemaker. Assen, the Netherlands: Royal VanGorcum, 1969; 125–297.
2. Barold SS, Ong LS, Heinle RA: Stimulation and sensing thresholds for cardiac pacing: electrophysiologic and technical aspects. Prog Cardiovasc Dis 1981; 24: 1–24.
3. Preston TA, Judge RD: Alteration of pacemaker threshold by drug and physiologic factors. Ann NY Acad Sci 1969; 167: 686–692.
4. Stokes K, Stephenson NL: The implantable cardiac pacing lead-just a simple wire? In: Barold SS, Mugica J, eds. The third decade of cardiac pacing. New York: Futura, 1982; 365–416.
5. Upton JE: New pacing lead conductors. In: Meere C, ed Cardiac pacing. Montreal: Pacesymp, 1979; 29–6.
6. Irnich W: Engineering concepts of pacemaker electrodes. In: Schaldach M, Furman S, in collaboration with Hein F, Thull R, eds Advances in pacemaker technology. New York: Springer-Verlag, 1975; 241–272.
7. Raber MB, Cuddy TE, Israel DA: Pacemaker electrodes act as highpass filters on the electrogram. In: Watanabe Y, ed Cardiac pacing. Amsterdam: Excerpta Medica, 1977; 506–509.
8. Timmis GC, Gordon S, Helland J: Enhanced electrode stability: The endocardial screw. In: Watanabe Y, ed. Cardiac pacing. Amsterdam: Excerpta Medica, 1977; 516–526.
9. Gordon S, Timmis GC, Ramos RG, Gangadharan V, Hauser J: Improved transvenous pacemaker electrode stability. In: Cardiac pacing. Meere C, ed Montreal: Pacesymp, 1979: 31–3.
10. Beanlands DS, Akyurekli Y, Keon WJ: Prednisone in the management of exit block. In: Meere C, ed Cardiac pacing. Montreal: Pacesymp, 1979: 18–3.
11. Timmis GC, Gordon S, Baer C. Goodfliesh R: Multiprogrammable pacemakers: noninvasive threshold tracking. American College of Physicians, Boyne, Michigan, October 10, 1981.
12. Berman ND, Dickson SE, Lipton IH: Acute and chronic clinical performance comparison of a porous and a solid electrode design. Pace 1982; 5: 67–71.
13. Guarda F, Galloni M, Assone F, Pasteris V, Luboz MP: Histological reactions of porous tip endocardial electrodes implanted in sheep. Int J Artif Organs 1982; 5[4]: 267–273.
14. Walker WJ, Elkins JT, Wood LW: Effect of potassium in restoring myocardial response to a subthreshold cardiac pacemaker. New Engl J Med 1964; 271: 597.
15. Kriett JM, Gornick CA, Stokes KL, Detloff BLS, Benditt DG: Cellular electrophysiologic effects of dexamethasone phosphate and sodium dexamethasone phosphate on isolated rabbit right atria. (In Press).
16. Folkman J, Long DM: The use of silicone rubber as a carrier for prolonged drug therapy. J Surg Res 1964; 4: 139–142.
17. Dziukm PJ, Cook B: Passage of steroids through silicone rubber. Endocrinology 1966; 78: 208–211.

Authors' address:
Dr. G. C. Timmis
William Beaumont Hospital
3601 West Thirteen Mile Road
Royal Oak 48072 Michigan
USA

A Steroid-Eluting, Low-Threshold, Low-Polarizing Electrode

K. B. Stokes, G. A. Bornzin, W. A. Wiebusch

Summary: A porous steroid-eluting electrode gives stable, low chronic thresholds without peaking in animal studies. Controlled steroid release at the tissue-electrode interface affects only a few myocardial cells, precluding systemic side effects. Human studies so far confirm the animal results. This will allow the use of much lower pulse generator voltage and pulse width without compromising safety. When combined with appropriate pacing circuits, the new electrode's low polarization characteristics may allow reliable capture detection.

Introduction

Our objective is to develop smaller, long-lasting pacing systems. This requires cardiac electrodes with stable chronic thresholds that do not rise appreciably after implant. Previous clinical studies have reported decreases in myocardial pacing threshold following systemic glucocorticosteroid administration but not without side effects. Thus, we have developed a porous cardiac pacemaker electrode which elutes a trace of glucocorticosteroid directly to the electrode-tissue interface. A small group of myocardial cells immediately surrounding the electrode are treated, avoiding systemic side effects. Chronic voltage thresholds in animals are about one-third those of solid electrode standards, and about one-half those of similar porous electrodes without steroid. As a result, pulse generators can now be used reliably with the new devices at significantly lower voltage amplitudes and pulse widths. Compared to standard leads, this can save up to 80% of the power source energy without compromising safety. In addition, since systemic glucocorticosteroids are known to be therapeutic for exit block, this new electrode may be useful for those patients with high threshold problems. Early human clinical data so far confirm animal results. The porous-steroid electrode is adaptable to reliable capture detection because of low polarization potentials.

Methods and Materials

Four electrodes were studied, (three with 8 mm^2 (geometric) surface areas and one 11 mm^2). The first, a porous drug-eluting device, was made by drilling a hole through the distal face of an approximately hemispherical titanium electrode. This communicated with a larger chamber within. Titanium particles were sintered on the surface and in the distal bore to form a less than 50 micron porosity and an approximately 8 mm^2 geometric surface area. A thin coating of platinum was applied to the distal surface by sputtering. Dexamethasone sodium phosphate particles were compounded with silicone rubber to form a monolithic controlled release device (MCRD). This was placed in the larger internal chamber. A small amount of dexamethasone sodium phosphate was also deposited on pore surfaces. Total steroid content was $\leqslant$ 1 mg. Both polyurethane and silicone insulated tined leads were studied (ventricular (V) Model 4003 and atrial (A) Model 4503). Results were compared against standard polyurethane insulated lead Models 6971 (V) and 6991U (A). The former has a solid 8 mm² ring-tip platinum electrode and the latter an 11 mm² canted cylindrical platinum tip. Control leads identical to Models 4003 and 4503 without steroid, Models IX397D (V) and IX053 (A) were also evaluated.

Methods

Two leads were implanted under general anesthesia in each canine (typically 20 kg). The electrode tips were placed in the right ventricular apex and right atrial appendage via the costocervical vertebral trunk vein subsequent to a right third intercostal thoracotomy. Fixation was achieved by firm ligation directly to the lead. Terminal ends were tunneled subcutaneously to a percutaneous access device (PAD). Some leads were continuously paced, most were not. Electrical monitoring was accomplished by use of specially-insulated needles to make percutaneous contact with the PAD. Leading edge voltage thresholds and resultant current were obtained with Medtronic pacing system analyzers (such as Model 5311) which measure amplitudes 90 μs into the pulse. Thresholds were obtained by increasing stimulus to the point where capture was consistently maintained (ten consecutive beats minimum). R- and P-wave amplitudes were measured with a storage oscilloscope (Tektronix Model 7000 series). Source impedance was measured using a decade resistance box and oscilloscope, reporting that resistance which attenuates the R- or P-wave amplitude by 50%. A Medtronic® Model 7000 pacing circuit and oscilloscope were used to generate stimuli and detect paced beats. Animal terminations were scheduled for 12, 52 and 104 weeks postimplant, sacrificing one-third of the original subjects at each point. After final monitor, the animals were heparinzed, then euthenized with an overdose of sodium pentobarbital (Beuthanasia). Thirty to sixty minutes postmortem, stimulation was resumed for a short period to obtain baseline photos where no paced beat complexes were possible. The animals were then subjected to necropsy. Electrode sites were photographed and specimens harvested for histopathologic analysis. Data from each experiment were analyzed separately, then models with the same electrode designs but different insulation materials were compared by a paired t-test. Given $P < 0.05$, data were combined resulting in four sets, steroid porous (N = 23 V, 12 A), porous (N = 3 each V and A), solid ring (V only, N = 8 and 9), and solid cylinder (A only, N = 12 and 13).

For polarization evaluation, the electrodes were immersed in 1/5 n-saline. A 1.8 ms constant current pulse was applied at 0.1 to 10 mA amplitudes. Using a storage oscilloscope, the polarization overvoltage was measured as shown in Figure 1.

Results

Ventricular leads with solid ring-tip electrodes have 0.5 ms thresholds that rise after implant to a 1.6 ± 0.32 V peak, then stabilize at a 12-week value of 1.5 ± 0.57 V. The porous electrode (without steroid) threshold rises to a 1.4 ± 0.25 V peak at 0.5 ms. This stabilizes at a chronic value of about 0.97 ± 0.45 V. The steroid-loaded porous electrode thresholds do not rise appreciably with time (p = 0.038 maximum) for a 12-week

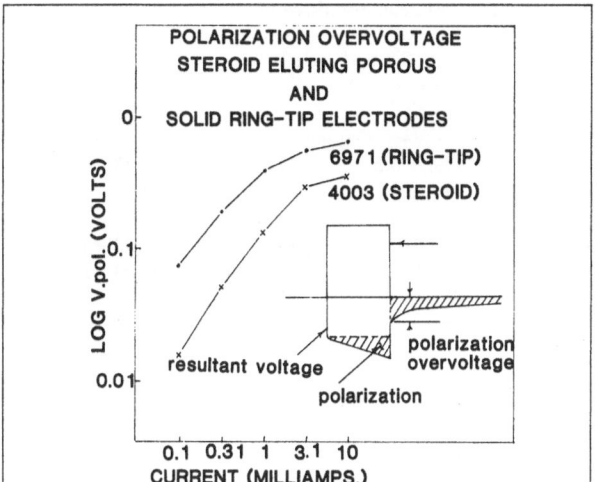

Fig. 1

value of 0.56 ± 0.18 V. These data represent a significant improvement over both ring-tip and the porous electrode (P < 0.001) at peak threshold. After 12 weeks, the porous-steroid electrode thresholds remain superior to the ring tip (P < 0.001) although the improvement over the porous only electrode is not as dramatic (P = 0.15). These data are summarized in Figure 2. Mean 12-week ventricular strength duration curves are shown in Figure 3. The steroid-eluting electrode gives a much lower curve compared to the ring-tip standard, with intermediate performance for porous tips without steroid. One can estimate rheobase (Rh) and chronaxie (Ch) by finding the pulse width (estimated Ch) at twice 1.8–2.0 ms voltage threshold (estimated Rh). The product of these two values is a convenient way to compare strength-duration curves (1). We find Rh · CH values of approximately 0.27 for the ring-tip, 0.22 for the porous and 0.09 for porous-steroid electrodes 12 weeks postimplant. Thus the porous-steroid electrodes chronic strength-duration curve is 2.4 times more favorable (lower) than the porous.

For all leads, (leading edge) pacing resistance drops to a minimum one-week postimplant, then rises to a more stable chronic value. The steroid-eluting electrode has a lower chronic pacing resistance (440 ± 66 Ω) compared to the ring tip (570 ± 47 Ω) or porous (650 ± 43 Ω) electrodes. In vitro polarization data for Models 4003 and 6971 are shown in Figure 1. Polarization overvoltage is much less for the former compared to the latter.

Intrinsic R-wave amplitudes and source impedances are shown in Table 1. Both porous only and porous-steroid electrodes sensed higher R-wave amplitudes than the solid ring-tip (P = 0.027 and 0.018 respectively). But the porous steroid electrode had lower source impedance than either control or standard (P < 0.001).

Atrial thresholds as a function of time are also presented in Figure 2. Again, the steroid-loaded electrode has significantly lower values at all monitor times except at implant (P < 0.001, for example, at 0.5 ms, 12 weeks). A small peak threshold is shown for the porous-steroid electrode one week postimplant in Figure 2. This is not statistically different from its implant value (P < 0.001). Chronic (12-week) pacing resistance was also reduced for the steroid-loaded device at 350 ± 72 Ω compared to 640 ± 49 Ω for the porous electrode and 550 ± 59 Ω for the canted cylinder. P-wave amplitudes were not im-

371

Table 1. Sensing of intrinsic Canine R-waves (peak-to-peak, oscilloscope).

Electrode	Parameter	Implant Time (Weeks)		
		0	1	12
Solid Ring[1])	Amplitude (mV)	32 ± 6.5	23 ± 3.3	23 ± 5.5
Porous[2])	Amplitude (mV)	34 ± 11	31 ± 8.0	31 ± 6.0
Porous-Steroid[3])	Amplitude (mV)	33 ± 5.5	29 ± 7.4	29 ± 6.8
Solid Ring[1])	Source Impedance (Ω)	1800 ± 490	1900 ± 410	1500 ± 360
Porous[2])	Source Impedance (Ω)	970 ± 150	700 ± 100	1000 ± 100
Porous-Steroid[3])	Source Impedance (Ω)	800 ± 210	640 ± 180	750 ± 130

[1]) Model 6971 (N = 5)
[2]) Model IX391 (N = 3)
[3]) Model 4003 (N = 23)

Fig. 2

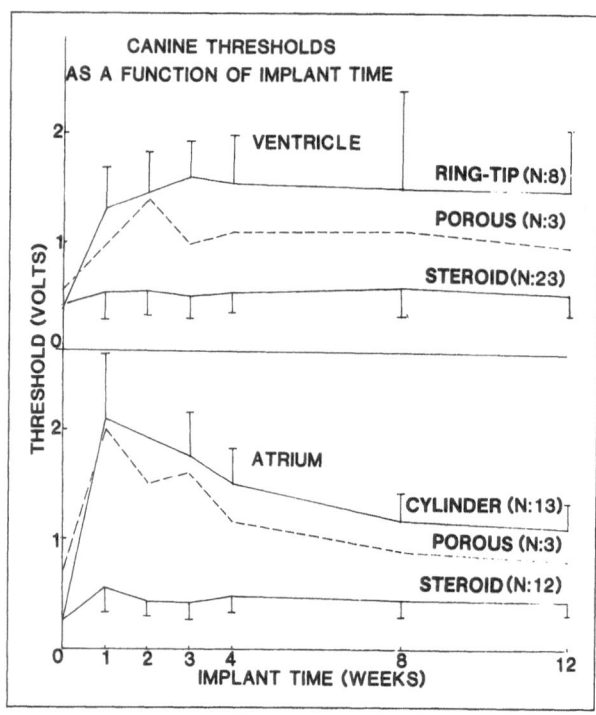

proved for the porous-steroid electrode over the cylindrical solid standard (P = 0.50), but source impedance was significantly lower (P < 0.001) (Table 2).

After a Model 7000 pacemaker spike in a dead animal, the "recharge" rises smoothly to baseline and stabilizes. In living animals, the steroid-loaded electrode shows clearly discernable paced R-, and T-wave amplitudes (Table 3). At high pacing rates and long pulse widths such as 130 bpm and 1.5 ms, Model 4003 mean RS amplitudes decrease to

Table 2. Sensing of intrinsic Canine P-waves (peak-to-peak, oscilloscope).

Electrode	Parameter	Implant Time (Weeks)		
		0	1	12
Solid Cylinder[1]	Amplitude (mV)	10 ± 4.1	4.1± 1.6	5.5± 2.5
Porous[2]	Amplitude (mV)	10 ± 3.0	5.3± 0.60	6.3± 1.5
Porous-Steroid[3]	Amplitude (mV)	7.5± 1.9	4.8± 1.7	5.6± 1.3
Solid Cylinder[1]	Source Impedance (Ω)	1300 ±230	1300 ±380	1400 ±310
Porous[2]	Source Impedance (Ω)	1100 ±400	500 ±200	800 ±300
Porous-Steroid[3]	Source Impedance (Ω)	780 ±270	570 ±170	580 ±130

[1] Model 6991U (N = 12)
[2] Model IX053 (N = 3)
[3] Model 4503 (N = 12)

zero two-weeks postimplant, then return quickly to detectable values. An acute transient capture detection loss might then be expected under such conditions. But under more commonly used conditions such as 70 bpm and 0.5 ms, canine capture detection appears to be reliable throughout the experiment. Using standard ring-tip electrodes, no paced R- or T-waves were discernable in chronic studies. Similar paced electrograms have not yet been obtained for porous-only electrodes. In the atrium, paced complexes were not as well defined, even for the porous-steroid electrode.

With one exception in our long-term studies (through one year), porous steroid thresholds, intrinsic and paced electrogram amplitudes, pacing and source impedances, etc., appeared to be essentially stable. The one exception was a polyurethane Model 4003 that developed low pacing resistance (250 Ω) and high threshold (1.1 V at 0.5 ms). At necropsy, one and one-half years postimplant, it was discovered that the endocardium was unusually smooth, devoid of trabeculae. The tines were unfixed. Fixation was accomplished only by fibrous ingrowth into the porous electrode. Due to constant rocking motion, a thick, dense, fibrous pedicle formed between the electrode and myocardium separating them by several millimeters. Five dogs with porous-steroid electrodes remain on long-term study. No significant differences have been observed between paced and unpaced leads (p < 0.05).

Discussion

Reoperation rates have been reduced from an estimated 40% in the early 1970s to 1% in 1983 by tined and screw-in leads. Good fixation allows the electrodes to do their job more reliably (2). With tined leads, high current density solid ring-tips have further improved efficiency and efficacy (3). But, the electrode's chronic performance remains a major factor in both generator design (size and longevity restrictions) and medical complications (exit block).

Pacing threshold is known to be altered by a variety of physiologic conditions and drugs (4–6). It can be increased by eating, sleeping, insulin, sodium and potassium infusions, and mineralocortacoids. Threshold is decreased by exercise, sympathomimetic drugs and

373

Table 3. Paced Peak-to-peak R-wave amplitudes using a model 7000* pacing circuit and oscilloscope (Porous-steroid electrode).

Implant Time (Weeks)	R-S Amplitudes	
	70 bpm 0.5 ms (mV)	130 bpm 1.5 ms (mV)
0	21 ±1.6	16 ±80
1	16 ±7.9	7.8± 5.3
2	9.8±1.5	0
3	18 ±2.9	7.5± 4.1
8	15 ±7.5	7.2± 6.4
12	13 ±8.4	4.2± 4.2

* Medtronic, Inc.

Fig. 3

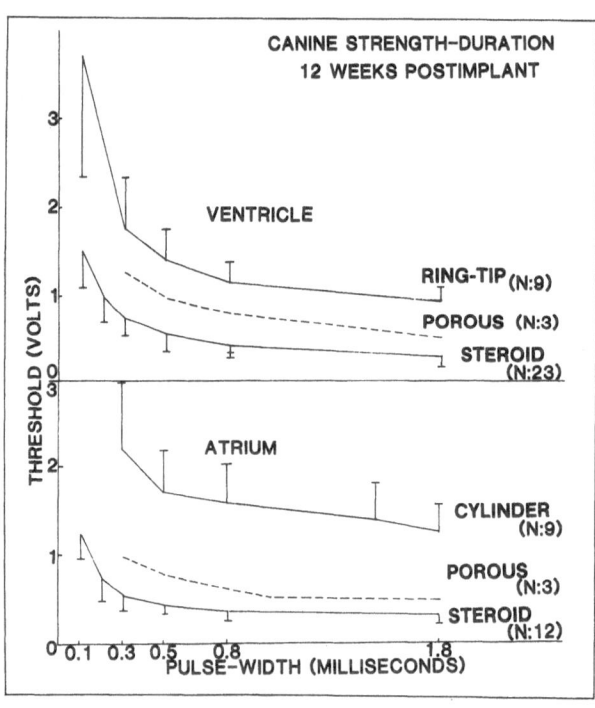

prednisone, a glucocortacoid. Following typical pacemaker implantation, pacing threshold is known to initially increase then peak or plateau within several weeks. Thus, the pulse generator must be designed to provide a safety factor. Safety factor at a given pulse width is defined as $V_{PG} \div (V_{Th} + 2SD) = SF(98)$, where the pulse generator's output is V_{PG}, threshold is V_{Th} and SD is one (threshold) standard deviation. Assuming a normal distribution, $V_{th} + 2SD$ estimates the voltage at which capture can be achieved in 98% of the population. The ring-tip electrode (as represented by Model 6971) has been very successful in its five-year human history, so we have chosen its performance as a standard. In canines we find Model 6971 to have SF(98) = 2.0 representing a 2 : 1 safety margin at 5.4 V, 0.5 ms. The porous-steroid electrode had a SF(98) of 2.4 at 2.7 V, 0.3 ms. In comparison, the porous electrode without steroid has SF(98) of 2.3 at 5.4 V, 0.3 ms – but $\leqslant$ 1.4 at 2.7 V and 0.5 ms. We thus can define the output characteristics for each lead where SF(98) $\geqslant$ 2.0 as approximately 5.4 V/0.5 ms (ring-tip), 5.4 V/0.3 ms (porous) and 2.7 V/0.3 ms (porous-steroid).

How does low threshold affect battery longevity in view of lower pacing resistance compared to the ring-tip or porous electrode without steroid? The energy (E) consumed by the lead is $V_{PG}^2 \cdot t \div R$ where t = pulse width and R = the pacing resistance. After 12 weeks implant, the energy consumed per pulse by Model 6971 at 5.4 V, 0.5 ms is approximately 25 μJ. The porous only electrode uses 13 μJ at 5.4 V, 0.3 ms; while the porous-steroid electrode at 2.7 V, 0.3 ms consumes only 5 μJ. Thus, the porous-steroid electrode used at 2.7 V, 0.3 ms can reduce battery consumption by 80% compared to the ring-tip or 60% compared to the porous electrode, while actually increasing patient safety factor.

Exit block, the failure of a normal pacemaker stimulus to elicit a propagated response due to an abnormally high threshold has been reported as the second leading cause of pacemaker failure (7). Several studies have reported successful resumption of pacing within 48–72 hours, in 50–80% of the patients following administration of prednisone, 40–80 milligram per day (7). But the development of steroid side effects eventually requires drug withdrawal. Thresholds then typically resume their upward course. So, systemic steroid therapy per se, is not a sufficient answer to achieve reliable chronic low-threshold performance. On the other hand, since the porous-steroid electrode treats only a few myocardial cells no systemic side effects can occur.

Reduced polarization improves the efficiency of the pacing pulse since less energy is wasted. Ordinarily, the discharging polarization overvoltage following a pulse interferes with and masks the paced electrogram (Figure 1). Reduced polarization, therefore, facilitates the sensing of paced beats. It also is reflected in low source impedance which means slightly less attenuation of signals by the sense amplifier.

Animal studies are necessary to establish the safety of a new device, but this does not assure comparable human efficacy. Human clinical studies are in progress under protocol control, with informed consent. So far, the new devices are performing extremely well. Mean ventricular pulse width thresholds are significantly lower than the ring-tip standard using a custom one-quarter amplitude (1.35 V) pulse generator (Spectrax SXT-L™) (9, 10). The threshold rise typically observed with standard leads has not been observed with the steroid-eluting electrode over $\geqslant$ 6 weeks study (N $\geqslant$ 25). In separate studies (as yet not reported), at least five patients with severe and repeated exit block problems have received the new device. All have remained symptom-free with low stable chronic thresholds for up to one year.

While the performance of this new electrode concept is indeed excellent, our studies suggest that the improvement is not secondary to a direct steroid membrane effect (11). Histologic studies on fibrous capsule thickness does reveal thinner membranes compared to controls. We tentatively conclude, therefore, that the drug is acting to reduce capsule thickness secondary to its anti-inflammatory action (11). Further research is in progress, both the deleniate the causes of normal fibrotic tissue formation and the action of corticosteroid in this device.

References

1. Irnich W: Comparison of Pacing Electrodes of Different Shape and Material Recommendations, Pace, 1983; 6: 422–426.
2. Stokes KB and Stephenson NL: The Implantable Cardiac Pacing Lead – Just a Simple Wire? In The Third Decade of Cardiac Pacing, Barold SS and Mugica J (Eds), Mount Kisko, NY, Futura, 1982: 365–416.
3. Pirzada FA and Seltzer J: Clinical Experience With the Medtronic 6971 Polyurethane Lead, Pace 1983: 6 (Abstract).
4. Preston TA and Judge RD: Alteration of Pacemaker Threshold by Drug and Physiological Factors. Ann NY Acad Sci 1969; 167: 686–692.
5. Sowton E and Barr I: Physiological Changes in Threshold. Ann NY Acad Sci, 1969; 167: 679–685.
6. Gettes LS, Shabetai R, Downs TA, et al: Effect of changes in potassium and calcium concentrations on diastolic threshold and strength interval relationships of the human heart. Ann NY Acad Sci, 1969; 167: 693–705.
7. Beanlands DS, Akyurekli Y and Keon WJ: Prednisone in the management of exit block. In Meere, C (ed) Proceedings of the VI World Symposium on Cardiac Pacing. Montreal, Pacesymp, 1979, Chapter 18–3.
8. Thiele G, Lachmann W, Eschemann et al: Zur Beeinflussung des Reizschwellenanstieges nach Herzschrittmacher Implantation durch Prednisolon. Zeitschrift für die gesamte Innere Medizin. 1980; 35: 863–866.
9. Gordon S, Timmis GE, Westveer DE, et al: A New Low Threshold Steroid-Eluting Pacing Lead. Proceedings, VII World Symposium on Cardiac Pacing.
10. Parsonnet V and Werres R: Clinical Experience With a Porous-Tip Steroid-Loaded Ventricular Pacing Electrode. Pace 1983; 6: 319 (abstract).
11. Stokes KB, Kriett JM, Gornick CA, et al: Low Threshold Cardiac Pacing Electrodes. Accepted for Proceedings – Fifth Annual Conference IEEE Engineering in Medicine and Biology Society, 1983.

Authors' address:
Kenneth Stokes
Medtronic, Inc.
3055 Old Highway Eight
POB 1453
Minneapolis, MN. 55440
USA

Resistive Equivalent of Lead Impedance

E. A. Astrinsky, S. Furman

Summary: The lead impedance "seen" by a pulse generator during the stimulating pulse varies over the pulse duration. It is a complex function of lead conductor resistance, tissue bulk resistance, and polarization phenomena which depend on electrode tip area and material, electrolyte concentrations, temperature, and stimulus intensity. Circuit models from resistors to non-linear series-parallel networks have been described. In 6 patients at pulse generator replacement, a Medtronic 5985 pulse generator was connected to the exposed proximal end of 4 types of chronic leads from 3 manufacturers. Stimulating pulse current and voltage waveforms were acquired and stored on floppy disks using a digital oscilloscope. The in-vivo charge per pulse, Qiv, mean pulse voltage, $\bar{V}$, and mean pulse current, $\bar{I}$, were calculated using the oscilloscope's computing capability. The mean equivalent impedance, $\bar{Z} = \bar{V}/\bar{I}$ were derived for pulse durations of 0.1, 0.5, 0.9 and 1.5 ms at 2.7 V and 5 V programmed pulse generator outputs. For the 36 measurements, $\bar{Z}$ ranged from 220 to 720 ohms and Qiv ranged from 0.5 to 14.5 μC. Resistive loads R' = $\bar{Z}$ were connected to the pulse generator programmed to the output used in determining $\bar{Z}$, and the charge, Qr, was measured as before. A graph of Qr vs Qiv was plotted. Using linear regression analysis it was found that Qr = 1.007 Qiv − 0.03 with a standard error of 0.003. Thus the charge per pulse measured when using a resistor equal to the magnitude of the mean impedance is very nearly equal to the charge per pulse delivered to a heart-electrode combination, provided the pulse generator is programmed to the same output settings. Hence a resistor equal to the mean equivalent impedance at a measured pulse generator output can be used to determine the charge per pulse, pulse generator battery current drain and estimated pulse generator longevity. Knowledge of the complex lead impedance is unnecessary.

Most implantable cardiac pacemakers have "constant voltage" capacitor coupled output circuits. The mean output current per pulse is determined primarily by the load impedance connected across the output terminals, decreasing as the load impedance increases. If the load is an in-vivo pacemaking lead, the impedance rises during the pacemaker output pulse due to electrochemical polarization effects occuring at the electrode electrolyte interface. Thus mean current per pulse falls with increasing pulse duration (Figure 1).

It has been shown that the charge per pulse is the electrical parameter primarily involved in the stimulation process (1). Charge per pulse at a pulse duration, t, can be calculated from the formula

$$Q(t) = \bar{I}.t \qquad [1]$$

where $\bar{I}$ is the mean current per pulse. Hence the impedance of the lead-electrode-heart combination determines the charge output of the pulse generator. If the output charge is above the threshold charge requirements at a particular pulse duration, then cardiac capture will result.

The impedance "seen" by the pulse generator during the stimulating pulse is a function of both linear and non-linear elements in the lead-electrode-heart circuit. Resistive portions of the circuit are the lead conductor resistance, and the bulk resistance of the return path of current from the stimulating cathodal electrode to the anodal indifferent electrode. The anode may form part of a bipolar lead or be the pacemaker can. Nonlinear and time dependent effects take place at the electrode-electrolyte interface where electron flow in the electrode changes to ionic flow in the electrolyte. A non-linear capacitor

Fig. 1. Graphs of mean voltage, $\overline{V}$, mean current, $\overline{I}$, and charge output per pulse, Q, as functions of pulse duration for the 5985 pulse generator programmed to 2.7 volt output. The mean equivalent impedance, $\overline{Z} = \overline{V}/\overline{I}$, increases as the pulse duration is increased.

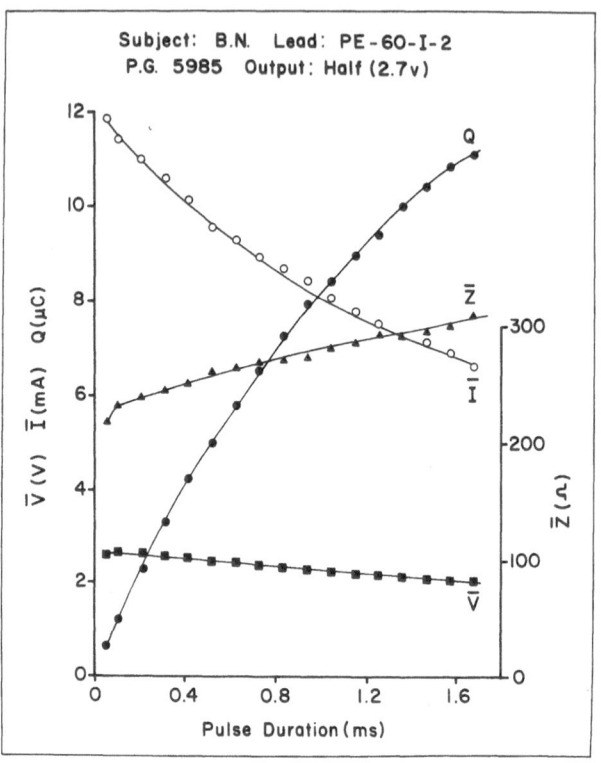

forms at the interface, influenced by current density, area of the electrode, electrode material, surface treatment of the electrode, and the electrolyte. In addition there are effects of temperature, ion concentration and electrolyte composition. Equivalent circuits comprising series and parallel combinations of electronic components including variable resistors, voltage dependent capacitors and Zener diodes have been used with varying success to model the behaviour of the electrode-electrolyte interface impedance (1, 2, 3, 4).

We have investigated the effects of resistive loading on output programmable pulse generators (5). This provided a method of estimating the pulse duration at which threshold occurs for a given heart-electrode combination connected to an output programmable pulse generator (6), as well as the effect of voltage and pulse duration variation on charge safety factor (7). A study was undertaken to test the validity of the assumption that a resistor equal in value to the mean equivalent impedance of the electrode-heart circuit (measured in vivo), results in equal charge per pulse output when either the lead or resistor are connected to an output programmable pulse generator. The mean equivalent impedance has been defined (8).

Mean electrode impedance during stimulation

$$= \frac{\text{Mean value of the stimulating voltage pulse}}{\text{Mean value of the stimulating current pulse}} \qquad [2]$$

$$\overline{Z} = \overline{V}/\overline{I} \qquad [3]$$

378

Materials and methods

In six patients undergoing pulse generator replacement a Medtronic* 5985 output programmable pulse generator was connected to the exposed proximal end of 4 models of
chronically implanted leads from three manufacturers. The circuit was completed by a 30
cm area stainless steel metal plate forming the indifferent electrode. The pulse duration
was decreased from 1.7 to 0.1 milliseconds (where possible) in 0.1 millisecond steps in
the "autothreshold" mode for programmed amplitudes of 5 V (Full) and 2.7 V (Half).
Output pulse voltage and current waveforms acquired at a 2 MHz sampling rate and with
12 bit precision were stored on floppy disks using a Nicolet** 4094 digital oscilloscope
(9). Using the 4094's waveform analysis programs and computing capability the mean
voltage per pulse, $\overline{V}$ in volts, and mean current per pulse, I in milliamperes, were found
by integrating the voltage and current waveforms and dividing these values by the pulse
duration. The area under the current waveform the charge per pulse for the in-vivo
measurements (Qiv) in microcoulombs. The mean equivalent impedance, $\overline{Z}$ was calculated
for each measurement using equation [3].

With the generator output programmed to the pulse duration and voltage used in each of
the above in-vivo measurements, a decade resistor box was connected in place of the
lead-electrode-heart load and adjusted to a resistance value R', where R' = $\overline{Z}$. The
charge per pulse (Qr) was then measured using the digital oscilloscope.

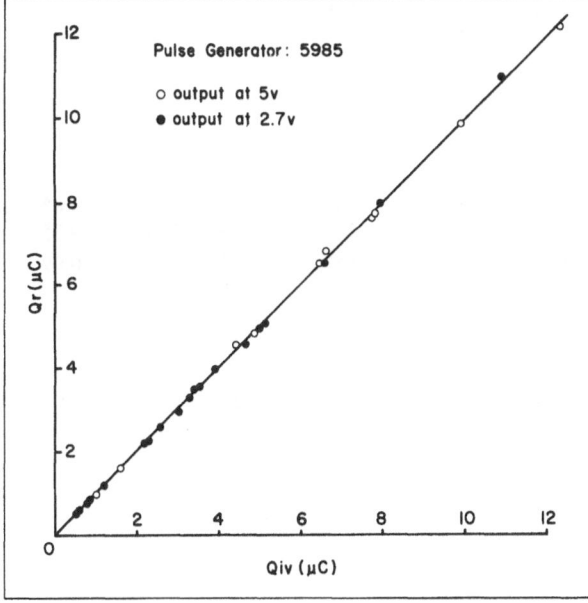

Fig. 2. Graph of charge per pulse with a resistive load, Qr, versus charge per pulse with an in-vivo pacemaking lead, Qiv. For both measurements the pulse generator was programmed to the same output amplitude (2.7 or 5 V) and pulse duration (0.1, 0.5, 0.9 and 1.5 ms) for the resistive load R' set equal to the mean equivalent impedance, $\overline{Z}$.

---

* Medtronic, Inc., Minneapolis, Minnesota
** Nicolet Instrument Corp., Madison, Wisconsin

Results

Table 1 lists the result of the above measurements. The regression line of the 36 values of Qr vs Qiv (Figure 2) for pulse durations of 0.1, 0.5, 0.9 and 1.5 ms at both Half and Full amplitudes was found to be:

Qr = 1.007 Qiv – 0.03 with a standard error of 0.003 μC.

Discussion

From the results it can be seen that the mean equivalent impedance of a given lead-electrode-heart combination, $\overline{Z}$, can be considered to be a pure resistance at any particular programmed pacemaker output pulse duration and amplitude. Connection of this re-

Table 1. Charge output from in-vivo and in-vitro measurements.

Subj.	Pulse Dura.	At "Half" Amplitude				At "Full" Amplitude			
		$\overline{Z}$	Qiv	R'	Qr	$\overline{Z}$	Qiv	R'	Qr
	ms	ohms	μC	ohms	μC	ohms	μC	ohms	μC
MD	0.1	335	0.87	330	0.87	328	1.62	330	1.60
	0.5	419	3.30	420	3.28	384	6.46	380	6.50
	0.9	466	5.11	470	5.07	431	9.87	430	9.88
DB	0.1	455	0.65	450	0.66	433	1.25	430	1.25
	0.5	626	2.30	630	2.27	538	4.79	540	4.75
	0.9	706	3.56	710	3.53	577	7.71	580	7.63
MF	0.1	–	–	–	–	441	1.23	440	1.22
	0.5	553	2.58	550	2.57	531	4.84	530	4.83
	0.9	641	3.90	640	3.87	573	7.76	570	7.75
MM	0.1	557	0.54	560	0.53	546	1.01	550	0.99
	0.5	648	2.20	650	2.21	575	4.41	570	4.52
	0.9	721	3.40	720	3.49	658	6.62	660	6.80
BD	0.1	372	0.79	370	0.78	341	1.56	340	1.55
	0.5	466	3.02	470	2.96	396	6.29	400	6.23
	0.9	526	4.64	530	4.57	430	9.86	430	9.88
	1.5	592	6.57	590	6.52	–	–	–	–
BN	0.1	232	1.21	230	1.21	216	2.35	220	2.30
	0.5	260	4.98	260	4.97	–	–	–	–
	0.9	270	7.94	270	8.00	260	14.5	260	14.6
	1.5	300	10.9	300	11.00				

$\overline{Z}$ is average impedance of lead-electrode-heart circuit
Qiv is charge per pulse measured with load of $\overline{Z}$
R' is resistive load equal to $\overline{Z}$
Qr is charge per pulse measured with resistive load R'
"Half" is 2.7 volt peak pulse generator output
"Full" is 5 volt peak pulse generator output

sistor to the output terminals will result in the same charge per pulse being delivered to the load and therefore should result in the same current being drawn from the pulse generator's power source.

The above does not imply that the impedance of the lead-electrode-heart combination is either linear or independent of pulse duration. The inference from the data is that the absolute value of the mean equivalent impedance found from actual simultaneous voltage and current waveform measurements can be modeled by an equivalent resistor to measure the effect of load variation on pulse generator output and longevity. This is useful when testing new pacemaker output circuits.

The variation in mean equivalent impedance with output amplitude, and pulse duration measured in this study, draws attention to the shortcomings involved in using 500 ohms as a standard test resistor for comparing pulse generator output and longevity.

References

1. Babotai I: Die elektrochemischen Impedanzen und die elektrische Reizschwelle des Herzens bei Stimulation mit Schrittmachern. Doctoral Thesis, Eidgenössische Technische Hochschule Zürich, Diss Nr. 1971, 4618.
2. Sluyters-Rehbach M, Sluyters JH: in AJ Bard (ed): Electroanalytical Chemistry. New York, Marcel Dekker, 1970, p. 3–128.
3. De Boer RW, van Oosterom A: Electrical properties of platinum electrodes: impedance and time-domain analysis. Med Biol Eng Comput 1978; 16: 1–10.
4. Fischler H: Polarization properties of small-surface-area pacemaker electrodes-implications on reliability of sensing and pacing. Pace 1979; 2: 403–416.
5. Astrinsky EA, Parker B, Furman S: Charge output of programmable pacemakers-effect of resistive loading. Pace 1980; 3: 362 (Abstract).
6. Astrinsky, EA, Parker B, Furman S: Graphical method for estimating pacing threshold. G. A. Feruglio (Ed): Cardiac Pacing – Electrophysiology and Pacemaker Technology. Padova, Piccin Medical Books, 1982, pp 109–111.
7. Astrinsky EA, Furman S: Pacemaker output programming for maximum safety and maximum longevity. Clin Prog Pacing Electrophysiol 1983; 1: 51–58.
8. Hammer E, Ohm OJ: The pacemaker electrode stimulating impedance and after potential. In Cardiac Pacing. C. Meere ed. Pacesymp Pub. Montreal, Chap 43–4 (1979).
9. Astrinsky EA, Furman S: Output programmable pulse generator adjustment: pulse duration or amplitude. Proc 7th World Symp on Cardiac Pacing. Vienna, 1983 (in press).

Authors' address:
E. A. Astrinsky, Ph.D.
Montefiore Medical Center
111 East 210th Street
Bronx, N.Y. 10467 USA

Effect of Pore Size on Threshold and Impedance of Pacemaker Electrodes

M. S. Hirshorn*, L. K. Holley*, M. Skalsky*, H. Mond**, A. Gale***,
S. Stewart *

Summary: The effect of pore size on threshold and pacing impedance of two sintered porous platinum electrodes was evaluated using non porous electrodes as controls.

Seventeen 8 mm² non-porous (NP), 17, 8 mm² large porous (LP) (200 micron diameter spheres) and 16, 8 mm² small porous (SP) (80 micron diameter spheres) were implanted, together with an Impedance and Threshold Measuring Pulse Generator in 32 male and 18 female patients with a mean age of 72 years. There was an attrition rate of 12% due to pacemaker unrelated death. No patients were treated with cardioactive drugs during the study.

The results indicate that there is no significant difference among the 3 electrode types over a 6 month period for threshold and pacing impedance. This study has shown that the porosity of pacemaker electrodes does not influence the acute or chronic values of threshold or pacing impedance.

Introduction

Over recent years, more sophisticated multiprogrammable and dual chamber pacemakers have gained acceptance. The increased complexity of their electronic circuitry has often resulted in a higher internal current drain. To offset the associated reduction in pulse generator lifetime, efforts have been made to increase the electrode pacing impedance by reducing the geometric surface area. However, the extent to which surface area can be reduced is limited by the resultant increase in sensing impedance (1, 2). As a step toward electrode optimisation, porous electrodes with an increased microsurface area have been developed (3, 4). The interconnecting channels within porous electrodes also augment attachment by tissue ingrowth. A reduction of stimulation threshold has also been reported in animals (4), but this has been disputed by a number of studies (5, 6) in humans. Limited data has been available on pacing impedance in humans.

The objective of this study was to evaluate the effect of pore size on threshold and pacing impedance of two sintered porous platinum electrodes using non-porous electrodes as controls, in humans.

Method

Two porous electrode tips were developed with an 8 mm² geometric area. Both were fabricated from sintered platinum spheres. One with a sphere diameter of 200 micron and the other with a sphere diameter of 80 micron.

---

* Bioengineering Research Centre, Telectronics, Sydney
** Royal Melbourne Hospital, Melbourne
*** St Vincents Hospital, Sydney

383

An Impedance and Threshold Measuring Pulse Generator (7, 8) was used to take measurements of the voltage threshold and pacing impedance at 1 and 2 days then at 1, 4, 13 and 26 weeks post implant. The frequent early measurements were taken to ensure documentation of the early threshold rise. All patients signed a consent form before admission to the study. The study was performed independently in two hospitals according to the same protocol.

Results

Seventeen 8 mm^2 non porous (NP), 17, 8 mm^2 large porous (LP) (200 micron diameter spheres) and 16, 8 mm^2 small porous (SP) (80 micron diameter spheres) were implanted, in 32 male and 18 female patients with a mean age of 72 years. The results of the acute and chronic threshold voltage and pacing impedance are shown in table 1. Using a one-way analysis of variance statistical test, there was no significant difference in voltage threshold or pacing impedance for the three electrode types at any post implant period.

Discussion and Conclusion

A number of studies in dogs have suggested that porous electrodes may result in a reduced stimulation threshold (3, 4). If confirmed in humans this would offer a potential reduction of pulse generator output requirements and consequently increased longevity. However, other studies have found no reduction in voltage threshold (5, 6). The availability of the impedance and threshold measuring pacemaker has made possible, the measurement of voltage threshold and pacing impedance with sufficient precision to enable an evaluation of the electrical properties of the three electrode types.

These results indicate that there is no significant difference among the two pore size and the non-porous electrodes over a 6 month period for threshold and pacing impedance.

A second result of interest, confirming some recent animal studies is that the threshold reaches a plateau rather than an acute "hump". The pacing impedance measurements

Table 1.

	Electrode type	Post implant time					
		1 day	2 days	1 wk	4 wks	3 mth	6 mth
Threshold	NP	0.48	0.67	1.41	1.41	1.49	1.60
voltage	LP	0.59	0.76	1.43	1.73	1.69	1.48
(volts)	SP	0.40	0.57	1.63	1.80	1.77	1.44
Pacing	NP	766	705	662	821	881	866
impedance	LP	754	674	622	785	866	910
(ohms)	SP	720	621	569	806	858	851

NP – non Porous
LP – large Porous
SP – small Porous

showed an impedance stabilization over the first 4 weeks of implant and little variation thereafter. The similar impedance values for the porous and solid tip electrodes confirm that the micro-surface area of the tip has negligible influence on pacing impedance.

Measurements of sensing impedance and attachment status are not possible with this system, but animal studies have shown an improvement in sensing and attachment characteristics for porous electrodes (9).

This clinical study has shown that the porosity of pacemaker electrodes does not influence the acute and chronic values of voltage threshold or pacing impedance.

Acknowledgement.

This project was assisted by the Department of Science and Technology, ACT, Australia.

References

1. Hughes Jr, HC, Brownlee RR, Tyers GFO: "Failure of Demand Pacing with Small Surface Electrodes", Circulation 1976; 54: 128.
2. Fischler H, "Polarization Properties of Small Surface Area Pacemaker Electrodes – Implications on Reliability of Sensing and Pacing", PACE, 1979; 2: 403.
3. MacGregor DC, Wilson GJ, Lixfield WL, Pilliar RM, Bobyn JD, Silver MD, Smardon S, Miller SL: "The Porous Surfaced Electrode – A New Concept in Pacemaker Lead Design", J Thorac Cardiovasc Surg 1979; 78: 281.
4. Amundson DC, McArthur W, Mosharrafa M: "The Porous Endocardial Electrode", PACE, 1979; 2: 40.
5. Breivik K, Ohm O-J, Dregelid E et al: "Electrophysiological characteristics of porous electrodes versus solid ones", PACE 1981; 4: A5 (Abstract).
6. Goioclea A, Serrano G, Wilhelm M et al: "Clinical evaluation of a porous tip electrode", PACE, 1981; 4: A48 (Abstract).
7. Hirshorn MS, Holley LK, Daly CM et al: "Impedance and Threshold Measuring Pulse Generator", PACE, 1981; 4: A88 (Abstract).
8. Daly CM, Hirshorn MS, Money DK, Holley LK: "Impedance Measuring Pacer", US Patent 4,337,776.
9. Hirshorn MS, Holley LK, Skalsky M et al: "Evaluation of Porous and Non-Porous Platinum as Cardiac Pacemaker Electrode Tips", PACE, 1981; 4: A88 (Abstract).

Authors' address:
Loraine K. Holley, m. App. Sc
Telectronics Pty. Ltd.
14 Mars Road
Sydney 2066
Australia

A Comparison Study of Chronaxie, Rheobase and Threshold Values for Solid, Porous and Carbon Tip Electrodes

Feliu Antúnez, Antonio Goicolea, Javier Belaza

Summary: The importance of strength duration (SD) curves as a method to asses (1) the electrical characteristics of different electrodes for pacing, as well as (2) the patient safety margin for stimulation with modern multiprogrammable units, has been recently reported by Irnich [1]. Various electrode designs to optimally match electrodes to pulse generators have been developed by several manufacturers; i.e. solid, ring, porous and carbon tip electrodes. To study the characteristics of these electrodes, one hundred electrodes of different types: 50 porous, 7.5–9 mm² surface (SA); 40 solid, 8–12 mm² (SA); 10 carbon tip have been implanted and evaluated using acute, voltage SD curves at various pulse widths ranging from 0.05 to 2.0 ms. A linear regression computer programm was used to calculate Chronaxie (C) and Rheobase (R) values. Acute and chronic thresholds (pulse width) were also obtained for most of the implanted electrodes. The correlation coefficient of linear regression for a majority of the SD curves was greater than 0.97. The smallest average chronaxie points from the SD curves were obtained with porous (0.30) and the smallest average Rheobase with the carbon tip electrode (0.16). Solid tip electrodes of smaller surface areas (8 mm²) exhibited lower chronaxie points as compared to solid electrodes with larger surface areas (12 mm²). Although porous electrodes acutely have lower thresholds as compared to solid electrodes, these differences were chronically statistically significant only for electrodes of different surface areas.
Chronaxie. Threshold measurements. Pacing electrodes.

Material and methods

One hundred implantation records were revised using a common protocol in our two hospitals. From the one hundred initially selected those who had not – enough points to calculate Chronaxie and Rheobase accurately were discarded. Also in order to compare only results from groups of a reasonably large sample size, those who had not more than five electrodes from the same manufacturer were discarded. As a consequence, the initial group was reduced to 80 electrodes. All electrodes studied were unipolar. The number and type of electrodes used is given in Table 1.
Thresholds were measured using a conventional pacing system analyzer (Cardiotest). All implantations were performed under local anesthesia. Measurements were taken using an indifferent plate electrode, placed in the pacemaker pocket and connected to the positive terminal. Output voltage initially set to 5 volts, was gradually decreased until one-to-one capture was lost and then increased to a value for which capture was consistent again, this value was taken as voltage threshold. Five to eight points were taken for most of the electrodes at different pulse widths ranging from 0.05 to 2.0 ms. Chronically for most of the electrodes implanted with a programmable pulse generator, pulse width stimulation threshold was measured by decreasing pulse width from the initial value to the minor pulse width in which a constant ventricular capture was reached. A linear regression computer program in BASIC was used to calculate Chronaxie and Rheobase from the acute voltage Strength-Duration curves. Correlation coefficient as well as estimated standard deviation, were calculated to evaluate the consistency of curve-fitting and measurements.

Table 1. Electrodes used

N	Manufacturer	Surface area	Tip
8	4110 CPI	12 mm²	solid
16	6971 Medtronic	8 mm²	ring
38	4116/4150 CPI	7.5-8 mm²	porous tined (4150)
7	2147 LOE Vitatron	7.6 mm²	ring
6	411S Siemens	12 mm²	carbon
5	Cordis porous	8.8 mm²	porous

Results

Results are presented giving average values and std.dev. for each group of electrodes for Chronaxie, Rheobase, Cr × Rh and chronic threshold if available for an average follow-up period greater than 12 months either in ms. or volts for those pulse generators using some type of non invasive voltage threshold such as Vitatron or Siemens "Vario" systems. After statistical comparison using Student's "t" test, the following results were obtained:

1. CPI porous had Chronaxie and Cr × Rh values significantly lower than CPI 4110 ($p < 0.05$ and $p < 0.01$).
2. Differences on Medtronic 6971 and CPI porous did not reach statistical significance.
3. Vitatron 2147 exhibit higher Chronaxie than CPI porous and Medtronic 6971, but lower Rheobase although there was no difference in the Cr × Rh products.
4. Siemens 411S exhibit only Rh value significantly lower than CPI porous.
5. Cordis porous electrode did not show any difference with either CPI porous or Medtronic 6971.

Although chronic threshold data was limited, CPI porous exhibited significantly ($p < 0.05$) lower thresholds than CPI 4110, but Medtronic 6971 values were not statistically different to those of CPI 4110.

Table 2. Results

Electrode	N	Cr	Rh	Cr × Rh	Chronic threshold
CPI 4110	8	0.37 ± 0.17	0.39 ± 0.17	0.16 ± 0.07.	0.11 ms. ± 0.06
CPI 4116/4150	38	0.30 ± 0.06	0.37 ± 0.09	0.11 ± 0.04	0.08 ms. ± 0.03 1.18 vol. for n = 3
Medtronic 6971	16	0.31 ± 0.06	0.34 ± 0.07	0.10 ± 0.02	0.08 ms. ± 0.05
Vitatron 2147 LOE	7	0.38 ± 0.15	0.23 ± 0.04	0.09 ± 0.03	1.82 volts ± 0.17
Siemens 411S	6	0.38 ± 0.21	0.16 ± 0.09	0.07 ± 0.04	1.2 volts for 2 electrodes
Cordis porous	5	0.36 ± 0.18	0.17 ± 0.09	0.07 ± 0.04	non available

Vitatron chronic voltage threshold was higher than both Siemens 411S and CPI porous electrodes (1.82 vs 1.2 and 1.18 volts respectively). The porous chronic average voltage threshold is in accordance with other studies (Amudson 1.1 volts [2], and Herbinger 1.3 volts [3]). Pulse width used in all cases was 0.5 ms.

Discussion

Different approaches have been used by several manufacturers to improve the electrical characteristics of electrodes. As it was pointed out by Irnich during last Cardiostim Congress in Paris [4] several factors should be considered for the ideal electrode:
1. Low Chronic Threshold.
2. Moderate threshold elevation during the maturation process.
3. Low tendence to displace.
4. Low sensing impedance.
Threshold values are related to different electrode characteristics such as tip surface area, [5, 7, 8], shape, microstructure (rough, porous), material and stress to the myocardium wall. These factors led to a specific fibrotic-capsule thickness that can be estimated by the well known relationship [9]:

$$d = r_0 \left(\sqrt{\frac{V_{cr}}{V_{ac}}} - 1 \right) \tag{1}$$

Being r_0 the electrode radium and V_{cr}, V_{ac} the chronic and acute voltage threshold respectively.
From a practical point of view, with modern multiprogrammable units we are mainly concerned about adjusting pulse width and voltage output values to have a "known" pacing system margin avoiding unnecessary loss of energy and increasing pulse generator longevity. Although Chronaxie and Rheobase are known from the beginning of this century. An excellent review of its potential importance was recently presented [4]. Neither its full meaning, nor its real clinical application has been totally recognized.
Unconsistency of threshold data available has probably contributed to the former situation. However, several studies have shown that electrodes of smaller surface areas exhibit lower Chronaxies and so pulse width can be reduced without a significant loss of safety [1, 6, 10].
As we are using only constant voltage generators, we are only concerned about voltage Chronaxie for different electrodes. Acute Chronaxies can easily be calculated from strength-duration curves using either a progammable calculator or a personal computer implementing a least-squares linear regression program.
The Chronaxie – Rheobase formula to describe the voltage threshold pulse width relationship is:

$$V(t) = Rh \left(1 + \frac{Cr}{t} \right) \tag{2}$$

with: V(t) the voltage threshold
Rh the Rheobase
Cr the Chronaxie
and t the pulse duration, being Rh the lowest voltage threshold for an infinite pulse duration and Cr the pulse duration at which threshold voltage is twice that of the Rheobase.

Although the hyperbolic function plot is similar to the strength-duration curve, practical use and understanding of the Cr and Rh meanings is not so evident. We have decided to use instead a different way to – present Cr and Rh values and meanings in a more clear representation in our opinion. Using the change of variable

$$z = \frac{1}{t}$$

(3)

(2) can be expresed as

$$V(z) = Rh\,(1 + z.\,Cr)$$

(4)

The meaning of Rh and Cr is given in Figure 1, with V_o the output voltage of the pulse generator and t_h the corresponding pulse width threshold value. The relationship between $V(z)$ and z is linear with a slope given by $Cr \times Rh$ which as we will show later is a very important factor when comparing electrical characteristics for pacing of different electrodes. Also a least-squares linear regression algorithm can easily be applied to (3).

If the strength-duration curve is accurately described by the hyperbolic function (2) and if V_o is the value of the output voltage for a given pacemaker, the pulse width threshold t_h can be estimated by:

$$t_h = \frac{Cr \times Rh}{V_o - Rh}$$

(5)

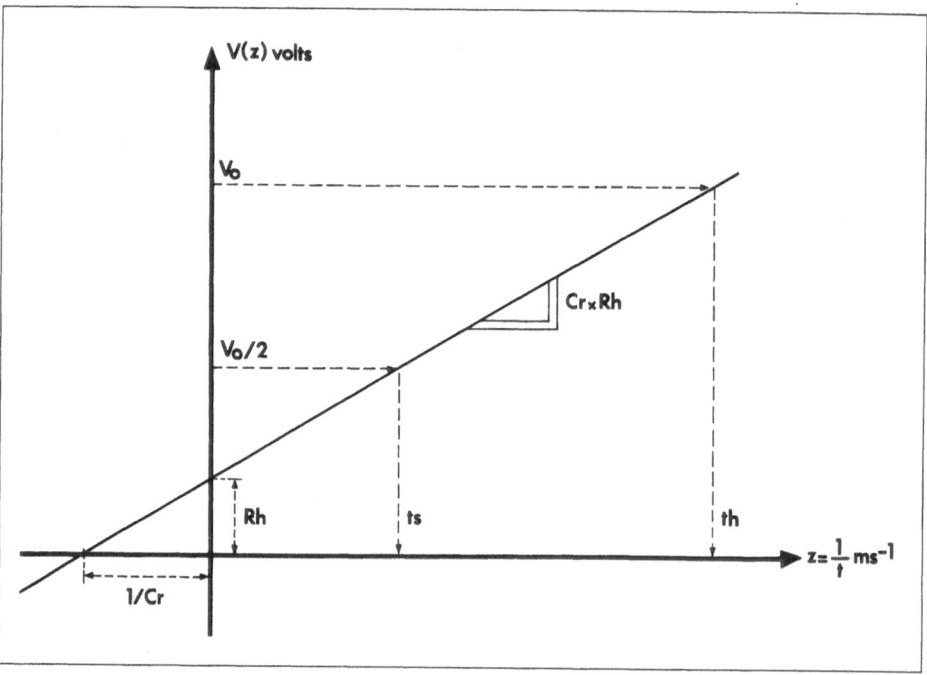

Figure 1: Linear representation of V(z) including Cr = Chronaxie, Rh = Rheobase, Cr × Rh = slope (Chronaxie – Rheobase product), th = pulse width threshold for V_o and ts = 100% safety margin pulse width.

As it can be easily deduced from (5), the Cr × Rh product works as a "quality factor" for a given electrode because t_h would be smaller for smaller Cr × Rh values [4]. So it is not only the Chronaxie value which is important to evaluate the pacing characteristics of an electrode but both Chronaxie and Rheobase and their product. Using same definition of $t_s = 100\%$ safety pulse duration as Irnich [1], Figure 1, and (5) t_s can be calculated by:

$$t_s = \frac{2\,Cr}{\dfrac{Cr}{t_h} - 1} = \frac{2 \cdot Cr \times Rh}{V_o - 2 \cdot Rh} = \frac{Cr \times Rh}{\dfrac{V_o}{2} - Rh} \tag{6}$$

In general, if we define f_s as a safety factor, knowing the "chronic" values for Rheobase and Chronaxie and the output voltage, the pulse width for a "real known safety margin" can be determined as

$$\overline{C} = \frac{Cr \times Rh}{\dfrac{V_o}{f_s} - Rh} \tag{7}$$

As a numeric example if Rh = 0.92 volts
Cr = 0.44 ms., $V_o = 5$ volts.
Using the same representation as in Figure 1, we can see the relationship among different factors; Figure 2.
For $\overline{C} = 0.1$ ms. capture would be lost for 5 volts output.

With $\overline{C} = 0.26$, voltage threshold would be 2.5 volts and so $f_s = \dfrac{5}{2.5} = 2$ that gives a

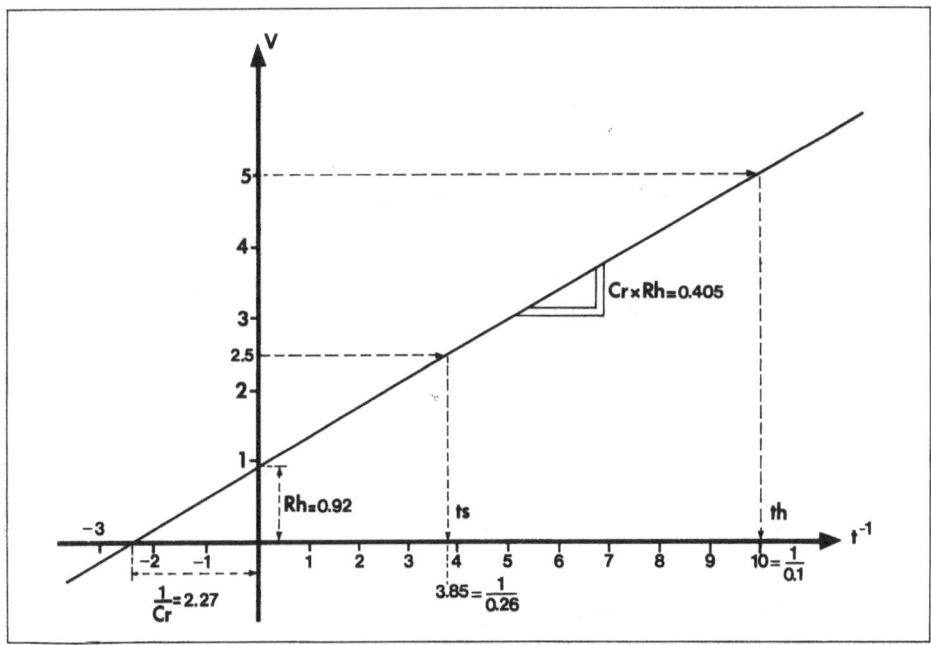

Figure 2: Calculation of th and ts for Rh = 0.92 and Cr = 0.44.

100% safety margin. If the pulse width used was $\overline{C} = 0.6$ ms. $f_s = 3.13$; 56% higher but 2.31 times energy consumption. This agrees with the fact that pulse widths greater than the Chronaxie lead to a greater consumption without reaching a similar increase in safety margin and as a consequence with an unnecessary loss of longevity. Normalized plot of the safety factor $f_s \cdot \dfrac{Rh}{V_o}$ versus the pulse width divided by the Chronaxie $\overline{C}/Cr$ is given in Figure 3.

$$f_s = \frac{V_o}{V(\overline{C})} = \frac{V_o}{Rh\left(1 + \dfrac{Cr}{\overline{C}}\right)} \rightarrow \frac{f_s \cdot Rh}{V_o} = \frac{\overline{C}/Cr}{1 + \overline{C}/Cr} \tag{8}$$

Regions I and II in Figure 3 correspond respectively to pulse width ranges with and without a steep increase of the safety factor; that makes pulse width right of the Chronaxie point very inefficient. Two important conclusions can be reached from the former discussion:

1. Both Chronaxie and Rheobase as well as its product, are very important factors to compare electrical characteristics for pacing of different electrodes. Mainly, the Chronaxie – Rheobase product can be used as a "quality factor" to compare different electrodes, the smaller the better would be the safety factor and the smaller the 100% safety pulse width t_s (6), [1].

2. The calculation of the most adequate pulse width for a given electrode pulse generator combination with a known safety margin maintaining a good pacing efficiency can be done by means of (7) if the values of Chronaxie, Rheobase and output voltage could be evaluated Chronically.

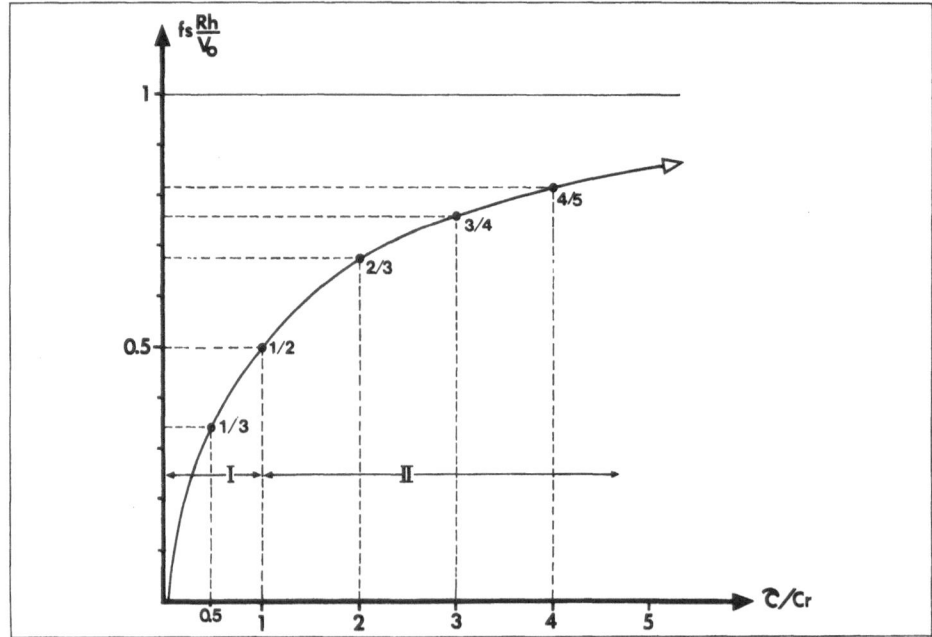

Figure 3: Normalized safety factor.

From our results CPI porous exhibit the lowest acute Chronaxie in ms. of all electrodes. Siemens Carbon tip electrode had the lowest acute Rheobase although we must point out the small sample size in this case. As far as acute Cr × Rh is concerned, no statistically significant difference was found except between the largest solid tip electrode CPI 4110 (12 mm²) and CPI porous electrode. Although the chronic data is limited, CPI porous exhibited significant lower pulse width threshold than CPI 4110. Medtronic 6971 pulse width threshold were not statistically different from CPI porous. Vitatron 2147 LOE although had a low acute Cr × Rh, chronically exhibited a voltage threshold higher than both Siemens and CPI porous electrodes. From our experience, CPI 4116/4150, Siemens 411S and Medtronic 6971 electrodes gave both acute and chronic low values compared with the rest of electrodes.

The most important conclusion of this study has been the outstanding importance of Chronaxie, Rheobase and its product using a new graphic representation to calculate pulse width for a given safety margin.

References

1. Irnich W: The Chronaxie time and its practical importance. Pace 1980; 3: 292–301.
2. Amudson DC, MCarthur W, Mosharrafa M: The porous endocardial electrode. Pace 1979; 2: 40.
3. Herbinger W, Habacher W, MacCarter D: Invasive Subchronic assessment of porous endocardial electrode performance in humans. Pace 1981; 4: A 51.
4. Irnich W: Comparison of Pacing electrodes of different shape and materialrecommendations. Pace 1983; 6: 422–426.
5. Furman S, Parker B, Escher DJW: Endocardial threshold of Cardiac response as a function of electrode surface area. J Surg Res 1968; 8: 161.
6. Kleinert M, Irnich W, Beer P: Comparative studies of threshold after implantation of pacemaker leads of different size. Z Kardiol 1977; 66: 191–197.
7. Smyth NPD, Tarjan PP, Chernoff E, Baker N: The significance of electrode surface area and stimulating thresholds in permanent cardiac pacing. J Thorac Cardiovasc Surg 1976; 71: 559–565.
8. Furman S, Garvey J, Hurzeler Ph: Pulse duration variation and electrode size as a factor in pacemaker longevity. J Thorac Cardiovasc Surg 1975; 69: 382–389.
9. Irnich W: Engineering concepts of pacemaker electrodes. In M Schaldach, S Furman (Eds). Advances in pacemaker technology. New York, Springer Verlag, 1975 pp 241–272.
10. Captal AP, Ribot A: Statistical survey of strength-duration threshold curves with endocardial electrodes and long-term behaviour of these electrodes. In C Meere (Ed): Cardiac Pacing. Montreal, Pacesymp, 1978, Chap 21–2.

Author's address:
F. Antúnez, M.D.
Hospital Sagrado Corazón
Viladomat 288
Barcelona/Spain

An Even More Physiological Pacing: Changing the Sequence of Ventricular Activation

E. de Teresa, J. L. Chamorro, L. A. Pulpón, Carmen Ruiz, Isabel R. Bailón, J. Alzueta, M. de Artaza

Summary: Physiological pacing includes preservation of A-V sequential stimulation and adaptation of heart rate to body requirements. However the sequence of ventricular activation (VA) is also important. In four patients with aortic valvular disease, LBBB and HV ⩾ 70 msec a Medtronic Versatrax DDD pacemaker was implanted at the time of aortic valve surgery. The ventricular electrode was placed in the free wall of the LV. With differents pulse generator A-V intervals (PG-AV), we obtained: A) LBBB morphology when PG-AV was > A-V conducted interval (C-AV); B) "RBBB" morphology when PG-AV < C-AV, and C) intermediate ("fusion") morphology when PG-AV ≃ C-AV. A mean delay of 70 ± 5 msec between beginning of the spontaneous activation of RV and arrival of stimulation to ventricular electrode in LV favoured these fusion beats. The sequence of mechanical ventricular emptying was non-invasively assessed by radioisotopic (Tc-99 m Pyp labelled red blood cells) study of the "wave of emptying" and of phase histograms, using the Fourier's analysis. The most "normal" pattern was found in C. LV ejection fraction (radioisotopic cineangiogram) was 0.59 ± 0.035 in C versus 0.51 ± 0.047 in B (p < 0.001) and 0.47 ± 0.045 in A (p < 0.001). We conclude than an appropriate placement of ventricular electrode besides a correct programation of A-V delay in DDD pacemakers allows for a more synergistic ventricular activation in patients with LBBB, improving their ventricular performance.

Introduction

The aim of achieving an artificial heart stimulations as "physiological" as possible has until now focused in sequential atrioventricular activation and in the modification of heart rate in accordance with the body requirements (1). The use of dual chamber systems (VDD, DVI and DDD modes) offers a reasonable way of solving the problems derived from dissociated atrioventricular activation, an even some new investigational devices may adjust the pulse generator rate to instantaneous variations in QT interval, thus allowing automatic variations of heart rate in response to autonomic nervous tonus, even in absence of normal sinus function (2).

The sequence in which both ventricles are activated seems to have also some importance (3), although this is not easily proved because of the methodological difficulties of analyzing "in vivo" ventricular activation (VA). Recently a computerized analysis of radionuclide cineangiogram (RCA), based in the application of Fourier's Analysis for studying cyclic functions, has been used as a non-invasive method of assessing VA (4). Using this technique we have tried, in selected patients with left bundle branch block (LBBB), to obtain a pattern of VA closer to "normal" and to assess its influence on the "wave of emptying" (WOE) and on left ventricular function. The results of this study are presented here.

Patients and methods

Four male patients (mean age 39.2 years; range 27–52) with severe aortic valve disease and advanced A-V conduction disturbance were studied; the conditions required for admittance were the following:

– LBBB
– First degree infrahissian block with a H-V interval of at least 70 msec.
– Documented episodes of 2nd or 3rd degree A-V block and/or syncopal attacks.
– Absence of wall motion abnormalities (akinesia or diskynesia) in the left ventriculogram.
– Absence of retrograde ventriculoatrial conduction at the time of electrophysiological study.

During the surgical procedure for replacement of the aortic valve with a mechanical prosthesis (in three cases, Björk-Shiley; in one, St Jude Medical) a Medtronic Versatrax 7000 universal pacemaker system was implanted. The atrial lead (Medtronic 4951) was placed high in the right atrium; the ventricular electrode (Medtronic 6917) was placed in the free lateral wall of the left ventricle (LV). The mean delay between unipolar electrograms at the apex of the right ventricle (RV) and the ventricular electrode in the LV, recorded by means of a hand-hold electrode probe, was 70 ± 5 msec (mean $\pm$ SD).

In the postoperative period, and using the Medtronic 9701-A programmer, the pulse generator A-V interval (PG-AV) was set at different values in order to obtain three different ECG morphologies:

– LBBB when PG-AV was greater than A-V conduction time through the conduction system (C-AV). This implies that the ventricular activation must reach the ventricular electrode before the pulse generator elicits the stimulus to the LV in order to inhibit it. So, PG-AV must be greater than the sum of conduction time to the RV plus RV-LV delay (R-L D) (Fig. 1 A).
– RBBB-like ECG when PG-AV is shorter than conduction time to RV (Fig. 1 B).
– Intermediate morphologies when PG-AV is equal to, or greater than conduction time to RV apex, but shorter than the sum of this time and R-L D (Fig. 1 C). In this situation, the possible explanation is a dual and near-simultaneous activation of both ventricles.

All patients underwent ECG-gated cardiac blood pool imaging. After "in vivo" labelling of red blood cells with 20–25 mCi of 99-mTc Pyp, 16-frame gated studies in 64×64 matrix were recorded with a standard Anger camera in the left anterior oblique projection in order to obtain the best visualization of the interventricular septum (usually 30 °) and stored in a commercial nuclear medicine computer system.

The ejection fraction was calculated using a program based on three regions of interest: end-diastolic, end-systolic and peri-systolic background.

The temporal Fourier transform at the fundamental frequence (the heart rate) was obtained on a pixel-by-pixel basis, according to the method previously described by Links et al. (4). The transform data were represented in two ways:

– Distribution histograms of the pixel phase values. The abscissa represents phase angles (10° per channel) and the ordinate, number of pixels. Only those pixels whose amplitude at the fundamental frequence was above a certain threshold (usually a 10% of the maximum amplitude) were counted, so that background activity did not contribute to the histogram.

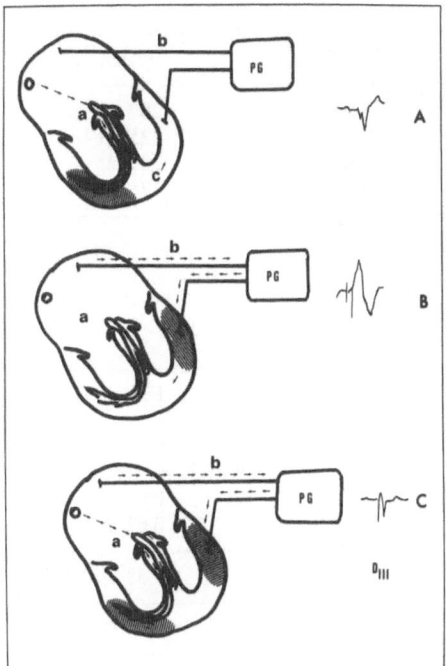

Fig. 1. Hypothesis to explain the different morphologies found in the ECG. In A (LBBB) the excitation wave travels faster down the conduction system than through the pulse generator (PG). In order to inhibit it, b must be greater than a plus c. In B, b is shorter than a, resulting in pacemaker induced "RBBB" morphology. In C there is a near simultaneous activation of both ventricles.

– A 16-frame cinematic display of the WOE as it spreads over the cardiac chambers. In each frame, the pixels corresponding to the maximal activity are depicted in black. Here, again, only those pixels representing at least 10% of the maximum amplitude were considered.

Results

The PG-AV required for every ECG pattern are reflected in Table 1. The analysis of the WOE in the RCA revealed:

A) In LBBB the activation begins in the paraseptal and apical RV, progressing to the RV outflow tract and finally, through the IV septum, to the LV (Fig. 2 A). These data are in accordance with those previously reported by Rosenbuch et al. (5).

B) In pacemaker induced RBBB the activation begins in the free lateral LV wall, spreading across the LV and septum to the RV (Fig. 2 B).

C) In the intermediate morphologies both ventricles are activated almost simultaneously, the RV usually preceding the LV (Fig. 2 C).

These patterns were essentially uniform in all four patients with only minor variations from patient to patient.

Phase histograms were wider in A and B (in three cases, A wider than B; in one, B wider than A) than in C, reflecting a more synchronic ventricular contraction in the latter situation (Fig. 3).

397

Table 1. Pacemaker A-V interval in different ECG patterns.

Case No	LBBB	"RBBB"	Fusion
1	225 ms	175 ms	200 ms
2	250 ms	200 ms	225 ms
3	225 ms	175 ms	200 ms
4	200 ms	150 ms	175 ms

Table 2. Left ventricular ejection fraction.

Case No	LBBB	"RBBB"	Fusion
1	0.40	0.44	0.53
2	0.50	0.53	0.61
3	0.47	0.51	0.60
4	0.52	0.57	0.62
Mean ± SD	0.47 ± 0.045 (1)	0.51 ± 0.047 (1)	0.59 ± 0.035

(1) p < 0.001

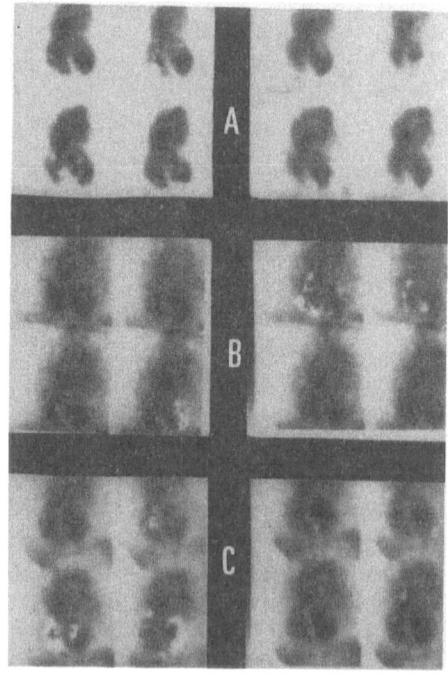

Fig. 2. Cinematic representation of the "Wave of Emptying". Only the first eight photograms are shown. A, basal LBBB; B, pacemaker induced "RBBB" and C, "fusion" beat.

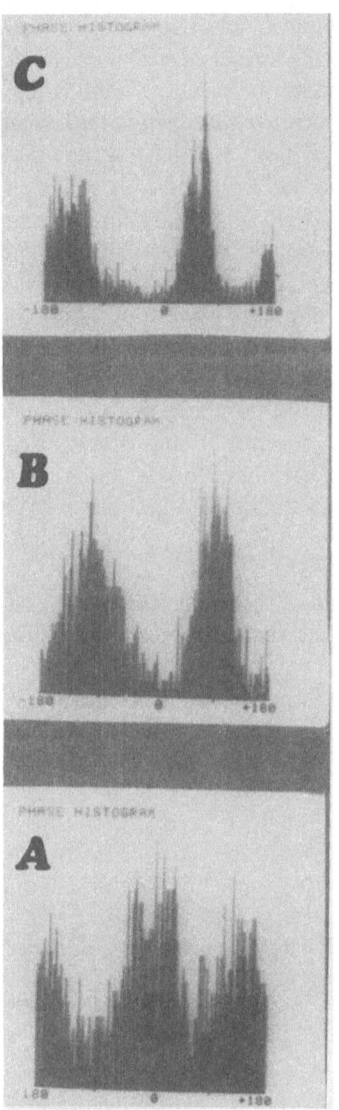

Fig. 3. Phase Histograms (same case than in Fig. 2). The histogram corresponding to ventricular activation is wider in A (LBBB) than in B or C ("fusion" beat). The differences of situation respect to 0 ° depend on the electrical signal used as gating; in A, the R-wave peak; in B and C the pacemaker artifact.

The LV ejection fraction is reflected in Table 2. It was 0.47 ± 0.045 in A versus 0.51 ± 0.047 in B ($p < 0.001$) and 0.59 ± 0.035 in C ($p < 0.001$).

Discussion

In LBBB patients with an implanted DDD pacemaker system, it is possible, if the ventricular lead is placed in the LV, to obtain different QRS patterns by varying the PG-AV. Some of these patterns show an intermediate morphology between basal LBBB and the

399

ECG resulting of pure LV stimulation. This is only possible if an adequate delay between the beginning of spontaneous ventricular activation and the arrival of excitation to the ventricular electrode exists, because the device used (Medtronic Versatrax 7000) is only able of varying A-V interval in 25 msec steps. However, to prove that these intermediate morphologies indeed represent simultaneous activation of both ventricles would have been quite difficult in the absence of the new radionuclid derived techniques. The analysis of the WOE, a technique that applies Fourier analysis to RCA, allows a noninvasive assessment of the sequence of ventricular contraction; in our cases this method confirmed the hypothesis of a close activation of both ventricles in the supposed "fusion" ECG pattern. In this situation, the LV ejection fraction improves significantly over the basal LBBB or the pure pacemaker induced stimulation. The reasons for this are not clear, because the way in which the LV is activated when it is paced from its free lateral wall is not much more normal than the LV activation in LBBB. The role of varying A-V intervals cannot be discarded (6) but a possible clue is the movement of the interventricular septum contributing, when it is simultaneous to that of the rest of the LV, to LV function improvement over those situations where there is a temporal gap between septum and lateral LV contraction.

We concluded that:

– In selected LBBB patients a near simultaneous activation of both ventricles may be obtained by means of a "physiological" pacemaker with the ventricular electrode placed in the LV and an adequate PG-AV.
– This may be the cause, at least in part, of a significative improvement in LV function.
– The RCA-based analysis of the "Wave of Emptying" provides an easy non-invasive method of assessing ventricular activation.

References

1. Obel IWP: Physiological Pacing. London: Pitman Medical, 1981: XIII-XV.
2. Rickards AF, Donaldson RM, Thalen HJTh: The use of QT interval to determine pacing rate: early clinical experience. Pace 1983; 6: 346–353.
3. Schlant RC: Normal physiology of the cardiovascular system. In: Hurst JW ed. The Heart. Tokyo: McGraw Hill Kogakusha Ltd, 1974; 89.
4. Links JM, Douglass KH, Wagner HN: Patterns of ventricular emptying by Fourier analysis of gated blood pool studies. J Nucl Med 1980; 21: 978–982.
5. Rosenbuch SW, Rugie N, Turner DA, Von Behren PL, Denes P, Fordham EW, Groch MW, Messer JV: Sequence and timing of ventricular wall motion in patients with bundle branch block. Assessment by radionuclide cineangiography. Circulation 1982; 66: 1113–1119.
6. Chandraratna PAN: Impact of atrioventricular delay on cardiac output in patients with atrioventricular sequential pacemakers: assessment by Doppler computer. Abstract Book, 2nd Central Pacific Symposium on Cardiac Pacing, 1983; 52.

Authors' address:
Eduardo de Teresa, M.D.
Clinica Puerta de Hierro
San Martin de Porres N. 4
Madrid 35/Spain

Fifteen Year Experience with Atrial Electrodes and Pacing

J. Venditti, Jr., T. Z. Lajos, S. T. Raza, A. N. Lewin, J. N. Bhayana, A. B. Lee, Jr., R. Kohn

Summary: Two hundred and twelve patients were treated in our institution, since 1968, with long term atrial and atrio/ventricular sequential pacing utilizing different atrial electrodes. Indications included, 1. atrial/ventricular arrythmia (16 pts.), 2. sick sinus syndrome with bradycardia (54 pts.), 3. sick sinus syndrome with brady/tachycardia (32 pts.), 4. intermittent heart block (73 pts.), 5. conversion from DVI to DDD pacing (8 pts.), 6. following open heart surgery (21 pts.), 7. miscellaneous (7 pts.). Forty-one (19%) of the 212 pts. had pre-existing congestive heart failure. Since 1968, a variety of atrial electrodes have been used; 1. epicardial electrodes: a) modified (Lajos, 27 pts.), b) conventional (17 pts.), 2. transvenous electrodes; a) standard "J" (102 pts.), b) Mark I Lajos (14 pts.), and c) Mark II Lajos (52 pts.). Electrode related complications include, 7 instances of atrial dislodgement, 8 instances of pectoral muscle stimulation and 8 instances of diaphragmatic stimulation. Reprogramming was extensively employed with 64 instances of changes in rate (24), sensitivity, (8) output, (2) pulse width, (9) pulse interval (2) or modes (19). Atrial threshold characteristics were 1.53 ± 0.8911 mVolts, 3.17 ± 2.1909 mAmps, P wave 3.26 ± 2.3569 mVolts at time of implantation. Based on our experience, the evolution of modern electrode technology has provided safe and long term atrial and A-V sequential pacing. Contraindications are limited to refractory atrial flutter or fibrillation. The utilization of the single pass, double electrode combined with a multiprogrammable unit has added to our armamentarium, a new method of treating patients when pacing is required.

Introduction

The era of modern cardiac pacing was initiated in 1960, with the implantation of the first self-contained long lasting ventricular pacemakers for complete heart block. (1) While ventricular pacing to be a most effective way of treating patients with complete heart block, it soon became apparent that the patient physiologically has lost the atrial transport mechanism to cardiac output entirely. This loss of atrial component to the cardiac output is adequately compensated for only in patients with good ventricular compliance (2, 3). It became advantageous, therefore, to develop a mode in which the atrial "kick" could be preserved. Fifteen years ago in 1968 we have started atrial pacing and atrial synchronous pacing (VAT) via atrial attached electrodes, at first, by direct atrial fixation and later by transvenous approach. The topic of this paper is to discuss our fifteen years experience with the use of different atrial electrodes.

Materials and Methods

From 1968 until 1982, 212 patients, 132 male and 80 female, underwent implantation of pacemakers with either and atrial electrode or an atrial ventricular electrode system. (Average age mean 67 years; range 22–99 years.) Various lead systems, as well as pulse generators, were employed during this period reflecting our philosophy at that time. The lead system and pulse generator was determined by the implanting physician at the time of implantation.

From 1968 to 1980 mostly epicardial electrodes were used; the Lajos modification of either the Cordis or the Medtronic epicardial (4) lead (18 pts.). Transvenous leads employed were the standard "J" lead (1 pt.) by Medtronic; the Lajos Mark I lead (5) (Fig. 1) (14 pts.) or the Lajos Mark II (6) (Fig. 2) in one patient. Pulse generators employed during that time period were either the Cordis Atricor (VAT) or VVI pacers attached to single or double atrial electrodes.

From 1980 to 1982 the following electrodes were used: 1. *Epicardial leads:* a) modified Lajos (9 patients) and b) conventional (17 patients). 2. *Transvenous leads:* a) standard "J" lead in 101 patients b) the Lajos Mark II lead in 51 patients (Fig. 2). A variety of pulse generators were employed: 1. Intermedics (Cyberlith or Avius), 2. Pacesetter, 3. Cordis (Sequicor) and 4. Medtronic (Byrel, Versatrax).

Applicable threshold measurements were taken using a Medtronic PSA 3600 analyser.

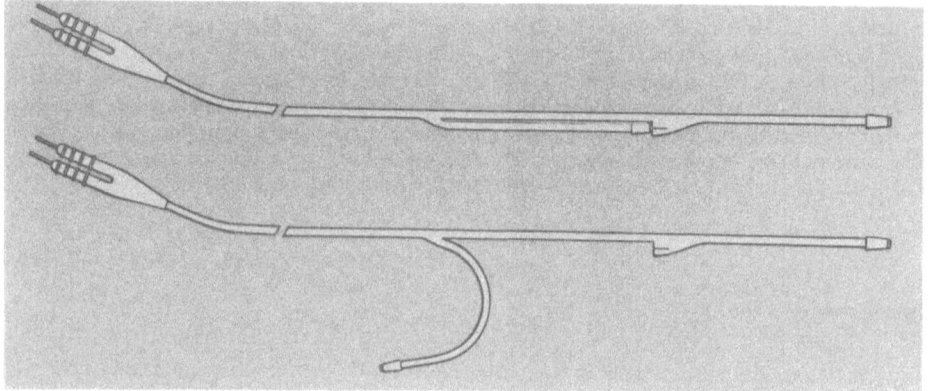

Fig. 1. This A-V transvenous electrode is incorporated into one body and has the mechanical advantages of double fixation and atrial or ventricular sensing or pacing.

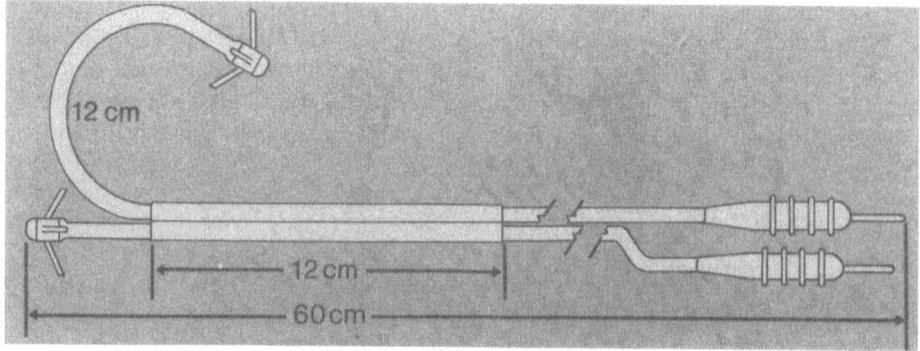

Fig. 2. The sliding atrioventricular electrode is also based on the concept of common body. The two electrodes are attached to each other by a sleeve which will promote stabilization of the atrial and ventricular components, but let them slide in the sleeve for ease of manipulation.

Operative Procedures

Epicardial leads were placed by a right parasternal mediastinotomy with an attachment to the right atrial appendage. From 1980 to 1982 the epicardial approach was used only when there was concommittent open heart surgery.

Transvenous electrodes were passed via: 1. cephalic vein cutdown procedure and 2. direct subclavian stick utilizing the Potts introducer.

Computations

Statistical analysis was carried out using the null hypothesis for comparison of the standard error of the mean. Statistical significance is taken to equal P (equal to or less than) 0.15. Actuarial survival curve is constructed utilizing the actuarial method of Anderson, Bonchek, Grunkemeier, et al. (8).

Results

Indications

Examination of our changing trends in implantation and indications for atrial pacing is reflected by dividing the study period into two groups. One from 1968 to 1980 and the second from 1980 to 1982.

Thirty-four implants were placed in the first group of patients, from 1968 to 1980. Pacemakers were implanted for atrial/ventricular arrythmia (1 pt.), sick sinus syndrome with bradycardia (9 pts.), sick sinus syndrome with brady/tachycardia (12 pts.), heart block (11 pts.), and miscellaneous (1 pt.). Eight of 34 patients suffered congestive heart failure at the time of implantation (23%).

In comparison, from 1980 to 1982, a total of 178 patients were involved. Pacemakers were implanted for atrial ventricular arrythmia (15 pts.), sick sinus syndrome with bradycardia (45 pts.), sick sinus syndrome brady/tachycardia (20 pts.), heart block (62 pts.), conversion of DVI pacemaker (8 pts.), at open heart surgery (21 pts.) and miscellaneous (7 pts.). Of the total 178 patients, 33 patients had congestive heart failure at the time of implantation (18%) (Table 1).

Analysis of electrodes

From 1968 to 1980, 18 *epicardial* electrodes were employed. In all instances, the previously described Lajos modification was employed (4). The *transvenous* electrode was employed 16 times. The predominant electrode used was the Lajos Mark I (5) (14 pts.). The standard "J" and the Mark II electrodes were each used once.

From 1980 to 1982, the *epicardial* approach was utilized 26 times; Modified Lajos (4) (9 pts.) and the conventional epicardial lead (17 pts.). The transvenous electrode was employed in 152 patients: standard "J" electrode (101 pts.) and the Lajos Mark II electrode (6) (51 pts.) (Table 2)

403

Table 1. Atrial electrode experience, N – 212 patients.

	1968–1980 N – 34			1980–1982 N – 178		
	# PTS	CHF	NO CHF	# PTS	CHF	NO CHF
Atrial / Ventricular Arrhythmia	1	–	1	15	1	14
A-V Sequential:						
"SSS bradycardia"	9	6	3	45	8	37
"SSS brady/tachycardia"	12	2	10	20	1	19
Heart-Block (Type II, III)	11	–	11	62	14	48
"Preserve atrial kick"						
a) Conversion				8	4	4
b) O.H.S.				21	5	16
Miscellaneous	1	–	1	7	–	7
Total	34	8 (23%)	26 (77%)	178	33 (18%)	145 (82%)

Table 2. Electrodes used for atrial pacing, N – 212 patients.

	1968–1980	1980–1982	Total
Epicardial:			
a) Modified (Lajos)[1]	18	9	27
b) Conventional	–	17	17
Transvenous:			
a) Standard "J"	• 1	101	102
b) Mark 1[2]	14	–	14
c) Mark 11[3]	1	51	52
No. of electrodes	34	178	212

Threshold characteristics

In 178 patients undergoing implantation of a pacemaker from January 1980 to December 1982, the atrial threshold characteristics were 1.53 ± 0.8911 mVolts; 3.17 ± 2.1909 mAmps; and a P wave of 3.26 ± 2.3569 mVolts. The ventricular characteristics were 0.92 ± 0.7597 mVolts; 1.79 ± 1.5360 mAmps; and an R wave of 9.27 ± 4.1957.

In the 212 patients comprising this study group since 1968, 27 patients had a Modified Lajos epicardial electrode placed. Atrial thresholds at time of implantation were 1.5 mVolt and 3.1 mAmp with ventricular thresholds of 1.5 mVolt and 1.9 mAmp. In the transvenous group, of the 212 patients, 102 patients had the standard "J" lead implanted. In this group atrial threshold were 1.44 ± 0.47 mVolts; 2.85 ± 1.19 mAmps; with a Pwave of 3.63 ± 1.94 mVolt.

Fifty-two patients had implantation of the Lajos Mark II single pass electrode. Atrial thresholds in this group were 1.41 ± 0.68 mVolts compared to a 1.61 ± 0.96 mVolt recorded in the total series minus the Mark II electrode (102 patients with transvenous electrodes) (P.10); 2.74 ± 1.84 mAmps compared to a 3.53 ± 0.287 mAmps recorded in the total series minus the Mark II electrode (P.05); and P wave of 3.13 ± 1.96 mVolt compared to 3.19 ± 1.51 mVolts recorded in the total series minus the Mark II electrode (Table 3).

Electrode complications

Two main complications occurred with the electrode placement: 1. dislodgement and 2. muscle twitching. There were seven documented atrial dislodgements (4 in 1968–1980) and 3 ventricular dislodgements. 2. In the muscle twitching group, there were eight documented instances of pectoral muscle stimulation and eight documented instances of diaphragmatic stimulation. During this period there were, also, three instances of infection of the pocket (1.4%) and one miscellaneous complication necessitating change of the pacemaker unit because of a faulty screw connection.

Table 3. Atrial threshold characteristics, 1/80–12/82, N – 154 patients, with transvenoua electrodes.

	Sliding – mark 11 electrode N – 52 Pts.		Total series minus mark II N – 102 Pts.
V	1.41 ± 0.68	P 0.10	1.61 ± 0.96
mAmp.	2.74 ± 1.84	P 0.05	3.53 ± 2.87
P wave	3.13 ± 0.96		3.19 ± 1.51

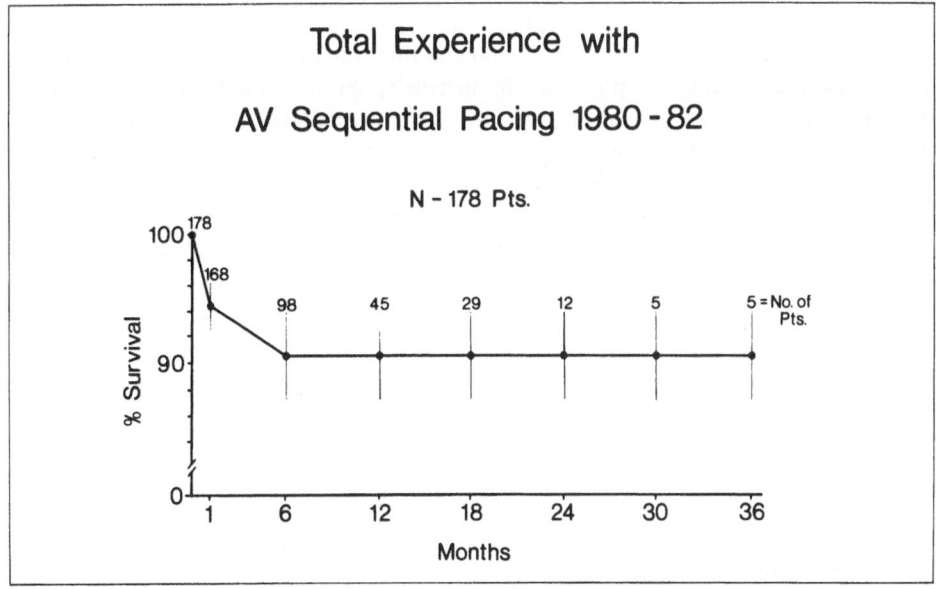

Fig. 3. Actuarial survival curve of our patients with AV sequential pacemakers. Mean follow-up of 13.3 months.

405

Survival

Actuarial survival curve was constructed and plotted on the 178 patients with a follow-up period of 1 to 36 months; a mean period of 13.3 months. There were ten perioperative deaths and six late deaths. The ten deaths in the perioperative group were not attributed to pacemaker implantation. These patients had pacemaker implantation at the time of open heart surgery when difficulty arose coming off the bypass pump. Subsequently they expired in the postoperative period. They had pre or perioperative acute myocardial infarction and A-V sequential pacing was instituted in the hope of optimizing the cardiac output. In the six late deaths, all patients died of their initial underlying cardiac rhythm disturbance. Examination of Fig. 3 shows that after the initial drop off in the first six months, (94.3%) the survival curve stays essentially unchanged all the way to 36 months with a 36 month survival of 90%.

Discussion

With the broadening indications for pacemaker implantation, the ability to efficiently pace the atrium became a necessity. In the 23 patients initially treated with atrial electrode placement from 1968 to 1980, the indications varied but the great majority of these patients had intact atrial/ventricular conduction and, therefore, adequate atrial pacing resulted in normal conduction and ventricular response.

Long term atrial pacing could be achieved by two methods; 1. the *transvenous* approach, in which initial electrode stability was at times a problem (4/7), and 2. Before the suggested modification by Lajos, the *epicardial* approach had been plagued with increasing thresholds and loss of pacing. It was due to the instability of the transvenous approach in the earlier days that lead the authors to advocate a "mini" mediastinotomy to place the atrial electrode, and fix it to the right atrium and that way to avoid the complication of a dislodgement. To obviate the problem with increasing thresholds in these epicardial leads the authors modified the standard Cordis or Medtronic epicardial electrode in such a way that the sleeve of insulating silcone rubber, around the coiled wire was removed. The coiled wire was then bent parallel to the electrode. When fixed in place in this manner, there was a better contact made between the atrium and the electrode. Pacing the atrium with this method, the problem of increasing threshold was no longer experienced and acceptable threshold characteristics were obtained for a long time (5). Commercial production of this electrode modification is well known (Cordis, Medtronic, etc.).

A single pass transvenous double electrode was developed at our institution to reduce the problems of implantation and stability. This electrode (Lajos Mark I) could be inserted as a single electrode and then opened up and uncoiled in the right atrium. Fourteen implantations of this electrode were carried out in the time period from 1968 to 1980 with satisfactory long term results. The main draw back to this electrode was that it was cumbersome to introduce and there were problems with dislodgement since anatomy tended to vary from person to person. (Distance from atrial appendage to tip of right ventricular varied) (6).

Nevertheless, the idea of a single pass double electrode was valid. The second generation single pass double electrode was devised: A "J" electrode was attached to the standard

406

transvenous ventricular electrode, by means of a sheath which allowed the electrodes to glide upon one another (7).

With the development of this sliding Mark II electrode from 1980 to 1982, the group at our hospital still relayed heavily on the standard "J" atrial electrode; 101 transvenous "J" electrodes were implanted. Examination of the threshold characteristics of the standard "J" electrode shows quite acceptable thresholds and lends itself for a comparison to the 51 implantations of the single pass double electrode (Lajos Mark II electrode). Threshold characteristics of the Mark II electrode have shown that current measurements were consistently superior to the rest of the series, to a P value of 0.05 (Table 3).

The ten perioperative deaths between 1980 to December 1982, were not directly pacemaker related. All these were the sequelae to myocardial infarction. Examination of this actuarial survival curve also (Fig. 3) substantiates the fact that heart block associated with an acute ischemic episode (myocardial infarction) will represent a worse prognosis in the first 6 months compared to patients with heart block of other etiology (9, 10).

The development of dual chamber pacemakers has been equally important with the development of new atrioventricular electrode technology. From 1980 to 1982 all of the pacemakers placed were of the dual chamber multiprogrammable variety (33.8% of total pacemaker implanted (178/527) in the same study period). The use of multiprogrammability was employed 64 times to make postoperative implantation adjustments of rate (24), sensitivity (8), output (2), pulse width (9), or pulse interval (2). There were 19 instances of mode changes enablying us to treat such varying conditions as retrograde conduction and transient atrial fibrillation and/or flutter in the postimplantation period (4). There were three instances of postimplantation atrial fibrillation thus the unit had to be programmed to a VVI mode. The patients were then treated with high doses of antiarrythmics and once the fibrillation was converted back to a sinus rhythm, the pacemaker was then reprogrammed to a DDD or a DVI mode.

References

1. Chardack WM, Gage AA, and Greatbatch W: A transistorized, self-contained, implantable pacemaker for the long term correction of complete heart-block. Surgery 48: 643, 1960.
2. Raza ST, Lajos TZ, Bhayana JN, Lee AB, Lewin AN, Gehring B, RN, and Schimert G: Abstract: Optimizing the advantages of AV sequential pacing with afterload reduction therapy in patients with low cardiac output. Pace 5: 302, 1982.
3. Raza ST, Lajos TZ, Bhayana JN, Lee AB, Jr, Lewin AN, Gehring B, and Schimert G: Improved cardiovascular hemodynamics with atrioventricular sequential pacing compared to ventricular demand (VVI) pacing: In Print: VIIth World Symposium on Cardiac Pacing, Vienna, Austria, May 1983.
4. Lewin AN, Vinditti J, Lajos TZ, Bhayana JN, Raza ST, Lee AB, and Schimert G: Physiologic pacing: An analysis of indications, clinical results and survival characteristics in 117 patients: Poster Session, VIIth World Symposium on Cardiac Pacing, Vienna, Austria, May 1983.
5. Lajos TZ, and Wanka J: Epicardial atrial pacing: Annals of Thoracic Surgery 25: 64, 1978.
6. Lajos TZ: Transvenous atrial pacing with a new electrode. Journal of Thoracic and Cardiovascular Surgery 69: 575, 1975.
7. Lajos TZ: Transvenous physiological pacing – A new atrioventricular electrode. Pace 5: 264, 1982.
8. Anderson RP, Bonchek LI, Grunkemeier GL, Lambert E, and Starr A: The analysis and presentation of surgical results by actuarial methods. Journal of Surgical Research 16: 221, 1974.

9. Hindman MC, Wagner GS, JaRo M, Atkins JM, Scheinman MM, DeSanctis RW, Hutter AH, Yeatman L, Rubenfire M, Pujura C, Rubin M, and Morris JJ: The clinical significance of bundle branch block complicating acute myocardial infarction: 1. Clinical characteristics, hospital mortality, and one-year follow-up. Circulation 58: 4, 1978.
10. Hindman MC, Wagner GS, JaRo M, Atkins JM, Scheinman MM, DeSanctis RW, Hutter AH, Yeatman L, Rubenfire M, Pujura C, Rubin M, and Morris JJ: The clinical significance of bundle branch block complicating acute myocardial infarction: 2. Indications for temporary and permanent pacemaker insertion. Circulation 58: 4, 1978.

Author's address:
Thomas Z. Lajos, M.D.
100 High Street
Buffalo, New York 14203

An A-V Data Lead System for Electrogram Detection[1])

H. C. Hughes[2]), R. R. Brownlee[3])

Summary

Some telemetrically monitored pacemakers are capable of detecting and transmitting either the P- or R-wave, however, none are able to transmit the complete electrogram (EGM) during normal and paced rhythms. A new lead system has been developed that, when used in conjunction with a tele-metrypacemaker system, permits the transmissionof the complete EGM and is not adversely affected by pacemaker outputs or afterpotentials. Detecting electrodes are placed in both right atrium and ventricle in order to optimize EGM detection. Electrically separate from the pacing-sensing electrodes, the A-V Data probes are structurally part of a transvenously placed ventricular lead no larger than a conventional bipolar lead (2.3 mm). The EGM telemetry system is also compatible with telephone monitoring systems. The A-V data lead has consistently demonstrated its ability to accurately detect the EGM during normal sinus rhythms as well as during atrial, ventricular, and A-V sequential pacing. In addition, this system can detect and transmit EGM abnormalities such as ectopic beats and retrograde conduction. Eight A-V data lead, telemetry monitored VVI pacemakers have been implanted in dogs for over two years. This system has provided the means to noninvasively detect and telemetrically record the entire normal and abnormal EGM, even in pacer dependent patients.

Introduction

The advances in telemetric monitoring have made it possible to continue to examine many pacemaker functions including rate, output current and voltage, pulse width, pacing energy, battery voltage, lead and battery impedance, sensing margin, etc. after implantation (1, 2, 3). However, the one highly critical factor that cannot presently be telemetrically monitored is the intracardiac electrogram (EGM). Although the EGM can be examined with relative ease during surgery, it cannot be detected once the pacemaker is connected. Furthermore, the EGM is obscured during pacing by the high outputs and afterpotentials of the electrical stimuli from either the pacing systems analyzer or the pacer itself, even at threshold levels. Therefore, with the multitude of highly sophisticated devices now available for pacemaker monitoring, the examination of its performance and capture still ultimately relies on the surface electrocardiogram (ecg). Not only can these ecg's changes be difficult to monitor and interpret, but the increased use of dual chamber (DDD and DVI) pacing has added even further to the difficulties of interpretation of the ecg for proper pacemaker function (4). Retrograde conduction, fusion, pseudo-

---

[1]) Supported, in part, by grants from USPHS (R01 HL-13988 and K04 HL-00586) and Cardiac Control Systems.

[2]) From the Department of Comparative Medicine, The Milton S. Hershey Medical Center, The Pennsylvania State University, Hershey, PA.

[3]) Cardiac Control Systems, Inc., State College, PA.

fusion, and confusion concerning programmed setting continue to plague the monitoring physician. Even capture is often not readily apparent.

The purpose of this study was to examine a new pacemaker lead system that permits the detection of the complete intracardiac electrogram and is not adversely affected by pacemaker outputs and afterpotentials. When used in conjunction with telemetrically monitorable pacemakers, transmission of the complete paced and nonpaced EGM is possible.

Materials and methods

The A-V Data Lead (CCS Model BB-102D) is designed for transvenous right ventricular placement. The lead is in either the coaxial configuration with the central wire being used for both pacemaker functions of pacing and sensing through a 9.0 mm² platinum-irridium (Pt-Ir) tip, or side-by-side with one side holding the tip electrode and the other the rings. The A-V Data Probe portion is composed of two separate Pt-Ir rings (50 mm² each) tied electronically together in parallel. These rings are positioned along the body of the lead so that the distal ring is in the right ventricle 1.0 cm from the tip for optimum R-wave detection. The proximal ring, in the leads used for animal studies, was positioned 8–10 cm from the tip so that it laid in close proximity to the S-A node for P-wave detection. The lead insulation is a segmented polyether polyurethane (CCS/Urethane) and is made so that the insulation material is bonded to the wires to produce a smooth, strong, thin (< 2.3 mm diameter), low friction, biocompatible system. The tip is tined for fixation.

In acute studies, dogs (n = 15) were anesthetized with pentobarbital, intubated and maintained on positive pressure ventilation. The right jugular vein was exposed and isolated 10 cm from the thoracic inlet. A right thoracotomy was done to visualize the heart. The A-V Data Lead was passed transvenously into the right ventricle so that the lead tip was lodged firmly in the apex. Atrial J-leads were passed through the same vein and their tips were placed in the right atrium. The positions of both leads were confirmed by direct observation and palpation.

Fig. 1. This is a schematic representation of the A-V Data Lead, VVI Pacemaker, and associated telemetry system. The EGM tracing is from a dog that has had the system implanted for over a year. Due to the dog's normal sinus arrhythmia, both pacer capture (arrows) and intrinsic beats are present in this strip.

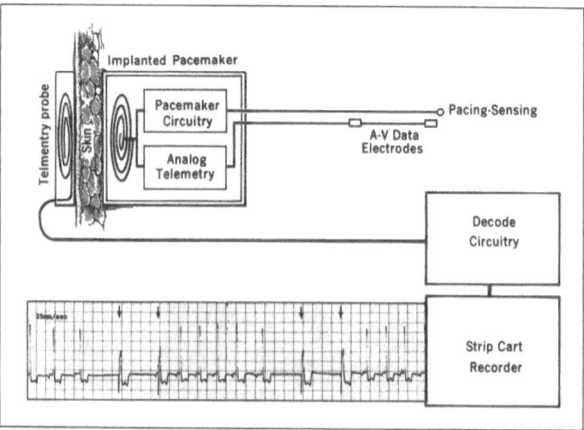

In chronic studies, eight dogs (35–40 lbs) were anesthetized and prepared for sterile surgery. The right jugular vein was isolated and the A-V Data Lead was passed transvenously into the right ventricle under a fluoroscope.

Electrophysiological measurements were done similarly in all animals. An E for M, VR-6 Recorder was used for the EGM measurements. All measurements were done using a 50 cm² subcutaneous ground plate as the indifferent. The EGM for the right ventricle was determined for the tip electrode in the unipolar mode. The EGM from the A-V Data Probe was examined separately, also in the unipolar mode. Continuous recordings were made at 100 mm/sec and triggered sweeps were photographed at 250–1000 mm/sec. Pacing thresholds were determined using a custom-designed square wave stimulator at five pulse durations from 0.1–1.0 msec (5). Threshold voltage and currents were determined using an oscilloscope. Electrograms were recorded from the A-V Data probe during atrial, ventricular, and A-V sequential pacing as well as during sinus rhythm. In the chronic studies, the A-V Data Leads were connected to telemetrically monitored VVI pacemakers following operative electrophysiologic measurements (Fig. 1).

Results

The A-V Data Lead handled like an ordinary coaxial lead. With the guidewire in place, it passed easily through the venous system and into the right ventricle. The position of the tip was confirmed visually and by palpation in the acute animals. Stability and lodgement were similar to other tined ventricular leads. The ability of the tip to detect R-waves and to pace the heart were identical to other unipolar ventricular leads of similar surface area. Acute R-wave potentials were 26 ± 6.7 mV with a duration of 9.8 ± 4.2 msec. Pacing thresholds are shown in Table 1.

Examination of the EGM detected from the A-V Data rings showed that it was similar in configuration to the lead II ecg but had a 5–6 times greater amplitude (Fig. 2). When compared to the EGM taken individually from the atrial and ventricular leads, there was a 25–50 percent attenuation of the signal.

After pacing was initiated, the EGM could not be detected on the lead doing the pacing because of the pacer spike and afterpotentials. Detection of the EGM from the A-V Data probes, however, was easily visible regardless of pacing site (Fig. 2). In comparison to the ecg, the individual waveforms were more easily recognized. In lead II, the P-waves were often obscured by T-waves (Fig. 2, 1st paced complex) and R-waves as atrial depolarization walked through the ecg. Similarly, the P-wave from the atrial lead EGM, tend-

Table 1. Pacing Thresholds for the Tip Electrode of the A-V Data Lead.

	0.1	0.2	0.5	0.8	1.0
Volts	0.84 ± 0.17	0.58 ± 0.20	0.36 ± 0.23	0.24 ± 0.3	0.19 ± 0.02
Milliamps	1.68 ± 0.45	1.10 ± 0.48	0.60 ± 0.40	0.39 ± 0.21	0.30 ± 0.17

Mean ± standard deviation.

411

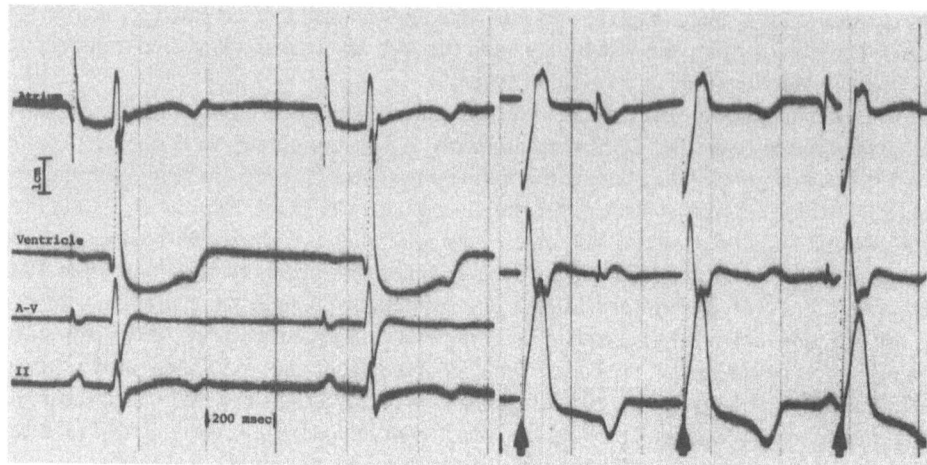

Fig. 2. This strip chart recording (first two sinus beats) shows a comparison of the unipolar EGM's from the atrium (2 mV/cm) ventricular tip (5 mV/cm), and A-V Data Lead (5 mV/cm) with the Lead II ecg (1 mV/cm) during sinus rhythm. During ventricular pacing (arrows), the EGM from the ventricle was obliterated by the pacer spike, therefore, only the atrial (upper), A-V Data Lead (middle), and Lead II (lower) tracings are visible. The A-V Lead shows all waveforms distinctly. In the first paced complex, the T-wave was obscured by the P-wave on the atrial lead EGM, and in the surface lead II ecg the P-wave was obscured by the T-wave.

Fig. 3. A high speed (250 mm/sec : 2 mV/cm) A-V Data Lead EGM during A-V sequential pacing. Determinations of atrial and ventricular capture, the A-V delay, Q-T intervals, S-T segments, analysis as well as other measurements of electrophysiologic phenomena are all readily accomplished using this lead system.

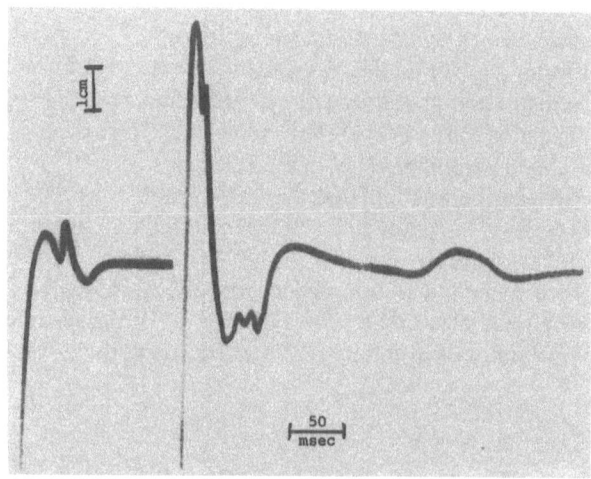

ed to obscure the T-wave during ventricular pacing. In contrast, the A-V Data Lead EGM always detected clear distinct individual waveforms (P-, R- and T-waves).

During atrial pacing, the ventricular tip electrode detected an entirely satisfactory R-wave. The P-waves detected by the ventricular lead, however, were of such low amplitude that determination of atrial capture was not always possible. With the A-V Data

412

Lead, there was excellent differentiation of waveforms. The pacer artifact was clear and P-waves were distinct. Accurate measurements of stimulus to P-wave and P-R intervals could be made. When A-V sequential pacing was initiated, the EGM from both the atrial and ventricular tip leads were not detectable due to the relatively high amplitude spikes and afterpotentials. With the A-V Data Lead, P-, R- and T-waves were readily detectable following the pacemaker stimuli, as were the other electrophysiologic parameters that are normally measured (Fig. 3).

In the chronic studies, A-V Data Leads have been functioning with telemetry units for over two years. Simply by placing an external telemetry coil in the vicinity of the internal telemetry system, intrinsic and paced intracardiac EGM's were easily detectable (Fig. 1). P-, R- and T-waves, premature beats, arrhythmias and EGM intervals were all easily identifiable. In one animal that had had previous chest surgery, a myocarditis and its associated arrhythmias were detected with this system before obvious clinical signs had occurred. There have been no lead or telemetry related failures.

Discussion

The evaluation of pacemaker function is considered mandatory for the health and well-being of the patient (6). As pacemaker longevity increases, better and more sophisticated follow-up methods become available. The telemetric monitoring of such diverse pacemaker functions as output voltage and current, rate, end-of-life indicators, refractory periods and delays, to name a few, are becoming common. The ordinary surface electrocardiogram is still relied upon to differentiate the arrhythmias produced by the pacemaker from abnormal pacemaker function. This seemingly simple task has become increasingly complex with the development of dual chamber and the so-called physiological pacemakers (4, 6). The multiple modes of pacing and having pacers being "committed" and "non-committed" have produced a wide array of ecg changes which can make interpretation of pacemaker function difficult. Monitoring has progressed from the simple lead II ecg to a minimum of six leads for ventricular pacing to a full 12 lead ecg for dual chamber pacers. Echocardiographs have even needed to be used to aid in determination of capture in some difficult cases (7). All are time-consuming and expensive for the patient and the physician.

The ability of pacing electrodes to sense and detect normal intrinsic cardiac electrical activity is not in question. These electrodes are adequate, in most instances, for the detection of the normal non-paced EGM. Telemetry systems incorporating such systems have already been used (8). They cannot, however, be used to detect the EGM immediately following a stimuli originating from that electrode. The high output spike, afterpotential, and electrode-tissue polarizations render the electrode blind to the induced EGM. Furthermore, since the sensing circuit gain is tuned for the relatively low voltages of the heart (3–4 mV for the atrium; 10–20 mV for the ventricle), the thousand-fold higher output levels produced by the pacemaker must be blocked from the sensing circuit by blanking and refractory periods so that the pacer is not disabled to subsequent electrical activity. This is somewhat analogous to dark-adapted eyes being suddenly blinded by a very bright light. Without protection temporary blindness will occur. It is not possible to try to even determine a capture EGM until long after the intrinsic waveform has moved well away from the pacing electrode. Thereafter, a system which uses the same electrode for pacing, sensing, and telemetry may only function when the pacemaker is not pacing. This negates the use of such a one electrode telemetry-pacing system in all single chamber and any dual chamber pacer where both chambers may be paced (DDD).

The use of a single, separate electrode for the detection of the EGM has been previously proposed (9, 10). Although this system was capable of detecting the EGM during both intrinsic and paced beats, it lacked the ability for high resolution EGM detection from both chambers simultaneously. The system described in this report is completely separate and independent of all pacemaker functions and is capable of high resolution EGM detection during all phases of the cardiac cycle. Two separate rings are electrically tied together and are placed for optimum EGM detection. The ventricular ring is 1 cm from the tip and the atrial ring in the dog test leads was 8 cm from the tip. Some cancellation of the signal, primarily the R-wave, does occur due to electrode loading and detection of far field signals on the ring in the nonactive chamber. This resulted in the 25–50% reduction in R-wave amplitude as compared to a single ring.

The A-V Data Lead is capable of detecting and transmitting the entire EGM from both chambers of the heart. The pacing EGM, whether it is single or dual chamber, is equally as clear and straightforward as is the intrinsic EGM. The pacer output spikes are clear and these are followed by distinct P- or R-waves. The T-wave and P-waves are not obscured by pacing or other electrical events occurring in the other chamber. Capture, fusion, pseudofusion, and non-capture are all readily identified. Similarly, the measurement of all electrophysiological intervals is possible.

The size (< 2.3 mm) and handling characteristics of this lead are similar to those of the standard bipolar leads. The polyurethane (CCS/Urethane) assures long-term biocompatibility and stability. When used in conjunction with telemetry pacing systems, this lead will add significantly to the long-term care and diagnostic ease in the pacemaker patient. Clear, concise EGM recordings will be available by transtelephonic monitoring systems (Fig. 1).

References

1. Brownlee RR, Hughes HC, Tyers GFO, Neff PH: Monitoring systems for cardiac pacemakers. Trans Am Soc Artif Inter Organs 1977; 23: 65–71.
2. DelMarco CJ, Tyers GFO, Brownlee RR: Lithium pacers with self-contained multiparameter telemetry: First year follow-up. In: Meere C, ed Proc VIth World Symposium on Cardiac Pacing. Pacesymp Montreal 1979; Chapter 28, Section 1.
3. Gorman IM, O'Neill MJ, Tyers GFO, Brownlee RR: A preliminary report on telemetric monitoring of pacemaker electrode impedance. In: Meere C, ed Proc VIth World Symposium on Cardiac Pacing. Pacesymp Montreal 1979; Chapter 28, Section 4.
4. Barold SS, Falkoff MD, Ong LS, Heinle RA: Interpretation of electrocardiograms produced by a new unipolar multiprogrammable "committed" A-V sequential demand (DVI) pulse generator. Pace 1981; 4: 692–708.
5. Hughes HC, Tyers GFO: Effect of stimulation site on ventricular threshold in dogs with complete heart block. Am Heart J 1975; 89: 68–73.
6. Zipes D: Current Clinical Applications of Dual Chamber Pacing. Minneapolis: Medtronic Inc, 1982.
7. Levine PA, Brodsky SJ, Seltzer JP: Assessment of atrial capture in committed atrioventricular sequential (DVI) pacing systems. Pace 1983; 6: 616–623.
8. Lathrop T: Medtronic's spectrax-sxt and the intracardiac electrogram. Medtronic News 1981; 11: 20–21.

9. Hughes HC, Brownlee RR, Tyers GFO: Failure of demand pacing with small surface area electrodes. Circulation 1976; 54: 128–132.
10. Hughes HC, Brownlee RR, Bertolet RD, Neff P, Sluetz J, Tyers GFO: The effects of electrode position on the detection of the transvenous cardiac electrogram. Pace 1980; 3: 651–655.

Authors' address:
Howard C. Hughes, M.D.
Department of Comparative Medicine
The Milton S. Hershey Medical Center
The Pennsylvania State University
500 University Drive
Hershey, PA 17033
USA

Rates and Modes of Failure for Eight Lead Types in 703 Implants: A Four-Year Structured Study

S. Furman, F. Pannizzo, I. Campo

Summary: To compare the ability to achieve and maintain satisfactory transvenous pacing, 8 commercially available unipolar leads were used on a strict rotation basis in 703 initial implants over a four year period. Implants were randomly distributed between the two surgeons normally performing these procedures, and pulse generators were also randomly distributed. Failure could occur during a procedure when attempt at use of a lead was abandoned and another was used, or following implant. Total (intra and post-operative) failures for the eight leads were: 1 mm 7/121 (5.8%), 6971 3/66 (4.5%), 6961 7/122 (5.7%), IE-65-I 12/136 (8.8%), 6907 7/76 (9.2%), CL 7/76 (9.2%), 4116 6/60 (10.0%), MIP-2000 9/45 (20.0%). The implants were performed during 3 major observation periods with follow-up from 9–54 months. The exposure of two lead types was abbreviated when the failure rate became clearly prohibitive. No correlation of failures with time of implant was found. Significant differences exist between the highest and lowest failure rates and between the lowest and the group of the remaining leads. No clear benefit was found for newer methods of gripping the endocardium, such as porous-tip, active fixation and tined leads.

Although transvenous pacing accounts for more than 90% of all permanent implants performed (1), there have been few studies comparing electrodes of various designs. Most studies are either retrospective analyses of modes and rates of failure or are structured studies involving only one or two lead types (2, 3, 4). Although in vitro and animal studies are valuable in predicting lead behaviour in humans, only clinical human use involving actual chronic observation periods can assess the reliability and utility of the various electrode types of lead designs available today.

The study described here is a direct comparison of eight lead types. The implants were performed in three series. The first two series involved four lead models each, and have been previously reported (5, 6). The third series contained three lead types. All three series are reported here in a combined presentation of eight lead models. Some lead types were continued from one series to another. Since the procedure and personnel were identical in each series, all three have been included in this report as a single study.

The chief purpose of the study was to compare the relative ability of the various electrode designs to achieve and maintain satisfactory pacing.

Materials and methods

Eight unipolar, ventricular transvenous leads were used in this study and all were commercially available. The Cordis Continuous Lead (CL) is a "standard tip" (ball-tip) lead having an electrode surface area of 8 mm². The Medtronic 6907 is also a passive fixation lead having a flat tip and electrode surface area of 11 mm². The Vitatron MIP-2000 is an active fixation lead, having four nylon bristles projecting from the electrode tip. The electrode surface area is 18 mm². The Biotronik IE-65-I has two fine, retractable, metal wires. These grasp the endocardium and are attached to a movable pin placed within a metal cylinder, the maximum diameter of which, with the insulating silicone rubber, is 3.5 mm. The tip of the cylinder is 2.8 mm², and the hooks are 0.22 mm in diameter and 3.0 mm long. The total electrode surface area is 12 mm². The IE-65-I is 85 cm in length. The Medtronic 6961 has four soft 2.5 mm long silicone rubber tines immediately proximal to the tip which enable the lead to be entrapped in the trabeculae. The conductor is a space-wound multifilar design. The electrode has a surface area of 8 mm². The Cardiac Pacemakers, Inc. (CPI) 4116 has an 85–90% porous platinum-iridium tip to allow tissue ingrowth to hold the lead tip to the endocardium. The conductor is a double-wound helical coil in a silicone rubber sheath, with a lead length of 59 cm. The external surface area (effective pacing area) is 7.5 mm². The Cordis 1 mm electrode is a "standard" solid tip (rounded, but not ball-tip), with an electrode surface area of 8.8 mm². The conductor is coil-wound Elgiloy. The Medtronic 6971 has silicone tines and an electrode surface area of 8 mm. The lead is 58 cm long.

Thresholds were determined using a calibrated Biotronik ERA-3, while the pacing was monitored on an Electronics-for-Medicine (E for M) DR-12 or VR-8.

The methods and personnel were identical to those in the previously reported studies (5, 6). All cases were initial implants – that is each pacemaker was the first ever received by that patient. Intraoperative lead failures were replaced by a lead that attained satisfactory pacing, was coded a failure (unable to pass) and the replacement lead not considered in the study. All implants were on a strict rotation basis with each lead being used in turn. Pulse generators were, in effect, randomized, and no effort was made to use any particular generator with any particular lead. An extremely wide variety of pulse generators is used at this center. All implants were performed under fluoroscopy using standard implant techniques.

The reasons for failure to pace satisfactorily soon after permanent implant are many and not always apparent. Two mechanisms commonly cited are macro- and micro-displacement. In macro-displacement, a radiographically apparent change in position of the lead occurs, and failure to pace or sense cardiac activity satisfactorily is obviously related (7). Micro-displacement is said to be present when failure to pace is not associated with visible displacement, perforation of the ventricle or other apparent cause. As a diagnosis by exclusion, it is difficult to ascertain the nature of micro-displacement and its causes and methods of treatment; yet in two-thirds of instances, a single electrode revision of an initial failure of any kind produces continued satisfactory pacing (8). Leads designed to grasp the endocardium and reduce early failure to pace rates had become available. Their evaluation was deemed important.

All patients having initial transvenous implants were considered. A revision of an earlier implant, whether originally done at our institution or elsewhere, permitted any approach or lead considered satisfactory. Failure of the lead under evaluation might occur either during the process of implant or post-implant. If a lead were deemed a failure during or after implant, any suitable lead was then used. Failures were calculated intraoperatively as well as cumulatively intra- and postoperatively. If a patient required special pacing, such as atrial or A–V sequential, for arrhythmia termination, or a bipolar electrode for any reason, such implant was performed as necessary and the sequence of unipolar leads continued thereafter.

Results

The failure rates are subdivided (Figure 1 and Figure 2) into the causes of failure that were observed for this study. The unweighted mean total failure rate (mean of failure rates) was 9.2 ($\pm$ 4.5)%, while that for the post-operative failure rate was 6.0 ($\pm$ 2.9)%. Total failures (intra- and post-operative) equaled 58/702 or 8.3%, while post-operative failures for all leads were 39/687, or 5.6%.

Although there is a fourfold range of failure rates in both total and post-operative results, the statistical tests do not yield the highly significant probability (p) values that might be expected. The 1 mm and MIP-2000, the "best" and "poorest" performers in total fail-

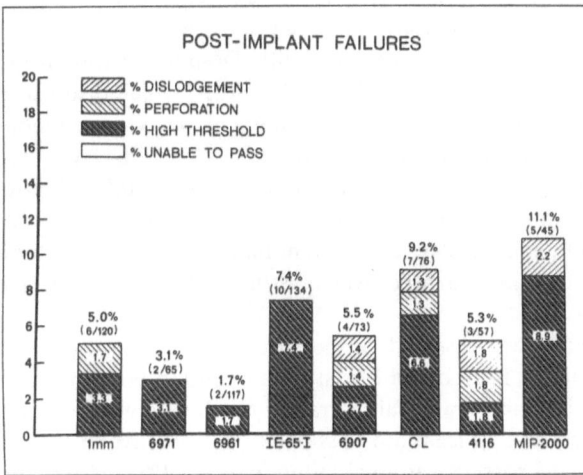

Fig. 1. Total failure rates: Intra and post implant

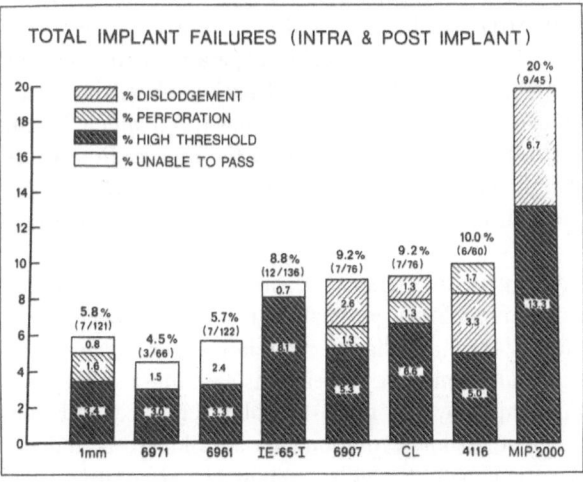

Fig. 2. Post-operative failure rates

ures, respectively, are clearly significantly different (p = 0.01). The same is true for the "second best" 6971 and the MIP-2000 (p = 0.025). The MIP-2000 is significantly different from the other seven leads taken as a group (p = 0.005). In the case of postoperative failures, the "best" and "poorest" performers – the 6961 and the MIP-2000 are significantly different (p = 0.025), while all other comparisons, grouped or individual are either "borderline" or clearly non-significant.

Discussion

Post-operative lead failure was divided into three varieties: displacement, in which radiographic movement was visible; ventricular perforation, in which endocardial electrograms existed which demonstrated perforation (9) and high threshold of unknown origin for all other failures. For the intra-operative failures, a fourth category, unable to pass, was added to describe the failure to attain a satisfactory pacing and sensing position. Micro-displacement was not considered as a diagnostic possibility. Despite the widespread belief in its existence, no diagnostic criteria or definitive findings exist which distinguish micro-displacement from other, perhaps equally ill-defined, failure modes. One commonly used expression for inability to stimulate the lead is "exit block" (10). This term, too, is ill-defined; for example, a pulse generator with a maximum output of 0.5 ms pulse duration at 5.0 volts and current limited at 10 mA (25 microjoules) may cease to stimulate the heart while a generator with equal voltage and current limits but a pulse duration of 2 ms (100 microjoules) may continue to pace over a rising and eventually stable threshold (11).

Although a wide range of failure rates was observed for these leads, significant differences resulted only between those having the highest and lowest failure rates in both total and post-operative situations. The highest and lowest failure rates in each case were attained for leads that are active fixation leads. If all leads are classified as either active or passive fixation and grouped accordingly, the passive lead total failure rate is 8.1% (27/333) and the active fixation total failure rate is 8.4% (31/369). There was also no difference in the mode of failure, high threshold or dislodgement. There is clearly no significant difference here. Postoperative failure rates for passive fixation leads was 6.1% (20/326), while that for active fixation leads was 5.3% (19/361), which again yields no significant difference.

The IE-65-I was a useful lead as a replacement in cases of intraoperative failure of other leads. The metal hooks apparently enabled the attainment of pacing where other leads would not. The IE-65-I lead has metal prongs attached to a collar (ring) which is fitted around the lead shaft near the electrode tip. The movement of the myocardium causes movement of the prong/collar assembly on the shaft, resulting in varying electrical potentials due to the motion of these metal surfaces. These potentials are capable of inhibiting VVI pacemakers.

The problem of lead caused electromagnetic interference was not resolved by the passage of time. Three patients with ventricular inhibited pacemakers required replacement because of symptomatic pacing pauses. One immediately after implant, another several months later and the third 50 months after implant. Other units continue to have lesser and asymptomatic pauses years after implant. The IE-65-I displayed the second highest rate of high threshold failures including threshold evolution over a prolonged period after implant. Examination of the 112 patient records available shows 15 (13.4%) had high threshold (above 25 uJ), 22 (19.6%) had electrode caused interference and 3.6% had both problems. This prompted the compilation of thresholds of all IE-65-I implants and pulse generator changes (acute and chronic thresholds) for 0.5 ms. This was compared to two leads with which this center has extensive experience – the 6907 and CL – both passive fixation leads (Figures 3A, 3B). All thresholds in the data base were included, whether they were or were not from implants in this study.

As can be seen in the graphs, the IE-65-I shows a considerably higher mean threshold than either the 6907 or CL in both the acute and chronic cases. The proportional differ-

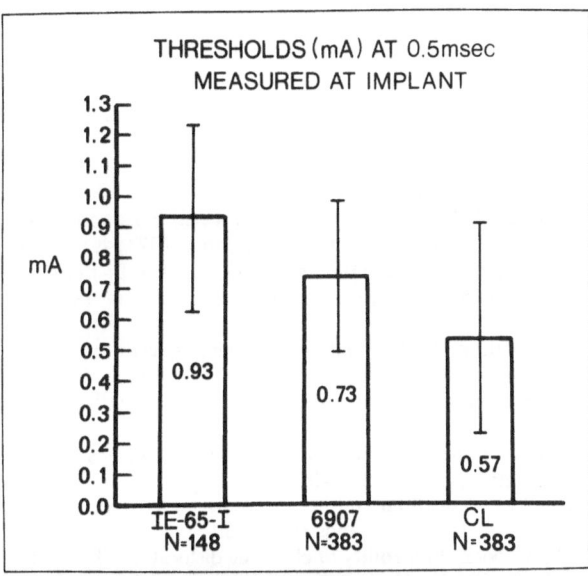

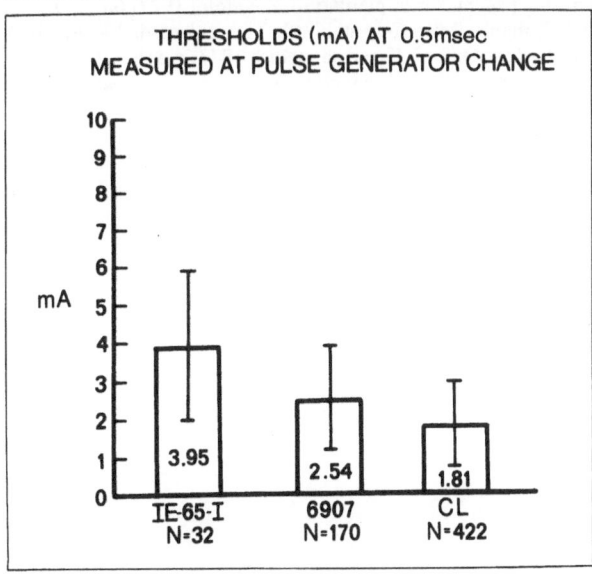

Fig. 3. Comparison of acute current thresholds at 0.5 ms for three leads (A); Comparison of chronic current thresholds at 0.5 ms for three leads (B)

ence is greater for the chronic case. These thresholds are not significantly different and may be due to the larger effective surface area of the IE-65-I, rather than any tissue damage from the metal hooks. The difference in threshold is not proportional to the surface area difference. This difference may be in agreement with previous studies concerning all passive leads which differ chiefly in surface area (12, 13). It must be noted, however, that any relationship between threshold and area must take stimulating pulse duration into account.

Although some new lead designs do yield better results than "standard" electrodes, there is no demonstrable significant advantage shown in this study for any of the tested lead types.

References

1. Charles RG, Clarke LM, Drysdale M, Sequeira RF: Endocardial pacing electrodes design and rate of displacement. Br Heart J 1977; 39: 515.
2. Wende U, Schaldach M: Neue intrakardiale Schrittmacherelektrode zur Vermeidung von Dislokationen bei stark dilatiertem Ventrikel. Dtsch Med Wschr 1970; 40: 2026.
3. Brenner AS, Wagner GS, Anderson ST et al: Transvenous, transmediastinal, transthoracic ventricular pacing: a comparison after complete two years follow-up. Circulation 1974; 49: 407.
4. Parsonnet V, Bilitch M, Furman S, Fisher JD, Escher DJW, Myers G, Cassady E: Early malfunction of transvenous pacemaker electrodes–A three center study, Circulation 1979; 60: 590–596.
5. Furman S, Pannizzo F, Campo I: Comparison of active and passive adhering leads for endocardial pacing. Pace 1979; 2: 417–427.
6. Furman S, Pannizzo F, Campo I: Comparison of active and passive leads for endocardial pacing-II. Pace 1981; 4: 78.
7. Irnich W, Bleifeld W, Effert S: Permanente transvenose Elektrostimulation des Herzens mit einer myokardial-fixierten Elektrode. Thoraxchirurgie 1972; 20: 440.
8. Thalen HJTH: Pacemaker electrodes: Past, present and future. In J Norman, A Rickards (eds): Proc of the pacemaker colloquium. Arnhem, The Netherlands 1975; p 39.
9. Renyi-Vamos FJ, Solti F, Gyongy T, Szabo Z: Probability of electrode dislocation: The importance of threshold measurements during pacemaker implantation. Z Kardiol 1977; 66: 310.
10. Timmis GC, Gordon S, Helland J: Enhanced electrode stability: The endocardial screw. In Y Watanabe (ed): Cardiac pacing. Amsterdam/Oxford, Excerpta medica 1977; p 516.
11. Furman S, Pannizzo F: Output programmability and reduction of secondary intervention after pacemaker implantation. J Thorac Cardiovasc Surg 1981; 81: 713–717.
12. Furman S, Parker B, Escher DJW, Solomon N: Endocardial threshold of cardiac response as a function of electrode surface area. J Surg Res 1968; 8: 161.
13. Furman S, Parker B, Escher DJW: Decreasing electrode size and increasing efficiency of cardiac stimulation. J Surg Res 1971; 11: 105.

Authors' address:
S. Furman, M.D.
Montefiore Medical Center
111 East 210th Street
Bronx, New York 10467, USA

Flexibility of Permanent Intracardiac Electrode Leads. Achieving a Balance between Perforation and Displacement

Grzegorz Opolski, Marian Pieniak, Roman Steckiewicz, Tadeusz Kraska

Summary: The three models (Biotronik IE-85-K-10-0, Tesla LES 165, Vitatron MIP 2147 LOES) of standard intracardiac electrodes with varying degrees of flexibility were tested in 655 patients during postoperative period. Twenty two cases (8.3%) of displacement and one case (0.3%) of myocardial wall perforation were observed in 264 patients with Biotronik leads. Fourteen displacements (4.2%) and six perforations (1.6%) occurred in 328 patients with Tesla leads. Eight perforations (12.6%) and one displacement (1.5%) were observed in 63 patients with Vitatron leads. The flexibility of the leads was determined by measurements of the bending and buckling forces in a developed mechanical model and by evaluation with Young's modulus and electrode unit pressure. It seems evident that in the case of the less flexible leads, higher number of perforations and a lower incidence of displacements may be expected. Accurate evaluation of the bending and buckling forces and a determination of electrode unit pressure is also useful for a comparison of the flexibility of different leads and a prediction of the eventual clinical complications.

Statement of Purpose

Does the degree of flexibility of the intracardiac lead have an influence on the displacement and perforation of the myocardial wall?

Material and Methods

The study examined 655 patients after insertion of intracardiac leads. The patients ranged in age from 17 years to 91 years, mean age of 69,6 years. The following leads were implanted 264 Biotronik IE-85-K-10-0 leads, 382 Tesla LES 165, and 63 Vitratron MIP 2147 LOES. The correct positioning for each electrode in the apex of the right ventricle was established under fluoroscopic TV ctrol, threshold measurements and intracardiac electrogram recording.

The rates of displacement and perforation were analysed for each model of lead during postoperative period. In each case the perforation was documented by an intracardiac electrogram recording (1, 4).

An attempt was made to determine qualitatively, the flexibility of the different models of leads and to compare the results with clinical observations. Mechanical studies of leads included the measurement and calculation of Young's modulus, bending force, buckling force, and electrode unit pressure.

Young's modulus and bending force were determined by using a simple mechanical model in which the 5 cm long segment of each type of lead was fixed at one end. The bending force necessary to deflect the tip at a constant distance was measured (Fig. 1).

Young's modulus was calculated by using the formula $X = \dfrac{Fl^3}{3\,EJ}$ where $J = \dfrac{\pi\,d^4}{64}$

The buckling force was determined by applying vertical force to the top of the free end of the lead (a 10 cm long segment was used in the experiment). Minimal force, which caused deflection of the segment, was defined as the buckling force (Fig. 2). It was assumed that the buckling force, as defined by the formula

$F = \dfrac{\pi^2 EJ}{l^2}$, corresponds to the stress resulting from the electrode pressing against the heart

wall. Additionally electrode unit pressure was calculated by dividing the buckling force by the cross-section of the electrode tip in contact with heart tissue.

Results

1. Clinical observations

In a total of 655 intracardiac implantations of the three tested models of leads, the different rates of displacement and perforation were observed during hospitalisation of the patients (Table 1).

Fig. 1.

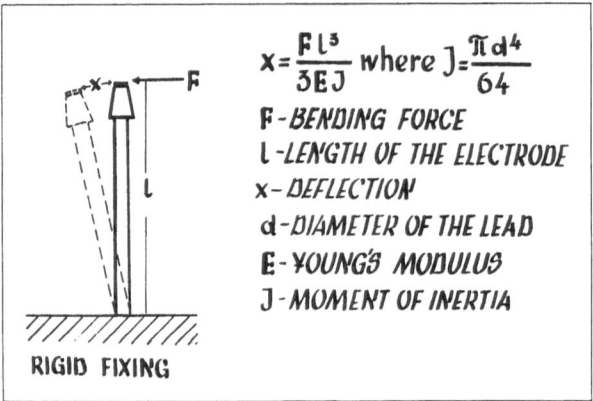

$$x = \frac{F\,l^3}{3EJ} \text{ where } J = \frac{\pi d^4}{64}$$

F - *BENDING FORCE*
l - *LENGTH OF THE ELECTRODE*
x - *DEFLECTION*
d - *DIAMETER OF THE LEAD*
E - *YOUNG'S MODULUS*
J - *MOMENT OF INERTIA*

RIGID FIXING

Fig. 2.

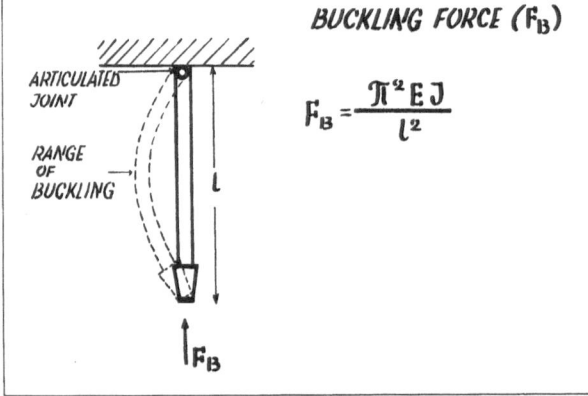

BUCKLING FORCE (F_B)

ARTICULATED JOINT

RANGE OF BUCKLING

$$F_B = \frac{\pi^2 EJ}{l^2}$$

F_B

Table 1.

Lead model	Total	Displacement	Perforation
Biotronik IE-85-K-10-0	264	22 (8,3%)	1 (0,3%)
Tesla LES 165	328	14 (4,2%)	6 (1,6%)
Vitatron MIP 2147 LOES	63	1 (1,5%)	8 (12,6%)

Table 2.

Lead model	Young's modulus (lead with stylet) $\left[\frac{N}{m^2} \cdot 10^6\right]$	Young's modulus (lead without stylet) $\left[\frac{N}{m^2} \cdot 10^6\right]$	Bending force $[N \cdot 10^{-3}](G)$	Buckling force $[N \cdot 10^{-3}](G)$	Electrode unit pressure $\left[\frac{N \cdot 10^{-3}}{mm^2}\right]\left[\frac{G}{mm^2}\right]$	
Biotronik IE-85-K-10-0	101	5,4	6,01 (0,61)	7,27 (0,74)	1,30	(0,17)
Tesla LES 165	942	16,6	10,62 (1,1)	12,85 (1,3)	3,01	(0,30)
Vitatron MIP 2147 LOES	147	17	26,95 (2,7)	32,6 (3,3)	5,69	(0,57)

2. Model studies

The values of Young's modulus, bending force, buckling force, and electrode unit pressure for the three models of tested leads are presented in Table 2:

Discussion

Transvenous pacing of the heart is, today, the dominant mode of permanent pacemakers, accounting for more than 90% of all permanent implants performed. Perhaps the major problem of transvenous pacing is the early post-implant lead failure rate. The reported failure rate varies from under 5% to almost 20% and is a significant source of morbidity and mortality (1, 3, 5). The majority of early lead malfunctions result from displacement and ventricular perforations. Although the incidence of dislodgement has fallen with the use of the active and tined leads, nevertheless, the problem remains (2, 3).

In this study three models of conventional leads, placed by the same personnel, had different rates of displacement and perforation. An attempt was made to determine, qualitatively, the flexibility of the three models of leads and to compare the results with clinical observations. The flexibility of the leads was determined by the measurements of bending and buckling forces in developed mechanical model and by evaluation of Young's modulus and electrode unit pressure.

The highest rate of perforation (12.6%) and the smallest rate of displacement (1.5%) were observed in the less flexible leads (Vitatron MIP 2147 LOES). On the contrary, in the more flexible leads (Biotronik JE-85-K-10-0), we found the highest rates of displacement (8,3%) and the smallest rates of perforation (0.3%).

The flexibility of the lead was significantly influenced by the stylet. In this study, Young's modulus of three types of the leads, with stylet, was found to be from 9 to 57 times higher than without stylet. Our study confirms clinical observations, that the usual cause of myocardial perforation is the positioning of the permanent pacemaker electrodes at the apex of the right ventricle, with the stylet fully inserted. The less flexible lead can easily penetrate a thin myocardial wall (3).

It seems evident that in the case of less flexible leads, a higher number of perforations and a lower incidence of displacements may be expected.

For a comparison of the flexibility between different types of leads, the measurement of the bending force, buckling force, and especially the calculation of the electrode unit pressure is of substantive value.

Knowing the amount of electrode unit pressure can be helpful in predicting displacement and perforation. Therefore, it may be useful in selecting the optimal lead for individual patients.

Conclusions

The rates of displacement and perforation depend on the degree of flexibility of the leads. For less flexible leads, a higher number of perforations and a lower incidence of displacement was observed.

It seems that for a comparison of the flexibility of different types of leads, the measurement of the bending force, buckling force, and especially the calculation of the electrode unit pressure is of substantive value.

References

1. Barold SS, Center S: Electrocardiographic diagnosis of perforation of the heart by pacing catheter electrode. Amer J Cardiol 1969; 24: 274.
2. Furman S, Pannizzo F, Campo J: Comparison of active and passive adhering leads for endocardial pacing. Pace 1979; 2: 417.
3. Mond H, Sloman G: The small-tined pacemaker lead – absence of dislodgement. Pace 1980; 3: 171.
4. Mond HG, Stuckej JG, Sloman G: The diagnosis of right ventricular perforation by an endocardial pacemaker electrode, Pace 1978; 1: 62.
5. Parsonnet V, Bilitch M, Furman S: Early malfunction of transvenous pacemaker electrodes: a three center study. Circulation 1979; 60: 590.

Authors' address:
G. Opolski, M.D.
Department of Cardiology
Medical Academy in Warsaw
4, Lindley'a, St. Build 3
02-005, Warsaw, Poland

Four Years Experience with the Bisping Transvenous Pacemaker Electrode

W. Stenzl, K.-H. Tscheliessnigg, D. Dacar, W. Hermann, F. Iberer

Summary: From October 1978 to March 1983 843 Bisping transvenous screw in pacemaker electrodes have been implanted at the surgical University Clinic of Graz/Austria. The Medtronic 6957 polyurethane coated electrode is placed into the right ventricle or atrium with the screw retracted in the insulating cover. When the desired electrode position is reached, the screw at the electrode tip is protruded by application of a torque at the external end of the conductor coil. In the ventricular position, stimulation threshold was a mean 0.7 V at 0.5 msec impulse width, the incidence of electrode instability was 1.1%. Reintervention for exit block became necessary in 2.0%. In atrial position (96 cases) the mean stimulation threshold was 1.1 V at 0.5 msec impulse width, the rate of lead dislocation was 3.1%. When extraction of the electrode became necessary in 8 cases due to infection, the screw at the electrode tip could be retracted in all cases, up to 6 months after implantation. In 3 cases, however, permanent traction of 50–100 grams for up to 72 hours had to be applied to remove the lead tip from the superior caval vein. In a group of 17 patients, in whom implantation was carried out before March, 1979, no electrode related problems were observed. Until now, we did not observe a single case of electrode dysfunction due to damage of the polyurethane cover or because of fracture of the unifilar conductor coil. The Bisping transvenous pacemaker electrode has largely reduced the risk of electrode dislocation and thus has contributed to safety in ventricular, atrial and bifocal pacing.

Electrode dislocation has been one of the most common complications after implantation of transvenous pacemaker electrodes. Especially in patients with dilated right ventricle and rarefied trabeculae, or with recurrent arrhythmia, a stable electrode position can be difficult to obtain. On the other hand serious complications such as ventricular rupture have been observed after implantation of sutureless epimyocardial leads using a subxyphoidal pericardiotomy (1). Moreover, the need for a reliable electrode function is emphasized by an increasing number of bifocal pacemaker implantations. In recent years various efforts to meet the problem of electrode instability have been made and electrode types utilizing nylon or metal barbs, coils or screws for active fixation in the myocardium have been designed (2). This report deals with our experience with 843 Bisping* endocardial leads which were implanted between October 1978 an March 1983.

Materials and Methods

The Medtronic 6957® transvenous screw-in pacemaker electrode (3) is placed into the right ventricle with the screw retracted in the insulating cover. When the desired posi-

---

* Medtronic 6957®

tion is reached, the screw is protrudedd by application of a torque at the external end of the conductor coil. The protrusion of the screw at the electrode tip can be ascertained by fluoroscopy. After fixation of the electrode, threshold and R-wave potential measurements are taken. The fastening corkscrew is identical to the stimulating area. After eventual measurement of unsatisfactory threshold or R-wave values, the screw can be retracted and the fixation procedure repeated in a new position for several times. The screw length is 2 mm, stimulation area is 10 mm², electrode diameter is 2.3 mm (3.4 mm at the tip). With the 58 cm electrode, an average of 6 turns is necessary to protrude the screw and to fasten the lead tip. Between October 1978 and March 1983, 843 leads were implanted in 765 patients. 669 electrodes were implanted for ventricular pacing (VVI), 14 electrodes were used for atrial pacing (AAI). For bifocal pacing (DDD, DVI, VAT) 78 electrodes were implanted into the right ventricle and 79 into the right atrium. 3 leads were used in antitachycardia devices.

Ventricular pacing:

In 669 patients, the electrode was used for ventricular pacing (VVI) only. In this group, access to the right ventricle was feasible via the cephalic vein in 475 cases (71%), in 63 cases (9.4%) the external jugular vein and in 19 cases (2.8%) the internal jugular vein was used. From 1981, the subclavian puncture technique was applied regularly for electrode insertion, when a cephalic vein was not available. In ventricular pacing, mean age was 72 years (range 8 to 94 years). The mean stimulation threshold was 0.7 V at 0.5 msec impulse width, mean R-wave potential was 7.5 mV (cases of asystolia or immeasurable R-wave potential excluded).

Complications – ventricular position:

747 electrodes were implanted in ventricular position for ventricular (VVI) or bifocal (DDD, DVI, VAT) pacing. The total rate of complications requiring reoperation was 3.1%. After ventricular implantation 8 dislocations (1.1%) were observed occurring between 5 hours and 6 months after implantation. In one patient, the electrode penetrated through an infarction area during implantation and caused a lethal hemopericardium. Exit block was observed in 22 cases (3%). In 7 cases (1.0%) it was responsive to conservative treatment, in 15 cases (2.0%) electrode repositioning and/or implantation of a high output or programmable pulse generator was carried out. In 10 of the 15 cases requiring reoperation for exit block, stimulation thresholds at the initial stimulation were higher than 1.5 V. Only 2 cases of exit block were observed more than 6 months after the initial implantation.

Electrode removal after ventricular implantation

In 8 cases electrode removal became necessary due to infection between 1 and 30 months after the initial implantation. In all cases it was possible to retract the screw and to withdraw the electrode tip from the ventricular cavity. In 3 cases, however, a slight permanent

428

traction (50–100 grams for up 3 days) had to be applied to remove the electrode tip from the superior caval vein.

Ventricular pacing – lead durability:

In 17 patients (mean age 64 years, range 8–84 years) the electrode was implanted before March 1979, in 83 patients it was implanted before March 1980. At that time, the electrode usually was implanted in patients who had suffered from intraoperative or postoperative electrode problems with conventional leads. In this group no electrode related technical problems became evident.

Atrial position:

91 standard Medtronic 6957® electrodes and 5 specially J-shaped Bisping electrodes (Medtronic 6957) were implanted, Mean stimulation threshold was 1.1 V at 0.5 msec impulse width (range 0.3–2.0 V), mean p-wave potential was 4.9 mV (range 1.8–8 mV). With both electrode types, implantations were carried out using straight and J-shaped guidewires. Preferred placement site was in the right atrial appendage.

Complications after atrial implantation:

3 cases of electrode dislocation (3.1%) requiring electrode repositioning were observed 24 hours up to 12 months after the initial implantation. Stimulation of the right phrenic nerve occurring in a female patient 6 months after implantation of a bifocal pacemaker disappeared after repositioning of the atrial electrode.

Discussion

The Bisping transvenous screw-in electrode (3) offers a logical approach to the problem of electrode instability in dilated ventricles with diminished trabecular structure, as the fixation is carried out by protrusion of a small screw right into the myocardium. We started to use this electrode in 1978 in patients who had a previous dislocation of a conventional electrode. Before, threshold measurements in animal experiments (4) yielded data similar to those of conventional electrodes. After encouraging initial clinical results, we implant the electrode now as a standard lead. In our opinion, the electrode offers several positive aspects in clinical pacing.

Electrode-tip dimensions are similar to those of conventional electrodes (Fig. 1). In our experience, insertion via the cephalic vein was possible as frequently as with conventional electrodes. When implantation is carried out correctly, the corkscrew leaves the insulating cover when the site of stimulation is reached. Therefore, electrode related traumatization of tricuspid valvular tissue or electrode entrapment are very unlikely to occur. The active fixation mechanism allows a wide choice of electrode positions to obtain optimal pacing conditions, as, at fixation the conductor coil rotates round the guidewire,

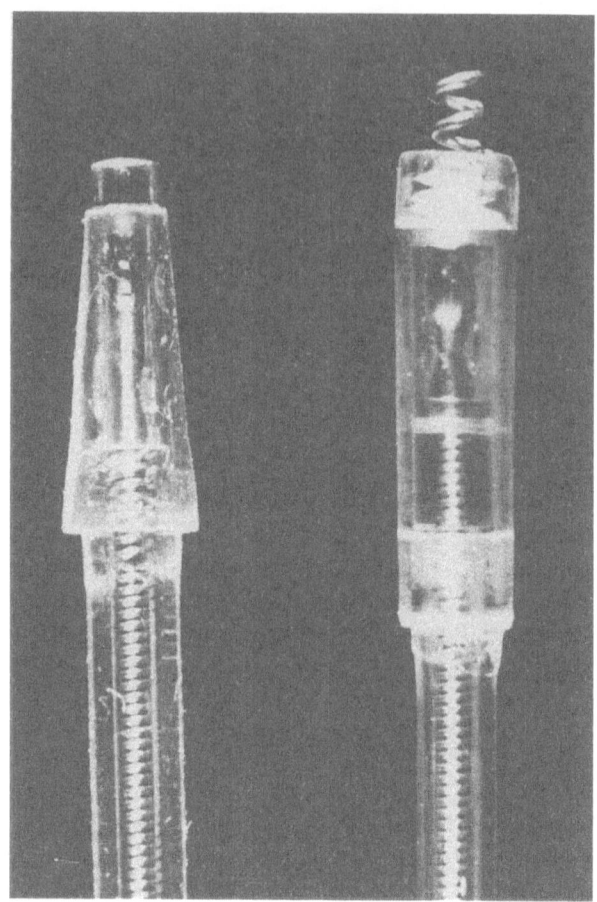

Fig. 1. The Bisping transvenous electrode (right, screw protruded), in comparison a conventional electrode (left)

which can be shaped in advance. In children, the probability of growth related electrode dysfunction can be diminished by formation of an intracardiac loop. For bifocal pacing, insertion of both electrodes into the same cephalic vein was possible in 25 cases (31%). When the cephalic vein could not be used for introduction of one or both electrodes, the subclavian-puncture technique (5) was applied. Before 1981 lead insertion were carried out using the cephalic and jugular veins exclusively. Until now, no cases of electrode dysfunction due to damage of the polyurethane insulating cover or due to fracture of the unifilar conductor coil have been observed in 4½ years with a total of 843 implantations.

In this regard it seems to be important to mention that before 1981 lead insertions were carried out using the jugular veins (82 patients) when a cephalic vein was not available. Even in the highly-stressed jugular region, electrode defects were not observed. With the Medtronic 6957 electrode we have observed a decrease of intra- and postoperative dislocations with threshold and R-wave potential measurements being similar to those of conventional electrodes (6). In the atrial position, too, the Bisping electrode has led to a decrease of complications an thus has enhanced the indication to bifocal pacing.

References

1. Hermann W, Gutschi S, Stenzl W, Rigler B: Myocardschraubelektrode. Acta Chir Austriaca 1975; 7: 131.
2. Gutschi S, Hermann W, Stenzl W, Tscheliessnigg KH: Die chirurgische Therapie nach Schrittmacherelektrodendislokation. Zbl Chir 1979; 104: 100.
3. Bisping HJ, Rupp H: A new transvenous electrode for fixation in the atrium. 5th Internat Symposion on Cardiac Pacing, Tokyo 1976.
4. Stenzl W, Hermann W, Tscheliessnigg KH, Rigler B, Gutschi S, Bisping HJ: Experimentelle Untersuchungen mit einer neuen transvenös fixierbaren Schrittmacherelektrode. Kongr Ber 18. Tagung der Österr Ges f Chir Graz 1977, p. 877.
5. Sterz H, Prager H, Koller H, Pachinger J: Percutaneous Implantation of Permanent Pacemakers. Pace 1981; 4: 175.
6. Dittrich H: Herzschrittmacher-Implantation. Chirurg 54, 1983: 143–148.

Authors' address:
Dr. W. Stenzl
Universitätsklinik für Chirurgie
Auenbruggerplatz
A-8036 Graz/Österreich

Management of Pacemaker Patients – Basic Concepts

S. Furman

Summary: Management of patients who require implantation of a pacemaker involves knowledge of the basic rhythmic disturbance and a decision concerning whether to pace in the single chamber atrial or ventricular modes, the AV universal mode or the physiologically responsive mode. Once implanted long term observation in the pacemaker clinic and by transtelephonic monitoring (TTM) is required. Extensive knowledge of the operation and eccentricities of a variety of pulse generators is required as is knowledge of the behaviour of the model pacemaker implanted. Pacemakers should be implanted for the diagnosis of heart block but only when sinus node dysfunction is associated with symptoms. An implanted pacemaker should not be competitive with the chamber that it paces so that dual chamber pacemakers should sense in both chambers.

Management of pacemaker patients can be considered from the perspective of the individual patient and from that of the patient population. In managing a pacemaker patient, he/she must therefore be considered individually and as part of the group of pacemaker patients and as part of the group with the specific pacemaker model implanted.

Before implantation, and during selection of the best equipment the patient's underlying cardiac rhythmic disturbance must be analyzed. Questions should be asked:
1. Is atrial fibrillation or flutter a prominent feature?
   If so it may be that atrial involvement in pacing is inappropriate.
2. Is the critical arrhythmia, bradycardia or tachycardia sufficiently frequent so that dual chamber pacing and restoration of the normal AV sequence is beneficial?
   If not, is single chamber pacing adequate to deal with infrequent episodic bradycardia?
3. Is the atrial rate so slow or is the ventricular response slow and fixed so that a pacemaker responsive to physiologic stimuli other than the atrium is desirable?
4. Is the critical bradycardia so infrequent that a recording should be made of the event? Is a tachycardia present so that its occurrence must be recorded to assist in management by medication?
   If so a pacemaker with memory should be used.
5. Is atrial function reliable so that dual chamber pacing is useful?
6. Is the procedure a pulse generator replacement in a stable patient so that flexibility and programmability are less required?
   If so, consider a single rate or simple programmable ventricular inhibited pacemaker.
7. Are the leads in use made of silicone rubber or polyurethane?
   If polyurethane, consider the possibility that deterioration of the material may occur.

The operating surgeon should consider the availability, in his clinic, of several manufacturers as no one manufacturer has available, at any given time, a full range of hardware which will meet the therapeutic needs listed above. By limitation to only one manufacturer it is unlikely that some features of dual chamber function, interrogatability, multi-programmability or memory will be available to a specific patient when needed. Conversely, only the largest clinics should use more than several manufacturers because of the confusion caused by a plethora of pulse generators. Even if only few models are used at any one time the total number of different models being followed will be cumulative and over several years great in variety.

Record keeping

Record keeping concerning implantable cardiac pacemakers is especially possible because of the numerical specificity of pacemaker hardware and functions. Pulse generators and leads are specifically identified by model and serial number; atrial and ventricular stimulation thresholds and electrograms are numerically defined; AV delay and atrial and ventricular refractory periods are all numerical; pulse generator end of life is by specific rate decline. The duration of a pacemaker in a specific patient is measured numerically in months and compared to the expected longevity for that design (1).

The Pacemaker Clinic

The pacemaker clinic consists of three different capabilities:
A) The ability to analyze pacemaker function by multichannel ECG; ambulatory telemetry of patient and hardware data; ECG monitoring; programming of all pacemaker functions. Only direct pacemaker analysis can determine thresholds, wound status and the general state of patient well being (2).
B) Radiography for identification of unknown pacemakers, lead and pulse generator position and the possibility of lead fracture (3).
C) Transtelephonic monitoring (TTM) of pacemaker function is the best technique for long term follow-up of stable pacemaker function, in which battery depletion or unanticipated sudden failure may occur. It is also the best method of follow-up of large groups of patients (4). Frequent face to face clinic follow-up for pacemaker analysis for large groups is not feasible.

The pacemaker physician should be acquainted with general events concerning his pacemaker patients. Recalls occur and unusual events and pacemaker eccentricities which may seem abnormal but represent normal function should be known (5). Specific records of the patient's pacemaker function should be kept separate in a defined area so that they are readily available.

If possible, computerized statistics should be available to the physician concerning his own patient population. That may be derived from an institutional data base, a commercial data base, i.e. from the manufacturer or as part of a national registry. Patients should be provided with adequate data on their person to allow a physician away from the patient's home to know the pacemaker and its state of function, when necessary. An identification card or a pacemaker "passport" is desirable (6) (Table 1).

Table 1A. Pulse Generator Replacements – 1982.

Electronic Failure	12
Mercury (2)	
Lithium (10)	
Battery Exhaustion	40
Mercury (21)	
Lithium (19)	
Recall	18
Total	70

Table 1B. Pulse generator replacements – 1982 (Electronic/Battery).

Mean Longevity (All)	52.1 ± 17.4 months
Mean Longevity (Lithium)	46.1 ± 18.7 months
Mean Longevity (Mercury)	60.0 ± 11.9 months
Mean Recall (Lithium)	31.1 ± 4.9 months

Table 2. Pacemaker Implantation Indications.

Heart Block	
Acquired	– on diagnosis
Congenital	– signs/symptoms
Sinus Node Dysfunction	
Sinus Bradycardia	– signs/symptoms
Sick Sinus Syndrome	– signs/symptoms

Indications for Pacemaker Implantation

Two broad areas of indication for implantation exist. One is that of episodic, frequent or fixed heart block punctuated by episodes of asystole or ventricular tachycardia. The second is the sick sinus syndrome (sinus node dysfunction) in which episodes of sinus bradycardia, sinus arrest or supraventricular tachycardia exist. At present, all other indications account for no more than 5–10% of all implantations. The indications for implantation of a pacemaker are different in the two groups (Table 2).

Acquired heart block is of well known evolution. Unless the episode of block has been associated with a reversible condition, such as (but not limited to) severe drug intoxication, posterior wall myocardial infarction, etc., pacemaker implantation should be performed. The presence of symptoms is not required. For patients with congenital heart block, symptoms are the indication, as some with congenital heart block can live a normally active existence of normal duration. Atrial fibrillation with slow ventricular response is better considered as part of heart block rather than sick sinus syndrome and implantation performed if pauses of three seconds or more appear or if the cardiac rate is persistently below 50 per minute.

Sinus node dysfunction is uncommonly a lethal cardiac condition; heart block is frequently lethal. Patients with sinus node dysfunction should therefore be implanted if they are symptomatic or give signs of impairment of cardiac function, and not implanted in the absence of such symptoms. Patients may be unaware of a significant degree of disability which may be apparent to those about them. In that case the signs apparent to others should determine the need for implant (7).

The question of the duration of a pause which, without associated signs or symptoms, should be managed by pacing is a difficult issue. In general, a well documented single pause of three seconds or more in duration requires further careful documentation and several such pauses should be treated. The sinus node is sensitive to many commonly used medications such as beta blockers and to electrolyte disturbances so that even multiple episodes of sinus arrest during a single period of illness may not be an indication for implantable pacing. Sinus bradycardia or sinus arrest may occur only during drug intoxication or electrolyte imbalance but electrolyte stability may be so difficult to achieve in a particular patient that implantable pacing may yet be required. Asymptomatic sinus bradycardia recorded during sleep, even at a continuing rate of 30 bpm, unassociated with escape ventricular arrhythmias, is not an indication for pacing.

Carotid sinus massage is a simple, rapid test which may be very useful. The carotid artery should be investigated by auscultation and palpation to assure that partial arterial compression will not produce neurologic symptoms. An induced sinus pause of more than 3 seconds, or the appearance of AV block can correlate with otherwise undiagnosed syncope. A positive finding in a symptomatic patient is an indication for implantable pacing (Fig. 1).

Sinus bradycardia above a rate of 40 beats per minute, not punctuated by slower periods or episodes of sinus arrest, is generally asymptomatic. This is not always the case. Some persons will have signs and symptoms of reduced cardiac output, lassitude, easy fatiguability and even lesser mental symptoms all based on sinus bradycardia. Though such patients are not at risk of life they have a bona fide need for cardiac pacing. Despite the relative restriction of indications to patients who are significantly symptomatic, the lesser symptoms may, nevertheless, be disabling and the physician should be able to recognize the patient who has reduced cardiac output caused by sinus bradycardia.

Temporary cardiac pacing is helpful in distinguishing the patient who is minimally symptomatic, but it should be of the atrium. Ventricular pacing, even at an accelerated rate is likely to decrease cardiac output, produce a reversal of the atrio-ventricular sequence and cause the unpleasant sensation of cannon waves in the neck and chest (8). As two-thirds of patients with chronically slow sinus rhythms will have such retrograde conduction it is wisest to plan for dual chamber pacing in all such patients. It must be remembered that retrograde conduction may be well maintained even when antegrade conduction is partially or wholly impaired. The state of antegrade conduction on the

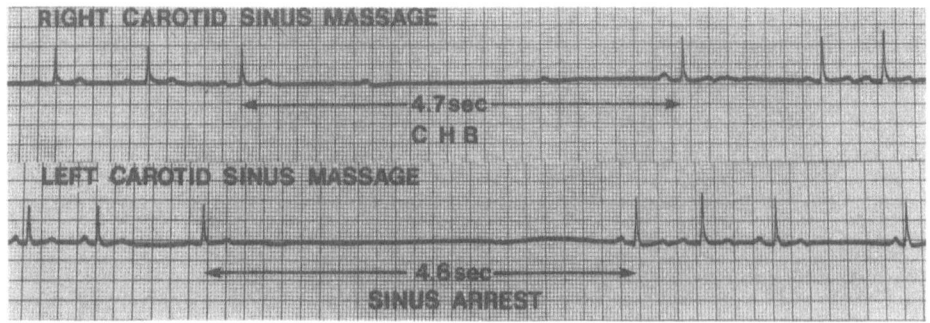

Fig. 1. This patient had had recurrent episodes of syncope. Two 24 hour ambulatory ECGs had been unrevealing. Right sided carotid sinus massage produced complete AV block and left sided massage produced sinus arrest. Following pacemaker implant syncopal episodes ceased.

ECG may be an inadequate clue to the state of retrograde conduction. If the patient frequently has an adequate sinus rhythm punctuated by episodic sinus arrest, it may be acceptable to pace the atrium, if AV conduction is stable and reliable. If it is not and ventricular pacing is required, then a slow paced rate, adequate to prevent asystole and syncope but one which will be usually inhibited, is useful. Pacemaker hysteresis is also valuable if it will allow the ventricular rate to fall to levels at which pacing is required and then pace at a more rapid rate. Dual chamber pacing is the best mode of all.

In any event, careful documentation of the rhythm which necessitated pacing is mandatory. That ECG, frequently lost, is critically important for later patient management and pacemaker selection. The physician who implants the pacemaker should see to it that this documentation is preserved.

Pulse Generators

Pulse generators should be bipolar whenever possible to avoid electromagnetic interference (EMI) including that from pectoral muscle artifacts (9). This is especially important when considering atrial pacing which requires higher sensitivity levels. Most dual chamber pacemakers are, however, unipolar and at present it may be difficult to find a dual chamber pacemaker which is adequately flexible and which can operate as a bipolar device.

A pulse generator should be widely programmable in output, rate and sensitivity. These are the three basic functions which require manipulation to provide patient safety and secure pacing. If the pacemaker selected is dual chamber, then rate, output and sensitivity should be independently programmable as should the delay between atrial and ventricular activity. If atrial sensing exists (as it should) the atrial refractory period and upper rate limit should be programmable. Lead failure rates vary, but are lowest for any lead when used with a multiprogrammable pacer because of the ability to override temporary threshold and sensing problems.

Attempt to restore the normal AV sequence if that is possible. Well placed and satisfactorily functioning dual chamber pacemakers should be able to respond adequately in both atrium and ventricle. If the atrial rate is slow and fixed (or if the patient has fixed atrial fibrillation) and retrograde conduction does not exist, a physiologically responsive single chamber pacemaker can be considered (10). Should a dual chamber pacemaker become available which responds to physiologic stimuli in addition to the atrium it should be used.

No pacemaker should be competitive or potentially competitive in a chamber it paces (Figure 2). This may be especially true for the atrium in which competition can readily cause atrial fibrillation, possibly more readily than ventricular competitive stimulation causes ventricular fibrillation (11) (Fig. 3). Stimulation of the atrium should not compel pacing of the ventricle and pacing of the ventricle should not force stimulation during a more rapid atrial rate. Cross talk between the two channels should be managed by a blanking period as short as possible. In a bipolar pacer the blanking period may be absent. The longer the blanking period, the greater the likelihood of an unsensed cardiac event, atrial or ventricular, and a competitive arrhythmia.

Always select the pulse generator of maximum projected longevity if it meets physiologic needs. It will be cheapest in the long run and in the broadest group of patients. Estimat-

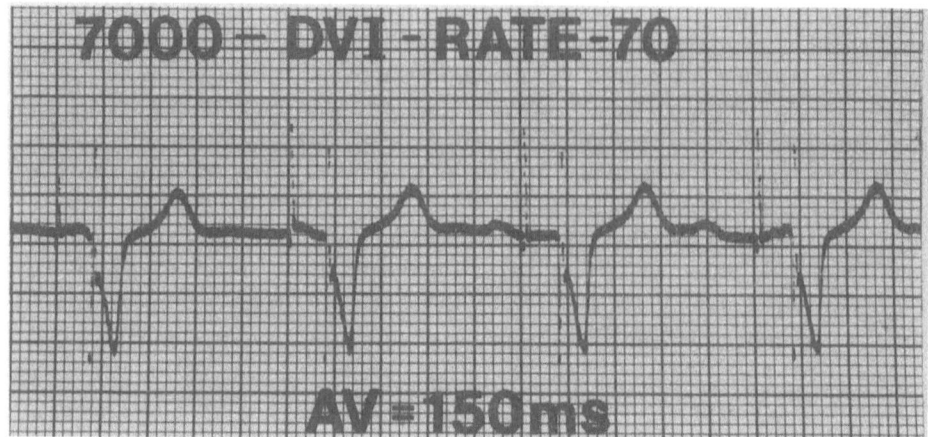

Fig. 2. The DVI pacemaker is potentially competitive with atrial activity during normal function. The first complex has a paced P wave. The next three atrial stimuli are competitive with spontaneous P waves. The final atrial stimulus produces an early second atrial contraction.

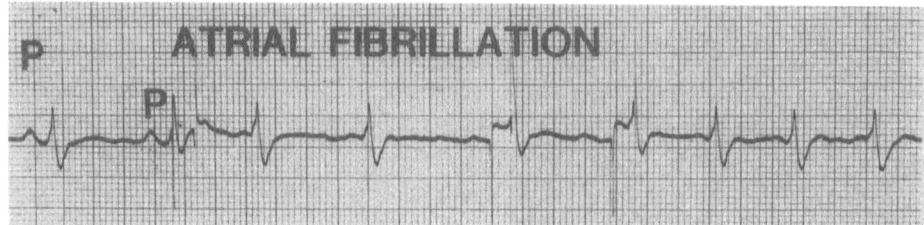

Fig. 3. Competition between pacemaker atrial stimulus and the P wave can, in the vulnerable atrium, produce atrial fibrillation. The first P wave has no pacemaker competition, an atrial stimulus competes with the second P wave and produces sustained atrial fibrillation.

ing projected longevity of a group of individual patients is unrewarding. Do not implant pulse generators with a memory of stimulating events in an effort to gain information required to legitimize the implant. Very likely some of the patients will never have needed a pacemaker. Pursue preoperative evaluation to reasonable lengths.

Post-Implant

The patient should be seen within a month after implant and 2–3 times yearly thereafter. He/she should always have the ability to contact the pacemaker clinic as necessary. Transtelephonic monitoring should be begun at the latest possible time. In several models of short duration dual chamber pacemakers this may mean onset of monitoring at eighteen months; for longer lasting models monitoring should begin at about three years after implant. For patients who are remote, monitoring should be begun early after implant. Each patient should be clear about the division of follow-up unless the pacemaker center

438

intends both pacemaker and cardiologic follow-up. A clearly defined cardiologic and medical follow-up should be designated apart from the pacemaker follow-up.

Management of patients with an implanted pacemaker is a complex undertaking involving the patient, his physiologic response to pacing and the function and durability of the hardware. Managment of the pacemaker is best accomplished in a specialized center. That center may not be equipped to provide total cardiologic management. Then, cardiologic and other attention should be carried out by another physician.

References

1. Bilitch M, Hauser RG, Goldman BS, Furman S, Parsonnet V: Performance of cardiac pacemaker pulse generators. Pace 1982; 5: 139–144.
2. Furman S: Cardiac pacing and pacemakers VIII. The pacemaker follow-up clinic. Am Heart J 1977; 94: 795–804.
3. Sorkin RP, Schuurmann BJ, Simon AB: Radiographic aspects of permanent cardiac pacemakers. Radiology 1976; 119: 281.
4. Pennock RS, Dreifus LS, Morse DP, Watanabe Y: Cardiac pacemaker function. JAMA 1972; 222: 1379.
5. Astrinsky EA, Furman S, Florio J: Asystolic episodes during pacemaker implantation. Circulation 1981; 63: 1379–1382.
6. Rickards A, Norman J: Clinical classification of generator and electrode failures. Pace 1980; 3: 17–23.
7. Shaw DB, Holman RR, Gowers JI; Survival in sinoatrial disorder (sick-sinus syndrome). Br Med J 1980; 280: 139.
8. Ogawa S, Dreifus LS, Shenoy PN, Brockman SK, Berkovits BV: Hemodynamic consequences of atrioventricular and ventriculoatrial pacing. Pace 1978; 1: 8–15.
9. Secemsky SI, Hauser RG, Denes P, Edwards LM: Unipolar sensing abnormalities: Incidence and clinical significance of skeletal muscle interference and undersensing in 228 patients. Pace 1982; 5: 10–19.
10. Rickards AF, Norman J: Relation between QT interval and heart rate, new design of physiologically adaptive cardiac pacemaker. Br Heart J 1981; 45: 56–61.
11. Furman S, Cooper JA: Atrial fibrillation during A-V sequential pacing. Pace 1982; 5: 133.

Authors' address:
S. Furman, M.D.
Montefiore Medical Center
111 East 210th Street
Bronx, New York 10467 USA

Techniques for Permanent Transvenous Pacemaker Implantation: Personal Preferences

V. Parsonnet

Summary: Every experienced surgeon eventually develops unique techniques that, in his hands, facilitate the operation. I have outlined a number of my own methods that are designed, in general, to enhance pacing reliability and avoid reoperation, and to simplify reoperations should they become necessary. These methods may prove useful to others.

Introduction

More than 95% of today's pacemakers are implanted by the transvenous route (1). Although most physicians who implant pacers are quite familiar with the basic principles of their operation, some evidence of differences in quality of care came to light in the 1981 United States Pacemaker Survey reported elsewhere at this Congress. From that study it appeared that technical sophistication of pacemaker implantation was not universal. Over the years experience has taught us techniques that, in our own hands, have proved to be most reliable and simple. This report describes some of these personal preferences. The reader may refer to other sources for details of basic transvenous implantation techniques (2–5).

Basic Implantation Principles

In any transvenous electrode implantation certain essentials for positioning the electrodes in either atrium or ventricle must be followed. For ventricular lead placement, preliminary advancement of the electrode into the pulmonary artery followed by slow pull-back into the right ventricle virtually assures that the definitive position will be in the right ventricle rather than in the coronary veins. In the atrium, a synchronous to-and-fro, right-to-left movement of the electrode is almost diagnostic of a proper location in the atrial appendage.

After achieving what appears to be a satisfactory anatomical position of the electrode fluoroscopically, various confirmatory threshold tests must be done. If the tests fail to establish a perfect functional location the lead must be repositioned (Table 1). We make all measurements oscilloscopically to avoid the inherent inaccuracy and variability of the commercial pacemaker systems analyzers.

The Electrode Introducer

I am *not* in favor of *routine* use of the introducer technique, because its apparent simplicity predisposes to its cavalier employment and the lurking complications. We should be

441

Table 1. Tests Performed at Implant and Desired Results (See Text).

Test	Range of Desired Findings	
	Atrium	Ventricle
Stimulation thereshold at a pulse duration of 1.5 msec	0.3–0.5 V*) 0.3–0.5 mA	0.2–0.4 V*) 0.2–0.4 mA
Electrogram amplitude**) "ST Deviation"	0.8–3 mV Present	5.0–12.0 mV ⩾ 2 mV
Pace at maximum output of external pulse generator (15–20 mA)	No twitch of right hemidiaphragm	No twitch of left hemidiaphragm
Pulse generator voltage output, open-circuit with a 1000-Ohms load; voltage and current with heart load	Nominal	Nominal

*) Values vary widely with electrode design. Leading-edge impedance may be calculated from these figures.
**) "Slew rates" not measured.

reminded that in contrast to the cephalic vein cutdown technique, which is associated with few serious complications, the introducer method has many known complications, at least four of which are potentially lethal (see asterisks in Table 2). Therefore, after making the preliminary incision, the deltopectoral groove is explored. If the cephalic vein is large it is used for the introducer. If not, the introducer is passed into the subclavian vein. Table 3 lists several precautions that have been most helpful in avoiding introducer complications.

Selection of Atrial Leads

Atrial lead unreliability has been a problem for many years, recently solved by the development of the screw-in atrial (Bisbing Remove) lead*. Actuarial survival analysis of these and other leads confirm their superior performance (Fig. 1). Therefore, for the sake of simplicity and uniformity I have begun to use the Bisbing polyurethane ventricular and atrial screw-in leads in all cases. Polyurethane degredation, a problem only in the earliest series of leads, no longer occurs and therefore I have seen no reason to discontinue using them (Table 4). In my own hands, electrode malfunctions due to perforation, malposition, or dislodgement have virtually disappeared as post-operative complications. It is also for this reason that I can continue the practice of shortening the leads to the desired length.

---

* Medtronic 5957 and 5957J electrodes, Medtronic, Inc., Minneapolis, Minnesota, USA.

Table 2. Complications That May Occur with Introducer Technique (See Text).

*Pneumothorax	Osteomyelitis
*Air Embolus	Septic Arthritis
*Hemothorax	AV Fistula
*Hemopneumothorax	Catheter "Embolus"
Hemomediastinum	Tracheal Perforation
Pneumomediastinum	Hematoma
Vein Thrombosis	Catheter or Stylet Knots
Brachial Nerve Trauma	Phrenic Nerve Injury
Thoracic Duct Tear	Catheter in Pleural Cavity
Air in Pacer Pocket	Guide Wire "Embolus"
	Lung Laceration

Table 3. Procedures That are Helpful in Avoiding Complications (See Text).

Precautionary Maneuver	Result
Elevate legs (or Trendelenberg position)	Distends vein for easy puncture; Avoids air embolization
Use cephalic vein for introducer	Avoids trama to lung (pneumothorax, tension pneumothorax) or subclavian artery hemorrhage (hemothorax)
"Retained-guidewire technique" for dual-chamber pacing (7)	Avoids second subclavian vein puncture
Sedate the restless patient	Avoids deep inhalation while introducer is in place (air embolization)
Pinch off introducer whenever it is not occluded by an electrode	Avoids air embolization
Loose double-ligature loop around introducer site	Eliminates intraoperative venous bleeding

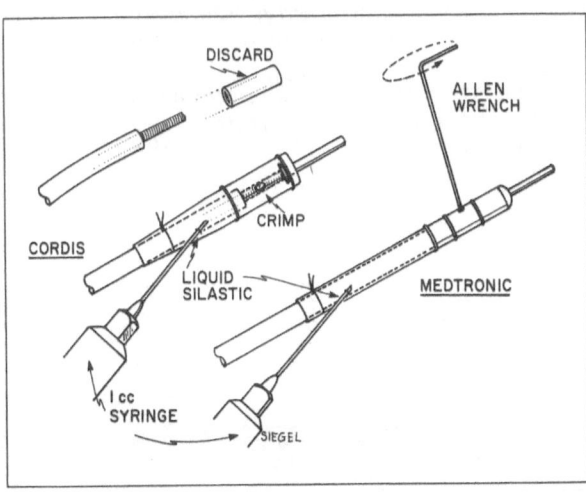

Fig. 1. The techniques for shortening wires and attaching Medtronic* or Cordis* connectors; *Medtronic, Inc., 3055 Old Highway Eight, P.O. Box 1453, Minneapolis, Minnesota, 55440, USA; **Cordis Corporation, P.O. Box 525700, Miami, Florida, 33152, USA

443

Wire Shortening

Once positioned, most leads are too long, and 20–40 cm of superfluous length must be wrapped around the pacemaker or stuffed into the pacer pocket. This practice, especially in two-lead systems, effectively makes the pacemaker larger; it also complicates the reoperation by the need to dissect out a tangle of wires. A technique for shortening wires is shown in the diagrams in Fig. 2. The only potential drawbacks to this technique are the resultant difficulty in reinserting a stiffening wire in case a reoperation for lead malposition is required, and the dangers of disruption of the insulation or fracture of the wire at the splice. As stated, electrode malfunction is now so rare that the former problem is no longer an issue. Regarding splice fractures or defects, analysis of our most recent experience with 117 shortened leads (57 atrial and 70 ventricular) over a mean follow-up period of 17 months reveals no fractures or structural defect. Therefore, I feel confident in continuing this practice. Unfortunately, lead shortening will not be practical with bipolar wires. One hopes that the manufacturers will provide wires of more appropriate lengths when the time comes.

Table 4. Polyurethane Implants in which Environmental Stress Corrosion (ESC) has been Identified.

Date of Implant	Number	Polyurethane ESC Number (%)
Before Jan. 1981	122	4 (3.3%)
Since Jan. 1981	444	0
Total	566	4 (0.7%)

Fig. 2. Cumulative survival curves for atrial leads. Note the improvement in results seen in the Medtronic 6990Pu and 5957J models.

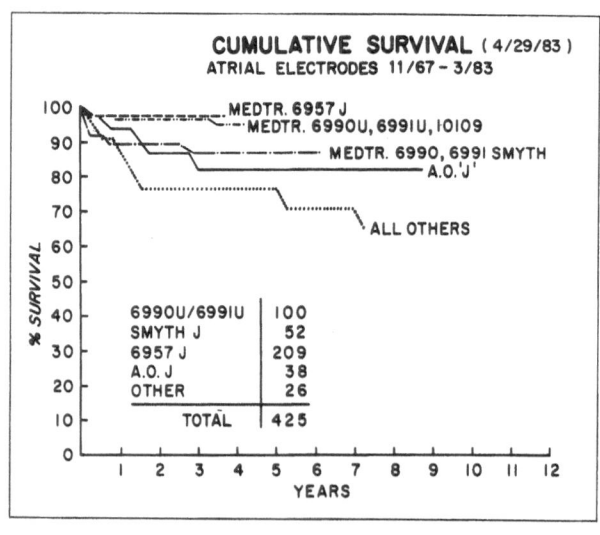

444

Splicing of Broken Wires

The technique for wire shortening evolved from the more compulsory method of splicing a broken wire. Although these splices could be accomplished reliably, refractures tended to occur at the splice or, in some cases, in entirely new areas of the wire (Fig. 3). These data suggest that for whatever reason, perhaps manufacturing variability, some wires become brittle and prone to fracture. For example, in one case simple traction on the bared wire produced repeated fractures, reminiscent of a piece of uncooked spaghetti. Therefore, for a first fracture, whenever the fracture can be reached (almost always made possible by the simple expedient of reducing the redundancy within the heart and vena cava), the procedure should be to splice this wire. If the wire breaks again in any location it should be replaced.

Pacemaker Pouch

For 15 years I have covered the implanted pulse generator with a stretchable polyester (Dacron) pouch*). The original motivation for this was to prevent migration and skin extrusion of the larger pulse generators of the day. Now, however, with small pulse generators we find the benefits of the pouch to be those listed in Table 5.

The pouch becomes an integral part of the pocket, and can be ignored at subsequent pacemaker operations. A second pouch is *never* used within the first. If an infection oc-

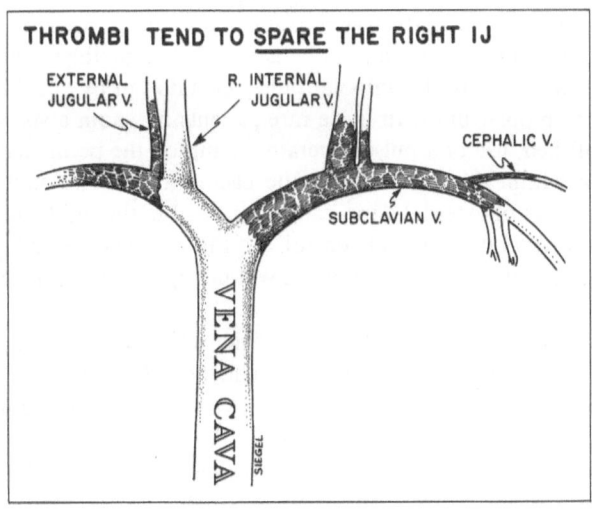

Fig. 3. Patterns of venous thrombosis that may occur after implant, suggesting that the right side is the preferred site for a primary implant.

---

*) USCI Surgical Products, Division of C. R. Bard, Inc., Concord Road, P.O. Box M, Billerica, MA 01821.

Table 5. Advantages of the Cloth Pouch.

Precludes Rotation (twiddling)
Prevents Migration
Reduces Extrusion
Promotes Hemostasis (?)
Decreases Muscle Twitch (?)

---

curs (which should happen rarely), the pouch must be removed entirely to prevent the development of a persistent foreign-body sinus. Overall the pouch is of considerable benefit.

It has been suggested that the pouch will prevent a local pocket twitch that is seen from time to time with unipolar pacers. Twitching occurs extremely rarely in our hands but I believe that it is not related to the use of the pouch, but rather to the practice of locating the pacemaker as *medially* as possible, away from the major mass of the pectoral muscles and nerves.

Pacemaker Reoperations

Two problems in pacemaker replacement deserve special comment: patient dependency on the pacemaker and thrombosis of the subclavian vein. Dependency can almost always be managed without preliminary temporary pacemaker implantation by intermittent pacing with the implanted unit, gradually increasing the pacing interval to as long as 2000 msec until spontaneous ventricular activity begins (sometimes called "weaning" the patient from the pacemaker). Intermittent pacing can be accomplished by the simple expedient of touching the opened wound with the unipolar pulse generator, or by opening and closing a connector in uni- or bipolar units. In those rare patients in whom a spontaneous rhythm cannot be established, use of a pulse generator clamp on the permanent unit allows continued dissection within the pocket while the pacing function is maintained (6). Alternatively a separate set of external wires can be attached to the implanted leads so that pacing can be continued under external control. All this can be done safely with a little forethought on the part of the surgeon on how he will manipulate the various wires, leads, ground plates, etc.

When a pacing lead must be added or replaced, thrombosis of the subclavian vein may make this impossible. Useful steps to insert a new electrode include the following:

1. Use the right side for a primary implant. Should subclavian vein thrombosis occur, the right external or internal jugular veins may still be patent. A primary implant on the left side may produce thrombosis of the innominate vein, as well as the internal jugular which enters it, thereby requiring replacement of the pacemaker on the opposite side (Fig. 4).
2. If the subclavian vein cannot be entered with the introducer needle, the vein may be located fluoroscopically by following the course of the existing lead.
3. Place a transverse incision high enough along the clavicle to facilitate exposure of the subclavian vein or its branches, or, if necessary, the internal jugular vein.

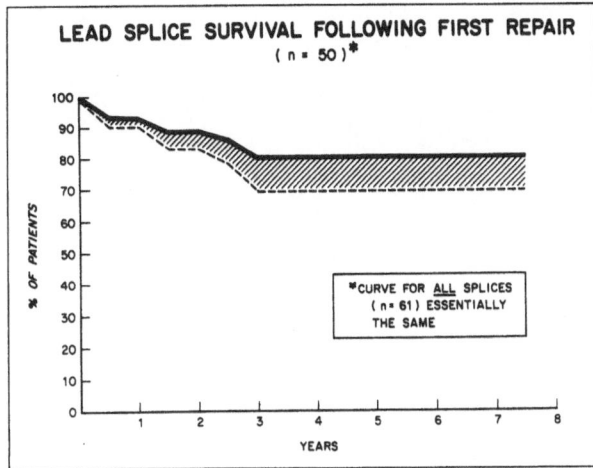

Fig. 4. Cumulative survival of leads after a splice for a wire fracture becomes necessary. Subsequent wire fractures at sites remote from the splice suggest that there may be a basic structural defect in the wire coil.

4. If in doubt about patency of the venous system perform a phlebogram through any available vein in the arm, shoulder or pectoral area. Watch for late filling of the major veins on the outside chance that one of the veins will be large enough to strike with an introducer needle beyond the obstruction site.

Acknowledgement

The author wishes to thank Jane Cort, Mark Widman, Ralph Gallagher, and Teddy Schwarz, MD, for their help in gathering the data, and Alan D. Bernstein, Eng.Sc.D. for his review of the manuscript.

References

1) Parsonnet V, Crawford C: United States survey on cardiac pacing. Proceedings of the VIIth World Symposium on Cardiac Pacing, Vienna. Pace 1983; 6: A-21 (Abstract).
2. Parsonnet V: Technics for implantation and replacement of permanent pacemakers, in Cohn L (ed): Modern Technics in Surgery, New York, Futura Publishing Co, 1979, pp 12-2 to 12–22.
3. Parsonnet V: Pacemaker implantation, in Effler DB (ed): Blade's Surgical Disease of the Chest, Saint Louis, C. V. Mosby Co, 1978; pp 699–758.
4. Alpert J, Gilbert L, Parsonnet V, Zucker IR: A protective clip lead for the changing of cardiac pacemakers. J Thor Cardiovasc Surg 1969; 57: 151–152.
5. Byrd C: Pacemaker Implantation Techniques (Pt. I). Medtronic News, Minneapolis, Minn., March, 1983; pp 7–10.
6. Furman S, Escher DJW: Principles and Techniques of Cardiac Pacing, New York, Harper and Rowe, 1970; chapt 6; pp 113–124.
7. Belott PH: Retaining guidewire, introducer technique for unlimited access to the central circulation: A review. Clin Prog Pacing Electrophysiol 1983; 1: 59–69.

Authors' address:
V. Parsonnet, M.D., Director of Surgery,
Newark Beth Israel Medical Center, 201 Lyons Avenue, Newark, N.J. 07112,
USA

447

Dual Chamber Pacing
Pacing Modes

B. Dodinot

Summary: The availability of tined or screw in leads is now making possible reliable long term atrial pacing and/or sensing. Progress in circuits and battery design lead to a reappraisal of dual chamber (DC) pacing. 3 methods are commonly used:

– *VAT pacing:* is the oldest method designed in 1963. The absence of ventricular sensing is the major disadvantage of VAT pacing with, as a consequence, possible ventricular vulnerable zone stimulation and VOO pacing in case of atrial sensing failures. The low cost and long refractory period of VAT pacemakers resulting in an extremely low risk of Electronic Reentry Tachycardias (ERT) are however advantages which maintain the existence of this obsolete mode of DC pacing.

– *VDD pacing* combines the theoretical advantages of VAT and VVI pacing. Like VAT, VDD pacing results in fixed rate ventricular pacing if the minimal ventricular pacing rate becomes superior to the sinus rate. A modified version of the VDD mode called RS (Rate Sensitive) aims to roughly adjust the ventricular rate to the sinus rate without providing true A-V synchrony.

– *DVI pacing* is offered in 2 versions: – non-committed: ventricular stimulation occurs only if no spontaneous QRS is present following atrial stimulation; – committed, when ventricular stimulation always follows atrial stimulation: the absence of atrial sensing results in possible atrial vulnerable zone stimulation – in the absence of spontaneous variation of the ventricular rate, a major limitation. DVI pacing is generally considered as the 2nd choice mode of DC pacing.

– *DDD pacing* is the most sophisticated mode of DC pacing, with the theoretical advantages of the previous DC pacing systems providing in all instances A-V synchrony.

Dual chamber pacing includes practical disadvantages; some are provisional: artificially high cost, faulty circuit design with risk of pacemaker induced tachycardias, theoretical limited longevity compared to VVI pacing. Some are structural: useless or even dangerous behaviour in the presence of atrial arrhythmia, the need for 2 electrodes, a more complex implantation technique and follow up.

Hence, DC pacing should not be considered as ideal but as a method to be carefully evaluated by sophisticated pacemaker Centers in the years to come.

Introduction

Dual chamber pacing is now celebrating its 20th anniversary: the first implantation of a pacemaker capable of synchronizing its ventricular stimuli on sinus "P" waves was indeed performed in 1963 by a Miami Group (1). In spite of obvious hemodynamic advantages, this physiological mode of pacing, then considered as theoretically ideal for the treatment of complete heart block with normal sinus activation, was almost completely abandoned with the advent of "demand pacemakers" and long term endocardial pacing.

More recently, in 1969, another approach of dual chamber pacing was designed by a Boston Group (2), the purpose of this new method being to pace sequentially both the atrium and the ventricle, the pacemaker being inhibited by the spontaneous ventricular activity. This method especially designed for the treatment of combined S-A and A-V block did not gain much success, the need of an additional electrode and the bulkiness of the pulse generators being usually considered as prohibitive disadvantages.

In the early 80's, progress in leads, batteries and circuit design has led to a reappraisal of dual chamber pacing which, from less than 1% of the implantations has reached 2 to 20% and even over 50% in some particularly advanced pacemaker Centers.

1. Electrodes

Two electrodes must be used for providing atrial and/or ventricular pacing and/or sensing. They most commonly consist of 2 independent leads, 99% endocardial.

– *Choice of the vein:* both electrodes can be introduced in the same vein, most frequently the cephalic if its diameter is sufficient; this is often the case if thin polyurethane leads are used, this material being in addition much smoother than silicone rubber. Subclavian per-or subcutaneous puncture is a more recent and also an excellent approach for introducing the atrial lead or both.

– *The atrial lead:* several types of leads are presently available. Tined J shape polyurethane leads are probably the most popular. Standard tined leads can only be placed in the atrial appendage using a preshaped stylet. Screw in retractable or non-retractable leads have the advantage of possible positioning in any site of the atrium or atrial appendage. Single A-V leads have been successfully used, the so called "crown of thorns" being used for both atrial and ventricular sensing and pacing (3), the orthogonal bipolar lead being designed for atrial sensing only (4).

2. The Various Pacing Modes

For purposes of simplicity, the world-wide accepted 3 letter code (5) will be used. It must be kept in mind that each pacing mode may be selected via programmability with the most advanced multi-programmable dual chamber pacemakers which are presently available.

A) *VAT pacing*

The purpose of this early mode of dual chamber pacing was to reestablish a link between the atrium and ventricle. The pacemaker senses every sinus "P" wave occurring between two, minimal and maximal, intervals, either preset or programmable, when the maximum limit is reached a 2/1 A-V block appears; when the minimum limit is reached, a pacemaker escape, acting like a true ventricular ectopic focus prevents a drop of the ventricular rate below the preset value. This type of pacemaker does not include a ventricular sensing circuit. In the presence of a spontaneous A-V conduction, ventricular stimulation will always occur inducing either fusion or pseudo-fusion beats. PVC's will not be sensed leading to occasional "T" wave stimulation. Loss of atrial sensing results in fixed rate (VOO pacing).

In 1983, this mode of dual chamber pacing is considered as outdated but is not entirely abandoned for two reasons: the relatively low price of the VAT pacemakers, the extremely small risk of inducing Electronic Reentry Tachycardia (ERT), a negative but important advantage of this primitive DCP mode including a long atrial refractory period. This is why VAT pacing may be still selected for the treatment of complete heart block with normal sinus activity.

B) *VDD pacing*

The only difference between VAT and VDD pacing is the presence of an additional ventricular sensing circuit. Therefore, VDD pacing includes theoretically the advantages of standard VVI pacing: absence of ventricular stimulation in the presence of spontaneous ventricular activation and of VAT pacing: presence of a ventricular stimulus if the A-V interval becomes superior to the preset or programmed A-V delay. Like VAT pacing, VDD pacing results in asynchronous ventricular stimulation with possible retrograde activation if the minimal ventricular escape rate is superior to the sinus rate; this may originate E.R.T. if the atrial refractory period of the pacemaker is too short (Fig. 1). This is the major practical disadvantage of VDD pacing in its 82–83 version.

Another modified mode of VDD pacing should be mentioned: the RS (rate sensitive) mode aiming not to establish a A-V true synchronization but to adjust the ventricular pacing rate roughly to the atrial rate, via a single A-V lead including two orthogonal intra-atrial sensing leads. The advantages of this mode of VDD pacing are: – the need of a single A-V lead with bipolar atrial sensing, – the absence of the risk of inducing ERT The disadvantages are related to concept: – absence of true A-V synchronization. Compared to DDD pacing, VDD pacing has few advantages. It may be indicated when additional atrial pacing cannot be performed for technial reasons (rise of threshold, muscle stimulation).

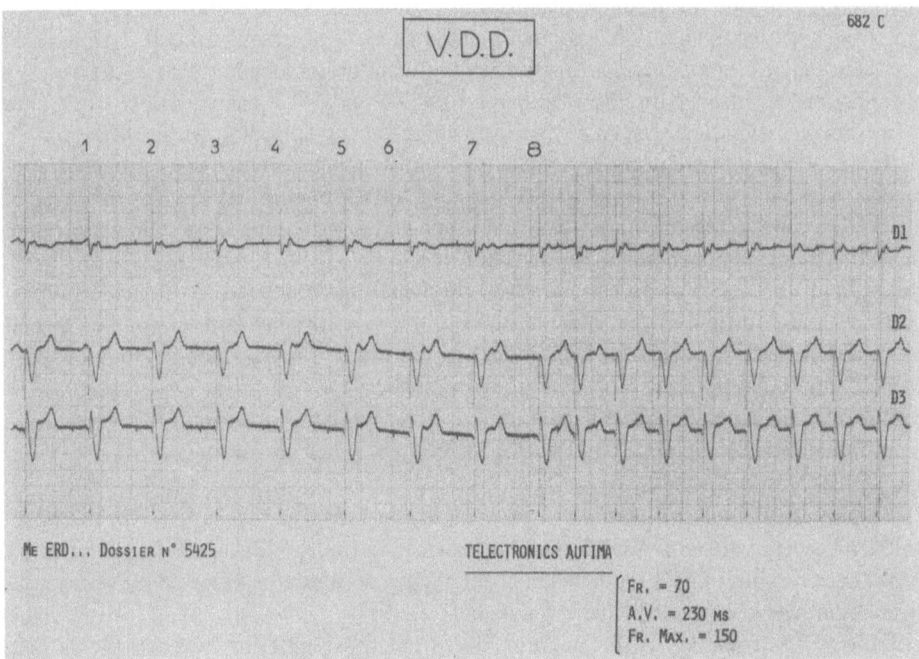

Fig. 1. The presence of an escape pacing rate faster than the sinus rate results in fixed ventricular pacing and retrograde "P" waves. "P" appearing 280 ms after beat 8 is sensed, the pacemaker starting an ERT.

C) DVI pacing

The purpose of this mode of pacing is to add a atrial pacing but not sensing circuit to standard VVI circuit, thus providing a normal A-V sequence in case of atrial bradycardia. Two types of DVI pacing modes are available:

– *The non-committed mode,* originally designed by Berkovitz. Atrial pacing is followed by ventricular stimulation in the absence of spontaneous QRS sensed during the preset or programmed A-V delay.

– *The committed mode:* every atrial stimulus is always followed by a ventricular stimulus; the ventricular refractory period includes the entire A-V delay which cannot be over 150 ms to minimize the risk of "T" wave stimulation. The only advantage of committed DVI pacing is the elimination of possible inhibition by cross talk. The semi-committed type of pacemaker acting as a committed one in the presence of early ventricular sensing immediately following atrial pacing (< 100 ms) and non-committed when ventricular sensing is less premature, is designed to combine both advantages of these two modes of DVI pacing.

In 1983, DVI pacing is generally considered as a 2nd choice mode of DC pacing which can be selected when DDD pacing cannot be safely achieved. This was too frequently the case in 1982.

D) DDD pacing

The presence of one atrial and ventricular lead makes it possible and desirable to pace and sense both chambers. DDD pacing is designed as "universal" since it is capable of providing the best hemodynamic treatment of all conduction disturbances in the absence of permanent atrial arrhythmias. Compared to VDD and VAT pacing, DDD pacing has the advantage of maintaining A-V synchronization during episodes of sinus bradycardia, therefore avoiding asynchronous ventricular pacing with possible atrial retrograde conduction (see Fig. 1). Compared to DVI pacing, DDD pacing has the superiorities of avoiding stimulation in the atrial vulnerable zone and of providing automatic variation of the ventricular rate depending upon the sinus rate.

The normal function of a pacemaker set in the DDD mode depends on many variables: the atrial and ventricular rate, the duration of the P-R interval and, of course, special electronic features varying from one model to the other, programmability inducing individual modification of the most common parameters:

– *absence of atrial and ventricular stimulation:* if the spontaneous atrial rate is superior to the minimal atrial escape rate and the P-R interval shorter than the programmed A-V delay,

– *exclusive ventricular stimulation:* if the spontaneous atrial rate is superior to the minimal atrial escape rate and the P-R interval longer than the A-V delay, the only exception being the committed DDD mode when atrial pacing or sensing is followed by ventricular stimulation whatever the P-R interval may be

– *exclusive atrial pacing:* if the spontaneous atrial rate is inferior to the minimal programmed atrial rate and the P-R interval inferior to the A-V delay,

– *sequential atrio-ventricular pacing:* if the spontaneous atrial rate is below the minimum programmed atrial rate and the P-R interval longer than the A-V delay.

It is most probable that in the near future all dual chamber pacemakers will be DDD models, programmability making possible selection of less sophisticated modes of pacing namely DVI, VVI or DOO.

E) *Exceptional Dual Chamber Pacing Modes*

By playing with the 3 letters of the code, it is possible to create 28 dual chamber pacing modes! Some of them such as ADI, VDO, VDT have a purely intellectual interest. Others may be inadvertently created by loss sensing in one chamber (DAI) or available via programmability (VAD). Others are considered as having diagnostic and therapeutic interest (6): dual demand, improperly named DVO pacing, is the best known of these exceptional pacing modes (7).

F) *The Ideal Pacing Mode*

DDD pacing is presently the most advanced mode of pacing available. Should it replace in a near future less advanced pacing modes just as VVI pacing replaced VOO pacing 15 years ago? In our opinion, the greatest caution should be exhibited before replacing a reliable, simple and relatively cheap mode of pacing by a complex and costly system with an obvious and unquestionable theoretical superiority but with practical major disadvantages as well. Some of these disadvantages can be considered as provisional:
– *their artificially high price:* in the near future, the cost of a DDD and a VVI circuit will become identical,
– *their present major disadvantage:* the risk of ERT will be prevented by better design of the electronic circuit, the purpose of a DDD pacemaker being to mimic normal conduction and not to create an electronic bundle of Kent,
– *their reduced potential longevity,* noticeable only in the rare patients with permanent S-A and A-V block resulting in permanent dual chamber pacing.
Some of the disadvantages are however structural:
– *the presence of atrial arrhythmias* making useless or even dangerous the use of dual chamber pacing,
 the occasionally low voltage of the atrial potentials making atrial sensing harzardous,
– the need of 2, atrial and ventricular, electrodes,
– the more complex implantation technique,
– problems of ECG follow up,
– the occasional poor tolerance of an excessively high ventricular rate.

Conclusion

Dual chamber pacing, particularly DDD pacing, offers major theoretical advantages but its practical and clinical value should be carefully evaluated in the years to come.
Dual chamber pacing may result in catastrophic results if patient and pacemaker selection, pacemaker implantation and follow up, are not correctly performed. Dual chamber

pacing should be performed in true pacemaker Centers, the notion of which has not been defined and accepted to date.

References

1. Nathan DA, Center S, WU CY, Keller W: "An implantable synchronous pacemaker for the long term correction of complete heart block" Amer J Cardiol, 1963; 11: 362–367.
2. Berkovits BV, Castellanos A Jr, and Lemberg L: "Bifocal demand pacing" Circulation, 1969; 39 (suppl. III): 111–44.
3. Wainwright R, Crick J, Sowton E: "Clinical evaluation of a single-pass implantable electrode for all modes of pacing. The "crown of thorns" lead." Pace, 1983; 6: 210–220.
4. Goldreyer BN, Olive AL, Leslie J, Cannom DS, and Wyman NG: "P synchronous pacing. A new orthogonal approach to "P" wave sensing." Am J Cardiol 1981; 47: 434.
5. Dodinot B: "Code à 3 lettres" Stimucoeur Medical, 1982; n° 1: 51–54.
6. Levine AP, Brodsky SJ, Seltzer JP: "AVI pacing, a new diagnostic and therapeutic pacing modality" Pace, 1983; 6: A 35.
7. Berkovits BV, Castellanos A, Dreifus LS, Lemberg L, Levy S, Mandel WJ, Obel JWP: "Double demand sequential pacing for the termination of paroxysmal reentry tachyarrhythmias" Pace, 1979; 2: A 15.

Authors' address:
Dr. B. Dodinot
Clinique Cardiologique
CHU Nancy-Brabois
Vandoeuvre/France

Symptom Control and Psychosocial Rehabilitation of Chronic Pacemaker Patients with Different Pacing Modes

G. Neumann, E. Grube, Ilona E. Leschhorn, Astrid Hussain, P. Stangier

Summary: 266 consecutive pacemaker patients had a psychological examination followed by a questionnaire after 6 months. They underwent telemetry at intervals performing everyday adjusted work, a chest x-ray and a standard clinical investigation besides pacemaker control.
All data were compiled to estimate subjective symptom control, professional and psychosocial rehabilitation, arrhythmia control and possible differences between different pacing modes. Syncope control was the most reliable effect of pacing without differences between the modes. Physiological systems controlled dizziness significantly better than VVI systems. Angina and respiratory, distress, however, were hardly influenced by either of the modes. Tachyarrhythmia problems and poor sleep occurred to a much higher degree with pacing, again without difference between the modes.
40% of the patients showed psychological alterations with pacing, half of them persistently with a significant level of depression. 30% of all patients terminated all social contacts after pacemaker implantation. The majority of the patients retired prematurely from their jobs. The dominating cause was the pacemaker implantation itself without further consideration of disease or age. Again there was no difference between the systems.
In spite of poor psychosocial rehabilitation many patients did much better in everyday life performance, at least as far as physical work was concerned. Hobbies became more active, physical activity increased in general. In both parameters physiologically paced patients did considerably better than VVI patients. Exercise performance was limited by ventricular arrhythmias. Rate responsiveness in all modes was the most important factor for optimal physical performance and arrhythmia control.

Bradycardia pacing is developing into a highly sophisticated differential therapy optimizing problems of hemodynamic performance and arrhythmia control. There are without doubt many publications, which underline the efficacy of these approaches (1, 2, 3, 4). However comparably few data cover the problems of subjective symptom control, psychosocial rehabilitation and everyday life performance of pacemaker patients (5, 6, 7). The purpose of this study therefore was to collect data allowing the estimation of these parameters of therapeutic efficacy and to find out possible differences between different modes of pacing.

Patients and Methods

266 consecutive patients of our outpatient pacemaker clinic under the average age of 67 years, having been paced for 6 months were included in the study. New, independent and postoperative cardiovascular events such as myocardial infarctions or cerebrovascular strokes, diabetic or hypertensive decompensations were exclusion criteria for participation. 52 patients were physiologically paced, e.g. under sinus rhythm with physiological devices.

455

All patients filled in a standard psychological questionnaire covering 64 items: Pacemaker influence on mood, social interactions, professional engagement and everyday life activities were analysed by the comparison of pre- and postoperative subjective judgements. 6 months later the patients answered a second questionnaire covering the same topics to verify the chronic persistence of the findings and to clarify possible misunderstandings during the first investigation. In order to be able to quantify the data a score system of physical activities and intensities of social interactions was filled out by the patients under the supervision of the investigator.

All patients underwent a thorough clinical investigation besides the psychological investigation. This included all clinical criteria of cardiovascular disease, a thorough analysis of medical history, a drug consumption protocol, chest x-rays and a standard pacemaker control.

An medium-term, two-channel, telemetric ECG test under controlled conditions of everyday life-adjusted work performance was carried out on all the patients. During this test the patients had to walk along a floor at their personal limit without inducing the symptoms, and climb stairs under the same criteria. These types of exercise were interrupted by random sequences of rest periods in standing or sitting position. Working capability was roughly calculated according to the distances walked and the number of stairs climbed. Symptoms limiting the physical capabilities were documented together with the time of occurrence in a symptom protocol. All telemetric observations were on-line controlled for artefacts, registered on tapes and, together with the analysis of the performance protocol, were analysed by two independent investigators for arrhythmia patterns.

All other earlier available patient data and the data from this study were compiled to answer the questions concerning the quality of the patients everyday life and the chronic influence of pacemaker therapy. In order to compare the physiologically paced patients with VVI patients, a matched group of VVI patients was selected with corresponding age distribution, cardiothoracic ratio, blood pressure, NYHA grading, basic cardiac diseases and arrhythmias responsible for pacing.

Results

The dominating preimplantation symptoms of all patients were syncope, dizziness, angina and respiratory distress. Their occurrence before and after implantation is shown in Fig. 1. It is evident from this diagram, that one of the consequences of pacemaker insertion is a highly reliable syncope control. There was no difference in the relative efficacy of VVI of physiological systems with respect to this parameters alone, but there was a significant difference statistically, between the control of dizziness and the combined control of both symptoms.

In spite of the expected improvements of hemodynamics, neither VVI type bradycardia control nor physiological pacing really induced a significant reduction of angina or respiratory distress problems. There was no quantitative difference between the systems. Surprisingly, both systems led to a considerable increase of sleeping problems and of tachyarrhythmias.

Looking at the chronic development of cardiothoracic ratios. 9% of the VVI patients and 11% of the physiologically paced patients deteriorated significantly over time, again without quantitative difference between the systems. These patients all had chronic atrial fi-

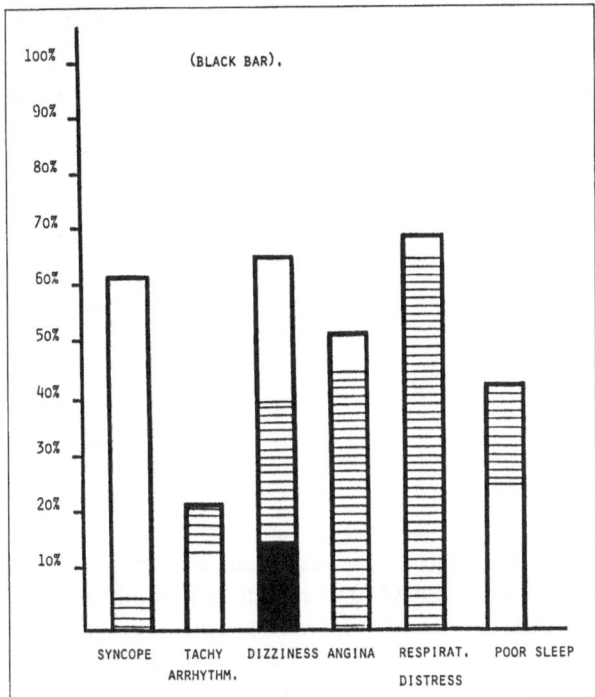

Fig. 1. Occurrence of main symptoms in the whole patient population before (open bars) and after PM implantation (lined bars). Dizziness control is the only significant difference between physiological and VVI groups (P = 0.05) (black bar).

brillation after 28 + 4 months and 29 + 5 months of pacing for VVI and physiological groups respectively. The cardiothoracic ratios of these two subgroups were 0.54 + 0.03 and 0.6 + 0.04 after the elapsed pacing period. There was no clinically significant difference between VVI and physiologically paced patients in these clinically poor subgroups.

All patients reduced their professional activities significantly after pacemaker implantation, again without difference between the pacing modes. More than 70% of the workers, 55% of the people with independent professions and roughly 40% of the employees had to retire prematurely after the implantation. The most surprising and inexplicable fact is, that pacemaker implantation by itself, without further consideration of age of specific disease was the dominating reason of early retirement from professional life. From the change in the degree of professional engagement postoperatively as estimated by the patients themselves, it becomes evident, that the higher the degree of engagement preoperatively is, the higher the percentage of the decrease of engagement postoperatively. In fact, the rate of professional rehabilitation after pacemaker implantation is rather low.

33% of the patients reported an almost complete cessation of all preoperative social activities. Of the remaining 67%, the percentage of social interaction remained roughly the same as in the preoperative situation (Table 1).

The main subjective reasons to explain the tendency of social isolation were "shame of being prosthesis dependent", fear of technical complications due to environmental factors, fear of involving other people too much in one's own severe problems and overprotection by the family. There was a considerable number of patients, who were disappointed when they compared their preoperative expectations with the postoperative results.

Table 1. Degrees of social interaction of all patients investigated. 30.9% of all patients judged themselves as dependant upon assistance of other people (In the majority family members). 33% of all patients experienced a total cessation of all social contacts after PM implantation. Score calculated personally after standard questions e.g. concerning No. of social contacts, types of activities, No. of average social events.

Degree of dependence		Higher	Lower
		2.3%	0.7%
Intensity of social interaction		31.1%	25.7%
Social interaction activity score	I	31.9%	15.7%
	II	16%	19.3%
	III	30.4%	41%
	IV	21.7%	15.8%

Only roughly 60% of the patients, who had expected no more than partial relief of their problems were really satisfied, while none of those who had expected a total alleviation of the symptoms reported this, and a considerable percentage of patients (40%) reported either no relief or even a deterioration of their preimplant problems. Again there was no difference between the pacing modes.

In the patients' subjective score of everyday life physical activity, quantifying activities such as housekeeping, shopping, walking, gardening, dancing, jogging, there was a significant difference when the matched groups of VVI and physiologically paced patients were compared. While 63% of the physiologically paced patients scored themselves at least one degree higher, this occurred in only 37% of the VVI patients, with an unproportionally high percentage, of 85%, of rate responsive VVI patients, as compared to a total of 56% in the physiologically paced patients.

There was a highly significant difference between patients, who reported having tested their personal limits and those avoiding to do this in both groups. Without doubt, physiologically paced patients scored themselves higher than VVI patients again, and were in higher activity grades in a combined judgement of subjective scoring and work performance (Fig. 2). If the hobby activities are analysed in detail it becomes clear that about the same percentage of patients in VVI and physiological groups engaged themselves in hobby activities. There was an overall increase in engagement of roughly 8% in both groups. Characteristically, physiologically paced patients had higher levels of actively performed and physically engaged hobbies than VVI patients (Fig. 3).

Looking at the telemetric arrhythmia control data and the grading of physical exercise capacity, two things are evident. Firstly, there is a considerable increase in ventricular arrhythmias with the different intensities of everyday life adjusted work. It became evident, that in the Lown grading scheme, which served as a descriptional system, there were much higher grades of arrhythmias to be observed during stair climbing than during floor walking or rest periods. Rate acceleration during exercise, be it by spontaneous rate responsiveness in VVI systems or by atrial triggered ventricular sinus rates, is the important factor in the suppression of ventricular ectopics during heavy physical work (Table 2).

458

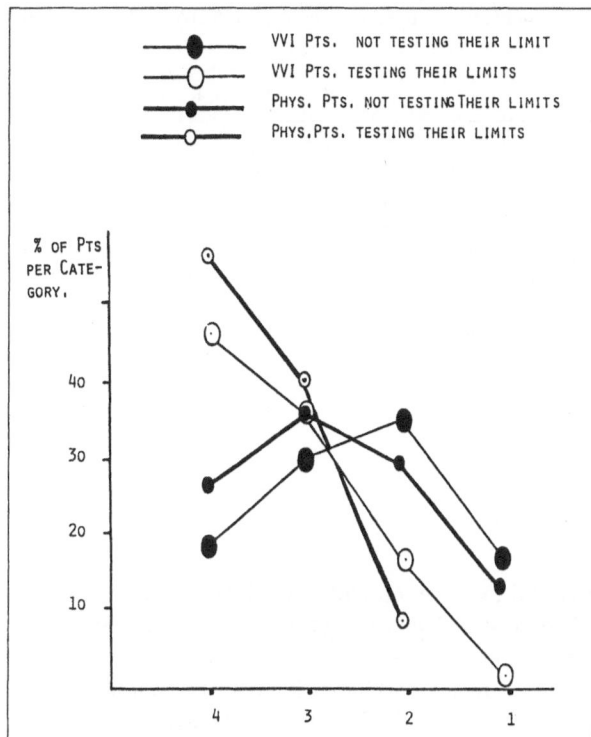

Fig. 2. Grades of intensity of physical performance calculated after comfortable walking and stair climbing and personal grading of everyday performance.

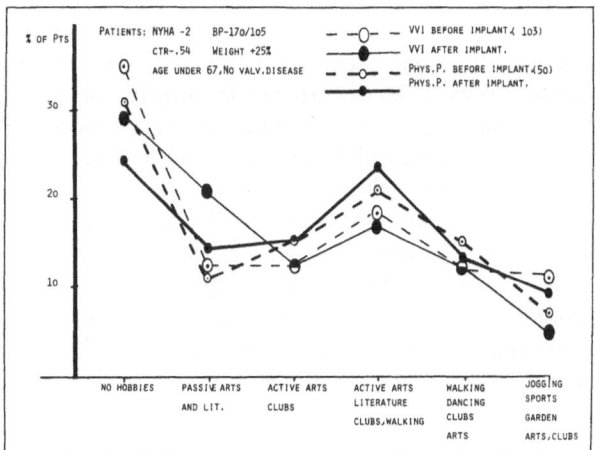

Fig. 3.

While 44% of the non rate responsive VVI patients had no ventricular arrhythmias at all, and 59% of them none under exercise, 20% showed Lown grade 3–5 and serious atrial arrhythmias in this condition. In comparision, 78% of the rate responsive VVI patients

Table 2. Ventricular arrhythmias of PM patients under telemetric control. NYHA grade 4 and atrial fibrillators excluded.

	*	+	°	#	*	+	°	#	*	+	°	#
Lown 5	–	–	–	–	–	–	2	–	6	2	2	–
Lown 4	–	2	–	–	7	2	–	–	10	1	4	–
Lown 3	2	3	8	–	4	2	6	3	4	–	6	3
Lown 1/2	6	11	10	12	12	9	11	10	21	19	24	14
No Arrh.	92	85	82	88	77	87	81	87	59	78	66	83
	Rest				Walking				Climbing stairs			

Not rate responsive VVI pts.	= *	(n = 52)
Rate responsive VVI pts.	= +	(n = 65)
Not rate Responsive Phys. pts.	= °	(n = 21)
Rate responsive Phys. p.	= #	(n = 26).

had no arrhythmia at all under maximal exercise. 66% of physiologically paced patients with insufficient rate acceleration had no ventricular arrhythmias at all, and 58% no arrhythmias even under maximal effort. Roughly 20% again showed grade 3–5 ventricular arrhythmias and atrial tachyarrhythmias in this condition. None of the rate responsive physiologically paced patients however had grade 3–5 ventricular arrhythmias or atrial tachyarrhythmias at all during maximal everyday life adjusted exercise, and 85% of these patients had no arrhythmia at all.

The physical performance grades in a score of 0–5 with increasing working capacity show that VVI patients without rate response scored 2.9 + 0.8 and VVI patients with rate response scored 2.93 + 0.6, and that physiologically paced patients without rate response scored 3.3 + 0.5 and physiologically paced patients with rate response scored 3.3 + 0.3, which shows that the difference between the two groups was insignificant.

The subgroups with minor grade arrhythmias (Lown 1–2 and atrial premature beats) scored 2.7 + 0.5, 2.7 + 0.4, 2.7 + 0.3 and 2.7 + 0.15, which again was neither significantly different to the nonarrhythmic subgroups nor in the slightly arrhythmic subgroups. However, all subgroups with Lown grade 3–5 arrhythmias and atrial tachyarrhythmias were graded 1.2 + 0.4 in the non rate responsive VVI group, 1.2 + 0.4 in the rate responsive VVI group and 1.3 + 0.2 in the non rate responsive physiological group.

To summarize, arrhythmias in physiologically paced patients decreased by a small degree with a slightly increased maximal working capacity, while evidently proper rate adjustment was of maximal importance in the control of these parameters.

Conclusions

As the data of this study show, the psychosocial rehabilitation of pacemaker patients without any regard to the pacing modality is very poor: Patients retire early from work, their social contacts decrease, they become socially isolated to an unexpected and not at all justified degree. Insufficient public education and knowledge, insufficient psychological patient training and education seem to be the dominating factors of these poor results. As far as bradycardia control is concerned, symptom control is evidently good, as expected. Physiological pacing proves to be much better in the combined control of dizziness and syncope.

References

1. Chapter in book: Neumann G, Funke H, Kirchhoff PG, Schaede A: Clinical experience with the universal DDD pacemaker in The Third Decade of Cardiac Pacing. Ed Barold S and Mugica J (Futura Publ Co 1982); 225–247.
2. Journal: Kruse I, Ryden L: A comparison of physical work capacity and systolic time intervals with ventricular inhibited and atrial synchronous ventricular inhibited pacing. Br Heart J: 1981; 46: 129.
3. Journal: Sutton R, Citron P: Electrophysiological and hemodynamic basis for application of a new pacemaker technology in sick sinus syndrome and atriaventricular block. Br Heart J 1979; 600.
4. Journal: Karlof I: Hemodynamic effect of atrial triggered vs. fixed rate pacing at rest and during exercise in complete heart block. Acta med Scand 1975; 197: 195–206.
5. Journal: Sabin G, Welter FL: Psychischer Befund und soziales Umfeld bei Schrittmacherträgern. Herz-Kreisl 1979; 11.5: 225–228.
6. Journal: Goble R, Gowers J, Morgan D, Kline P: Artificial pacemaker patients treatment outcome and the sixteen personality factor questionnaire. J of Psychosom Res 22: 467–472.
7. Doenecke P, Flöthner R, Bette L: Medizinische und soziale Rehabilitation von Schrittmacherträgern. Mü Med Wschr 1979; 113: 1712.

Authors' address:
Priv.-Doz. Dr. Gert Neumann
Medizinische Klinik
Gotenstr. 1
5650 Solingen

Follow-up of Pacemaker Patients

Hugo E. Ector, Hilaire De Geest

Summary: The patient-pacemaker combination requires a specific follow-up with important techno-logical implications. Capture and inhibition remain the basic functions to be assessed. Sophisticated devices are changing and complicating follow-up.

An appropriate rehabilitation of the patient will permit a return to a virtually normal life but vigor-ous exercise should be avoided. A subgroup of pacemaker dependent patients requires special atten-tion. Potential hazards for paced patients are: ionizing radiation, interference by internal and exter-nal sources. Even damage or destruction of a pacemaker can occur. Interference of muscular origin is common in unipolar systems. It can be prevented by the adjustment of sensitivity or by the use of bi-polar leads.

The actual reliability and longevity of lithium-powered pacemakers allow a convenient surveillance schedule.

Electrical pacing of the heart has still something magic which accompanied its introduc-tion 25 years ago. The side-effect of magic is panic. An appropriate follow-up of the pacemaker patients has nothing magic and must prevent panic as well in the individual case as in the community.

Lampadius (1) suggested that the check-up possibilities in a pacemaker clinic must cover 3 aspects: (1) the patient together with his pacemaker; (2) the pacemaker as a single unit; (3) the pacemaker as a series product.

The Pacemaker as a Single Unit and as a Series Product

Table 1 gives an overview of the different testing aspects in the follow-up of pacing sys-tems.

Table 1. Tests of the pacemaker as a single unit and as a series product.

Capture	Magnet	– Telephone monitoring
Inhibition	ECG	– Self-check
Waveform analysis	Oscilloscope	– Information from central registry on "current" pacing failures
Röntgen analysis	Chest X-Ray	
Interrogation of the pacemaker	Telemetry	

– proper programmability and
  proper programming: pacer longevity depends on setting of output and battery drain
– for each pacemaker-patient combination the remaining functional time of the pacer must be
  determined

Pacemakers are manufactured in large quantities by companies which meet stringent standards of quality control. Nevertheless, the series products, called pacemakers, have proven in the past that premature failures can occur. For this reason every pacemaker clinic should be in contact with a central registry providing information on current pacing failures. The first goal of a follow-up system is to determine at regular intervals the remaining functional time of the pacer. Knowledge of the specific end-of-life indicators becomes difficult with the increasing variety of pacing devices.

Capture and inhibition

Capture and inhibition are the major functions to be assessed on each control examination. For this purpose we only need an ECG and a magnet. The magnet activates the pacemaker when it is inhibited by the intrinsic heart rhythm. ECG and pacemaker spike can be recorded directly on an ECG recorder or transmitted by telephone.

Photoanalysis, Telemetry

If we want to perform waveform analysis we need an oscilloscope. Waveform analysis has been an enthusiasming topic in the 1970s. We assessed the exclusive contribution of waveform analysis in 231 consecutive pacemaker replacements. A diagnosis exclusively made by photoanalysis only occurred in 9% of the replacements: battery depletion in 11 cases, lead malfunction in 9 cases and electronic failure in 1 case (2). As pacemakers and leads became more reliable the specific contribution of waveform analysis will decrease. Furthermore interrogation of the pacemaker by telemetry will become a more accurate method for the assessment of the different parameters that we tried to measure by photoanalysis. Anyway I feel that in a pacemaker clinic and especially in a teaching hospital waveform analysis can still function as an independent control of the more sophisticated telemetric and programming functions.

Surveillance: techniques and guidelines

In the next years follow-up will change considerably. Most attention will go to the proper programmability and the proper programming of the pacing device. The longevity of the pacemaker will largely depend on the setting of output and battery drain.
A chest X-ray is useful for recognition of dislocation, perforation and fracture of a lead. In some instances connector faults can be visualized.
New pacemakers will not eliminate surveillance but will merely change and probably further complicate the system (3). An acceptable schedule for follow-up must be one that reduces the chance of undetected pacemaker failure, and at the same time does not increase cost unreasonably (3). Transtelephone pacemaker monitoring in this respect offers certain advantages for some patients (4). The application of telephone in the follow-up will primarily depend on local, national, geographic and socioeconomic factors. Dodinot (5) emphasizes that self-check is an important follow-up technique. It gives patients safety without making them slaves of a pacemaker clinic, either by telephone or by

coming for a photoanalysis. Self-check can be performed by simple electronic devices and also by taking the pulse daily or weekly. At the time of mercury-zinc batteries our patients were advised to take the pulse daily. Now we recommend that they take their pulse at least weekly.

Hopefully the quality of pacemakers and the skill of the implanting physician will permit the surveillance system summarized in Table 2. A significant increase in risk of pacing failure nowadays is an indication for elective replacement. With the actual longevity of pacemakers there is no more place for weekly or monthly controls of suspect pacemakers, as we used to do for mercury-zinc pacemakers.

Evaluation of the Patient together with his Pacemaker

Full attention must go to the interaction pacemaker-patient. There are side effects as erosion, infection, pain and thrombosis. In a few instances we face a diagnosis of pacemaker syndrome. Muscle stimulation can cause considerable discomfort. An excellent discussion on the malfunctioning pacemaker-patient system is given by Mond and Sloman (6).

Rehabilitation and recommendations for daily life

Patient longevity will depend primarily on associated heart disease. Psychological problems and a difficult rehabilitation are frequent. We have to advise on medicolegal implications as there are in some countries: for example, the regulations for holding a driving license. Employment of the patient and re-employment after pacemaker implantation will depend on national and individual socioeconomic factors. We studied employment conditions in 35 consecutive pacemaker patients younger than 60 years and without sig-

Table 2. Hopefully the quality of pacemakers and the skill of the implanting physician will permit the following surveillance schedule.

Procedure	New pacing system	Replacement
Day 1–6	ECG daily	
Day 7	Complete check-up	
Discharge from the Hospital	after 4 to 7 days	after 1 day
ECG	every 3 months	every 3 months
Check-up in a pacemaker clinic		
month 1–40	every 8 months	every 8 months
40–64	every 6 months	every 6 months
64–..	every 3 months	every 3 months
Self-check		
month 1–60	weekly	weekly
60–..	daily	daily

Elective replacement, when some considerations would suggest monthly or weekly check-ups.

nificant associated disease (7). Seven patients were unemployed before pacemaker implantation. Only 12 of 28 employed patients resumed work after pacemaker implantation. If sufficient benefits are provided by insurance plans a return to normal professional activities can become unneccessary and unattractive. In our hospital we ask for restriction in physical exercise for the first two months. After 2 months the patient is allowed to drive a car and he is encouraged to work normally. He is allowed to do physical exercise as walking, bicycling, swimming and jogging. In our opinion vigorous exercise should be avoided, as many pacemaker patients cannot increase their heart rate. They must increase their cardiac output by increasing their stroke volume. Patients are always strongly advised against competitive sports.

Pacemaker dependence

Another important feature in the follow-up of a pacemaker patient is awareness about pacing dependence. Many patients have a deficient underlying heart rhythm. Underlying heart rhythm or escape rhythm can be demonstrated by inhibiting a VVI pacemaker. Inhibition is obtained by chest wall stimulation or by programming. Underlying heart rhythm is deficient in 40 to 50% of patients with AV block (8, 9). Absence of escape rhythm is a rare finding in patients with sick sinus syndrome (9). There are important implications in the case of pacemaker dependence. Malfunction of the pacing system should be detected early by increasing the follow-up frequency. If any malfunction, the pulse generator and/or lead must be replaced without delay. Especially in this group of patients, we must consider elective replacement rather than waiting for "end-of-life" indicators.

Potential Hazards for paced patients.

Table 3 lists a number of possible causes of pacemaker interference, damage and even destruction. This enumeration is certainly not exhaustive. In the future more complicated problems can be expected for systems with an increased sensitivity as atrial pacers, special sensing circuits as used in antitachycardia pacers and in implantable defibrillators. There is also a real danger from ionizing radiation. I refer to clear statements of Calfee (10). Any CMOS device can fail when exposed to sufficiently high doses of therapeutic radiation. Diagnostic radiation levels are not high enough to be of concern. The pacemaker has to be shielded from therapeutic radiation and, if shielding is not possible, the pacemaker should be moved to another site. Since the dose of radiation is cumulative the pacemaker performance should be monitored throughout the course of the radiation therapy. The effects of electromagnetic interference will depend on the circuitry of the pacemaker, the waveform of the interfering current and the frequency of the magnetic, electric and radiated fields. The inhibition-reversion changeover frequency varies over wide limits. Bipolar pacers are less sensitive than unipolar systems (11). Until today no fatalities due to interference have been reported. The situations in which interference has been noted have not had serious consequences (11). Interference is an emotionally charged issue. We must avoid burdening the patient with too many rules (12).

466

Table 3. Potential hazards for paced patients interference, damage, destruction.

Ionizing radiation: CMOS devices can fail when exposed to therapeutic radiation,
– Defibrillators, electrosurgery

Interference by internal sources: myopotentials, afterpotentials, repolarization artifacts, autointerference

Electromagnetic interference by external sources:
– chest wall stimulation, electrical acupuncture, waving magnets, nerve stimulators
– electric motors & stoves, ARC welding, radio and television transmitters, microwave ovens, citizen's band radio, radar
– refrigerator doors, mechanic's magnets, lifting electromagnets, theft detectors, high power lines, airport security magnetometers
– leakage current from any powerline connected device

Future problems:
Implantable cardiac defibrillators, antitachycardia pacers, systems with increased sensitivity (atrial pacers), spurious programming

---

Myopotentials

Interference of muscular origin occurs in 40 to 70% of patients with unipolar pacing systems (13, 14, 15). It can only provoke symptoms in patients with deficient underlying heart rhythm. In a few instances myopotential inhibition resulted in serious ventricular arrhythmias (16). Possible solutions for the problem of interference by myopotentials are the external adjustment of sensitivity and the return to bipolar systems. Hauser (17) definitely prefers bipolar leads because they provide a satisfactory signal for sensing and because they are immune to interference. Otherwise Mugica (18) states that unipolar stainless steel electrodes behave better than bipolar ones. False inhibition by false signals has been reported to occur also in bipolar lead systems (19). Possible reasons for this type of false inhibition are: heart motion related potentials, minor conductor defects, friction between two coaxial wires. If we add the thinnest sophisticated leads to the multiprogrammable pacers we risk creating new and interesting phenomena, for which we can hope to find a non-invasive programmable solution.

Pacemaker patient societies

The membership of a patient society can support the emotional and psychological needs of pacemaker recipients. If helps patients understand the use and purpose of pacemakers. Information was obtained about regular activities of several organizations (20). In the USA: International association of pacemaker patients with the publication "Pulse"; Pacemakers Unlimited, Inc.; Mended Hearts, Inc; several hospital clubs. In Sweden: Swedish National Heart and Lung Association. In France: the association Stimucoeur with the journal Stimucoeur. Groups are being formed in Italy, Portugal, The Netherlands and Belgium. At this moment complete information is lacking on other pacemaker patient societies.

This review of follow-up in pacing ends with a request to send information on pacemaker patient societies to the authors of this article.

467

References

1. Lampadius MS: Pacemaker follow-up methods. In Thalen JH, Harthorne JW, eds. To pace or not to pace. The Hague: Martinus Nyhoff, 1978; 367.
2. Ector H, Haeseldonckx C, Staessen J, Vermeersch L, De Geest H: Relatief belang van impuls-analyse in de pacemakerkliniek. Tijdschr voor Geneeskunde 1980; 36: 305–308.
3. Parsonnet V, Myers GH, Manhardt M: A review of pacemaker surveillance, 1978. In: Thalen HJ, Meere C, eds. Fundamentals of cardiac pacing. Martinus Nyhoff, 1979: 248–251.
4. Furman S: Transtelephone pacemaker monitoring. In: Thalen JH, Harthorne JW, eds. To pace or not to pace. The Hague: Martinus Nyhoff, 1978; 381–388.
5. Panel discussion, In: Thalen HJ, Harthorne JW, eds. To pace or not to pace. The Hague: Martinus Nyhoff, 1978; 196.
6. Mond HG, Sloman JG: The malfunctioning pacemaker system. Pace 1981; 4: 49–60; 168–181; 304–312.
7. Lambrechts C, Ector H, De Geest H: Psychosociale aspecten van pacemakertherapie in België. Tijdschr voor Geneeskunde 1975; 31: 318–319.
8. Grendahl H, Miller M, Kjekshus J: Overdrive suppression of implanted pacemakers in patients with AV block. Br Heart J 1978; 40: 106.
9. Staessen J, Ector H, De Geest H: The underlying heart rhythm in patients with an artificial cardiac pacemaker. Pace 1982; 5: 801–807.
10. Calfee RV: Therapeutic radiation and pacemakers. Pace 1982; 5: 160–161.
11. Exworthy KW: Pacemaker Interference. In: Varriale P, Naclerio EA, eds. Cardiac Pacing Philadelphia: Lea & Febiger, 1979: 325–348.
12. Pannizzo F, Furman S: Pacemaker and patient response to the "Point of Sale" terminal as an actual and simulated electromagnetic interference source. Pace 1980; 3: 461–469.
13. Breivik K, Ohm OJ: Myopotential inhibition of unipolar QRS-inhibited (VVI) pacemakers, assessed by ambulatory Holter monitoring of the electrocardiogram. Pace 1980; 3: 470–478.
14. Symposium on electromagnetic interference of muscular origin. Pace 1982; 5: 1–37.
15. Secemsky SI, Hauser RG, Denes P, Edwards LM: Unipolar sensing abnormalities; incidence and clinical significance of skeletal muscle interference and undersensing in 228 patients. Pace 1982; 5: 10–19.
16. Iesaka Y, Pinakatt T, Gosselin AJ, Lister JW: Bradycardia dependent ventricular tachycardia facilitated by myopotential inhibition of a VVI pacemaker. Pace 1982; 5: 23–29.
17. Hauser RG: Bipolar leads for cardiac pacing in the 1980s: a reappraisal provoked by skeletal muscle interference. Pace 1982; 5: 34–37.
18. Mugica J, Rollet M, Lazarus B, Henry L, Duconge R, Laxenaire P, Dubois MT: Long term behaviour of pacing electrodes, a twelve years survey (6032 cases). Stimucoeur 1982; 10: 272.
19. Ector H, Emmerechts C, De Schepper S, De Geest H: Results of follow-up study in cardiac pacing at St-Raphael University Hospital in Leuven. Acta Cardiol 1976; suppl 21: 85–95.
20. Personal information from Lee Seligman, Intermedics, Inc, Freeport, USA
21. Barold SS, Levine PA: Autointerference of demand pulse generators. Pace 1981; 4: 274–280.

Authors' address:
Hugo E. Ector
Department of Cardiology
University Clinic St.-Raphael
B-3000 Leuven, Belgium

Dual Chamber Pacemakers-Follow Up

L. Rydén, B.-E. Kristensson, I. Kruse

Summary: A description is given of the protocol for follow up of patients with dual chamber pacemakers at the Central Hospital, Skövde, Sweden. Based on experiences of 111 patients followed during 1–71 months some ideas are given on clinical problems with dual chamber pacing systems. The importance of checking of different parameters is outlined.

Introduction

During the last years improved techniques for atrial pacing and sensing (1, 2) together with the development of advanced pacemaker technology (3, 4) have made dual chamber pacing increasingly more common (5). The benefits of incorporating and utilizing the correctly timed atrial contraction in the paced cardiac cycle "physiological pacing" have been reported (6, 7) but attention has also been directed to the lack of information on long-term clinical follow up (8). Such experiences should document the possible limitations and drawbacks in clinical practise together with suggestions of how to manage the problems with dual-chamber systems. They should also result in a feasable and realistic schedule for patient and pacemaker control. Based on our own experience the present report contains some advices concerning the clinical follow up of and trouble-shooting in patients with dual chamber pacemakers.

Table 1. Patients with dual chamber pacemakers in Skövde 1977–1983 (March 31st).

Type	No	Dead	Change of mode	Paced 31/3-83	Pacemakers			Observation time (months)		
					Med-tronic 213	Cordis	Elema 674	Σ	Range	Mean ± SD
VDD	69	6	3 VVI (1) DDD(2)	60	60[1]	0	0	2322	3–71	34 ± 21
DDD	28	4	2 VDD(2)	22	16[2]	1	5	339	1–44	12 ± 11
DVI	6	1	1 DDD	4	4[3]	0	0	229	26–48	38 ± 7
VAT	8	4	4 VDD(4)	0	0	0	0	174	1–65	22 ± 22
Total	111	15	10	86	80	1	5	3064	1–71	–

[1] 5993; 2409; 7100
[2] SP 69; 7000
[3] 5992

Material

Since 1977 111 patients have received VAT, DVI or VDD-pacemakers at our hospital. At the end of March 1983 ninetyfive of them are still alive with dual-chamber pacemakers and have been followed at the out-patient pacemaker clinic during a total of 3064 months (Table 1). The distribution of different pacemaker types are also presented in this table. All atrial and ventricular leads are transvenous (Medtronic Inc). During the last years the same type of straight lead has been used in both ventricle and atrium (SP 34; 9).

Methods

Time and protocol for the routine follow up of our dual-chamber pacemaker patients are shown in Tables 2 and 3. When testing the VDD-pacemakers a telemetry read out of programmed parameters together with a marker channel and an endocardial electrogram have been most helpful (Fig. 1–3, 4).

Experiences and Comments

In the following our experiences will be reported under different headings focusing on problems appearing during the follow up period.

Hospital care

Uncomplicated patients are followed according to the routine outlined. Since many patients in addition to the reason for pacing have concomitant cardiovascular and other diseases appointments for clinical follow up may be more frequent than what is necessary

Table 2. Time schedule and measures for the follow up of patients with dual pacemakers.

	Time after implantation	Measure
Hours	{ 0–48	ECG monitoring (telemetry)
	~ 3–4	Final programming pacemaker control
Days	{ 3–4	Hospital discharge
	10–14	Surgical control: sutures, PM-pocket Clinical control: Subjective Feeling
Weeks	{ 4–6	Clinical control Pacemaker control
Months	{ 6, 12, 24, 36......	Clinical control Pacemaker control

Table 3. Protocol for dual chamber pacemarker control.

Case history	General condition; Daily life exercise capacity; Palpitations Dizziness/fainting

Recordings	ECG
	    Spontaneous; Magnet applied
	Telemetry*)
	    Programmed parameters; R-waves; Marker channel

Measurements	Pulse width; Pulse intervals (± Magnet); Stimulation threshold
	    autothreshold; vario*)
	P-wave amplitude
	    indirect via P-sensitivity; programming

*) When available.

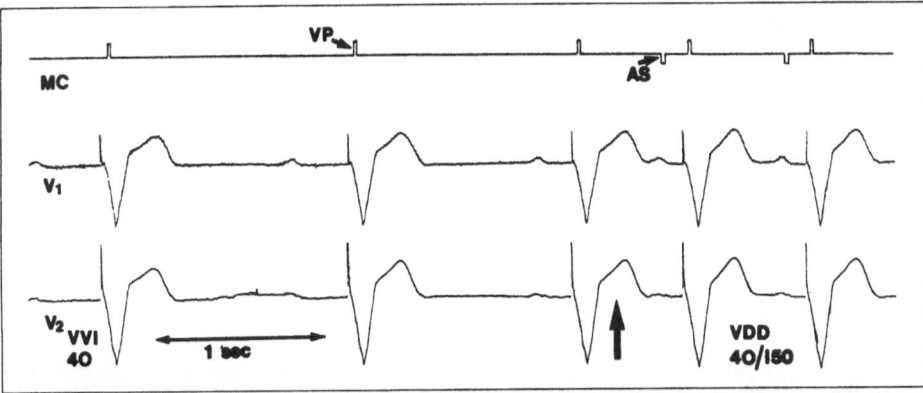

Fig. 1. ECG (V1, V2) and marker channel (MC) during reprogramming from VVI-pacing (40 ppm) to VDD-pacing (back up rate 40 ppm, upper rate limit 150 ppm). The programming is done at the arrow activating the atrial sensing amplifier (AS = atrial sense, VP = ventricular pace). Note: marker channel pulses are inverted in this example.

for pacemaker control. To determine whether dual-chamber pacing cause increased number of hospital admissions compared to single chamber systems we reviewed the 54 VDD-paced patients who had been observed for a time period exceeding 12 months (mean 39 ± 17; range 12–69). In this survey we excluded hospital admissions for pacemaker surgery or scientific investigations. Observations for and/or treatment of arrhythmias was the major indication (14 pats = 26%). The second most common reason to hospital admission was congestive heart failure (8 pats = 15%). These findings were not surprising since 24% of the patients have ischemic heart disease, 22% hypertension and 11% paroxysmal atrial tachyarrhythmias in addition to the conduction defect. Fifty per cent of the patients were never admitted apart from the pacemaker implant.

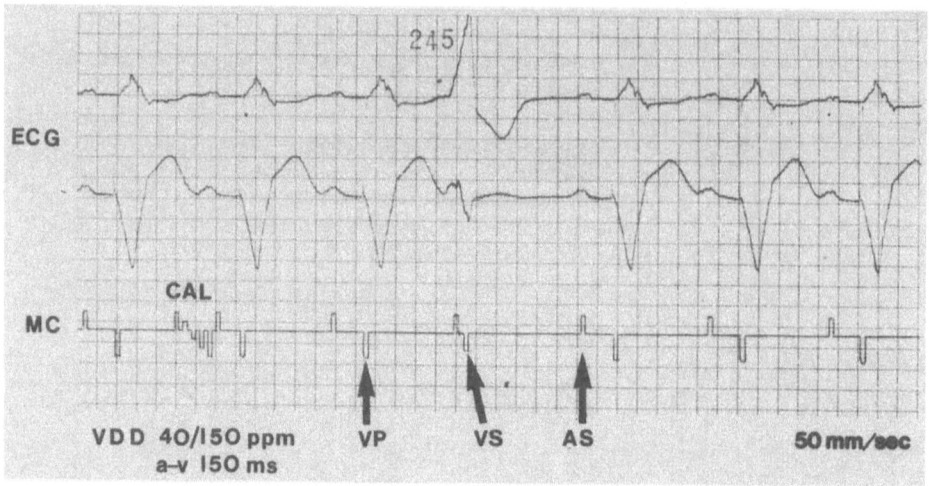

Fig. 2. Pacemaker program: VDD-mode; AV-interval 150 ms. In complex 4 a normal P-wave is followed by a premature ventricular contraction. Sensing of this (VS = ventricular sense) resets all timing intervals and prevents pacing 150 ms after the sensed P-wave. Note also the calibration signal (CAL) of the marker channel.

Fig. 3. The Wenckebach like upper limit behaviour of a VDD-pacemaker is initiated during exercise at a work load of 150 watts. The AV-delay is gradually increased from the programmed 150 ms to 340 ms during beat 1–5. The sixth P-wave is not sensed as it occurs during the atrial refractory period initiated by beat 5. Consequently next ventricular stimulus is dropped and next AV-delay (beat 6) returns to 150 ms. In this example an atrial rate of 138 bpm results in an average ventricular rate of 115 bpm with the pacemaker programmed to an upper rate limit of 125 ppm. Every sixth atrial contraction is not sensed. This recording obtained during heavy exercise also demonstrates the possibility to obtain exact information about the timing of sensing and pacing events in the pacemaker through the marker channel (MC) when the ECG (V1, V2) is distorted by muscle artefacts.

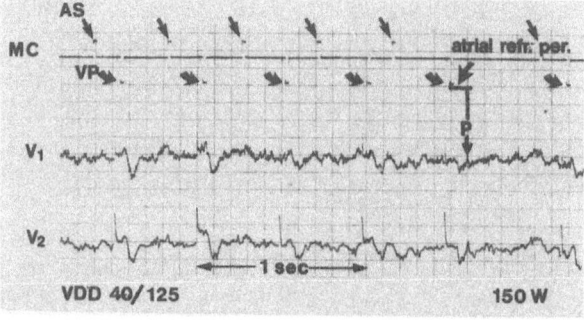

Leads

Concerning ventricular leads no problems caused by or of any particular importance to the dual-chamber pacemakers occurred. Regarding atrial leads some observations may be of interest. Since 1977 we have implanted a total of 122 atrial leads. Dislodgements have been rare (3%) and occurred within the first 24 hours following lead insertion. Late

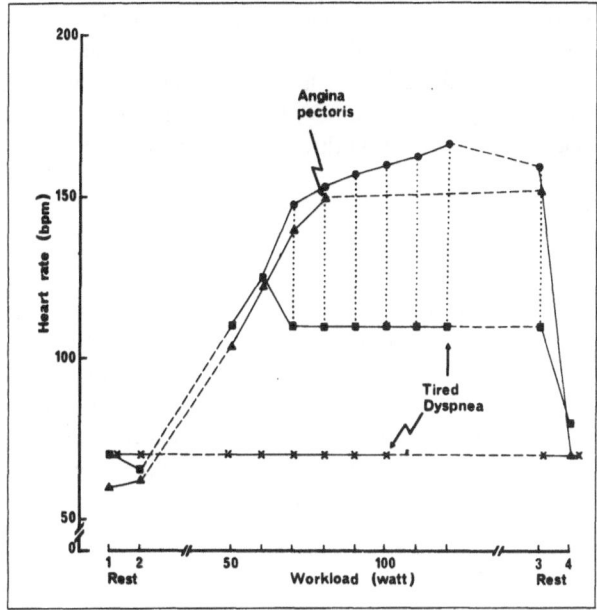

Fig. 4. Results of repeated exercise tests in a male patient, 58 years old. See text for details.
VVI-pacing: x——x = ventricular rate June 79 and February 80.
VDD-pacing: ▲——▲ = atrial and ventricular rate June 79
■——■ = ventricular rate
●——● = atrial rate when exceeding ventricular rate February 80.
Dotted line indicates the gap between atrial and ventricular rate due to blocking in the pacemaker.
1 and 2 = supine and sitting at rest.
3 and 4 = directly after and four minutes after exercise.

loss of atrial sensing has occurred in three patients. In two of these atrial sensing/pacing was abandoned one and 24 months after implant and in one the lead was repositioned six months after implant. Loss of atrial sensing in one patient twice parallelled an increase in heart size due to exacerbation of congestive heart failure. The VDD-pacemaker was temporarily programmed to VVI but as soon as the heart size had been normalized atrial sensing was reestablished and VDD-pacing reinstituted. This particular VDD-pacemaker had a fixed atrial-sensitivity of 0,75 mV. It is believed that the dilation of the right atrium caused a decrease in the amplitude and/or the slew rate of the P-wave. It is important to recognize such a phenomenon in order to avoid unnecessary attempts to reposition the lead. The second case of temporary loss of atrial sensing illustrates the importance of a careful case history when solving pacing problems. DDD-pacing had been instituted due to a combined sinus and atrioventricular node disease. However, occasional symptoms suggestive of bradycardia continued. Holter monitoring revealed periods of normal VDD-pacing intermingled with episodes of bradycardia at the programmed escape rate of 50 ppm. Intermittent loss of atrial sensing was suspected but when exploring the electrode peak to peak amplitude of P-waves were 3.3–4.7 mV i.e. well above the programmed atrial sensitivity of 1.5 mV. It was however noted that loss of atrial sensing only occurred in the upright position when the patient was bending forward. Following reprogramming of atrial sensitivity to 0.75 mV there was no further loss of atrial sensing. An unusually great variability of P-wave amplitudes appeared to be the reason for the intermittent loss of atrial sensing. In order to avoid similar problems one may advocate a constant programming of a high atrial sensitivity. This may on the other hand cause oversensing problems. In one of our patients the last part of the QRS-complex was sensed by the atrial amplifier when atrial sensitivity was set to 0.75 mV but never at a setting of 1.5 mV. A too high atrial sensitivity might also result in interference from inappropiate sig-

473

nals like muscle noise. We believe that atrial sensitivity should be investigated and programmed accordingly at pacemaker controls. So far there are no available pacemaker where P-waves as well as R-waves can be noninvasively telemetered. Until now we have not noted any problems with atrial pacing among our DVI- and DDD-patients. The measurements have revealed reasonably low stimulation thresholds less than 1.7 V.

Pacemakers

Except for two early DDD-devices (one Medtronic and one Siemens-Elema) showing occasional self-inhibition we have not had any malfunctioning DDD-pacemakers. The VDD-pacemakers have also functioned well disregarding a few problems with some early Medtronic 2409 generators. These failures are considered dependent on the investigational hand-made design of the first series of those pacemakers. It may be mentioned that we have had a number of DC-conversions performed on patients with VDD-pacemakers. They were always checked afterwards for possible phantomprogramming and failures, but without any untoward findings.

Atrial tachyarrhythmias

Tachyarrhythmias induced by dual chamber pacemakers will be dealt with separately during this symposium. This is an important problem during follow up and our experiences of atrial tachyarrhythmias is briefly reported in Table 4. There is a limited number of pacemaker induced atrial reentry tachycardia. All of them were successfully treated and so far we have not been forced to abandon atrial synchronous pacing due to atrial reentry tachycardia in any patient.

Exercise testing and Holter monitoring

Sometimes and in particular when dealing with patients with ischaemic heart disease it is important to investigate not only at rest but also during exercise (10). Fig. 3 contains

Table 4. Clinically significant atrial tachyarrhythmias among 111 patients on VAT, VDD, DDD or VDI pacing.

	Arrhythmia	No	%	Treatment
Spontaneous:	Par fibr	5	4.5	Conventional:
	Par tach	2	1.8	Digoxine, Quinidine
				DC-conversion
Pacemaker related:	Reentry	6	5.4	Digoxine 3
				Verapamil 1
				AV-delay ↑ 1
				AV-delay ↓
				+ Digoxine 1

474

an example of such a patient and it can clearly be seen that a proper upper rate programming is of crucial importance for a successful result of atrial synchronous pacing.

Follow up of dual chamber pacemaker patients should at least once include an exercise test to certify the pacemaker and patient behaviour during work and during the recovery period. Holter monitoring is of special value in those cases where symptoms are rare and not related to exercise but still give reason to suspect improper pacemaker-function.

Concluding remarks

Any center responsible for patients with dual-chamber pacemakers must'have a round the clock possibility of and instructions for programming the pacemaker to VVI 70 ppm. Thereafter the patient awaits referred to a physician with knowledge of both the patients and the pacemaker for adequate treatment. The major objective of pacemaker follow up is to continuously adapt the pacemaker to the needs of the patient to achieve the best possible quality of life.

References

1. Kruse I, Rydén L, Ydse B: Clinical and electrophysiological characteristics of a transvenous atrial lead. Br Heart J 1979; 49: 595–602.
2. Kruse I, Rydén L, Ydse B: A new lead for transvenous atrial pacing and sensing. Pace 1980; 3: 395–405.
3. Kruse I, Duffin E, Rydén L: Clinical evaluation of atrial synchronous ventricular inhibited pacemakers. Pace 1980; 3: 641–650.
4. Kruse I, Markowitz T, Rydén L: Timing markers showing pacemaker behaviour to aid the follow up of a physiological pacemaker. Pace, 1983. In press.
5. Sutton R, Perrins J, Citron P: Physiological cardiac pacing. Pace 1980; 3: 207–219.
6. Karlöf I: Haemodynamic effect of atrial triggered versus fixed rate pacing at rest and during exercise and complete heart block. Acta Med Scand 1975; 197: 195–206.
7. Kruse I, Arnman K, Conradson T-B, Rydén L: A comparison of acute and lontterm haemodynamic effects of ventricular inhibited and atrial synchronous ventricular inhibited pacing. Circulation 1982; 65: 846–855.
8. Parsonnet V: The proliferation of cardiac pacing: Medical, technical and socioeconomical dilemmas. Circulation 1982; 65: 841–845.
9. Kruse I, Peters P, Rydén L: A new transvenous lead for atrial and ventricular sensing and pacing. Pace, 1983. In press.
10. Kruse I, Rydén L: Comparison of work capacity and systolic time intervals with ventricular inhibited and atrial synchronous ventricular inhibited pacing. Br Heart J 1981: 46: 129–136.

Authors' address:
L. Rydén,
Department of Medicine
Central Hospital
S-541 85 Skövde, Sweden

Dual Chamber DDD Pacing: Initial and Early Follow-Up Assessments. Problems, Complications and Limitations

R. J. Eastway, Jr.; J. D. Maloney; L. W. Castle; J. Yiannikas; J. C. Cooper, V. A. Morant

Summary: Since the implantation of our first dual chamber DDD pacing system in August of 1981, our experience has expanded to include more than 150 units. Our first 70 patients were followed for a mean period of 8.8 months. Major indications for pacing included heart block and sick sinus syndrome. Fifty five of the 70 patients were studied electrophysiologically including an assessment of retrograde VA conduction. Retrograde conduction was present in 73% of those studied. No clinical or ECG findings enabled us to predict the presence or absence of retrograde conduction. Pacemakter related tachycardia was our most frequently encountered problem. A programmable atrial refractory period offered a solution to this problem. Other problems included lead dislodgement and transient atrial sensing abnormalities. We conclude that DDD pacing is safe, reliable and affords symptomatic relief in a broad spectrum of patients.

Introduction

Since the introduction of the first implantable cardiac pacemaker in 1958 (1), significant technological advances have expanded our capabilities from single chamber asynchronous pacing to dual chamber universal pacing (2). The past two decades have been especially productive when one considers the reduction in pulse generator size, the increase in battery longevity, the development of multiparameter multiprogrammability, and improvements in lead-electrode system.

Currently available dual chamber DDD pulse generators are able to sense and pace in both the atrium and ventricle. An intrinsic atrial rate below a programmed minimum pacing rate results in an atrial paced event. Atrial rates between the programmed minimum and maximum pacing rates are sensed and tracked appropriately. Atrial rates above a programmed maximum pacing rate are handled differently by each particular pulse generator utilizing various atrial tachycardia response modes. An atrial sensed or paced event initiates an AV delay during which the ventricular sensing circuit awaits an inherent QRS complex. Sensing of an inherent QRS complex during the programmed AV delay results in suppression of the ventricular pacing artifact. When no ventricular activity is sensed during the programmed AV delay, a ventricular paced event occurs.

One of the major problems with implantation of a pulse generator capable of sensing an atrial event (sinus impulse, atrial premature impulse or retrograde impulse utilizing either the His-AV nodes axis or an accessory atrioventricular connection) and following with a ventricular paced event, is that the pacemaker system itself may act as an "iatrogenic" accessory atrioventricular connection. Consequently, when retrograde ventriculoatrial conduction is present, endless loop tachycardias can occur with the pacemaker system functioning as the antegrade limb of a macro-reentrant circuit.

477

This report describes our initial and early follow-up assessment, problems, complications and limitations in 70 patients who received dual chamber DDD pacing systems. Table I outlines the diagnoses and/or conduction system disturbances necessitating permanent pacemaker implantation.

Materials and Methods

Since the implantation of our first dual chamber DDD pacing system in August of 1981, our experience has expanded to include over 150 such devices. Devices utilized included the Cordis 233 D in 31 patients, the Telectronics 2251 in 24 patients and the Medtronic model 7000 in 15 patients. All units are multiparameter multiprogrammable units. A comparison of the programmable parameters is outlined in Table 2.

Electrophysiologic Studies

Utilizing several multipolar electrodes catheters passed percutaneously via the right femoral vein approach, electrophysiologic studies were performed on 55 of the 70 patients. The sinoatrial node, atrioventricular node and His-Purkinje systems were evaluated in the usual manner. Retrograde ventriculoatrial conduction was assessed utilizing both right ventricular pacing at various pacing basic cycle lengths and programmed ventricular stimulation to introduce premature ventricular beats. Recordings were obtained from at

Table 1. Underlying conduction system disturbances and/or diagnosis necessitating permanent pacemaker implantation

Rhythm Disturbance	Cordis 233D (31)		Telectronics 2251 (24)		Medtronic 7000 (15)	
	No.	*Percent	No.	*Percent	No.	*Percent
Sinus node dysfunction	15	48	7	29	5	33
Trifascicular block	5	16	5	21	1	6.7
Carotid sinus hypersensitivity	3	9.7	1	4.2	4	26.7
Intra/infra His block	3	9.7	2	8.4	1	6.7
Drug induced symptomatic bradycardia	1	3.2	1	4.2		
Postoperative heart block						
AVR	1	3.2	3	12.5	1	6.7
ACBG	1	3.2	1	4.2		
Type I aortic dissection					1	6.7
Non-operative heart block						
Complete	2	6.4	4	16.7		
High grade	3	9.7	1	4.2	4	26.7
Intermittent			1	4.2		
Pacemaker syndrome	1	3.2				

* Some patients had more than one diagnosis

Table 2. Programmable parameters

	Cordis 233D (Sequicor)	Telectronics 2251 (Autima)	Medtronic 7000 (Versatrax)
Mode	DDD, DVI, DAD, VDD, VAT, VVI, DOO, VOO, VET	DDD, DVI, VDD, VVI, DOO, VOO	DDD, DVI, VVI
Minimum pacing rate	50, 60, 70, 80 ppm	60, 65, 70, 75, 80, 90, 100, 110 ppm	§ 40–80 ppm (steps of 10 ppm)
Maximum pacing rate	100, 130, 160, 180 ppm	120, 130, 150 ppm	100, 125, 150, 175 ppm
AV delay	80, 120, 165, 250 msec	0, 50, 80, 110, 140, 170, 200, 230 msec	25– 250 msec (steps of 25 msec)
Atrial sensitivity	Off, 7.0, 1.5, 0.8 mV	1.0, 0.5 mV	Asynchronous, 3.0, 1.5 0.75 mV
Ventricular sensitivity	Off, 2.5, 1.5, 0.8 mV	*2.7 mV	Asynchronous, 5.0, 2.5 mV
Atrial output pulse width	Off, 0.5, 1.0, 1.5 msec	*0.5 msec	0.05, 0.1, 0.2,...1.5 msec
Ventricular output pulse width	0.5, 1.0, 1.5, 2.0 msec	*0.55 msec	0.5, 0.1, 0.2,...1.5 msec

* Non-programmable
§ DDD mode

least two different sites within the right atrium. Low septal right atrial activity was recorded with a catheter positioned across the tricuspid valve and high right atrial activity was recorded from a catheter in the right atrial appendage area. Recordings were obtained on either a Siemens-Elema mingograph model 82 recorder filtered at 50–550 Hz at paper speeds of 100 mm/sec or a Gould ES 1000 recorder filtered at 30–500 Hz at similar paper speed. Pacing and stimulation were performed with a Medtronic 5325 programmable stimulator. Intact retrograde VA conduction was defined as the ability to conduct at least one impulse retrogradely from the right ventricle to the atria utilizing the His-AV node axis.

Lead Electrode Systems

Lead electrode systems were transvenous in 69 patients and epicardial in one patient. The single subclavian venepuncture route was utilized in 60 patients and the cephalic cutdown approach in 10 patients. In general, no particular lead electrode system was chosen to match a particular pulse generator. Leads with large connector pins were generally used with the Cordis 233D pulse generator to avoid the use of an adaptor. Active fixation endocardial screw in leads were used in patients whose atrial appendage had been truncated by previous open heart surgery.

Follow-Up

Follow-up consisted of continuous bedside monitoring for the first 24 hours, 24 hour ambulatory monitoring and thorough pacemaker clinic evaluation (including fluoroscopic visualization) prior to hospital discharge. Six week, six months, and one year pacemaker clinic visits were required as well as periodic evaluation by a telephone transmission device.

Results

Retrograde conduction
Retrograde VA conduction was present in 40 of the 55 (73%) patients studied electrophysiologically. Twelve patients had no evidence of retrograde conduction. Of the 15 patients not studied electrophysiologically, six patients had antegrade complete heart block and we initially assumed that retrograde conduction would be absent.
Our experience and that of others suggests that retrograde VA conduction utilizing the His-AV node axis is not a static, but rather a dynamic process behaving physiologically like antegrade conduction, being influenced in a similar manner by such things as exercise, drugs, catecholamine state and pacing rate. Indeed retrograde conduction can be absent one day and present the next. Because retrograde conduction is a dynamic process, we chose not to assign an absolute number to retrograde conduction times, but to look upon retrograde conduction as being either intact or absent. We were unable to find any clinical or electrocardiographic parameters which enabled us to predict the presence or absence of retrograde conduction. In general though, patients with normal antegrade AV nodal conduction at electrophysiologic study tended to show poor or absent retrograde conduction.

Pacemaker Related Tachycardia (endless loop tachycardia)

The most frequently encountered problem was pacemaker related tachycardia. Twenty-one of our 70 patients experienced pacemaker related tachycardia. PRT occurred more frequently during our initial experience, which consisted of 20 Cordis 233D devices. Sustained episodes of PRT occurred prior to hospital discharge when this unit was initially programmed to function in the fallback atrial tachycardia response mode. A short atrial refractroy period when programmed to the fallback atrial tachycardia response mode rendered patients particularly susceptible to the development of PRT. Reprogramming to the 2 : 1 AV block response mode with a low maximum pacing rate lengthened the atrial refractory period offering a solution to the problem. Although not as frequent a problem with the Telectronics 2251 or Medtronic 7000, reprogramming to DVI mode was required in those patients experiencing PRT.

Pacemaker related tachycardia occurred in 15 of the 40 patients who had intact retrograde conduction at the time of electrophysiologic study. No PRT was encountered in the group of 15 patients with absent retrograde conduction. Four of six patients with antegrade complete heart block in whom retrograde conduction was assumed absent developed PRT.

Complications

Lead dislodgement requiring reoperation occurred in four patients. Two atrial and two ventricular leads dislodged acutely (within the first 24 hours). Additional programmability involving atrial output and/or pulse width in the Telectronics 2251 may have saved one reoperation.

A single small pneumothorax not requiring chest tube insertion resolved spontaneously.

An episode of PRT, which went unrecognized by night house staff unfamiliar with the potential problems of DDD pacing, resulted in an acute myocardial infarction in one patient. An uneventful recovery ensued.

Transient failure to sense in the atrium occurred in six patients (8.5%). Five of these six patients had sick sinus syndrome and all five had P wave amplitudes at implant of 2.0 mV – 2.6 mV, which was considerably less than our mean value of 3.2 mV for all patients. Sensing function returned to normal in all patients prior to discharge. The etiology of the atrial sensing problems remains unknown.

Discussion

Although the concept of physiologic pacing is not new, interest in dual chamber physiologic pacing systems has been rekindled because recent technological advances have eliminated some of the previously existing historical barriers to both atrial and dual chamber pacing.

Until the introduction of polyurethane insulation, atrial leads have been relatively large and the passage of two leads through a single vein has been difficult. Long term reliability of both atrial pacing and sensing has been lacking and until the development of active fixation as well as tined tipped passive fixation leads, dislodgement has been a significant problem. The decrease in pulse generator size, increase in battery longevity, improvements in lead electrode systems and the development of microprocessor based circuitry have also contributed to the increasing interest in utilizing dual chamber pacing systems.

A physiologic pacing system may be defined as a pacing system which allows the heart rate to increase or decrease according to the patient's needs while maintaining AV synchrony. Although not currently available, it would be ideal to have the AV delay shorten slightly as the heart rate increases and to allow ventricular depolarization to occur in as normal a sequence as possible.

Our experience and that of others has resulted in an increasing number of physicians becoming convinced of the hemodynamic and electrophysiologic benefits of dual chamber physiologic pacing. Recent data has clearly shown dual chamber DDD pacing is safe, reliable and is hemodynamically superior to single chamber VVI pacing (3, 4).

After a detailed analysis of our first 70 implants we conclude that DDD pacing is safe, reliable and affords symptomatic improvement in a broad spectrum of patients with symptomatic bradycardia.

References

1. Furman S, Robinson G: Use of intracardiac pacemaker in correction of total heart block. Surgical Forum 1958: 9, 245.
2. Sutton R, Citron P: Electrophysiological and haemodynamic basis for application of new pacemaker technology in sick sinus syndrome and atrioventricular block. Br Heart J 1979: 41, 600.
3. Eastway RJ, Esper WA, Maloney JD, Tsai AR, Yiannikas J, Morant VA, Castle LW, Dorfman PM: Investigational dual chambered pacing systems functioning in DDD mode — Initial experience. (Abstract) Circulation 66 (Supp II): II-218, 1982
4. Morley C, Chan S, Sutton R: A randomized controlled trial of physiologic versus ventricular pacing. (Abstract) Circulation 66 (Supp II): II-218, 1982

Author's address:
Lon W. Castle, M.D.
Cleveland Clinic Foundation
9500 Euclid Ave
Cleveland, Ohio 44106
USA

Survival after Pacemaker Implantation

R. G. Hauser, J. Jones, K. Moss, L. M. Edwards, J. V. Messer

Summary: The prognosis of 968 patients who were paced for bradyarrhythmias which were not complicated by ventricular tachycardia was assessed by actuarial and proportional hazards analysis. The average age at implant was 67.8 ± 16.2 years and the mean implant time was 41 months (range 1 mo to 18 yrs). The number of patients and the number of years when 50% of patients (pts) could be expected to survive were:
1. complete AV block – 373 pts, 11.8 yrs;
2. second degree AV block – 88 pts, 6.3 yrs;
3. sinus bradyarrhythmia – 301 pts, 8.8 yrs;
4. sinus bradyarrhythmia/atrial fibrillation or supraventricular tachycardia – 172 pts, 7.8 yrs;
5. all indications – 968 pts, 8.9 yrs.
Highly significant (p < 0.001) predictors of mortality were age at implant > prior myocardial infarction > congestive heart failure > congenital heart disease > chronic renal failure. Conclusions:
1. pacing systems which provide optimum physiologic support should last 10 years;
2. advanced age and associated cardiovascular disease are not necessarily prudent reasons for withholding long-lived multiprogrammable and/or dual chamber pacemakers.

Introduction

In a previous communication we reported that patients who are paced for bradyarrhythmias complicated by ventricular tachycardia (VT) have a high mortality rate (1). Among the group of 60 such patients, more than half were dead at the end of one year and the presence of VT as a clinical problem at the time of pacemaker implantation was found to be a stronger predictor of subsequent mortality than a history of prior myocardial infarction or congestive heart failure. Since the prevalence of VT in the paced population will have a significant impact on survival, we initiated a study to assess the prognosis of patients who have undergone permanent pacemaker implantation for bradyarrhythmias which were not complicated by ventricular tachycardia. Our data suggest that previous reports (2–5) have underestimated the survival of patients who have sinoatrial disease, and that the outlook for individuals who are paced for atrioventricular (AV) block is largely determined by the type of conduction disturbance and the severity rather than the simple coexistence of underlying cardiac disorders.

Methods

Subjects. The study population consisted 968 patients who underwent pacemaker implantation for the reasons shown in Table 1 and who were followed in our pacemaker clinic between July 1, 1975 and December 31, 1982. None of those patients had a history of VT at the time of pacemaker insertion. At the end of the study period, 621 (64%) patients were alive, 294 (30%) had expired, and no contact had been established with 53 individuals (6%) for more than one year. The mean age at implant was 67.8 ± 16.2 years

Table 1. Reason for pacing

	No.		% Total
Complete AV Block		373	39%
Acquired	335		35%
Surgical	30		3%
Congenital	8		1%
2° AV Block		88	9%
Sinoatrial Disease		468	48%
Bradyarrhythmia	301		31%
Brady + Tachy	172		18%
Carotid Sinus Syndrome		18	2%
IV Conduction Defect		16	2%
Total		968	100%

Fig. 1. Associated cardiovascular conditions and the proportion of patients who were dead at the end of the study period.

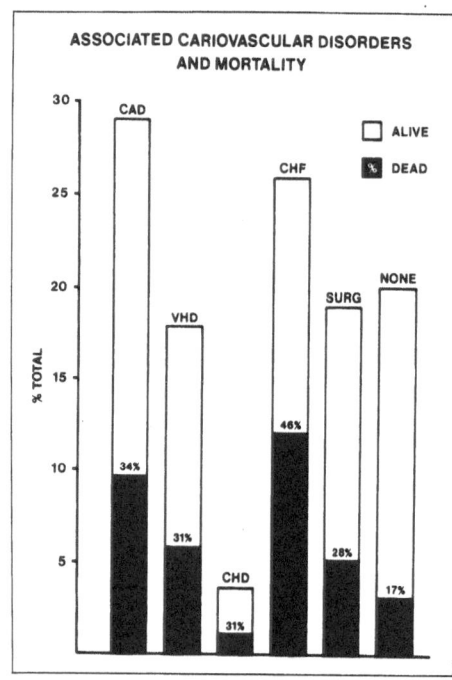

ASSOCIATED CARIOVASCULAR DISORDERS AND MORTALITY

(range: 1 day to 99 years), 53% of the population was male, and the average duration of pacing was 41.1 mos (range: 1 mo to 18 years). Ventricular pacing was used in 97% of cases and the vast majority received transvenous pacing systems. The incidences of associated cardiovascular disorders for the entire population are shown in Figure 1. Only 20% of patients did not have an underlying cardiovascular disorder and 19% had undergone cardiac surgery; these observations are consistent with the referral population served by our medical center. Coronary artery disease (CAD), manifested by either ischemic heart disease or electrocardiographic evidence of prior myocardial infarction, was present in 39% of patients and congestive heart failure (CHF) requiring medication was seen in nearly 26% of cases. There were no significant differences in the prevalence of these disorders based on the reason for pacing except that patients who were paced for bradycardia-tachycardia had a higher than expected incidence of valvular heart disease.

Statistical analysis. Actuarial survival probabilities were calculated using the method of Cutler and Ederer (6) and the comparison of survival between groups was performed by the chi square method (7). Stepwise proportional hazards analysis was used to weigh predictors of mortality (8). Categorical data was compared using the chi square statistic.

Results

The overall survival of the 968 patients is shown in Figure 2 where it is compared to that of 66 patients whose paced bradyarrhythmias (10 AV block, 56 sinoatrial disease) were complicated by ventricular tachycardia. In the absence of VT, the anticipated longevity of the average paced patient was nearly 75% at three years, 50% at 10 years, and in excess of 25% at 15 years after implantation. When the 66 VT patients were grouped with the patients without VT, the average (50%) survival was decreased from 10 to 8.9 years.

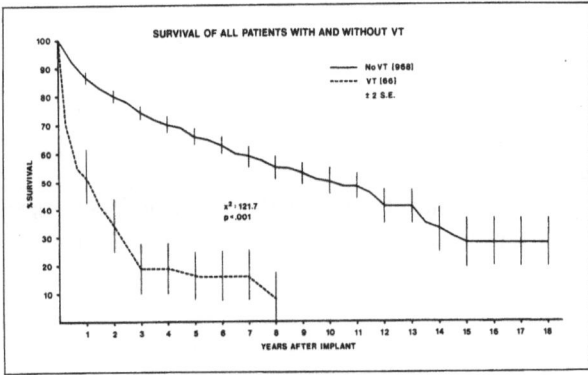

Fig. 2: Actuarial survival of the 968 patients who were paced for bradyarrhythmias which were not complicated by ventricular tachycardia. Also shown is the survival curve of 66 patients whose paced bradyarrhythmias were accompanied by ventricular tachycardia.

Table 2. Predictors of mortality for all patients

	χ^2	r	p
Age at Implant	51.9	0.11	<0.001
Prior Myocardial Infarction	37.2	0.08	<0.001
Congestive Heart Failure	30.6	0.07	<0.001
Congenital Heart Disease	27.1	0.06	<0.001
Chronic Renal Failure	25.1	0.06	<0.001
Valvular Heart Disease	10.6	0.03	<0.05

485

The significant predictors of mortality based on proportional hazards analysis are shown in Table 2. The most powerful predictor of death after pacemaker insertion was the age at implant, but other significant prognostic indicators included electrocardiographic evidence of prior myocardial infarction and congestive heart failure requiring medical therapy; these observations are consistent with the data illustrated in Figure 1, which shows that the highest mortalities for this population were found in the groups with CAD (34%) and CHF (46%). A history of cardiac surgery *per se* did not affect prognosis, but both congenital heart disease and valvular heart disease were significant predictors of mortality.

Atrioventricular Block

The survivial of patients who were paced for AV block is shown in Figure 3A. The longevity of patients who had complete AV block was significantly better than those individuals who received pacemakers for second degree AV block (p < 0.001). The average patient who had second degree AV block could be expected to live only five years, while more than 50% of patients who were paced for complete AV block survived more than 10 years. The poor prognosis of the group with second degree AV block could not be explained by underlying cardiac disease (Table 3), although there was a slightly higher mortality in a subgroup of individuals with second degree AV block who had coronary artery disease. However, even when second degree AV block patients without CAD were compared to a like group of patients who were paced for complete AV block, the longevity of the former was still significantly less (χ^2 = 5.7, p < 0.025). The only significant cardiovascular predictor of mortality in the complete AV block population was prior myocardial infarction (Table 3).

Sinoatrial Disease

The survival of patients who were paced for sinus bradyarrhythmias alone, including sinus arrest, sinus exit block or severe sinus bradycardia, is shown in Figure 3B. The 301

Fig. 3. A) Survival of patients who were paced for complete or second degree AV block.

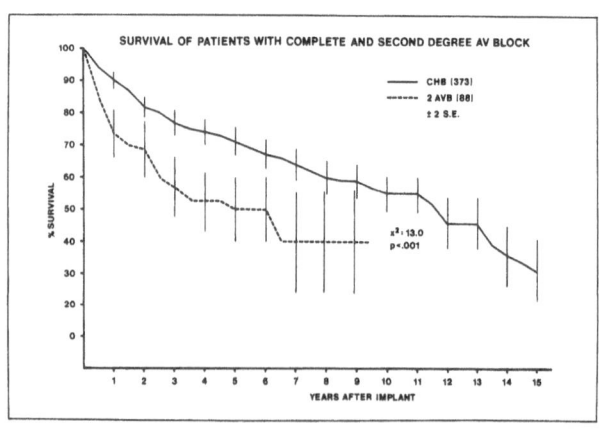

Table 3. Cardiac predictors of mortality

Reason	Condition	χ^2	p
Complete AV Block	Prior M.I.	44.6	<0.001
2° AV Block	None		
Sinoatrial Disease			
Bradyarrhythmia:	CHF	12.6	<0.001
	Congential H.D.	7.3	<0.01
	Valvular H.D.	5.6	<0.05
	Prior M.I.	4.9	<0.05
Brady + Tachy:	Prior M.I.	9.0	<0.01
	CHF	5.2	<0.05

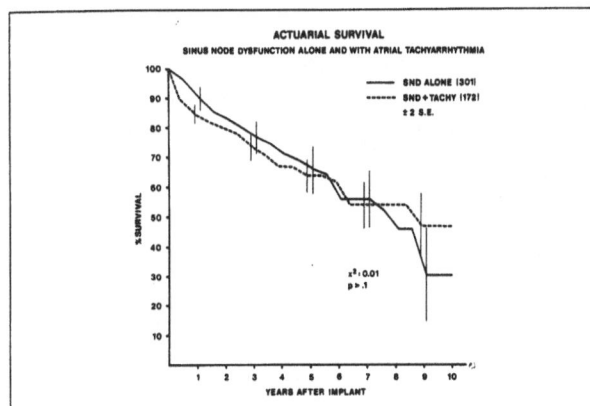

Fig. 3. B) Survival of patients who were paced for sinus bradyarrhythmia alone or for bradycardia-tachycardia.

patients in this group were older (mean: 71.8 ± 11.3 SD years) than the average age (67.8 years) of the study population as a whole and, in contrast to patients who had AV block, the prognosis was less favorable for patients who were 75 years or older at the time of implant. Of 132 patients who were over 75 years of age when first paced for sinus bradyarrhythmia, less than half could be expected to survive five years; however, 50% of individuals who were 60 to 74 years at implant would be alive after eight years, and the difference in longevity between the two age groups was very significant ($\chi^2 = 9.6$, $p < 0.005$). Cardiac predictors of mortality for patients who were paced for sinus bradyarrhythmia alone are given in Table 3. These individuals had more significant cardiac risk factors than any other group.

Patients who were paced for sinus bradyarrhythmia complicated by paroxysmal or established atrial fibrillation, atrial flutter, or other supraventricular tachyarrhythmias (bradycardia-tachycardia) exhibited a pattern of survival which was similar to that of sinus bradyarrhythmia alone (Fig. 3B). While mortality was significantly higher during the first 6 months after implant for the bradycardia-tachycardia group ($p < 0.05$), their overall survival compared to that of patients with sinus bradyarrhythmia was not significantly different ($p > 0.1$). In contrast, age at implant was less of an influence on longevity for the bradycardia-tachycardia patient; no significant difference in survival was found for

487

individuals 60 to 74 years of age compared to those who were older than 75 years when they were originally paced. Significant predictors of death for the bradycardia-tachycardia group included a history of prior myocardial infarction and the presence of congestive heart failure (Table 3).

Carotid Sinus Hypersensitivity

Only 18 patients were paced for symptomatic carotid sinus hypersensitivity. Longevity in this group was excellent with a cumulative survival probability of $92 \pm 7\%$ after 42 implant months.

Intraventricular Conduction Defects

The 16 patients paced for intraventricular conduction defects had a one year mortality of 20% and a five year cumulative survival of $44 \pm 17\%$. Fifty percent of these individuals had coronary artery disease and 25% were being treated for congestive heart failure at the time of pacemaker insertion.

Discussion

The excellent prognosis of patients who are paced for complete AV block has been recognized and reported by others (9, 10). Except for age, only a history of prior myocardial infarction truely influenced survival. In the absence of myocardial infarction or ischemic heart disease, a patient who is paced for complete AV block may be expected to live nearly 12 years after pacemaker implantation. Even the very elderly who have complete AV block will usually survive more than seven years and the outlook is even more favorable in the absence of clinically apparent cardiovascular disease.

Unfortunately the optimistic prognosis of complete heart block treated by pacing does not apply to patients who are paced for second degree AV block. Not only do these individuals fare poorly as a group, but even those patients who do not have prior myocardial infarction or ischemic heart disease exhibit decreased survival; of 60 patients in the latter category, nearly half were dead by the end of the sixth year. As noted earlier, the only apparent reason for the higher mortality associated with second degree AV block was the association of more severe underlying cardiac disease. However, such an explanation is largely inferential and clearly additional studies are required to identify those factors which specifically affect the clinical course of patients who have symptomatic second degree AV block which requires pacemaker therapy.

The group of patients who were paced for sinoatrial disorders, including those with bradycardia-tachycardia, did not differ greatly in regard to longevity from the population with complete AV block. The average patient with sinoatrial disease may be expected to live between eight and nine years, and their longevity is only slightly less favorable than that of the complete AV block group ($p < 0.05$). This finding contrasts sharply with those reported by others (3–5), but the high mortalities which they observed were probably due to the impact of ventricular tachycardia in their study populations. Patients who had VT were excluded from the present study because we have already shown that it is a stronger predictor of mortality in the paced population than age or coronary artery disease.

Clinical Implications

This study shows that the majority of patients may be expected to live nine years after pacemaker implantation. Therefore, physicians should select pulse generators and leads which may be anticipated to provide maximum clinical benefit and technical performance over a decade of use. Neither advanced age nor the existence of associated cardiovascular disease may be justifiably used as a reason for denying most patients the potential advantages of multiprogrammable and/or dual chamber pacing systems. Moreover, the cost of pacing wil be reduced if battery longevity matches that of the paced population; current dual chamber models will probably require replacement during the lifetime of the average patient.

References

1. Hauser RG, Jones J, Denes P, Messer JV: Prognosis of patients paced for bradyarrhythmias complicated by ventricular tachycardia. Pace 1982; 5: 300.
2. Van Hemel NM, Schaepkens van Riempst ALE, Bakema H, Swenne CA: Long-term follow-up after pacemaker implantation in sick sinus syndrome. Pace 1980; 4: 8–13.
3. Aroesty JM, Cohen SI, Morkin E: Bradycardia-tachycardia syndrome: results in 28 patients treated by combined pharmacologic therapy and pacemaker implantation. Chest 1974; 66: 257–263.
4. Chokshi DS, Mascarenhas E, Samet P, Center S: Treatment of sinoatrial rhythm disturbances with permanent cardiac pacing. Am J Cardiol 1973; 32: 215–220.
5. Simon AB, Janz N: Symptomatic bradyarrhythmia in the adult: natural history following ventricular pacemaker implantation. Pace 1982; 5: 372–383.
6. Cutler SJ, Ederer F: Maximum utilization of the life table method in analyzing survival. J Chron Dis 1958; 8: 699–712.
7. Peto R, Pike MC, Armitage P, Breslow NE, Cox DR, Howard SV, Mantel N, McPherson K, Peto J, Smith PG: Design and analysis of randomized clinical trials requiring prolonged observation of each patient II. analysis and examples. Br J Cancer 1977; 35: 1–39.
8. Cox DR: Regression models and life tables. J Royal Statist Soc 1972; 34: 187–220.
9. Furman S: Results of cardiac pacing. In: Samet P, El-Sherif N, eds, Cardiac Pacing, 2nd edn, New York: Grune and Stratton, 1980: 271–293.
10. Bette L, Doenecke P, Rettig G, Flothner R: Results of permanent cardiac stimulation therapy. In: Schaldach M, Furman S, eds. Advances in pacemaker technology. New York: Springer-Verlag, 1975; 75–90.

Authors' address:
Robert G. Hauser, M.D.
1753 West Congress Parkway
Chicago, IL 60612
USA

Long-Term Follow-up of Patients with Reused Implanted Pacemakers

S. Amikam, S. Feldman, B. Boal, E. Riss, H. N. Neufeld

Summary: The reuse of previously implanted pulse generators (PG) has been an accepted practice in Israel. This survey summarizes the long-term follow-up of 132 pts in whom reused PGs were implanted during the years 1976–1982 in 2 of the main medical centers in Israel. Sixty-four PGs were removed post-mortem and 68 from living pts who required reoperation for pouch or electrode problems. The preparation of the units included verifying normal function using a pacemaker (PM) analyzer, thorough cleansing and gas sterilization. During the yrs 1976–1979, the used PGs were implanted only in pts who were over the age of 75 or who suffered from chronic diseases and had predicted short life span, but since 1980 they were used also in younger pts without additional diseases. These reimplanted PGs have been in use for mean period of 18 mos per pt (range: 6 mos to 40 mos) and have contributed until now 2239 mos of pacing. Forty-six PGs are still functioning and 39 have been replaced (mostly the mercury cell units). Forty-two pts died during the follow-up and 5 were lost to follow-up. None of the deaths have been attributed to PG malfunction. In 2 cases pouch infection developed following implantation. No systemic infections, immunological reactions or hepatitis resulted from this procedure.

Introduction

As medical services in Israel are provided on a socialized basis, the entire cost of pacemaker implantation including hospitalization is carried by the government. Spiraling inflation and budget restriction on one hand and the commitment to implant a pacemaker to every patient who required this therapy on the other hand, led us to introduce a policy of reusing pulse-generators. Many patients who have had a pacemaker implanted are elderly and suffer from concomitant diseases. A high proportion of these patients die shortly after the implantation. Since most pulse-generators are nowadays with a life expectancy of six years or more, reuse of these pacemakers would yield major financial savings. In this paper we summarize the experience with reused pulse-generators which was gained in two of the main medical centers in Israel.

Material and methods

In the six year period 1976–1982, a total of 132 reused pulse-generators (PG) were implanted at the Chaim Sheba Medical Center at Tel-Hashomer and at the Rambam Medical Center in Haifa. The PG had been previously in use in other patients: 64 were removed from deceased patients who died in hospital from causes other than pacemaker malfunction and 68 were removed from living patients, during reoperations for either electrode malfunction or pouch problems, including infection. In several patients the PG were removed when the mode of pacing had to be changed (to programmable, high output, atrial pacemaker).

Our experience with reused pacemakers started in 1976 when the Mercury-cell batteries were still in use. Mercury-cell PG were reused only if they had been in use in the initial

491

implantation for less than one year and nowadays with lithium-cell PG only if they have been in use for less then two years (for lithium-cell models with expected longevity of more than 5 years). The time lapsed between the removal of the pacemaker and its reimplantation – the shelf time, was considered as a period of continuous use.

86 pulse-generators were reused during first implant and 46 in replacements. In all new implantations new electrodes were used. We have never reused electrodes that were implanted previously.

From 1976 until 1979 reused pulse-generators were used only in elderly patients over the age of 75 years, whose natural life expectancy is considered relatively shortened especially in those patients who suffered also from severe diseases like advanced renal failure, malignancy, organic-mental syndrome and severe congestive heart failure which further reduced their life expectancy. After our excellent initial experience we extended the reuse of pacemakers since 1980 also to younger patients suffering no additional diseases. The age of the patients ranged from 52 years to 92 (mean 78). 102 patients suffered from atrio ventricular block, 20 patients from sick sinus syndrome and 10 patients received this therapy for other indications.

The preparation of the used PG before their reimplantation consisted of three steps: 1. A thorough cleaning of the PG with special emphasis on the removal of an adherent organic material and clotted blood (this included the immersion of the PG for 48 hours in a detergent and antiseptic solution – "Detergicide"). 2. The verification of normal functioning of the PG with the aid of a pacemaker analyser (Medtronic model 5300). 3. Gas sterilization of the PG (Ethylene-Oxide). All patients were treated prophylactically with antibiotic therapy for at least seven days after the implantation.

All patients remained under a close surveillance at the pacemaker clinics of both hospitals, several patients being monitored weekly by telephone ECG transmission.

Results

Until September 1982, the mean period of function of the 132 reused PG was 18 months and they contributed 2239 patient pacing months. Forty-six units are still in function and 39 have been replaced. Forty-two patients died and 5 pts are lost to follow-up. Among the patients who died, in no case could we find any evidence of pulse-generator malfunction as the cause of death. Usually the cause of death was due to the underlying disease or heart failure.

In 39 pts the reused units had been replaced for the following reasons: In 12 patients electively, in 18 because of normal PG end of life, in 1 patient for pouch infection, in 2 for skin erosions, in 4 for fracture of electrode, in 1 for high threshold and in 1 for malsensing. Depletion of batteries in the reused pulse-generators did not occur earlier than in primary used PG of the same models. Pouch infection appeared in 2 patients who received reused units, in one patient post-operatively and it was treated medically and successfully and in the other patients later on during the follow-up. In this case the unit had to be replaced. This incidence of pouch infection was not higher than the incidence in our primary implanted units. There were no systemic infection, immunological diseases or reactions, or clinical hepatitis during the long-term follow-up of these patients.

Discussion

In recent years the reuse of PG has received more attention and it is widely employed in many countries like Italy (1), Sweden (2), Australia (3), Israel (4), France and the United Kingdom. Today's PG have longer projected life-time and are being hermetically sealed in metal cases, and therefore are more suitable for resterilization and reuse.

The sources for the reused units are either from patients in whom early removal was employed because of electrode or pouch problems or from patients who died early following implantation from causes unrelated to the pacemaker function. Since the introduction of the new universal dual-chamber pacemakers (VDD, DDD), many single-chamber units are being prematurely explanted because of a change to dual-chamber mode of pacing and are available for reuse. These new universal PG are not only sophisticated and "physiologic" but also very expensive, and if they are to be explanted earlier for any reason, surely they should be reused.

Previous studies which included large number of patients who were treated with reused PG (1–4), showed that this procedure entails no problems of pacemaker malfunction or infections. This present study also proves that there are no long-term adverse reactions like immunological reactions or diseases or clinical hepatitis, which were connected with the reuse of PG.

It is concluded that the reuse of PG is a safe and reliable procedure without any particular short or long-term complications, provided that adequate cleaning and sterilization methods are employed: By adopting this policy, a limited budget for pacemaker implantations, will make this therapy available for a larger number of patients who are in need of it. This is especially justified nowadays since the introduction of the new sophisticated and very expensive dual-chamber units.

References

1. Feruglio GA, Petz E, Zanuttini D: Pacemaker re-utilization: A seven multicenter experience in Italy. In: Meere C, Proceedings of the 6th World Symposium on Cardiac Pacing, Montreal, 1979: Chap. 39-2.
2. Aren C, Larsson S, Reuse of Lithium-powered pulse generators. In: Meere C, Proceedings of the 6th World Symposium on Cardiac Pacing, Montreal, 1979: Chap. 39-3.
3. Mond H, Sloman G, Tartaglia S, Cole A: The refurbished pulse-generator. In Meere C, Proceeding of the 6th World Symposium on Cardiac Pacing, Montreal, 1979: Chap. 39-4.
4. Amikam S, Feldman S, Riss E, Neufeld HN: Clinical experience with reused pulse-generators. In Meere C, Proceedings of the 6th World Symposium on Cardiac Pacing, Montreal, 1979: Chap. 39-1.

Authors' address:
S. Amikam, M.D.
Rambam Medical Center,
Dept. of Cardiology,
Haifa 34601, Israel

The Isotopic Cardiac Pacemaker: A Ten-Year Clinical Experience

N. P. D. Smyth, J. M. Keshishian, Mary L. Millette

Summary: In the past, the battery has been the main cause of pacemaker failure. We were interested in seeing whether or not the isotopic powered cardiac pacemaker would provide greater reliability and longevity than pacemakers powered by chemical batteries.

We studied 79 isotopic pacemakers in 75 patients for up to 10 years. Four types of Plutonium 238 powered pacemakers were studied. They included 5 VOO, 51 VVI, 14 VVIP, and 9 VVIM pacemakers. A more diverse group of 93 VVI, VVIP and VVIM pacemakers, powered by chemical batteries, were studied as controls.

During the study the mercury zinc battery has become obsolete. The initial promise of increasd longevity of the lithium powered pacemaker has been compromised by the demands firstly of smaller size, and later of more complex circuits.

The longevity and reliability of the isotopic pacemakers has been found to be superior to pacemakers powered by chemical batteries.

There may be a need for the greater longevity provided by isotopic power for the increasingly complex circuits required for dual chamber pacemakers.

The Isotopic Cardiac Pacemaker: A Ten-Year Clinical Experience

The development of the isotopic cardiac pacemaker began in 1965 with a joint effort by the United States Atomic Energy Commission and "NUMEC" (later ARCO Medical Products Company) to develop the device. The first unit was implanted in a dog in April 1969 (1) and in patient in April 1973 (2). The Medtronic-Alcatel unit was developed independently and was first used clinically in France in April 1970 (3).

Since then a world-wide clinical experience with isotopic pacers has been accumulated (2–10) The Promethium-147 (Biotronik) unit was soon rendered obsolete by lithium batteries and has been discontinued. Only the Plutonium-238 powered pacers remain, and of the original five companies (ARCO, Medtronic, Biotronik, Coratomic and Cordis), only one (Coratomic) remains in production. The others have discontinued production of isotopic pacers.

Our clinical experience began in June 1973 with the implantation of five ARCO Nu-5 pulse generators. Subsequently, we implanted six Medtronic 9000 units, fifty-four Coratomic C-100, C-101 and C-101P units and fourteen Cordis units. The seventy-nine units have been implanted in seventy-five patients.

Supported in part by The Potomac Fund for Cardiovascular Research and The Research Foundation of the Washington Hospital Center, Washington, D.C.

Materials and Methods

The ARCO Nu-5 pulse generator is a fixed rate unit (VOO) (11). The Medtronic 9000 is a VVI unit (11). The Cordis is a VVIP unit (12). It is programmable in rate and output. The Coratomic C-100 and C-101 are VVI units and the Coratomic C-101-P is a VVIM unit (12), programmable in rate, output and sensitivity (10).

These units have been illustrated and their function described in detail in previous publications (1–10, 13–16). The Coratomic C-101-P, the only unit now available, is illustrated in Figure 1.

In June 1973, five ARCO Nu-5 pulse generators were implanted as replacement units in patients all of whom had been paced for several years and were known to be in stable complete heart block. The clinical protocol required that the pacers be implanted in patients with complete heart block only since the ARCO Nu-5 unit is a fixed rate unit. Patients must have a life expectany of at least ten years. A control series of patients using conventional pacemakers was required, one for each nuclear pacer implanted. It was not possible to find at that time a group of patients that would provide a strictly comparable control group (Table 1).

Later in 1973 six Medtronic 9000 pulse generators were implanted in patients with complete heart block and sick sinus syndrome. Three were new implants and three were re-

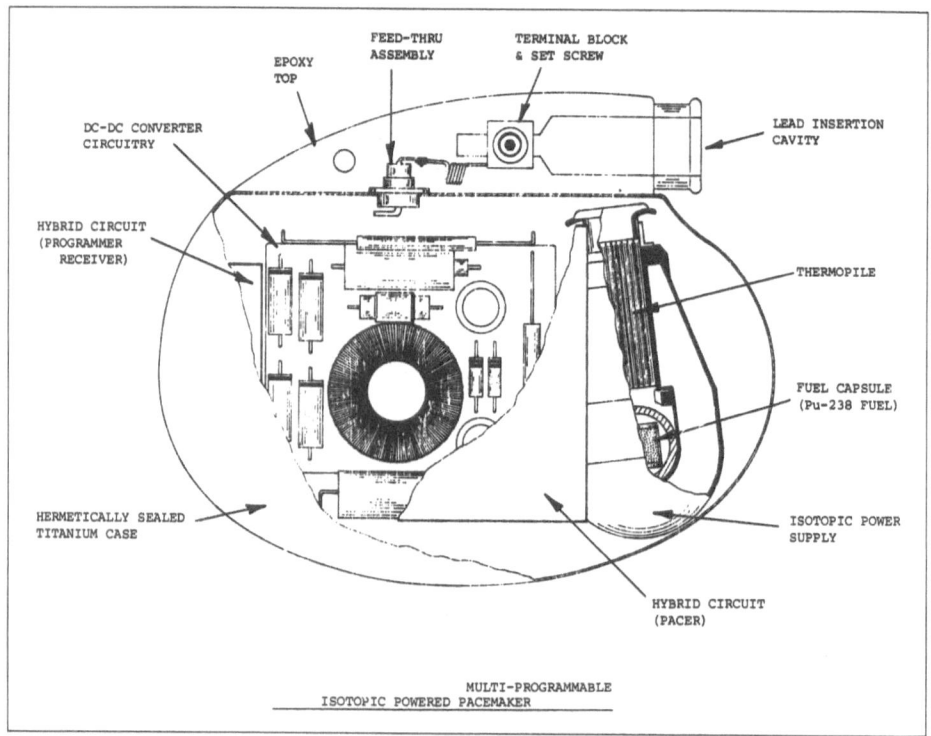

Fig. 1. Multi-programmable Isotopic Powered Pacemaker

placements. In all cases, the bipolar unit was converted to the unipolar mode using and anodal ground plate adjacent to the pulse generator. This was done to maintain comparability with the ARCO series and with a series of control patients in whom unipolar pulse generators were implanted. The Medtronic protocol required that the patient must have a life expectancy of ten years or more. A control series was required of four patients with conventional battery-powered pulse generators for each one receiving a nuclear unit. In our series, twenty-four patients were followed in the control group. Their ages and range of disease matched the nuclear test series more closely than was possible in the ARCO

Table 1. Summary of data on ARCO test group (five patients) and control group (five patients).

Group	Age range (years)	Diagnosis	I	R	Pulse generator	Status	
						Patients	Pacemakers
Test	40–68	Complete heart block, 5	0	5	ARCO Nu-5	Alive, well 3. 10 yrs.	Functioning 3. 10 yrs.
Control	68–83	Sick sinus syndrome, 3 Complete heart block, 2	0	5	Coris Stanicor (Hg. Zn.)	Alive, well 1. 10 yrs.	Functioning 0. 10 yrs.

I = Initial insertion
R = Replacement

Table 2. Summary of data on Medtronic 9000 test group (six patients) and control group (twenty-four patients).

Group	Age range (years)	Diagnosis	I	R	Pulse generator	Status	
						Patients	Pacemakers
Test	39–67	Complete heart block, 5 Sick sinus syndrome, 1	3	3	Medtronic 9000	Alive, well 4. 10 yrs.	Functioning 4. 10 yrs.
Control	48–85	Complete heart block, 16 Sick sinus syndrome, 7 Atrial fibrillation with bradycardia, 1	8	16	Medtronic 5494 (Hg. Zn.)	Alive, well 8. 10 yrs.	Functioning 0. 10 yrs.

I = Initial insertion
R = Replacement

control group. The control series was homogeneous in one sense, in that all the patients received the mercury-zinc battery powered Medtronic 5945 pulse generator (17). (Table 2).

The first clinical implant of a Coratomic C-100 pulse generator was carried out by us at the Washington Hospital Center, Washington, D.C., in October 1974.

The clinical protocol for the Coratomic pacers C-100 series (C-100, C-101 and D-101-P) differs from those previously referred to, in both test and control patients. One control patient is required for each nuclear implant as in the ARCO protocol, but the indications for implantation are broader in the test group and more specific in the control series (13). Patient selection in the test series is defined, in part, as follows:

... In certain other cases, the physician may judge the use of the C-100 to be paramount in prolonging life in an older patient who has had many previous operations, or is resistant to frequent operations, or is not mentally capable of handling a rechargeable unit. In these cases, expected to be a small percentage, the physician may use his discretion in implanting the C-100 unit.

Table 3. Summary of data on Coratomic C-100, C-101 and C-101p test group (fifty patients) and control group (fifty patients).

Group	Age range (years)	Diagnosis	I	R	Pulse generator	Status	
						Patients	Pacemakers
Test	31–74	Sick sinus syndrome, 16 Complete heart block, 27 Atrial fibrillation with bradycardia, 1 Vaso-vagal syndrome, 1 Second degree heart block, 4	34	16	C-100, 17 C-101, 26 C-101p, 9	Alive, well 41. 1–9 yrs.	Functioning 41. 1–9 yrs.
Control	50–85	Sick sinus syndrome, 20 Complete heart block, 28 Atrial fibrillation with bradycardia, 1	27	23	CPI 301-UD, 13 Coratomic L-500, 15 Medtronic 5951, 8 Medtronic 5973, 2 Biotronic IDP-44, 2 Cordis Omni Stanicor, 2 Biotronic 1E-60K, 1 Medtronic Xyrel, 1 Coratomic Ovalith P, 3 Medtronic Spectrax, 2 Intermedics Cyberlith 253–04, 1 (Hg. Zn. and Lithium)	Alive, well 28. 1–9 yrs.	Functioning 9. 1–3 yrs.

I = Initial insertion
R = Replacement

The control group is defined in part as follows:

... An attempt should be made to include in this group pacer systems using lithium or rechargeable nickel cadmium batteries to provide comparative data on other potentially long lived systems. The numbers of patients in this group should be equal to the C-100 group...

Since October 1974 a total of fifty-four Coratomic C-100, C-101 and C-101-P pacers have been implanted in fifty patients. The indications included various degrees of heart block, spontaneous and post-surgical; atrial fibrillation with slow ventricular response; vaso-vagal syncopal attacks and sick sinus syndrome. In thirty-three cases the units were initial implants and in sixteen cases replacements.

The indications for pacemaker insertion in the control series of fifty patients were similar but there were not constraints relative to patient age (Table 3).

Since November 1976 a total of fourteen Cordis nuclear pacers have been implanted heart block, second degree heart block and sinus syndrome. Nine were initial implants and five were replacements.

The indications for pacing in the control series of fourteen patients were complete heart block, sick sinus syndrome, and atrial fibrillation with slow ventricular response (Table 4).

Results

In general there were no infections and no erosions in the one hundred and sixty-eight patients in the test and control series. There were three early lead displacements and one

Table 4. Summary of data on Cordis test group (fourteen patients) and control group (fourteen patients).

Group	Age range (years)	Diagnosis	I	R	Pulse generator	Status	
						Patients	Pacemakers
Test	46–67	Sick sinus syndrome, 5 Complete heart block, 8 Second degree heart block, 1	9	5	Cordis Nuclear Omni-Stanicor	Alive, well 12. 2–7yrs.	Functioning 11. 2–7 yrs.
Control	55–84	Sick sinus syndrome, 8 Complete heart block, 5 Atrial fibrillation with bradycardia, 1	9	5	Coratomic L-500, 8 Coratomic Ovalith-P, 3 Cordis Multicor γ, 1 Intermedics 253–04, 1 Biotronic Nomos, 1 (Lithium)	Alive, well 11. 2–7 yrs.	Functioning 6. 1–3 yrs.

I = Initial insertion
R= Replacement

case of early exit block. Each required lead replacement, using the same pulse generator. Specific problems are addressed under the relevant group heading.

All patients were studied one week post-operatively, one month post-operatively, and at three-monthly intervals for one year, and six-monthly office visits, with two monthly telephone transmissions thereafter. Follow-up has been 100% in both test and control series.

A complete study of the pacer parameters was carried out on each occasion. These tests have been described in detail elsewhere (9). All patients demonstrated normal pacing initially.

In all patients in the test (isotopic) series who died, the pulse generator was recovered and returned to the manufacturer.

Test Series

There were no problems in the ARCO Nu-5 group. Three of the five patients are alive and well ten years post-operatively. Two died of causes not related to their pacemakers.

In the Medtronic 9000 group there was one apparent malfunction: In this patient the pulse generator and lead were removed after a chest injury in the area of the pacemaker pocket with immediate loss of pacing. It was not at first clear what was the cause of the pacing failure. A new system (C-101) was inserted on the left side. Subsequent study showed that a lead pin fracture had occurred in the old lead. The explanted pulse generator functioned normally on testing at the factory.

On pulse generator was removed at another hospital because of a minimal muscle twitch at the anode plate. The twitch persists with the replacement rechargeable unit. The explanted unit was functioning normally. Four of the patients are alive and well ten years post-operatively. Two died of causes not related to their pacemakers.

In the Coratomic C-100, C-101 and C-101-P series a sensing problem was encountered in one patient. This patient had a low voltage $(+2 - 2v.)$ biphasic R wave with a slow slew rate. In rare cases this type of R wave has not always been sensed by the C-100 (8). Sensing has been satisfactory since the pulse generator was replaced by the more sensitive C-101 unit.

In one patient a C-100 unit was replaced by a C-101 unit for apparent malfunction – a rate change – which could not be duplicated in the explanted unit at the factory.

There were two C-100 failures, one due to a fracture of the feedthrough tab weld and the other due to failure of a capacitor. A C-101 unit was used for replacement in one patient and a C-101-P unit in the other. There was one failure, unusual in that it was "postmortem". This pulse generator, at the time of the patient's death from a massive myocardial infarction, was functioning after five defibrillation shocks. Twenty-four hours later a check at the factory (Coratomic) showed no output. Breakdown analysis showed destruction of the zener diode by heat resulting from the multiple defibrillation shocks.

Ten patients died of causes not related to their pacemakers. Forty-one of the fifty patients are alive and well, one to nine years post-operatively.

There was one problem in the Cordis test series. One of the units was erroneously removed for a presumed sensing problem not found on later testing. The unit was replaced by a lithium pulse generator because an isotopic unit was not immediately available.

Two of the patients died of causes not related to their pacemakers. Twelve are alive and well, two to seven years post-operatively.

Control Series

There are no patients remaining in the control series for the ARCO Nu-5 group. Four of the patients died and in all the pulse generators were replaced (Table 1).

There are no patients remaining in the control series for the medtronic 9000 group (Table 2). One pulse generator was removed because of a pacer induced bigeminy caused by retrograde conduction. The patient's effective rate slowed and he became symptomatic. The replacement programmable pacer set at a faster rate eliminated the problem.

One pulse generator was removed two and one-half years post-opeatively, during a radical mastectomy for carcinoma in the adjacent breast. The pulse generator was functioning normally, but the opportunity was taken to replace it to avoid another operation later. One pulse generator was removed for malfunction two years post-operatively. Fifteen pulse generators were removed either at end of life or electively close to end of life. Sixteen patients died of causes not related to their pacemakers. Eight patients are alive and well.

In the Coratomic C-100, C-101 and C-101-P control group twelve pulse generators were removed for premature failure. On was replaced because of diaphragmatic pacing. Seven pulse generators were replaced at end of life. Twenty-two patients died of causes not related to their pacemakers. Twenty-eight patients are alive and well (Table 3).

In the Cordis group, five pulse generators were removed for premature failure. One was replaced at end of life. Three patients died of causes not related to their pacemakers. Eleven patients are alive and well (Table 4).

Discussion

No statistical analysis of these groups is possible. There are too many variables such as patient age, type of disease, number of controls, types of test and control pulse generators, different power sources in control units, dates of insertion and others. Certain comparisons and conclusions are permissible, however.

Malfunction. In the entire test series of isotopic pulse generators there were two documented pulse generator failures.

In the control group there were sixteen, mostly due to premature battery depletion.

Power source depletion (end of life). In the test series there were none.

In the control series there were sixty-two.

Pulse generator longevity. In every group, as shown in the Tables, the number of functioning pulse generators n the test (isotopic) series exceeds that in the control group.

Fifty-eight out of seventy-five test (isotopic) pulse generators remain (77%). Fifteen out of ninety-three remain in the control group (16%). Although many of these patients are alive, their pulse generators have been replaced and they are therefore no longer followed in the control group.

Patient longevity. In every group, as shown in the Tables, the number of living patients in the test (isotopic) series exceeds that in the control group. The results are skewed, however, by the choice, required by protocol, of younger patients with a ten year life expectancy for the test group. The control group contains many much older and sicker patients.

Fifty-nine out of seventy-eight patients survive in the test (isotopic) series (75%); forty-eight out of ninety-three in the control series (51%).

It is of interest that all of the sixteen patients in the test (isotopic) group who died, died with their original nuclear pacemaker in place. Their pacemaker was in fact a lifetime unit and they never required a second operation. It is also of interest that the nuclear pulse generators removed from patients who died would probably still be functioning but this cannot be definitely established. In the ARCO series the returned units were tested, found to be working normally and were then dismantled and the fuel cells returned to Oak Ridge, Tennessee. In the Medtronic, Coratomic and Cordis groups the same initial testing was carried out but the pulse generators have been stored subsequently, and are not checked for continuing function.

Statements by patients in the two environmental impact studies filed by the Atomic Energy Commission (18, 19) indicate there is no reason to fear the minimal radioactivity of these pulse generators. None of our patients has had any concern about this. In fact, they are proud of their "unconventional" pacemakers and are confident in the projected increase in longevity. We have many disappointed patients who would like to have a nuclear pacer but who do not fit the current protocols because of age or associated disease likely to limit their life span.

It is clear in many cases the isotopic pulse generator has proved that it will last ten years and that it can be a life time pacer for many people.

While lithium powered pulse generators may last ten years, there has been a trend in recent years towards smaller, lighter and thinner pulsed generators, with, in many cases, reduction in life expectancy to half the original goal, or less. Furthermore, the high current

Fig. 2. Comparative performance of pulse generator performance by power source. Note that performance of isotopic power source is significantly better than that of the chemical batteries (20).

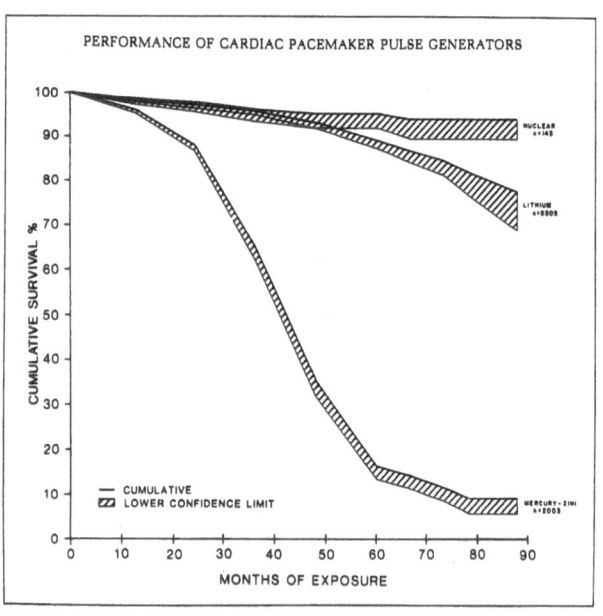

drain of the complex circuitry of modern DDD pulse generators has in at least one case reduced the battery life expectancy to two years.

In spite of the onerous regulations and paperwork imposed on manufacturer and physician alike by the Nuclear Regulatory Commission it may be necessary to re-examine Plutonium-238 as a power source, especially for complex dual chamber (DDD) pacing systems. Certainly the isotopic pacer should be considered for any adult patient requiring conventional ventricular pacing whose life expectancy is ten years or more. There may be some reservation about usng a nuclear device in an infant or child because of the remote chance of carcinogenesis due to low-dose irradiation, but for the adult at least the isotopic powered pacer has proved its dependability and longevity in our experience and that of others (20) (Fig. 2), and that for many it is a life time pacer – a goal long sought in the field of cardiac pacing.

References

1. Morrow, AG, Levitsky S, Frommer TL et al: Experimental evaluation of a radioisotope powered cardiac pacemaker. Jour Thor Cardiovasc Surg 1970; 60: 836.
2. Parsonnet V, Myers GH, Gilbert L et al: Clinical experience with nuclear pacemakers. Surg 1975; 78: 776.
3. Laurens P, Piwnica A, Reidemeister C et al: Clinical results of the implantation of an isotopic pacemaker. In Thalen HJTh, ed: Cardiac Pacing, Proceedings of the IV International Symposium, Assen, The Netherlands, 1973, Van Gorcum & Company, pp 198–208.
4. ARCO nuclear technical memorandum, Report VI on the status of the clinical studies of the ARCO nuclear pacemaker, No 5, Leechburg, Pa, 1975; Apr 15.
5. Huffman FN, and Norman JC: Nuclear fueled cardiac pacemakers, Chest 1974; 65: 667.
6. Kahn AR, Hixon JD, Puffer JE et al: Three years clinical experience with radioisotope powered cardiac pacemakers, IEE Trans Biomed Eng 1973; 29: 326.
7. Smyth NPD, Hernandez T, Deitz R et al: Clinical experience with radioisotopic-powered pacemakers. Maryland State Medical Journal, Apr. 1975.
8. Smyth NPD, Magovern GJ, Cushing WJ et al: Preliminary clinical experience with a new radioisotope-powered cardiac pacemaker. Jour Thor Cardiovasc Surg 1976; 71: 262–267.
9. Smyth NPD, Keshishian JM, Garcia JM et al: Clinical experience with the isotopic cardiac pacemaker. Anns Thor Surg 1979; 28: 14–21.
10. Smyth NPD, Purdy D, Sager D et al: A new multiprogrammable isotopic powered cardiac pacemaker. Pace 1982; 5: 761–766.
11. Parsonnet V, Furman S, and Smyth NPD: Implantable Cardiac Pacemakers. Status Report and Resource Guideline – Report of the Inter-Society Commission for Heart Disease Resources, Circulation 1974; 50: A-21.
12. Parsonnet V, Furman S, and Smyth NPD: A revised code for pacemaker identification. Pace 1981; 4: 400.
13. Human Clinical Protocol for the Coratomic C-100 Radioisotope Powered Cardiac Pacer, Coratomic Inc, Indiana, Penna, Aug 1, 1974.
14. Master Protocol for Clinical Evaluation of the Programmable Cordis Nuclear Omni-Stanicor Pacemaker.Cordis Corporation, Miami Fla, October 1974.
15. Purdy DL, Magovern GJ, and Smyth NPD: A new radioisotope-powered cardiac pacer. Jour Thorac Cardiovasc Surg 1975; 69: 82–91.
16. Parsonnet V, Myers GH, Hursen TF et al: The American nuclear powered pacemaker. Ann Cardiol d'Angeiol. 1971; 20: 405.
17. Smyth NPD, Alferness F, Shearon L et al: Clinical evaluation of a new pulse generator with narrow pulse width for conservation of battery energy. Jour Thorac Cardiovasc Surg 1974; 68: 471–478.

18. Final generic environmental statement on routine use of Plutonium powered cardiac pacemakers, July 1976. US Nuclear Regulatory Commission, Office of Nuclear material, Safety and Safeguards. NUREG-0060.
19. Final generic environmental statement on routine use of Plutonium powered cardiac pacemakers, May 1979. US Nuclear Regulatory Commission, Office of Standards Development. NUREG-0060, Supplement I (update of information on power sources for pacemakers.)
20. Bilitch M, Hauser RG, Goldman BS et al: Performance of cardiac pacemaker pulse generators. Pace 1982; 5: 139.

Authors' address:
Nicholas P. D. Smyth, M.D.
106 Irving Street, N.W.
Suite # 220
Washington, D.C. 20010

Arrhythmias Caused by Dual-Chambered Pacing

S. S. Barold, M. D. Falkoff, L. S. Ong, R. A. Heinle

Summary: The recent release of DDD (and VDD) pulse generators with relatively short atrial refractory periods has set the stage for the development of endless loop or electronic reentry tachycardias because of the frequent occurrence of retrograde VA conduction in patients requiring permanent pacing. The absence of VA conduction during electrophysiologic testing at the time of implantation does not necessarily predict protection against endless loop tachycardia because VA conduction may occasionally become manifest only after implantation. Programmability of the atrial refractory period constitutes the most important pacemaker characteristic for the prevention of endless loop tachycardia. We have found chest wall stimulation a useful technique for the verification of the programmed upper atrial tracking rate, duration of the pacemaker atrial refractory period, and characterization of the predicted response to the upper programmed rate. Chest wall stimulation can initiate and terminate endless loop tachycardia in patients predisposed to this arrhythmia.
Potentially serious repetitive ventricular firing or tachycardia may occasionally be caused by a normally functioning DVI or DDD pulse generator. The problem of cross-talk or self-inhibition is unique to dual-chambered pacemakers and remains a potential problem despite the incorporation of a ventricular blanking period.

Arrhythmias Caused by Dual-Chambered Pacing

Dual-chambered pulse generators have created new problems in the interpretation of pacemaker function and arrhythmias. The term arrhythmia as applied to pacing has always been rather loose and unclear and often used to describe normal function. So-called pacemaker arrhythmias are best classified as either pacemaker-induced or pacemaker-mediated arrhythmias.

1. Endless Loop Tachycardia

The first generation of VAT pulse generators released many years ago rarely sensed retrograde P waves because they were designed with a relatively long atrial refractory period after the ventricular stimulus. The recent release of DDD (and VDD) pulse generators with relatively short atrial refractory periods (150–200 msec after a ventricular event) has set the stage for the development of endless loop or electronic reentry tachycardia because of the frequent occurrence of retrograde VA conduction (average VA conduction interval 200–350 msec) (1) in patients requiring permanent pacing. Sensing of a retrograde P wave triggers the ventricular output and thereby initiates a self-perpetuating mechanism (2–4). The tachycardia cycle length is equal to the upper rate limit interval or the sum of the VA conduction time and the AV interval, whichever is greater. The initiating mechanisms of endless loop tachycardia include: 1. A lower (escape) pacemaker rate faster than the sinus rate (applicable to VAT and VDD units only). 2. Ventricular and atrial extrasystoles. 3. Myopotential oversensing by the atrial channel, thereby triggering a ventricular stimulus. 4. Undersensing of P waves: loss of sensing of sinus P waves may be associated with normal sensing of retrograde P waves. 5. Application and withdrawal

505

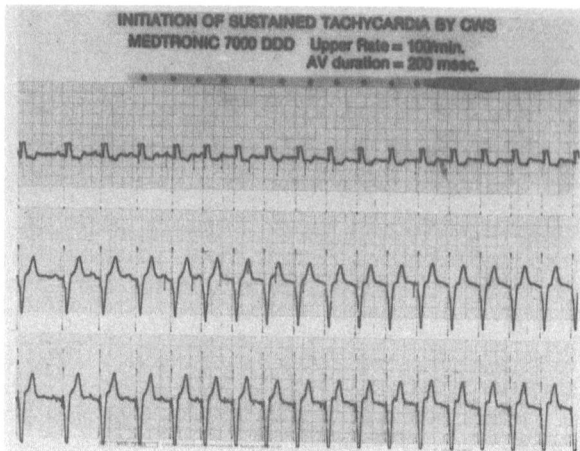

Fig. 1A. Initiation of endless loop tachycardia by chest wall stimulation (black dots).

of the magnet. 6. Chest wall stimulation (Fig. 1A). The absence of VA conduction during electrophysiologic testing at the time of implantation does not necessarily predict protection against endless loop tachycardia because VA conduction may occasionally become manifest only after implantation. Several methods have been tried to minimize or prevent endless loop tachycardia, but many are obviously unsatisfactory.

Methods other than Programmability of the Atrial Refractory Period used for the Preventation of Endless Loop Tachycardia:

1. VAT and VDD pulse generators. Reduce the lower or minimal ventricular escape rate.
2. Shortening of the AV interval may prevent VA conduction.
3. Adjustment of maximum or upper rate. Progranming to a higher rate may cause VA block.
4. Pharmacological intervention to block VA conduction. This may, however, aggravate the problem by prolonging VA conduction.
5. Decreasing the atrial sensitivity if retrograde P waves are smaller than sinus P waves.
6. Reprogramming to DVI or VVI mode.
7. DVI (rather than VVI) escape mode following a ventricular extrasystole.
8. Lengthening of the atrial refractory period following a ventricular extrasystole.
9. After a sudden increase in rate (either after a ventricular extrasystole or predetermined number of events), the pacemaker drops an atrial event to interrupt the tachycardia circuit.

Programmability of the atrial refractory period constitutes the most important pacemaker characteristic for the prevention of endless loop tachycardia. Programming a long atrial refractory period will, however, limit the upper tracking rate of the pulse generator. Because the atrial refractory period starts with an atrial event, the longer the AV interval, the longer the atrial refractory period. For example, if the AV interval is 200 msec and the atrial refractory period is 350 msec after a ventricular event, the total duration of the atrial refractory period is 550 msec. An interval of 550 msec corresponds to a rate of 110 per minute and represents the maximum tracking rate. Some pulse generators now incorporate an automatic extension of the atrial refractory period after a sensed ventricular event so as to contain a delayed retrograde P wave. The atrial refractory extension feature is important because it avoids reducing the maximum (tracking response) rate of the pulse generator. One design uses a relatively simple technique for terminating a tachycardia once it has begun because endless loop tachycardia usually occurs at the upper programmed ventricular tracking limit. Thus when the atrial rate equals the ventricular tracking limit for 15 beats, the pacemaker circuit will automatically drop a single ventricular pulse, thereby terminating pacemaker mediated tachycardia.

2. Chest Wall Stimulation in the Evaluation of DDD Pulse Generators

VA conduction may be evaluated by programming the pulse generator to the VVI mode at various rates. In the DDD mode, application of the magnet or programming the atrial output to subthreshold levels may also initiate endless loop tachycardia. We have found chest wall stimulation a useful technique for the verification of some of the programmable functions of pulse generators such as the programmed upper atrial rate, duration of the pacemaker atrial refractory period, and characterization of the predicted response to the upper programmed rate. This is particularly important in devices without telemetry. Even with sophisticated telemetry, maneuvers such as chest wall stimulation or exercise provide the only certain way of verifying the programmed upper rate. The demonstration of tolerance to maximal tracking rates may be important in some patients, especially those with coronary artery disease. Chest wall stimulation therefore provides a simple technique to test the clinical safety of the upper programmed rate, a determination otherwise requiring treadmill stress testing which is often impractical or impossible in the elderly population.

Chest wall stimulation in our series of 25 patients easily induced reentry loop tachycardia in predisposed patients who exhibited the arrhythmia spontaneously. Moreover, the characteristics of the tachycardia (rate, sustained or unsustained) induced by chest wall stimulation correlated with the ones documented clinically. The ease with which endless loop tachycardia can be initiated in predisposed patients provides a very simple way of determining the optimal pacemaker characteristics for its prevention, particularly in pulse generators with a programmable atrial refractory period. In addition, chest wall stimulation allows determination of the duration of the new programmed atrial refractory period. In one commercially available DDD pulse generator (Autima I – Telectronics) application of the magnet does not convert the pulse generator to the DOO mode and cannot terminate an endless loop tachycardia. Chest wall stimulation provides an immediate way of breaking the tachycardia by inhibiting the ventricular output (Fig. 1B). In some cases of DDD pacing, it may be difficult to determine the actual programmed mode of pacing (e.g., DVI or DDD) during continuous atrial and ventricular stimulation. Chest wall stimulation provides an easy way of determining the pacing mode because atrial tracking can only occur in the DDD mode.

Fig. 2B. Chest wall stimulation (black dots) terminating sustained endless loop tachycardia.

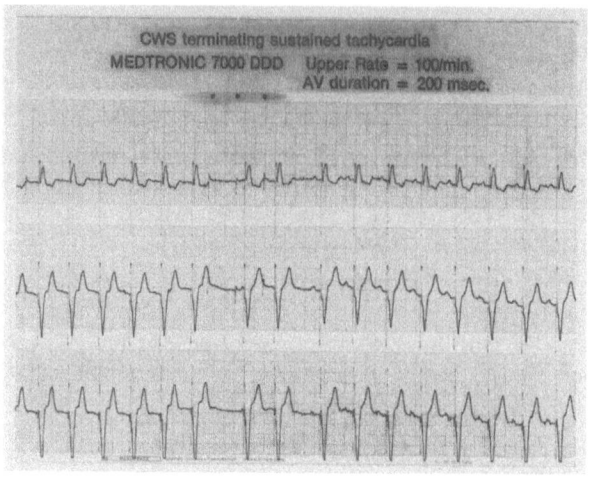

3. Arrhythmias Related to Stimulation in the Atrial or Ventricular Vulnerable Period

Furman and Cooper recently documented a case of atrial fibrillation induced by asynchronous atrial pacing with a DVI committed pulse generator (5). Because atrial fibrillation occurs as a consequence of the natural history of sick sinus syndrome, further studies are required to determine whether asynchronous atrial pacing truly increases the incidence of atrial fibrillation. Potentially serious ventricular arrhythmias may occur with normally functioning dualchambered systems. Recently Luceri et al. (6) documented the induction of ventricular tachycardia-fibrillation in a patient with a committed DVI pulse generator when the second or ventricular stimulus was delivered in the ventricular vulnerable period. Stimulation in the vulnerable period may also be observed with normally functioning DDD pulse generators. Potentially serious repetitive firing or ventricular tachycardia may be caused by sensing of an early retrograde P wave, particulary if the atrial refractory period of the pulse generator is relatively short and the AV sequential time is also short (7). This may allow the delivery of a ventricular stimulus in the ventricular vulnerable period. This is another reason for the need of a programmable atrial refractory period, to avoid sensing of an early P wave, AV synchrony and the delivery of a pacemaker stimulus in the ventricular vulnerable period.

4. Cross-Talk or Self-Inhibition

Cross-talk or self-inhibition refers to sensing of the atrial output stimulus by the ventricular sensing amplifier (8, 9). This problem is far more important in unipolar than in bipolar systems because of the size of the pacing stimulus. Despite sophisticated circuitry, cross-talk may still be observed clinically with DDD pacemakers and should be suspected under the following circumstances:
a) Unexpected prolongation of AV interval or atrial spike – QRS interval (Fig. 2).
b) Increase in the atrial pacing rate (Fig. 3).

508

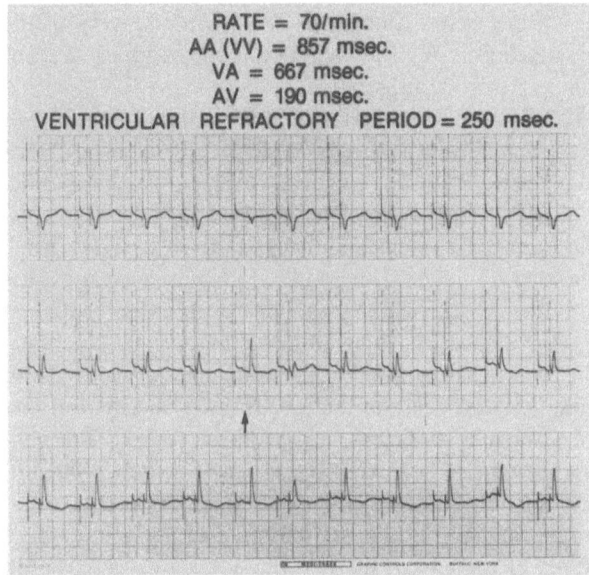

RATE = 70/min.
AA (VV) = 857 msec.
VA = 667 msec.
AV = 190 msec.
VENTRICULAR REFRACTORY PERIOD = 250 msec.

Fig. 2. Cross-talk in DDD pulse generator. Specifications are shown above the electrocardiogram. Note the unexpected prolongation of atrial spike – QRS interval (arrow) due to cross-talk.

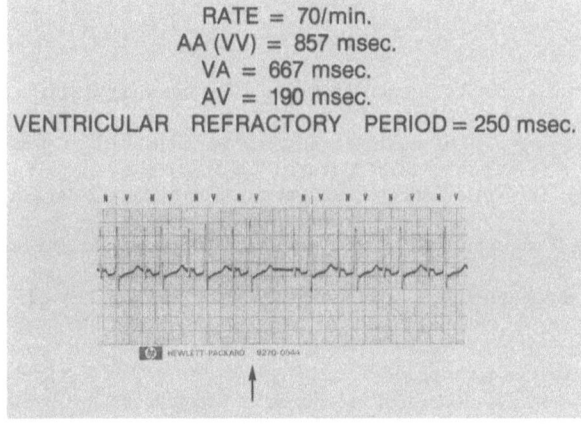

RATE = 70/min.
AA (VV) = 857 msec.
VA = 667 msec.
AV = 190 msec.
VENTRICULAR REFRACTORY PERIOD = 250 msec.

Fig. 3. Cross-talk in DDD pulse generator. Same patient and DDD pulse generator as in Figure 2. The programmed parameters are shown above the electrocardiogram. Note the increase in the atrial pacing rate with the AA spike intervals equal to the programmed VA interval. Lengthening of the AA spike interval at the arrow may be explained as follows: All the atrial stimuli are sensed by the ventricular electrode, whereupon a ventricular refractory period of 250 msec is initiated by sensing of the atrial stimulus. The first three spontaneous QRS complexes fall within the ventricular refractory period and are therefore unsensed. Because of a very slight prolongation of the PR interval, the fourth QRS complex falls just beyond the ventricular refractory period and is therefore sensed by the ventricular electrode and recycles the pacemaker according to the programmed VA interval. Cross-talk was eliminated by reducing the atrial output voltage and decreasing the ventricular sensitivity.

c) AA spike intervals equal to the programmed VA interval (Fig. 3).
There are several ways to minimize or eliminate cross-talk.
a) Use of a bipolar system.

509

b) Initiation of the ventricular refractory period immediately with the delivery of the atrial stimulus and encompassing the entire AV interval. This is the hallmark of committed DVI pacing systems (10).

c) Ventricular blanking period. All DDD pulse generators contain a circuit that blanks or turns off the ventricular sensing amplifier starting with the delivery of an atrial stimulus. The ventricular blanking period may be considered a short refractory period. Ideally the blanking period should be as short as possible because a long period predisposes to undersensing of ectopic ventricular events and firing in the vulnerable period, particularly in the presence of a long AV interval. Because DDD pulse generators are multiprogrammable with programmable ventricular sensitivity, atrial pulse width and amplitude, the blanking period should ideally by programmable for optimal function.

d) Ventricular safety pacing or the incorporation of a "non-physiologic AV delay" also avoids the problem of cross-talk. This provides an additional safety mechanism and implies that blanking may not always be sufficient to prevent cross-talk. The non-physiologic delay is shorter than the normal AV delay and is usually around 100–110 msec. If a ventricular sensed event (polarization phenomena, QRS complexes, interference, etc.) occurs after blanking but during the non-physiologic delay interval, a ventricular pulse will be delivered at the end of the non-physiologic delay 100–110 msec after the atrial stimulus, thereby shortening the AV interval but preventing inappropriate ventricular inhibtion and retaining some degree of AV synchrony.

References

1. Hayes DL, Furman S: Atrio-ventricular and Ventriculo-atrial conduction times in patients undergoing pacemaker implant. Pace 1983; 6: 38–46.
2. Tolentino AO, Javier RP, Byrd C, Samet P. Pacer-induced tachycardia associated with an atrial-synchronous ventricular-inhibited (ASVIP) pulse generator. Pace: 1982; 5: 251–259.
3. Bathen J, Gundersen T, Forfang K: Tachycardias related to atrial synchronous ventricular pacing. Pace 1982; 5: 471–475.
4. Furman S, Fisher JD: Endless loop tachycardia in an AV universal (DDD) pacemaker. Pace 1982; 5: 486–489.
5. Furman S, Cooper JA: Atrial fibrillation during AV sequential pacing. Pace: 1982; 5: 133–135.
6. Luceri RM, Ramirez AV, Castellanos A, Zaman L, Thurer RJ, Myerburg RJ: Ventricular tachycardia produced by a normally functioning AV sequential demand (DVI) pacemaker with "committed" ventricular stimulation. J Am Coll Cardiol 1983; 1: 1177– 1179.
7. Freedman RA, Rothman MT, Mason JW: Recurrent ventricular tachycardia induced by an atrial synchronous ventricular-inhibited pacemaker. Pace 1982; 5: 490–494.
8. Furman S, Reicher-Reiss H, Escher DJW: Atrioventricular sequential pacing and pacemakers. Chest: 1973; 63: 783–789.
9. DenDulk K, Lindemans FW, Bär FW, Wellens HJJ: Pacemaker related tachycardias. Pace 1982; 5: 476–485.
10. Barold SS, Falkoff MD, Ong LS, Heinle RA: Interpretation of electrocardiograms produced by a new unipolar multiprogrammable "committed" AV sequential demand (DVI) pulse generator. Pace 1981; 4: 692–708.

Authors' address:
Dr. S. Serge Barold
The Genesee Hospital
224 Alexander Street
Rochester, New York 14607
USA

Method to Assess and Avoid Re-Entrant Tachycardias with Dual Chamber Sensing Pacemakers

D. L. Hayes, S. Furman

Summary: Pacemaker mediated re-entrant tachycardias have been seen frequently during use of dual chamber sensing pacemakers and are dependent on the presence of intact retrograde (ventriculo-atrial) conduction. The status of a patient's retrograde (VA) conduction cannot be determined from the surface electrocardiogram. At the time of pacemaker implant the state of antegrade conduction should be determined at incremental atrial pacing rates, the exact timing measured from the intracardiac electrograms, i.e. from the intrinsic deflection of the atrium to the intrinsic deflection of the ventricle. With this information obtained in 110 patients, determination was possible of which patients could safely receive dual chamber sensing pacemaker devices, the appropriate pacemaker atrial refractory period setting to avoid pacemaker mediated tachycardias in those patients with intact retrograde conduction, and the optimal timing for programming the pacemaker's AV delay. Patients who have been studied in this manner and who were felt to be suitable for a dual chamber sensing device have not displayed pacemaker mediated re-entrant tachycardias. Forty-five percent of all patients who require pacemaker implant have VA 1 : 1 conduction; 67% of those with sinus node dysfunction and 14% of those with complete antegrade block have VA conduction at a mean interval of 235 ± 50 ms (range 110–380 ms).

The present generation of dual chamber pacemakers which allow sensing in both the atrium and the ventricle have brought to our attention the importance of retrograde or ventriculo-atrial (VA) conduction. Implantation of an AV synchronous (VDD) or AV universal (DDD) pacemaker is the eqivalent of creating an artificial accessory pathway. If the patient has intact retrograde conduction, placement of an artificial antegrade pathway via the pacemaker will allow an "endless loop" or pacemaker mediated tachycardia via conduction through the intact retrograde pathway and sensing of the retrograde atrial activity. A pacemaker mediated tachycardia is dependent on the integrity of the bypass tract, the existance of the retrograde conduction, the duration of the refractory of the two tracts, and the rate of conduction. The potential of reciprocating rhythms was postulated as early as 1913 (3) and many subsequent authors have described ventriculo-atrial conduction in the genesis of arrhythmias (4, 5, 6, 7, 8, 9, 10). In those patients receiving dual chamber sensing pacing devices, the status of the VA conduction has now become critical information.

During evaluation of patients undergoing implantation of dual chamber pacemakers, data has been gathered concerning the incidence of VA conduction and the duration of VA and AV conduction intervals involved. The method of measurement of these intervals is specific so that the data may be correctly derived.

Methods and materials

The endocardial or epicardial electrogram (EGM) is the electrical signal emitted by the heart and detected from within or upon its surface. Both atrial and ventricular electrograms are readily determined via the implanted lead system. It is the EGM and not the electrocardiogram which an implanted pacing device senses and from which the pacemaker circuitry is timed. The intrinsic deflection (ID) is that portion of the EGM which corresponds to passage of the depolarization wave througout the electrode. It is characterized by the most rapid movement, the greatest amplitude, the greatest slew rate and highest frequency content (11). It is the intrinsic deflection which is sensed by the implanted pulse generator. Exact measurements of AV and VA conduction times can only be determined by recording and comparing the atrial and ventricular EGM from one intrinsic deflection to the other. It is, therefore, necessary to record the atrial and ventricular electrograms during paced and unpaced cardiac activity. Each of the intervals determined is important for the proper programming of the implantable dual chamber pacemaker.

A total of 107 patients who underwent pacemaker implant at Montefiore Hospital and Medical Center between February 1, 1982 and January 1, 1983 were assessed intraoperatively for timing of antegrade (AV) and retrograde (VA) conduction. In those patients in whom single chamber pacing was intended preoperatively, the implantable lead was first placed, either in the right atrial appendage or right ventricular apex, and a temporary pacing lead was passed alongside the permanent lead to the cardiac chamber from which permanent pacing was not intended. Therefore, intracardiac recordings were available from both chambers. Electrode positions were as follows: In the ventricular position, recordings were made from the right ventricular apex in 108 patients and recordings were made with a temporary lead along the interventricular septum in two patients. The atrial electrogram was obtained with the lead in the right atrial appendage in 64 patients, in the high right atrium in 8 patients, in the mid-right atrium in 37 patients, and in the low right atrium in 1 patient. With leads in place, the following measurements were made on a multichannel recorder with oscilloscope and hard copy recordings:

Fig. 1. A diagramatic example of how the leads are connected at the time of pacemaker implant for intraoperative measurement of the intervals described.

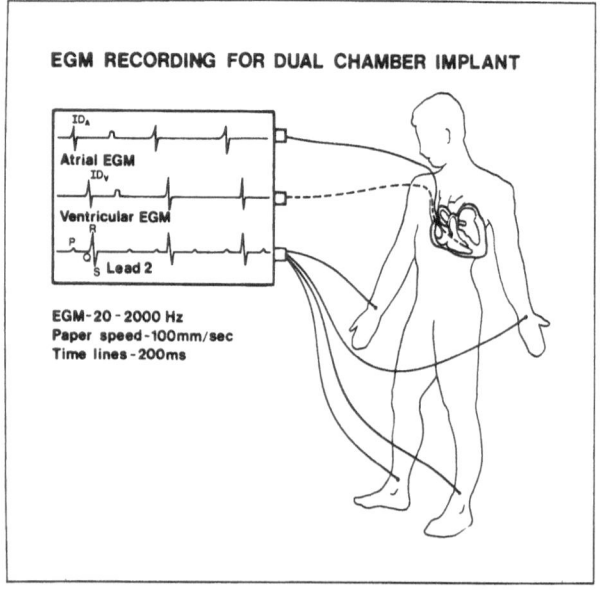

1. interval from intrinsic deflection of the atrial depolarization ID_A to intrinsic deflection of the ventricular depolarization (ID_V ($ID_A \rightarrow ID_V$) (Fig. 1);
2. the interval from the atrial pacemaker stimulus St to the intrinsic deflection of ventricular depolarization ID_V ($St_A \rightarrow ID_V$); optimally patients were paced at rates of 60, 80, 100, 120 and 140 beats per minute and atrioventricular conduction time assessed and the rate for onset of AV block ascertained;
3. the interval from the ventricular pacing stimulus St_V to the intrinsic deflection of atrial depolarization ID_A ($St_V \rightarrow ID_A$); again, patients were paced at 20 beat increments from 60 to 160 beats per minute and ventriculo-atrial conduction intervals assessed and the rate for onset of VA block ascertained. Retrograde (VA) conduction can only be evaluated adequately when the ventricular rate (paced or unpaced) is more rapid than the atrial rate (Fig. 3);
4. routine measurement of atrial and/or ventricular stimulation thresholds:
5. recording and measurement of the atrial and ventricular electrograms independently.

On examining the recordings with ventricular pacing, the absence of orderly atrial depolarization, i.e. atrial depolarization which occurred independently of any ventricular activity, documented the absence of retrograde conduction. Conversely, atrial pacing without orderly ventricular depolarization documented the absence of antegrade conduction.

Medications were withheld the morning of pacemaker implantation. Otherwise, patients were maintained on any cardiac drugs, i.e. digoxin, beta blockers or antiarrhythmic medications as the clinical situation demanded. All procedures were performed under Lidocaine local anesthesia.

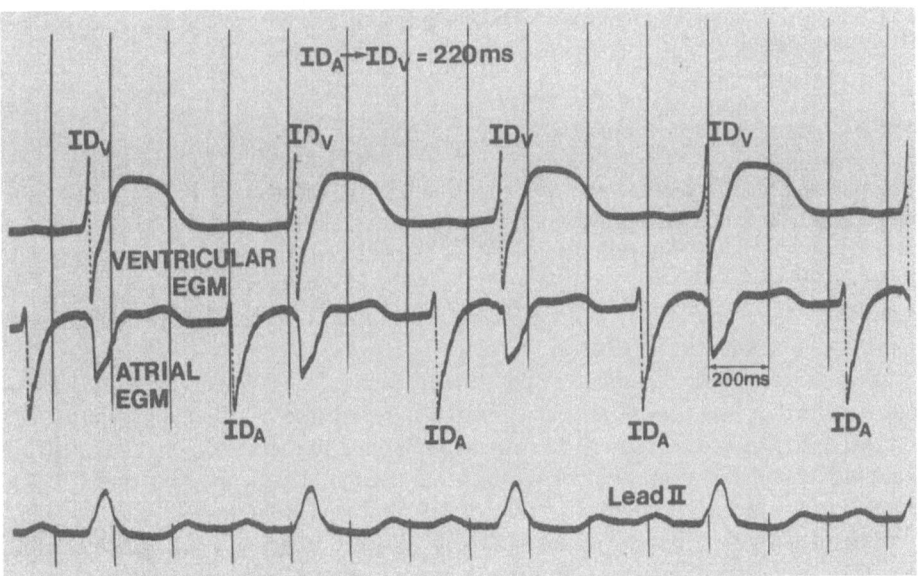

Fig. 2. The pacemaker senses only the intrinsic deflection of either the atrium (ID_A) or the ventricle (ID_V). The time between the two is the PR interval for the pacemaker. In this recording, the intrinsic deflections were sensed from the right atrial appendage and the right ventricular apex, both referenced in lead II.

513

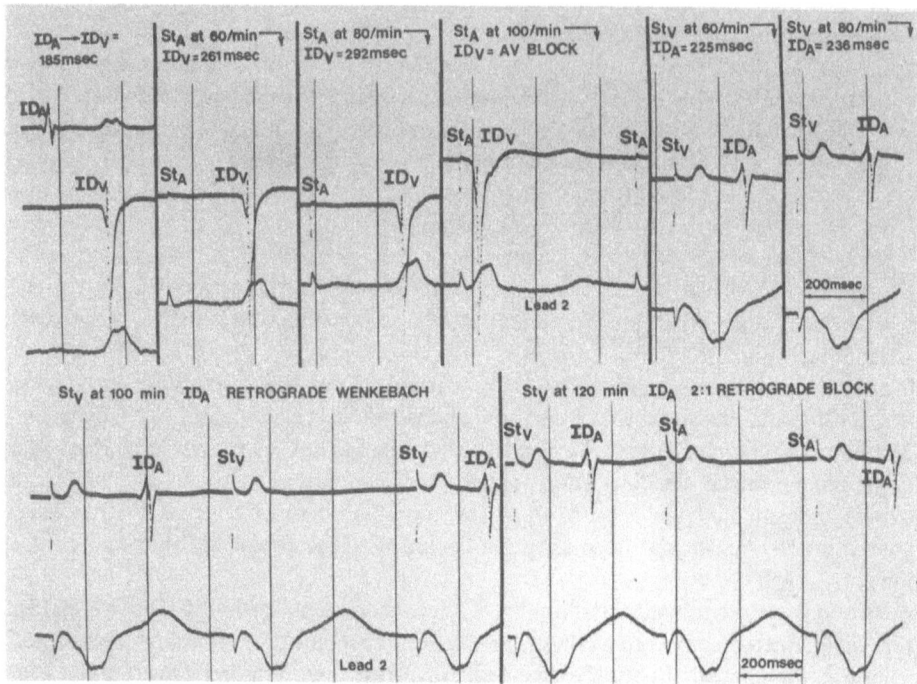

Fig. 3. A complete intraoperative study from one patient. Measurements include the intrinsic atrial (ID$_A$) to intrinsic ventricular (ID$_V$) deflection, atrial pacing at rates of 60, 80 and 100 beats per minute with antegrade block occurring at 100 and incremental ventricular pacing at rates of 60, 80, 100 and 120 beats per minute with retrograde Wenckebach occurring at 100 and 2 : 1 retrograde block at 120 beats per minute.

Results

In 67 patients the mean antegrade conduction interval at rest (ID$_A$ → ID$_V$) was 222 ± 30 msec (range 100 to 420 ms) prolonging to a mean interval (St$_A$ → ID$_V$) of 332 ± 60 msec at the highest atrial pacing rate before AV block occurred. Five patients developed AV block pacing rate of 80 beats per minute; 11 developed AV block at 100 per minute; 16 patients at 120 per minute; 17 patients at 140 per minute; 14 patients at 160 per minute; 4 patients did not develop AV block.

A variety of retrograde conduction responses were found. In 48 patients (45%) 1 : 1 retrograde conduction was present at some ventricular paced rate, 3 patients had retrograde Wenckebach (3%) and 56 of the 107 patients (52%) had retrograde block. Of the 34 patients with complete antegrade block during atrial pacing, 11 patients (32%) had 1 : 1 VA conduction at a mean VA conduction time of 229 msec (range 110 to 380 msec).

Considering all indications for pacing, 45% (48/107) had intact 1 : 1 retrograde conduction. The proportion of patients with intact VA conduction varied considerably when patients were analyzed by rhythm disturbance (Table 1). In those patients with sinus node dysfunction (defined as demonstrating both tachycardia and bradycardia) 62% had intact VA conduction and 53% of patients with sinus bradycardia or sinus arrest had intact VA conduction. Thirty-six percent of patients with incomplete atrioventricular block and

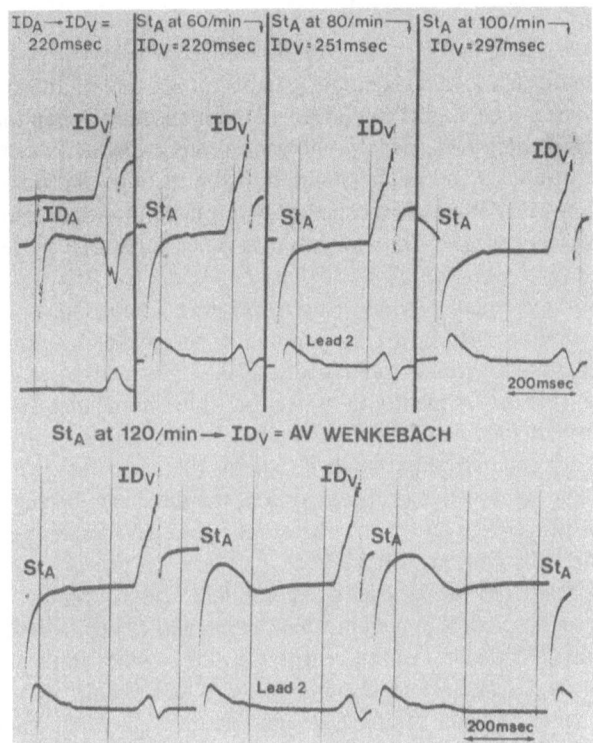

Fig. 4. The pacing rate at which Wenckebach AV block occurs is determined during implant by incremental atrial pacing at 60, 80, 100, 120, and 140 beats per minute. The unpaced conduction interval $ID_A \rightarrow ID_V$ is at the upper left. $ST_A \rightarrow ID_V$ prolongs and Wenckenbach conduction occurs at 120 per minute.

Table 1. Retrograde conduction. Status by underlying rhythm disturbance.

Primary diagnosis	No.	VA conduction	
		% 1 : 1 at any rate	Time (ms) at lowest rate
Sick sinus syndrome	13	61.5	244
Sinus bradycardia or sinus arrest	32	53	211
Incomplete AV block	22	36	265
Complete AV block	34	32	229
Misc conduction disturbances	6	67	263

32% of patients with complete atrioventricular block (spontaneously and during atrial pacing) had intact VA conduction. Six additional patients were paced for miscellaneous conduction defects. Four of the 6 patients had intact 1 : 1 retrograde conduction (3 patients were paced for an unstable junctional rhythm; 2 were paced for episodes of ventricular asystole and 1 had trifascicular conduction disease).

tion defects. Four of the 6 patients had intact 1 : 1 retrograde conduction (3 patients were paced for an unstable junctional rhythm; 2 were paced for episodes of ventricular asystole and 1 had trifascicular conduction disease).

515

Discussion

The interaction between the 2 chambers of a dual chamber pacemaker is based on the appropriate pacing and sensing of 2 chambers and of the setting of the intervals between the atrial and ventricular channels. A variety of refractory and sensing intervals then determine the means of dealing with atrial and ventricular premature contractions and minimum and maximum atrial tracking rates. We have recognized that 3 intervals are of critical importance to successful management of an implanted pulse generator which senses in 2 chambers.

The first measurement is that of the spontaneous AV conduction time if antegrade conduction exists. This allows the optimal setting for the automatic pacemaker rate and atrioventricular delay which will permit sensing spontaneous atrial activity and permit AV conduction to drive the ventricle as frequently as is feasible. Measurement of the atrial paced interval to the intrinsic deflection of the ventricle ($St_A \rightarrow ID_V$) is determined by 2 distinct timing events. These are the atrial pacemaker stimulus (St_A) and the ventricular intrinsic deflection (ID_V). The significance of recognition of the difference between the spontaneous AV conduction rate ($ID_A \rightarrow ID_V$) and the atrial paced AV conduction rate ($St_A \rightarrow ID_V$) is in maintenance of a constant PR interval. As there is a latent period of atrial stimulation and as all pacemaker timing cycles begin with a sensed event or a stimulus, always followed by a latent period, it is obvious that the interval of intrinsic deflection of the atrium to the intrinsic deflection of the ventricle is shorter than from the atrial pacing stimulus to the ventricular intrinsic deflection. In order to maintain a constant PR interval, the dual chamber pacemaker timing cycle must be different when sensing the P wave than when pacing the atrium. No pulse generator now provides the different timing intervals to provide a constant PR interval. Paced and sensed PR intervals are, therefore, of different duration.

The last measurement made was that of the interval for retrograde (VA) conduction following a ventricular stimulus. It is the presence of intact retrograde conduction that allows a pacemaker mediated tachycardia to occur and, therefore, the determination of the presence and duration of VA conduction is required. It was apparent early that few conclusions can be drawn from the surface electrocardiogram as it was also apparent that retrograde AV nodal conduction could not be predicted from knowledge of the state of antegrade conduction. Although previous work makes generalizations about the state of retrograde conduction (13) and the electrophysiolgic literature also contains a great deal of information about retrograde conduction (14, 15, 16), little data exist on the exact determination and timing of retrograde conduction in the context of dual chamber pacemaker implantation.

As described, in our patients all retrograde (VA) conduction intervals were determined from the ventricular stimulus (St_V) to the atrial intrinsic deflection (ID_A) following the ventricular stimulus. In order for an artificial re-entry tachycardia or endless-loop tachycardia to occur, the most important interval is the time during which the atrial channel will be refractory after a paced or sensed ventricular event. As 45% of all patients who require pacemaker implantation and 32% of those whose indication was complete antegrade (AV) block have intact 1 : 1 retrograde conduction, the importance of retrograde conduction becomes apparent. The duration of the VA conduction time demonstrates that a short atrial refractory period after a ventricular event allows sensing of the retrograde P wave. Therefore, if an implanted pulse generator does not have the capability of extending the atrial refractory period beyond the retrograde conduction time measured, a pacemaker-mediated tachycardia will occur. The effect of medication on retrograde conduction has been investigated in other contexts but a careful delineation within the context of cardiac pacemakers and the atrial refractory period is still needed.

If a pacemaker-mediated tachycardia does occur, termination of such tachycardia depends on ending the retrograde P waves. This may be accomplished by fatigue of the retrograde limb, by application of a magnet to produce atrial and ventricular insensitivity, the prolongation of the atrial refractory period beyond the retrograde VA conduction time, and programming to atrial intensitivity such as the AV sequential (DVI) mode with or without ventricular sensing or ventricular sensing only.

With this patient population and information derived from the intraoperative studies, we conclude that with the limitations of the current initial generation of dual chamber sensing pacemakers and the inability to draw conclusions from a surface electrocardiogram, each patient requires intraoperative study to assess the parameters discussed above. Although newer pulse generators may provide an adequate range of atrial refractory programmability that will allow for atrial refractoriness for those patients with the longest retrograde conduction times, and also allow an extension of atrial refractoriness after a premature ventricular contraction, until these devices are available the intraoperative measurements described above allow the implanting physician to choose the pulse generator most appropriate for a given patient.

References

1. Tolentino AO, Javier RP, Byrd C, Samet P: Pacer-induced tachycardia associated with an atrial synchronous ventricular inhibited (ASVIP) pulse generator. Pace 1982; 5: 251–258.
2. Furman S, Fisher JD: Endless loop tachycardia in an AV universal DDD pacemaker. Pace 1982; 5: 486–489.
3. Mines GR: On dynamic equilibrium in the heart. Arch J Physiol 1913; 46: 349–383.
4. Kastor JA, DeSanctis RW: Reciprocal beating from artificial ventricular pacemaker. Circulation 1961; 35: 1170–1173.
5. Barold S, Linhart J, Samet P: Reciprocal beating induced by ventricular pacing. Circulation 1968; 38: 330–340.
6. Kistin AD: Retrograde conduction to the atria in ventricular tachycardia. Circulation 1961; 24: 236–249.
7. Castillo C, Samet P: Retrograde conduction in complete heart block. Br Heart J 1967; 29: 553–558.
8. Drury AN: Paroxysmal tachycardia of an A-V nodal origin, exhibiting retrograde heart block and reciprocal rhythm. Heart 1924; 11: 405–411.
9. Louvros N, Costeas F: Retrograde activation of atria in auriculoventricular block. Arch Intern Med 1965; 116: 778–779.
10. Scherf D, Cohen J, Orphanos RP: Retrograde activation of atria in atrioventricular block. Am J Cardiol 1964; 13: 219–225.
11. Furman S, Hurzeler P, DeCaprio V: The ventricular endocardial electrogram and pacemaker sensing. J Thorac Cardiovasc Surg 1977; 73: 258–266.
12. Furman S, Hurzeler P, DeCaprio V: Cardiac pacing and pacemakers III. Sensing the cardiac electrogram. Am Heart J 1977; 93: 794–801.
13. Akhtar M: Retrograde conduction in man. Pace 1981; 4: 548–562.
14. Schuilenburg RM: Patterns of VA conduction in the human heart in the presence of normal and abnormal AV conduction. In HJJ Wellens, KI Lie, MJ Janse (eds): The Conduction System Of The Heart. Philadelphia. Lea Febiger. 1976; p 485–503.

15. Goldreyer BN, Bigger JT, Jr: Ventriculo-atrial conduction in man. Circulation 1970; 41: 935–946.
16. Narula OS: Retrograde pre-excitation. Comparison of antegrade and retrograde conduction intervals in man. Circulation 1974; 50: 1129–1143.

Authors' address:
David L. Hayes, M.D.
Mayo Clinic,
Rochester, Minnesota 55905,
USA

A Method for Predicting the Potential for Pacemaker-Induced Reciprocating Tachycardias in Patients with DDD Pulse Generators

M. E. Irwin, T. K. Lee, W. R. St. Clair

Summary: Irwin, Me., et al: Intra-operative analyses of ventricular-atrial conduction (VAC) was studied as a means of predicting subsequent development of pacemaker-induced reciprocating tachycardia (PIRT) in 20 patients selected for DDD pulse generator implants. At the time of lead implantation right atrial electrograms were performed while pacing the ventricle at varying cycle lengths. Patients were followed up post implantation at one and three weeks and then at six weekly intervals over a twelve month period. On-going analyses were conducted on atrial and ventricular stimulation and sensing thresholds and sinus triggering capabilities at slow and accelerated sinus rates. Programming sequences to provoke and terminate VAC and sustained PIRT were studied. The effects of myopotential sensing on pacemaker function including initiation of PIRT were also assessed. Eight of 11 patients with Sick Sinus Syndrome (SSS) and 2 of 9 patients with Atrio-ventricular Block (AVB) manifested intra-operative VAC. Follow-up showed that 7 of the 8 SSS patients and both of the AVB patients with VAC developed PIRT, either spontaneously or on provocation. Of the remaining 10 patients without intra-operative manifestation of VAC only one developed PIRT (p < 0.001). This study suggests that intra-operative analysis of VAC is an effective predictor of subsequent PIRT, whereas its absence suggests minimal potential for PIRT post implantation of a DDD pulse generator.

Treatment for symptomatic sinus node disorders and atrial ventricular blocks, uncomplicated by atrial ectopy or atrial fibrillation/flutter now commonly involves the use of pulse generators (PG) which pace and sense both right atrial and right ventricular chambers in sequential manner (1–4). The electrophysiologic and hemodynamic benefits that can be achieved by synchronizing atrial and ventricular stimulation have been well documented (5–7). Reports have shown that cardiac output can increase from 14 to 20 percent when the atrial chamber is allowed to contribute to ventricular filling (1, 8). This increase in cardiac output is accomplished by

1. timing of the closure of the atrioventricular (A-V) valves before ventricular contraction,
2. addition to ventricular filling and
3. preventation of retrograde Ventricular-Atrial (V-A) conduction (9, 10). By maintaining A-V synchrony the events which develop into "pacemaker syndrome" are eliminated (8, 11–13).

The DDD pacing system is one in which both pacing and sensing occurs in the right atrial and right ventricular chamber (14). The improvements in lead technology have lead to very stable lead systems which pace at very low threshold levels and maintain adequate sensing thresholds for inherent atrial and ventricular depolarizations (8, 15–17). Advances have also been made in surgical implantation techniques of the atrial and ventricular leads (18).

The DDD PG functions in such a way that should the intrinsic atrial rate fall below the programmed lower rate limit (LRL) of the PG, the outcome is A-V sequential pacing at that chosen LRL when normal A-V conduction is prolonged and, is atrial pacing alone when A-V conduction is intact. If the intrinsic atrial rate is faster than the LRL of the PG the result is complete inhibition of the atrial stimulus (STa) and ventricular stimulus (STv), if intrinsic A-V conduction is intact and is of shorter duration than the programmed A-V interval of the PG. If, however, A-V conduction is longer than the programmed A-V interval of the PG, atrial synchronous pacing is initiated. The PG paces the ventricle synchronously with the atrial until such time as the atrial rate limit (ARL) is reached (1, 19).

With normal A-V synchrony, intrinsic or paced, it is highly unlikely that ventricular atrial conduction (VAC) will occur, due to the conduction tissue being refractory following normal atrial ventricular (A-V) conduction (20, 21). When retrograde conduction does occur following a normal A-V sequence, it may occur via anomalous pathways, e.g. bundle of Kent (22). Retrograde conduction is most likely to occur as a result of a ventricular event, intrinsic or paced, which is not preceded by an atrial event (21, 23, 24). A-V synchrony is lost and the normal conduction tissue can then be utilized for VAC because the conduction tissue is no longer refractory. During such episodes the heart's own tissue may act as the retrograde limb, and the pacemaker circuitry provides the anterograde limb, of a re-entrant loop (25). With a PG in the DDD mode, if A-V synchrony is lost the outcome is ventricular pacing with the possible development of VAC. A retrograde intrinsic atrial depolarization (IDa) may be detected by the PG's atrial sensing amplifier, should it arrive after the atrial refractory period following the ventricular paced event (ARP) (26). This retrograde IDa triggers a ventricular paced event and the circus movement begins with the result being a pacemaker-induced reciprocating tachycardia (PIRT), which we define as a salvo of 4 or more ventricular paced beats occurring under the above circumstances.

It was necessary to develop a method for predicting the potential for PIRT in patients with PG in the DDD mode.

Methods and materials

Study Population

Twenty consecutive patients chosen for atrial-ventricular pacing, were studied (2). Eleven manifested sinus node disorders (SND), (6 male, 5 female, mean age 66 yrs.) the remaining 9 manifested atrial ventricular block (AVB) (5 male, 4 female, mean age 70 yrs.) (Ta-

Table 1. Sample and indications for DDD cardiac pacing (N = 20).

	No.	M/F	Age
Sinus Node Disorders	11	6/5	48–85 (Mean – 66)
Atrio Ventricular Block	9	5/4	55–85 (Mean – 70)

ble 1). Ten of the total patients studied had initially been paced in the VVI mode, however, "pacemaker syndrome", was symptomatically described in each of these patients and documented by the use of simultaneous surface electrocardiogram and intra-arterial blood pressure recordings (10, 11).

Procedures

At the time of PG and lead implantation and under general anaesthetic, each patients right atrial electrogram (RAE) was recorded while pacing the ventricle (27). The ventricular pacing cycle lengths (PCL) were varied with the intent to override and pace beyond the inherent sinus rate. Ventricular PCL from 850 ms to 600 ms were employed, while recording the RAE simultaneously with surface recordings of lead II and modified VI (Fig. 1).

The patient's systolic blood pressure, if recorded as falling with this maneuvre, was the limiting factor in proceding with decreasing PCL's. Fig. 2 demonstrates the surface recording revealing Stv, designated by the arrows, with subsequent depolarization. Upon termination of ventricular pacing 2 junctional escape beats are recorded, followed by 2 sinus beats with normal A-V conduction. The corresponding RAE depicts in the first 3 pacing cycles retrograde IDa, designated by the stars, resulting from ventricular pacing. Compared with the sinus IDa, designated by the triangles, in the last 2 sinus complexes. In Fig. 3 showing complete AVB, the surface recording on the lower channel shows cessation of ventricular pacing revealing atrial depolarizations without A-V conduction. Simultaneous RAE showing the corresponding sinus IDa. When ventricular pacing, designated by the arrows, begins in the last 3 cycles, there is no apparent relationship between the Stv and the IDa. There is continuation of the sinus IDa, as depicted by the triangles, thus representing complete anterograde and retrograde block.

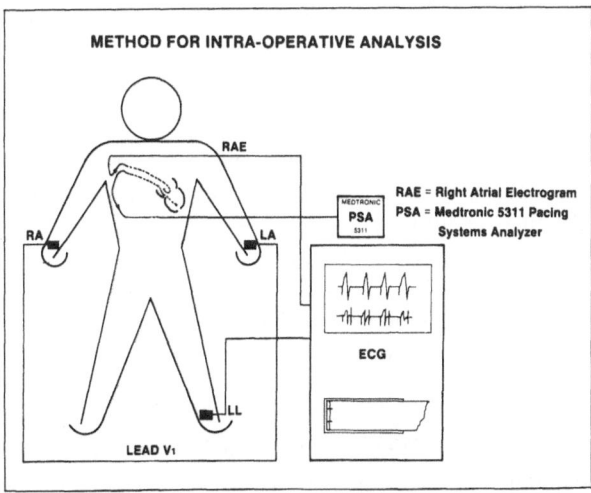

Fig. 1. The intraoperative method by which the ventricles are paced and the right atrial electrogram is recorded simultaneously with surface recording, on hard copy printer and visual display on 2 channel osciloscope. E.C.G. = Mennen Greatback 4 channel oscilloscope with double channel hard copy recorder. RAE = right atrial electrogram. PSA = Medtronic 5311 pacing systems analyzer.

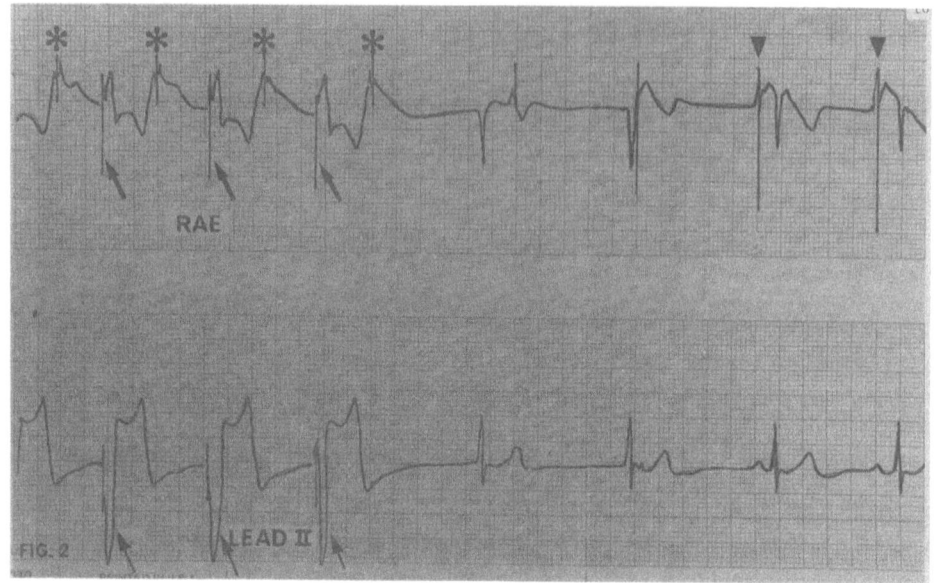

Fig. 2. Intraoperative assessment of 1 : 1 VAC. Lead II surface ECG shows ventricular pacing for the first 3 cycles, simultaneous RAE shows retrograde IDa as a result of ventricular pacing. The last 2 deflections are sinus complexes with normal A-V conduction with the simultaneous RAE showing sinus IDa.

★ = retrograde intrinsic atrial deflection (IDa) as a result of VAC.

▼ = sinus intrinsic atrial deflection.

↘ = ventricular stimulus. RAE = right atrial electrogram.

The patients who were already being paced in the VVI mode, underwent new atrial lead implants while keeping their previous ventricular leads. The remaining received new atrial and ventricular leads. All underwent analysis and documentation of atrial/ventricular stimulation thresholds and atrial/ventricular sensing thresholds, be means of the Medtronic 5309 and 5311 pacing systems analyzer (17).

Follow-up Procedures

Each patient was followed up post PG implant at 1 and 3 weeks, and then at 6 weekly intervals. Ongoing analysis has extended over at least 18 months. For all patients, each individual's stimulation threshold being determined using the 9701A Medtronic programmer. Progressive programmed shortening of the atrial and ventricular pulse durations allow us to ascertain at which pulse duration loss of capture occurs. The threshold is determined as that pulse duration at which capture was regained.

Atrial sensing was analyzed on each patient by progressively decreasing the atrial sensitivity until loss of atrial sensing occurred. The sensitivity was then programmed to twice that at which the loss occurred.

Patients were also assessed by serial ECG's, DCG's and occasional exercise tolerance tests, with PG's in the DVI (14) and DDD modes. In the latter mode, we were able to do-

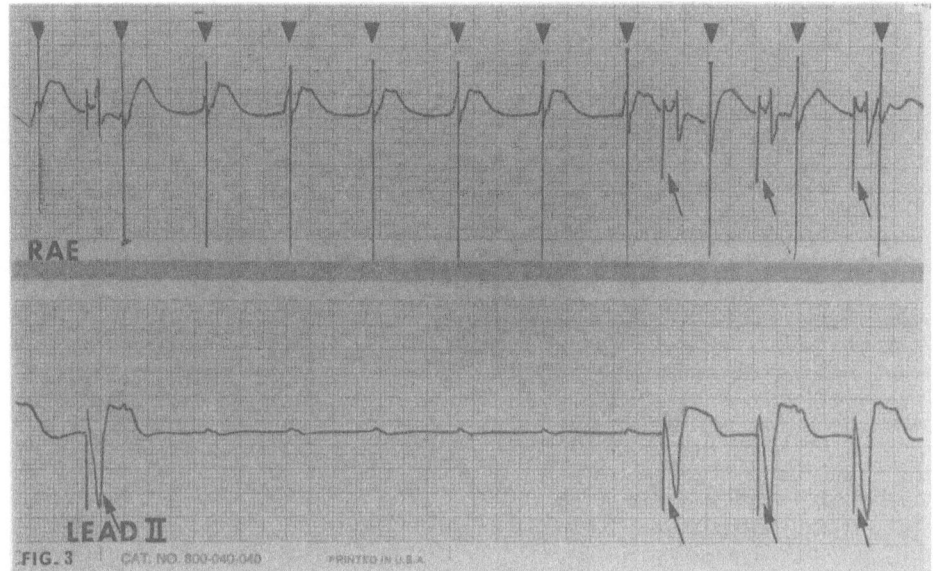

Fig. 3. Intraoperative assessment of complete antrograde and retrograde block. Cessation of ventricular pacing reveals complete A-V block with sinus depolarizations seen on surface ECG lead II at an interval of 720 ms. Initiation of ventricular pacing does not induce VAC, but dissociation of sinus atrial deflections and ventricular pacing is seen. Simultaneous RAE reveals the sinus IDa dissociated from ventricular pacing.

▼ = sinus intrinsic deflection. RAE = Right atrial electrogram. ⟍ = ventricular stimulus.

cument the causes for spontaneous development of PIRT and make appropriate assessments of pacing, sensing and triggering capabilities of the PG.

Provocation of PIRT

Programming sequences were routinely followed on each patient with the intent being provocation of VAC with development of PIRT. The induction of VAC was accomplished in the following ways:

1. Programmed loss of atrial capture (LOAC), with atrial sensing maintained (Fig. 4a).
2. Myopotential Triggering (MPT) produced by varying durations of isometric exercise using the pectoral musculature in the region in which the PG was housed, and the programming of the atrial sensing amplifier to the most sensitive setting (Fig. 4b).
3. Myopotential Inhibition (MPI) as a result of similar isometric exercise, after programming the ventricular sensing amplifier to the most sensitive setting (28).

Each of these sequences gives rise to the potential for ventricular pacing without a preceding atrial depolarization, intrinsic or paced. With the loss of the atrial depolarization and maintenance of ventricular pacing, at shorter cycle lengths than the sinus cycles, the atrial chamber is susceptible to depolarization by retrograde impulses. The final result, if the ARP is shorter than the VAC interval, is PIRT (23, 25, 29–31).

523

Fig. 4a: Lead II rhythm strip obtained during provocation of VAC due to LOAC. Following the 5th pacing cycle there is STa without atrial capture followed by STv with ventricular depolarization and VAC. The STv-P' interval of 200 ms and P'-STv interval of approximately 400 ms is equivalent to a PCL of 600 ms. LOAC has left the atrium receptive to VAC with the result being PIRT. A modified ladder diagram is shown below the tracing. Horizontally hatched areas (V) represent ventricular depolarization by STv. Solid black rectangles indicated ARP of the PG (155 ms). Vertically hatched areas represent pacemaker A-V delay of 150 ms. Stippled areas indicate ARL of 600 ms. Note that the retrograde P-waves (P') fall outside the ARP, and are therefore sensed. The atrial events (A) occur within the ARL, hence, the STv are delivered at the end of this period (29).

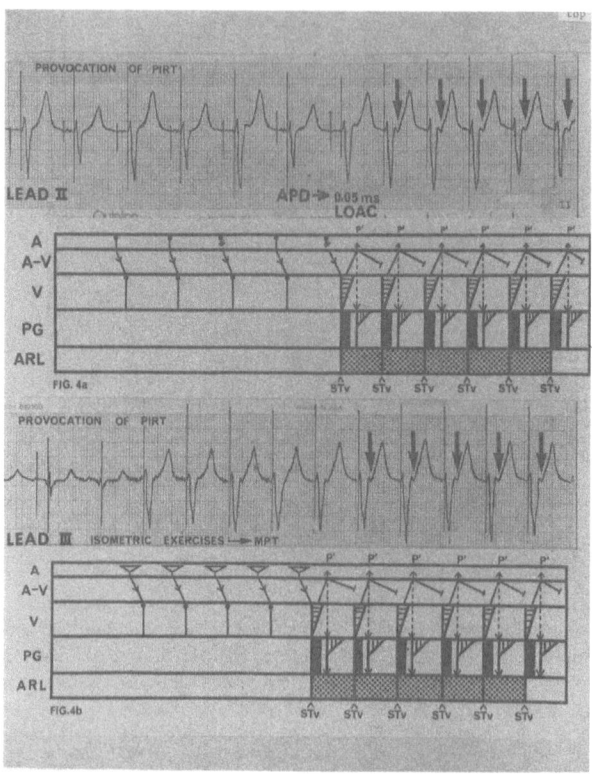

Fig. 4b: Lead II rhythm strip obtained during provocation of PIRT by MPT. The atrial amplifier senses the myopotentials and the result is ventricular pacing after the programmed A-V interval of 150 ms, as seen in the 2nd to 6th pacing cycles. Ventricular pacing without preceding atrial depolarization again leaves the atrium receptive to VAC which results in PIRT.

The STv-P' interval of 180 ms and the P'-STv interval of approximately 420 ms is equivalent to a PCL of 600 ms. A modified ladder diagram is shown below the tracing. The open triangles represent myopotential sensing with the programmed A-V interval of 150 elapsing before ventricular pacing, represented by the solid dot. Horizontally hatched areas (V) represent ventricular depolarization by STv. Solid black rectangles indicated ARP of the PG (155 ms). Vertically hatched areas represent normal pacemaker A-V delay of 150 ms. Stippled areas indicate ARL of 600 ms. Note that the retrograde P-waves (P') fall outside the ARP, and are therefore sensed. However, atrial events (A) occur within the ARL, hence, the STv are delivered at the end of this period (29).

Results

Eight of the 11 patients with SND, and 2 of the 9 patients with AVB manifested intra-operative VAC.

524

Seven of the 8 patients with SND showing VAC developed PIRT. The 8th patient was lost to follow-up shortly after PG implantation. Of the 2 AVB patients with intraoperative VAC, both subsequently developed PIRT (p < 0.001) (Fig. 5). One patient in the SND group not showing VAC spontaneously developed an episode of 3 beats of atrial synchronous ventricular pacing at ARL. We attribute this to being a salvo of atrial ectopy (which the patient had also demonstrated on preimplant serial ECG's and DCG's), and do not believe it to be PIRT. There has been no recurrence with the patient on antiarrhythmic agents.

Of the SND patients with VAC, 1 spontaneously developed PIRT as a result of MPT, and 3 spontaneously developed PIRT as a result of ventricular ectopy (24). Of the AVB patients with VAC, both spontaneously developed PIRT, 1 as a result of LOAC and 1 as a result of MPT (Fig. 6).

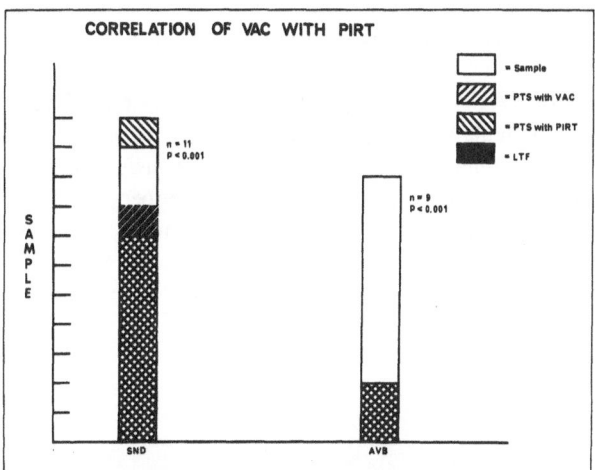

Fig. 5. Correlation of the patients with intraoperative VAC and the subsequent development of PIRT post implantation of the PG. AVB = Atrial ventricular block, LTF = lost to follow-up, PIRT = pacemaker-induced recdiprocating tachycardia, PTS = patients studied, SND = sinus node disorders, VAC = ventricular atrial conduction.

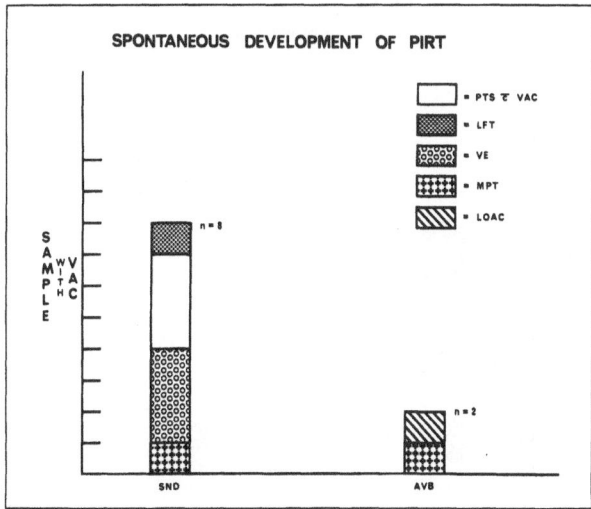

Fig. 6. Sample studied with VAC, showing spontaneous development of PIRT and the mechanism by which it is triggered, while undergoing ambulatory monitoring. AVB = atrial ventricular block, LOAC = loss of atrial capture, LTF = lost to follow-up, MPT = myopotential triggering, PIRT = pacemaker-induced reciprocating tachycardias, PTS = patients studied, SND = sinus node disorders, VAC = ventricular atrial conduction, VE = ventricular ectopy.

Attempts to provoke PIRT were made on every patient on each visit post PG implantation, as outlined previously. Of the 7 SND patients with intraoperative VAC, all could be provoked into a sustained PIRT, 3 as a result of MPT and all 7 as a result of LOAC. Of the 2 AVB patients with VAC, both could be provoked into a sustained PIRT as a result of LOAC, and 1 of the 2 as a result of MPT (Fig. 7).

The remaining 10 patients in the study who did not show intraoperative VAC, also did not spontaneously develop PIRT, nor could each be provoked into a VAC with resultant PIRT (Fig. 5) ($p < 0.001$).

Discussion

Treating patients with a PG in the DDD mode maintains A-V synchrony, with long-term hemodynamic benefits now being well documented (5–7). If, however, this synchrony is not maintained due to some anomalous and/or normal response mechanism of the pulse generator resulting in VAC which may result in PIRT, patients may be left in a compromised situation, as well as present with symptoms relating to this mode of PG behaviour (29–32).

By means of intraoperative studies of VAC while pacing the ventricle and recording an atrial electrogram we assessed those patients with potential for VAC. Subsequent to PG placement close follow-up for the development of PIRT, either spontaneously or on provocation, was conducted. Virtually all patients who demonstrated intraoperative VAC, also developed PIRT spontaneously or on provocation during post implant follow-up. As a result, each patient could also be given the proper PG modality with the proper stimulation and sensing parameters to achieve effective A-V pacing, and at the same time eliminate the possibility of PIRT.

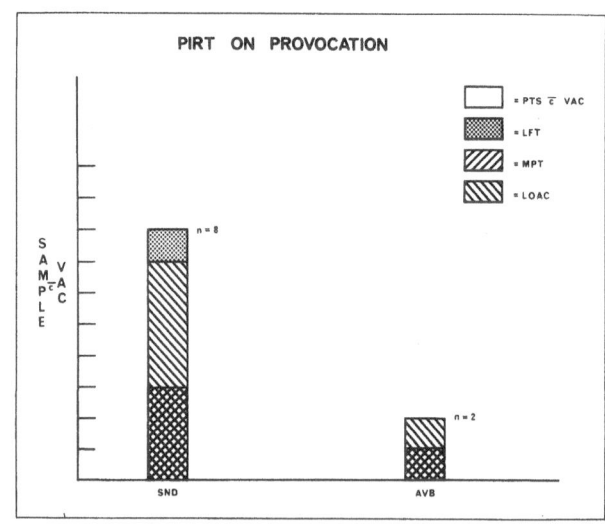

Fig. 7. Sample studied with VAC, showing development of PIRT upon provocation and the mechanisms by which it is provoked. AVB = atrio-ventricular block, LTF = lost to follow-up, LOAC = loss of atrial capture, MPT = myopotential triggering, PIRT = pacemaker-induced reciprocating tachycardias, PTS = patients studied, SND = sinus node disorders, VAC = ventricular atrial conduction.

In conclusion, the data suggests that intraoperative analysis of VAC is an effective predictor of subsequent development of PIRT, whereas its absence suggests minimal potential for the development of PIRT in patients with a PG in the DDD mode.

Acknowledgement

The author is indebted to Medtronic of Canada for their technical support. Mr. Herman Went in the Photography Department at the Edmonton General Hospital and Ms. Ruth Doram for the typing of this manuscript.

References

1. Sutton R, Perrins J, Citron P: Physiological Cardiac Pacing Pace 1980; 3: 207.
2. Harthorne, JW: Indications for pacemaker insertion: Types and modes of pacing. Prog Cardiovasc Dis 1981; 23: 393.
3. Rogel S and Mahler Y: Experience with artificial pacing of the heart. Comparison of synchronized and nonsynchronized pacers. Israel J Med Sci 1965; 1: 1022.
4. Funke H: Cardiac pacing with the universal DDD pulse generator. In S Barold and J Mugica (eds): The Third Decade of Cardiac Pacing. Mt Kisco, New York, Futura Publishing Company, Inc 1982; pp 191–223.
5. Sutton R and Citron P: Electrophysiological and haemodynamic basis for application of new pacemaker technology in sick sinus syndrome and atrioventricular block. Br Heart J 1979; 41: 600.
6. Kappenberger L, Gloor HO, Babotai I, Steinbrunn W and Turina M: Hemodynamic effects of atrial synchronization in acute and long-term ventricular pacing. Pace 1982; 5: 639.
7. Hartzler GO, Maloney JB and Curtis JJ: Hemodynamic benefits of atrioventricular sequential pacing after cardiac surgery. Am J Cardiol 1977; 40: 232.
8. Nishimura RA, Vlietstra RE, Maloney JDD and Merideth J: Early follow-up of lead performance in atrioventricular sequential systems. Pace 1982; 5: 694.
9. Ogawa S, Dreifus LS, Shenoy PN, Brockman SK and Berkovits BV: Hemodynamic consequences of atrioventricular and ventriculoatrial pacing. Pace 1978; 1: 8.
10. Nishimura RA, Bersh BJ, Vlietstra RE, Osborn MJ, Ilstrup DM and Holmes DR: Hemodynamic and symptomatic consequences of ventricular pacing. Pace 1982; 5: 903.
11. Erbel R: Pacemaker syndrome. Am J Cardiol 1979; 44: 771.
12. Goldreyer BN: Physiologic Pacing: The role of AV synchrony. Pace 1982; 5: 613.
13. Lewis M, Sung RJ, Alter BR et al: Pacemaker-induced hypotension. Chest 1981; 79: 354.
14. Inter-society Commission for Heart Disease Resource Code. Am J Card 1974; 34: 487.
15. Sutton R: P-wave sensing, unipolar vs bipolar. In I.W.P. Obel (Ed): Physiological Pacing, London, Pitman Medical, 1981, p. 27.
16. Snow N: Elimination of lead dislodgement by the use of tined transvenous electrodes. Pace 1982; 5: 571.
17. Barold SS, Ong LS and Heinle RA: Stimulation and sensing thresholds for cardiac pacing: Electrophysiologic and technical aspects. Cardiovascular Diseases 1981; 24: 1.
18. Miller FA Jr, Holmes DR Jr Gersh BJ, et al: Permanent transvenous pacemaker implantation via the subclavian vein. Mayo Clin Proc 1980; 55: 309.
19. Furman S: Physiologic pacing. Pace 1980; 3: 639.
20. Van Mechelen R, Hagemeijer F, De Boer H and Schelling A: Atrioventricular and ventriculoatrial conduction in patients with symptomatic sinus node dysfunction. Pace 1983; 6: 13.
21. Akhtar M: Retrograde Conduction in man. Pace 1981; 4: 548.
22. Akhtar M, Damato AN, Caracta AR et al: A comparative analysis of antegrade and retrograde conduction patterns in man. Circulation 1975; 52: 766.
23. Barold S, Linhart J and Samet P: Reciprocal beating induced by ventricular pacing. Circulation 1968; 38: 330.

24. Kistin AD and Landowne M: Retrograde conduction from premature ventricular contractions: A common occurrence in the human heart. Circulation 1951; 3: 738.
25. Den Dulk K, Lindemans FW, Bar FW and Wellens HJJ: Pacemaker related tachycardias. Pace 1982; 5: 476.
26. Medtronic 7000 (Versatrax) manual, Medtronic, Inc.
27. Hayes DL and Furman S: Atrio-ventricular and ventriculo-atrial conduction times in patients undergoing pacemaker implant. Pace 1983; 6: 39.
28. Levine PA, Caplan CH, Klein MD, Brodsky SJ and Ryan TJ: Myopotential inhibition of unipolar lithium pacemakers. Chest 1982; 4: 461.
29. Tolentino AO, Javier RP, Byrd C and Samet P: Pacer-induced tachycardia associated with an atrial synchronous ventricular inhibited (ASVIP) pulse generator. Pace 1982; 5: 251.
30. Bathen J, Gundersen T and Forfang K: Tachycardias related to atrial synchronous ventricular pacing. Pace 1982; 5: 471.
31. Freedman RA, Rothman MT and Mason JW: Recurrent ventricular tachycardia induced by an atrial synchronous ventricular-inhibited pacemaker. Pace 1982; 5: 490.
32. Parsonnet V and Bernstein AD: Cardiac pacing in the 1980s: Treatment and techniques in transition. Am J Cardiol 1983; 1: 339.

Authors' address:
Marleen E. Irwin, R.R.T., C.V.T.
Edmonton General Hospital
11111-Jasper Ave.
Edmonton T5K OL4,
Canada

Eccentricities of DDD (AV Universal) Pacemakers

R. M. Luceri, A. Castellanos, V. Medina-Ravell, L. Zaman, R. J. Thurer, R. J. Myerburg

Summary: The widespread use of dual chamber cardiac pacemakers, specifically the AV universal (DDD) devices, has resulted in the recognition of operational patterns which could be interpreted as pacemaker malfunction. These "eccentricities" include the Wenckebach-like period of upper rate limit response, endless loop tachycardia, physiologic and non-physiologic AV delays, and various response patterns to ventricular extrasystoles. The ultimate recognition of these phenomena requires detailed knowledge of the pulse generators' characteristics. The pacemaker industry, in turn, should attempt to standardize basic DDD characteristics in order to facilitate proper utilization of these sophisticated devices.

Introduction

The recent increase in the use of dual chamber cardiac pacemakers, specifically AV universal (DDD) pulse generators, has resulted in the recognition of specific electrocardiographic and operational patterns. Since the engineering design of these pulse generators is extremely complex, there have resulted several phenomena which provide an interface between "artificial" mechanical operation and its relationship to the normal conduction system of the heart. It is therefore appropriate to label these phenomena as "eccentricities", defined as variations of normal function (anticipated or not) which may lead to erroneous pacemaker analysis, and which generally result from incomplete interpretation of the operating characteristics of a particular pulse generator. A description of some eccentricities observed in AV sequential (DVI) pacemakers has been reported (1). In this communication, an effort will be made to describe and analyze those eccentricities of DDD (AV universal) pacemakers. Although each manufacturers' model has specific eccentricities, the subject will be addressed in a generic sense, although individual specific characteristics will be detailed when appropriate.

In any case, it is important to recognize that pacemaker eccentricities are associated with normal pacemaker function (2). Indeed, it is exceedingly rare for the pacemaker to be truly malfunctioning; the errors usually lie in misinterpretation of normal operating characteristics.

Potential Sources of Error in Analyzing DDD Pacemakers

The many functions of AV universal DDD pacemakers have left us with a compendium of new terms to describe pacing limits, AV intervals, atrial and ventricular refractory periods, etc. The scope of this presentation will be limited to the description of four phenomena or eccentricities which may, in particular, lend themselves to misinterpretation during routine pacemaker analysis.

529

A) Wenckebach-like Periods of AV Synchronization

The Wenckebach type response to attainment of upper rate limit is an artificially engineered mechanism for protecting against sudden changes in ventricular paced rates in response to sensed atrial rate increases. Thus, at the programmed upper rate limit, the ventricular rate is limited to that programmed value. At atrial rates which are higher than the programmed upper rate, there is progressive increase of the total AV interval. This is represented (Figure 1) by gradually increasing AV interval which in effect equals the sum of the normal programmed AV delay plus a waiting period. The latter represents the interval necessary to "time out" the upper rate limit counter for ventricular pacing. As in the figure shown, the intervals between the P waves and the following paced ventricular complexes gradually lengthen, until a dropped QRS occurs. The blocked P wave (preceding the dropped QRS complex) is actually governed by the refractoriness of the ventricular channel. Since the P wave comes progressively closer to the preceding paced QRS complex, at the end of a Wenckebach cycle it falls within the atrial refractory period of the pacemaker. It is therefore, correctly non-sensed and thus does not result in a subsequent ventricular paced stimulus. As long as the atrial rate is above the programmed upper rate limit, the Wenckebach sequence will continue. If the atrial rate surpasses the sum of the atrial refractory period and the AV delay, a 2 : 1 AV block pattern results. This is

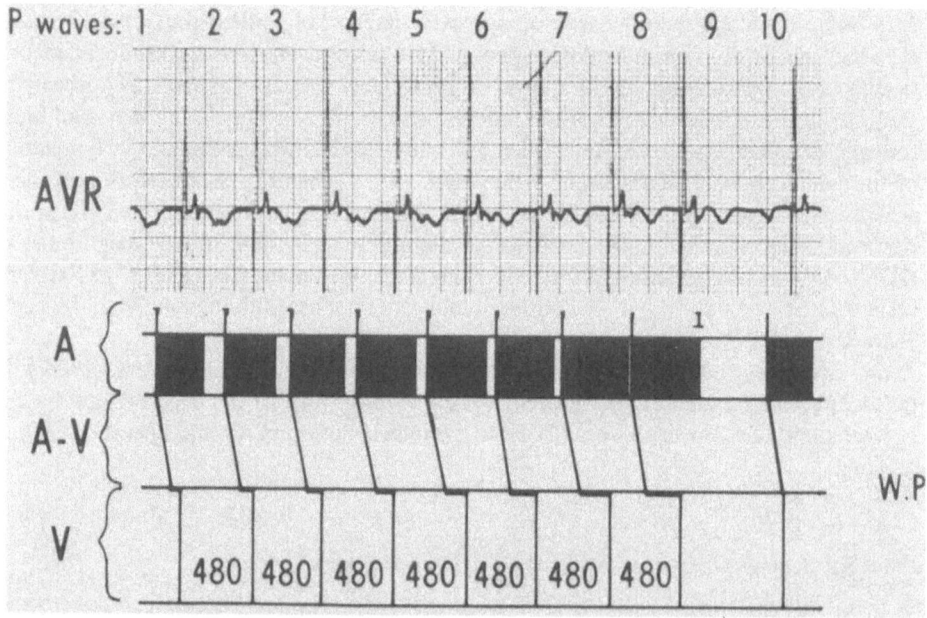

Fig. 1. Wenckebach-like period, (ECG lead AVR). The maximum rate is set at 480 ms (125 Bpm). Since the atrial rate is slightly faster than the maximum rate, the total AV intervals are increasingly prolonged. This is accomplished by the addition of "waiting periods" to the fixed AV interval in order to withhold subsequent ventricular stimulation until the upper rate counter (480 ms) has "timed out". A = Atrium; A-V = AV interval; WP = waiting period; V = ventricle.

530

similar to Mobitz Type II block in which the artificial AV interval preceding the first blocked P wave has a constant and fixed value.

In analyzing this type of phenomenon, it should be understood that differences do exist between artificial and natural phenomena. In spontaneous AV Wenckebach periods, it is unusual for the R-R intervals to remain as constant as they do in this artificial cycle. In addition, the electrocardiogram of the Wenckebach-like period revealed an AV dissociation pattern. In contrast to spontaneous AV dissociation where atrial and ventricular events are unrelated, in pacemaker mediated Wenckebach-like periods, there is a definite relationship between the preceding P wave and the following ventricular stimulus.

B) Endless Loop Tachycardia

The implantation of DDD pacemaker has been likened to the placement of an artificial bypass tract (3). Although the potential for AV reciprocating tachycardia to occur was recognized as early as 1969 (4), attention has been focused on this phenomenon since the increased frequency of implantation of VDD or DDD pacemakers. Endless loop tachycardia, a term coined by Furman (5), generally occurs when a paced (or spontaneous) ventricular stimulus is followed by retrograde atrial activation (Fig. 2). The atrial impulse, which is sensed, triggers an AV delay followed by another ventricular stimulus. This in turn generates still another retrograde atrial impulse, which again is sensed, and followed by a ventricular stimulus. The process repeats itself until either natural events (block) or mechanical intervention occurs. Endless loop tachycardia may be initiated by several mechanisms (6). These typically include ventricular premature complexes with retrograde atrial conduction, electro-mechanical interference whereby "noise", or myopotentials may be misinterpreted for atrial signals, undersensed P waves, and atrial premature complexes. The frequency of occurrence of endless loop tachycardia has been the subject of several recent reviews. In general, the incidence is directly related to whether retrograde ventriculo-atrial conduction is present. The latter occurs typically in instances where antegrade AV block does not occur. Thus, for example, in patient who receive permanent pacemakers for sick sinus syndrome or carotid sinus hypersensitivity, there is ap-

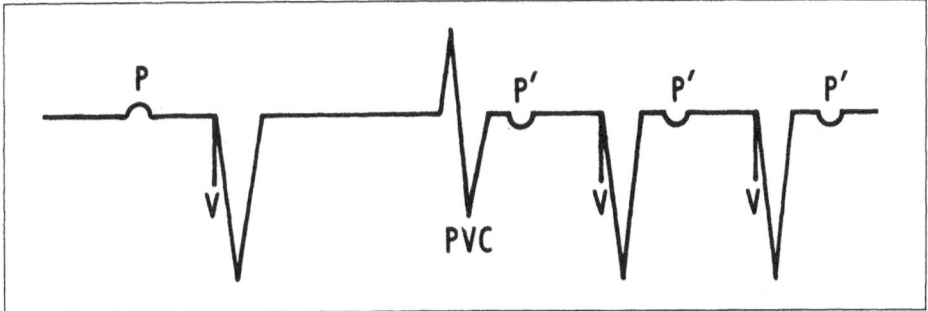

Fig. 2. Endless loop tachycardia during DDD pacing. Following the ventricular extrasystole (PVC) is a retrograde P wave (P') which is sensed by the atrial channel. An AV interval ensues and is followed by ventricular stimulation. The process repeats itself, and the tachycardia rate (V-V) is governed by the programmed upper rate limit.

proximately a sixty-five percent incidence of retrograde conduction (7). In contrast, when complete AV block occurs, the incidence of retrograde ventriculo-atrial conduction decreases to approximately 10 or 15 percent. The incidence of retrograde conduction has been extensively reviewed (7–9).

The tachycardia rate (in endless loop) is determined by retrograde conduction time and antegrade AV delay. This is under the control of the programmable upper rate limit of the pacemaker and is mediated through pacemaker delay of the AV interval. In endless loop tachycardias, the ventricular rate will always be at the upper rate limit. This is in contrast to the previous description of Wenckebach-like periods in which ventricular pacing rate will vary according to the Wenckebach cycle.

The acute management of endless loop tachycardia requires application of an external magnet for immediate conversion to asynchronous dual chamber (DOO) pacing. Long term management includes extension of the atrial refractory period (through programmability) of the pacemaker. This serves to render the atrial channel insensitive to retrograde activation. In general, drugs which block ventriculo-atrial conduction are not advised since they may lead to secondary effects (6). Philosophically, the burden lies on choosing the correct pacemaker rather than adding antiarrhythmic agents to alter its performance.

C) Physiologic and non-physiologic AV delays

The differences between committed and non-committed DVI pacing have been reported in detail and will not be the subject of review in this text (10, 11). However, efforts have been made to divide the AV delay into a non-physiologic and a physiologic interval (Fig. 3). In the Medtronic* Versatrax Model 7000 pacemaker, for example, an atrial paced event triggers the onset of the AV interval. The first part of the AV interval is represented by a non-physiologic period of 110 ms, during which time ventricular sensing triggers a ventricular pace at the end of 110 ms, (12). The purpose of the "noise sensitive" period is to avoid the chance occurrence of an asynchronous ventricular stimulus falling at the end of an abnormal QRS complex, thus potentially allowing for ventricular repetitive response. After the 110 ms noise sensitive period, the remainder of the programmed AV delay would operate in a normal physiologic mode (non-committed), whereby sensed ventricular events would completely inhibit ventricular out put. Thus, triggered ventricular sensing may occasionally be seen in DDD pacing utilizing this type of AV delay.

D) Pacemaker response to sensed ventricular extrasystoles

One of the greatest sources of confusion in interpreting DDD electrocardiograms is the behavior of the DDD pulse generators of sense extrasystoles whether they are premature or spontaneous. Depending upon whether or not the ectopic ventricular complex is followed by retrograde activation, the pulse generator will respond in a different manner.

---

* Medtronic Inc, Minneapolis MN, USA

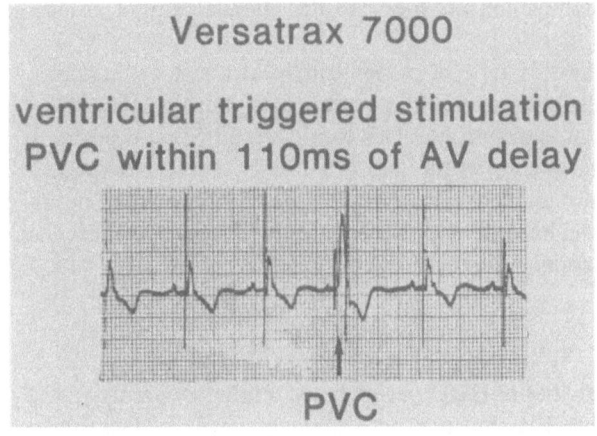

Fig. 3. Example of the triggered ventricular stimulus which occurs when the ventricular channel senses "noises" or a PVC within the first 110 ms of the AV interval. The ECG appearance is therefore that of "committed" ventricular stimulation at an AV delay which is 110 ms.

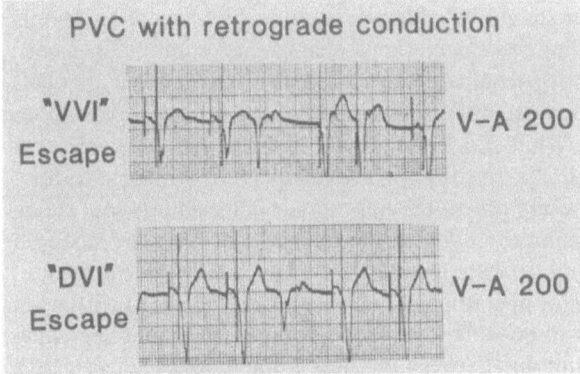

Fig. 4. DDD function following a ventricular extrasystole. Both strips are from the same patient (at the same settings) with a Versatrax 7000 pulse generator. Top strip: a PVC is followed by a retrograde P wave at a V-A interval of 200 ms (retrograde conduction time). The subsequent impulse is ventricular paced. Bottom strip: a PVC with a retrograde P at the same conduction interval (200 ms is followed by a paced AV sequential (DVI) impulse. The explanation for this, although ambiguous, is presumably due to the fact that in the top strip, the P wave fell during a period (155–342 ms following the PVC) in which the AV counter was disabled. This prolonged the refractory period so that the expected atrial output did not occur prior to the ventricular escape interval. In the bottom strip, however, despite "normal" appearances, the "DVI escape" must be considered true malfunction since it does not act according to specifications.

The confusion occurs in the interpretation of surface electrocardiograms, since little distinction can be made between retrograde conduction times. As is shown in the example in figure 4, two similarly appearing ventricular premature complexes occur with retrograde atrial activation in a Versatrax 7000 pacemaker in DDD mode. However, the complexes or escape beats following the ventricular ectopic beat are ventricular in one (top strip) and AV sequential in the other (bottom) strip), despite the fact that retrograde conduction time is similar. The explanation lies in the fact that one retrograde P wave fell within a period in which the AV counter was disabled by the ectopic ventricular complex (between 155 and 342 ms following the PVC). This prolonged the atrial refractory period so much so that an expected paced atrial stimulus was not delivered before the completion of the programmed ventricular escape interval. Thus, the escape beat is ventricular (VVI). In the bottom strip, however, despite "normal" appearances, one must conclude that the "DVI escape" is pacer malfunction according to the manufacturing specifications.

Despite the ambiguity generated by this type of response to ventricular extrasystoles, there are efforts to design DDD pulse generators with an automatic extension of atrial refractory periods following ventricular extrasystoles. This would serve two purposes: 1. It would avoid competitive ventricular pacing in the face of an early sensed retrograde P wave; and 2. the extension of atrial refractory period would generally prevent the occurrence of endless loop tachycardia which is initiated in the majority of cases by ventricular extrasystoles with retrograde atrial conduction.

Discussion

Several remarks concerning eccentricities of DDD pacing based on the previously shown examples can be made. It is evident that with the increasing complexity of these pulse generators, analysis of "normal" function is indeed complex (13). It would be even more distressing to imagine the complexities which might occur in the presence of true pacemaker malfunction. A second point should be addressed specifically to the manufacturing community. Information regarding these operational characteristics and the behavior of the pacemakers in the face of arrhythmias, etc., is lacking. The implant manuals either do not mention or show rather incomplete description of the various eccentricities of these advanced pulse generators. While it is evident that individual manufacturers will maintain some form of personalization with their respective units, this advanced technology is of no benefit to physician users unless the appropriate information concerning pacemaker function in all known clinical circumstances is provided. An issue has been raised concerning standardization of operating features (13–14). From a clinical point of view, industry-wide standardization of operating features would be welcomed with open arms. However, since it is virtually impossible to expect it occurrence, again the emphasis must be placed on intimate relationship between physicians and industry regarding the design and analysis of advanced pulse generators.

Finally, the following points are offered in the spirit of advice and concern: 1. It is imperative for the physician to know in detail the operating characteristics of the particular DDD pacemaker in question; 2. in hospitals or centers exposed to relatively small numbers of DDD implants, it may be beneficial to avoid the use of several different types of pulse generators. The complexities of one model may require a lengthy learning period, so much so that it would be impractical to implant many different models in relatively small numbers; 3. an eventuality facing modern pacing is the development of central or satellite pacing centers specifically equipped to follow "complex" pulse generators. The evolution of cardiac pacing towards a broader prescription of devices for tachycardia control would render this type of center necessary and useful from a practical point of view; 4. finally, the ultimate reaction to the complexity of modern pacemakers would be a return to the use of single chamber (VVI, AAI) devices. If misunderstanding prevails, a return to single chamber pacing would not be completely inappropriate.

Conclusion

The eccentricities of DDD pulse generators represent variations of normal functions which may lead to misinterpretation of pacemaker function. In general, these eccentricities are all associated with normal pacemaker function. Intimate knowledge of the operating characteristics of each pulse generator is mandatory for successful management and interpretation of data generated by complex AV universal (DDD) pacemakers. Efforts on the part of the pacemaker industry, as well as continuing efforts on the part of physicians and pacing organizations, are required in order to provide practical information for successful pacemaker follow and avoid misinterpretation and even inappropriate explantation of these sophisticated devices.

References

1. Luceri RM, Ramirez AV, Medina-Ravell V, Thurer RJ, Castellanos A, Myerburg RJ: Ventricular tachycardia and atrioventricular reciprocation produced by, and myopotential inhibition of, normally-functioning DVI (AV sequential) pacemakers. Amer J Card (Abstr) 1982; 49: 953.
2. Furman S: Pacemaker eccentricity. Pace 1981; 4: 261.
3. Furman S: Arrhythmias of dual chamber pacemakers. Pace 1982; 5: 469.
4. Castellanos A, Lemberg L: Electrophysiology of pacing and cardioversion. New York: Appleton-Century-Crofts; 1969: p 54.
5. Furman S, Fisher JD: Endless loop tachycardia in an AV universal (DDD) pacemaker. Pace 1982; 5: 486.
6. Luceri RM, Castellanos A, Zaman L, Myerburg RJ. Arrhythmias of dual chamber cardiac pacemakers and their management. Ann Int Med 1983; 99: 354.
7. Schuilenburg RM: Patterns of VA conduction in the human heart in the presence of normal and abnormal AV conduction. In: Wellens HJJ, Lie KI, Janse MJ, eds. The conduction system of the heart. Structure, function and clinical implications. Philadelphia: Lea and Febiger, 1976: p 485.
8. Levy S, Corbelli JL, Labruine P, et al: Retrograde (ventriculo atrial) conduction. Pace 1983; 6: 364.
9. Akhtar M: Retrograde conduction in man. Pace 1981; 4: 548.
10. Barold SS, Falkoff MD, Ong LS, Heinle RA: Characterization of pacemaker arrhythmias due to normally functioning AV demand (DVI) pulse generators. Pace 1980; 3: 712.
11. Barold SS, Falkoff MD, Ong LS, Heinle RA: Interpretation of electrocardiograms produced by a new unipolar multiprogrammable "committed" AV sequential demand (DVI) pulse generator. Pace 1981; 4: 692.
12. Versatrax, Model 7000 Universal AV pacemaker. Medtronic, inc Minneapolis MN (USA), 1981.
13. Hauser RG: The electrocardiography of A-V universal DDD pacemakers. Pace 1983; 6: 399.
14. Parsonnet V, Bernstein AD: Pseudomalfunctions of Dual-Chamber Pacemakers. Pace 1983; 6: 376.

Authors' address:
Richard M. Luceri, M.D.
University of Miami School of Medicine
Division of Cardiology (D-39)
P.O. Box 016960
Miami, Florida 33101
USA

Diaphragmatic Myopotential Inhibition in Multiprogrammable Unipolar and Bipolar Pulse Generators

S. S. Barold, M. D. Falkoff, L. S. Ong, R. A. Heinle

Summary: Diaphragmatic myopotential inhibition in multiprogrammable pacemakers was tested in 119 patients with implanted devices from six different manufacturers. There were 105 VVI pulse generators (46 bipolar and 59 unipolar) and 14 unipolar DVI pulse generators. Diaphragmatic myopotential inhibition was tested by observing the effect of a maximal deep inspiration in the supine position with the pulse generator programmed at various sensitivities. Inhibition was demonstrated in four of 46 bipolar VVI units (8.7%) and twelve of 59 unipolar VVI units (20.3%). Inhibition was also demonstrated in four of 14 unipolar DVI systems from the one manufacturer (28.6%).

This form of interference appears to be a benign clinical problem and rarely if ever leads to prolonged asystole. It should be considered in the differential diagnosis of pacemaker pauses, particularly in patients with multiprogrammable pulse generators programmed at higher sensitivities.

Despite spectacular improvements in pacemaker technology, the incidence of myopotential (musculoskeletal) inhibition of unipolar pulse generators has remained basically unchanged over the last ten years. In contrast to this well-known type of interference, usually arising from the deltopectroal muscles, oversensing of diaphragmatic myopotential is considered rare and documented in isolated instances with unipolar or bipolar VVI pulse generators[1-4]. The recent widespread availability of multiprogrammable pacemakers with programmable sensitivity may set the stage for the more frequent development of this unusual form of interference. We therefore evaluated the incidence of diaphragmatic myopotential oversensing in 119 patients with multiprogrammable pulse generators from

Table 1. Diaphragmatic myopotential inhibition
(The number of pulse generators exhibiting inhibition is shown in parentheses.)

1. VVI pulse generators – Total number = 105

	Unipolar	Bipolar
Intermedics (Cyberlith & Quantum)	22 (9)	20 (3)
Medtronic (Spectrax)	5 (0)	7 (0)
CPI (Command 5)	17 (0)	0
Pacesetter (Programmalith)	11 (1)	10 (0)
Siemens Elema (688)	4 (2)	8 (0)
Telectronics (Optima)	0	1 (1)
Total	59 (12)	46 (4)
Percentage	20.3%	8.7%

2. DVI pulse generators
Intermedics (Cyberlith IV): 14 unipolar DVI units (4) – 28.6%

six different manufacturers (Table 1). This study was prompted by the observation of un-explained pauses in the Holter recording of two patients with bipolar VVI pulse genera-tors programmed to the highest sensitivity.

Material and methods

A total of 119 multiprogrammable pulse generators from six different manufacturers were evaluated (Table 1). There were 105 VVI pulse generators (46 bipolar and 59 unipolar) and 14 unipolar DVI pulse generators. Diaphragmatic myopotential inhibition was test-ed at several programmed sensitivities by recording long rhythm strips, usually on a three-channel electrocardiograph, during maximal inspiration in the supine position (Fig. 1, 2). This was repeated at least five times after the patients became familiar with the procedure. Diaphragmatic myopotential inhibition was also evaluated in the same way on two subsequent follow-up visits.

Diaphragmatic myopotential inhibition was considered positive when pacemaker pauses (exceeding the automatic interval by more than 450 msec.) were reproduced on at least three occasions at the same sensitivity. The presence of oversensing was confirmed by ap-plication of the magnet which eliminated the pauses.

Results (Table 1)

Diaphragmatic myopotential inhibition was demonstrated in four of 46 bipolar VVI units (8.7%) and twelve of 59 unipolar VVI units (20.3%). Inhibtion was also demonstrated in four of 14 unipolar DVI systems from the same manufacturer (28.6%).

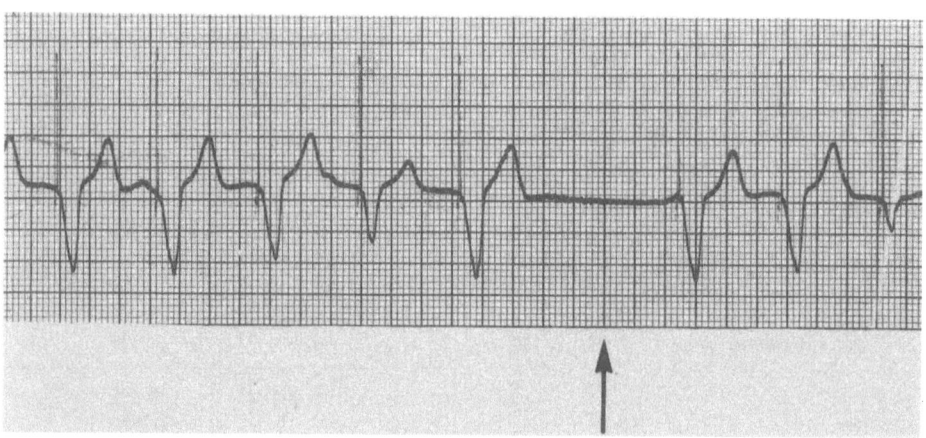

Fig. 1. Unipolar Cyberlith (Intermedics) VVI pulse generator with automatic interval of approxi-mately 680 msec., showing pause of 1440 msec. with deep inspiration. The sensitivity was pro-grammed to 0.8 mV.

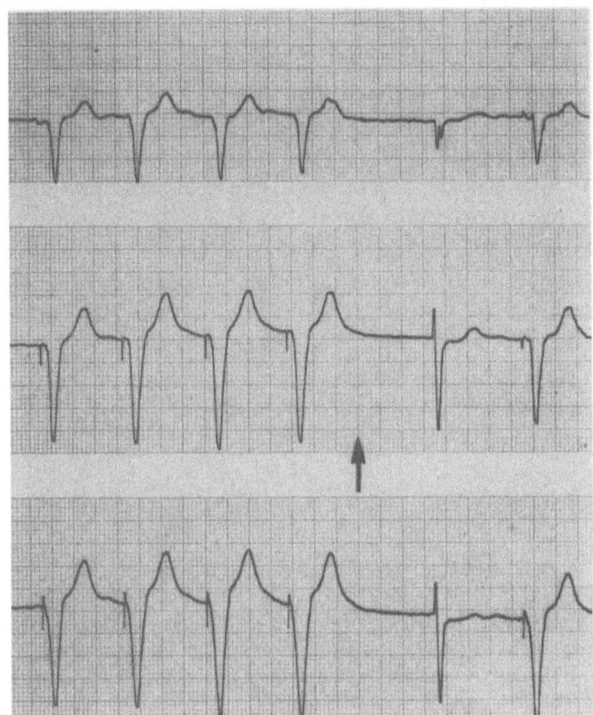

Fig. 2. Bipolar Cyberlith (Intermedics) VVI pulse generator with automatic interval of approximately 760 msec., showing pause of 1320 msec. with deep inspiration. The sensitivity was programmed to 0.8 mV.

Diaphragmatic myopotential inhibition was observed at sensitivities higher than nominal value in all the cases except for two pulse generators that were inhibited when programmed at nominal sensitivity – one unipolar and one bipolar VVI pulse generator. Diaphragmatic myopotential inhibition was reproduced during follow-up visits in all the patients except four at the same programmed sensitivity that had previously demonstrated inhibition.

Discussion

Our observations in 119 patients with multiprogrammable pulse generators suggest that diaphragmatic myopotential inhibition may not be uncommon when pulse generators are programmed to higher sensitivities. Oversensing of diaphragmatic myopotentials depends on several factors: (1) The characteristics of the sensing amplifier that may vary widely from manufacturer to manufacturer. The relatively high occurrence of diaphragmatic myopotential interference observed with the units of one manufacturer probably reflects circuit design, bandpass characteristics, and selection of rather high sensitivity settings unavailable from other manufacturers. Indeed a relatively high sensitivity may occasionally be advantageous in the presence of a very low intracardiac signal. In this context, it should be remembered that the optimal sensitivity for the treatment of undersensing always represents a trade-off between oversensing and undersensing. (2) Body build. It is our impression that diaphragmatic myopotential interference is more easily demonstrable in patients capable of greater diaphragmatic excursion. (3) Diaphragmatic myopotential inhibition is more common with unipolar than bipolar VVI pulse generators. The smaller incidence with bipolar pulse generators may be related to the delivery of extraneous signals of essentially similar amplitude to the two poles of bipolar pacing catheters. Because a bipolar system detects the potential difference between two electrodes in close proximity, the effective myopotential signal may be smaller compared to that delivered to a unipolar electrode. In this context it would be interesting to compare the incidence of diaphragmatic myopotential oversensing in the unipolar and bipolar modes in patients with pulse generators that have the capability of programming polarity. Although diaphragmatic myopotential inhibition appears to be a benign clinical problem, it should be considered in the differential diagnosis of pacemaker pauses, particularly in patients with multiprogrammable pacemakers programmed at a higher sensitivity.

References

1. Peter R, Harper R, Sloman G: Inhibition of demand pacemakers caused by potentials associated with inspiration. Brit Heart J 1976: 38, 211.
2. Barold SS, Ong LS, Falkoff MD, Heinle RA: Inhibition of bipolar demand pacemaker by diaphragmatic myopotentials. Circulation 1977: 56, 679.
3. Baggioni, GF, Antonoli GE: Cause apparentemente insolite diinibizione dei pacemakers unipolari a domanda. G Ital Cardiol 1978: 8, 61.
4. El Gamal M, VanGelder B: Suppression of an extenal demand pacemaker by diaphragmatic myopotentials: a sign of electrode perforation? Pace 1979: 2, 191.

Author's address:
S. S. Barold, M.D.
Division of Cardiology
Department of Medicine
The Genesee Hospital
Rochester, New York 14607, U.S.A.

Rectus Abdominis as a Source of Myopotentials Inhibiting Demand Pacemakers

J. Gialafos, A. Maillis, Ch. Kalogeropoulos, J. Kandilas, N. Koulizakis, D. Avgoustakis

Summary: The possibility of the Rectus Abdominis (RA) as a source of myopotentials inhibiting unipolar demand pacemakers was investigated in 205 consecutive paced patients, 110 males and 95 females.

ECG recordings were taken in all patients during rest and during effort in which maximal muscular strength from the RA and Pectoralis Major (PM) was required. In 72 of these 205 cases transient pacer inhibition was observed. In all 72, myopotentials from the RA and PM were recorded simultaneously at rest and during special effort. In 19 of the 72 cases pacer inhibition was caused by myopotentials generated mainly by the RA, although in 16 of the above 19 cases the generator was located superficially to the PM. In 10 cases the pacer inhibition lasted for more than twice the pacing interval (long), while in the remaining 9 cases it lasted for less (short). In 38 of the 72 cases there was pacer inhibition by myopotentials generated mainly from the PM (23 long and 15 short). In one of the PM long inhibition group the pacemaker was located superficially to the RA. In the remaining 15 cases the inhibition was evident as a clear synergetic effect from both muscle groups.

It is concluded that, apart from the PM, the RA has always to be considered as a main and serious source of myopotentials inhibiting unipolar demand pacemakers.

The problem of the transient inhibition of unipolar demand pacemakers by myopotentials has been studied quite extensively by a number of investigators over the past few years (1–11). The conclusion of these studies was that the Pectoralis Major (PM) was the main if not the single source of myopotentials causing this phenomenon of inhibition, except in two cases where participation by other muscles – diaphragm in one case, Rectus Abdominis (RA) in the other – was suspected.

However, Gialafos et al (12, 13), using simultaneous multi- and/or single-unit recordings from the RA and PM muscles, presented five cases with similar problems which were caused by myopotentials originating in the RA.

In this study we present our findings from 205 paced patients.

Material and method

Two hundred and five consecutive paced patients, with or without symptoms and in steady pacing rhythm, were included in this study. Of these 205 patients 110 were males and 95 females. In 198 cases the generator was located superficially to the PM and in 7 was superficial to the RA.

ECG recordings were taken in all patients during rest and during effort in which maximal muscular strength from the RA and PM was required. In 72 of these 205 cases, where

541

transient pacemaker inhibition was observed, a study of the myopotentials of the RA and PM muscles was carried out.

The myograms from the PM and RA, the ECG and two EEG tracings were recorded simultaneously on tracing paper using a Polygraph-SAN-El, model 1A–12. In all cases surface electrodes of 1 cm diameter were used coupled with the Tectronix type 122 preamplifier to record total muscle activity. In 5 cases, for comparison reasons, concentric needle electrodes having 0.4 mm tip diameter, coupled with a DISA 14A21 myograph, were used to record muscle activity. In all cases, the searching electrodes were recording muscle potentials at various distances from the pulse generator housing.

During these recordings, the patients were asked to perform certain movements. For the PM a variety of movements were applied, with support or against resistance, in order to obtain different strengths of muscle contraction from minimum to maximum. Similar measures were used for the RA muscle test: precautions were taken to minimise as far as possible the interference from other muscle groups (synergists – agonists) by assisting the patients during their efforts. While the patient was rising to the sitting position his feet were immobilised and assistance was given from behind in order to confine the muscular activity to the abdominal region. In all cases Valsava's tests excluded the possibility of diaphragm participation.

Results

The myopotentials recorded during muscle activity ranged from 0.5 mV to 5 mV in amplitude and varied in frequency from 5 to 20 impulses per second for the high amplitude peaks, depending on the muscle under investigation, the location of the recording electrodes and the strength of muscle contraction.

In all cases studied electrophysiologically with simultaneous recordings from the PM and RA muscles we found it practically impossible to separate out completely the activity of one muscle group while testing the other.

With respect to muscle contraction characteristics (strength) the EMG recordings can be classified into three main groups – maximal, intermediate and minimal. Thus, we were able to organise our results in terms of muscle group dominance in the pacing inhibition phenomenon into three main categories: RA dominant, PM dominant, and PM and RA synergy (Figures 1, 2, 3, respectively and Table 1).

Table 2 shows the same groups as Table 1 in relation to the type of pacemaker implanted and the duration of pacing inhibition.

As Tables 1 and 2 show, in 72 (35.1%) of the 205 cases studied transient pacing inhibition was observed.

In 38 of these 72 cases (first group) there was pacing inhibition by myopotentials generated mainly by the PM muscle. In 23 cases the pacing inhibition lasted for more than twice the pacing interval (long), while in the remaining 15 cases the inhibition lasted for less than two intervals (short). In one case with long inhibition the pacemaker was located superficially to the RA muscle.

In 19 of the 72 cases (second group) pacing inhibition was caused by myopotentials generated mainly by the RA (10 long and 9 short), although in 16 of these 19 cases the generator was located superficially to the PM.

In the remaining 15 cases (third group) the inhibition was evident as a clear synergetic effect from both muscle groups (12 long and 3 short). In all these 15 cases the generator was located superficially to the PM muscle.

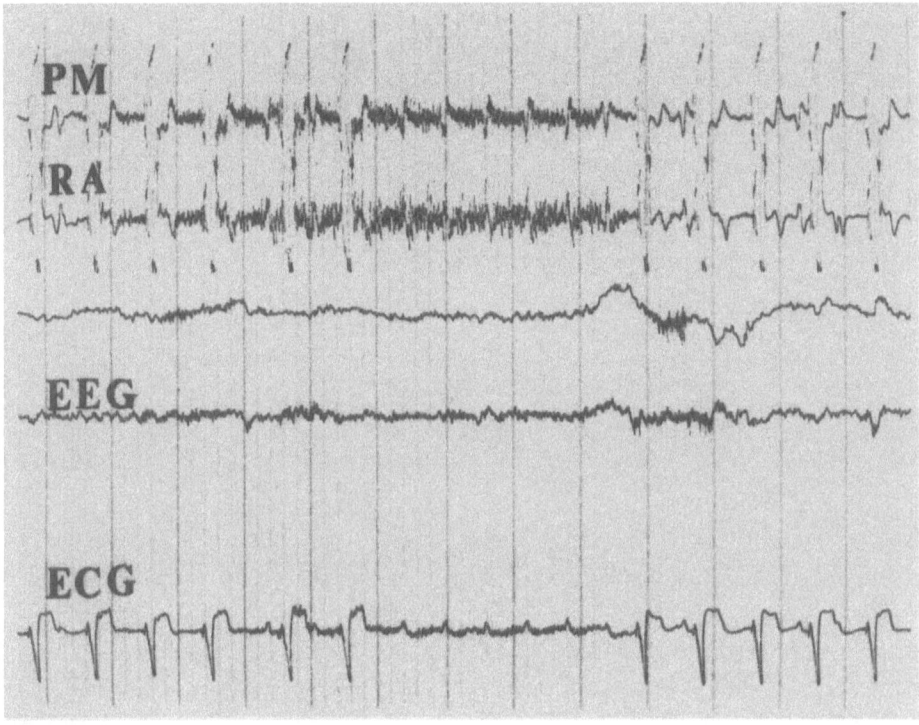

Fig. 1. Simultaneous recordings of myopotentials from Pectoralis Major (PM) and Rectus Abdominis (RA) muscles with electrocardiogram (ECG) in a case with dominant RA myopotentials although the pacemaker is located superficially to the PM muscle. Long pacing inhibition appears as the RA myopotentials increase. Sensitivity 2 mV/cm and recording speed 15 mm/sec.

Table 1. Site of pacemakers and source of inhibiting myopotentials.

Area of pacemaker location	No.	Pacing inhibition by myopotentials		Muscle group myopotentials dominant in pacing inhibition		
		No.	%	RA	PM	Synergy of PM and RA
Pectoralis Major (PM)	198	68	34.3	16	37	15
Rectus Abdominis (RA)	7	4	57.1	3	1	–
Total Number	205	72	35.1	19 (26.4%)	38 (52.8%)	15 (20.8%)

Among the total of 45 cases with long inhibition 18 exhibited pacing inhibition lasting between 2.5 and 8.5 seconds.

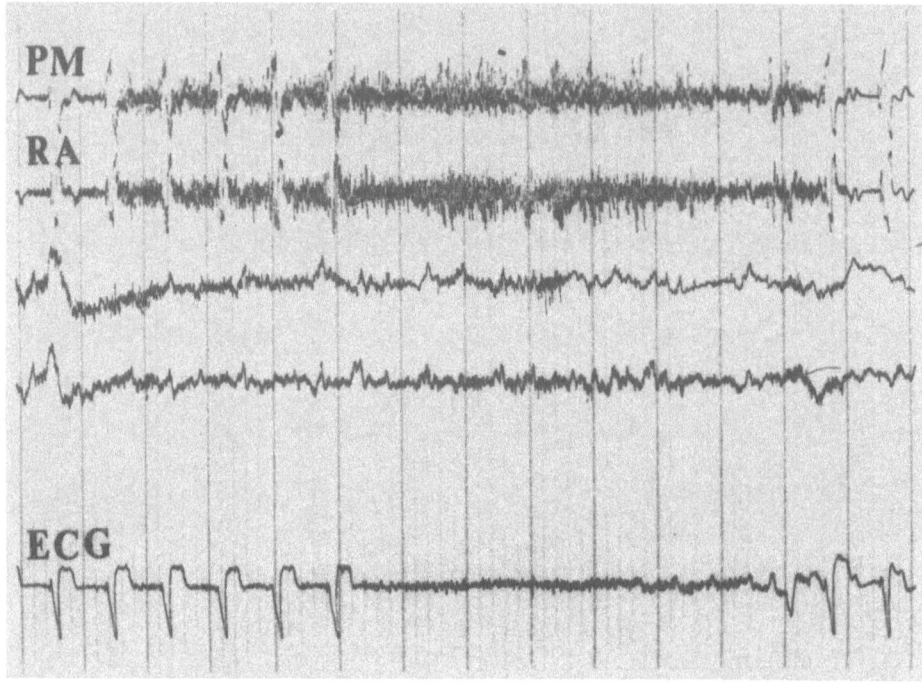

Fig. 2. Synergetic effect of myopotentials from PM and RA in a case with the pacemaker superficial to the PM muscle. The inhibition appears only after the simultaneous increase of myopotentials from both muscle groups. Sensitivity 2 mV/cm and recording speed 15 mm/sec.

Table 2. Origin of Myopotentials and Type of Pacemaker Affected.

Type	No. of implantations	Dominant RA myopotential inhibition long/short	Dominant PM myopotential inhibition long/short	RA and PM synergy long/short
Intermedics	120	6/4	15/12	11/3
Medtronic	45	1/2	2/1	–
General Electric	23	1/2	4/1	1/–
Siemens Elema	8	1/1	–	–
Telectronics	3	–	1/–	–
CPI	2	–	1/–	–
Digikon	2	–	–/1	–
Biotronik	1	–	–	–
Sorin	1	1/–	–	–
Total	205	10/9	23/15	12/3

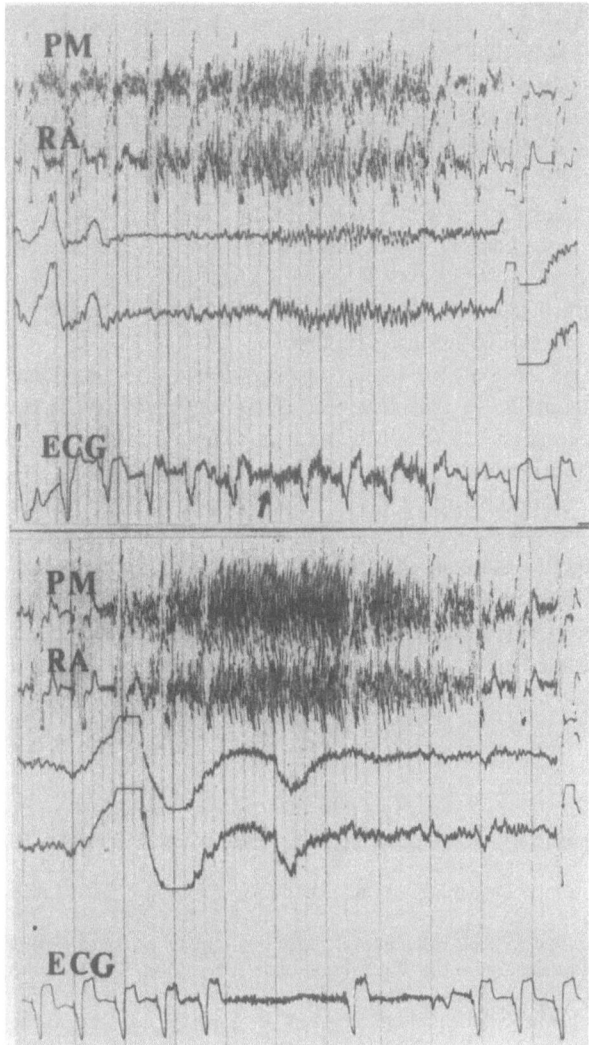

Fig. 3. Dominant PM myopotentials in a case with the pacemaker superficial to the RA muscle. Note (upper trace) the short inhibition by qualitatively almost equal myopotentials from the PM and RA muscles. As there is an increase of PM myopotentials (lower trace) a longer pacing inhibition appears. Sensitivity 1 mV/cm and recording speed 15 mm/sec.

Discussion

Our results show that pacing inhibition by myopotentials occurs in 35% of unipolar demand pacemakers, which results are in agreement with those reported by others (2, 10). The higher incidence of failure among those pacemakers implanted on the abdominal wall (4 out of 7) is worth considering, although the small number of cases does not permit us to draw any conclusions.

The results of this study corroborate the observations and conclusions reported by Gialafos et al [13] where paced patients exhibited symptoms of dizziness during postural changes which, although originally giving the impression of labyrinthine vertigo, proved to be due to inhibiting myopotentials generated by the RA, whether the pacemaker was located superficially to either the PM or the RA muscle.

The advantage of the simultaneous recordings employed in our study was that we were able to detect the origin of myopotentials and their contributory role in pacing inhibition. Thus, by means of this technique, our findings were classified into three main groups as shown in Table 1.

In the first group of 38 cases (37 over PM, 1 over RA) the pacing inhibition was caused by PM myopotentials. This is in agreement with previous observations (2, 3, 5, 10, 14). In the second group of 19 cases (16 over PM, 3 over RA) the RA was the main source of inhibiting myopotentials. In the third group of 15 cases (all over PM) the inhibition was evident only as a clear synergetic effect of both muscle groups.

From the above groups only the 38 cases in the first group conform to the "classical" type of inhibition by PM myopotentials. In the remaining thirty-four cases of the two other groups (47% of the failing pacers and 16.6% of the total cases tested) pacing inhibition appeared only with the contribution of the RA muscle.

Our results show that the results reported by others (2, 3, 5, 10, 14) who did not use double recording techniques and did not mention a contribution by the RA have resulted in an overestimation of the role of the PM as the main source of inhibiting myopotentials.

It is concluded that the RA muscle has always to be considered as a serious source of myopotentials which can interfere with the function of unipolar demand pacemakers, irrespective of whether they are located on the abdominal or thoracic wall.

References

1. Wirtzfeld A, Lampadius M, Ruprecht ED: Unterdrückung von Demandschrittmachern durch Muselpotentiale. Dtsch Med Wochensch 1972; 97: 61.
2. Mymin D, Cuddy TE, Sinha SN, Winter DA: Inhibition of demand pacemakers by skeletal muscle potential. JAMA 1973; 223: 527.
3. Wirtzfeld A, Lampadius M, Schmück L: The influence of muscle potentials on synchronised pacemakers. In: Cardiac Pacing: Proceedings of the 4th International Symposium, Van Gorcum, The Netherlands, 1973; 169–174.
4. Barold SS, Keller JW: Sensing problems with demand pacemakers. In: Samet P, ed, Cardiac Pacing. New York and London: Grune and Stratton, 1973; 385–412.
5. Olm OJ, Bruland H, Pedersen OM, Wearness E: Interference effect of myopotentials on function of unipolar demand pacemakers. Br Heart J 1974; 36: 77.
6. Wickam GG: Preventing myocardial inhibition of the unipolar demand pacemaker. In: Cardiac Pacing: Proceedings of the 5th International Symposium, Tokyo, 1976; 340–343.
7. Jacobs LJ, Kerzner JS, Diamond MA, Sprung CL: Myopotential inhibition of demand pacemakers: detection by ambulatory electrocardiography. Am Heart J 1981; 101: 346.
8. Furman S: Electromagnetic interference. From The Editor, Pace 1982; 5: 1.
9. Daly JE, Wite AA: Non-invasive analysis of simulated pacemaker failure available in multiprogrammable pulse generators. Pace 1982; 5: 4.
10. Secemsky SI, Hauser RG, Denes P, Edwards LM: Unipolar sensing of skeletal muscle interference and undersensing in 228 patients. Pace 1982; 5: 10.
11. Echeveria HJ, Luceri RM, Thurer RJ, Castellanos A: Myopotential inhibition of unipolar AV sequential (DVI) pacemaker. Pace 1982; 5: 20.
12. Gialafos J, Maillis A, Tsakiris M, Basiakos L, Skarpalezos S, Avgoustakis D: Inhibition of demand pacemaking by myopotentials. Hellenic Cardiological Review 1980; 21: 196.
13. Gialafos J, Maillis A, Basiakos L, Avgoustakis D: Rectus Abdominis as a source of myopotentials inhibiting demand pacemakers. Pace in press.

14. Levine PA, Klein MD: Myopotential inhibition of unipolar pacemakers: A disease of technologic progress. Editorial, Ann Int Med 1983; 98: 101.

Authors' address:
John Gialafos, M.D.
Department of Cardiology
Hippokration Hospital
114, Vas. Sophias Ave.
Athens 610,
Greece

Incidence and Significance of Muscle Potential Interference in Patients with Dual Chamber Pacemakers

M. Jost, M. Pfisterer, Doris Schelker, F. Burkart

Summary: To assess incidence, significance and mechanisms of muscle potential (MP) interference in dual chamber pacing, 33 consecutive patients (DVI 5 patients, VDD 6 patients, DDD 22 patients) were studied. MP interference was studied by stimulation manoeuvres, 24 hour Holter ECG monitoring and history of symptoms.

Stimulation manoeuvres revealed MP-interference in 42% of patients. Three patterns of interference were observed: 1. inhibition of atrial and ventricular impulses; 2. triggering of ventricular stimulation; 3. triggering and inhibition of pacemaker impulses. In the third group, the pattern of MP-interference varied with changing atrial sensitivity: in association with a high atrial sensitivity MP induced pacemaker triggering was seen whereas pacemaker inhibition was found with a low atrial sensitivity. In some patients, a mixed pattern of inhibition and triggering of ventricular stimulation was observed at high atrial sensitivities.

Despite this frequent laboratory finding, no episode of pacemaker interference due to MP could be detected during 24 hour Holter ECG monitoring and no patient complained of MP related symptoms.

Inhibition of demand pacemakers by skeletal muscle potentials has first been described by Wirtzfeld in 1972 (1). Since then, the incidence and significance of muscle potential interference during unipolar ventricular pacing (VVI, VVT) has been investigated by several authors (2–11). Inhibition of bipolar units by muscle potentials has also been reported (12–15).

In view of hemodynamic advantages associated with improvement in exercise tolerance and symptomatic benefit, dual chamber pacing is becoming more and more popular in patients with sick-sinus-syndrome and AV-block. Reports about muscle potential interference in dual chamber pacemakers (DVI, DDD, VDD), however, are still rare (6, 16). The purpose of the present study was, therefore, (a) to assess the incidence and significance of muscle potential interference in patients with dual chamber pacemakers (DVI, VDD, DDD) and (b) to describe the various interference patterns in patients with atrial synchronised pacemaker system (VDD, DDD).

Methods

33 consecutive patients with dual chamber pacemakers were prospectively evaluated for presence of muscle potential interference by stimulation manoeuvres in the laboratory, 24 hour Holter monitoring and history of symptoms. Patients' age ranged from 49 to 90 years, 16 were male and 17 female. The reason for implantation of the pacemaker was an AV-block in 24 patients and a sick-sinus-syndrome in 8 patients.

All patients had dual chamber pacemakers implanted subcutaneously in the right pectoral region and transvenous unipolar right atrial and right ventricular endocardial leads. The pulse generators included the following systems: DVI in 5 patients (Pacesetter AV

549

223), VDD in 6 patients (3 Medtronic ASVIP 2409 and 3 Medtronic 7100) and DDD in 22 patients (8 Medtronic 7000 and 14 Biotronik Diplos 03).

For study purposes the pulse generators were programmed to nominal and maximal ventricular as well as low and high atrial sensitivities.

Sensing of skeletal muscle potentials was assessed (1) by stimulation manoeuvres in the laboratory (2) by 24 hour Holter monitoring and (3) by history of symptoms. Stimulation manoeuvres in the laboratory included isometric hand-grip, pressing of one hand against the other, lifting of the right arm against resistance and pushing of the hand against the contralateral shoulder. These pectoral muscle exercises were performed during continuous recording of a six channel ECG (leads 1–3, aVR, aVL, aVF). During the 24 hour period of Holter monitoring, the patients performed routine daily activities; symptoms were recorded in a protocol. All ECG tracings were analysed manually by a cardiologist.

Results

Stimulation manoeuvres in the laboratory

Interference of the pacemaker with muscle potentials could be detected in 14 out of 33 patients (42%) during isometric pectoral muscle exercises at nominal ventricular sensitivity and various atrial sensitivities.

In 2 of 5 patients with DVI pacemakers, inhibition of atrial and ventricular impulses by muscle potentials could be provoked at nominal and maximal sensitivities.

Interference with muscle potentials was seen in 12 out of 28 patients with VDD or DDD pacemakers: in 6/14 patients with Biotronik Diplos 03, in 5/8 patients with Medtronic 7000, in 1/3 patients with Medtronic 7100 and in 0/3 patients with Medtronic 2409.

In these patients we could observe three different patterns of interference with muscle potentials:

1. Inhibition of atrial and ventricular impulses at various atrial sensitivities could be provoked by isometric exercises in 3 patients (atrial sensitivities 0.75 mV and 1.5 mV).
2. Acceleration of ventricular stimulation rate by atrial triggering, without inhibition, could be registered in one patient at an atrial sensitivity of 0.75 mV.
3. Triggering and inhibition of ventricular response to muscle potentials was detected in 8 patients. In these patients, the pattern of interference varied with changing atrial sensitivities:

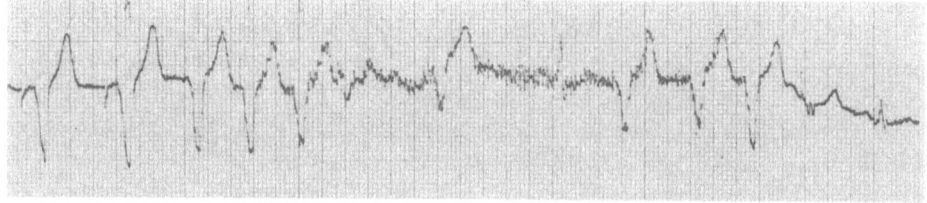

Fig. 1. Alternating acceleration and inhibition of ventricular stimulation (mixed pattern of atrial triggering and ventricular inhibition) by skeletal muscle interference (Biotronik Diplos 03).

a) alternating acceleration and inhibition of ventricular stimulation (mixed pattern of atrial triggering and ventricular inhibition) was observed in 3 out of the 8 patients (atrial sensitivity of 1.25 mV) (Fig. 1).

b) In 5 patients muscle potentials induced acceleration of the ventricular stimulation rate by atrial triggering in association with high atrial sensitivities (1.25 mV and 0.75 mV, respectively). At lower settings of atrial sensitivity (2.5 mV and 1.5 mV, respectively) isometric pectoral muscle exercises resulted mainly in inhibition of ventricular impulses. This interference pattern is illustrated by Fig. 2.

24 hour Holter ECG monitoring

Despite the frequent finding of muscle potential interference with isometric pectoral muscle exercises in the laboratory, no episode of pacemaker interference due to muscle potentials could be detected by 24 hour Holter monitoring during routine daily activities. In addition, none of our patients with dual chamber pacemakers complained of syncope or dizziness associated with exercises of the right arm or shoulder.

Discussion

Muscle potentials due to contraction of pectoral muscles may interfere with a normally functioning unipolar pacemaker. In their first report of skeletal muscle interference of pacemakers, Wirtzfeld (1) described inhibition of ventricular stimulation in unipolar VVI pacemakers as well as triggering of ventricular impulses in VVT systems. Since this original description, skeletal muscle interference of unipolar VVI pacemakers have been investigated extensively (2–11). Interference could be demonstrated in 11% to 85% of patients by isometric pectoral muscle exercise in the laboratory. Factors such as patient po-

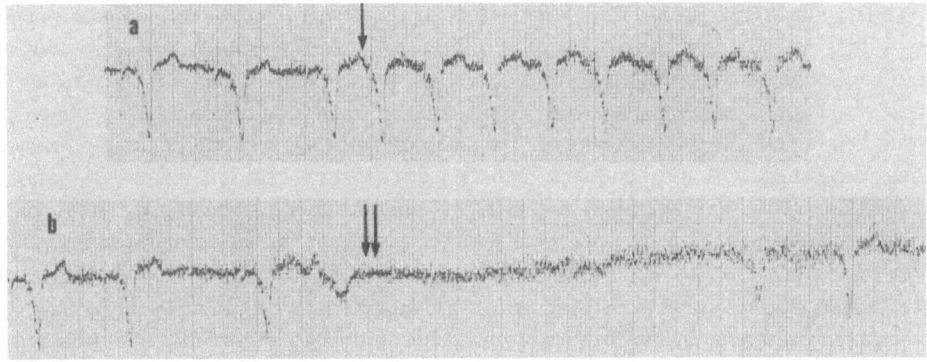

Fig. 2. a) Acceleration of ventricular stimulation rate by atrial triggering in association with atrial sensitivity of 1.25 mV (Biotronik Diplos 03).
Fig. 2. b) Inhibition of ventricular stimulation by skeletal muscle interference in the same patient (atrial sensitivity 2.5 mV).

pulation studied (age, profession, pacemaker dependency), sensing characteristics of the pacemakers used and methods applied to detect skeletal muscle interference in the laboratory may explain differences between the various studies. In addition, amplitudes (up to 10 mV) and frequencies (10–200 Hz) of muscle potentials may vary widely (8). Using systematic 24 hour Holter monitoring, Secemsky and co-workers (11) found skeletal muscle interference of VVI pacemakers in 14%; in some patients, interference due to inhibition of the pacemaker system was symptomatic. Interference of bipolar pacemakers by skeletal muscle potentials is comparatively rare (12–15). Inhibition of bipolar systems has been described in cases of battery leakage (14) and sensing of diaphragmatic myopotentials, possibly related to electrode perforation (15).

Dual chamber pacing has become an alternative to VVI pacing. Hemodynamic advantages, improvement of exercise tolerance and symptomatic benefit for many patients due to this pacing mode are now well recognised. A reevaluation of skeletal muscle interference in dual chamber pacing seemed mandatory for several reasons: 1. in dual chamber pacing, unipolar electrodes are used almost exclusively; 2. in the atrium, higher sensitivity levels are necessary to guarantee atrial tracking; 3. depending on the sensed event, acceleration and/or inhibition of ventricular stimulation is possible in DDD/VDD pacemaker systems. A higher incidence of skeletal muscular interference and more complex interference patterns could thus be expected in dual chamber compared to VVI pacing.

In the present study, skeletal muscle interference was found in 42% of patients with dual chamber pacemakers. This finding relates to standard muscular exercise in the laboratory using nominal settings of ventricular sensitivity. By more extensive pectoral muscle exercises and in a younger population, the incidence of muscle potential interference may have been even higher. The pattern of muscle potential interference in patients with DVI systems as previously described by Echeverria and co-workers (16), is essentially the same as in VVI pacemakers. In contrast, different patterns of muscle potential interference were recognised in VDD/DDD pacemakers in this study, depending on a) sensitivity levels of atrial and ventricular sensing circuits, b) relative sensitivity levels of atrial and ventricular electrodes, c) characteristics of pacemaker inhibition by ventricular events (committed ventricular stimulation in Biotronik Diplos 03; inhibition by ventricular events following atrial stimulation-sensing in other models used) and d) amplitude of muscle potentials.

Acceleration of ventricular stimulation by atrial triggering is expected if muscle potentials interfere only with the atrial sensing circuit (high atrial sensitivity, low amplitude of muscle potentials). Total inhibition of atrial and ventricular output may occur due to muscle potential interference with the ventricular sensing circuit if muscle potential amplitudes are high enough to be sensed by the ventricular sensing circuit (high amplitude of muscle potentials). If atrial and ventricular sensitivities are set at different levels, various amplitudes of muscle potentials may interfere either with the atrial sensing circuit only (triggering of ventricular stimulation) or with the ventricular sensing circuit (inhibition of ventricular stimulation), resulting in a mixed pattern of acceleration and inhibition of ventricular impulses (Fig. 1). In the present investigation, all these different patterns of pacemaker interference due to muscle potentials could be recorded. In certain patients (mainly with Biotronik Diplos 03 pacemakers, a DDD system with committed ventricular stimulation), atrial triggering with acceleration of ventricular stimulation due to muscle potentials was detected if atrial sensitivity was high. With low atrial sensitivities, inhibition of ventricular stimulation could be provoked due to interference of myopotentials with the ventricular sensing circuit. In these systems, low ventricular sensitivity should be chosen in case of symptomatic muscle potential interference to prevent complete pacemaker inhibition.

In this study, muscle potential interference was found only in the laboratory. It was not detected by 24 hour Holter ECG monitoring during normal daily activities on any of our patients. It has to be noted, however, that our study population was relatively old (40–90 years) with few still working; in younger and more physically active patients with dual chamber pacemakers, the clinical significance of skeletal muscle interference might be more important.

References

1. Wirtzfeld A, Lampadius M, Schmuck L: Unterdrückung von demand-Schrittmachern durch Muskelpotentiale. Dtsch Med Wschr 1982; 97: 61–66.
2. Andersen ST, Pitt A, Withford JA, Davis BB: Interference with function of unipolar pacemaker due to muscle potential. J Thorac cardiovasc Surg 1976; 71: 698–703.
3. Berger R, Jacobs W: Myopotential inhibition of demand pacemakers: etiologic, diagnostic and therapeutic considerations. Pace 1979; 2: 596–602.
4. Breivik K, Ohm OJ: Myopotential inhibition of unipolar QRS-inhibited pacemaker assessed by ambulatory Holter monitoring of the electrocardiogram. Pace 1980; 3: 470–478.
5. Hurvitz RJ, Tucker BL, Lindermith GG, Stiles RR, Hughes RK, et al: Skeletal muscle potential inhibition of demand pacemakers. In: Proceedings of the 6th International Symposium of Cardiac Pacing. Montreal, 1978; p 35.
6. Jost M, Schelker D, Steinmann E, Hoffmann A, Burkart F: Inhibierung und Triggerung von Herzschrittmachern durch Muskelpotentiale. Schweiz med Wschr 1982; 112: 1588–1591.
7. Mymin D, Cuddy IE, Sinha SN, Winter DA: Inhibition of demand cardiac pacemakers by skeletal muscle potentials. J Amer med Ass 1973; 233: 527–529.
8. Ohm OJ, Bruland H, Pedersen OM, Waerness E: Interference effect of myopotentials on function of unipolar demand pacemakers. Brit Heart J 1974; 36: 77–84.
9. Piller LW, Kennelly BM: Myopotential inhibition of demand pacemakers. Chest 1974; 66: 418–420.
10. Vrints C, Lambrecht A, Bossard L, Snoeck J: Myopotential inhibition of unipolar ventricular inhibited pacemakers: prevention by an insulated-sheat. Acta cardiol 1981; 36: 167–174.
11. Secemsky SI, Hauser RG, Denes P, Edwards LM: Unipolar sensing abnormalities: incidence and clinical significance of skeletal muscle interference and undersensing in 228 patients. Pace 1982; 5: 10–19.
12. Widlansky S, Zipes DP: Suppression of a ventricular inhibited bipolar pacemaker by skeletal muscle activity. J Electrocardiol 1974; 7: 371–374.
13. Barold SS, Ong LS, Falkoff LD, Heinle RA: Inhibition of bipolar demand pacemaker by diaphragmatic myopotentials. Circulation 1977; 56: 679–683.
14. Amikam S, Peleg H, Lemer J, Riss E: Myopotential inhibition of a bipolar pacemaker caused by electrode insulation defect. Br Heart J 1977; 39: 1279–1281.
15. El Gamal M, Van Gelder B: Suppression of an external demand pacemaker by diaphragmatic myopotential: a sign of electrode perforation? Pace 1979; 2: 191–195.
16. Echeverria HJ, Luceri RM, Thures RJ, Castellanos A: Myopotential inhibition of unipolar AV sequential (DVI) pacemaker. Pace 1982; 5: 20–22.

Authors' address:
M. Pfisterer, M.D.
Division of Cardiology
Department of Internal Medicine
University Hospital
CH-4031 Basle/Switzerland

Influence of Myopotentials on Implanted DDD-M Pacemakers

L. M. van Gelder, M. I. H. El Gamal

Summary: The influence of myopotentials on pacemaker function was studied in a group of 32 patients with implanted DDD-M pacemakers. (Medtronic 7000, Versatrax.) Twenty four patients had their pulse generator implanted subcutaneously in the pectoral region (group A), seven had their pulse generator implanted in the abdominal region (group B).

The influence of myopotentials was assessed by instructing the patient to contract his pectoral or abdominal muscles, while the electrocardiogram was continuously recorded. When the ventricular input sensitivity was set at 2.5 mV the following observations were made in group A:
1. Total inhibition of the pulse generator in 11 pts (46%)
2. Acceleration of the ventricular stimulation rate by artificial atrial triggering in 6 pts. (25%)
3. Alternating inhibition and acceleration 5 pts (21%)
4. Initiation of artificial circus movement tachycardia (A.C.M.T.) in 1 pt (4%)
5. No influence in 1 pt. (4%)

Three out of the eleven patients with total inhibition were symptomatic. When the ventricular sensitivity was programmed to 5 mV, inhibition was only observed in two out of the eleven patients. The remaining 9 now showed acceleration of the stimulation rate by artificial atrial triggering. This resulted in A.C.M.T. in 2 patients, one sustained and one self terminating. In group B, pulse generators were not affected during contracture of the abdominal muscles.

Since the first publication of Wirtzfeld (1) in 1972 there have been several reports on the influence of skeletal myopotentials on implanted pacemakers. The majority of these papers describe the incidence and clinical significance of undesired inhibition in unipolar single chamber pacemaker (2, 3, 4, 5, 6, 7, 8, 9, 10). There are only a few reports on the influence of myopotentials on bipolar pacing systems (11, 12, 13, 14). There is a single case report of myopotential inhibition of a unipolar AV-sequential (DVI) pacemaker (15), but the mechanism of inhibition actually does not differ from that in VVI pacemakers.

Because of the dual sensing mechanism in DDD-pacemakers and the different mode of reponse to a sensed event in the atrial and ventricular input amplifiers, there are various modes of reaction after sensing myopotentials. This communication describes the influence of myopotentials studied in a group of 32 patients with implanted DDD-pacemakers.

Patient material and methods

Thirty-two patients, 19 males and 13 females with implanted DDD-M pacemakers (Medtronic 7000, Versatrax) were investigated during a regular out patient follow up. The mean age was 63.5 years (range 45–80). Twenty four patients had their pulse generator implanted subcutaneously in the pectoral region, twenty two in the right, two in the left (Group A). All patients had transvenous atrial and ventricular leads, implanted via the subclavian vein.

555

Seven patients had their pulse generators implanted subcutaneously in the upper abdominal region. The majority of these patients had epicardial atrial and ventricular leads, implanted during open heart surgery (Group B). Influence of skeletal muscle potentials was assessed by instructing the patient to contract his pectoral or abdominal muscles, while a 3-channel electrocardiogram was continuously recorded. The power of muscle contraction was not calibrated and strongly depended on the physical state of the patient. The patients were encouraged to use their maximal strength during this exercise. All pacemakers were programmed in the DDD-mode. The programmed upper rate, lower rate and A-V interval were unchanged.

The atrial sensitivity was programmed to a sufficiently high level to ensure proper sensing of intrinsic atrial depolarisation. The atrial input sensitivity was at 0.75 mV for the majority of the patients. The ventricular input sensitivity was programmed to 2.5 mV for all patients. Patients who exhibited complete inhibition during contraction of their pectoral muscles, underwent reprogramming of the ventricular input sensitivity to 5.0 mV and the exercise was repeated.

Results

In patients with pacemakers implanted subcutaneously in the pectoral region (group A), the following observations were made when the ventricular input sensitivity was programmed to 2.5 mV.

1. Eleven patients (46%) showed total inhibition of the pacemaker during contraction of the pectoral muscle. During monitoring 3 of the 11 patients complained of dizziness at the time of inhibition. Pauses of 2.5, 3.6 and 4.2 s were recorded.
2. In 6 patients (25%) acceleration of the ventricular stimulation by artificial atrial triggering was observed (Fig. 1). In 5 of the 6 patients the ventricular stimulation rate was equal to the programmed upper tracking rate, in a single patient the acceleration was

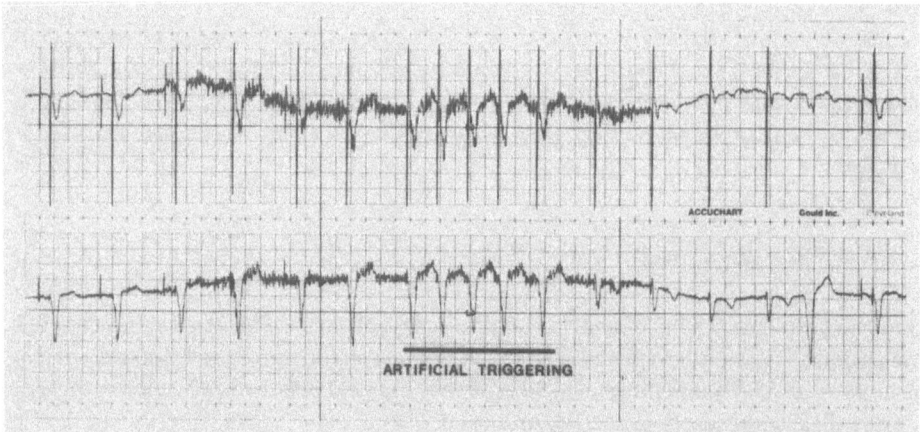

Fig. 1. Two channel ecg tracing showing acceleration of the ventricular stimulation rate by artificial atrial triggering during contraction of the pectoral muscle.

below the upper tracking rate. All patients were completely asymptomatic during the acceleration of the stimulation rate.

3. In 5 patients there were alternating short periods of inhibition and acceleration by artificial triggering. None of these patients were symptomatic (Fig. 2).

4. One patient developed an artificial circus movement tachycardia (16) by artificial atrial triggering (Fig. 3). The tachycardia was sustained and had to be interrupted by application of a magnet. During A.C.M.T. the patient was symptomatic and complained of palpitations (17).

5. Pacemaker function was not affected by contraction of the pectoral muscles in a single patient.

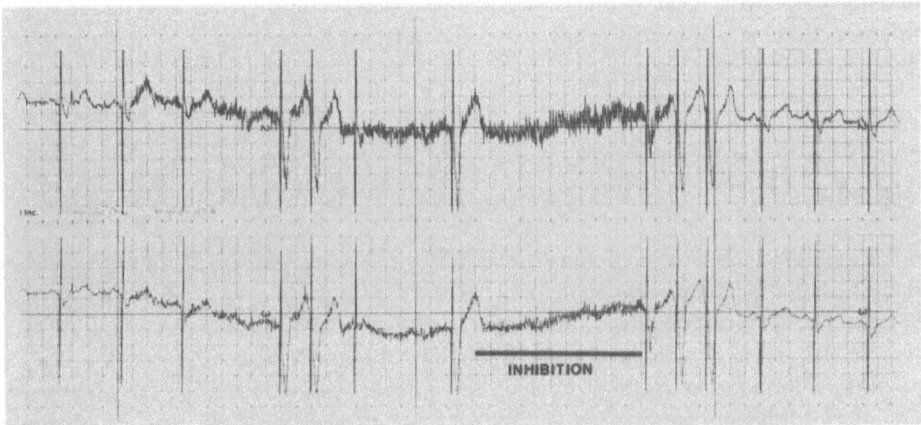

Fig. 2. Two channel ecg tracing showing alternating inhibition and artificial triggering during contraction of the pectoral muscle.

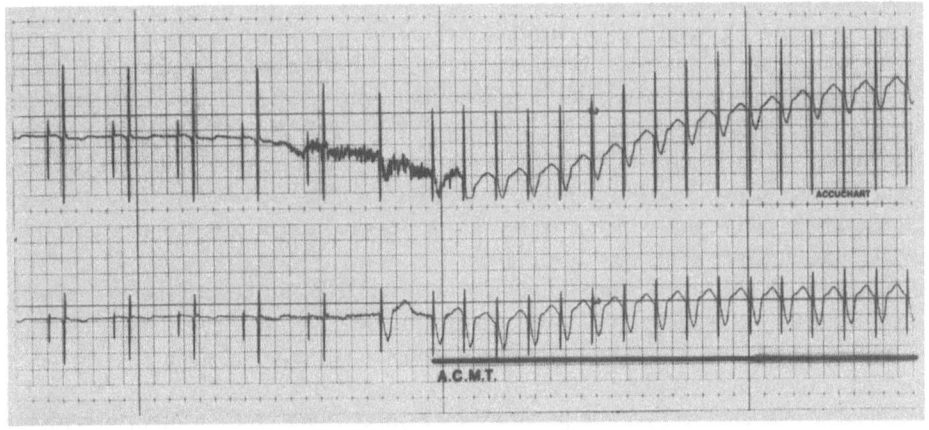

Fig. 3. Two channel ecg tracing showing initiation of artificial circus movement tachycardia after contraction of the pectoral muscle.

557

After these observations the ventricular sensitivity was programmed to 5 mV in the 11 patients, that showed inhibition of the pulse generator during contraction of the pectoral muscle.

Subsequently the same exercise was repeated while a 3-channel electrocardiogram was recorded. Inhibition was now observed in only 2 patients who were asymptomatic. The remaining patients showed acceleration of the ventricular stimulation rate by artificial atrial triggering.

The three patients who complained of dizziness during contraction of the pectoral muscle at 2.5 mV ventricular sensitivity, were asymptomatic when the exercise was repeated at 5.0 mV ventricular input sensitivity.

Two of them showed acceleration of the stimulation rate and one exhibited a short asymptomatic period of inhibition (1.4 s). One of the three patients had no ventricular sensing at 5.0 mV. After changing the ventricular sensitivity to 5.0 mV, two patients developed A.C.M.T. One was sustained, and the other self terminating after about 15 s.

In group B, none of the pulse generators were affected by contraction of the abdominal muscles.

Discussion

Since the introduction of non competitive pulse generators, numerous reports have been published on the influence myopotentials.

Wirtzfeld et al. and Mymin et al. described in 1972 and 1973 the phenomenon of inhibition and triggering of unipolar R-wave inhibited (VVI) and R-wave triggered (VVT) pulse generators. Provocative methods to study the influence of myopotentials in patients with unipolar pacemakers showed that pacemaker function was affected in 11–85% of the patients.

Only a small number however were symptomatic during these manoeuvres. The influence of myopotentials on dual chamber pulse generators with sensing through the atrial as well as the ventricular lead has not been previously described. Our results indicate that there is a variable reponse to muscular contraction, due to dual sensing properties of these pulse generators. The incidence of disturbance of pacemaker function is high (96%) for patients with a pulse generator implanted in the pectoral region. The percentage of symptomatic patients exhibiting inhibition with a nominal (2.5 mV) input sensitivity is relatively high (3 out of 11, 27%).

Inhibition with resulting symptoms can easily be prevented by programming the ventricular input sensitivity to a less sensitive level, which resulted however in loss of ventricular sensing in one of our patients. A wider range of programming ventricular sensitivity would make it easier to manage this problem.

Acceleration of the ventricular stimulation rate caused by artificial atrial triggering by myopotentials will be difficult to avoid, because of the high input sensitivity of the atrial amplifier. This however did not result in symptoms in our group of patients, with the exception of the patients who developed pacemaker mediated tachycardia.

Pacemaker mediated tachycardia provoked by myopotentials is still a problem with this pulse generator because of the short atrial refractory period after ventricular pacing (155 ms).

The incidence of pacemaker mediated tachycardia is higher if one tries to avoid inhibition of the system by changing the ventricular input sensitivity from 2.5 to 5 mV. With pulse generators having a longer atrial refractory period or a programmable atrial refractory the problem of pacemaker mediated tachycardia can be prevented in the near future. Although the influence of myopotentials on pulse generators implanted in the abdominal region is negligible, it is not a favourable site of implantation because of the widespread use of the subclavian route for implantation of dual chamber systems.

Acknowledgement

We gratefully acknowledge the support of the Foundation for Applied Cardiovascular Research, Eindhoven, The Netherlands and Mrs. J. van Kemenade-Driesen for the preparation of this manuscript.

References

1. Wirtzfeld A, Lampadius M, and Ruprecht EO: Unterdrückung von Demand-Schrittmachern durch Muskelpotentiale. Dtsch Med Wschr 1972; 97: 61.
2. Mymin D, Cuddy TW, Sinha SN, and Winter DA: Inhibition of demand pacemakers by skeletal muscle potentials. JAMA, 1973; 223: 527.
3. Piller LW, and Kennelly BM: Myopotential inhibition of demand pacemakers. Chest, 1974; 66: 418.
4. Ohm O-J, Brulnov DH, Pedersen OM, and Waerness E: Interference effect of myopotentials on function of unipolar demand pacemakers. Br. Heart J, 1974; 36: 77.
5. Anderson ST, Pitt A, Whitford JA, and Davis BB: Interference with function of unipolar pacemaker due to muscle potentials. J Thorac Cardiovasc Surg, 1976; 71: 698.
6. Ohm O-J, Hammer E, And Mörkrid L: Biological signals and their characteristics as a cause of pacemaker malfunction. In, Y Watanabe (Ed): Cardiac Pacing, Amsterdam/Oxford, Excerpta Medica, 1976; p. 401.
7. Breivik K, and Ohm O-J: Myopotential inhibition of unipolar QRS-inhibited (VVI) pacemakers assessed by ambulatory Holter monitoring of the electrocardiogram. Pace 1980; 3: 370.
8. Berger R, and Jacobs W: Myopotential inhibition of demand pacemakers: etiologic, diagnostic and therapeutic conclusions. Pace 1982; 2: 596.
9. Jacobs LJ, Kerzner JS, Diamond MA, Berlin HF and Sprung CL: Pacemaker inhibition by myopotentials detected by Holter monitoring. Pace 1982; 5: 30.
10. Secemsky SI, Hauser RG, Denes P and Edwards LM: Unipolar sensing abnormalities: Incidence and clinical significance of skeletal muscle interference and undersensing in 228 patients. Pace 1982; 5: 10.
11. Widlansky S, and Zipes DP: Suppression of a ventricular inhibition bipolar pacemaker by skeletal muscle activity. J Electrocardiol 1974; 7: 371.
12. Barold SS, Ong LS, Falkoff MD and Heinle RA: Inhibition of bipolar demand pacemakers by diaphragmatic myopotentials. Circulation 1977; 56: 679.
13. Amikam S, Peleg H, Lemer J, and Riss E: Myopotential inhibition of a bipolar pacemaker caused by electrode insulation defect. Br Heart J 1977; 39: 1279.
14. El Gamal MIH, and Van Gelder LM: Suppression of an external demand pacemaker by diaphragmatic myopotentials: A sign of electrode perforation? Pace 1979; 2: 191.
15. Echeverria HJ, Luceri RM, Thurrer RJ, and Castellanos A: Myopotential inhibition of unipolar AV sequential (DVI) pacemaker. Pace 1982; 5: 20.
16. Den Dulk K, Lindemans FW, Bär FW, and Wellens HJ: Pacemaker related tachycardias. Pace 1982; 5: 476.

17. Bathen J, Gundersen T, and Forfang K: Tachycardias related to atrial synchronous ventricular pacing. Pace 1982; 5: 471.

Authors' address:
Dr. L. M. van Gelder
Department of Cardiology,
Catharina Hospital, Michelangelolaan 2,
NL-5623 EJ Eindhoven,
The Netherlands

Early "Exit Block" or "Late" Myocardial Perforation? Clinician's Dilemma and What to Do?

M. Pieniak, T. Kraska, G. Opelski, R. Steckiewicz

Summary: We found eight cases of late perforations, i.e., up to several days after implantation had taken place, in 15 documented myocardial perforations, by intracardiac electrodes (out of a total of 655 new intracardiac insertions). These are analyzed in this study. In five of these patients, the same electrode was repositioned satisfactorily; in two patients, electrodes with more flexible leads, were introduced, and the former were removed. No signs of cardiac tamponade were observed. In one case, an "exit block" had been diagnosed and, after prednisone therapy was found to be ineffective, reoperation was attempted in the third week after insertion. Perforation was proved by a high threshold, ST elevation in an intracardiac electrogram and by resistance while trying to remove the electrode. It was finally abandoned, and a new electrode was inserted. An interesting case involved a 69 year old man, with brady-tachy syndrome, in whom ineffective pacing and undersensing appeared on the eleventh postoperative day. Effective pacing and normal sensing reappeared on the thirteenth day, without any pharmacological or surgical intervention. We concluded from this experience, that presumably in some cases that are recognized and treated as "exit block", the true cause of ineffective pacing may be late perforation of the right ventricular wall. In such cases, early reoperation is preferred to prednisone therapy.

Statement of Purpose

The purpose of this study is to give support to the hypothesis that a "late perforation" of the right ventricular wall may occur, even several days after implantation of an intracardiac electrode, and may be erroneously diagnosed and treated as a classical "exit block". This hypothesis is based on the analysis of the clinical course of the eight patients, and it is proved by intracardiac electrogram registrations taken while removing the electrodes.

Material and Methods

Three models of intracardiac electrodes were used in our study: Biotronik IE-85-K-10-0, Tesla LES 165, and *Vitatron Mip* 2147 LOEs. These were implanted into 655 patients. In each case, after passing the tricuspid valve, the stylet of lead was removed some 5 cm to avoid "acute perforation". All the necessary threshold measurements (ERA-2, Biotronik) and intracardiac registrations (Mingograf 34, Elema) were performed without a stylet. Oscillosynchroscopic examination was used as a routine during the postoperative period. X-ray examinations, in two projections (posteroanterior and lateral), were performed in each case, at the time of suspicion of perforation.

Out of 655 new intracardiac insertions, we found 15 perforations of the right ventricular wall. Eight cases of "late perforation" underwent special alteration.

For the purposes of this study, we define a " late perforation" of the right ventricular wall when an ineffective pacing appears after an intracardiac electrode had been placed in the apex of the right ventricle, and its correct fixation was proved by fluoroscopic TV

561

control, threshold measurement and intracardiac electrogram registration, the electrode fixed at the entrance of the vein, and the pacemaker implanted in its pocket. Thus, a "late perforation" depends, in our understanding, on a steady "interplay" between the electrode diameter, shape, and flexibility of the lead, which determines the force imposed on the right ventricular wall at the point of fixation, and the mechanical properties of the contracting wall itself.

Results

At the time of the first insertion of an intracardiac electrode, we did not find areas of diminished excitability in the right ventricular apex in any of our patients. None had histories of myocardial infarctions. The diagnosis of "late perforation" was established in seven cases, when all characteristic changes were present in a constant, intracardiac registration, while removing the electrode: the appearance and then disappearance of ST elevation and with the return of the electrogram to a normal right ventricular pattern (1). At this time, X-rays showed no signs suggestive of perforation.

In one case (patient J. M. 74), after appearance of ST elevation together with some mechanical resistance when we attempted to remove the electrode, we concluded that deeper penetration into the myocardium probably had taken place (involving the silicone conus), and we discontinued removal. Another electrode was inserted.

The clinical course of these patients is summarized in Table 1.

Discussion

The problem we defined as a "late perforation" of the right ventricular wall appeared in our pacemaker center with the introduction of some models of standard intracardiac electrodes with less flexible electrode leads. The clinical courses of the patients presented in Table 1 demonstrates the clinician's diagnostic and therapeutic dilemma arising when ineffective pacing and, very often, undersensing, appear in an early postimplantation period and available diagnostic techniques do not answer the question of why the pacing is ineffective. Usually, we think first about displacement of the electrode but an X-ray can easily exclude this possibility. Then we are apt to consider "microdisplacement" a diagnosis which is rather difficult and which involves the determining of what is required in the diagnosis of inexcitable endocardium. We have nover proved "microdisplacement" as a cause of ineffective pacing. A recent myocardial infarction involving the area under the electrode, in the early postoperative period, can explain ineffective pacing, but this was not the case with our patients.

Why not a "late perforation" of the right ventricular wall? This is probably the true "microdisplacement" of the intracardiac electrode slowly perforating the myocardium.

Because the critical current density (J_{Th}) needed to depolarize a myocardial tissue should be about 0.05 ma/mm², or 10 ms of the applied current (1) of presently available pacemakers, the distance ($r + \Delta$) from the centre of the electrode within which the depolarization is possible, achieves approximately 4 mm according to the equation (3):

Table 1.

Patient	Electrode Model	Initial ST Elevation (mV)	Initial Threshold (V)	Signs of Dilatation of right Ventricle (−) (+) (++)	Loss of Capture (postoperative day)	Undersensing (−) (+)	Prednisone Treatment 60 mg/$\frac{per}{day}$	Reoperation (day)	Final solution	Follow-up
M.M. ♀ 73. tachy-brady	TESLA LES 165	9.1	0.58	+	7	+	4 days	12	New electrode inserted (biotronic IE-85-K-10-O) LES 165 removed	o.k.
A.S. ♂ 81. tachy-brady	TESLA LES 165	8.2	0.6	++	4	+ intermittent	3 days	7	Reposition ot the same electrode	o.k.
J.M. ♀ 74. II/III degree A–V Block	TELSA LES 165	6.3	0.82	+	6	−	11 days	18	New electrode of the same model inserted (the former LES 165 abandoned)	o.k.
A.S. ♀ 69. intermittent CHB	VITATRON MIP 2147 LOE-S	12	0.48	+	9 intermittent	+ intermittent	12 days	21	Reposition of the same electrode	o.k.
N.L. ♀ 63. intermittent CHB	VITATRON MIP-2147 LOE-S	7.2	0.6	+	7 intermittent	+ intermittent	NO	8	Reposition ot the same electrode	o.k.
H.G. ♀ 60. tachy-brady	VITATRON MIP-2147 LOE-S	7	0.46	++	6	+	NO	7	Reposition of the same electrode	o.k.
A.O. ♂ 60. II/III degree A–V block	VITATRON MIP-2147 LOE-S	2.6	0.58	−	6	+ intermittent	NO	7	Reposition of the same electrode	o.k.
A.R. ♀ 83. CHB 6971–65)	TESLA LES 165	6.6	0.8	−	14 intermittent	−	NO	19	New electrode (inserted (Medtronic)	o.k.

$$/ r + \Delta / = \left(\frac{I}{J_{TH} \times 4\pi}\right)^{1/2} = \left(\frac{10}{0.05 \times 4\pi}\right)^{1/2} \approx 4 \text{ mm}$$

where: r – is the radius of the electrode

Δ – is the difference between the radius of the electrodes (r) and the radius of a spherical surface depending on the applied current (I).

The values of Δ for the electrode used in this study exceed 2,5 mm.

This means that even in the case of a perforation of the right ventricular myocardium, when the front of the electrode opposes the epicardial layer, the effective depolarization may still be present, constantly or intermittently. The final result depends probably on the thickening of the epicardium due to a fibrous tissue formation which sometimes prevents a progression of perforation. When the epicardial layer is perforated, probably the silicon rubber conus at the tip of electrode creates additional resistance.

We believe that the diagnostic "puzzle" of the 69 year old man mentioned in the summary, in whom intermittent, ineffective pacing and undersensing were observed between the eleventh and the thirteenth days after implantation, and disappeared without any pharmacological or surgical intervention, can best be explained by the "late" subendocardial perforation (a steady state was achieved when progression of perforation was stopped). The electrode used was a Vitatron 2147 LOE-S. Since the time when the summaries had been sent to the Symposium, we observed another patient who was 59 years old, with intermittent complete heart block, in whom intermittent ineffectiveness of pacing and undersensing appeared between the eight and eleventh days after electrode insertion (Vitatron 2147 LOE-S). Normal pacing and sensing returned without any intervention.

"Late" right ventricular wall perforation should be suspected when the loss of capture is observed in the first week and an X-ray does not show any evidence of dislocation of the electrode. In our opinion the operation, with necessary threshold measurements and electrogram registrations, is indicated as a method of choice.

In the second or third week after an electrode insertion, a true "exit block" is theoretically possible, thus prednisone therapy may be justified (2). We suggest, however, that this therapy should not be extended beyond four to five days, and that the patient be reoperated on if pacing and sensing does not return to normal. In such cases, we sometimes observe the patients, without prednisone therapy and under careful monitoring for a few days, before the decision of reoperation is made. This is possible when the patient's own cardiac rhythm is sufficient.

Conclusions

1. "Late perforation" of the right ventricular wall may be the true cause of ineffective pacing in some cases which are recognized and treated as an early "exit block".
2. In cases when "late perforation" is suspected, reoperation is justified more frequently than prednisone therapy.

References

1. Barold SS, Center S: Electrocardiographic diagnosis of perforation of the heart by pacing catheter electrode. Amer J Cardiol 1969; 24: 274.

2. Mowry FM, Judge RD, Preston TA, Morris JD: Identification and management of exit block in patients with implanted pacemakers. Circulation 1965; 32: 157.
3. Tarjan PP: Engineering aspects of implantable cardiac pacemakers. In P Samet (Ed): Cardiac Pacing, Grune and Stratton, New York 1973: 47.

Authors' address:
M. Pieniak, M.D.
Department of Cardiology
Medical Academy in Warsaw
4, Lindley'a, St. Build 3
02-005, Warsaw, Poland

Syncope in Pacemaker Patients: Diagnostic Value of Dynamic Electrocardiography

Leopoldo Bianconi, Maria Ambrosini, Roberto Serdoz, Salvatore Greco,
Giuseppe Saba, Mauro Mennuni, Michele Pistolese

Summary: We permanently electrostimulated 581 patients for symptomatic bradyarrhythmias in our institution during 1980–82. After PM implantation, during a mean follow-up period of 14 months, 40 pts. (6.9%) showed recurrence of syncopal or presyncopal episodes (SE), whose origins were not clarified by clinical examination, ECG or pacemaker control. All of these patients underwent dynamic electrocardiogram (DECG) for 24 or 48 hours.

During DECG 20 patients (50%) had syncopal episodes. In 15 patients (37.5%) the symptoms were related to: myopotential inhibition (3), insufficient pacing rate in programmable pacemakers (2), failure of pacemaker to capture (1), paroxysmal supraventricular tachycardia (2), or ventricular tachycardia (7); in the other five patients (12.5%) DECG was negative. Twenty patients were asymptomatic during DECG and six patients (15%) had negative DECG. Pathological events were found in 14 patients (35%). They were: seven pacemaker malfunctions (one sensing and two capture failures, four myopotential inhibitions) and seven ventricular premature beats Lown class 4 or 5 (2 ventricular tachycardias). These events, although not correlated with symptoms, can suggest a cardiac cause for SE.

Conclusion: DECG was of absolute diagnostic value in 50% of the cases studied, detecting or excluding a cardiac cause for the SE, supplied a diagnostic orientation in 35% and had no diagnostic usefulness in 15% of the cases. In the 15 cases of diagnostic DECG ventricular tachycardia was the most frequent cause of the symptom and was correlated with ischemic heart disease and a high rate of subsequent sudden death.

Patients with implanted pacemakers (PM) for symptomatic bradyarrhythmias may have recurrence of syncope or presyncope. Symptoms may be due to PM malfunction occurring at an early or late stage after implantation, tachyarrhythmias, or non-cardiac events. There are still insufficient data regarding the incidence of such episodes, either of cardiac or non cardiac origin, in PM patients (1–2).

A careful clinical and instrumental examination of the symptomatic patients may provide an accurate diagnosis. However, the usual control – because of the limited time for observation – may fail to detect intermittent abnormalities of the pacing system or arrhythmias may be the cause of the patient's symptoms. It is within this context that dynamic electrocardiography (DECG) has been found to be a valuable adjunct in detecting paroxysmal pathological events. Only a few reports in the literature deal with this problem (3, 4, 5, 6, 7).

The objective of the following study is to evaluate the diagnostic value of DECG in PM patients complaining of recurring syncopal or presyncopal episodes.

Methods

In the period from January 1980 to October 1982, 581 patients with symptomatic bradyarrhythmias underwent PM implantation in our Institute. They also attended the PM Clinic.

567

Table 1. Population data and ambulatory monitoring results.

Pt	Sex	Age	Heart disease	Rhythm disorder	PM	Months	DECG symptom	Results
1	M	84	idiop.	CAVB	VVI	22	+	m.p.i.
2	M	60	isch.	CAVB	VVI/P	18	+	m.p.i.
3	M	55	isch.	CAVB	VVI	3	+	m.p.i.
4	M	35	CM	SSS	VVI/P	5	+	i.p.r.
5	M	70	isch.	BFB	VVI/P	8	+	i.p.r.
6	F	77	isch.	SSS	VVI	27	+	c.f.
7	F	80	idiop.	BFB	VVI	2	+	VT
8	F	48	cong.	CAVB	VVI/P	1	+	VT
9	M	55	isch.	CAVB	VVI/P	25	+	VT
10	F	59	isch.	SSS	DVI	2	+	VT
11	M	70	isch.	CAVB	VVI	23	+	VT
12	M	68	isch.	BFB	VVI/P	27	+	VT
13	M	60	isch.	CAVB	VVI/P	5	+	VT
14	M	69	isch.	SSS	AAI/P	4	+	SVT
15	M	74	isch.	SSS	VVI	16	+	SCT
16	F	62	rheum.	CAVB	VVI/P	23	+	–
17	M	74	idiop.	CAVP	VVI/P	15	+	–
18	F	30	cong.	CAVB	VVI	24	+	–
19	M	47	idiop.	SSS	AAI/P	12	+	–
20	F	36	cong.	CAVB	VVI/P	20	+	–
21	F	60	CM	BFB	DVI	1	–	–
22	M	67	idiop.	CAVB	VVI	5	–	–
23	F	75	idiop.	CAVB	VVI	24	–	–
24	M	75	isch.	SSS	AAI/P	20	–	–
25	F	53	isch.	CAVB	VVI	18	–	–
26	F	77	idiop.	SSS	VVI	24	–	–
27	M	60	isch.	SSS	AAI/P	1	–	s.f.
28	F	74	idiop.	SSS	VVI	12	–	c.f.
29	M	68	idiop.	CAVB	VVI	32	–	c.f.
30	F	75	idiop.	CAVB	VVI/P	1	–	m.p.i.
31	M	52	idiop.	CAVB	VVI	26	–	m.p.i.
32	M	75	idiop.	CAVB	VVI	24	–	m.p.i.
33	M	47	isch.	CAVB	VVI/P	30	–	m.p.i.
34	M	70	CM	BFB	VVI/P	1	–	PVCs
35	F	80	isch.	CAVB	VVI	2	–	PVCs
36	M	83	idiop.	CAVB	VVI	18	–	PVCs
37	M	82	isch.	SSS	VVI	20	–	PVCs
38	F	71	isch.	CAVB	VVI/P	12	–	VT
39	M	90	idiop.	SSS	VVI/P	2	–	PVCs
40	M	61	isch.	BFB	VVI/P	5	–	VT

Abbreviations: PT: patient; PM: pacemaker; DECG: dynamic electrocardiography; M: male; F: female; idiop: idiopathic; isch.: ischemic; CM: cardiomyopathy; cong.: congenital; rheum.: rheumatic; CAVB: complete atrio-ventricular block; SSS: sick sinus syndrome; BFB: bifascicular block; months: implantation-system interval (months); m.p.i.: myopotential inhibition; i.p.r.: insufficient pacing rate; c.f.: capture failure; VT: ventricular tachycardia; SVT: supraventricular tachycardia; s.f.: sensing failure; PVCs: premature ventricular contractions.

Table 2. DECG results in 40 patients with syncope after PM implantation.

	PM malfunctions				Arrhythmias			nega-tive DECG	total patients
	MPI	IPR	capture failure	sensing failure	VT	SVT	PVCs		
Pts symptomatic during DECG	3	2	1	–	7	2	–	5	20
Pts asymptomatic during DECG	4	–	2	1				6	20

DECG: dynamic electrocardiography; PM: pacemaker; Pts: patients; MPI: myopotential inhibition; IPR: insufficient pacing rate; VT: ventricular tachycardia; SVT: supraventricular tachycardia; PVCs: premature ventricular contractions Lown Class 4 and 5.

The patients who complained of recurrent symptoms attributable to transient cerebral hypoperfusion (dizziness, light headedness, faintness, or syncope) underwent thorough clinical examinations which included blood pressure measurement in supine and upright postures, examination of neck movements for vertebro-basilar insufficiencies and carotid sinus node stimulation. The PM was tested electrocardiographically and electronically. Isometric arm exercises were performed to search for PM skeletal muscle inhibition. Also, chest x-rays were taken.

Despite careful examination of 40 patients (6.9% of population under control), in whom symptoms appeared from 1 to 32 months after PM implantation (mean 14 months), we could not discover the cause of these symptoms.

These patients – 26 males and 14 females, aged between 29 and 90 (mean age 65.2) – had been submitted to permanent pacing for: complete atrioventricular block in 22 cases, sick sinus syndrome in 12 cases, and symptomatic bifascicular block in 6 cases. The underlying heart disease was: ischemic (19 patients), idiopathic (14 patients), cardiomyopathic (3 patients), congenital (3 patients), and rheumatic (1 patient). The implanted PM-devices were: VVI (18), VVI/P (16), AAI/P (4), and DVI (2).

All patients underwent 24-hour ambulatory monitoring with a PM dedicated recorder (Ela Medical 21–24). If the patient did not exhibit symptoms during the first 24-hour recording, DECG was extended over 48 hours. Tape readings were carried out with Ela Medical Anatec Analysis System.

Results

Twenty (50%) of the 40 patients exhibited symptomatic events during monitoring: 2 had syncopes and 18 suffered dizziness or faintness. Twenty patients (50%) were asymptomatic for all 48 hours of recording.

Patients symptomatic during DECG

Ambulatory monitoring revealed electrocardiographic abnormalities related to the symptoms in 15 cases (37.5%), while in 5 patients (12.5%) no electrocardiographic abnormalities were found. The following electrocardiographic disorders were detected. Four PM malfunctions (three myopotential inhibition (Fig. 1), one intermittent capture failure), and nine symptomatic tachyarrhythmias (two paroxysmal supraventricular tachycardias and seven ventricular tachycardias). In two patients with bifascicular block and spontaneous rhythm, whose PM had been programmed at 40 bpm, the presyncopal events occurred during exertion, because of an inadequate pacing rate at the onset of transient complete atrioventricular block. The two Adams Stokes episodes were caused by capture failure with prolonged asystole in one case and ventricular tachycardia in the other (Fig. 2).

Patients asymptomatic during DECG

DECG was negative in six patients (15%), while it showed pathological events in 14 cases (35%): seven PM malfunctions (one sensing failure in AAI PM, two capture failures, four myopotential inhibitions), and seven ventricular arrhythmias Lown classes 4 or 5, including two ventricular tachycardias.

Underlying heart disease

Table 3 shows the correlation between the underlying heart disease and the DECG results. Excluding the patient with idiopathic bifascicular block and ventricular tachycardia

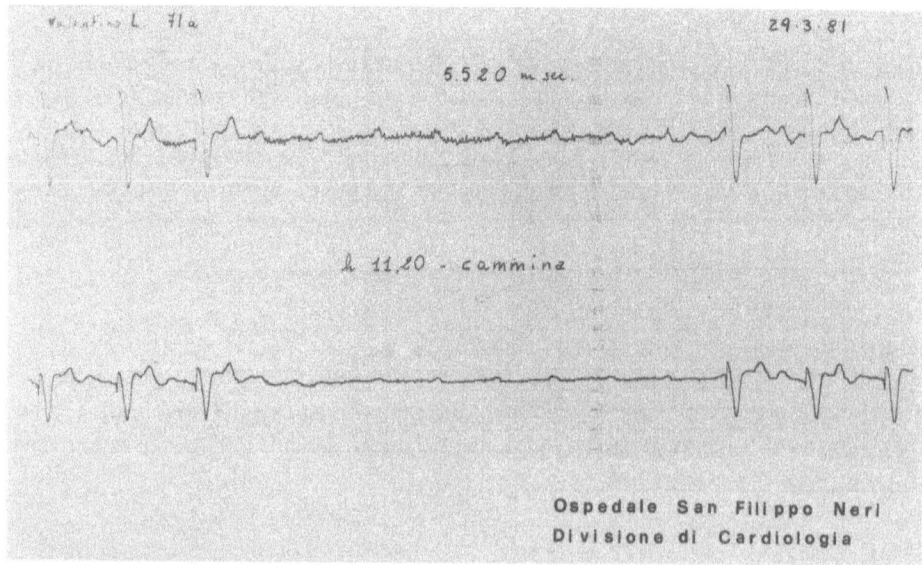

Fig. 1. Patient with PM VVI/P, implanted because of symptomatic bifascicular block. 18 months after implantation he complained recurrence of presyncopal events. Clinical and PM control were negative. Ambulatory monitoring showed, during walking, myopotential inhibition without spontaneous underlying rhythm.

570

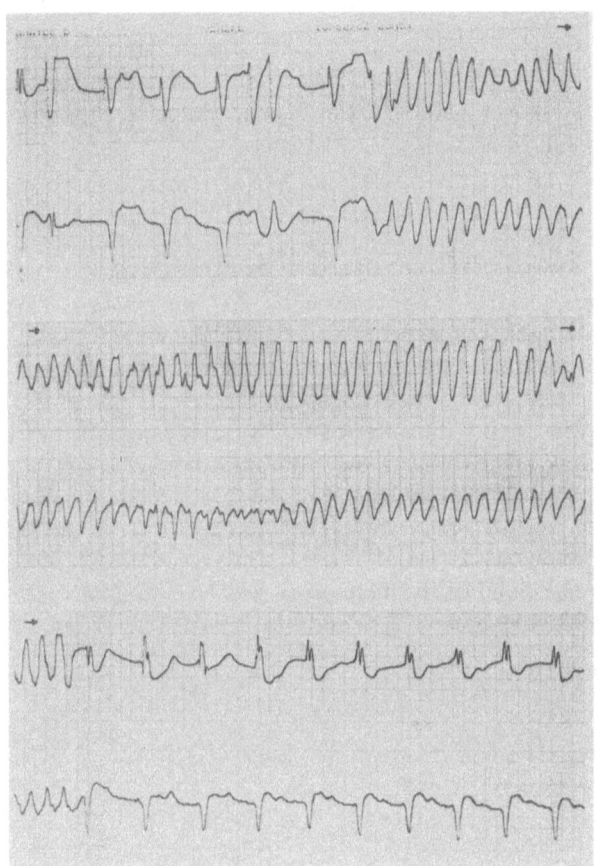

Fig. 2. Female patients with PM implanted for symptomatic bifascicular block. Two months after PM implantation she underwent DECG because recurrence of syncope. Ambulatory monitoring, during a syncopal episode, revealed sustained ventricular tachycardia.

Table 3. Relation between underlying heart disease and DECG results.

	negative DECG	VG	SVT	PVCs	PM malfunction	total patients
Ischemic heart disease	2	7	2	2	6	19
Non ischemic heart disease	9	2	–	3	7	21

DECG: dynamic electrocardiography; VT: ventricular tachycardia; SVT: supraventricular tachycardia; PVCs: premature ventricular contractions Lown Class 4a–5; PM: pacemaker.

caused by quinidine, ventricular tachycardias were found in 36.8% of ischemic patients and in 4.7% of patients with non-ischemic heart disease. The majority had idiopathic atrioventricular block. PM malfunctions were present in similar proportion in both groups (31.6 and 33.3). DECG was negative in 42.9% of non-ischemic patients and in only 10.5% of ischemic patients.

571

Follow-up

In all patients with ECG abnormalities – either symptomatic or asymptomatic during ambulatory monitoring – correction of PM malfunction or treatment of arrhythmias was carried out. The mean subsequent follow-up period was 8 months.

Patients with PM malfunction

One sensing and one capture failure occurred in devices recently after implantation. They were corrected by PM-reprogramming. In two patients with capture failure and PM implantation more than 2 years ago revision of the systems was required. Intraoperatively the threshold was elevated.

The myopotential inhibitions (seven cases) were corrected by PM reprogramming or replacement. In the two cases of inadequate pacing rate, the PM was set at a higher rate.

During follow-up all seven patients with previous symptomatic dysfunctions remained asymptomatic, while two of seven patients with asymptomatic dysfunctions complained again of presyncopal events.

Therefore in 12 patients (30%) the ambulatory monitoring was able to detect PM-malfunction. The correction eliminated symptoms in these 12 patients.

Fig. 3. Female patients with ischemic heart disease and complete AV block. One year after PM implantation she had two syncopal events. 48 hour DECG showed short asymptomatic runs of ventricular tachycardia (A). Then, in spite of successful Amiodarone therapy, she had recurrence of syncope. A subsequent ambulatory monitoring revealed a previously undetected episode of myopotential inhibition, symptomatic for presyncope (B).

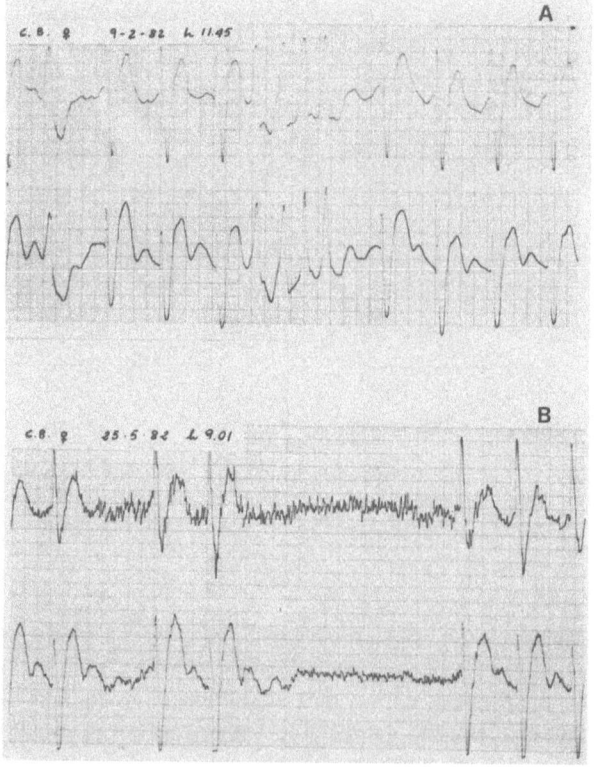

Patients with tachyarrhythmias

The drug was withdrawn from the one patient with quinidine related arrhythmias. All other patients were treated pharmacologically. Drug efficacy was assessed by subsequent ambulatory monitorings. The goal of at least 85% reduction of ventricular extrasystoles and disappearance of major arrhythmias was obtained in 14 patients (93%). However, only seven of these patients were asymptomatic during the follow-up. Five patients had recurring syncopal episodes. One of them exhibited a previously undetected symptomatic episode of myopotential inhibition in a subsequent ambulatory monitoring (Fig. 3). Only two of these patients were symptomatic during DECG.

Five patients died (two with recurrent syncopes despite treatment): one from non cardiac cause (lung carcinoma) and from myocardial infarction and three of sudden death. It is worth noting that out of six patients with symptomatic ventricular tachycardias, three (50%) died of cardiac causes (two of sudden death) within a short period in spite of antiarrhythmic treatment.

Patients with negative DECG

These patients underwent subsequent diagnostic procedures which were successful in six cases (four out of five patients with normal ECGs during a symptomatic period, two out of six asymptomatic patients). The diagnoses were: vertebrobasilar insufficiency (two patients), labyrinthic pathology (three patients) and neurosis (one patient).

In five cases diagnosis remained undertermined.

Discussion:

To the best of our knowledge, few data are available (8) regarding the incidence of syncope on presyncope in PM-patients, whose pathogenesis cannot be clarified by usual clinical and instrumental control.

In our experience, during a mean 14 months period following PM-implantation, we had to deal with this problem in 6,9% of the patients. Symptoms occurred in 50% of the patients during 48-hour ambulatory monitoring. DECG was therefore of absolute diagnostic value in all symptomatic cases. It made possible identification of the cardiac cause of the symptom in 37.5% of the patients. In the remaining 12.5% of patients the symptoms did not correlate with electrocardiographic abnormalities, and cardiac etiology of the symptoms was thereby excluded.

Nevertheless in asymptomatic patients during monitoring this technique was able to identify electrocardiographic events which could have been responsible for symptoms in 35% of the cases. Each of these events, though not symptom-correlated and therefore without absolute diagnostic value, can suggest a possible diagnosis especially in cases of dangerous arrhythmias or serious PM-malfunctions e.g. capture failure.

Only in 15% of the cases 48-hour ambulatory monitoring did not contribute to the diagnosis, as no symptoms nor significant ECG changes were present during recording (supraventricular or ventricular extrasystoles Lown class 1–3 found in four patients were not considered significant).

Follow-up after treatment of the supposed cause led to disappearance of the symptoms in nine out of 14 patients (64,3%), five out of seven patients with PM-malfunction, and four out of seven patients with asymptomatic tachyarrhythmias. These data confirm the diagnostic usefulness of DECG even in asymptomatic patients during monitoring and suggests the opportunity of undertaking treatment even for asymptomatic pathological events.

Among four of our patients with asymptomatic myopotential inhibition two continued to be symptomatic dispite the correction of PM malfunction. Taking into account the high frequency of myopotential inhibition in asymptomatic patients with unipolar lead PM – 69% in some reports (9) – and since in non-programmable PM the only way to solve this problem is generator replacement. The occurrence of short, asymptomatic periods of myopotential inhibition has to be judged cautiously. Therefore, every effort must be made in these cases to achieve a diagnosis reproducing the symptoms through muscle contraction and even performing, if necessary, daily ambulatory monitoring until symptoms occur. In our experience, DECG was able to detect myopotential inhibition in seven patients (three symptomatic) in whom clinical examinations failed. Actually, because of the high frequency of these phenomena during clinical controls, the findings have been considered responsible for the symptoms only if they are able to reproduce the symptoms. Moreover, it is possible that the kind of movements performed by the patients during control were not the same as those during ambulatory monitoring, which may have caused the inhibition. The analysis of the causes of syncope or presyncope are of interest in patients in whom DECG provided a diagnosis: tachyarrhythmias (45%), malfunctions or misprogramming of PM (30%), non-cardiac causes (25%). The incidence of malfunctions, namely of capture or sensing failures, is not elevated in our experience and is inferior to that of other reports (10).

Ventricular tachycardias resulted in the most frequent cause of syncopes or presyncopes (35%). These events were found to be significantly associated with ischemic heart disease: it was actually found in 36.8% of ischemic patients and only in 4.7% of others. Moreover, among the 7 patients who died during the follow-up period, four had ischemic heart disease and three had shown ventricular tachycardia during ambulatory monitoring. The number of patients is insufficient and the follow-up too limited to make these data statistically significant; anyway, the observation seems to be fortuitous and in agreement with other reports (11–12), in which mortality does not correlate to the progression of the block in patients with conduction disorders: Mortality relates to the underlying heart disease.

References

1. Escher DJW, Fisher JD, Furman S, Willig J, De Campos-Aranjo H, Kim SG: Dizziness in the paced patient: pacemaker malfunction or not. In: Proceedings of the VI World Symposium on Cardiac Pacing. Edited by Claude Meere MD, 1979: Chap 17–1.
2. Davies AB, Gould B, Balasubramanian V, Raftery EB: Persistent syncope despite permanent pacing. Pace 1981; 4: A46.
3. Baratto MT, Mazzocca G, Bongiorni MG, Pauletti M, Levorato D, Contini C: Holter monitoring in pacemaker patient. Pace 1981; 4: A31.
4. Kelen GJ, Bloomfield DA, Hardage M, Gomes JA, Khan R, Gopalaswamy C, El Sherif N: A clinical evaluation of improved Holter monitoring technique for artificial pacemaker function. Pace 1980; 3: 192–197.

5. Murray A, Jordan RS, Gold RG: Pacemaker assessment in the ambulant patient. Br Heart J 1981; 46: 531–538.
6. Lipsky J, Cohen L, Espinoza J, Motro M, Dack S, Domoso E: Value of Holter monitoring in assessing cardiac arrhythmias in symptomatic patients. Am J Cardiology 1976; 37: 102–107.
7. Steinbach K, Glogar D, Huber J, Joskowicz G, Weber H: Long term monitoring for detection of failure of the pacemaker/electrode system and arrhythmias. In: Presentations of 1st European Symposium of Cardiac Pacing London 1978.
8. Famularo MA, Kennedy HL: Ambulatory electrocardiography in the assessment of pacemaker function. Am Heart J 1982; 104 (5): 1086–1094.
9. Breivik K, Ohm OJ; Myopotential inhibition of unipolar QRS-inhibited (VVI) pacemaker, assessed by ambulatory Holter monitoring of the electrocardiogram. Pace 1980; 3: 470–478.
10. Ward D, Camm A, Spurrel R: Dynamic electrocardiography in patients with permanent pacemakers. In: Presentations of 1st European Symposium of Cardiac Pacing, London 1978.
11. Denes P, Dhingra RC, Wu D, Wyndham CR, Amat-y-Leon F, Rosen KM: Sudden death in patients with chronic bifascicular block. Arch Inter Med 1977; 137: 1005–1010.
12. Simon AB, Janz M: Symptomatic bradyarrhythmias in the adult: natural history following ventricular pacemaker implantation. Pace 1982; 5: 372–383.

Authors' address:
Dr. L. Bianconi
U.S.L. RM XIX
Piazza S. Maria della Pieta 5
I-00100 Roma
Italy

Uniformed Services Collaborative Study on Indications and Follow-Up of Pacemakers in Children

B. Guller, W. A. Todd, J. C. Hill, E. R. Alden

Summary: The current status of pacemaker therapy was evaluated retrospectively in 36 children and adolescents who were under care in Uniformed Service Hospitals between 1970 and 1983. Indications for permanent pacing included: Postoperative heart block 13, sick sinus syndrome 10, congenital heart block 9, tachyarrhythmias 2, digitalis toxicity 1, Kearns-Sayre Syndrome 1. Our patient population reflects the current trend toward pacing in children who are predominantly symptomatic from cardiac dysrhythmias rather than from underlying heart disease. Pacemaker lead implantation was epicardial in 29 and transvenous in 7. There were 23 reoperations in 12 patients with an average implant interval of 20.1 months. An analysis of risk factors revealed that children were at risk for reimplant in the first six postoperative months from infection (5 reoperations), in the first 24 months from rising myocardial threshold (7 reoperations), and between two to four years of followup from generator failure (11 reoperations). Other factors causing increased pacemaker morbidity were postpericardiotomy syndrome (5 patients) which was seen with epicardial leads and ventricular dysrhythmias which were seen with each lead system in one patient.

Due to improved generator and lead technology, the pacemaker morbidity and longevity in our patients was improved compared to previous reports. However, the occurrence of high chronic myocardial threshold levels (which were documented in 11 out of 12 reoperated patients) is of concern. High chronic threshold levels ranged from 4.5 to 13.3 mA. They were more prevalent in younger children and were associated with epicardial leads. Implantation of epicardial leads in children is by some considered to be a well-tolerated procedure with good long-term esults. Based on our experience, we caution against the use of epicardial leads and support the use of transvenous leads.

The opinions herein contained are those of the authors and do not necessarily represent those of the Department of Defense or the Department of the Army.

Cardiac pacing in children is rare. Data presented in 1979 at the VIth World Symposium on Cardiac Pacing indicated that in large institutions the average number of yearly pacemaker implants in children was six (1, 2). Reports from 1979 concern predominantly surgically acquired complete atrio-ventricular block (1, 2). At present complete heart block is rare after repair of the common cardiac malformations. However, due to improved surgical survival of children with complex congenital heart disease, pacemakers are required for other bradyarrhythmias, in particular for sinus node dysfunction following atriotomy (3–5). While the indications for pacing in surgically acquired complete atrio-ventricular block have been well established, the indications for pacing in children with sinus node dysfunction need to be further defined. The decision for pacing in pediatric patients not only depends on the presence of symptoms and coinciding electrocardiographic abnormalities, but also on the morbidity associated with currently used pacemaker-lead systems (6, 7). This morbidity is still significantly higher than in adults although problems related to body growth, pacemaker size and lead breakage have been reduced. We have analyzed the course of pacemaker implants in 36 pediatric and adolescent patients.

Materials and methods

Records of 36 children and adolescents with pacemakers who were under care in Uniformed Service Hospitals between 1970 and 1983 were reviewed. Nine institutions representing the United States Army, Navy and Air Force participated.

Ages of the patients at the time of implant ranged from 4 months to 24 years with a mean of 9.6 years. The following were tabulated: symptoms at the time of implant, indications for pacing, operative technique, electrical measurements at the time of the operation (current strength, current voltage, pulse width and lead impedance), pacemaker and lead model, and followup data. Epicardial leads were used in 29 patients and transvenous leads in 7. The epicardial leads were sutureless or of the screw-in type and were inserted with a thoracotomy in most instances, or with the subxiphoid technique. All pacemakers were demand operated and lithium powered.

Acute and chronic stimulation thresholds were measured at time of operation or reoperation and were expressed as current strength in mA. Current threshold is helpful in determining the integrity of the electrode tissue interface and reflects the density of current, which is thought to be the prime factor responsible for successful stimulation. 34 out of the 36 patients had constant voltage generators with pulse amplitudes of 5 volt or slightly higher. At the time of current threshold testing, the voltage applied to the lead system varied from one patient to another with settings ranging from 0.5 to 5 volt. Pulse width was 0.5 msec in most patients during determination of the pacing threshold, but in some it was as high as 0.8 msec. Only a few patients had programmable pacemakers allowing non-invasive changes in pulse width. The patients were followed in pacemaker clinics with recordings of pacemaker rate, magnet rate and pulse width and, in some instances, with additional measurements of lead and battery parameters. For the entire patient population, the length of followup varied form 0.3 months to 13 years with a mean of 2.8 years. Total length of followup was 107 patient years. The 7 patients with transvenous leads were followed for a total of 14 patient years with a mean followup of two years.

Indications for permanent pacemaker therapy were symptomatic bradyarrhythmias or the presence of potentially fatal dysrhythmias documented by Holter monitoring or intracardiac electrophysiologic study. Diagnosis of the patients is shown in Table 1.

Table 1. Indications for pacing.

Complete heart block		24
surgically acquired	13	
congenital*)	9	
Kearns-Sayre Syndrome	1	
Sinus node dysfunction		10
post-operative	8	
idiopathic	2	
Atrial tachyarrhythmia		2

*) Five of nine patients with congenital complete heart block had corrected transposition of the great arteries.

Results:

Symptoms disappeared in all patients after pacemaker implantation. There was, however, still a significant morbidity associated with pacemaker implants (Tables 2 and 3, Figures 1–3). Almost all complications occurred in patients with epicardial leads (Table 2). While the average followup period for epicardial and transvenous leads was similar, the mean age for patients with transvenous leads was higher and transvenous implants were only used in twenty percent of all patients.

There were five deaths (Table 2), three of which were unrelated to pacing (severe underlying heart disease 2, pancreatitis 1). Two early deaths were in part pacemaker related:

1. a four year old patient with Down's syndrome and complete atrioventricular canal died one month following implant of postpericardiotomy syndrome complicated by pneumonitis;
2. a 24 year old patient with corrected transposition of the great arteries had repair of associated intracardiac defects. She died suddenly 10 days after implant when epicardial leads became dislodged as a complications of post pericardiotomy syndrome.

Table 2. Pacemaker morbidity and mortality in 36 patients.

	Number of patients	Epicardial leads	Transvenous leads**)
Reoperations	12	12	0
Deaths*)	5	5	0
Post pericardiotomy syndrome	5	5	0
Ventricular dysrhythmia requiring countershock	2	1	1
Pacemaker syndrome	1	1	0

*) Two out of five deaths were pacemaker related.
**) Of the 36 patients 29 had epicardial leads and 7 transvenous leads.

Table 3. Cause of reoperation in 12 patients.

	Number of patients*)	Number of reoperations
Infection	2	5
Generator related		
elective	2	2
recall	1	1
drop in magnet rate	2	2
other	6	6
Lead related		
high pacing threshold	6	6
broken lead	1	1

*) There were 23 reoperations in 12 patients. Number of operations per patient ranged from 1 to 5.

There were 23 reoperations in 12 patients (Table 3). Average time interval between reoperations was 20 months. Longest followup without reimplantation was six years (Fig. 1). The time of reoperation was related to the cause of reoperation. Infection, which necessitated five reoperations, occurred within 6 months after implant. Generator failure (11 reoperations) occurred after a period of 12 to 48 months with a peak incidence between 42 and 48 months. In six patients reoperation was precipitated by a high chronic

Fig. 1. The number of implants and reimplants in relation to the year of operation is shown.

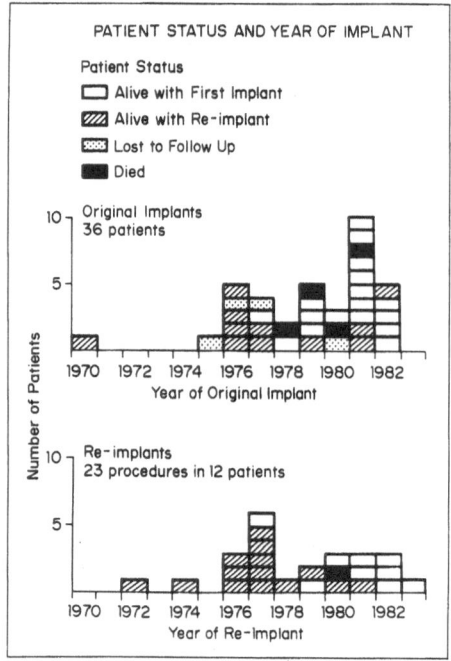

Fig. 2. Chronic pacing thresholds in children were higher than reported in adults. Several children had a progressive increase in threshold at each reoperation.

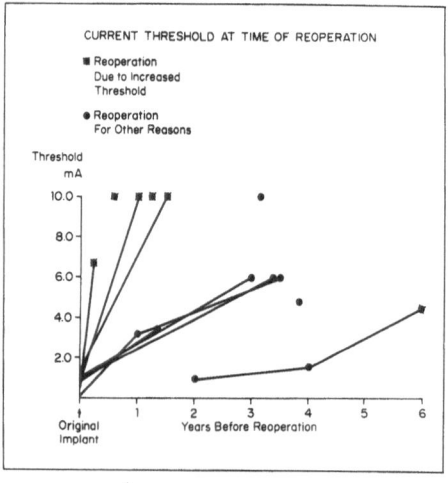

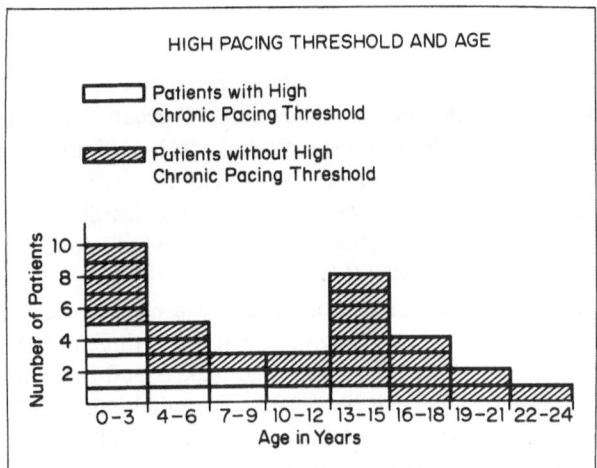

Fig. 3. The incidence of high chronic pacing threshold was inversely related to age. This finding could not be explained by differences in followup between patients with and without high threshold levels. Both of these patient groups had similar followup durations.

myocardial threshold. The latter produced exit block within 24 months. As shown in Fig. 2, chronic myocardial pacing threshold exceeded 4.0 mA in 11 patients at time of reoperation. The increase in threshold was progressive. As shown in Fig. 3, the occurrence of high chronic myocardial thresholds was inversely related to age.

Discussion

Indications:

Comparison of this study with previous reports indicates that fewer children are paced because of surgical complete atrioventricular block and more require pacing for surigically acquired or idiopathic sinus node dysfunction. Out of 448 pediatric patients paced between 1974 and 1980, 270 had surgical atrio-ventricular block and 41 sinus node dysfunction (5). In the present study sinus node dysfunction was the indication for pacing in approximately one third of the patients and was almost as prevalent as postoperative complete heart block (Table 1). With improvements in surgical technique, damage to the bundle of His or to the initial portion of the bundle branches can be avoided even in children with complex congenital heart disease. Atriotomy for complex intra atrial repair in contrary still carries a significant risk of impaired sino-atrial conduction either through progressive fibrosis in the area of the sinus node or through direct interruption of the atrial preferential pathways (8). In children with sinus node dysfunction pacemaker implantation should be restricted to symptomatic patients in whom periods of bradycardia coincide with symptoms (4, 7, 9). In asymptomatic patients with bradycardia, potentially dangerous escape rhythms should be documented electrocardiographically as evidence for pacing (4, 7, 9).

Mortality and Morbidity:

In children pacemaker related deaths occur between four to fifteen percent of all patients (5). Two of our 36 patients (six percent) had pacemaker related death. It occurred in conjunction with post pericardiotomy syndrome in both instances (see result section). Post pericardiotomy syndrome is known to occur in up to 25 percent of children with epicardial pacemakers (10). It was present in 15 percent of our patients with epicardial leads and required steroid therapy in some. Long term prognosis is usually good but late recurrences and constrictive pericarditis have been reported (11).

Two of our patients required countershock at the time of implant because of ventricular tachycardia and fibrillation. One of the two children developed exit block three months later. Countershock is usually well tolerated in patients with pacemakers and there are only sporadic reports of complications, including exit block and myocardial infarct (12). These complications can be minimized through applications of one of the paddles to the posterior chest (12).

Myocardial Stimulation Threshold:

Progressive rises in stimulation threshold level above the output capacity of a generator is the most unusual cause for failure of the electrode lead system in adults (13) and necessitates re-operation in only two to seven percent of patients (14). In this pediatric followup study, progressive rise in myocardial threshold was the cause for reoperations in 26 percent of all patients (Table 3, Fig. 2). Others have reported high myocardial threshold levels resulting in exit block in up to 28 percent of children (4, 6). These figures indicate that exit block due to a high chronic stimulation threshold is at present one of the most significant problems associated with pacing in children.

The methodology for measurement of stimulation threshold in children has been little addressed in previous reports. This hampers comparison of various electrode systems (15). Most pacemakers used in this study were constant voltage generators. For these pacemakers current strength is at present the parameter most widely used in obtaining threshold, but voltage, energy and other variables have been advocated (15). In this study current threshold in mA was used (Fig. 2). Current threshold rises initially after implant and reaches a chronic level after two to three months. Chronic current threshold levels above 4 mA are undesirable. As shown in Fig. 2, this level was exceeded in 11 out of 36 patients during evaluation of current threshold levels. The voltage applied to the lead-electrode system at the time of measurement and the pulse width should be known. Voltage applied must be within the safety margin required for constant voltage generators and pulse width should be approximately 0.5 to 1.0 msec in order to obtain a meaningful determination of current strength.

The cause for high chronic pacing thresholds in children has not been elucidated. As illustrated in Fig. 3 our data suggest that age is a risk factor in the development of high myocardial thresholds in children. The occurrence of high chronic pacing thresholds was inversely related to age. One may speculate that tissue reaction to the electrodes is age dependent, such as seen with bioprosthetic materials (16). This hypothesis would have to be confirmed by histologic study demonstrating more fibrosis at the site of the electrodes in young children.

582

Transvenous versus Epicardial Leads:

Pacemaker morbidity in our patients was almost exclusively associated with the use of epicardial leads (Table 2). This finding supports observations in adults where the lower morbidity of transvenous leads is widely accepted. It has been suggested that with the availability of active and newer passive endocardial fixation leads, transvenous pacing in children should become more widely accepted (17, 18). The morbidity associated with epicardial leads observed in this and other studies support the use of transvenous rather than of epicardial leads. In 10 children aged two to nine years, no lead dislodgements were reported with the use of actively adhering endocardial leads. In children below the age of two years, venous access still remains a problem (18).

References:

1. Nissen RG, Holmes DR, Maloney JD, Feldt RH, Danielson RG: Experience with permanent cardiac pacemakers in congenital heart disease. Pace, September–October 1979; 2: A-72.
2. Williams WG, Izukawa T, Trusler GA: Experience with permanent cardiac pacing in pediatrics. Pace, September–October 1979; 2: A-72.
3. Vetter VL, Horowitz LN: Electrophysiologic residua and sequelae of surgery for congenital heart defects. A J Cardiol 1982; 50: 588–604.
4. Simon AB, MacDonald D, Stern AM, Behrendt DM, Sloan H: Ventricular pacing in children. Pace, 1982; 5: 836–844.
5. Young D: Permanent pacemaker implantation in children: Current status and future considerations. Pace, 1981; 4: 61–66.
6. Williams WG, Izukawa T, Olley PM, Trusler GA, Rowe RD: Permanent cardiac pacing in infants and children. Pace, 1978; 1: 439–447.
7. Morris JH, Ott DA, Cooley DA, Gillette PC: Pacemakers-indications implantation, and follow-up. In: Gillette PC, Garson A, eds. Pediatric cardiac dysrhythmias. New York: Grune and Stratton, 1981: 421–436.
8. Bharati S, Lev M: Sequelae of atriotomy and ventriculotomy on the endocardium, conduction system and coronary arteries. Am J Cardiol 1982; 50: 580–587.
9. Dreifuss LS, Michelson EL, Kaplinsky L: Bradyarrhythmias: Clinical significance and management. J Am Coll Cardiol 1983; 1: 327–338.
10. Hayward R, Sommerville J, Rickards AF: Problems of permanent pacing in children. Pace, September–October 1979, A-72.
11. Peter RN, Scheinman MM, Raskin S, Thomas AN: Unusual complications of epicardial pacemakers. Recurrent pericarditis, cardiac tamponade and pericardial constriction. Am J Cardiol 1980; 45: 1088–1094.
12. Furman S: External defibrillation and implanted cardiac pacemakers. Pace 1981; 4: 503–506.
13. Furman S: Results of cardial pacing. In: Samet P, El Sharif N, eds. Cardiac pacing. New York: Grune and Stratton, 1981; 271–293.
14. Lawrie GM, Seale JP, Morris GC et al: Results of epicardial pacing by the left subcostal approach. Ann Thorac Surg 1979; 28: 561–567.
15. Barold SS, Ong LS, Heinle RA: Stimulation and sensing thresholds for cardiac pacing: Electrophysiologic and technical aspects. Prog Cardiovasc Dis 1981; 24: 1–24.
16. McGoon DC: Long-term effects of prosthetic materials. Am J Cardiol 1982; 50: 621–630.
17. Fraedrich G, Mulch J, Netz H, Scheld HH: Actively adhering endocardial leads for pacing in children. Thorac Cardiovasc Surgeon 1981; 29: 242–245.
18. Holmes DR, Maloney JD, Feldt RH: The use of percutaneous subclavian technique for permanent cardiac pacing in childhood. Mayo Clin Proc 1980; 55: 579–582.

Author's address:
Barbara Guller, M.D., LTC MC, Pediatric Cardiology
Box 686, Madigan Army Medical Center, Tacoma, Washington 98431

Long-Term Endocardial Pacing in Children With Postoperative Bradycardia-Tachycardia Syndrome Following the Senning, Mustard and Fontan Operations

James D. Maloney, Lon W. Castle, Robert J. Eastway, Jr., Richard Sterba, Douglas S. Moodie, Carl C. Gill, Michael D. McGoon

Summary: Permanent pacing in children, including those with postoperative bradycardia-tachycardia syndrome (BTS), remains compromised by devices, lead-electrode systems and implantation technics designed for the adult. Althogh recent technology and simplified implantation technics have reduced many of these barriers, children with congenital anomalies and intra-atrial cardiac operations are particularly prone to postoperative BTS and require special approaches to pacemaker therapy.

This report describes the use of endocardial atrial demand pacing, with antitachycardial burst pacing capabilities (either automatic or parent activated) in the treatment of three children following Mustard repair, one following a Fontan repair, and two following Senning operations. Ages ranged from 3 to 11 years. All had life threatening bradycardias and incapacitating tachyarrhythmias documented clinically. Devices utilized included the Intermedics 262–01 (Cybertach 60) in one patient, and the Medtronic 5984 (Spectrax SX) in five patients. Atrial endocardial pacing was accomplished using the subclavian venipuncture technique and active fixation endocardial leads.

This experience, with a follow-up of 3 to 24 months, suggests that atrial endocardial pacing in children with postoperative BTS and normal A-V nodal function reliably controls symptomatic bradycardia, restores A-V synchrony, appears to decrease the frequency of intra-atrial tachycardia, and with concurrent antiarrhythmic agents provides a means of safe, effective control or termination of tachycardia.

Introduction

Atrial hypertrophy and enlargement secondary to complex congenital heart disease, and direct surgical trauma subsequent to extensive atrial reconstructive surgery are common to children with several types of complex cogenital heart disease. Surgical correction of these anomalies frequently result in disordered sino-atrial impulse formation, and intra-atrial conduction delays. Sinus arrest, junctional escape rhythms, atrial ectopy, and paroxysmal intra-atrial reentry tachycardia (IAT) complicate these operations and present as the brady-tachy syndrome of sick sinus syndrome (BTS – SSS) (1) D-transposition of the great arteries (D-TGA), tricuspid atresia, and common ventricle are the anomalies most frequently requiring operations classified as intra-atrial reconstructive surgery. The Mustard repair and the Senning repair for D-TGA are the most comon causes for postoperative BTS (1). BTS is less frequently precipitated by the Fontan operation, repair of sinus venous atrial septal defect, or septation of common atrium.

The children comprising this report developed the brady-tachy syndrome following the Mustard operation, the Senning operation, and the Fontan repair. Despite attempts at modifying these operations to avoid traumatic disruption of atrial conduction pathways, the incidence of postoperative BTS is reported from 15 to 90 percent (2). For many of these children, the postoperative BTS is incapacitating because of the arrhythmias need for antiarrhythmic pharmacologic agents, life threatening episodes of severe bradyarrhythmias, recurrent IAT presenting as a atypical flutter with ventricular rates approaching 300 beats per minute, and BS drug-mediated vulnerability to ventricular fibrillation.

The approach to managing the BTS syndrome following atrial reconstructive surgery has generally required multiple antiarrhythmic agents (quinidine-like drugs, beta blockers, digitalis) to control the recurrent, sustained atrial tachyarrhythmias and their associated rapid ventricular rates. Pharmacologic control of the IAT invariably aggravates the bradyarrhythmias of sick sinus syndrome the combination of drug therapy plus backup-permanent pacing systems are frequently needed. Our experience and others (2) using these modes of therapy have been frustrating because of the difficulties in compliance and adverse drug side effects, frequent failure of past epicardial lead electrode systems used with standard VVI pacing in the pediatric patient, and persistence of disabling IAT aggravated because of bradycardia dependency, and persisting precursors (atrial ectopy, retrograde VA conduction with VVI pacing, compromised hemodynamics with nonphysiologic pacing systems).

After studying the postoperative electrophysiologic characteristics of selected children with BTS following Mustard and Senning operations, and recognizing the limitations of current therapy, we undertook a new approach to management that incorporated standard electrophysiologic techniques for tachycardia induction and termination applied to chronic maintenance therapy.

BTS following intra-atrial reconstructive surgery that proved refractory to standard therapy were managed as follows:

1. Documentation of spontaneous life threatening or incapacitating tachyarrhythmias (IAT) or bradyarrhythmias.
2. Invasive electrophysiologic testing to confirm the tachycardia-bradycardia mechanism, sinus node and A-V nodal function, and reliability for IAT induction and termination through programmed electronic burst pacing and other modalities.
3. Implantation of transvenous multi-programmable AAI pacing systems designed to prevent malignant bradyarrhythmias, suppress bradycardia-dependent precursors to paroxysmal IAT and provide manual or automatic antitachycardia burst stimulation for terminating IAT.

Our experience with this approach (1) confirmed the clinical feasibility of subclavian transvenous atrial pacing in postoperative Mustard and Fontan cases. The purpose of this report is to expand our initial experience to include two children with BTS following Senning operations managed in a similar way. The technical differences with transvenous pacemaker implantation following the Senning operation vs. the Mustard operation are reviewed. The late follow-up experience with all six children provide preliminary data regarding efficacy, safety, and limitations of these pacing technics in managing BTS.

Patient Population

Ages ranged from 3 to 11 years at the time of pacemaker implantation. There were two females and four males. The congenital cardiac anomaly was transposition of the great arteries and associated ventricular septal defect in 5 of the 6 patients. Three of these had associated atrial septal defect and two had pulmonary stenosis. One patient had tricuspid atresia with atrial septal defect and ventricular septal defect.

All of the children had a Blalock-Hanlon atrial septectomy or balloon septostomy prior to the Mustard or Senning operation. The brady-tachy syndrome was recognized during the initial early postoperative course in 3 of the 6 patients. The diagnosis was not made in the other three patients for 3 to 30 months post-operation. All children had recurrent episodes of syncopes or near-syncope. Paroxysmal tachycardia (IAT) resulted in hypotension, congestive failure, and chest pain. Three children had Stokes-Adams attacks, while two had documented episodes of ventricular fibrillation in the presence of complex antiarrhythmic agents and refractory BTS. Prior medical therapy included trials with digitalis, beta blockers, and quinidine-like drugs alone and in combination at near toxic levels. Dilantin was added to the medical program in two patients without benefit. Daily episodes of incapacitating IAT occurred in two children, while the tachycardia frequency in the remaining group varied from one per week to one per month.

Preimplant electrophysiologic evaluation

Using two or three multi-electrode recording catheters, electrophysiologic assessment of the sinus node function, A-V node, and mechanisms for tachycardia induction and termination were determined using the standard methods. All patients had abnormal sinoatrial impulse formation, with post pacing escape beats arising from the low atrium or junction. Normal A-V nodal conduction and refractoriness was present in all. This was reflected by a 1 : 2 A-V conduction at atrial pacing rates exceeding 200 beats per minute and spontaneously occurring IAT with ventricular rates recorded at 200 to 320 beats per minute.
Single and double premature atrial extrastimuli could induce the IAT in 5 of 6 patients. Burst pacing was required in the sixth patient. Single and double extrastimuli were unsuccessful in terminating IAT in five children. Burst atrial pacing during electrophysiologic study and at the time of permanent pacemaker implantation was effective in inducing and terminating IAT in all. Two patients developed induced atrial fibrillation which terminated spontaneously after several minutes. Tachycardia induction and termination was performed a minimum of 20 times per patient prior to utilization of the permanent pacing technic.

Pacemaker Implantation Technique

The left subclavian venipuncture technique was used for all. Five patients received the active fixation atrial endocardial lead, while one was managed with a passive tined atrial lead.
Atrial endocardial lead placement was directed away from the left atrial appendage (location of left phrenic nerve vulnerable to electrical stimulation and left diaphragmatic contraction). The anatomy of the Mustard repair required posterior medial atrial lead fixation. The anterior wall of the baffle was made of Dacron and not suitable for stimulation. Children with the Senning operation were equally susceptible to left phrenic nerve stimulation if the left atrial appendage was not avoided, but had both the anterior and posterior

wall of the intra-atrial baffle composed of myocardium. This permitted either an anterior or posterior site for lead fixation.

Another site effective atrial myocardial pacing in both the anatomic substrates would include the "roof of the morphologic left atrium".

The size of these children (smallest, 20 kg) did not preclude the transvenous approach and a pectoral pocket. Atrial sensing and capture electronic characteristics were satisfactory for all patients. Multiparameter programmability permitted adjusting the AAI mode to 80 beats per minute in two, and 90 beats per minute in one. This relative overdrive atrial (physiologic) pacing proved more effective in suppressing and preventing IAT than VVI demand rates of 60 and 70 beats per minute.

Early and Late Post Implant Experience

The follow-up period ranges from 5 to 28 months. One patient died due to severe congestive heart failure and incomplete surgical correction. Continuous ECG monitoring at the time of death excluded pacemaker related phenomenon.

One child developed late onset left phrenic nerve stimulation (second patient in the experience). This could not be effectively managed with output and pulse width programming. He also continued to experience mild episodes of altered consciousness despite normal atrial paced rhythm. This proved to be a temporal lobe seizures. Both factors resulted in explantation of the pacing device. Since explantation, the patient has had multiple episodes of IAT requiring hospitalization and intensive drug therapy. He has the least malignant bradyarrhythmia in this series.

The remaining four children continued to demonstrate normal pacemaker function, effective ventricular rate control through atrial stimulation, and suppression of IAT frequency. Two patients have had no further episodes of IAT. The remaining two patients have had a marked decrease in the frequency of tachycardia, as well as a marked decrease in the number and amounts of antiarrhythmic agents. Ambulatory ECG monitoring, analysis of the antitachycardia activation flag, and noninvasive pacemaker induction and termination "testing" have confirmed the efficacy safety, and reliability of the manual and automatic tachycardia detection and termination pacing modalities.

Conclusions

This experience further supports the feasibility of transvenous pacing in the pediatric patient and the need to correlate the anatomic-electrophysiologic substrate created by congenital heart disease and surgical repair to determine the mechanism and treatment of postoperative arrhythmias.

If additional experiences confirm our results with AAI transvenous pacing to suppress, prevent, and terminate bradycardia-dependent paroxysmal intra-atrial tachyarrhythmias, it seems reasonable to conclude that:

1. AAI MB pacing is an effective adjunct for management of postoperative BTS following Mustard, Fontan, and Sennng operations.
2. Atrial endocardial lead placement in a child with a Mustard repair should be directed posteriorly and medially in the morphologic left atrium. The posterior medial, and anteriology directed electrode site is suited for this Senning repair. Fontan repairs provide a generous right atrium for which the usual stimulation sites can be used.
3. Although transvenous lead-electrode durability in the postoperative child is not ideal, this late follow-up experience suggests that endocardial lead systems are superior to the recent epicardial ventricular lead experiences for postoperative children.
4. Multiparameter pacing systems that combine bradycardia therapy and antitachycardia therapy are an important adjunct to the treatment of BTS in children.
5. The safety and efficacy of this pacing modality is dependent upon the integrity of the patient's A-V conduction. Similar pacing technics may be applicable to patients with A-V block when smaller dual-chamber physiologic pacing systems, combined with antitachycardia modalities, are available.
6. Suppression and prevention of reentry supraventricular tachycardias through restoration of normal A-V synchrony may be appropriate for pacemaker management of all patients with tachy-brady syndrome.

References

1. McGoon MD, Maloney JD, McGoon DC, Danielson GK: Lont term endocardial atrial pacing in children with postoperative bradycardia-tachycardia syndrome and limited ventricular access. Am J Cardiol 1982; 49: 1750–57.
2. Greenwood RD, Rosenthal A, Sloss LJ, LaCorte M, Nadas AS: Sick sinus syndrome after surgery for congenital heart disease. Circulation 1975; 52: 208–13.
3. Nissen RG, Holmes DR, Maloney JD, Feldt RH, Danielson GK: Experience with permanent cardiac pacemaker in congenital heart disease. In: Meere C, ed Proceedings of the Sixth World Conference on Cardiac Pacing, Montreal, Canada. Pace Symp Oct 1979; 2–5: chap 23–1.
4. Maloney JD, Berkovits BU: Hemodynamic and antitachycardia value of dual chamber pacing: initial and followup assessment. Second European Symposium on Cardiac Pacing, May 1981.
5. Maloney JD, Medina-Ravell V, Pierett OH, Portillo B, Maduro C, Castellanos A, Berkovits B: Followup assessment of dual-demand, dual-chamber DVI-DVO pacing for automatic conversion, control and prevention of refractory paroxysmal supraventricular tachycardia, Second European Symposium on Cardiac Pacing, May 1981.

Authors' address:
Dr. Lon Castle
Cleveland Clinic Foundation
9500 Euclid Avenue
Cleveland, Ohio 44106
USA

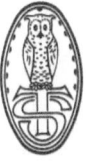

Cardiac Pacing in Children: A French Multicenter Study of 241 Patients

A. Vanetti, P. A. Chaptal, M. F. Lefebvre, M. Choussat, J. F. Godin,
B. Dodinot, V. Dor, J. F. Conso, G. Soots, D. Gaillard, F. Bourlon, L. Kubler,
P. Laurens †, Ch. Dubost

Summary: This study includes 241 children implanted from 1965 to March 1982 in 9 French Hospital centers.
Ages at first implantation are as follows: ≤ 5 years = 32.8%, from 6 to 10 years = 33.6%, over 11 up to 16.5 years = 33.6%.
Congenital heart block was present in 98 (40.7%) cases and post-surgical block in 136 (56.4%) of which 34 interventricular septal defects, tetralogy: 33, AV canal: 18. Symptoms leading to implantation were mainly: syncopes (67), bradycardia (92), heart failure (33). The main ECG indication was 3rd degree AV block, 66.8% of cases.
The abdominal profound location is chosen in 71.8% of cases. Energy sources of devices in service are, as of August 1982, lithium (74%) and isotope powered (26%) batteries.
Myocardial leads are placed in 93.4% of cases, among them 82.2% are Medtronic leads.
Early post-operative failures are mainly: infection (10), endocardial lead dislodgement (3), high thresholds (2). Late complications: lead fracture (19), and high thresholds (50).
Two-hundred and seven children are still alive and healthy. They required 341 PG's of which 90% were VVI mode devices. As of August 1982, 56.5% are programmable or multiprogrammable pacemakers.
In spite of remaining technical problems, myocardial approach was mainly and satisfactorily used in young children and infants. However endocardial approach seems to offer an alternative in children aged 5 years and above. It's likely that, in a near future, "physiological" devices will be more widely used in children in order to assure better haemodynamic conditions.

Introduction

Though significant advances in cardiac pacing occurred within the last few years, permanent pacemaker implantation in children is still burdened with numerous technical problems, especially in infants: their growth and the relatively large size of devices lead to repetitive surgical procedures.

Because there are few case reports in the literature, we had to collect the results of clinical experience in several Centers – mainly surgical ones. The data collected in this report are, in fact, those of earliest cases: this may account for the quite high number of technical problems, due to the equipment used.

Clinical Material

This study represents the data collection from 9 french Centers, with a total of 241 children operated on from 1965 to March 1982.

1. Distribution by age and sex

The distribution by age groups and sex is as follows:

	Male	Female	Total (%)
⩽ 1 year	13	14	27 (11.2%)
1–5 years	32	20	52 (21.6%)
6–10 years	44	37	81 (33.6%)
11–16.5 years	43	38	81 (33.6%)

Children age 1 to 10 years represent more than 50% of patients and one third of them are less than 5 years.

2. Aetiologies

Ninety-eight children have congenital heart block, either isolated (66 cases) or associated with congenital heart disease (32 cases). The heart block is acquired in 7 cases whereas 136 children have post-surgical block. Table 1 shows the distribution of the aetiologies.
We must note that most of post-surgical blocks occurred after correction of congenital heart defect including the closure of an either interventricular or interauricular septal defect (ostium secundum). On the other hand, post-operative block after surgical repair of valvular defect is rare.

3. Indication for surgery

Indications for implanting procedure were roughly distinguished between "clinical" and "electrocardiographic" indication, though they are obviously associated. Table 2 gives a summary of clinical findings which led to implantation of a pulse generator.
Symptoms most frequently encountered are: severe bradycardia (38.2%) and syncopes (27.8%) as well as heart failure (13.7%). In the group with congenital heart block (isolated), a history of syncope is the major indication for surgical procedure (50%).
We can roughly say that there is a permanent conduction disturbance in 66.8% of children, a paroxystic one in 32% of them (whilst 1.2% are symptom-free patients). These percentages are similar in the different age groups.
Table 3 shows ECG findings.
Conduction abnormalities are third-degree atrio-ventricular ones in most cases (66.8%). The conduction disturbance involves the atrial stage in 12.1% of cases.

4. Operative techniques

a) In most cases, myocardial leads were used at first implantation (225 children). They were placed either by left thoracotomy (110) or by subxiphoïdian, retrosternal approach (85), or by median sternotomy (28).

594

Table 1. Aetiologies.

1) Isolated congenital heart block	66 (27.4%)
2) Congenital heart block with congenital heart defect	32 (13.3%)
– Corrected transposition of the great vessels	8
– Interventricular septal defect (IVC)	3
– Atrioventricular septal defect (ostium primum)	3
– Atrioventricular septal defect (ostium secundum)	3
– Pulmonary stenosis	1
– Tetralogy	2
– Others	12
3) Post-operative block	136 (56.4%)
– Interatrial communication (ostium secundum)	2
– Interventricular Septal defect	34
– Tetralogy	33
– Atrioventricular septal defect (ostium primum)	18
– Corrected transposition + IVC	8
– Left corrected transposition	7
– Right corrected transposition + IVC	7
– Valvular surgery	6
– Rhythm disturbances	1
– Other reasons	20
4) Acquired heart block	7 (2.9%)
– Post-infection	3
– Systemic illness	2
– Others	2

IVC = Interventricular septal defect

Table 2. Clinical indications for pacing.

Total population		Patient population without associated congenital heart defect. n = 66
Syncope	27.8%	50.8%
Dizziness	4.1%	4.5%
Bradycardia	38.2%	30.3%
Tachycardia	2.5%	3.0%
Prophylactic	10.4%	3.0%
Heart failure	13.7%	7.6%
Miscellaneous	2.1%	
Unspecified	1.2%	

Table 3. Electrocardiographic indications.

Sinus rhythm		0.8%
First and second degree A–V block		10.1%
Third-degree A–V block		66.8%
with narrow QRS complex	35.3%	
with wide QRS complex	14.1%	
QRS unspecified	17.4%	
Bundle branch block		1.2%
Trifascicular block		2.9%
Sino-atrial block		7.1%
Sinus arrest		1.7%
Sick sinus syndrome		3.3%
Ventricular rhythm disturbance		1.2%
Unspecified indication		4.9%

A–V = atrio-ventricular.

The different lead models implanted are:

Medtronic 5814, 6917 A and others:	185
Telectronics "Jausseran":	33
Cordis:	2
Others:	5

They were placed either on the right ventricle (103 cases) or on the left ventricle (122 cases).

b) At initial implantation there were only 16 endocardial approaches. The lead brands used were mainly Medtronic (5) and Elema (3). Left veins were chosen in 9 cases and right ones in 7 cases.

c) Different locations of pulse generators have been chosen; pacemaker pockets were deep enough to avoid skin erosion, whilst external programming still could be performed.

At first implantation, pacemaker locations were as follows:

Abdominal location (186)

– sub-cutaneous	13
– under great or behind right muscles	137
– before left kidney	36

Thoracic location (55)

– thoracic wall	26
– intra-pleural	29

5. At first implantation, energy sources in the devices employed were mercury-zinc cells (21.2%), lithium cells (59.8%) nuclear batteries (18.3%) and others (0.8%).

The pacing modes of these devices were: VOO: 18, VVI: 213, VVT: 5, VAT: 3, DDD: 2.

In addition, it can be noted that 137 (35%) out of 387 pulse generators implanted were multiprogrammable devices. As of August 1982, 117 out of 207 alive and followed patients are paced by programmable or multiprogrammable devices, ie. 56.5%.

6. Non-lethal complications

a) 16 patients had a history of 17 complications: 10 infections, 3 important haematomae, 4 skin erosions.
b) 61 children (25.3%) had lead-related problems.
1. In the group with myocardial leads, 52 children had 86 incidents, of which 16 leadf fractures and 46 high thresholds (in 31 children).
In addition, we could also observe: early high thresholds (4), diaphragmatic stimulation (2), infection (2), insulation defects (3), sensing defects (2), systematic change (3) and others (8).
2. In the group with endocardial leads, 9 children had 17 lead-related incidents, of which 3 lead fractures, 7 lead dislodgements (in 4 children) and 2 high thresholds (in 2 children). One could also observe: insulation defects (2), permanent diaphragmatic stimulation (1) and systematic changes (2).
3. These complications were corrected by 46 lead replacements, 11 cases in which bipolar pacing was replaced by unipolar pacing; in 12 cases myocardial pacing was replaced by endocardial pacing, and in 10 cases the increase in pulse width was required in order to augment the energy.

7. One can see below the summary of the number of leads by child:

	Alive	Dead or lost to follow-up	Total
Children with one lead	156	29	185
Children with 2 leads	39	3	42
Children with 3 leads	5	1	6
Children with 4 leads	2		2
Children with 5 leads	4	1	5
Children with 6 leads	1		1

(a total of 283 either unipolar or bipolar leads were implanted in 207 children still alive today, and a total of 43 leads were used in the children dead or lost to follow-up).
The distribution of the 326 leads is: 287 myocardial leads and 39 endocardial ones.
The myocardial leads employed were mainly: Medtronic 6917 (120), 5814 (83), 6913 (8), 4951 (4) and Telectronics "Jausseran" (41).

8. Replacement of pulse generators

In the early years of pacing, these Centers experienced frequent pulse generator replacements due to the nature of power sources, i.e. mercuryzinc cells. Later on, marketing of nuclear-powered and lithium-powered pacemakers made them less frequent.
In this series, 70% of children had only one pacemaker; 17% had two devices, 7% had three and 8% three or more, with a maximum of seven pacemakers in three children.

9. Mortality

a) Ten children have died within the first post-operative month: 8 cases are congenital heart defect-related, 1 case is due to a systemic thromboembolic event, 1 case for unknown reason (5 children were less than 3.5 months).

b) Sixteen children have died after the first post-operative month (from 1.5 month to 14.6 years after surgery): 10 cases are congenital heart defect-related, 2 cases were accidental deaths, 2 were due to infection, and 2 occurred for unknown reasons.

10. Survival

These children as of August 30, 1982, were:

Alive	207	85.9%
Alive – lost to follow-up	4	1.7%
Alive – followed elsewhere	1	0.4%
Alive – pacing material removed	3	1.2%
Dead	26	10.8%

The mean follow-up is 1763.5 days (4.8 years) for the alive children (mean range: from 970.4 days to 2928.7 days – according to the different Centers). The survival range is from 0 day to 17.5 years.

Discussion

This multicenter study emphasizes the following points:

1. The need for permanent pacemaker implantation is relatively limited in children. Most of them are required in case of post-operative conduction disturbances (after surgical closure of interventricular or interauricular septal defect).

2. Cardiac pacing is an effective treatment, in spite of several repetitive surgical procedures for the early implanted children of this series.

3. Today, indications for surgery are well-known. In most cases, the indication is third-degree A-V block. In our series, the group of patients with severe post-operative heart failure must be examined separately. This concerns mainly children less than 1 year (10/27) and those aged 1 to 5 years (12/52); its incidence is, in male children twice the one of female children. It occurred frequently in one Center (28/76) and was in fact the major indication with bradycardia (35/76). In fact, this Center is a medico-surgical one, highly trained in heart surgery of infants. This probably accounts for the lower incidence of these indications in the other Centers.

4. The majority of children have myocardial leads. We personally prefer myocardial approach for the following reasons: good lead fixation – availability of physiological pacing – it allows for children's growth with a low risk of lead fractures.

Pulse generator location must be deeply performed in order to avoid skin erosion and to permit, if necessary, external programming of the devices.

Intra-pleural location in only admitted in the new-born child. Furthermore if a thoracic implantation has to be made, it's more advisable to locate the pulse generator between the pleura and the chest wall than in an intrapleural position. Most of the pulse generators are deeply placed in the abdominal wall or before left kidney.

The complications with a total of 287 myocardial leads occurred in 52 children who presented with 86 incidents.

a) *Lead fractures*

They only appear with the Medtronic Model 5814 leads, which have the longest follow-up. There are 7 (31.8%) fractures when the leads are on the left ventricle and 5 (8.2%) fractures when the right ventricle is chosen. Therefore, it seems preferable to implant myocardial leads on the right ventricle.

b) *High thresholds*

They occurred with the 3 types of leads employed. The incidence seems hihger with the left ventricular implantation but there is no statistically significant difference.

Complications can also be observed with endocardial leads. Nine children presented with 17 incidents (on a total of 39 endocardial leads). The prevailing complications are dislodgements (7 cases), fractures (3 cases) and high thresholds (2 cases).

5. The ratio between incidents and the total number of leads is 86/287, i.e. 29% for myocardial leads; for endocardial leads, this ratio is 17/39 i.e. 43.6%. This difference is not statistically significant.

6. It is therefore obvious that lead-related complications are less frequent with myocardial leads than with endocardial leads, mainly with the screw-in Medtronic Model 6917 lead, in which no fracture was observed.

The main cause for pacing failure is still late high thresholds, whatever the route chosen.

New lead models should therefore have – in addition to the usual mechanical and electrical performances – as small size as possible in order to take care fo areas where myocardial leads can be implanted.

7. In our opinion, myocardial approach is therefore a very interesting one in children; it's the only suitable one for infants and new-born. Endocardial approach may be considered for children aged 6 to 7 years and above. However, it is not without disadvantages, especially risks for veinous thrombosis, embolic migration, tricuspid valve insufficiency...

These incidents are likely to occur in case of dual-chamber pacing, when 2 pervenous leads must be inserted.

Though these complications remain relatively frequent, the benefits of long-term cardiac pacing in children are many. Because of its technological advances, physicians are less reluctant than years ago to use this treatment. However, prevention of post-operative heart block remains an important point; its occurrence could be controlled via a better knowledge of conduction pathways as well as of their per-operative identification.

We have extensively discussed the choice of implanting approach; as for the choice of pulse generator models, it would be advisable to implant at least multiprogrammable models, the best course to take being to dispose of physiological devices.

Authors' address:
A. Vanetti, M.D.
Hôpital Saint-Joseph
7, rue Pierre Larousse
75014 Paris
France

Clinical Reliability of Multiprogrammable Pacemaker in Pediatrics

J. Cabo Salvador, F. Moreno Granados, P. A. Sanchez, G. Cordovilla, P. Malo, J. M. Brito, F. Alvarez Diaz

Summary: In our experience the incidence of postsurgical complete heart block (PCHB) in children is less frequent than congenital complete heart block (CCHB) requiring permanent cardiac pacing (PCP). Only in 5 patients (pts) (0.2%) out of more than 2000 open heart corrections of congenital heart defects a pacemaker (PM) implantation was needed and only in 18 (27.7%) out of 65 pts with CCHB, PCP was required. In all, an epicardial approach, acute threshold measurement (voltage, current, resistance and R-wave) and multiprogrammable generator (MPG) implantation were performed. There was 1 death unrelated to the PM. Complications such as exit-block, sensing problems (oversensing) and wound complications could be found during the follow-up (12 months-8 years, mean 40 months). For anatomical reasons we prefered an epicardial approach, sutureless leads with a minimal myocardial penetration and small sized MPGs. Because of frequent exit-block in pediatrics we selected the site for permanent epicardial pacing (mapping) to measuring the acute threshold and using MPGs which allow the PM-adaptation to children's requirements.

Different forms and modes of artificial cardiac pacing obtained world wide acceptance in patients with permanent cardiac pacing (PCP). The availability of noninvasive multiparameter programmable pacing devices allows pacemaker's adaptation to patient's requirements as well as to test the function of the system. Programmability has proven its clinical effectiveness (1–4) in different aspects: reducing incidence of reoperations, increasing pacemaker longevity, allowing rate adjustments for the growing child, and increasing the energy output to permit cardiac capture in the presence of continuously rising stimulation thresholds. Therefore we found such multiprogrammable PM-devices specially indicated in the pediatric age group.

Clinical Material and Methods

Permanent cardiac pacing (PCP) with multiprogrammable generators was performed in 25 patients, 10 male and 15 females (Table 1). Out of 65 children with congenital complete heart block (CCHB) PCP was required in 18 patients (27.7%). The indications were: syncope (Adams-Stookes syndrome) in 13 cases, congestive heart failure with slow ventricular rate in 4 cases, rapid atrial (> 140 bpm) and slow ventricular (< 50 bpm) rate in 1 case. In two cases the pacemaker (PM) was implanted due to a drug resistant sinus nodal dysfunction.

Among more than 2000 open heart corrections of congenital heart defects (0.2%) a pacemaker (PM) was needed in five patients (Table 1) with a mean age of 22 months (6 days to 12 years). In 18 cases a temporal pacing was needed, previous to definitive implantation.

Epicardial pacing was performed in all instances, thoracotomy in 1 case and subxiphoid-subcostal in the remainder 24 cases. In all patients an epicardial screw-in lead (cork-

Table 1. Indication for permanent cardiac pacing.

Congenital complete heart block (N = 18)		No of cases
Syncope (Stockes-Adams syndrome)		13
Congestive heart failure with slow ventriculare rate		4
Rapid atrial (> 140) and slow ventricular rate (< 50)		1

Postsurgical complete heart block (N = 5)

Anatomi Defect	Type of Correction	
D-Transposition of the great arteries intact ventricular septum	Hemodynamic correction (Mustard technique	1
Complete atrioventricular canal defect, banding	Double patch technique, Bjork prosthesis, debanding	1
Atrioventricular canal ostium primum type	Total correction	1
Double aortic valvular lesion	Bjork valve prosthesis	1
L-Transposition of the great arteries, ventricular septal defect, patent ductus arteriosus, pulmonary hypertension	Total correction	1

Sinus nodal dysfunction

Bradycardia – Tachycardia (Short syndrome)		1
Total		25

screw electrode) with 3.5 mm depth-penetration and 6.6 mm² of surface area was employed.

PM-Implantation Technique

a) *Surgical approach:*

Through a left subcostal incision, extended from the xiphisternum to the left costal arch, the pericardial sac is exposed through the Larrey's space. An anterior pericardial incision carried down to the diaphragm and left laterally extension is performed. This approach offers various advantages: good access to the right ventricular diaphragmatic surface, left ventricular anterior wall and right atrial appendage, if needed; shorter operative and anesthetic times and the possibility of extubation at the end of the procedure.

b) *Electrophysiologic studies-Mapping:*

Prior to the definitive implantation a precise and carefull mapping and also an electrophysiologic study was performed with voltage, current, resistance, and R-wave measurements. A myocardial test probe was used to identify the implantation site. Acute stimulation and sensing threshold measurements were determined routinely. Measurements made at a pulse duration setting of 0.5 milliseconds by means of a Pacing System Analyzer that provided a readout of the intrinisc cardiac signal derived either from the myocardial testing electrode or from the sutureless epicardial lead.

c) *Electrode-implantation*

Once the epicardial electrode (sutureless) is anchored, the lead is looped inside the pericardium (Fig. 1A, 1B) to allow enlargement, so that the child's growth will not produce tension on the electrode or on the interface (Fig. 2A, 2B).

d) *Generator-implantation:*

The linea alba and the rectus sheath are opened. The rectus muscle is elevated from the posterior sheath and the PM is placed into the newly created space, a submuscularly pocket bounded anteriorly by the rectus and oblique muscles and posteriorly by the posterior sheath and transversalis muscle.

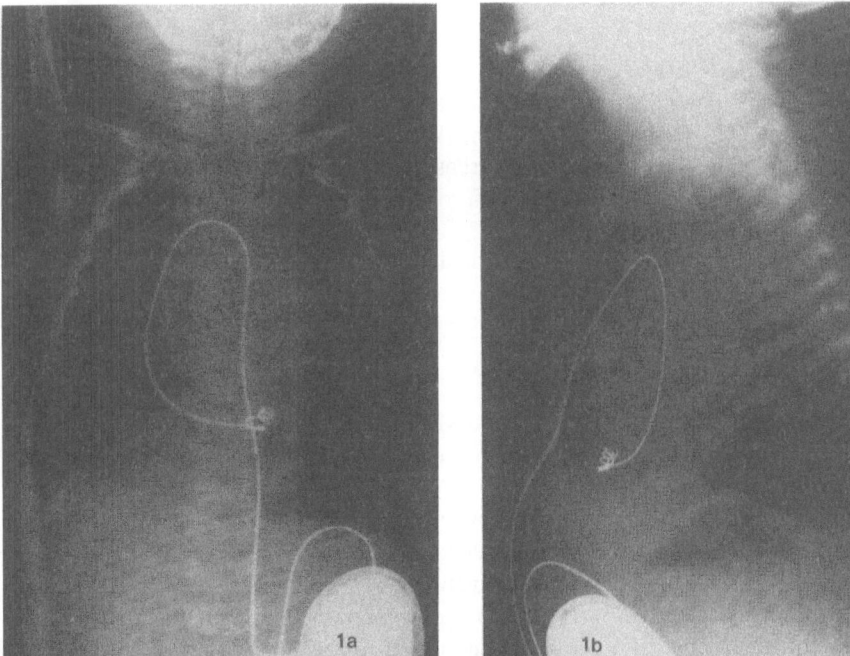

Fig. 1. A) Postero-anterior view of the loop inside the pericardium. B) A lateral view of the loop in the same patient.

603

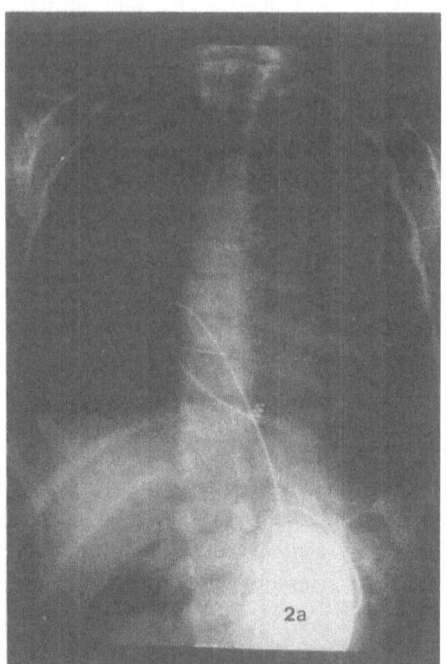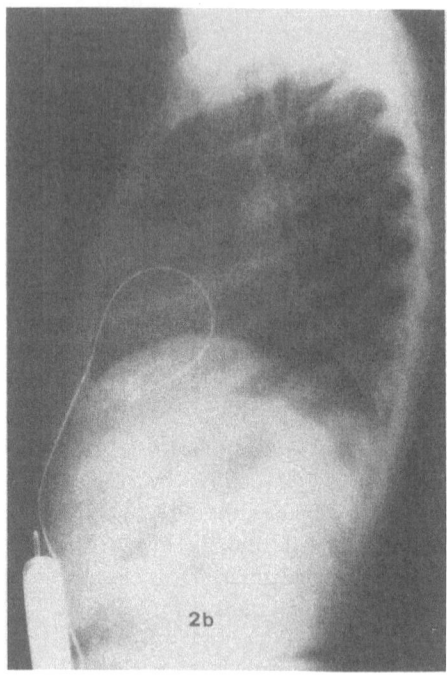

Fig. 2. The loop has decreased at the follow up. A) postero-anterior view. B) lateral view.

e) *Generator:*

It has been our policy to employ in all cases a lithium powered, noninvasive multipara-meter-programmable pacing device, in the VVI-mode. Programmable parameters in-clude: rate, pulse width and amplitude, sensitivity, refractory period and operational mode. Recently, in the last patients a multiprogrammable PM with telemetric data trans-mission has been implanted.

In all cases the pacing mode has been ventricular demand pacing (VVI).

Results

There was one only death unrelated to the PM-device. It occurred in the child with levo-transposition and pulmonary hypertension due to low cardiac output in the immediate postoperative period.

In the group of patients requiring temporary pacing due to transient postoperative PCHB, only in 5 patients a permanent PM was needed. Two neonates with CCHB received their first PM at the age of 2 and 7 years respectively.

During a follow-up ranging from 12 months to 8 years (mean 40 months) in 2 cases the PCP was retired. In one child with implantation at the age of 28 days, a first grade AV block with left anterior hemiblock (LAH) and right bundle branch block (RBBB) was ob-served 2½ years later. In the other child with implantation at the age of 3 years, an acceptable basic rhythm was found at the moment of elective generator replacement for battery depletion.

The mean values of acute threshold measurements (epicardial electrode) were: voltage, 0.91 ± 0.2 Vs; current, 1.35 ± 0.36 mA; resistance, 675 ± 171 ohms; R-wave, 9.04 ± 3 mv.

Chronic threshold measurements were available in 10 patients. The overage threshold values were: voltage, 2.30 ± 0.8 Vs; current, 3.42 ± 2 mA; resistance, 709 ± 132 ohms, with a mean interval-time between acute and chronic measurements of 72 months (Table 2).

Pacemaker replacement due to battery depletion was performed in five patients.

Leads system replacement was needed in 2 patients, due to high chronic myocardial thresholds both out of the unmapped group. The first one with PM implantation at the age of 3 years and sensing failure 3 months later required lead replacement at the age of 8 years (chronic threshold were: 4.5 Vs, and current, 27 mA). The second one with PM implantation at the age of 16 months required lead replacement at the age of 7 years (chronic threshold were: voltage, 7 Vs; current, 5.2 mA).

Wound complications such as infection and/or PM extrussion occurred in 3 patients, being the major indication for reoperation. One 6-days-old neonate with a submuscularly implanted generator (Fig. 3) had the PM partially exposed through the incision due to rectus muscular necrosis requiring an intrathoracic reimplantation.

One child developed sudden loss of ventricular capture and sensing due to iatrogenic into the componenets of the latter, which required a replacement of the unit. No wire fractures occurred in the entire series.

Discussion

PCP indications in children are different to those of adults (5–18).

In CCHB the indication for a permanent PM has to be carefully considered. At the present moment, we recommend PM-implantation in the following circumstances: a) children with syncopes or recurrent dizzines; b) at the time of surgical correction of associated cardiac anomalies; c) congestive heart failure due to a slow ventricular rate refractory to medical treatment; d) low cardiac output during exercise confirmed by ergometry tests; e) wide QRS complex > 0.08 ms as prophylactic procedure due to the high incidence of

Table 2. Threshold evolution at the follow-up. Acute and achronic measurements.

Threshold measurements at a pulse duration of 0.5 msec.
Interval-time between measurements = 72 months.

	Acute threshold (N = 25)	Chronic threshold (N = 10)
Voltage (Vs)	0.91 ± 0.2	2.3 ± 0.8
Current (mA)	1.35 ± 0.3	3.4 ± 2
Resistance (Ω)	675 ± 171	709 ± 132
R-wave (mv)	9 ± 3	6 ± 4

Fig. 3. Chest-X-ray of a neonate (6 days old). Although the unit was the smallest one available it can be appreciated the relation between PM and body surface.

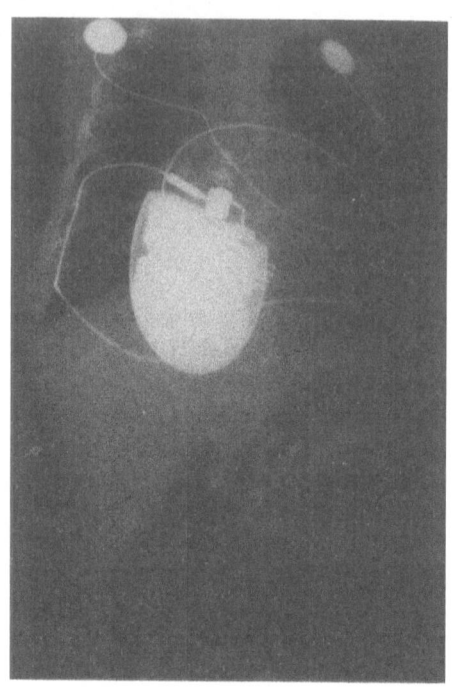

potential sudden death (7, 13); and f) neonates with a rapid atrial (> 140 bpm) and slow ventricular rate (< 50 bpm) with a poor prognosis without permanent stimulation (5, 13–15, 18).

PCHB is the most common and noncontroversial indication for PCP (5–12, 14, 16, 19–23), with an immediate postoperative mortality rate without treatment ranging between 60 to 100 percent (6, 9, 20, 21, 23). Due to better knowledge of the conduction system anatomy and due to the improvement of surgical techniques, the PCHB incidence has decreased considerably and few patients require PCP nowadays. (In our experience it has been only 0.2%.) At present, we indicate PCP when the PCHB persists for more than 2 weeks and the electrophysiologic study has shown an AV block within or below the His bundle level or the Holter monitoring demonstrates a persistent ventricular rate under 50 bpm at rest.

Sick sinus syndrome is frequently seen in children after repair of congenital heart lesions (7, 9–12, 17, 26), the transient form is probably due to the routinely use of cardioplegic solutions and to the tissue damage during surgical repair. Usually, these types of sinus node dysfunction dissappear in the immediate postoperative period without sequelae. In patients with persistent and symptomatic sick sinus syndrome, we perform electrophysiologic studies and Holter's monitoring to assess the sinus node function. The decision for PM implantation is difficult and problematic, being PCP indicated when syncope, recurrent or drug resistant sinus nodal dysfunction occurs and also when symptomatic postoperative bradycardia-tachycardia syndrome or other forms of arrhythmias such as incesant re-entry tachycardia are present (Table 3).

606

Table 3. Indication for permanent cardiac pacing in pediatrics.

Complete congenital heart block,
   Syncope or recurrent dizzines
   Associated to other cardiac anomalies
   Congestive heart failure (slow ventricular rate)
   Evidence of inadequate cardiac output (physiologic and stress testing)
   Wide QRS complex (more than 0.08 msc)
   Newborn with rapid atrial rate (more than 140 bpm) and slow ventricular rate (less than 50 bpm)

Sick sinus syndrome
   Symptomatic, with syncope or recurrent dizzines
   Drug resistant sinus nodal dysfunction
   Symptomatic postoperative bradycardia-tachycardia syndrome
   Incesant re-entry tachycardia

Postsurgical complete heart block
   Persistent more than 2 weeks with electrophysiologic study and block within or below the His bundle.
   Persistent ventricular rate at rest of less than 50 bqm.

As indicated by other groups (5, 7–12, 15, 17, 22, 24–28), we prefer epicardial versus endocardial approach, sutureless leads with a minimal depth penetration and with small size and low weight multiprogrammable generator (14, 18). Electrode and generator implantation techniques in infants lead to problems which are uncommon in adults. As a routine, we place the electrode through a subxiphisternum-subcostal approach with a morbidity as low as reported with either approaches (29–31). In addition, it provides a good access to the right ventricular diaphragmatic surface, which has been shown to be a suitable one for long term pacing (14, 18, 33). Displacement or lead-fracture resulting from the child's growth has been reported as a common cause of PM-failure (9, 11, 12, 16, 17, 27, 29–31).

In our experimence the large intrathoracic loop of the lead can avoid this problem as it has been proven during the follow-up. The loop decreases gradually while the child grows.

Due to the great tendency to exit-block in pediatrics (9, 11, 12, 16, 17, 27, 29–31) we think it is neccessary to select carefully the site for permanent epicardial pacing, performing an electrophysiological mapping of the heart with acute threshold measurements during PM implantation, which provides long term effectiveness of the system (14, 18, 32–34). In many of our patients the final threshold obtained with this technique was much better than measured initially (14, 18, 33).

Another problems in the pediatric patient is the site for PM implantation. The subcutaneous implantation (7) produces not only unacceptable esthetical results but it also can lead to skin necrosis and subsequently extrusion of the unit (11, 26). As other authors (24–26, 28, 35), we recommend the submuscular implantation of the generator under the rectus anterior abdominus muscle (14, 18).

During the follow up period it is necessary to assess the changes in the stimulation threshold and to vary the PM parameters obtained by the use of a multiprogrammable pulse generator. As consequence of the recent development of PM technology the spectrum of programmable functions has increased. Multiprogrammability represents a great advance in cardiac pacing allowing to variate the characteristics of pacing rate, pulse width and amplitude, refractory period, sensitivity and pacing mode according to patient requirements. The benefits of its use are well established (1–4).

The most common medical application of multiprogrammable generators are:

Rate programmability: a) for selection of appropriate pacing-rate according to phyisiological requirements leading to an optimal cardiac output and an efficient cardiac performance, b) for rate adjustments in the growing pediatric patient; c) for overdirve suppression of ventricular ectopic rhythm. In all our patients the rate was reprogrammed during the follow up period.

Pulse width programmability: During the early postimplant period the myocardial threshold increased with a subsequent decrease, because of tissue damage, fibrotic changes and foreign body reaction around the electrode tip. The avoid sensing and pacing failure due to this threshold increase we perform strength-duration curves increasing the pulse duration in milliseconds to double. Although the concept of output programmability was primarily introdùced in order to save energy, but it has also important clinical applications with the following possibilities: to obtain a noninvasive assessment of threshold- and electrode-status; to minimize energy delivery increasing PM longevity; to correct an anomalous muscle stimulation; and to eliminate temporarily intermittent loss of capture reobtaining cardiac stimulation in the presence of an exit-block with the use of a high pulse width which avoids the necessity of reoperation. All our patients had reprogrammed pulse width on the basis of threshold testing and strength-duration curves.

Sensitivity programmability: Which allows the two following possibilities: to increase the sensitivity to restore normal sensing, especially in the atrial pacing and in cases with poor

Table 4. Clinical application of programmability.

Rate
For rate-selection according physiologic requirements.
For adjustments in the growing pediatric patient.
For overdrive supression of ventricular ectopic rhythm.

Pulse width
Noninvasive assessment of threshold and electrode status.
Increase in pacemaker longevity.
Correction of anomalous muscle stimulation.
Elimination of intermittent loos of capture.

Sensitivity
Increase, to restore normal sensing.
Decrease, to eliminate abnormal T-wave sensing
Decrease, to eliminate electomagnetic interferences or false-recycling.

Refractory period
Reduction for effective sensing of premature ventricular or atrial ectopic beats.
Increase to avoid oversensing (afterpotentials).

ventricular electrogram, and to decrease the sensitivity to eliminate abnormal T-wave sensing or other sensing anomalies such as electromagnetic interferences or false recycling.

Refractory period program ability: a) for effective sensing of premature ventricular or atrial ectopic beats reducing the refractory period, and b) to avoid oversensing (afterpotentials, in one of our case) increasing the refractory period (Table 4).

Recently in the last patients we have implanted a multiprogrammable device with telemetry that displays the programmed settings in a noninvasive manner, checking the battery and transmitting the intracardiac electrogram continuously. The transmitted electrogram permits to assess the interface providing an accurate information of the position of the lead. Such electrograms could be obtained in two patients because they had underlying intrinsic rhythm. The full clinical usefulness of intracardiac electrogram can be obtained only in those patients with underlying intrinsic rhythm. Therefore, our opinion is that this device must be reserved to this special group of patients.

References

1. MacGregor DC, Furman S, Dreifus LS, Cuddy TE: The utility of the programmable pacemaker. PACE 1978; 1: 254–259.
2. Vera Z, Klein RC, Mason DT: Recent advances in programmable pacemakers. Am J Med 1979; 66: 473–438.
3. Furman S, Escher DJW, Fisher JD: Seven year experience with programmable pulse generator. Proceedings of the VI World Symposium on Cardiac Pacing. In Cardiac Pacing. C Meere Ed. Laplante + Langevin Inc Montreal 1979, chap 19–1.
4. Griffin JC: Pacemaker programmability: Its role in the maintenance of pacing system function. Proceedings of the Second European Symposium on Cardiac Pacing. In Cardiac Pacing. Electrophysiology and Pacemaker Technology. GA Feruglio Ed. Piccin Medical Books. Padova 1982: p 759–763.
5. Benrey J, Gillete PC, Masrallah AT, Hallman GL: Permanent pacemaker implantation in infants, children and adolescents. Lont term follow up. Circulation 1976; 53: 245–248.
6. Hofschire PJ, Nicoloff DM, Moller JH: Postoperative complete heart block in 64 children treated with and without cardiac pacing. Am J Cardiol 1977; 39: 559–562.
7. Furman S, Young D: Cardiac Pacing in children and adolescents. Am J Cardiol 1977; 39: 550–558.
8. Shearin RPN, Fleming WH: Fourteen years of implanted pacemakers in children. Ann Thorac Surg 1978; 25: 144–147.
9. Williams WG, Izukawa T, Olley PM, Trusler GA, Rowe RD: Permanent cardiac pacing in infants and children. PACE 1978; 1: 439–447.
10. Driscoll DJ, Gillete PC, Hallman GL, Cooley DA, McNamara DG: Management of surgical complete atrioventricular block in children. Am J Cardiol 1979; 43: 1175–1180.
11. Williams WG, Izukawa T, Trusler GA, Smith JM: Experience with permanent cardiac pacing in paediatrics. Proceedings of the VI World Symposium on Cardiac Pacing. In Cardiac Pacing. C Meere Ed. Laplante + Langevin Inc Montreal 1979: chap 23–7.
12. Nissen RG, Holmes DR, Maloney JD, Feldt RH, Danielson GK: Experience with permanent cardiac pacemakers in congenital heart disease. Proceedings of the VI World Symposium on Cardiac Pacing. In Cardiac Pacing. C Meere Ed. Laplante + Langevin Inc Montreal 1979: chap 23–2.
13. Gross DM, Izukawa T, Williams WG, Trusler GA, Freedom RM, Rowe RD: Use of artificial pacemakers in treatment of neonatal congenital complete heart block. Proceedings of the VI World Symposium on Cardiac Pacing. In Cardiac Pacing. C Meere ED. Laplante + Langevin Inc Montreal 1979: chap. 23–6.

14. Cabo Salvador J, Moreno Granados F, Sanz Galeote E, Borches Jacassa D, Cordovilla Zurdo G, Alvarez Diaz F: Estimulación cardiaca permanente en niños: Indicaciones y resultados. Estimulación Cardíaca 1981; 2: 237–242.
15. Karpawich PP, Gillete PC, Garson A Jr, Hesslein PS, Porter C, McNamara DG: Congenital complete atrioventricular block: Clinical and electrophysiologic predictors of need for pacemaker insertion. Am J Cardiol 1981; 48: 1098–1102.
16. Weber H, Eigster G, Wesselhoeft H, Ruschewski W, deVivie ER: A 17 year survey of permanent pacing in infants and children. PACE 1981; 4: A-26.
17. Vanetti A, Aubry Ph, Chaptal PA, Conso JF, Laurens P, Leca F, Lefebvre MF: Pacing in children under 15 years of age. PACE 1981; 4: A-77.
18. Cabo Salvador J, Cordovilla G, Sanz E, Borches D, Alvarez Diaz F: Pacemakers in infants and children with congenital heart block. Proceedings of the Second European Symposium on Cardiac Pacing. In Cardiac Pacing. Electrophysiology and Pacemaker Technology: GA Feruglio Ed. Piccin Medical Books. Padova 1982: p 439–441.
19. Wolff GS, Rowland TW, Ellison RC: Surgically induced right bundle-branch block with left anterior hemiblock: An ominous sign in postoperative tetralogy of Fallot. Ped Res 1972; 6: 348/88.
20. Moss AJ, Kylman G, Emmanouilides GC: Late onset complete heart block. Newly recognized sequela of cardiac surgery. Am J Cardiol 1972; 30: 884–887.
21. Zion MM, Marchand PE, Obel IWP: Long-term prognosis after cardiac pacing in atrioventricular block. Br Heart J 1973; 35: 359–364.
22. Daicoff GR, Aslami A, Tobias JA, Miller BL: Management of postoperative complete heart block in infants and children. Chest 1974; 66: 639–641.
23. Izukawa T, Trusler GA, Williams WG: Effect of transient heart block occurring at the time of closure of ventricular septal defects on the incidence of late complete heart block. Proceedings of the VI World Symposium on Cardiac Pacing. In Cardiac Pacing. C Meere Ed. Laplante + Langevin Inc Montreal 1979: chap 23–5.
24. Donahoo JS, Haller JA, Zonnebelt S, Neill C, Golt V, Brawley RK: Permanent cardiac pacemakers in children: Technical considerations. Ann Thorac Surg 1976: 22: 584–587.
25. Culliford AT, Isom OW, Doyle E: Pacemaker implantation in the extremely young. J Thorac Cardiovasc Surg 1978; 75: 763–764.
26. Amato JJ, Khan A, Payne D, Cleveland RJ: Pacemaker implantation in infants and children. In Proceedings of the VI World Symposium on Cardiac Pacing. In Cardiac Pacing. C Meere Ed. Laplante + Langevin Inc Montreal 1979: chap 23–1.
27. Hayward RP, Somerville J, Rickards AF: Problems of permanent pacing in children. Proceedings of the VI world Symposium on Cardiac Pacing. In Cardiac Pacing. C Meere Ed. Laplante-+ Langevin Inc Montreal 1979: chap 23–3.
28. Van Heeckeren DW, Borkat G, Clayman JA, Horrigan TP, Ankeney JL: Pacemaking in children. Proceedings of the VI World Symposium on Cardiac Pacing. In Cardiac Pacing. C Meere Ed. Laplante + Langevin Inc Montreal 1979: chap 23–4.
29. Hayes DL, Maloney JD, Neubauer SA, Ritter DG: Effectiveness of transvenous endocardial pacing in the pediatric age group. Proceedings of the Second European Symposium on Cardiac Pacing. In Cardiac Pacing. Electrophysiology and Pacemaker Technology. GA Feruglio Ed. Piccin Medical Books. Padova 1982: p. 441–446.
30. Siddons H: Transvenous pacing in the child. Ann Cardiol Angeiol 1971; 20: 445–450.
31. Whitman V, Berman W Jr, Tyers GFO: Pacemakers in young patients: 1977. J Pediatrics 1978; 92: 722–724.
32. Varriale P, Naclerio EA, Niznik J: Selection of the site for permanent epicardial pacing using myocardial testing electrode. NY State J Med 1977; 77: 1272–1275.
33. Cabo Salvador J, Rubio Alvarez J, Amaro Cendon A, Garcia Bengochea JB: Umbrales agudos y cronicos en la estimulación epicardica de la cara diafragmática del ventriculo derecho. Arch Inst Cardiol Mex 1981; 51: 221–225.
34. Garcia Bengochea JB, Rubio Alvarez J, Cabo Salvador J: Clinical experience with the sutureless epicardial lead using an intramyocardial probe detector for selection of the insertion site. 27th International Congress of the European Society of Cardiovascular Surgery (Proceedings). Lyon 1978.

35. Amato JJ, Payne D, Rheinlander HF, Cleveland RJ: Intermuscular abdominal implantation of permanent pacemakers in infants and children. Ann Thorac Surg 1978; 25: 243–247.

Author's address:
Dr. J. Cabo Salvador
Servicio de Cirugía Cardiovascular Infantil
Ciudad Sanitaria "La Paz"
Paseo de la Castellana, 261
Madrid – 34. Spain

His Bundle Recording and Electrical Programmed Stimulation

N. Shantha*), G. Fontaine**)

Summary: Since the introduction of His-bundle recordings in 1969 many different methods were developed for introduction and termination of various tachyarrhythmias: In supraventricular tachycardia sinus node reentrant tachycardia occurs either spontaneously or can be induced by atrial pacing or by the extrastimulus technique. The termination often is spontaneous mediated through the autonomic tone. To make the diagnosis, intraatrial mapping is required.

Careful analysis of the atrial sequence is needed to differentiate AV nodal reentry from a concealed bypass tract using the ventricular stimulation technique. Infrequently a reentry tachycardia originates from the His-bundle itself, which mostly demonstrates prolonged and split His-potentials.

A separation of ventricular tachycardia into reentry and focal may be arbitrary. It is not possible to rule out a micro-reentry. The initiation of VT by programmed ventricular stimulation is limited by the different methods used. Nevertheless this technique can induce in 80–90% of the patients with VT. The prognostic value is controversial. The extrastimuli technique will be also used in the evaluation of antiarrhythmic therapy ("Electrophysiologic drug testing").

Results are useful in the prediction of long term efficacy: In patients with CAD the recurrence rate of VT and sudden death was lower if VT cannot be induced. In the WPW-Syndrome programmed stimulation techniques allow assessment of conduction characteristics and refractoriness of the AV-node and the anomalous pathways.

The non-invasive techniques of an oesophageal lead can be used to differentiate SVT and VT. Oesophageal pacing can induce and terminate SVT, atrial flutter and can induce atrial fibrillation.

Intraoperative pacemapping involves stimulation of various sites of the heart until stimulation at a particular site produces a QRS configuration identical to the known VT. Ablation of this focus would abolish the arrhythmia.

In summary electrophysiologic methods enhanced our understanding of the mechanism of tachyarrhythmias.

Since the original technique for recording of His Bundle electrogram in AV block was described by Scherlag in 1969 (1), major advances have been made in clinical electrophysiology. Using multiple intracardiac electrode recordings and by using extrastimulus technique, it has been possible to reproduce supraventricular and ventricular tachyarrhythmias in a cardiac catheterization laboratory and to study systematically the effects due to one or more antiarrhythmic drug in the abolition of the tachyarrhythmia. More recently, more definitive methods of treatment like electrical ablation of the His bundle, accessory pathway and ectopic foci have become feasible (2, 3, 4). The purpose of this present paper is to cover briefly the methods used in the laboratory for induction and termination of various tachyarrhythmias.

In the electrophysiological laboratory, electrical stimulation of the heart requires placement of electrode catheters at different locations in the heart, depending on the type of ta-

*) State University of New York
**) Service de Rythmologie et de Stimulation Cardiaque

chycardia one is dealing with. The purpose of these catheters is not only to record bipolar electrograms at the local site but also for pacing. Conventionally three catheters are used. One is positioned in the right atrium close to its junction with the superior vena cava, the second across the tricuspid valve to record the His Bundle activation and the third at the right ventricular apex. Sometimes a catheter is placed in the coronary sinus to record left atrial activity when one is dealing with an AV bypass tract. Similarly, additional catheters can be positioned at the RV outflow tract or LV for pacing of the ventricles. For measuring intracardiac activation times, unipolar or bipolar recordings are obtained using an electrode catheter which can be manipulated to record from different sites in the atrium or ventricle.

The protocol used for initiation of tachycardia is different in different laboratories. Usually one or more extrastimuli are used during regular sinus rhythm, followed by regular pacing at different rates with the introduction of one, two or three extrastimuli after a fixed number of driven or paced beats. The prematurity of these extrastimuli is gradually increased until either tachycardia is initiated or until the tissue becomes refractory. Some have advocated the use of incremental pacing (at rates 80–250/min) to initiate tachycardia. However, in some patients in whom tachycardia is induced by this method, mechanisms other than reentry may be responsible. In the event of a tachycardia being initiated, it is important to evaluate the mode of termination. Usually, one or two extrastimuli are induced during the tachycardia and the coupling interval gradually decreased until the tachycardia is terminated. The other method than can be used to terminate a tachycardia is overdrive stimulation (5). The number of impulses used varies from 3 to pacing for a few seconds, the rate of the impulses in the train usually is increased gradually, starting with a rate 10 beats more than the tachycardia rate. One must remember that in some cases entrainment of the tachycardia may occur and in some the tachycardia rate may accelerate enough the cause hemodynamic embarressment (6, 7).

Supraventricular tachycardia

Paroxysmal supraventricular tachycardia may be due to enhanced automaticity of an ectopic focus or may be recurrent in nature. The site of reentry may be the sino-atrial node, atrium, AV node, accessory AV tracts or the His Bundle itself.

– *Sinus node reentrant tachycardia* can occur in all age groups, including in children. The majority of the patients are between 50 and 70 years of age. Association of paroxysmal sinus tachycardia with sinus node disease has not been well established, although some type of heart disease or hypertension is usually present in these patients (8, 9). It is usually suspected when there is a history of paroxysmal tachycardia and the ECG shows abrupt onset and termination of a tachycardia wherein the P waves are similar to those seen during sinus rhythm. Usually though, the diagnosis is made incidentally at the time of an electrophysiologic study undertaken to investigate other conduction or rhythm abnormalities. Sinus reentrant tachycardia often occurs spontaneously when there is a sudden shortening of the sinus cycle length, as during sinus arrhythmia. More frequently it can be induced by continuous atrial pacing or during extrastimulus technique. The tachycardia should be predictably induced over a zone of prematurity with the sequence of activation as described before. The tachycardia often shows slight variation in cycle length and is probably due to the extensive autonomic innervation of the peri-sinus tissue. The termination often is spontaneous and is probably mediated through changes in the autonomic tone to which the tachycardia is sensitive. In order to make the diagnosis, atrial activation should be mapped from different intraatrial recording sites and the pattern of activation must be similar to that of sinus beats, i.e. high to low and from right to left atrium. Minor changes in P wave morphology have been noted and are thought to be due to changes in the part of the sinus node which is used for antegrade conduction of the sinus impulse. The continuation of tachycardia during second degree block at the AV node is another proof that AV node is not a part of the reentrant circuit although it does not rule out intraatrial reentry. However, the morphology of the P wave and the slower tachycardia (often in the range of 80–142/min mean rate ± 105/min) usually differentiates it from the latter.

AV nodal reentrant tachycardia

Anatomical and electrophysiologic inhomogenity in the cells of the AV node favour reentrant rhythms. The reentrant pathway in a true AV nodal reentry is limited to the AV node and excitation of the atrium and ventricle are only incidental. The concept of dual AV nodal pathways was first described by Moe in 1956 and later popularised by Rosen and he explained it by functional dissociation of the AV node into a fast and slow pathway (alpha and beta) (10, 11). These two pathways have different refractory periods and have different conduction velocities. An initiating atrial impulse is blocked in the pathway with prolonged refractory period and conducts slowly through the other pathway (with a shorter refractory period but with prolonged conduction time) and if a sufficient delay is achieved, the impulse returns retrogradely up the fast pathway and initiates a reentrant tachycardia. The conduction time through the slow pathway must therefore exceed the refractory period of the fast pathway for the tachycardia to occur. The atrium is therefore activated retrograde (Ae) hence the sequence of activation is from the low atrium to the high atrium and the surface ECG shows negative P waves in leads II, III and aVF. Often the low atrial electrogram is buried in the ventriculogram or in some cases precedes the His deflection. Thus the short H.Ae time is pathognomonic for true AV nodal reentry.
Spontaneous changes in CL usually seen prior to termination of the tachycardia and in the interval between vagal manoeuvres produce changes in the antegrade limb i.e. Ae to His which is often the site of termination. Ventriculo-atrial conduction during ventricular pacing shows incremental conduction with block occuring in the AV node i.e. retrograde His not followed by atrial electrogram.

Reentrant tachycardias using concealed bypass tracts

The presence of bypass tracts which are utilised only for retrograde conduction from the ventricle to atrium (hence concealed in the surface ECG) was first described by Slama in 1973 (12). The reported incidence of PSVT due to the presence of concealed bypass tracts has been increasing in the last few years since most centers now use ventricular stimulation as a routine in their protocol for studying tachyarrhythmia patients.

615

In some patients a concealed Kent bundle may form the retrograde limb during tachycardia. Antegrade conduction is usually normal. During ventricular stimulation, the conduction is maintained up to fast pacing cycle lengths (usually retrograde conduction better than antegrade AV conduction).

– The VA time is constant at all pacing rates and with premature impulses. The atrial activation is eccentric and by recording atrial electrograms from different sites, one can judge the point of earliest atrial activation corresponding to the atrial end of the bypass tract. Often with premature impulses, one can demonstrate atrial activation occurring before the His Bundle depolarization i.e. sequence V-A-H, since the atrium is activated via the bypass tract.

– During tachycardia, atrial activation follows the ventriculograms when the QRS complex is narrow or may be superimposed on the ventriculogram when the QRS complex is aberrant. A VPB induced when the His Bundle is refractory can depolarize the atrium with identical atrial activation sequence. (Termination of tachycardia can sometimes be achieved.)

– When functional bundle branch block occurs during tachycardia, the cycle of the tachycardia may prolong if the BBB is ipsilateral as the concealed bypass tract, or may shorten if it is contralateral since ventricular activation is necessary for atrial activation, the tachycardia cannot continue if AV block occurs during the tachycardia. Vagotonic maneuvers may slow or block the antegrade limb during tachycardia.

In a large number of cases previously diagnosed as AV nodal reentrant tachycardia, it is possible that concealed atrio-His often formed the fast retrograde limb. The following criteria can be used to diagnose concealed bypass tracts (13):

– Usually, in these patients the antegrade conduction is normal.

– During ventricular pacing, the conduction time between the ventricle and atrium is constant and is usually shorter than the AV interval. An incremental delay is noted until block occurs in the retrograde limb or when the ventricle becomes refractory.

– The atrial activation sequence is normal, i.e. from low septal RA, high RA, distal coronary sinus.

– With premature ventricular beats, the VA time remains constant, the activation sequence being V-H-A.

– His-A time is short and does not increase in pacing with increase in prematurity and is unaffected by AV nodal depressant drugs.

– The bypass tract may join the proximal His Bundle and hence tachycardia can exist in the presence of 2° AV block distal to His.

– The presence of aberrant intraventricular conduction does not prolong the tachycardia cycle length, however the VA time may shorten.

Thus an awareness of the possible presence of a concealed bypass tract and careful analysis of the atrial sequence during ventricular extrastimulus techniques is needed to diagnose the role of these bypass tracts in the tachycardia.

Reentry within the His Bundle

His Bundle can under certain circumstances be the site for reentry. The presence of longitudinal dissociation in the His Bundle has been described by Narula and in some cases reentry has been demonstrated in the His Bundle (14, 15). Most of the cases had prolonged and split His potentials, HV time indicating a diseased His Bundle, predisposing to reentrant rhythms.

Ventricular tachycardia

By definition, in ventricular tachycardia, the tachycardia circuit is below the bifurcation of the His Bundle, however in some cases of macro-reentry involving the bundle branches, His Bundle may form part of the reentrant circuit. Reentry is assumed to be the mechanism whenever a tachycardia is predictably initiated and terminated by programmed stimulations. The division of ventricular tachycardia into focal or reentrant may be somewhat arbitrary, since in clinical studies it is not possible to rule out the presence of micro-reentrant circuit. Also the failure to initiate a tachycardia by programmed extrastimulus technique has its limitations, since tachycardia circuit may be far from the site of stimulation. Pacing at multiple sites and sometimes LV pacing (in the presence of tachycardia limited to LV) may be required before one excludes the possibility of a reentrant tachycardia. In some cases, tachycardia can be induced only with 3, 4, or 5 extrastimuli or after Isuprel infusion. However, the sensitivity and specificity of these techniques remains controversial.

Most forms of VT are believed to originate at the Purkinje muscle junction. Hence the His Bundle activation occurs retrogradely and often the His Bundle electrogram is buried in the ventriculogram. One of the difficult problems in clinical cardiology is to differentiate ventricular vs supraventricular origin when confronted with wide QRS. However, if normalisation of the QRS complex is seen during overdrive atrial pacing, one can infer that the tachycardia is ventricular in origin. However, during overdrive atrial pacing, 2° block may occur at the level of the AV node and differentiation between SVT and VT may be difficult (16).

Wellens et al. first described the use of programmed stimulation techniques in the evaluation of ventricular tachycardia (17). Usually in a patient with documented sustained ventricular tachycardia it is possible to induce tachycardia in about 80–90% of the cases with the ventricular extrastimulus techniques (18). In some cases, ventricular premature stimulation may cause repetitive ventricular response by either: 1. macroentry within the His Purkinje system (Re HPS) also referred to as bundle branch reentry (BBR) wherein the bundle branches and a portion of the His Bundle are involved in the circuit. 2. Micro-reentry also referred to as *intraventricular reentry* (IVR) in which the reentry is localised to more peripheral areas in the Purkinje muscle junction (19, 20, 21).

BBR or ReHPS is a physiologic phenomenon which occurs almost in 50% of cases studied by ventricular stimulation techniques, and in a smaller number of cases studied by atrial pacing. It occurs with equal frequency in patients with and without structural heart disease and in patients with or without arrhythmia. Often the phenomenon becomes more prominent after Procainamide due to slowing of conduction and or due to prolongation of the refractory period (22). However, IVR is considered to be an abnormal response, since it is seen more frequently in patients with underlying coronary heart disease. Both BBR and IVR occur more frequently during ventricular stimulation rather than during atrial stimulation and more so when 2 or 3 extrastimuli are used. Greene and co-workers reported a high incidence of RVR in patients with history of recurrent ventricular tachycardia and a high incidence of sudden death in those with RVR, when followed for a period of time (23). However, in other studies the incidence of IVR was not different in the population with or without prior MI, the incidence of IVR and BBR was low and sudden death dit not occur more frequently in patients with IVR or BBR (24, 25). Ruskin et al found that RVR was an insensitive index for detecting ventricular vulnerability to life threatening arrhythmias and that RVR to single ventricular extrastimuli during sinus rhythm or atrial pacing are rare (26).

Studies by Josephson et al in patients with chronic recurrent sustained ventricular tachycardia used induction of ventricular tachycardia as the end point (18). In their population of patients with VT, coronary heart disease was the most common underlying heart disease. Reentry as the mechanism for VT was suggested by reproducible initiation and termination of tachycardia by programmed stimulation. In 90% of patients VT could be induced by one or two ventricular extrastimuli, the tachycardia rate and morphology being similar to that seen during spontaneous VT. The initiation of the tachycardia was independant of the presence of retrograde His-Purkinje delay and was not related to the development of BBR. In some patients rapid ventricular pacing induced tachycardia probably due to the development of rate dependant block in the tissues responsible for the tachycardia. Ventricular premature depolarization induced during tachycardia did not terminate VT in some cases. In others, sinus captures on atrial pacing could normalize the QRS and not terminate VT suggesting that the site of reentry was limited to a small portion of the ventricle which was relatively protected from the rest of the ventricle.

Electrophysiological studies in nonstained ventricular tachycardia have been more difficult due to lack of consistant induction. Some studies have shown poor prognosis in patients with MI who have nonstained VT (23).

Ventricular tachycardia is sometimes seen in a different population with no identifiable heart disease. Usually, these patients had tachycardia with a LBBB configuration (27). The tachycardia often was unresponsive to conventioned medical treatment and on long term follow up, course was benign.

Another group of patients in whom recurrent VT does not have the benign course was described by our group (28, 29). The clinical entity referred to arrhythmogenic right ventricular dysplasia is common in young patients between the ages of 20 to 40 years with 2 : 1 male predominance. One third of the patients have intermittent partial or complete right bundle branch block and T wave is commonly inverted in the right precordial leads. High amplitude surface ECG recordings often show delayed activation of part of the right ventricular epicardium, manifest as post-excitation potentials. During VT, usually complexes show LBBB configuration with either a normal or right axis deviation when the VT is infundibular in origin and marked left axis deviation when VT arises from the apex or postero-diaphragmatic surface of right ventricle. Endocavitary electrophysiological studies show initiation and termination of the arrhythmia by programmed pacing. In some cases, delayed potentials have been recorded in the right ventricle starting after the end of the rapid ventricular potential. When medical treatment fails in these patients, epicardial and endocardial mapping followed by surgery offers the best solution.

The therapeutic implication of the extrastimulus techniques is debatable. On one hand, electrophysiologic drug testing has provided an objective basis for choosing proper therapy since clinical episode of ventricular tachycardia and fibrillation are unpredictable in their occurence. In a recent study Spielman et al evaluated multiple invasive and non invasive variables in 84 of 120 patients studied for recurrent ventricular tachycardia. Using non-inducibility of VT as the manifestation of a successful medical response, they

618

found certain indices which prognosticated good medical response: age < 45 years, EF > 50%, absence of heart disease and when hypokinesis was only contraction abnormality (30).

Chronic recurrent VT is a potentially lethal arrhythmia and often difficult to control medically. The selection of an appropriate drug or a combination of drugs is time consuming. The drug testing was simplified since the use of programmed stimulation in evaluation of drug therapy. When VT is inducible reproducibly by extrastimulus technique, a drug is given intravenously and the studies repeated. If VT is not inducible, the drug is considered to be successful in abolition and given in an oral form on chronic basis. If however, VT is still inducible, a second drug is tried on successive days until a suitable drug or combination is found. In this way Horowitz reported success in 13/54 patients with VT followed up 3–27 months (31).

Mason found that using catheter techniques an effective drug to prevent can be identified in 71% of patients (32). When the acute drug administration prevented VT in the lab, the drug was usually effective when given orally a long period of time. In three patients, drugs failed to suppress VT acutely when given over a chronic period in the same combination successfully prevented VT. This is specially true of the newer drug, amiodarone which is effective when given orally for a long term management of VT. However, acute intravenous administration of amiodarone often does not prevent induction of tachycardia. On the other hand, chloracetyl ajmaline is effective only when given intravenously in the treatment of VT and is not useful when given in an oral form. Thus one of the drawbacks of invasive testing is the possiblity of spontaneous variability in inducibility of ventricular tachycardia. No data concerning the variability in relation to time and progress of the patients heart disease is available at the present time and this may be an important factor in analysing results of drug studies in managment of chronic ventricular tachycardia.

In conclusion, however, some of the long term results based on serial electrophysiologic studies done in 310 patients followed for a long time (6 centers in US and 3 centers FRG) should be discussed (3). There is unequivocal evidence that the results of the serial testing are useful in predicting long term efficacy. In patients with CAD, the recurrence rate of arrhythmia and sudden death were lower in patients in whom VT was not inducible as compared to those in whom VT was inducible. In some patients, the drug may fail to prevent acute attack but may be useful when given over a chronic period, probably because blood levels may be different from that in the myocardium. However, failure to respond to one Class I drug does not mean failure to another Class I agent. Failure to respond to intravenous drug does not mean failure to chronic oral therapy.

Bypass tracts

Pre-excitation of the ventricles resulting in a short PR interval, a delta wave and a slurred wide QRS complex constitute the electrocardiographic changes associated with WPW syndrome. Incidence of WPW in general population varies between 0.1–3.0./1000 (34). The clinical importance of this syndrome is the high association of PSVT due to the presence of the bypass tract. Tachycardias associated with this condition can be of many types.

1. PSVT utilizing the AV node, HPS and ventricular myocardium for anterograde conduction and the bypass tract for retrograde conduction to the atrium. The QRS complex during tachycardia is therefore narrow.

2. PSVT utilizing the bypass tract and the myocardium for antegrade conduction and the HPS, AV node for retrograde conduction. The QRS complex then is wide with BBB morphology depending on which side the bypass tract is present.

3. Atrial flutter or fibrillation with antegrade conduction through AV node and/or the bypass tract. Atrial fibrillation appears to be frequent in patients with WPW syndrome. Some patients can develop many highly life-threatening ventricular rates due to exclusive atrioventricular conduction over the AP, resulting sometimes in ventricular fibrillation. The shortest RR interval obtained during atrial fibrillation appears to correlate well with the ERP of the anomalous pathway (35).

Programmed stimulation techniques allow assessment of conduction characteristics and refractoriness of the AV node and anomalous pathways and to assess the effects of various drugs on the reentrant pathways. An estimation of effective refractory period of the anomalous pathway allows one to distinguish the patients at high risk or sudden death, i.e. those with short ERP of the anomalous pathway.

During electrophysiologic studies, not only can one study the physiological characteristics of these accessory pathways, but also the anatomical location of the bypass tract by mapping and the site of early activation at the atrial and ventricular end.

Oesophageal pacing

One of the noninvasive methods to record atrial activity is with the use of an electrode positioned in the esophagus and is often used at the bedside to differentiate SVT from VT. Transoesophageal pacing has been known for the last fifteen years. Recent studies by Gallagher et al. have shown that stable atrial pacing of the atrium can be obtained by using an electrode catheter with a wide interelectrode distance (36). Using a pulse wave of 9,9 ms duration (mean threshold of 11 mA) stable atrial pacing was obtained in all the 38 patients studied by them. This method has been used to induce and terminate supraventricular tachycardia, to induce atrial flutter and fibrillation and terminate flutter (36, 37). Thus, in patients with recurrent tachyarrhythmia, undergoing serial drug testing, this method can be used to induce and terminate tachycardia and for measurement of refractory periods. The technique of transesophageal pacing appears to offer an additional valuable bedside diagnostic and therapeutic tool in patients with tachyarrhythmias.

Value of exercise testing

Most attacks of VT in young people are triggered by exertion. Thus the frequency of VT and the results of drug treatment can be assessed by treadmill testing.

Recently Frank et al have described a method of inducing tachycardia during exercise testing to evaluate the efficacy of drug treatment in patients with WPW syndrome (38). Since in WPW the conduction velocity, refractoriness are variable with changes in autonomic tone, this appears to be the method of choice in evaluating the conduction characteristics of the anomalous pathway and the effect of drug therapy.

Pacemapping

Intra-operative pacemapping has been proposed as a method to identify the origin of ventricular tachycardia (39, 40). Experimental studies have shown that the epicardial breakthrough during ventricular tachycardia, does not necessarily correlate with the site of origin of the tachycardia and that the electrocardiographic pattern is not specific for the site of origin but nearly represents the pattern of activation of the entire ventricle. Josephson et al in a study of 75 pts with VT, in whom endocardial mapping was done, found presystolic or sometimes continuous activity in all cases (40). Stimulation during the tachycardia demonstrated capture of large areas of the ventricle with persistance of the arrhythmia. These data show that in tachycardia associated with CAD, the reentrant circuit is small and is near or involves the endocardium or both.

Because mapping of VT before or during surgery requires complex electrophysiological devices and the ability to initiate reproducible stable VT, the indirect technique of pacemapping is used as an alternative.

This technique involves stimulation of various preselected sites of the heart at the time of surgery until stimulation at a particular site produce a QRS configuration identical to that seen in the spontaneous tachycardia. The assumption is that this site from which the ECG of spontaneous or induced VT is the same, identifies the site of origin of the tachycardia. Thus ablation of this focus would ablate the arrhythmia. The procedure has some advantages: it decreases the time needed for cardiopulmonary bypass and that the tachycardia need not be induced at surgery. In a study of 12 pts, pacing at the area of the earliest recorded activity was accomplished in all. Pacing from the area of earliest activity usually produced a QRS pattern similar to that of the spontaneous or induced VT. However, certain limitations were noted:

1. The electrocardiogram alone was not specific for the site of origin of tachycardia. In both normal patients and in those with heart disease, pacing at adjacent sites could result in changes in QRS configuration from left to right BBB pattern.

2. The 12 lead ECG obtained preoperatively could not be compared with the one obtained during surgery when the chest was open.

3. The QRS configuration of VT is most closely related to the epicardial breakthrough and a subsequent pattern of ventricular activation whereas the VT may originate from subendocardial regions several cms away (41).

4. Pacemapping involved pacing at multiple epicardial and endocardial sites and hence did not conserve time during CP bypass. Thus in their experience, pacemapping was neither easy, nor accurate or quicker than during localization by mapping during VT.

Significant progress has been made in the field of electrophysiological testing in the last decade, and has improved our understanding of the mechanisms of tachyarrhythmia. Long-term follow-up is needed however in trying to evaluate the efficacy of various procedures that have been developed in the management of tachyarrhythmia.

References

1. Scherlag BJ, Lau SH, Helfant RH, Berkowits WP, Stein E, Damato AN: Catheter technique for recording His Bundle activity in man. Circulation 1969; 39: 13.

2. Gallagher JJ, Svenson RH, Kasell JH, Germand LD, Bardy GH, Broughton A, Critelli G: Catheter technique for closed-chest ablation of the atrioventricular conduction system. New Engl J Med 1982; 306: 194–200.
3. Brodman R, Fisher JD: Evaluation of a catheter technique for ablation of accessory pathways near the coronary sinus using a canine model. Circulation 1983; 67: 923–929.
4. Fisher JD, Brodman R, Kim SG, Matos JA: Wolff-Parkinson-White syndrome: Nonsurgical Kent Bundle ablation via the coronary sinus. (Abstract). Pace 1983; 6: 547.
5. Waldo AL, MacLean WAH, Karp RB, Kouchoukos NT, James TN: Continous rapid pacing to control recurrent or sustained supraventricular tachycardias following open heart surgery. Circulation 1976; 54: 245–250.
6. Waldo AL, MacLean WAH, Karp RB, Kouchoukos NJ, James TN: Entrainment and interruption of atrial flutter with atrial pacing studies in man following open heart surgery. Circulation 1977; 56: 737.
7. Fisher JD, Mehra R, Furman S: Termination of ventricular tachycardia with bursts of rapid pacing. Amer J Cardiol 1978; 41: 94.
8. Dhingra RC: Sinus node response to atrial extrastimuli in patients without apparent sinus node disease. Amer J Cardiol 1975; 36: 445.
9. Curry PVL, Evans TR, Krikler DM: Paroxysmal Reciprocating sinus tachycardia. Europ J Cardiol 1977; 6: 199.
10. Moe GK, Preston JB, Burlington H: Physiologic evidence for a dual AV transmission system. Circ Res 1956; 4: 357.
11. Denes P, Wu D, Dhingra RC, Chuquimia R, Rosen KM: Demonstration of dual A-V nodal pathways in patients with paroxysmal supraventricular tachycardia. Circulation 1973; 48: 549.
12. Slama R, Coumel P, Bouvrain Y: Les syndromes de WPW de type a inapparents ou latents en rythme sinusal. Arch Mal Coeur 1973; 66: 639.
13. Narula OS: Paroxysmal Supraventricular tachycardia due to reciprocating via concealed accessory pathways. In – Cardiac Arrhythmias. Electrophysiology, Diagnosis and Management – OS Narula Ed, Williams and Wilkins Pub. Philadelphia 1979: p 318–346.
14. Narula OS: Longitudinal dissociation in the His Bundle: Bundle branch block due to asynchronous conduction within the His Bundle in man. Circulation 1977; 56: 996.
15. Shantha N, Alboni P, Towne W, Narula OS: Reentry due to longitudinal dissociation in the His Bundle (abstract). Amer J Cardiol 1979; 43: 389.
16. Easley RM, Goldstein S: Differentiation of ventricular tachycardia from junctional tachycardia with aberrant conduction: The use of competitive atrial pacing. Circulation 1968; 37: 1015.
17. Wellens HJJ, Schuilenburg RM, Durrer D: Electrical stimulation of the heart in patients with ventricular tachycardia. Circulation 1972; 46: 216.
18. Josephson ME, Horowitz LN, Farshidi A, Kastor JA: Recurrent sustained ventricular tachycardia I-mechanisms. Circulation 1978; 57: 431–440.
19. Akhtar M, Damato AN, Batsford WP, Ruskin JN, Ogunkelu JB, Vargas G: Demonstration of reentry within the His-Purkinje system in man. Circulation 1974; 50: 1150.
20. Farshidt A, Michelson EL, Greenspan AM, Spielman SR, Horowitz LN, Josephson ME: Repetitive responses to ventricular extrastimuli: Incidence, mechanism and significance. Amer Heart J 1980; 100: 59.
21. Gomes J, Kang PS, Matheson M, Kelen G: The repetitive ventricular response in man. A prospective study of its incidence reproducibility and significance. Clinic Res 1980; 28: 194-A.
22. Reddy CP, Damato AN, Akthar M, Dhat M, Gomes JA, Calon T: Effect of procainamide on reentry within the His Purkinje system in man. Amer J Cardiol 1977; 40: 957.
23. Greene HL, Reid PR, Schaeffer AH: The repetitive ventricular response in man. A predictor of sudden death. New Engl J Med 1978; 299: 729.
24. Mason JW: Repetitive beating after single ventricular extrastimuli: Incidence and prognostic significance in patients with recurrent ventricular tachycardia. Amer J Cardiol 1980; 45: 1126.
25. Heger JJ, Prystowsky EN, Jackman WM, Naccarelli GV, Zipes DP: Repetitive ventricular tachycardia: Clinical and electrophysiologic characteristics (abstract). Circulation 1980; 62 Sup-III: 321.
26. Ruskin JN, Dimarco JP, Garan H: Repetitive responses to single ventricular extrastimuli in patients with serious ventricular arrhythmias: Incidence and clinical significance. Circulation 1981; 63: 767.

622

27. Pietras R, Bauerfeind RA, Lam W, Wyndham CRC, Rosen K: Right ventricular function and angiography in patients with right ventricular tachycardia without ischemic heart disease. Amer J Card 1980; 45: 405 (Abs).
28. Fontaine G, Guiraudon G, Frank R, Cabrol C, Grosgogeat Y: The arrhythmogenic right ventricular dysplasia syndrome. Excerpta Medica Int Cong Series 1979; 470: 955.
29. Marcus FI, Fontaine G, Guiraudon G, Frank R, Laurenceau JL, Malergue MC: Right ventricular dysplasia. Clinical experience with 22 adult cases (Abstract). Circulation 1980; 62: 491.
30. Spielman SR, Schwartz S, Mac Carthy DM: Predictors of the success or failure of medical therapy in patients with chronic recurrent sustained ventricular tachycardia. J Amer Coll Cardiol 1983; 1: 401–408.
31. Horowitz LN, Josephson ME, Farshidi A, Spielman SR, Michelson EL, Greenspan AM; Recurrent sustained ventricular tachycardia. 3. Role of the electrophysiologic study in selection of anti-arrhythmic regimens. Circulation 1978; 58: 986.
32. Mason JW, Winkle RA: Electrode-catheter arrhythmia induction in the selection and assessment of anti-arrhythmic drug therapy in recurrent ventricular tachycardia. Circulation 1978; 58: 971.
33. Breithardt G, Borggrefe M, Seipel L: Present status of serial electrophysiologic testing for predicting anti-arrhythmic drug efficacy in patients with ventricular tachycardia. In: new aspects in the medical treatment of tachyarrhythmias. Role of amiodarone – G Breithardt and F Loogen Ed. Urban and Schwarzenberg Pub 1983: p 112.
34. Chung KY, Walsh TJ, Massie E: Wolff-Parkinson-White syndrome. Amer Heart J 1965; 69: 16.
35. Wellens HJJ, Farre J, Bar FW: Wolff-Parkinson-White syndrome: Value and limitations of programmed electrical stimulation. In: Innovations in Diagnosis and Management of Cardiac Arrhythmias – OS Narula Ed. Williams & Wilkins Pub Baltimore 1979: p 589.
36. Gallagher JJ, Smith WM, Kerr CR, Kasell J, Cook L, Reiter M, Sterba R, Harte M: Esophageal pacing: A diagnostic and therapeutic tool. Circulation 1982; 65: 336.
37. Kerr CR, Gallagher JJ, Smith WM, Sterba R, German LD, Cook L, Kasell JH: The induction of atrial flutter and fibrillation and the termination of atrial flutter by esophageal pacing. Pace 1983; 6: 60–72.
38. Frank R, Fontaine G, Tonet JL, Grosgogeat Y: Electrophysiological studies at exercise in patients with atrioventricular accessory pathway (abstract). Pace 1983; 6: 540.
39. Waxman HL, Josephson ME: Ventricular activation during ventricular endocardial pacing. I: Electrocardiographic pattern related to the site of pacing. Amer J Cardiol 1982; 50: 1.
40. Josephson ME, Waxman HL, Cam ME, Gardner MJ, Buxton AF: Ventricular activation during ventricular endocardial pacing. II: Role of pacemapping to localize origin of ventricular tachycardia. Amer J Cardiol 1982; 50: 22.
41. Spielman SR, Michelson EL, Horowitz LN, Spea JF, Moore EN: Limitations of epicardial mapping as a guide to the surgical therapy of ventricular tachycardia. Circulation 1978; 57: 666–676.

Authors' address:
Dr. N. Shantha
State University of New York
Downstate Medical Center
Brooklyn, New York 11203
USA

Assessment of Ventricular Vulnerability by Holter ECG, Programmed Ventricular Stimulation and Recording of Ventricular Late Potentials

H.-W. Höpp, V. Hombach, H.-J. Deutsch, A. Osterspey, U. Winter, H. H. Hilger

Summary: In a total of 40 patients, 10 females and 30 males, aged 42 to 65 years (mean: 53 ± 6 years) the diagnostic accuracy of three methods that might indicate left ventricular vulnerability, has been tested. These methods comprise the spontaneous occurrence of complex ventricular arrhythmias (Lown's classes IVa and b and ventricular tachycardias), the recovery of ventricular late potentials within the signal averaged surface ECG, and the induction of repetitive ventricular response during programmed right ventricular stimulation. The "gold standard" was the out-of-hospital documented spontaneous occurrence of ventricular tachycardias and/or fibrillation in each of these 40 patients, 21 of whom had to be resuscitated by DC shock.

When comparing the results of the three methods, in 22/40 patients complex VEA was present, but only 16/22 patients had ventricular late potentials, too, and only 13/22 patients with complex VEA also had repetitive ventricular response (RVR). Only 10/14 patients with VLP had RVR and none of them had complex VEA. There were 3 patients with RVR, but without VLP and complex VEA. In 4 patients completely negative results were obtained.

Based on these results the sensitivity and specificity of each of the methods alone and in combination were calculated. Sensitivity of VLP was highest (75%) as well as specificity (86%), and RVP had a similar specificity (86%) as the recovery of VLP. When combining the three methods sensitivity decreased to 32%, but specificity increased to 100%. The positive predictive value for sudden death was highest with VLP (26%) and with RVR (24%), and could be increased to 30% by combining VLP and RVR, and to 31% when combining the three methods.

From these data we conclude that each of the three methods described is suitable for detection of ventricular vulnerability. The highest sensitivity is obtained with VLP and the highest specificity with combination of all three methods. The predictive value of these methods is fairly low, perhaps it might be considerably increased when the functional role of VLP in the initiation of ventricular tachycardia can be elucidated in each patient by the method of continuous beat-by-beat registration of VLPs from body surface.

Introduction

In an increasing number of patients with cardiovascular diseases the occurrence of sudden cardiac death represents a major epidemiologic and medical problem (1). Based on clinical studies, the majority of patients that are threatened by sudden cardiac death are those with Coronary Heart Disease (CHD) and in particular those with left ventricular contraction abnormalities (2, 3). Spontaneously occurring complex and frequent ventricular ectopic activity (VEA) or ventricular tachycardias are considered as an additional risk factor, though the independent role of VEA, as detected by Holter ECG monitoring, as a

---

*) Supported by the Deutsche Forschungsgesellschaft, SFB 68 Cologne.

prognostic factor remains controversial (4). If compared to both criteria, the predictive value of resting and exercise ECG seems to be low (5).

From the view of preventive medicine the most important question, as to how those patients prone to sudden death can be identified, remained unanswered up to now. Some studies showed a high correlation between left ventricular dysfunction and VEA of Lown's classes IVa/b or ventricular tachycardias and the incidence of sudden death (6, 7). However, the specificity of these criteria is relatively low and does not allow an exact differentiation between patients threatened by sudden death and those that are not.

Consequently in recent years new techniques have been developed in order to identify and predict left ventricular vulnerability in those patients more precisely: recording of ventricular late potentials (VLP) within the signal averaged high gain amplified surface ECG, and provocation of repetitive ventricular response (RVR) by programmed ventricular stimulation (8), namely. From animal experiments VLP have been shown to represent local conduction delays within certain ischemic areas of the myocardium, that may favor the initiation of re-entry excitation with the consequence of single ventricular ectopic beats or runs of ventricular tachycardias. The diagnostic value of non-invasively recorded VLPs has been reported in several studies (9, 10, 11). Thus, in Coronary Heart

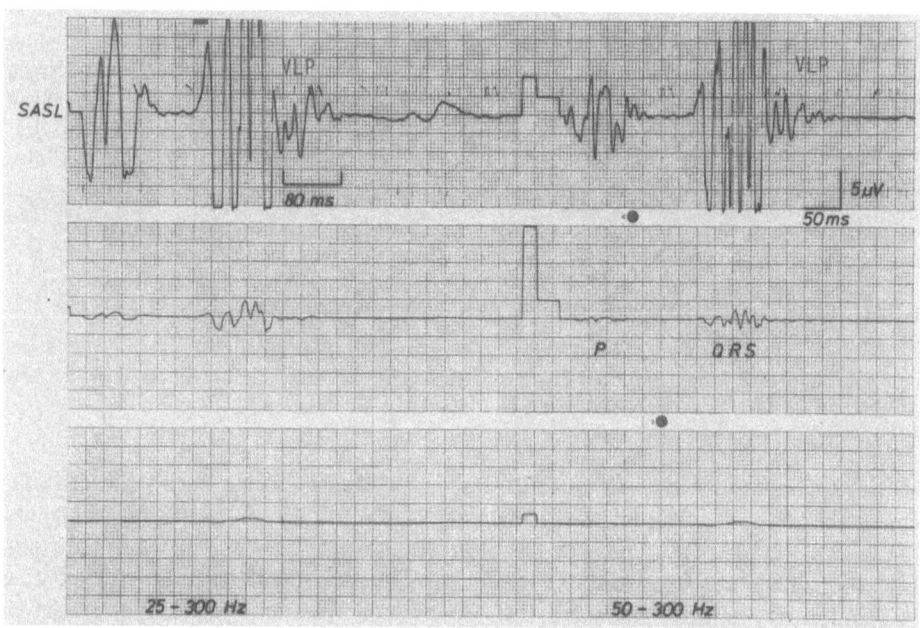

Fig. 1: Signal averaged high gain surface electrocardiogram (SASL) of a 56-years old patient with CHD and anterior wall aneurysm with recurrent attacks of non-sustained and sustained ventricular tachycardias.

Bottom trace: reference low amplified ECG, medium trace: amplification of 20-fold, upper trace: amplification of 400 fold the bottom trace. The averaged complexes are printed out with 25–300 Hz (left panel) and 50–300 Hz (right panel) frequency range. Paper speed: 100 mm/sec, VLP: ventricular late potential.

Disease patients a relatively high correlation between the incidence of VLPs and the degree of left ventricular dysfunction, and the occurrence of repetitive ventricular ectopic beats was found (12, 13). However, the predictive value of each of the methods for assessing left ventricular vulnerability for sudden cardiac death has not been clarified, as yet, and also the question remained unanswered, whether the combined use of the three methods altogether might improve the diagnostic impact of complex VEA, of VLPs and of RVR.

Patients

A total of 40 patients, 10 females and 30 males, with ages from 42 to 65 years (mean: 53 ± 6 years) with angiographically or scintigraphically documented CHD were studied by Holter ECG, by recording of the signal averaged surface ECG and by programmed ventricular stimulation. All of these patients had documented ventricular tachycardias (n = 30) or ventricular fibrillation (n = 10) prior to admission, and these events had occurred without concomitant myocardial ischemic episodes or myocardial infarction. 21/40 patients had been successfully resuscitated, in part by external DC shock.

Methods

During a drug-free period in each patient a Holter ECG was obtained, the monitoring period lasted 48.0 ± 8.7 hours as a mean. The patients were also studied with a signal averaging ECG computer (MAC I, Marquette electronics) in order ot obtain VLPs, and they were subjected to a programmed right ventricular stimulation at one to three stimulation sites (right ventricular inflow tract, apex and outflow tract) with a basic driven rhythm of 100, 120 and 140 stimuli/min and single and double extrastimuli delivered with steadily decreasing coupling intervals until right ventricular effective refractory period was reached.

During programmed stimulation the occurrence of equal or more than three consecutive ventricular echo beats or non-sustained or sustained ventricular tachycardias were considered as to be positive (RVR). During Holter ECG monitoring the identification of complex ventricular ectopic activity, i.e. pairs, salvos or ventricular tachycardias, was noted as positive for increased left ventricular vulnerability, since the "gold standard" in these patients were documented ventricular tachycardias or fibrillation outside the hospital. VLPs were considered to be true signals, if they outlasted the QRS complex in the reference low gain amplified ECG by more than 10 ms (to exclude possible filter ringing with the digital finite impulse response filters incorporated within the MAC-I signal averaging computer, D. Mortara: personal communication) in at least three or more of the high gain amplified and averaged leads, and the amplitude of VLPs had to equal or exceed twice the amplitude of diastolic background noise.

Results

Complex VEA was observed within the Holter ECG in only 22/40 patients (55%) with out-of-hospital documented VT/VFib, and VEA of Lown's class IVb or VTs were only documented in 33% of patients. On the other hand VLPs were detected in 30/40 patients (75%), and repetitive ventricular response could be initiated in 29/40 patients (72%). Patients with documented ventricular fibrillation represented a separate group, since VLPs were present in only 50% of cases, and RVR was inducible in only 4/10 VFib-patients (40%).

A composite view of the discrepancies of results obtained with the three methods is given in Fig. 2. Only 16/22 patients (73%) with spontaneous complex VEA within the Holter ECG had VLPs and a comparable number (16/22 patients) the phenomenon of RVR. In 3 patients with complex VEA and initiation of RVR the phenomenon of VLPs could not be observed. On the other hand, 14 patients with VLPs and 13 patients with inducible RVR (10 of whom with concomitant VLPs) did not have complex VEA within the Holter ECG. Positive results with all three methods (complex VEA plus VLP plus RVR) were obtained in only 13/40 patients (32%), and in 4/40 patients (10%) completely negative results were observed.

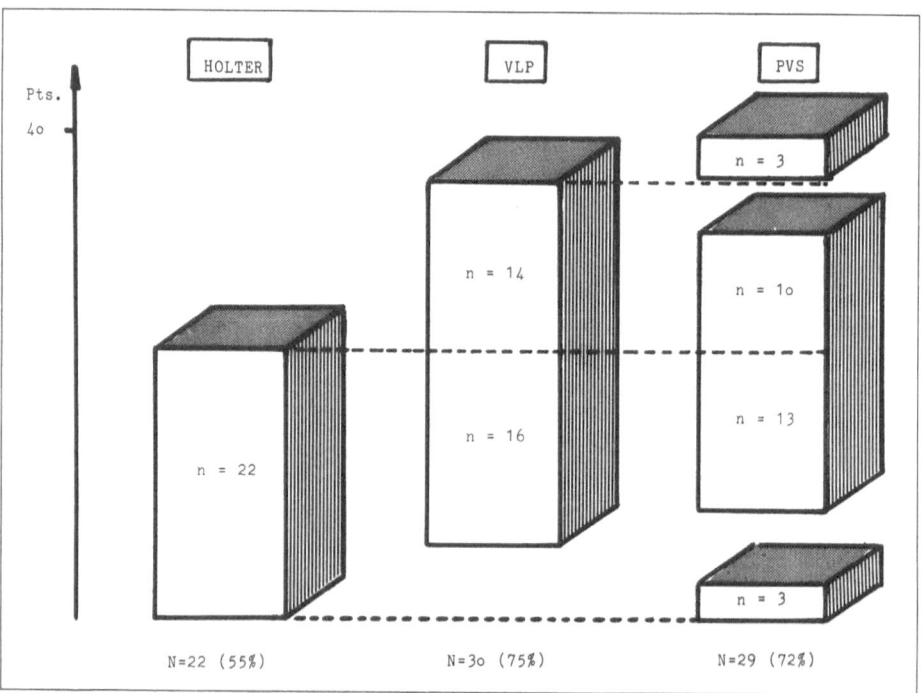

Fig. 2. Positive findings for assessment of previously documented ventricular vulnerability (out-of-hospital documented spontaneous VT/VFib) by applying Holter ECG (left), recovery of ventricular late potentials (VLP) with the signal averaging technique (center), and by initiation of repetitive ventricular response on programmed ventricular stimulation (PVS, right).

Based on these results the sensitivity of each of the methods alone or in combination to each other could be calculated (Table 1). With application of each of the tests alone, the highest sensitivities were obtained with detection of VLPs (75%) and with the initiation of RVR (72%). When combining two or even all three methods, the highest sensitivity was found for recovery of VLPs plus induction of RVR (57%), whereas combination of the three methods provided the lowest sensitivity (32%). Specificity of the tests mentioned could be calculated by studying a control group of 25 patients with various supraventricular tachycardias, in whom for diagnostic purposes all three methods were applied. None of these patients were suffering from CHD. It was quite interesting to note that specificity was increasing with the combination of two methods (96%), and when combining the three methods specificity was 100%. These discrepancies cannot be solely explained methodologically or by the known phenomenon of spontaneous variability of complex VEA, and further studies on larger patients groups have to be awaited in order to exclude spontaneous variability and to further elucidate the role of complex VEA in the assessment of left ventricular vulnerability.

Follow-up

All patients were followed up to now, the mean follow-up period was 18 ± 3 months (Fig. 3). During this time 3 patients were provided with an automatic antitachycardial pacemaker (Cyber-Tach 60, Intermedics) because of drug-resistant sustained VTs, and a total of 7 patients were operated (5/7 aneurysmectomy with aortocoronary bypass grafting in 2 patients, in 2/7 solely aorto-coronary bypass grafting). One of these 7 operated patients died from sudden cardiac death 11 months post-operatively. 23/30 patients treated medically survived, consequently 7/30 patients died, all of whom with signs of sudden death within one hour.

The sudden death victims were treated by antiarrhythmic drugs alone, and in 18 patients drug efficacy was controlled by Holter ECG monitoring, in the remaining 12 patients by means of programmed ventricular stimulation. Interestingly mortality rates in the Holter ECG controlled group were much higher (5/18 = 28%) than those in the stimulation controlled group (2/12 = 17%), however, these differences were not statistically significant.

VLPs were present in all of the 8 sudden death patients, in 7 of them RVR had been inducible, whereas in only 4/8 sudden death patients complex VEA was detected within

Table 1. Sensitivity and specificity of diagnostic parameters of ventricular vulnerability. (HM: Holter ECG monitoring, VLP: ventricular late potentials, PVS: programmed ventricular stimulation).

VT/VF	Sensitivity	Specificity
Hm	55%	66%
VLP	75%	86%
PVS	72%	86%
Hm + VLP	40%	96%
Hm + PVS	40%	96%
VLP + PVS	57%	96%
HM + VLP + PVS	32%	100%

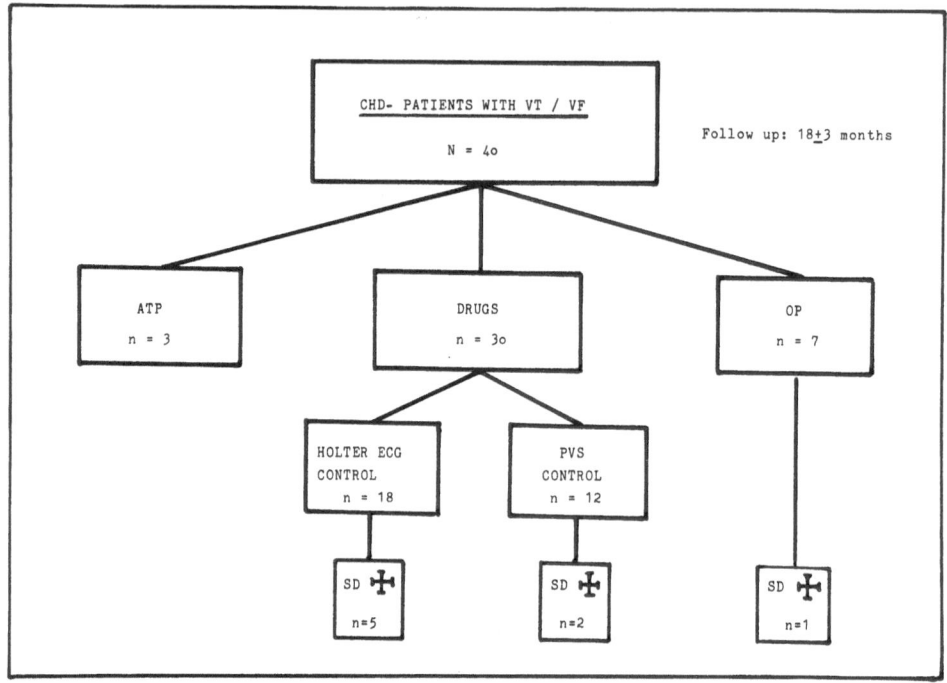

Fig. 3. Follow-up of the 40 patients with documented VT/VFib. and underlying CHD.

Table 2. Predictive value of the parameters of ventricular vulnerability. (HM: Holter ECG monitoring, VLP: ventricular late potentials, PVS: programmed ventricular stimulation).

SD	Predictive value
HM	18%
VLP	26%
PVS	24%
HM + VLP	25%
HM + PVS	25%
VLP + PVS	30%
HM + VLP + PVS	31%

the Holter ECG. In 4/8 patients all three parameters of left ventricular vulnerability were recorded, in 3/8 VLPs plus RVR were present, and only 1/8 patients had VLPs without RVR and complex VEA.

Thus, the predictive value of sudden death was highest (30%) with the combined group of VLPs plus RVR, and it was only slightly increased to 31%, when all three methods for assessment of left ventricular vulnerability were considered (Table 2). When using the single methods for calculation the predictive value for sudden death was highest with the demonstration of VLPs (26%).

630

Conclusions

Based on the results in this highly specialized group of Coronary Heart Disease patients, in whom out-of-hospital documented VT/VFib were taken as the "gold standard" to evaluate the diagnostic accuracy of three methods for assessing ventricular vulnerability (complex VEA within the Holter ECG, VLPs within the signal averaged high gain amplified surface ECG, and RVR with programmed right ventricular stimulation), we may draw some conclusions:

1. Each of the three methods seems to be suitable to detect ventricular vulnerability
2. The highest sensitivity may be obtained with the detection of ventricular late potentials, whereas the highest specificity may be expected with the combination of all three methods
3. The prognostic value in predicting a high risk of sudden death seems to be best with the demonstration of repetitive ventricular response on programmed ventricular stimulation plus recovery of ventricular late potentials or the combined use of all three methods

In general, due to the limited number of patients and the relatively short follow-up period further valid prognostic statements of stronger diagnostic impact are not warranted. However, the relatively high predictive value of VLPs in CHD patients remains to be emphasized. Whether beat-to-beat registration of ventricular late potentials (17) with recovery of dynamic changes of heart rhythm and demonstration of complex VEA or ventricular tachycardias to be triggered by late potentials will be a better and more sensitive method for predicting the patient's risk of the fatal event of ventricular fibrillation, remains to be clarified in the future.

References

1. Todesursachenstatistik (Cause-of-death statistics). DMW 1981; 106: 157–158.
2. Schulze RA, Strauss HW, Pitt B: Sudden death in the year following myocardial infarction. Relation to ventricular premature contractions in the late hospital phase and left ventricular ejection fraction. Am J Med 1977; 62: 192–99.
3. Bethge KP, Lichtlen PR: Ventricular arrhythmias in relation to the extent of coronary lesions and left ventricular function. In: Macfarlane PW (ed) Progress in electrocardiology. London: Pitman, 1979; 126–132.
4. Cats VM, Lie KI, Capellen FJL van, Durrer D: Limitations of 24 hour ambulatory electrocardiographic recording in predicting coronary events after acute myocardial infarction. Am J Cardiol 1979; 44: 1257–62.
5. Vedin UA, Wilhelmson CE, Wilhemsen L, Bjure J, Ekström-Jodal B: Relation of resting and exercise – induced ectopic beats to other ischemic manifestations and to coronary risk factors. Am J Cardiol 1972; 30: 25–31.
6. Bethge KP, Lichtlen PR: Risikoprofil plötzlich verstorbener bzw. reanimierter Patienten. Z. Kardiol 1980; 69: 200.
7. Geltman EM, Ehsani AA, Campbell MK, Schechtmann K, Roberts R, Sobel BE: The influence of location and extent of myocardial infarction on long-term ventricular dysrhythmia and mortality. Circulation 1979; 60: 805.
8. Breithardt G, Seipel L, Loogen F: Der akute Herztod – Bedeutung elektrophysiologischer Stimulationsverfahren. Verh Dtsch Ges Herz- u Kreislaufforschg 1980; 46: 38–64.

9. Hombach V, Höpp HW, Braun V, Behrenbeck DW, Tauchert M, Hilger HH: Die Bedeutung von Nachpotentialen innerhalb des ST-Segmentes im Oberflächen-EKG bei Patienten mit koronarer Herzkrankheit. DMW 1980; 105: 1457–1462.

10. Berbari EJ, Scherlag BJ, Hope RR, Lazzara R: Recording from the body surface of arrhythmogenic ventricular activity during the ST segment. Am J Cardiol 1978; 41: 697–702.

11. Rozanski JJ, Mortara D, Myerburg RJ, Castellanos A: Body surface detection of delayed depolarizations in patients with recurrent ventricular tachycardia and left ventricular aneurysm. Circulation 1981; 63: 1172–1178.

12. Breithardt G, Becker R, Seipel L, Abendroth R-R, Ostermeyer J: Non-invasive detection of late potentials in man – A new marker for ventricular tachycardia. Eur Heart J 1981; 2: 1–11.

13. Höpp HW, Hombach V, Braun V, Tauchert M, Behrenbeck DW, Hilger HH: Kammerarrhythmien und ventrikuläre Spätpotentiale bei akutem Myokardinfarkt. Herz/Kreislauf 1982; 3: 11–120.

14. Spielberg C, Leitner E-Rv, Andresen D, Schröder R: Prognostische Bedeutung komplexer tachykarder ventrikulärer Rhythmusstörungen im 24-Stunden-Langzeit-EKG. Z Kardiol 1982; 71: 271–277.

15. Heger JJ, Prystowsky EN, Jackman W: Comparison between results obtained from electrophysiologic testing, exercise testing and ambulatory ECG recording. In: Wenger et al. Ambulatory electrocardiographic recording. Year Book Medical Publishers 1981: 379–389.

16. Leitner E-Rv, Andresen D, Oeff M, Spielberg C, Schröder R: Nichtinvasive und invasive Arrhythmiediagnostik bei Patienten mit malignen tachykarden ventrikulären Herzrhythmusstörungen. Z Kardiol 1982; 71: 201.

17. Hombach V, Kebbel U, Höpp HW, Winter HU, Braun V, Deutsch H, Hirche H, Hilger HH: Fortlaufende Registrierung von Mikropotentialen des menschlichen Herzens. DMW 1982; 51/52: 1951–1956.

Authors address:
H.-W. Höpp, M.D.
Medical Center and Policlinic III
and Department of Cardiology
University of Cologne
5000 Köln

Activation Mapping and Functional Properties of Single Premature Ventricular Beats in Asymptomatic Patients: Electrophysiologic Evidence of Supernormal Conduction and Latency

Pietro Santarelli, Fulvio Bellocci, Francesco Loperfido

Summary: Conduction times (CT) of single premature ventricular beats (PVBs) delivered at the right ventricular apex (RVA) and outflow tract (RVOT) were measured at different right ventricular sites in seven asymptomatic patients during sinus rhythm. CT were similar during RVA and RVOT stimulation. Ventricular conduction curves were constructed by plotting coupling interval against CT at all recording sites (including that close to the stimulation site). Two types of curves were observed: in type I, CT of PVBs was constant until 35–105 msec before the effective refractory period, when a progressive delay of appearance of activation was observed at all recording sites; this phenomenon was called latency and was observed in all patients. In type II curve, a decrease of CT of PVBs with a coupling interval ranging between 470 and 320 msec was observed and lasted 50–150 msec; this phenomenon was thought to represent supernormal conduction, and was observed in four patients. We concluded that in asymptomatic patients: 1. homogeneity of right ventricular endocardial activation of single PVBs is independent of site of origin and coupling interval; 2. latency, not conduction delay, is responsible for the delayed appearance at distant sites of early PVBs; 3. supernormal conduction can be observed in the right ventricle.

Although it has been extensively studied in animal experiments (1–8) little is known about the electrophysiologic characteristics of artificially induced premature ventricular beats (PVBs) in man. Some characteristics, which have been determined experimentally, such as latency (6) and supernormal conduction (9–14), could be relevant in the interpretation of clinical electrophysiological studies. The purpose of this investigation was to study, the conduction characteristics of single PVBs in the right ventricle, utilizing standard intracardiac recording techniques, having no clinical evidence of organic heart disease in patients.

Material and methods

The study group consisted of seven patients (five males and two females) ranging in age from 29 to 52 years (41 ± 8.3, mean = SD). Clinical diagnosis was paroxysmal supraventricular tachycardia in four patients, paroxysmal atrial flutter in one patient, and sick sinus syndrome in two patients. Clinical history, physical examinations, ECGs, chest x-rays, echocardiograms, and stress tests were otherwise unremarkable. After informed consent forms were obtained, three quadripolar catheters (Josephson multipurpose electrode catheters, 6 F, USCI) with an interelectrode distance of 5 mm were positioned under fluoroscopic control in the right ventricle (RV). Three locations were selected: the outflow tract, apex, and inflow tract. The outflow tract (RVOT) was identified as the site where electrical activity first appeared during withdrawal of the catheter from the trunk of the pulmonary artery. The right ventricular apex (RVA) was reached by advancing the catheter to the most distal portion of the body of the RV. The right ventricular inflow tract (RVIT) was identified by withdrawing the catheter to the position just below the tricuspid valve where a His bundle recording was obtained. The position of the catheters was frequently checked during the study. Filtered (40–400 Hz) bipolar electrograms were recorded simultaneously with three surface leads at a paper speed of 200 mm/sec.

After the catheters were positioned and stable, single PVBs were delivered at the RVA after every eighth sinus beat, beginning at a coupling interval of 600 msec; the cycle was scanned at 5–10 msec intervals until the effective refractory period (ERP) was reached. The same procedure was performed at the RVOT. The spontaneous sinus cycle length ranged from 710 to 900 msec (790 ± 79 msec). Ventricular stimulation was performed with a programmable, constant current stimulator (Medtronic 5325) that delivered rectangular pulses of 2 msec duration and at twice the diastolic threshold. The distal pair of electrodes were used for recording RV electrograms except when they were used for pacing (in this case the proximal pair was used for recording). The following intervals were measured from the stimulus (St) artifact to the first rapid deflection of each electrogram (V) when PVBs were delivered at the RVA: St-RVA, St-RVOT, and St-RVIT. When PVBs were delivered at the RVOT, the intervals measured were: St-RVOT, St-RVA and St-RVIT. Measurements were performed independently by two of the authors. Cases in which the interobserver variations were ± 5 msec or greater were excluded from the study. In each patient, either for RVA or RVOT pacing, ventricular conduction curves were constructed by plotting the St-V of each PVB (ordinate) at the three recording sites against coupling interval (abscissa). Student's t test was used for statistical analysis. Values are expressed as mean ± SD.

Results

Activation mapping

The conduction time (CT) of single PVBs at the selected RV sites are presented in Table 1. When PVBs were delivered at the RVA, CT was 15.9 ± 9.6 msec at the RVA, 29.9 ± 11.6 msec at the RVOT, and 32.6 ± 11.3 msec at the RVIT. When PVBs were introduced at the RVOT, CT was 16.9 ± 10 msec at the RVOT, 32.4 ± 13.5 msec at the RVA, and 36.5 ± 15 msec at the RVIT. No significant differences were found between CT of PVBs delivered at the RVA and RVOT.

Table 1. Conduction of single premature ventricular beats at selected right ventricular sites.

	RVA	RVOT	RVIT
RVA stimulation	15.9 ± 9.6	29.9 ± 11.6	32.6 ± 11.3
RVOT stimulation	32.4 ± 13.5	16.9 ± 10	36.5 ± 15

Abbreviations: RVA = right ventricular apex; RVOT = right ventricular outflow tract. RVIT = right ventricular inflow tract. Values are expressed in milliseconds.

Two types of ventricular conduction curves were observed. In type I (Fig. 1) CT of PVBs was constant throughout the diastole until the PVB was close to the ERP, when a sudden increase of CT was observed. In all seven patients, the increase of CT was evident either during RVA or RVOT stimulation at all three recording sites (an increase of the St-V interval was always recorded at the stimulation site): this phenomenon was called latency. A type II curve (Figs. 2 and 3) was observed in four patients in whom PVBs with a cou-

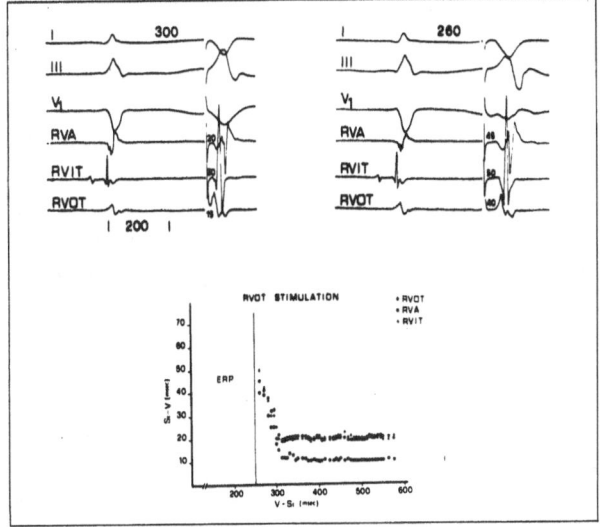

Fig. 1. Conduction time of two premature ventricular beats delivered at the right ventricular outflow tract (top) showing normal conduction (left) and latency (right). Surface leads I, III and V_1 and the ventricular intracardiac electrograms at the right ventricular apex (RVA), inflow tract (RVIT), and outflow tract (RVOT) are shown. The ventricular conduction curve is also shown (bottom). See text for details.

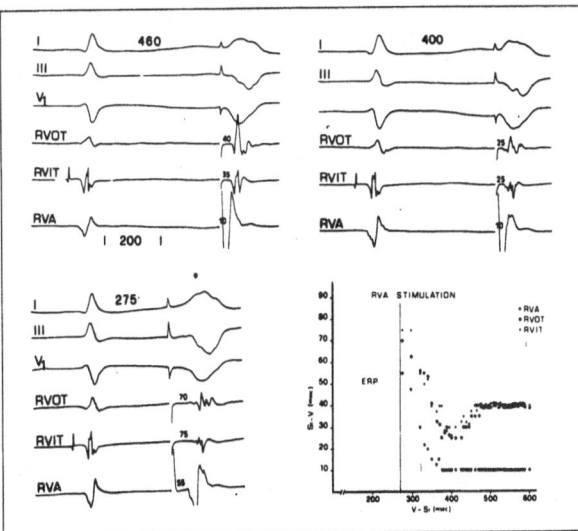

Fig. 2. Conduction time of premature ventricular beats delivered at the RVA at three coupling intervals (460, 400, and 275 msec) showing normal conduction, supernormal conduction, and latency. The corresponding ventricular conduction curve is also shown. See text for details.

Fig. 3. Conduction time of premature ventricular beats delivered at the RVOT at three coupling intervals (480, 350, and 275 msec) showing normal conduction, supernormal conduction, and latency in the same patient of Fig. 2. The corresponding ventricular conduction curve is also shown. See text for details.

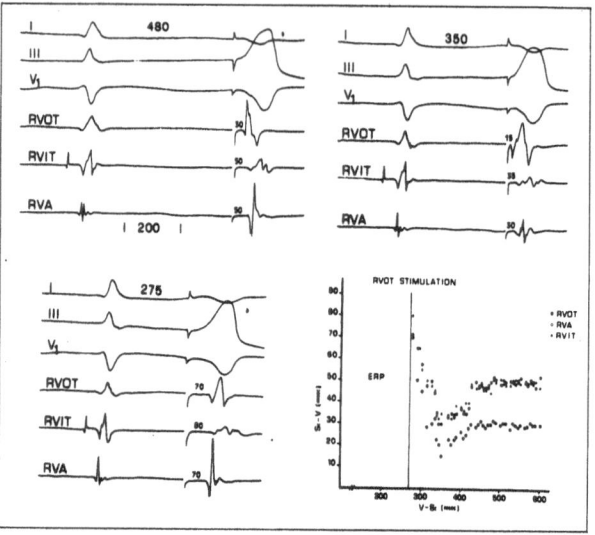

pling interval ranging between 470 and 320 msec had a shorter CT than that of late PVBs. This was thought to represent supernormal conduction.

Latency

The duration and peak values (maximum increase of CT) of latency, measured during RVA and RVOT stimulation at all three recording sites, are shown in Tables 2 and 3. During RVA stimulation (Table 2), latency lasted 71 ± 18 msec (range 50–105) at the RVA, 61 ± 11 msec (range 50–80) at the RVOT, and 66 ± 19 msec (range 50–95) at the RVIT. The peak values were 47 ± 11 msec (range 35–70), 37 ± 13 msec (range 25–65), and 39 ± 12 msec (range 25–60), respectively. During RVOT stimulation (Table 3), latency lasted 60 ± 13 msec (range 35–75) at the RVOT, 59 ± 12 msec (range 40–75) at the RVA, and 56 ± 11 msec (range 40–75) at the RVIT. The peak values of latency were 40 ± 5 msec (range 30–45), 36 ± 12 msec (range 25–50), and 40 ± 10 msec (range 30–50), respectively.

Supernormal conduction

A phase of supernormal conduction was observed in four patients at a coupling interval of PVBs ranging between 470 and 320 msec. The duration and peak values (maximum decrease of CT) of supernormal conduction during RVA and RVOT stimulation, at all three recording sites, are shown in Tables 2 and 3. During RVA stimulation (Table 2), supernormal conduction lasted 93 ± 43 msec (range 60–150) at the RVOT and 76 ± 31 msec (range 50–120) at the RVIT. Supernormal conduction was not observed close to the stimulation site during RVA stimulation. The peak values were 17 ± 2 msec (range 15–20) and 15 ± 2 msec (range 12–17), respectively. During RVOT stimulation (Table

636

Table 2. Values of latency and supernormal conduction at selected right ventricular sites during stimulation at the right ventricular apex.

Case no	RVA					RVOT				RVIT			
	ERP	LAT dur	LAT max	SN dur	SN max	LAT dur	LAT max	SN dur	SN max	LAT dur	LAT max	SN dur	SN max
1	270	105	45	–	–	80	30	100	15	95	35	75	12
2	240	60	70	–	–	50	65	–	–	90	60	–	–
3	260	70	50	–	–	50	30	–	–	70	50	–	–
4	320	80	40	–	–	60	30	150	17	50	25	120	15
5	305	70	40	–	–	70	40	60	15	60	40	60	15
6	275	50	35	–	–	60	25	–	–	50	35	–	–
7	300	60	50	–	–	55	40	60	20	50	30	50	17
Mean	281	71	47			61	37	93	17	66	39	76	15
±SD	±28	±18	±11			±11	±13	±43	±2	±19	±12	±31	±2

Abbreviations: ERP = effective refractory period; LAT = latency; SN = Supernormal conduction; dur = duration; max = peak value. All values are expressed in milliseconds. Other abbreviations as in Table 1.

Table 3. Values of latency and supernormal conduction at selected right ventricular sites during stimulation at the right ventricular outflow tract.

Case no	RVOT					RVA				RVIT			
	ERP	LAT dur	LAT max	SN dur	SN max	LAT dur	LAT max	SN dur	SN max	LAT dur	LAT max	SN dur	SN max
1	270	35	40	90	15	40	20	100	20	40	30	100	15
2	250	60	40	–	–	70	40	–	–	60	50	–	–
3	250	60	30	–	–	60	25	–	–	60	30	–	–
4	290	75	45	–	–	65	35	75	15	50	30	60	15
5	315	70	40	–	–	50	30	50	15	60	40	70	17
6	290	60	45	–	–	75	50	–	–	75	50	–	–
7	300	60	40	–	–	50	50	50	12	50	50	50	17
Mean	281	60	40			59	36	69	16	56	40	70	16
±SD	±25	±13	±5			±12	±12	±24	±3	±11	±10	±22	±1

Abbrevations as in Table 1 and 2.

3), supernormal conduction lasted 69 ± 24 msec (range 50–100) at the RVA and 70 ± 22 msec (range 50–100) at the RVIT). The peak values were 16 ± 3 msec (range 12–20) and 16 ± 1 msec (range 15–17), respectively. During RVOT stimulation, supernormal conduction was observed at the RVOT in only one patient.

Discussion

The conduction velocity of a PVB is related to its coupling interval. Early premature beats, that occur at a time when the membrane potential of the preceding impulse is not completely repolarized, show delayed conduction (2). Surawicz et al. (3), in isolated perfused rabbit hearts, have demonstrated that PVBs induced multiple responses by slowing conduction in the ventricular myocardium and shortening the ERP. On the other hand, Moe et al. (4) and Van Dam et al. (5) found no differences between the time of arrival of the activation at different points on the ventricular surface distally to the stimulating electrodes in the early and late premature beats. Both groups of investigators concluded that conduction velocity, distally to the stimulating electrodes, was not altered by the times of stimulation.

In all of our seven patients, the arrival time of the PVBs at the RVOT during RVA stimulation and at the RVA during RVOT stimulation, was similar, suggesting that in the normal right ventricle the pathways involved in the activation process are the same and independent of the site of origin of the PVB (Table 1). Obviously, the values obtained were dependent on the areas in wich stimulation and recording were performed and should not be regarded as absolute values of conduction. Furthermore, in all patients, the arrival time of the PVBs at distant sites (either during RVA or RVOT stimulation) was independent of their coupling interval. As shown in Figs. 1–3, when PVBs were delivered close to the ERP, a delayed appearance of the excitation process at the distant sites was observed: a similar delay was recorded a few millimeters distal to the stimulation site. The relationship between the conduction time at the sites distal and close to the stimulating electrodes remained fairly constant throughout the cycle. This suggests that the delayed appearance of the excitation process, in the area surrounding the stimulation site, was responsible for the apparently delayed conduction at the distal sites of early PVBs. This phenomenon has been ascribed to latency (6) and reflects the increasing difficulty of activating partially refractory cells when the extrastimulus approaches the ERP. Other factors have been suggested, such as true decrease of conduction velocity (7) and differences in refractoriness between the ventricular muscle and the distal Purkinje fibres (8). Our data suggest that, if conduction delay is present, this is a local phenomenon around the stimulation site: once the activation process is started, its propagation is as fast as it is during late PVBs.

The analysis of the ventricular conduction curves in four of our patients showed, for coupling intervals ranging between 470 and 320 msec, a decrease of CT of PVBs. Supernormal conduction, defined as shorter CT of premature beats with respect to normal conduction of later stimuli (9), has been demonstrated in the canine (10) and human atria (11), the isolated His bundle branch system of the dog (12), and canine (13) and human ventricle (14). Two different forms of supernormal conduction have been described. The first appears at the end of the relative refractory period and corresponds to the supernormal phase of excitation (15): during this period, the lower threshold allows electrotonic currents to stimulate the cell membrane for greater distances and conduction velocity is increased. The second form of supernormal conduction begins after excitability has returned to normal and corresponds to the maximum level of the membrane potential (2, 16). The decrease of CT observed in our four patients is likely a true electrophysiologic event rather than an artifactual finding. The characteristics of this phenomenon, such as duration and degree, were similar in the same patient at different recordings and from different stimulation sites. The coupling intervals of PVBs at which supernormal conduction was observed and the degree of supernormal conduction, were similar to those previously reported.

The nature of the phenomenon has been discussed. For example, Castellanos et al (17), in two patients, found that there was a part of the cycle during which premature impulses reached the recording electrode with less delay than driven impulses. The duration of the corresponding QRS complexes was also shorter. These changes were not attributed to intraventricular supernormal conduction but to inhomogeneity of excitability related changes in the conduction pathways occurring during the end of the period of incomplete recovery. In our cases, the decrease of CT appeared 100–210 msec before the ERP was reached when the cell should be completely repolarized.

Finally, the limitations of our study deserve some comments. The use of standard recording techniques introduces a significant source of error: catheter movements with heart motion and difficulty in defining the onset of the ventricular electrogram may cause incorrect measurement of the arrival time of excitation at the recording sites. Consequently, the phenomena here described should be considered as a qualitative, not a quantitative, assessment of the characteristics of conduction of single PVBs and their clinical relevance in the interpretation of clinical electrophysiologic studies should be further evaluated.

References

1. Singer DH, Lazzara R, Hoffman BF: Interrelationship between automaticity and conduction in Purkinje fibres. Cir Res 1967; 21: 537–558.
2. Weidman S: The effect of the cardiac membrane potential on the rapid availability of the sodium carrying system. J of Physiol 1955; 127: 213–224.
3. Surawicz B, Gettes LS, Ponce-Zumino A: Relation of vulnerability to ECG and action potential characteristics of premature beats. Am J Physiol 1966; 212: 1519–1528.
4. Moe GK, Harris AS, Wiggers CJ: Analysis of the initiation of fibrillation by electrocardiographic studies. Am J Physiol 1941; 134: 473–492.
5. Van Dam RT, Durrer D, Van der Twell LH: Origin and porpagation of extrasystoles resulting from stimulation during diastole and during the refractory period of the dog's heart. Acta Physiol Pharmacol Neerl 1960; 9: 431–442.
6. Hoffman BF, Cranefield PF: Electrophysiology of the heart. New York: McGraw-Hill 1960: 249.
7. Van Dam RT, Hoffman BF, Stuckey SH: Recovery of excitability and impulse propagation in the in situ canine conducting system. Am J Cardiol 1964; 14: 184–192.
8. Myerburg RJ, Stewart JW, Hoffman BF: Electrophysiologic properties of the canine peripheral AV conducting system. Cir Res 1970; 26: 361–378.
9. Schamroth L: The disorders of cardiac rhythm. Oxford: Blackwell, 1974: 271.
10. Childers RW, Meredith J, Moe GK: Supernormality in Bachman's bundle. An in vitro and in vivo study in the dog. Cir Res 1973; 22: 363–370.
11. Agha AS, Castillo CA, Castellanos A jr, Myerburg RS, Tessler MP: Supernormal conduction in the human atria. Circulation 1972; 46: 522–527.
12. Spear JF, Moore EN: Effect of potassium on supernormal conduction in the bundle branch-Purkinje system of the dog. Am J Cardiol 1977; 40: 923–929.
13. Puech P, Guimaud C, Nadeau R, Morena H, Molina L, Matina D: Supernormal conduction in the intact heart. In Narula O: Cardiac Arrhythmias. Electrophysiology, diagnosis and management. Baltimore 1979: 40.

14. Harper RW, Ollsson SB: Effect of Mexiletine on conduction of premature ventricular beats in man: a study using monophasic action potential recordings from the right ventricle. Cardiovasc Res 1979; 13: 311–319.
15. Van Dam RT, Moore EN, Hoffman BF: Initiation and conduction of cardiac impulses in partially depolarized cells. Am J Physiol 1963; 204: 1133–1144.
16. Hoffman BF, Singer DH: Progress in Cardiovascular Disease. 1974; 7: 231–248.
17. Castellanos A jr, Befeler B, Myerburg RJ, Castillo CA, Agha AS, Vagueiro MC: Functional properties of the ventricular muscle and distal conducting system during right ventricular stimulation, with special reference tothe RBBB pattern in V_1, supernormal intraventricular conduction and physiologic gate. Eur J Cardiol 1973; 1: 41–48.

Authors' address:
Dr. P. Santarelli
Ospedale Policlinico Gemelli Roma
Via della Camilluccia 589/2
I-00100 Roma
Italy

Methods for Non-Invasive Detection of Ventricular Late Potentials – A Comparative Multicenter Study

M. Oeff*), E.-R. v. Leitner*), R. Sthapit*), G. Breithardt**), M. Borggrefe**), U. Karbenn**), T. Meinertz⁺), R. Zotz⁺), W. Clas⁺),V. Hombach⁺⁺), H.-W. Höpp⁺⁺)[1])

Summary: To evaluate the methodological problems of the non-invasive registration of delayed depolarizations the results obtained with four different averaging systems in the same 109 patients (pts) (80 with coronary artery disease, 29 with dilative cardiomyopathy) were compared. The high-resolution-ECG was obtained from the body-surface, high-gain amplified and filtered. The signal-to-noise ratio was improved with the averaging technique.

The following systems were used:

1. Modified Princeton Signal Averager Model 4202, 6 bipolar precordial leads, gain 10 000- to 25 000fold, bandpass-filtering (100–300 Hz, 6 dB/okt.), 127–200 cycles. Visual interpretation with (method B) and without (method D1) regard to the QRS-width obtained from reference leads. Occurrence of depolarizations more than 10 msec after QRS is a positive result.

2. Signal averager described by Simson et al., 3 bipolar orthogonal leads, 25 Hz highpass prefiltering, gain 1000- to 5000fold, bidirectional digital filtering, calculating of the vector magnitude. With automatic interpretation a vector magnitude less than 25 μV in the last 40 msec of the QRS is a positive result (method D2).

3. MAC I (Marquette electronics), 12 bipolar leads, bandpass-filtering (100–300 Hz, 18 dB/okt.), visual interpretation. A positive result is the occurrence of depolarizations in at least 5 leads more than 10 msec after QRS obtained from reference leads (method M/K).

Delayed depolarizations were registered in 12 to 21% of the pts. Corresponding positive results were obtained in 5.5%, corresponding negative results in 68.8% of the pts. Differences in comparison to the other 3 were seen 12 times for D2, 5 times for D1 and 2 times for B. In 10% of the pts two methods showed the same results.

The discrepancies between methods B, D1 and M/K were mainly due to the differences in visual interpretation and not to differences in recording methodology. Method D2 using an automatic interpretation resulted in quite controversial findings, mostly registering a positive result.

Introduction

The non-invasive registration of delayed depolarizations from the body-surface is possible using the signal-averaging-technique to improve the signal-to-noise-ratio.

These delayed depolarizations have been detected mostly in patients with left-ventricular wall motion abnormalities and malignant ventricular tachyarrhythmias (1–13).

Various types of devices are available for their registration and this – besides the selection of the patients –may be the reason for the different results of the studies mentioned above. To evaluate the methodoligical problems we compared the results of the registration with four different averaging-systems obtained in the same patients.

---

[1]) Medical Hospitals of the Universities of Berlin Steglitz*), Düsseldorf**), Mainz⁺) and Köln⁺⁺)

Method:

109 patients (97 men and 12 women) with angiographically proven coronary artery disease (n = 80) or dilative cardiomyopathy (n = 29) were investigated with four different averaging devices. In the individual patient all registrations were done within two hours.

The high-resolution-ECG was obtained from the body surface, high-gain amplified and filtered.

The signal-to-noise-ratio was improved with the signal-averaging-technique. The characteristics of the devices are as follows:

1. The method B (Berlin) and D1 (first method used in Düsseldorf) is using a modified Princeton Signal Averager Model 4202. 127 to 200 QRS-cycles are registered from 6 bipolar precordial leads with high amplification (10 000- to 25 000fold) and bandpass-filtering (100 to 300 Hz, 6 dB/okt.).

The slope-trigger has a jittering of $\pm$ 0.5 msec.

While method D1 only analyses the terminal part of the QRS-complex and the ST-segment, with method B a delay – unit allows additional registration of the pre-trigger part of the QRS, i.e. the beginning of the QRS-complex.

The tracings are stored in a microcomputer for further processing and plotting.

The interpretation of the tracings is visually.

Fractioned depolarizations more than 10 msec after maximum QRS-duration determined from 6 low-resolution reference leads represent positive findings (5).

With method D1, a positive result is present when fractioned depolarizations are detected at the end of the QRS or within the ST-segment that have a 2fold magnitude with respect to the background noise irrespectively of the QRS-duration (8).

2. Method D2, the second device used in Düsseldorf, is identical to the one described by Simson (6). Approximately 150 cycles from 3 bipolar orthogonal leads are amplified with a gain of 1000 to 5000, prefiltered and digitally stored in a HP 9825 B microcomputer. The tracings are bidirectionally filtered with a 3 dB corner frequency of 25 Hz. The

vector magnitude is calculated as $Vi = \sqrt{Xi + Yi + Zi}$ with X, Y and Z being

the magnitude of the corresponding orthogonal lead at time i.

The interpretation is automatical. A delayed depolarization is present when the vector magnitude during the last 40 msec of the QRS-complex is less than 25 μV.

3. With method M/K, as used in Mainz and Köln, the high-resolution-ECG is obtained with the averager MAC I (Marquette Electronics, Milwaukee, USA) (2).

With this device 4 bipolar leads are recorded and further 8 calculated. The filter-settings are 50 to 300 Hz and 100 to 300 Hz (18 dB/okt.).

The interpretation is visual.

A positive result is present when a fractioned depolarization is detected more than 10 msec after QRS (obtained from 12 low-resolution leads) in more than 5 high-resolution leads.

This evaluation method differs from the one used in the studies published so far by the Köln-group (2, 11).

The association between the results of the 4 methods was examined using Pearson's contingency coefficient and the Guttman's prediction measure (14).

Results:

The incidence of delayed depolarizations registered in the same patients with the different methods and the conformity of the results are shown in Table 1.

13 of 109 (12%) patients showed a late potential with method B, 23 (21.1%) with D1, 23 (21.1%) with D2 and 15 (13.8%) with M/K. All four methods gave corresponding results in 72.5% of the patients, 5.5% positive and 68.8% negative findings.

In 4 of 109 patients (3.7%) one method failed to demonstrate delayed depolarizations and in 15 (13.8%) only one of the methods detected one.

In 11 (10.1%) two methods detected delayed depolarizations and two did not.

In the group with one different negative or positive result it was mainly the method D2 which differed from the others (Table 2).

The association between all four methods is statistically significant. The Pearson's contingency coefficient (Table 3) shows the measure of association. The higher the value, the better is the association of two methods.

The smallest values were found for method D2.

Figure 1 shows the delayed depolarizations detected with all four methods in a patient with coronary artery disease and recurrent sustained ventricular tachycardia.

Method B as well as method M/K is registering a fractioned electrical activity of 4 μV maximum 50 to 80 msec after the end of QRS. It is well distinguished from the background noise.

With D2 the magnitude of the tracing during the last 40 msec is 2.35 μV, which also is a pathological finding.

Table 1

Registration of delayed depolarizations

Method		
B	13/109	(12.0%)
D 1	23/109	(21.1%)
D 2	23/109	(21.1%)
M, K	15/109	(13.8%)

Conformity of positive findings:

4 methods	6/109	(5.5%)
3 methods	4/109	(3.7%)
2 methods	11/109	(10.1%)
1 method	15/109	(13.8%)

Conformity of negative findings:

4 methods	73/109	(67%)

Table 2

Discrepancies in the findings:

Method B	2/19
Method D 1	5/19
Method D 2	12/19
Method M, K	0/19

Table 3

Pearson's contingency coefficient

	B	D 1	D 2	M, K
B	1	0.64	0.49	0.72
D 1		1	0.39	0.76
D 2			1	0.5
M, K				1

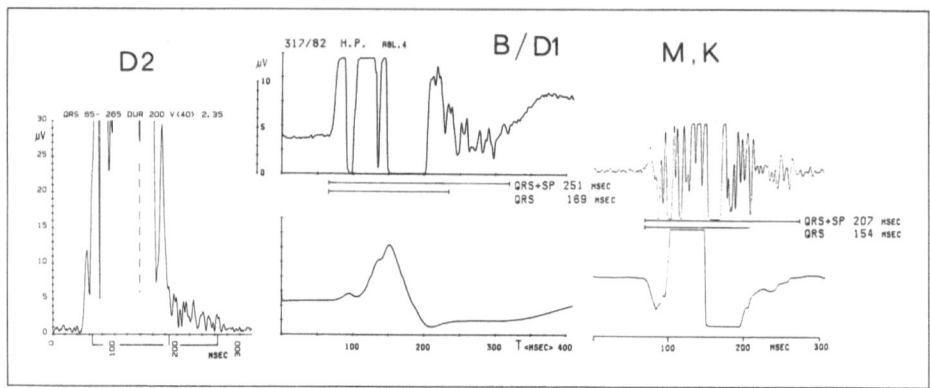

Fig. 1. Delayed depolarizations registered with all four methods in a patient with coronary artery disease and a history of ventricular tachycardia. Fractioned electrical activity in the tracings B, D1 and M/K, magnitude of 2.35 μV in the last 40 msec of QRS in D2.

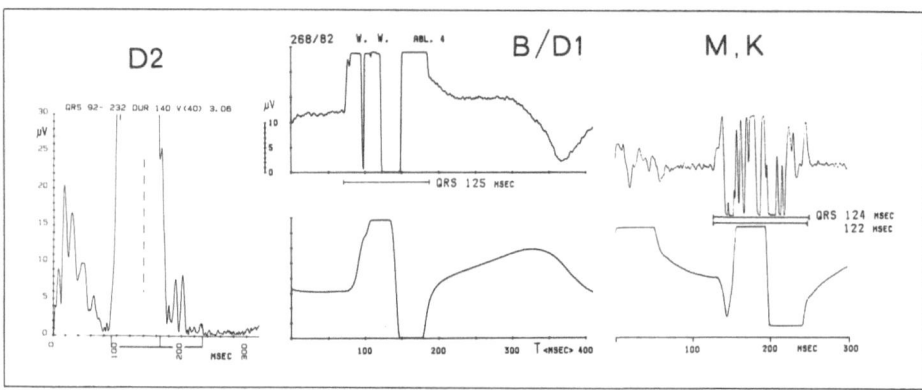

Fig. 2. No fractioned electrical activity is registered with B, M/K and D1, but positive finding with D2 (3.06 μV in the last 40 msec of QRS).

In the tracings shown in Figure 2 fractioned electrical activity is not distinguishable from background noise with B, M/K and D1, but with the D2-system a low-amplitude-part of 3.06 μV in the last 40 msec is recognized.

Figure 3 shows a delayed depolarization with the systems B, D1 and M/K, but not with D1.

Discussion

Delayed fragmented depolarizations can be recorded from the ischemic myocardium in the animal experiment (15–22) or with endo- or epicardial mapping in patients with ventricular arrhythmias (23–28). These areas of delayed electrical activity may be part of a reentrant circuit of ventricular tachycardia or the origin of ventricular ectopic beats.

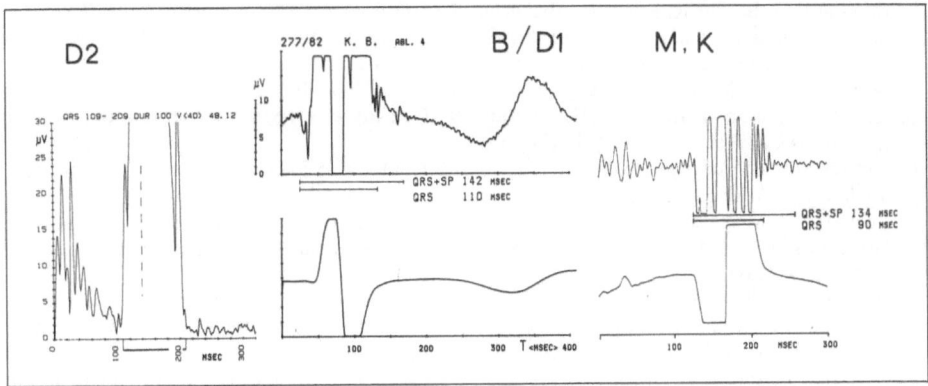

Fig. 3. Delayed depolarizations are detected with the systems B, D1 and M/K, but no low-amplitude-signal in the last part of QRS with D2.

The beat-to-beat-registration of these delayed depolarizations from the body surface is possible, when appropriate recording equipment and shielding from background noise is used (29, 30).

Non-invasive beat-to-beat-recording of these potentials seem to be well correlated to the endocardial signals (31), whereas the specific low-amplitude part on the signal-averaged electrogram as obtained with the Simson-method is unrelated to epicardial events (32). After high amplification and filtering the signal-to-noise-ratio is improved with the averaging technique. Various devices are in use with different modes of amplification, triggering, filtering and evaluation, which were compared in this study (1, 2, 4, 5, 6, 7).

All four systems that are evaluated in this study were able to register delayed depolarizations from the body surface in 12 to 21% of the patients with coronary artery disease or dilative cardiomyopathy. In 72.5% of the patients all four systems gave corresponding findings, 67% of which were negative and 5.5% were positive.

Detailed analysis of the tracings showed that the discrepancies between methods B, D1 and M/K were mainly due to differences in visual interpretation than to differences in recording methodology.

Method D2 using a completely different approach gave quite controversial results in a number of patients, mostly registering a positive finding.

Thus results published in the literature that use method B, D1 and M/K should be comparable to one another.

In the individual patient those obtained by method D2 may not be totally comparable to the results of methods B, D1 and M/K.

References

1. Berbari EJ, Scherlag BJ, Hope RR, Lazzarra R: Recording From the Body Surface of Arrhythmogenic Ventricular Activity During the ST-segment. Amer J Cardiol 1978; 41: 697.
2. Hombach V, Höpp H-W, Braun V, Behrenbeck DW, Tauchert M, Hilger HH: Die Bedeutung von Nachpotentialen innerhalb des ST-Segmentes im Oberflächen-EKG bei Patienten mit koronarer Herzkrankheit. Dtsch Med Wschr 1980; 105: 1457.

3. Breithardt G, Becker R, Seipel L, Abendroth R-R, Ostermeyer J: Non-invasive detection of late potentials in man – a new marker for ventricular tachycardia. European Heart J 1981; 2: 1.
4. Breithardt G, Becker R, Seipel L, Abendroth R-R: Nicht-invasive Registrierung ventrikulärer Spätpotentiale – Methodik und erste Erfahrungen. Z Kardiol 1981; 70: 1–7.
5. Oeff M, v Leitner E-R, Loock D, Schröder R: Non-invasive registration of late potentials in man. European Heart J 1981; 2: 15 (Suppl A).
6. Simson MB: Use of Signals in the terminal QRS Complex to Identify Patients with Ventricular Tachycardia After Myocardial Infarction. Circulation 1981; 64: 235–242.
7. Rozanski JJ, Mortara D, Myerburg RJ, Castellanos A: Body surface detection of delayed depolarizations in patients with recurrent ventricular tachycardia and left ventricular aneurysm. Circulation 1981; 63: 1172.
8. Breithardt G, Borggrefe M, Karbenn U, Abendroth R-R, Yeh S-L, Seipel L: Prevalence of late potentials in patients with and without ventricular tachycardia: correlation with angiographic findings. Am J Cardiol 1982; 49: 1932.
9. Oeff M, v Leitner E-R, Brüggemann T, Andresen D, Sthapit R, Schröder R: Methodische Probleme bei der Registrierung ventrikulärer Spätpotentiale. Z Kardiol 1982; 71: 204.
10. Borggrefe M, Karbenn U, Breithardt G: Spätpotentiale und elektrophysiologische Befunde bei ventrikulären Tachykardien. Z Kardiol 1982; 71: 627.
11. Höpp H-W, Hombach V, Braun V, Tauchert M, Behrenbeck DW, Hilger HH: Kammerarrhythmien und ventrikuläre Spätpotentiale bei akutem Myokardinfarkt. Herz/Kreislauf 1982; 3: 111.
12. Kruck I, Oeff M, Schwietzer U, v Leitner E-R, Biamino G, Andresen D, Friedrich T, Gast D, Meister B, Spielberg C, Schröder R: Besteht eine Beziehung zwischen dem Auftreten von ventrikulären Spätpotentialen und Wandbewegungsstörungen in der 2D-Echokardiographie nach Myokardinfarkt? Z Kardiol 1982; 71: 600.
13. Denes P, Santarelli P, Hauser RG, Uretz EF: Quantitative analysis of the high-frequency Components of the terminal portion of the body surface QRS in Normal Subjects and in Patients with ventricular Tachycardia. Circulation 1983; 67: 1129–1138.
14. Goodman LA, Kruskal WH: Measures of Association for Cross Classifications. New York, Heidelberg, Berlin 1979.
15. Boineau JP, Cox JL: Slow ventricular Activation in acute Myocardial Infarction, a source of Reentrant Premature Ventricular Contractions. Circulation 1973; 48: 702–713.
16. El-Sherif N, Scherlag B, Lazzarra R, Hope RR: Re-entrant ventricular arrhythmias in the late myocardial infarction period. 1. Conduction characteristics in the infarction zone. Circulation 1977; 55: 686.
17. El-Sherif N, Hope RR, Scherlag BJ, Lazzarra R: Re-entrant ventricular arrhythmias in the late myocardial infarction period. 2. Patterns of initiation and termination of re-entry. Circulation 1977; 55: 702.
18. Euler DD, Moore EN: Continuous fractionated electrical activity after stimulation of the ventricles during the vulnarable period: Evidence for local reentry. Am J Cardiol 1980; 46: 783.
19. El-Sherif N, Smith RA, Evans KE: Canine ventricular arrhythmias in the late myocardial infarction period 8. Epicardial mapping of reentrant circuits. Circulation Research 1981; 49: 255.
20. Wit EA, Allessie MA, Bonke FIM, Lammers W, Smeets J, Fenoglio JJ: Electrophysiologic mapping to determine the mechanism of experimental ventricular tachycardia initiated by premature impulses. Amer J Cardiol 1982; 49: 166.
21. Brachmann J, Kabell G, Scherlag B, Harrison L, Lazzarra R: Analysis of Interectopic Activation Patterns During Sustained Ventricular Tachycardia. Circulation 1983; 67: 449–456.
22. Mehra R, Zeiler RH, Gough WB, El-Sherif N: Reentrant Ventricular Arrhythmias in the Late Myocardial Infarction Period. 9. Electrophysiologic-Anatomic Correlation of Reentrant Circuits. Circulation 1983; 67: 11–24.
23. Josephson ME, Horowitz LN, Farshidi A, Kastor JA: Recurrent sustained ventricular tachycardia. II. Endocardial mapping. Circulation 1978; 57: 440.
24. Josephson ME, Horowitz LN, Farshidi A: Continuous local electrical activity, a mechanism of recurrent ventricular tachycardia. Circulation 1978; 57: 659.
25. Fontaine G, Guiraudon G, Frank R: Intramyocardial conduction defects in patients prone to chronic ventricular tachycardia. I. The post-excitation syndrome in sinus rhythm. In: Sandoe E, Julian DG, Bell JW (ed): Management of ventricular tachycardia – role of Mexiletine. Amsterdam – Oxford 1978.

26. Horowitz LN, Josephson ME, Harken AH, Kastor JA: Ventricular resection guided by epicardial and endocardial mapping for treatment of recurrent ventricular tachycardia. N. Engl J Med 1980; 302: 589.

27. Wiener I, Mindich B, Pitchon R, Pichard A, Kupersmith J, Estioko M, Jurado R, Camunas R, Litwak R: Epicardial activation in patients with coronary artery disease: Effects of regional contraction abnormalities. Circulation 1982; 65: 154.

28. Klein H, Karp RB, Kouchoukos NT, Zorn GL, James TN, Waldo AL: Intraoperative electrophysiologic mapping of the ventricles during sinus rhythm in patients with a previous myocardial infarction. Identification of the electrophysiologic substrate of ventricular arrhythmias. Circulation 1982; 66: 847.

29. Oeff M, v Leitner E-R, Erné SN, Hahlbohm HD, Lehmann HP, Schröder R: Einzelschlag-Registrierung ventrikularer Spätdepolarisationen von der Körperoberfläche koronarkranker Patienten. Z Kardiol 1982; 71: 627.

30. Hombach V, Kebbel U, Höpp H-W, Winter U-J, Braun V, Deutsch H, Hirche H, Hilger HH: Fortlaufende Registrierung von Mikropotentialen des menschlichen Herzens. Dtsch med Wschr 1982; 107: 1951.

31. Oeff M, v Leitner E-R, Erné SN, Hahlbohm HD, Lehmann HP, Schröder R: Einzelschlag-Registrierung ventrikulärer Spätdepolarisationen und arrhythmogener diastolischer Potentiale von der Körperoberfläche koronarkranker Patienten. Verh Dtsch Ges Innere Med 1983: in press.

32. Josephson ME, Simson MB, Harken AH, Horowitz LN, Falcone RA: The Incidence and Clinical significance of epicardial late potentials in patients with recurrent sustained ventricular tachycardia and coronary artery disease. Circulation 1982; 66: 1199.

Authors' address:
Dr. M. Oeff
Freie Universität Berlin
Universitätsklinikum Steglitz
Kardiopulmologische Abteilung
Hindenburgdamm 30
D-1000 Berlin 45

Reproducibility of Measurements Made by Signal Averaging the Body Surface Vectorcardiogram

D. A. Richards*), W. R. Dassen, V. van Ommen, C. de Zwaan, H. J. Wellens

Summary: The aim of this study was to quantify the interduplicate variability of measurements made by signal averaging and digital filtering at 25 Hz and 50 Hz, the body surface vectorcardiogram. Measurements of QRS duration ms (QRS) and root mean square voltage uV during the terminal 40 ms of QRS (V40) were made on separate days in 20 control subjects without heart disease (21 to 34 years, Group I), and 15 patients (33–70 years, Group II) 1 to 3 days and 4 to 7 days after myocardial infarction.
For Group I at 25 Hz and 50 Hz, the mean differences in QRS duration ± standard deviation (SD) were 2 ± 5 ms and 1 ± 6 ms, and the mean differences in V40 ± SD were 4 ± 36 uV and 2 ± 14 uV respectively. For Group II, mean differences in QRS and V40 at 25 Hz and 50 Hz were 0 ± 11 ms, 1 ± 10 ms and -13 ± 64 uV, -11 ± 23 uV respectively.

Conclusions:

1. On the average, interduplicate differences in QRS were small in control subjects, and patients 1 to 3 and 4 to 7 days after infarction.
2. Interduplicate differences in V40 were sometimes large, particularly in patients after myocardial infarction.
3. Care must be taken before attributing differences in QRS and V40 to medical or surgical perturbations.

Introduction

Signal averaging has been used for several years to facilitate accurate measurements of QRS onset and offset (1–7). It has been observed that low amplitude signals extending into the ST segment occur commonly in ischaemic heart disease patients with recurrent spontaneous ventricular tachycardia, but occur uncommonly in patients without ventricular tachycardia.

Denniss et al. (7) recently reported that QRS prolongation observed at signal averaging within one month of myocardial infarction, was a highly sensitive predictor of subsequent spontaneous ventricular tachycardia, in a cohort of patients without previous spontaneous ventricular tachycardia. However, the prognostic significance of changes in measurements made after signal averaging has yet to be determined.

*) Dr. Richards is the recipient of Overseas Research Fellowships of The National Heart Foundation of Australia and The Royal Australasian College of Physicians.

In the present study we made duplicate recordings on separate days, of signal averaged vectorcardiograms in normal control subjects, and patients 1 to 3 and 4 to 7 days after acute myocardial infarction. Digital filtering and computer algorithms were used to determine total QRS duration, and root mean square voltage in the terminal 40 ms of QRS.
The aim of this study was to quantify the interduplicate variability of measurements of QRS duration and amplitude in the terminal part of the QRS complex.

Methods

The study population comprised two Groups: I, Twenty control subjects without heart disease, aged 21 to 34 years, and II, Fifteen survivors of acute myocardial infarction (8 anterior, 7 inferior), aged 33 to 70 years. Two Group II patients exhibited spontaneous ventricular tachycardia (more than 48 hours after acute myocardial infarction in the absence of further ischaemia). None of the study population had evidence of left ventricular hypertrophy or bundle branch block on standard 12 lead electrocardiogram, and each was in normal sinus rhythm when signal averaged recordings were made. Whereas no Group I subject was receiving any cardioactive medication, all Group II patients were receiving cardioactive medications at some stage during the study. Duplicate signal averaged vectorcardiogram recordings were made on separate days from each Group I subject and on two occasions (1 to 3 and 4 to 7 days) after acute myocardial infarction from each Group II patient.
The signal averaged vectorcardiogram was recorded using previously published techniques (4). Bipolar leads X, Y and Z were serially digitized along with fiducial point markers obtained from a reference lead via an analogue trigger for 133 seconds. Ectopic and excessively noisy beats were rejected by a template algorithm. Averaged complexes (100 to 150 beats) were computed for each bipolar lead, then filtered digitally using a bi-directional digital technique. High pass filter frequencies were 25 and 50 Hz.
Each set of 3 averaged, filtered bipolar recordings was then combined into a vector magnitude "filtered QRS complex" ($[X^2 + Y^2 + Z^2]^{0.5}$). Two parameters (QRS ms, V40 uV) from each filtered QRS complex were measured, and used for subsequent analysis. QRS duration was defined as total duration of filtered QRS determined by computer algorithm, and V40 as root mean square voltage during the last 40 ms of the filtered QRS complex.
Student's t tests for paired samples were used to determine the significance of differences between duplicate recordings, and between recordings at different filter settings.

Results

Table 1 summarizes the results. The "Values" for QRS and V40 were calculated by pooling duplicate recordings at each filter setting in each Group. The "Differences" for QRS and V40 represent the differences between duplicate recordings (second minus first recording) at each filter setting in each Group.
QRS tended to shorten as high pass filter frequency was increased but this trend was only significant in Group I ($p < 0.05$). In contrast V40 was less at 50 than at 25 Hz in both Groups ($p < 0.001$). Overall, the ranges of QRS and V40 for control subjects and infarct

650

Table 1. Filtered QRS duration and voltage in the last 40 ms of filtered ORS complex.

Filter (Hz)		Values		Differences	
		QRS (ms)	V40 (uV)	QRS (ms)	V40 (uV)
Group I Control subjects					
25	Mean ± SD	99± 8	61± 31	2± 5	−4±36
	(range)	82 – 113	17 – 181	−10 – 10	−134 – 64
		*	**		
50	Mean ± SD	96± 8	26± 14	1± 6	2±14
	(range)	82 – 122	8 – 81	−10 – 15	−39 – 41
Group II Infarct Patients					
25	Mean ± SD	98± 12	61± 55	0±11	−13±64
	(range)	76 – 120	9 – 296	−15 – 20	−203 – 61
	NS		**		
50	Mean ± SD	97± 11	28± 24	1±10	−11±23
	(range)	78 – 119	5 – 124	−14 – 12	−76 – 10

Differences = Differences between duplicate recordings (second recording minus first recording)
Filter = High pass filter frequency
QRS = Filtered QRS complex duration
Values = Pooled data from duplicate recordings
V40 = Root mean square voltage in last 40 ms of filtered QRS
* = $p < 0.05$
** = $p < 0.001$
NS = not significant

patients were similar. Although the absolute variations between interduplicate recordings tended to be greater amongst the infarct population than the control population, this tendency was not statistically significant.

Reproducibility in Group I

In Group I the mean differences in QRS duration measured at 25 Hz and 50 Hz were 2 ms and 1 ms respectively (2% and 1% of mean QRS durations respectively). The standard deviations of these differences were 5 ms and 6 ms respectively (5% and 6% of mean QRS durations respectively). Therefore 95% of individual interduplicate differences would be expected to fall within ± 10 ms and ± 12 ms of initial recordings made at 25 Hz and 50 Hz respectively.

The mean differences in V40 amplitude measured at 25 Hz and 50 Hz were 4 uV and 2 uV respectively (7% and 8% of mean V40 amplitudes respectively). The standard deviations of these differences were 36 uV and 14 uV respectively (59% and 54% of mean V40 amplitudes respectively). Thus the variation in V40 amplitude was very much more considerable than the variation in QRS duration among control subjects.

Fig. 1 illustrates a high level of reproducibility of recordings made in a control subject. Note that QRS durations and V40 amplitudes were similar in both recordings (104 ms, 29 uV, and 105 ms, 33 uV at 25 Hz; 98 ms 14 uV, and 97 ms, 15 uV at 50 Hz). Further, note that QRS durations were shorter after filtering at 50 Hz than after filtering at 25 Hz (98 ms versus 104 ms, and 97 ms versus 105 ms respectively); and that V40 amplitudes were less after filtering at the higher frequency (14 uV versus 29 uV, and 15 uV versus 33 uV, respectively).

Fig. 2 illustrates the recordings and measurements made in another control subject. In this case, as in the example shown in Fig. 1, QRS morphology and vector magnitude plots were generally comparable at initial and duplicate recordings. However, when filtered at 25 Hz, QRS duration was longer and V40 amplitude was less at the duplicate recording than at the initial recording. The source of this difference is apparent when one inspects the terminal portion of the filtered QRS complex in the centre panels. The computer algorithm has detected significant energy extending to 107 ms after QRS onset, on the right, but only to 98 ms on the left. This sort of variation in "QRS end detection" will occur whenever the transition from "high energy QRS" to "low energy ST segment" is gradual and only just above threshold for end detection (1 uV using the present algorithm). The reduction in V40 in the duplicate recording compared with the initial recording is a direct consequence of the later QRS end detection.

Note that QRS duration and V40 amplitude are more reproducible after filtering at 50 Hz than after filtering at 25 Hz (100 ms, 26 uV, and 102 ms, 29 uV versus 98 ms, 102 uV, and 107 ms, 80 uV).

Fig. 1. Records from a control subject. Left panels from initial study, right panels from duplicate study. Upper panels are truncated tracings of the averaged X, Y and Z leads. Centre panels are the vector magnitude plots derived from the traces illustrated at the top, filtered at 25 Hz. Lower panels are the vector magnitude plots derived from the traces illustrated at the top, filtered at 50 Hz. QRS durations and V40 amplitudes are shown in each of the lower 4 panels. Broken lines above depict QRS onset and offset determined by computer algorithm, after filtering at 25 Hz. Broken lines below depict QRS onset and offset determined by computer algorithm, after filtering at 50 Hz.

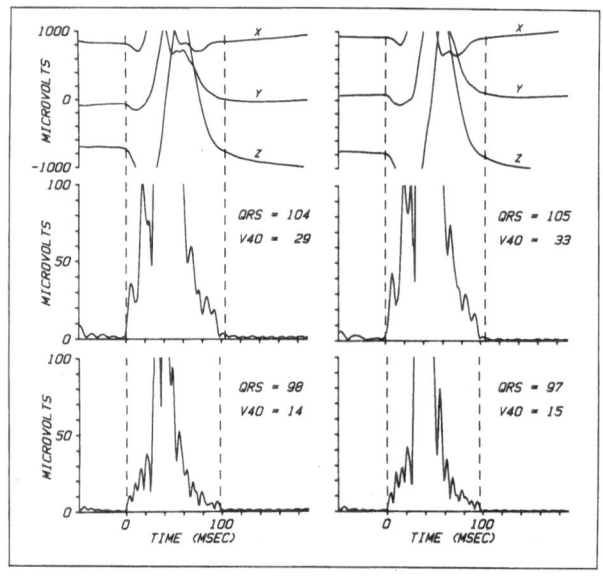

652

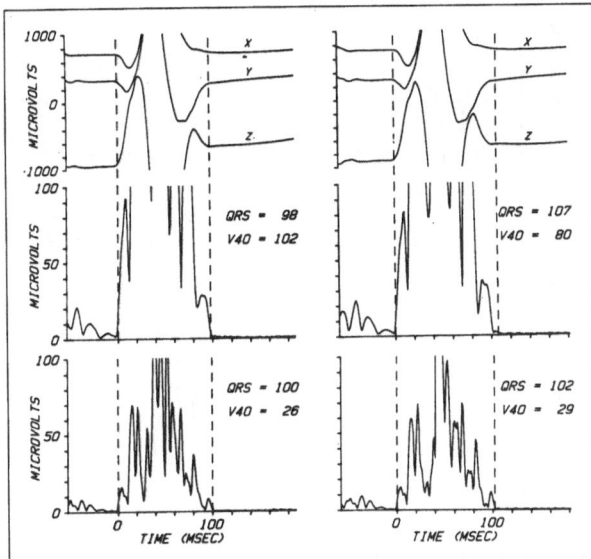

Fig. 2. Records from another control subject, illustrating a source of variation in QRS and V40 measurements. See text for details. Layout is the same as in Figure 1.

Reproducibility in Group II

In Group II the mean differences in QRS duration measured at 25 Hz and 50 Hz were 0 ms and 1 ms respectively (0% and 1% of mean QRS durations respectively). The standard deviations of these differences were 11 ms and 10 ms respectively (11% and 10% of mean QRS durations respectively). Therefore 95% of individual interduplicate differences would be expected to fall within ± 22 ms and ± 20 ms of initial recordings made at 25 Hz and 50 Hz respectively.

The mean differences in V40 amplitude measured at 25 Hz and 50 Hz were 13 uV and 11 uV respectively (21% and 39% of mean V40 amplitudes respectively). The standard deviations of these differences were 64 uV and 23 uV respectively (105% and 82% of mean V40 amplitudes respectively). As with Group I, Group II variation in V40 was very much more considerable than variation in QRS duration.

Fig. 3 illustrates a source of variation in QRS duration and V40 amplitude in a patient with inferolateral myocardial infarction (Q waves in X and Y). The panels of this figure are arranged similarly to those of Figures 1 and 2. Note the low amplitude signals in the terminal part of the QRS, particularly well seen in leads X and Y, in the upper right panel (duplicate) not seen in the upper left panel (initial). These differences in QRS duration are reflected in the measurements made not only after filtering at 25 Hz but also after filtering at 50 Hz.

Discussion

We have used a signal averaging and bidirectional digital filtering system to measure QRS duration and root mean square voltage in the terminal 40 ms of QRS filtered at 25 Hz and 50 Hz.

653

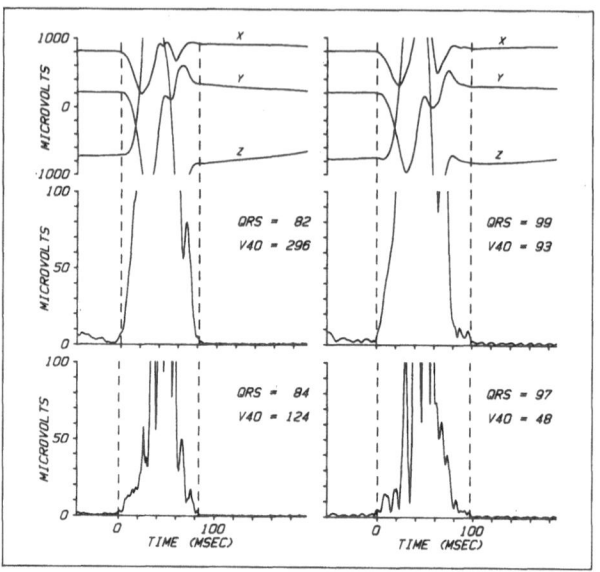

Fig. 3. Records from an infarct patient, illustrating another source of variation in QRS and V40 measurements. See text for details. Layout is the same as in previous figures.

On the average, QRS durations, measured at each filter setting were highly reproducible (≤ 2%). However, the ranges of QRS duration differences (between duplicate recordings) in normal subjects and infarct patients were considerable (10% to 20%). In all cases, measured QRS duration depends on a computer algorithm for "QRS end detection". Variation in "QRS end detection" will occur whenever the transition from "high energy QRS" to "low energy ST segment" is gradual and only just above threshold for end detection (1 uV in the present report).

In infarct patients "biological changes" in QRS morphology and duration (Fig. 3) may produce variation in measured QRS duration. On the other hand, variations in QRS duration, of the type illustrated in Fig. 2 are less likely to occur at higher filter frequencies (lower panels) because of greater "dampening" of signals, in this case between 25 Hz and 50 Hz.

Measurement of V40 is highly dependent upon "QRS end detection". As QRS offset is moved later, away from peak voltage, V40 falls. Therefore a small change in QRS offset determination may produce a large change in V40 measurement (at either filter setting). The optimal high pass filter cutoff frequency for measurement of QRS duration remains to be determined, but should probably be of the order of 50 Hz.

Another potential (technical) source of variation in measurements of QRS duration and V40 amplitude is variation in location of lead placement. The system used in this study utilizes simple bipolar leads (4), unlike others (1, 7) which use a "balanced" resistive network to approximate the gains of the resultant orthogonal leads (8–10). Formal studies of lead systems and lead placement may be useful to determine the clinical relevance of these potential sources of interduplicate variation.

Conclusions

1. On the average, interduplicate differences in QRS duration measured on different days were small, both in control subjects, and in patients studied 1 to 3 and 4 to 7 days after myocardial infarction. However, individual interduplicate differences in QRS durations, up to 20%, were observed.
2. Measurement of V40 amplitude was dependent upon determination of QRS offset and was subject to considerable variation, up to 100%.
3. Technical and biological sources of variation should be considered before attributing differences in measurements of QRS duration and V40 amplitude to medical or surgical perturbations.

Acknowledgements

The authors gratefully acknowledge the provision of equipment by Arrhythmia Research Technology (USA), and the expert technical assistance of Adri van den Dool.

References

1. Uther JB, Dennett CJ, Tan A: The detection of delayed activation signals of low amplitude in the vectorcardiogram of patients with recurrent ventricular tachycardia by signal averaging. In: Sandoe E, Julian DG, Bell JW, eds. Management of Ventricular Tachycardia – Role of Mexiletine. Amsterdam: Excerpta Medica, 1978; 80–82.
2. Berbari EJ, Scherlag BJ, Hope RR, Lazarra R: Recording from the body surface of arrhythmogenic ventricular activity during the ST segment. Am J Cardiol 1978; 41: 697–702.
3. Briethardt G, Becker G, Seipel L, Abendroth RR, Ostermeyer J: Non-invasive detection of late potentials in man – A new marker for ventricular tachycardia. Eur Heart J 1981; 2: 1–11.
4. Simson MB: Use of signals in the terminal QRS complex to identify patients with ventricular tachycardia after myocardial infarction. Circulation 1981; 64: 235–241.
5. Rozanski JJ, Mortara D, Myerburg RJ, Castellanos A: Body surface detection of delayed depolarizations in patients with recurrent ventricular tachycardia and left ventricular aneurysm. Circulation 1981; 63: 1172–1178.
6. Josephson ME, Simson MB, Harken AH, Horowitz LN, Falcone RA: The incidence and clinical significance of epicardial late potentials in patients with recurrent sustained ventricular tachycardia and coronary artery disease. Circulation 1982; 66: 1199–1204.
7. Denniss A, Richards D, Farrow R, Davison A, Uther J: Use of the signal averaged vectorcardiogram to predict ventricular electrical instability after myocardial infarction. Circulation 1982; 66 Suppl II: II-16 (abstr).
8. Frank E: An accurate clinically practical system for spatial vectorcardiography. Circulation 1956; 13: 737–749.
9. McFee R, Parungao A: An orthogonal lead system for clinical electrocardiography. Am Heart J 1961; 62: 93–100.
10. Gau GT, Smith RE: The effect of electrode position on a modified Frank electrocardiographic lead system. Mayo Clinic Proc 1971; 46: 536–543.

Authors' address:
David A. Richards, M.D.
Department of Cardiology
University of Limburg
Annadal Hospital Maastricht
The Netherlands

Electrophysiological Studies at Exercise in Patients with Accessory Atrioventricular Pathways

R. Frank, G. Fontaine, J. L. Tonet, N. Shantha, Y. Grosgogeat

Summary: 14 patients, 7 with bidirectional, 7 with unidirectional retrograde atrioventricular (AV) conduction through an AV accessory pathway, were submitted to bicycle exercise test from 20 to 140 watts, with 6 minutes and 30 watts steps. Left atrium was paced through a temporary coronary sinus quadripolar electrode. Measurements were done in the supine, sitting position and for each step of the exercise: 1. Atrial (ARP), Kent (KRP) and AV nodal (NPR) effective refractory periods (ERP) on spontaneous rate, and when possible on paced rate at 90 and 130/mn. 2. Shortest atrial cycle conducted 1/1 to the ventricles. 3. AV conduction time in sinus rhythm and orthodromic tachycardia, and VA time in orthodromic tachycardia. Results: 1. ERP constantly shortened with exercise: At 80 watts, compared to the supine values, ARP decreased 62 ± 30 ms, KRP 94 ± 19 ms, NRP 68 ± 34 ms. The shortest 1/1 AV cycle conducted through the AV node shortened 85 ± 31 ms, and 60 ± 25 ms through the Kent bundle. 2. Kent conduction time did not change in an appreciable way. AV nodal conduction time constantly shortened in sinus rhythm (40 ms at 80 watts) as in orthodromic tachycardia (95 ± 10 ms at 110 watts). It explains less marked preexcitation in sinus rhythm, and faster heart rate in orthodromic tachycardia at exercise. 3. These data show the importance of humoral factors on refractory periods and conduction times. They have to be considered when only supine provocative techniques are used to assess effectiveness of anti-arrhythmic therapy.

Introduction

Clinical electrophysiological studies are widely used to identify tachyarrhythmia mechanism and to assess effectiveness of anti-arrhythmic therapy. These sophisticated studies are usually done while the patient is supine, and their results are supposed to be applicable to the patient in other situations. In fact, electrophysiological parameters can be modified with changes in posture (1) and exercise (2), but the importance of these factors is not well known. This study was done to evaluate modifications due to exercise on electrophysiological parameters in patients with accessory atrioventricular pathways (Kent bundles) in sinus rhythm.

Population

14 patients, 10 men and 4 women, age 45 ± 16 years, without any congenital or acquired heart disease were included in the study. 7 had a WPW syndrome with permanent anterograde conduction, 5 left lateral, 2 right lateral. 7 had a Kent bundle with only retrograde conduction at the time of the study, 2 right lateral, 5 left lateral. Despite the fact that anti-arrhythmic drugs were stopped in all patients, two patients

657

with WPW had been on Amiodarone until one month prior to the study, and therefore could have some residual effect due to the drug therapy.

Method

Electrophysiological studies were done under basal state to measure refractory periods and conduction properties of AV nodal and bypass tract. A quadripolar lead inserted via a left subclavian vein was positioned in the coronary sinus and left after the study. The following day an ergometric bicycle test was done, starting from 20 watts up to the point of exhaustion, in steps of 30 watts, each of 6 mn duration.

Measurements were done with the patient supine, when the patient was sitting on the bicycle, and at each step of exercise, starting 1 minute after the beginning of the step.

An 11 lead ECG and unipolar coronary sinus potential were recorded, at paper speed of 50 and 100 mm/sec. The accuracy of the measurement was in the range of 5 to 10 ms.

Left atrium was paced using the other coronary sinus electrodes.

The following measurements were made for each step of exercise:

- Blood pressure, sinus rate, PR interval.
- Effective and functional refractory periods of left atrium, AV node and Kent were measured using the extrastimulus technique during sinus rhythm and during atrial paced rate of 130/mn.
- Maximal atrial rate conducted 1/1 to the ventricles.
- Tachycardia cycle length and AV and VA time during orthodromic tachycardia.

Refractory periods of the retrograde VA conduction was not measured since only one catheter was used, positioned in the coronary sinus. Care was taken to avoid induction of atrial fibrillation.

Results

The complete protocol could not be completed on each patient. Exercise could only be done up to 50 watts in all patients, up to 80 watts in 10 patients, and only 3 completed 140 watts exercise. The functional refractory period was a limiting factor in the measurement of AV nodal refractory periods and of the Kent bundle in some cases. In some cases, a short Kent bundle refractory period prevented determination of AV nodal refractory period. 1/1 AV conduction rates above 250/mn were avoided, since they could not be tolerated by the patients.

The mean values and standard deviations are represented on Table 1.

With exercise, systolic blood pressure rose from 120 ± 10 to 160 ± 30 at 100 watts. Mean heart rate increased from 75 ± 14/mn while supine to 147 ± 23/mn at maximal exercise.

PR interval shortened in patients with concealed pre-excitation from 175 ± 25 ms at rest to 110 ± 10 ms at 140 watts. The mean decrease was 40 ms at 80 watts. PR interval was stable in all but one patient with pre-excitation. In that patient, pre-excitation disap-

Table 1. For each parameter, is given, on the first line: Mean values; Standard deviation; Number of patients. On the second linie: Mean decrease form the supine values and standard deviation.

	Supine	Seated	20 Watts	50 Watts	80 Watts	110 Watts	140 Watts
Pr	175+/–	160+/–	155+/–	141+/–	140+/–	125+/–	110+/–
	26 (7)	20 (7)	11 (7)	14 (7)	15 (5)	12 (4)	14 (2)
		16+/–14	22+/–13	34+/–21	38+/–21	55+/–15	60+/–28
ARP SC	270+/–	252+/–	242+/–	228+/–	211+/–	195+/–	176+/–
	36 (14)	32 (14)	30 (12)	22 (12)	31 (9)	28 (7)	25 (3)
		21+/–27	33+/–27	49+/–29	+/–62+/–30	64+/–33	70+/–17
ARP 130	247+/–	235+/–	217+/–	206+/–	190+/–	182+/–	–
	21 (11)	27 (13)	23 (12)	21 (9)	25 (7)	21 (5)	
		21+/–23	36+/–18	48+/–20	71+/–24	80+/–30	
KRP SC	334+/–	295+/–	274+/–	247+/–	230+/–	217+/–	200 (1)
	61 (7)	58 (7)	56 (7)	44 (7)	43 (5)	28 (4)	160
		35+/–19	57+/–26	80+/–23	94+/–19	122+/–28	
KRP 130	278+/–	258+/–	256+/–	253+/–	253+/–	240+/–	–
	30 (6)	23 (6)	20 (5)	25 (3)	25 (3)	20 (3)	
		20+/–20	34+/–20	35+/–23	35+/–23	56+/–5	
NRP SC	290+/–	274+/–	248+/–	250+/–	218+/–	200+/–	–
	43 (13)	42 (12)	38 (9)	37 (9)	29 (6)	25 (4)	
		19+/–24	40+/–23	51+/–24	68+/–34	85+/–47	
NRP 130	300+/–	246+/–	235+/–	244+/–	230+/–	197+/–	–
	41 (8)	31 (11)	24 (6)	23 (5)	33 (4)	25 (4)	
		44+/–38	60+/–39	60+/–48	80+/–50	112+/–55	
AVN 1/1	364+/–	339+/–	285+/–	284+/–	271+/–	250 (3)	–
	46 (9)	48 (8)	30	37 (5)	18 (5)	127+/–38	
		28+/–14	56+/–17	62+/–23	85+/–31		
AVK 1/1	302+/–	278+/–	269+/–	259+/–	252+/–	–	–
	48 (4)	46 (4)	46 (4)	38 (4)	31 (4)		
		23+/–5	40+/–28	60+/–32	60+/–25		
ORT RR	387+/–	364+/–	354+/–	322+/–	295+/–	274+/–	–
	47 (10)	49 (12)	54 (11)	35 (11)	39 (7)	46 (5)	
		27+/–16	36+/–19	63+/–30	86+/–9	95+/–10	

PR: PR interval; RPSR: Refractory period on sinus rate; RP 130: Refractory period on 130/min paced beat; A: Atrial; K: Kent; N: Nodal; AVN 1/1: Shortest atrial cycle lenght with conduction 1/1 through the AV node; AVK 1/1: Shortest atrial cycle length with conduction 1/1 through the Kent bundle. ORT RR cycle in orthodromic reciprocal tachycardia values in milliseconds.

peared at a 50 watts exercise; however the delta wave was visible after an atrial extra-stimulus.

Refractory periods of the left atrium decreased from 270 ± 36 to 176 ± 25 ms. The mean decrease was 49 ± 29 ms at 50 watts and 70 ± 17 ms at 140 watts. Kent bundle refractory periods decreased from 334 ± 61 ms to 247 ± 44 at 50 watts and to 217 ± 28 at 110 watts. The mean decrease was 80 ± 23 ms at 50 watts, and 160 ms at 140 watts.

AV nodal refractory period was limited by the atrial refractory period, or by the Kent bundle refractory period. It decreased from 290 ± 43 ms supine to less than 200 ms (110 watts). In mean decrease was 51 ± 24 ms at 50 watts and 85 ± 47 at 110 watts.

The shortest atrial cycle length with 1/1 conduction through the AV node averaged 360 ms when supine to <250 ms at 110 watts. The shortest atrial cycle length conducted 1/1 through the Kent bundle decreased from 302 ms to less than 240 ms.

The cycle length of orthodromic tachycardia shortened in every case from 387 ± 47 ms at rest to 275 ± 46 ms at 110 watts. The mean decrease was 27 ± 16 ms when seated and 95 ± 10 ms at 110 watts. The decrease was primarily due to shortening of AV nodal conduction time in each case.

Comments

The changes in refractory periods and conduction velocity due to exercise are well known, but little documented. The mechanisms by which these changes are mediated include sympathetic stimulation, vagal depression and the effect of the rate in itself.

There is shortening of atrial refractory period with the increase of the atrial rate (3). Refractory period shortens also at constant driven rate if the degree of effort is increased, demonstrating the effects of humoral factors. In fact, these effects seem to be the predominant factor in shortening refractory periods, as the difference between refractory periods at rest and for a given exercise step is in the same range when measured during sinus rhythm rate, and during pacing at 130/mn (Table 1).

The refractory period and the conduction time of the AV node are both prolonged at rest, when the atrial rate is increased by pacing (3). Exercise enhances that conduction. In 1965 (2), Lister showed that in man, increase of sinus rate by exercise was associated with a decrease in AV conduction time with an AV 1/1 conduction for higher atrial rate. In 1978 (1), Curry demonstrated that changes in posture shortens AH time, and allows 1/1 AV conduction at higher rate. This is consistent with our findings where the PR interval in patients without anterograde pre-excitation, the nodal refractory period and the shortest atrial cycle length which allowed 1/1 through the AV node, shortened with exercise. Again, the humoral factors seemed to be predominant rather than the effect of the faster sinus rate.

The Kent bundle refractory periods are shortened by a faster atrial rate (4). These values were shortened even more with exercise in our 7 cases. This is consistent with studies evaluating the effect of exercise on the RR interval during atrial fibrillation (5, 6), as it has been shown to correlate with Kent refractory period (7). In our series, shortening in effective refractory period of the Kent was seen in all patients, the degree of shortening increasing with the level of exercise. For a given step, the degree of shortening differed from patient to patient, but did not correlate with the initial value (8): for instance at 50 watts, the refractory period shortened by 40 to 130 ms. The 2 patients with initial values of 260 ms exhibited 90 and 50 ms shortening. Those with 300 and 310 ms showed a shortening at 90 and 40 ms respectively. In the cases where refractory period was longer (360, 380 and 460 ms) a decrease of 130, 80 and 120 ms was noted. This is not consistent with the effect of Isoproterenol on Kent refractory periods as demonstrated by some authors (6, 8). The 2 last patients had been treated with amiodarone and their Kent refractory period did not lower less than the others, but starting from a larger refractory period they stayed at 300 ms at 50 watts exercise. However, these values were limited by the left atrial refractory period in 5/7 patients during exercise, whereas they could be measured in the supine position. This implies that a shorter refractory period could be found for a higher atrial rate. The·shortest atrial cycle length conducted 1/1 to the ventricle by the Kent bundle overcomes that limitation as the data brought by inducting atrial fibrillation.

The Kent bundle conduction time, did not change, in an appreciable way, during the study. This is in contrast with the constant shortening of the AV nodal conduction time. This will change the balance in ventricular activation between two pathways, and explain the observation of less marked pre-excitation (8, 9), or its disappearance with exercise. Such a phenomenon occurred only in one patient in our series, and cannot be attributed to a block in the Kent bundle, since a premature atrial stimulus restored the full pre-excitation. Strasberg (9) and Levy (10) proposed that sudden disappearance of pre-excitation at exercise, could be an indication of a prolonged Kent bundle refractory period longer as compared to the AV nodal refractory period, at rest. But in this serie (10) Kent bundle refractory period averaged 300 ± 65 ms in 9 patients which is different from the data of Strasberg where the abrupt disappearance of Kent bundle conduction was observed in 4 patients, with a mean refractory period of 368 ± 28 ms. In our series the patient in whom the pre-excitation disappeared with exercise had at rest a refractory period of 420 ms during the sinus rhythm and 360 ms at the paced rate of 90/mn. All the other patients had a Kent bundle refractory period on sinus rate or at the paced rate of 90/mn, larger than the AV nodal refractory period, between 380 ms and 260 ms and the pre-excitation did not disappear at exercise. This does not make the test very sensitive in detecting Kent bundle with long refractory periods.

Conclusion

Constant shortening of refractory periods and conduction time was induced by exercise in all our patients. These data must be considered when electrophysiological studies are aimed at the treatment of arrhythmia, like assessing the effectiveness of anti-arrhythmic drugs, or determining the need for anti-tachycardia pacemaker. As the electrophysiological parameters appear to change with the patient activity, effect of therapy may not be the same with changes in posture and activity, allowing relapses of tachycardia and faster tachycardia rates.

References

1. Curry PVL: The hemodynamic and electrophysiological effects of paroxysmal tachycardia. In: Cardiac arrhythmias. Electrophysiology, Diagnostic and Management. O Narula Ed, Williams and Wilkins Pub, Baltimore 1979: p 364.
2. Lister JW, Stein E, Kossoowsky BD, Lau SH, Damato AN: Atrio-ventricular conduction in man: Effect of rate, exercise, isoproterenol and atropine on the P-R interval. Amer J Cardiol 1965; 16: 516.
3. Cagin AN, Kunstadt D, Wolfish P, Levitt B: The influence of heart rate on the refractory period of the atrium and AV conducting system. Amer Heart J 1973; 85: 358.
4. Frank R: Apport des investigations endocavitaires et des cartographies epicardiques dans l'etude des syndromes de pre-excitation ventriculaire. Theses Paris 1974.
5. Crick JCP, Davies DW, Curry PVL, Sowton E: Wolff-Parkinson-White syndrome. Effect of exercise on ventricular response to atrial fibrillation (Abstract). J Am Coll Cardiol 1983; 1: 634.

6. German LD, Gallagher JJ, Broughton A, Guarnieri T, Trantham JL: Effects of exercise and iso-proterenol during atrial fibrillation in patients with Wolff-Parkinson-White Syndrome. Amer J Cardiol 1983; 51: 1203–1206.

7. Castellanos A Jr, Iyengar R, Agha AS, Castillo CA: Wenckebach Phenomenon within the atria. Brit Heart 1972; 34: 1121.

8. Wellens HJJ, Brugada P, Roy D, Weiss J, Bar FW: Effect of isoproterenol on the Anterograde Refractory period of the accessory pathway in patients with the Wolff-Parkinson-White Syndrome. Amer J Cardiol 1982; 50: 180–184.

9. Strasberg B, Ashley WW, Wyndham CRC, Bauernfeind RA, Swiryn SP, Dhingra RC, Rosen KM: Treadmill exercise testing in the Wolff-Parkinson-White syndrome. Amer J Cardiol 1980; 45: 742–748.

10. Levy S, Broustet JP, Clementy J, Vircoulon B, Guern P, Bricaud H: Syndrome de Wolff-Parkinson-White. Correlations entre l'exploration electrophysiologique et l'effect de l'epreuve d'effort sur l'aspect electrocardiographique de preexcitation. Arch Mal Coeur 1979; 72: 634.

Authors' address:
Service de Rythmologie et de Stimulation Cardiaque
du Professeur Y. Grosgogeat
Hôpital Jean Rostand
39 rue Jean Le Galleu
94200 Ivry (France)

Diagnostic and Prognostic Significance of Ventricular Late Potentials in Patients with Coronary Heart Disease

A. Osterspey, H.-W. Höpp, V. Hombach, H.-J. Deutsch, U. Winter,
D. W. Behrenbeck, M. Tauchert, H. H. Hilger

Summary: A total of 250 patients 41 females and 209 males, aged 37–70 years (mean: 55 ± 6 years) with Coronary Heart Disease (50 patients with acute myocardial infarction, 200 patients with chronic CHD) were studied by Holter ECG monitoring for recording of ventricular arrhythmias, by signal averaging of the high gain amplified surface ECG for retrieval of ventricular late potentials, and in a subgroup by programmed ventricular stimulation to evaluate repetitive ventricular response as a tool for testing effectiveness of antiarrhythmic agents.

During acute myocardial infarction the incidence of ventricular late potentials (VLP) was relatively low, whereas that of ventricular tachycardia was high. Four weeks after AMI the incidence of VIP increased and that of VT decreased. During follow-up 12 patients with VLP died from sudden death, in contrast to one non-sudden death in the patients without VLP.

In patients with chronic CHD 54% had VLP, there was a close correlation between the incidence of VLP and left ventricular contraction abnormalities and between the incidence of VLP and of ventricular arrhythmias. During follow-up 15 patients with VLP died from sudden death, in contrast to 4 non-sudden deaths in the group of patients without VLP.

Our data suggest that, besides the occurrence of complex ventricular arrhythmias, the incidence of ventricular late potentials may serve as an additional parameter for the identification of CHD patients with an increased risk of sudden cardiac death.

Introduction

According to clinical experiences patients with Coronary Heart Disease (CHD) are particularly threatened by sudden cardiac death, which in most cases is initiated by an acute ventricular instability with consecutive ventricular flutter and fibrillation (1). A special disposition seems to exist for CHD patients with left ventricular contraction abnormalities and with spontaneously occurring complex ventricular arrhythmias of Lown's class IV a and b and ventricular tachycardias (2, 3). Thus, methods for assessing left ventricular performance (echocardiography, radionuclide angiography, coronary and left ventricular angiography) and of spontaneous left ventricular vulnerability with complex ventricular arrhythmias (Holter ECG) are currently in a wide clinical use.

In recent years newer techniques such as the signal averaging method or the high resolution beat-by-beat registration of ventricular late potentials have been developed (4, 5, 6), and the role of ventricular late potentials within the ST segment as a marker of increased ventricular vulnerability has been principally accepted. Since late potentials may represent ischemic and late depolarized myocardial areas, as has ben convincingly shown in animal experiments, they may intrinsically provide the depressed pathway of intraventricular re-entry circuits, that can initiate single or complex ventricular arrhythmias or

---

*) Supported by the Deutsche Forschungsgemeinschaft, SFB 68, Cologne.

sustained forms of ventricular tachycardias. In some studies a high correlation between the incidence of ventricular late potentials and the occurrence of complex ventricular ectopic beats as well as the incidence of repetitive ventricular response phenomena during programmed ventricular stimulation as another, sign of increased ventricular vulnerability has been observed (7, 8).

The aim of this study was to discover the incidence of ventricular late potentials and of complex ventricular arrhythmias in a larger group of patients with either acute myocardial infarction or with chronic stable CHD, and to evaluate the predictive value of late potentials with respect to sudden cardiac death during longer follow-up periods.

Patients and methods

A total of 250 patients, 41 females and 209 males, with ages from 37–70 years (mean: 55 ± 6 years) with angiographically and/or scintigraphically documented CHD were studied. 50/250 patients were followed from the first day of myocardial infarction after admission to the hospital, and the remaining 200 patients were suffering from chronic stable CHD.

Each patient was studied by coronary and left ventricular angiography, by Holter ECG monitoring (mean recording period: 42 ± 5 hours) and by registration of the high gain amplified, signal averaged surface ECG, using the MAC-I (Marquette electronics, USA) averaging computer. The technical specifications of this system have been extensively described elsewhere (9). Ventricular late potentials were considered as to be true signals, if they outlasted the QRS complex by more than 10 ms in at least three or more of the high gain amplified and averaged leads, and the amplitude of late potentials had to equal or exceed twice the amplitude of diastolic baseline noise.

The patients with acute myocardial infarction were followed within certain intervals (first, seventh, fourteenth day, fourth and twelvth week, and six, twelve and twentyfour months) by clinical examination, surface ECG, Holter ECG and signal averaged surface ECG. The patients with chronic Coronary Heart Disease were investigated by these methods at their entrance into the study and thereafter followed for a period of 20 ± 5 months. The follow-up period of patients within both groups was 22 ± 4 months.

Results

During the early phase of acute myocardial infarction (1.–6th day) ventricular arrhythmias were observed in 40/50 patients (80%), and ventricular salvos or tachycardias were seen in 15/50 patients (30%). 7/50 patients died during the acute phase from intractable ventricular tachycardia-fibrillation episodes, and all patients had demonstrable ventricular late potentials. Within the whole group, however, ventricular late potentials were relatively rare during the first stage of illness (in 17/50 patients = 34%).

During further follow-up (2nd to 4th week) the incidence of ventricular arrhythmias slightly increased (86% of patients), however, the number of patients with ventricular tachycardias steadily decreased to 6/50 patients (12%). In contrast, the incidence of ventricular late potentials increased during follow-up, and 4 weeks after the acute phase of myocardial infarction late potentials were recorded in 23/42 patients (55%). It should also be mentioned that up to the 8th week after myocardial infarction about 90% of late potentials showed an increasing distance to the corresponding QRS complex, when the time interval to the acute phase of myocardial infarction was more and more increasing (Fig. 1). This increasing QRS-late potential interval has been interpreted as representing most likely an increasing conduction delay within the border zone of the infarcted myocardium (10).

All late potentials that were demonstrable 4 weeks after myocardial infarction, could be reproducibly recovered during further follow-up, in contrast to reports of other groups (11), and they differed only with respect to the time interval to the corresponding QRS complex, not with respect to their shape. The amplitude of the late potentials was 8 μV as a maximum, and the QRS-late potential interval was 138 $\pm$ 9 ms as a mean (as measured from the beginning of QRS complex to the end of the late potential).

When comparing the incidence of ventricular late potentials and of ventricular arrhythmias we observed that only few patients with ventricular arrhythmias within the acute phase of infarction had ventricular late potentials (17/50 = 43%). 7/17 patients with late potentials died during the acute stage of illness (Figure 2). Correlations were found more significant 4 weeks and 3 months following acute myocardial infarction: in 23/39 patients (59%) at 4 weeks and in 24/36 patients at 12 weeks after myocardial infarction late potentials were present, and this accounted only for patients with ventricular arrhythmias of Lown's classes II-IV b and ventricular tachycardias, whereas patients with Lown's class I did not have late potentials. These results may support the hypothesis that

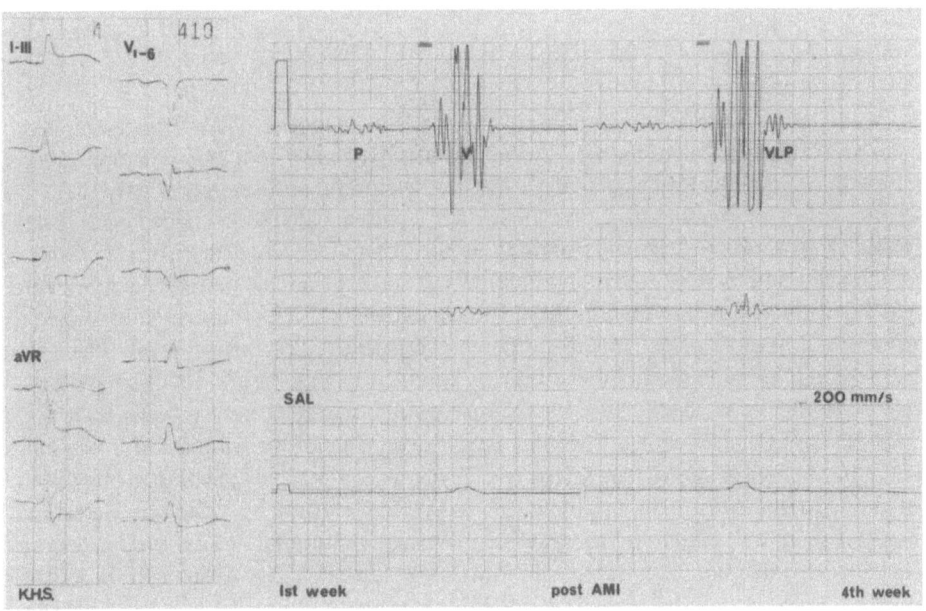

Fig. 1. Surface ECG (left panel) and signal averaged high gain amplified surface ECG (right panel) of a patient with acute anterior wall myocardial infarction. During first week no late potential within the ST segment was demonstrable, however, 4 weeks following the acute stage of illness a ventricular late potential (VLP) was present at the end of the QRS complex merging into the ST segment.

665

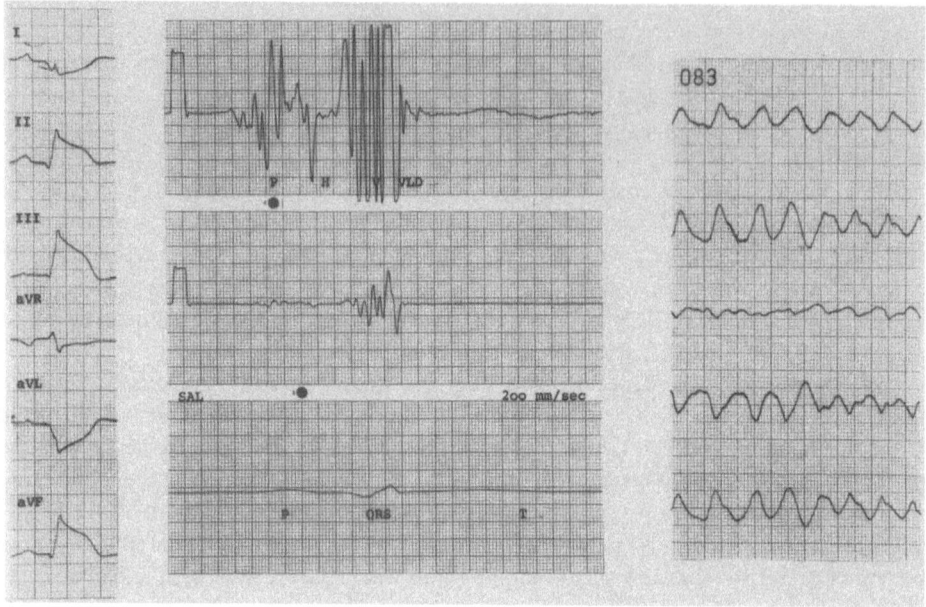

Fig. 2. Surface ECG (left and right panel) and signal averaged high gain amplified surface ECG (center) of a patients with acute posterior wall myocardial infarction. This patient with a large area of infarction had a ventricular late potential at the beginning of the ST segment (VLD), which is an uncommon finding in patients with AMI. This patient died from intractable ventricular tachycardia-fibrillation episodes (right panel). P: P-wave, H: His bundle potential

during acute myocardial infarction focal mechanisms may lead to life-threatening ventricular arrhythmias, besides the well known re-entry pathways, that may be more responsible for initiation of ventricular tachycardias in the chronic post-infarction state (12).

During follow-up (maximum 2.5 years) further 5 patients died from sudden cardiac death (Table 1). In all of these patients ventricular late potentials were demonstrable within the ST segment, and the QRS-late potential interval in these patients was considerably longer (164 ± 12 ms as a mean) than in the surviving patients (131 ± 8 ms as a mean), because of the small number of patients this difference was statistically insignificant. These findings resemble those found in other studies (7), indicating that base width of late potentials may be of functional significance for the ease of initiating re-entrant ventricular arrhythmias. Each of the sudden death victims had also ventricular arrhythmias of Lown's class I-IVa, but none had ventricular salvos or tachycardias. 4/5 sudden death patients were set on antiarrhythmic drugs, in 3 patients antiarrhythmic efficacy was tested by Holter ECG monitoring, in one patient by programmed ventricular stimulation. All suddendeath patients had considerable left ventricular contraction abnormalities with an EF of less than 50%.

All patients with ventricular tachycardias 4 weeks following myocardial infarction survived, though in all of them ventricular late potentials were retrieved. 2 of these patients were provided with an automated antitachycardial burst pacemaker (Cyber-Tach, Intermedics, USA) for control of drug-refractory ventricular tachycardias.

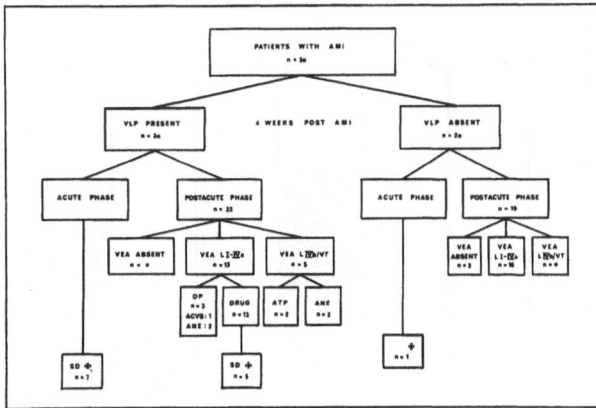

Table 1. Follow-up (mean follow-up period: 24 ± 5 months) of 50 patients with acute myocardial infarction (AMI), beginning at the first day of admission to the hospital. Patients were divided into two subgroups, in those having ventricular late potentials 4 weeks after AMI and in those that did not show ventricular late potentials within the signal averaged surface ECG. There were 12 sudden deaths in the group of 30 patients with ventricular late potentials, in contrast to one non-sudden death in the group of 20 patients without ventricular late potentials, this difference in sudden death rate was statistically significant ($p < 0.01$). VLP: Ventricular late potential, VEA: Ventricular ectopic activity, ACVB: Bypass graft, ANE: aneurysmectomy, ATP: antitachycardial pacemaker, SD: sudden death.

In contrast to patients with ventricular late potentials, none of the patients without demonstrable late potentials died from sudden cardiac death, only one of them suffered from re-infarction and died from subsequent myocardial pump failure. When considering only patients, who survived up to the 28th day following acute myocardial infarction and were not operated later on, the following parameters for characterization of patients at risk for sudden death could be calculated: ventricular late potentials: sensitivity 100%, positive accuracy 65%, predictive value 23%; ventricular arrhythmias of Lown's class IVa and b as well as ventricular tachycardias: sensitivity 53%, positive accuracy 74% and predictive value 43%.

Patients with chronic coronary heart disease

In 108/200 patients of this group one year after myocardial infarction ventricular late potentials were present (54% of cases). This incidence closely resembles that found in patients with acute myocardial infarction 4 weeks after the acute stage of illness. As compared to a group of patients without CHD, ventricular late potentials were significantly correlated to patients with manifest CHD (4% of non-CHD patients, 54% of CHD patients). These results are in agreement with those obtained by other investigators (7).

Ventricular late potentials were significantly correlated to the incidence of left ventricular contraction abnormalities. Late potentials were detected in 2/51 patients with normokinesis (4%) and in 106/149 patients with contraction abnormalities (71%). In addition, in only 9/52 patients (17%) without ventricular arrhythmias late potentials were detected, wheras of 148 patients with ventricular arrhythmias within the Holter ECG 99 individuals (67%) had late potentials, and 29/34 patients (84%) with ventricular salvos or tachycardias within the Holter ECG had ventricular late potentials (Fig. 3).

During follow-up of 20 ± 5 months as a mean 20/200 patients (10%) died, 15 with the clinical course of sudden death, and 4 patients with myocardial failure during re-

Fig. 3. Incidence of left ventricular contraction abnormalities (left panel) and correlation between the incidence of ventricular arrhythmias and of ventricular late potentials (right panel) in the group of 200 patients with chronic Coronary Heart Disease.

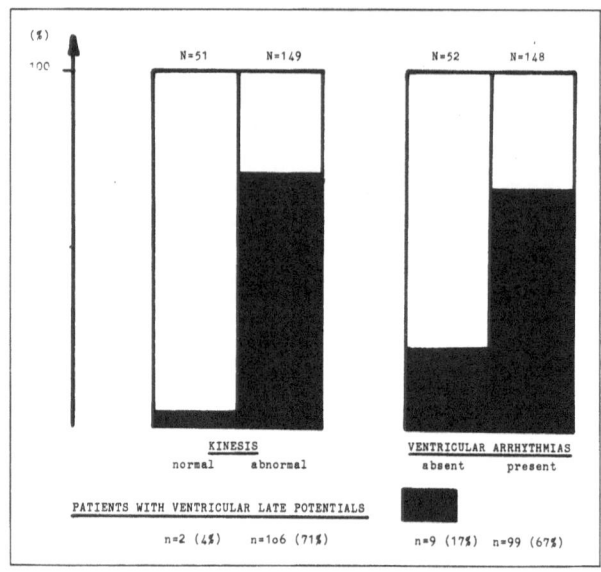

Table 2. Follow-up (mean follow-up period of 20 ± 5 months) of 200 patients with chronic Coronary Heart Disease. Patients were divided in two subgroups of those having ventricular late potentials and those devoid of ventricular late potentials within the signal averaged surface ECG. There were 15 sudden and one death from myocardial failure during re-infarction in the group of patients with demonstrable late potentials, whereas in those patients without ventricular late potentials 4 non-sudden deaths

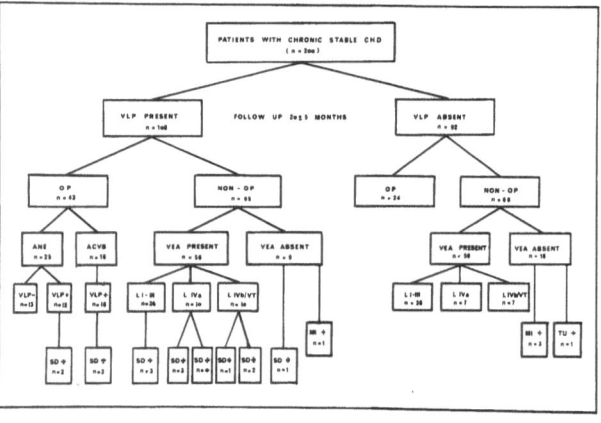

occurred, this difference in sudden death rates were statistically significant (p < 0.01). VLP: ventricular late potential, ANE: aneurysmectomy, ACVB: Bypass graft, L: Lown-class, MI: myocardial infarction, TU: tumor disease, SD: sudden death.

infarction, whereas one patient died from a tumor disease. Each of the sudden death victims, including the 5 patients that had been operated prior to the sudden death episode, had demonstrable ventricular late potentials. On the other hand, repetitive ventricular arrhythmias could be detected by Holter ECG monitoring in only 10/15 sudden death victims (Lown's class IVa: 5 patients, IVb and ventricular tachycardias: 5 patients). 4 patients with sudden death had ventricular arrhythmias of Lown's class I–III, and one patient had a completely regular rhythm. The differences in sudden death rates between patients with late potentials and those without late potentials were statistically significant (p < 0.01, Chi-square test).

It is interesting to note that only 3/13 patients set on antiarrhythmic drugs with control of drug efficacy by programmed ventricular stimulation died from sudden death, in contrast to a death rate of 6/11 patients, whose drug efficacy was controlled by Holter ECG monitoring. Because of the small number of observations this difference was not statistically significant. From the data reported the following parameters for identification of patients at high risk of sudden death within the group of chronic stable Coronary Heart Disease could be calculated: presence of ventricular late potentials: sensitivity 100%, positive accuracy 51%, predictive value 15%, ventricular repetitive arrhythmias within Holter ECG: sensitivity 16%, positive accuracy 85%, predictive value 17%. The patients who were operated were not included in this calculations.

From our results we may summarize and conclude: In contrast to ventricular arrhythmias ventricular late potentials are relatively uncommon during the acute phase of myocardial infarction. With progression of organization of the infarcted myocardium late potentials may be retrieved in 50% of patients, and these abnormal depolarisations reveal an increasing distance to the corresponding QRS complex with further time interval to the acute phase of myocardial infarction. 8 weeks following myocardial infarction a significant correlation between the incidence of late potentials, of ventricular arrhythmias and of left ventricular contraction abnormalities may be observed, as is true for patients with chronic stable Coronary Heart Disease, too.

Follow-up data in both groups of CHD patients reveal a high sensitivity of late potentials in the identification of sudden death victims (100% of 15 sudden death patients), whereas the sensitivity of complex ventricular arrhythmias is lower (40% of sudden death victims had couplets, 20% had salvos or ventricular tachycardias). Specificity and predictive values of late potentials are relatively low, due to the high number of fals positives (with respect to prediction of sudden death). In addition, longer follow-up periods may increase the predictive value of both late potentials and complex ventricular arrhythmias.

At present ventricular late potentials as a non-invasive parameter may serve as an additional indicator of increased ventricular vulnerability and thus, of an increased risk of sudden death. The value of combined use of other parameters of increased ventricular vulnerability such as complex ventricular arrhythmias and of repetitive ventricular response during programmed ventricular stimulation in predicting sudden death in patients with Coronary Heart Disease remains to be clarified by future more extended studies.

References

1. Lown B: Sudden cardiac death: the major challenge confronting contemporary cardiology. Amer J Cardiol 1979; 43: 313.
2. Bigger JT, Dresdale RJ, Heissenbuttel RH, Weld FM, Wit AL: Ventricular arrhythmias in ischemic heart disease: mechanism, prevalence, significance and management. Progr Cardiovasc Dis 1977; 14: 255.
3. Calvert A, Lown B, Gorlin R: Ventricular premature beats and anatomically defined coronary heart disease. Amer J Cardiol 1977; 39: 627.
4. Uther JB, Dennett CJ, Tan A: The detection of the late activation signals of low amplitude in the vectorcardiogram of patients with recurrent ventricular tachycardia by signal averaging. In:

Sandoe E, Julian DG, Bell JW (eds) Management of ventricular tachycardia – Role of Mexiletine. Amsterdam/Oxford, Excerpta Medica 1978; 80–82.

5. Simson MB: Use of signals in the terminal QRS complex to identify patients with ventricular tachycardia after myocardial infarction. Circulation 1981; 64: 235–242.

6. Hombach V, Kebbel U, Höpp HW, Winter U-J, Braun V, Deutsch H, Hirche H, Hilger HH: Fortlaufende Registrierung von Mikropotentialen des menschlichen Herzens. DMW 1982; 51/52: 1951–1956.

7. Breithardt G, Borggrefe M, Karbenn U, Haerten K, Ostermeyer J, Seipel L: Die mögliche Bedeutung von Spätpotentialen für die Identifizierung von Patienten, die einer antiarrhythmischen Therapie bedürfen. In: Schlepper M, Olsson B (eds) Kardiale Rhythmusstörungen; Diagnose, Prognose; Therapie. Berlin Heidelberg, Springer 1983; 39–57.

8. Höpp HW, Hombach V, Braun V, Behrenbeck DW, Tauchert M, Hilger HH: Ventricular delayed depolarisations in patients with chronic stable coronary heart disease and with acute myocardial infarction. In: Hombach V, Hilger HH (eds) Signal averaging technique in clinical cardiology. Stuttgart–New York 1981; 233–251.

9. Hombach V, Braun V, Höpp HW, Gil-Sanchez D, Scholl H, Behrenbeck DW, Tauchert M, Hilger HH: The applicability of the signal averaging technique in clinical cardiology. Clin Cardiol 1982; 5: 107–124.

10. Höpp HW, Hombach V, Braun V, Tauchert M, Behrenbeck DW, Hilger HH: Kammerarrhythmien und ventrikuläre Spätpotentiale bei akutem Myokardinfarkt. Herz/Kreislauf 1982; 3: 111–120.

11. Haerten K, Borggrefe M, Weyers FJ, Breithardt G: Langzeitverhalten ventrikulärer Spätpotentiale bei Patienten nach Infarkt. Z. Kardiol 1982; 71/3: 205.

12. Boineau SB, Cox JL: Slow ventricular activation in acute myocardial infarction: a source of reentrant premature ventricular contraction. Circulation 1973; 48: 702–13.

Authors' address:
A. Osterspey, M.D.
Medical Clinic and Policlinic III
and Department of Cardiology
University of Cologne
5000 Köln

Influence of Current Strength and Length of Basic Drive on Atrial Refractoriness in Man

A. Michelucci, L. Padeletti, G. A. Fradella, R. M. Lova, D. Monizzi, A. Giomi, P. Seniori*, G. Berni*, F. Fantini

Summary: An analysis of the influence of current strength and length of basic drive on atrial refractoriness has not been performed sistematically in the human atrium. We studied 29 patients (24 males and 5 females), ranging in age from 23 to 78 yrs. Atrial effective (ERP) and functional (FRP) refractory periods were measured during atrial pacing (100/min) using: a) variable current strengths (2, 3, 4, 5, 7, 10, 15 mA) and introducing extrastimuli after the eight paced complex of the basic drive; b) a constant current strength (5 mA) and introducing extrastimuli after 8 beats, 1 minute and 3 minutes of the basic drive. A bipolar stimulation, with the distal pole as cathode was performed. In all patients the increase of both current strength and basic drive length produced a reduction of ERP and FRP. At current strengths higher than 7 mA ERP and FRP became nearly fixed. We conclude that: 1. as stimulation occurs earlier in the cardiac cycle, more current and/or a longer previous basic drive are required to initiate a response. This is noteworthy considering that the ability to initiate or terminate reentrant arrhythmias by programmed stimulation is dependent on the refractoriness of the limbs of the reentrant circuit; 2. the relation between stimulus strength and atrial refractoriness is non linear. This could imply that if refractoriness is determined at a single current strength, it would be more appropriate to do so at a current strength (> 7 mA) at which minimal changes in refractoriness are observed; 3. 8 beats of atrial pacing are not sufficient to achieve a steady state of atrial refractoriness.

Introduction

Determination of refractoriness is routinely employed as a measurement of excitability in clinical electrophysiology using single extrastimulus introduced after every eight beat of a regular basic driven rhythm. In performing this technique: a) current strength ranging from threshold to twice diastolic threshold is used; b) it is assumed that after 8 beats at the new driving frequency re-setting and stabilization of refractory period occurs.

However, it has been affirmed that the refractory period is a measurement that is meaningful only when related to the strength of the stimulus (1). Further a cumulative effect of up to 16 preceeding cycles on atrial refractoriness following an abrupt alteration of frequency has been described in animals (2).

Based on this and considering that an analysis of the current and length of basic drive dependence of refractoriness has not been done systematically in the human atrium, we decided to explore this problem.

Material and Methods

We studied 29 patients (24 males and 5 females) ranging in age from 23 to 78 yrs, undergoing electrophysiologic evaluation for clinical indications. Atrial stimulation was per-

---

Cardiology Unit, University of Florence; *Arcispedale of S.M. Nuova, Florence, Italy.

formed in all subjects in the nonsedated postabsorptive state after informed consent had been obtained. All cardioactive drugs had been withdrawn for at least 5 halflives. All patients were in sinus rhythm at the start of the study. A quadripolar catheter (1 cm inter-electrode distance), introduced percutaneously by way of an antecubital vein, was positioned under fluoroscopic control in the high right atrium. Stimulation was achieved using the distal electrode pair (with the distal pole as a cathode), while an atrial electrogram was recorded from the proximal pair. The atrial electrogram and multiple electro-cardiographic leads, usually leads I, II, III and V_1 were recorded on a Elema-Schonander Mingograph 62-6 channel ink-jet at paper speed of 100 mm/sec. Overdrive and premature atrial stimulation were performed using an electrically isolated battery-powered Medtronics 5325 stimulator. The pulse width was 2 msec. Atrial effective (ERP) and functional (FRP) refractory periods determinations were made during atrial pacing (100/min) using: a) variable current strengths (2, 3, 4, 5, 7, 10, 15 mA) and introducing extrastimuli after the eight paced complex of the basic drive; b) a constant current strength (5 mA) and introducing extrastimuli after 8 beats, 1 minute and 3 minutes of the basic drive.

The determination of the effects of length of basic drive was performed at least 10 minutes after that of increasing current strength. The value at 5 mA after 8 beats at b) was determined just before increasing the length of basic drive.

The coupling interval of extrastimulus was reduced by 5–10 msec decrements until it failed to initiate an atrial response. FRP was the shortest coupling interval recorded on the atrial electrogram. ERP was the longest interval between the stimulus artefact (atrial pacing) and the extrastimulus failing to propagate. Values are expressed in msec and as mean ± 1 standard deviation. Refractoriness at different current strengths and lengths of basic drive was compared with a paired t-test. $p < 0.05$ was considered significant.

Results

Effects of changes in current strength

In all patients both ERP and FRP decreased with increasing current. The ERP (Table 1) at 2 mA ranged from 220 to 380 msec (mean 305 ± 42), at 3 mA from 210 to 350 msec (mean 286 ± 40), at 4 mA from 210 to 350 msec (mean 282 ± 39), at 5 mA from 210 to 340 msec (mean 273 ± 36), at 7 mA from 210 to 340 msec (mean 260 ± 35), at 10 mA from 190 to 330 msec (mean 256 ± 33), at 15 mA from 190 to 310 msec (mean 250 ± 31). The difference was significant at each increase of current strength (2 vs 3 mA, $p < 0.0005$; 3 vs 4 mA, $p < 0.05$; 4 vs 5 mA, $p < 0.005$; 5 vs 7 mA, $p < 0.0005$; 7 vs 10 mA, $p < 0.025$; 10 vs 15 mA, $p < 0.025$).

The same behaviour was observed for FRP (Table 1), which at 2 mA ranged from 240 to 400 msec (mean 326 ± 45), at 3 mA from 240 to 400 msec (mean 311 ± 43), at 4 mA from 230 to 390 msec (mean 303 ± 43), at 5 mA from 230 to 390 msec (mean 298 ± 42), at 7 mA from 220 to 390 msec (mean 286 ± 42), at 10 mA from 210 to 360 msec (mean 282 ± 40), at 15 mA from 210 to 340 msec (mean 275 ± 38). Again the difference was significant at each increase of current strength (2 vs 3 mA, $p < 0.0005$; 3 vs 4 mA, $p < 0.005$; 4 vs 5 mA, $p < 0.05$; 5 vs 7 mA, $p < 0.0005$; 7 vs 10 mA, $p < 0.05$; 10 vs 15 mA, $p < 0.0025$).

Table 1. Range of single values, mean value of ERP and FRP at each current strength and statistical significance at each increase of current strength.

Current strength		2 mA	3 mA	4 mA	5 mA	7 mA	10 mA	15 mA
ERP (msec)	range	220–380	210–350	210–350	210–340	210–340	190–330	190–310
	mean	305±42	286±40	282±39	273±36	260±35	256±33	250±31
	p <		0.0005	0.05	0.005	0.0005	0.025	0.025
			(2 vs 3)	(3 vs 4)	(4 vs 5)	(5 vs 7)	(7 vs 10)	(10 vs 15)
FRP (msec)	range	240–400	240–400	230–390	230–390	220–390	210–360	210–340
	mean	326±45	311±43	303±43	298±42	286±42	282±40	275±38
	p <		0.0005	0.005	0.05	0.0005	0.05	0.025
			(2 vs 3)	(3 vs 4)	(4 vs 5)	(5 vs 7)	(7 vs 10)	(10 vs 15)

ERP = effective refractory period; FRP = functional refractory period.

Table 2. Range of single values, mean value of ERP and FRP at each length of basic drive and statistical significance at each increase thereof.

Length of basic drive		8 beats	1 minute	3 minutes
ERP (msec)	range	210–330	200–300	190–300
	mean	274±37	257±31	250±32
	p <		0.0005	N.S.
			(8 bts vs 1 min)	(1 vs 3 min)
FRP (mesc)	range	230–400	220–350	210–340
	mean	300±42	288±35	281±34
	p <		0.0025	0.0025
			(8 bts vs 1 min)	(1 vs 3 min)

ERP = effective refractory period; FRP = functional refractory period.

The relation between atrial refractoriness and current strength was non linear. At low current strengths large changes were observed both in ERP and FRP whereas at higher current strengths (≥ 7 mA) the changes in atrial refractory periods were small and the strength-refractoriness curve became steep.

Effects of length of basic drive

Mean value of ERP and of FRP after 8 beats did not differ significantly from those obtained during the increase of current strength.
ERP (Table 2) after 8 beats ranged from 210 to 330 msec (mean 274 ± 37), after 1 minute from 200 to 300 msec (mean 257 ± 31), after 3 minutes from 190 to 300 msec (mean

250 ± 32). The difference was statistically significant between 8 beats and 1 minute ($p < 0.0005$) and between 8 beats and 3 minutes ($p < 0.0005$) while not between 1 and 3 minutes.

FRP (Table 2) after 8 beats ranged from 230 to 400 msec (mean 300 ± 42), after 1 minute from 220 to 350 msec (mean 288 ± 35), after 3 minutes from 210 to 340 msec (mean 281 ± 34). The difference was statistically significant between 8 beats and 1 minute ($p < 0.0025$); 1 minute and 3 minutes ($p < 0.0025$); 8 beats and 3 minutes ($p > 0.0005$).

Discussion

Effects of changes in current strength

Previous studies on atrial tissue of animals evidenced that the period of excitability shortens as the strength of the applied extrastimulus is increased (3, 4). A non linear relation between stimulus strength and refractory period has been observed. This relation had the characteristic that at low current strengths small changes in current cause large changes in refractoriness, whereas at high current strengths changes in refractoriness with similar change in current approach O. We have shown that these conclusions hold in the human atrium using bipolar stimuli of 2 msec duration, delivered through a transvenous intracardiac electrode catheter with an interelectrode distance of 1 cm.

The shape of the current strength-refractory period curve is similar to the strength-interval curve observed in animals. Even in our patients, in fact, at low current strengths large changes in refractoriness were observed, whereas at high current strengths (generally $\geqslant 7$ mA) ERP and FRP became nearly fixed.

There is evidence that the increase in the intensity of the driving stimuli results in liberation of autonomic mediators (5), which are able to influence recovery of atrial excitability (6–9).

A progressively greater release of autonomic mediators, increasing current strength, could explain the behaviour of the current strength-refractory period curve. At high current strengths ($\geqslant 7$ mA) this release might be nearly complete as indicated by the minimal changes of refractoriness observed during the steep portion of the curve.

Effect of length of basic drive

Recently it has been suggested that in man fewer beats at the given cycle length may give refractory period determinations similar to those found after a longer basic drive in the atrium (10). Nevertheless a cumulative effect of up to 16 preceeding cycles on atrial refractoriness, following an abrupt alteration of frequency, has been described in intact heart of dogs (2).

Our results indicate that 8 beats of atrial pacing are not sufficient to achieve a "steady state" of atrial refractoriness because its reduction was observed after a longer basic drive. On this basis a cumulative effect of more than 8 beats on human atrial refractoriness could be suggested.

We used 8 beats as a control state because this is the number commonly used in clinical electrophysiologic studies. It is assumed that this number is sufficient to iron out preceeding fluctuations in electrophysiological state and to stabilize refractory periods and conduction velocities (11).

Our data do not support this conclusion. Atrial pacing (at a constant rate) leads to a release of autonomic mediators (4, 12). As for the increase of current strength it is possible to suppose that the greater is the duration of atrial pacing the major is the release of autonomic mediators. Therefore 8 beats of atrial pacing would not be sufficient to exhaust this effect as indicated by the reduction of atrial refractoriness obtained after a longer basic drive.

Importance to clinical electrophysiology

We have shown that as stimulation occurs earlier in the cardiac cycle, more current an/ or a longer preceeding basic drive are required to initiate a response in the atrium. Our results have implications for the performance and interpretation of stimulation studies. The presence of a non linear relation between stimulus strength and atrial refractoriness could imply that if refractoriness is determined at a single current strength it would be more appropriate to do so at a current strength (≥ 7 mA) at which, minimal changes in refractoriness are observed. The assumption that eight beats of atrial pacing are sufficient to avoid the consequences of preceeding fluctuations in electrophysiological state, should be reconsidered. Our data indicate that eight beats are not sufficient to achieve a steady state of atrial refractoriness. Single stimuli can be used to initiate or terminate episodes of reentrant arrhythmias. This technique requires that an impulse penetrate a reentrant circuit. Refractoriness of the intervening tissue can limit the ability of an impulse to reach the reentrant circuit. Thus, any manipulation that could modify refractoriness of the intervening tissue and permit an impulse to reach and penetrate the circuit might allow an increased success rate for initiation or termination of arrhythmia by single stimuli. In this regard determination of the behaviour of the atrial functional refractory period as well as the effective refractory period with current strength and length of basic drive is pertinent, since the functional refractory period determines the critical atrial coupling interval that can be achieved to influence the reentrant circuit.

References

1. Arnsdorf MF: Membrane factors in arrhythmogenesis: concepts and definitions. Prog Cardiovasc Dis 1977; 19: 413–429.
2. Han J, Moe GK: Cumulative effects of cycle length on refractory periods of cardiac tissues. Am J Physiol 1969; 217: 106–109.
3. Dawes GS, Vane JR: The refractory period of atria isolated from mammalian hearts. J Physiol 1956; 132: 611–629.
4. Azuma T, Hayashi H, Kanno T, Matsuda K: Effects of intensity of driving stimulus on the shape of membrane action potential of the heart. Nature 1961; 192: 1295–1296.
5. Furchgott RF, De Gubareff T, Grossman A: Release of autonomic mediators in cardiac tissue by suprathreshold stimulation. Science 1959; 129: 328–329.
6. Benfey BG, Varma DR: Interactions of sympathomimetic drugs, propranolol and phentolamine, on atrial refractory period and contractility. Br J Pharmacol 1967; 30: 603–611.
7. De Elio FJ: The action of acetylcholine, adrenaline and other substances on the refractory period of the rabbit auricle. Brit J Pharmacol 1947; 2: 131–142.

8. Govier WC, Mosal NC, Whittington P, Broom AH: Myocardial alpha and beta adrenergic receptors as demonstrated by atrial functional refractory-period changes. J Pharmacol Exp Ther 1966; 154: 255–263.

9. Pappano AJ: Propranolol, insensitive effects of epinephrine on action potential regolarization in electrically driven atria of the guinea pig. J Pharmacol Exp Ther 1971; 177: 85–95.

10. Wiener I, Kunkes S, Rubin D, Kupersmith J, Packer M, Pitchon R, Schweitzer P: Effects of sudden change in cycle length on human atrial, atrioventricular nodal and ventricular refractory periods. Circulation 1981; 64: 245–248.

11. Curry PVL: Fundamentals of Arrhythmias: Modern Methods of investigation. In: Krikler DM, Goodwin JF eds. Cardiac Arrhythmias. The modern electrophysiological approach. London: WB Saunders Company Ltd, 1975: 39–80.

12. Lange G: Action of driving stimuli from intrinsic and extrinsic sources on in situ cardiac pacemaker tissues. Circ Res 1965; 17: 449–459.

Authors' address:
Dr. Antonio Michelucci
Via Bronzino 163
I-50 100 Firenze
Italy

Intraoperative Spectral Analysis of Ventricular Potentials During Sinus Rhythm and Ventricular Tachycardia

S. Saksena, W. Craelius, S. M. Hussain, D. Pantopoulos, V. Parsonnet

Summary: We determined the frequency spectra of ventricular potentials obtained in patients with recurrent sustained ventricular tachycardia (VT) undergoing cardiac electrosurgery. Recordings were obtained from direct myocardial bipolar electrodes inserted at locations distant from the site of arrhythmogenesis. Analyses of standard filtered (30–500 Hz), and wideband (0.5–2500 Hz) recordings were performed using a FFT analyser during sinus rhythm and VT.

In eleven patients studied, the spectra of standard recordings during sinus rhythm consisted of a broad peak having a center frequency between 20 and 30 Hz, with an average of 24 ± 4 Hz. Spectra of wideband recordings was substantially lower due to the large T wave component. During VT the spectral peaks of ventricular potentials shifted to lower frequencies, with an average for standard recordings of 18 ± 5 Hz. The observations are consistent with a reduction of myocardial conduction velocity during VT or delayed activation at local or distant sites.

Introduction

Several features of electrical signals recorded directly from the heart have been used to identify areas of arrhythmogenesis. Epicardial and endocardial activation time analysis has been used to localize the site of origin of ventricular tachycardia (1–3). The presence of delayed activation potentials or continuous electrical activity is used as a marker for abnormal impulse conduction in sites of reentry (3–5). Experimental studies have correlated the morphology of epicardial signals with the speed and direction of impulse propagation (6).

While there is much information on ventricular potentials within the time domain, there is little corresponding knowledge within the frequency domain. Myers et al. analyzed the frequency spectra of endocardial potentials recorded with catheter electrodes and reported a major spectral peak for the R wave of approximately 30 Hz (7). A premature ventricular contraction was found to have somewhat lower frequency. Kleinert et al. reported similar results (8). The present study extends the characterization of cardiac signals within the frequency domain, to determine whether such analyses can offer new insight into signal patterns in diseased states.

Methods

Patient Selection

Patients with recurrent sustained ventricular tachycardia (VT) undergoing cardiac electrosurgery for arrhythmia ablation with or without aorto-coronary bypass surgery were studied. All patients had inducible sustained VT during clinical electrophysiologic studies and were refractory to conventional and experimental drug therapy. Catheter endocardial mapping was performed preoperatively to localize the site of arrhythmia origin prior to surgery.

Recording Techniques

After median sternotomy and adequate cardiac exposure, two myocardial wire electrodes were placed in normal appearing ventricle at a site distant from the preoperatively determined arrhythmogenic region. The electrodes were placed sub-epicardially 1–2 mm, spaced less than 5 mm apart. Another pair of bipolar myocardial wire electrodes were placed on the right ventricular apex or anterior wall for pacing.

Standard ECG leads I, aVF, and V5, and bipolar myocardial wire electrograms were recorded using a standard multichannel recording system (Electronics for Medicine VR-12, White Plains, N.Y.). Filter settings for bipolar leads were either 30 to 500 Hz (standard) or 0.5 to 2500 Hz (wideband). Recordings were stored on analog FM tape. Recordings were obtained during sinus rhythm and after induced sustained VT, prior to hypothermia, cardioplegia, or ventriculotomy. Some patients required partial cardio-pulmonary bypass for hemodynamic stability.

Frequency spectra of ventricular potentials were obtained with a fast Fourier transform analyser based on a 16 bit microprocessor (Ono Sokki, Tokyo, Japan). The sampling rate was 2.56 times the selected bandwidth and thus ranged from 256 to 512 samples per second. Spectra of some signals were obtained using a QRS window circuit to eliminate signals other than those within the QRS from the spectra. Statistical significance of results was determined using the paired t-test.

Results

Patient Population

Eleven patients, ten males and one female, with ages ranging from 48 to 70 (mean 62) years, satisfied the selection criteria. All patients had recurrent sustained VT and coronary artery disease. Ten patients had triple vessel disease, and one had two vessel disease. LV aneurysms were present in 9 patients, and four patients had intraventricular conduction defects, with QRS durations greater than 100 msec. The duration of VT was 4 to 24 (mean 8) months and all patients had failed to respond to conventional and one or more experimental drugs. At the time of surgery, no patient was receiving antiarrhythmic therapy.

Spectral Analysis

Typical ventricular potentials recorded with and without high-pass filtering are shown in Figure 1 A. There is a large T wave present in the wideband recording (lower panel), and a fewer number of deflections within the QRS as compared with the filtered recording (upper panel). The corresponding spectra of these potentials are shown in Figure 1 B. Both spectra have a single broad peak frequency that is 25 Hz for the filtered potentials,

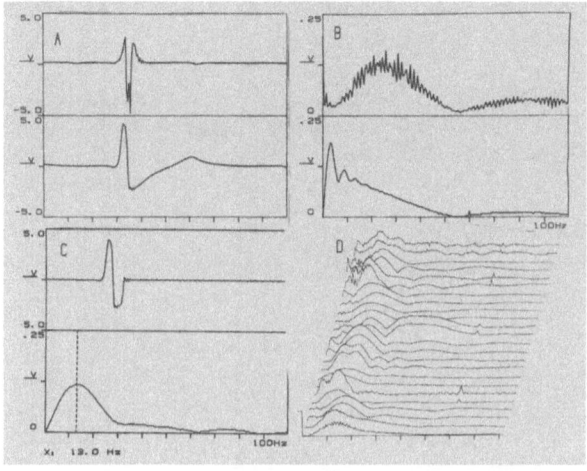

Fig. 1. Spectral analysis of ventricular potentials during sinus rhythm.

A. Upper panel shows ventricular potential during sinus rhythm potential recorded from left ventricle with filter settings 30–500 Hz. Lower panel shows the same potential occurring a few beats later, with filter settings at 0.5–2500 Hz.

B. Corresponding spectra of filtered and wideband recordings as seen in (A).

C. At top, a wideband recording of the ventricular potential seen in (A) using the QRS window circuit is shown. Lower panel shows spectrum of the depolarization.

D. Each horizontal line represents the frequency spectrum of a filtered ventricular potential recorded from a patient during sinus rhythm. Eleven patients are represented with two adjacent spectra shown for each patient.

and 3 Hz for the wideband recordings. Both spectra reach minimal values at approximately 55 Hz. It can be seen that high pass filtering tends to suppress the T wave, and increase the frequency within the QRS by electronic differentiation.

Figure 1 C shows a spectral analysis of a ventricular potential, recorded wideband, with the T wave and other non-QRS potentials removed using a QRS window circuit. The potential thus represents a pure ventricular depolarization, whose spectrum has a peak of 13 Hz and reaches a minimum at 50 Hz. Comparing Figures 1 B and C, it can be inferred that the prominent peak of 3 Hz seen in Figure 1B is primarily due to the T wave.

Figure 1D presents spectra obtained on filtered recordings during sinus rhythm for all patients. Each spectrum contains a single major peak, whose value usually lies between 20 and 30 Hz.

Spectra during Ventricular tachycardia

Figure 2A shows spectral analysis of filtered ventricular potentials during VT recorded from the same patient represented in Figure 1. The peak amplitude of the signal during VT is increased slightly, but its overall morphology is similar to that observed in sinus rhythm. The spectrum is also similar in appearance, but the peak frequency is lowered to 16.5 Hz. Spectra from another patient, recorded sequentially during sinus rhythm and VT, are shown in Figure 2B. Note the uniformity of spectra from beat to beat in both sinuus rhythm and VT. There is a shift to lower peak frequencies during VT. Summarized results for all patients are presented in Figure 3. Ten out of eleven patients had lower peak frequencies in VT compared with sinus rhythm, and one patient showed no change. The frequency shift ranged from 0 to 12 Hz, with a mean frequency during sinus rhythm of 24 ± Hz and a mean of 18 ± 6 Hz during VT ($p < 0.05$). Preliminary analyses of

Fig 2. Spectral analysis of ventricular potentials during VT.
A. Upper panel shows ventricular potential recorded during VT from the same patient represented in Fig. 1. Lower panel shows averaged spectrum of 8 potentials as shown above.
B. Spectra obtained on filtered potentials in sinus rhythm from another patient are displayed in the lower portion, and spectra obtained during VT begin at the arrow. Note the regularity of peaks at 22.5 Hz obtained during sinus rhythm and the shift to 13 Hz during VT.

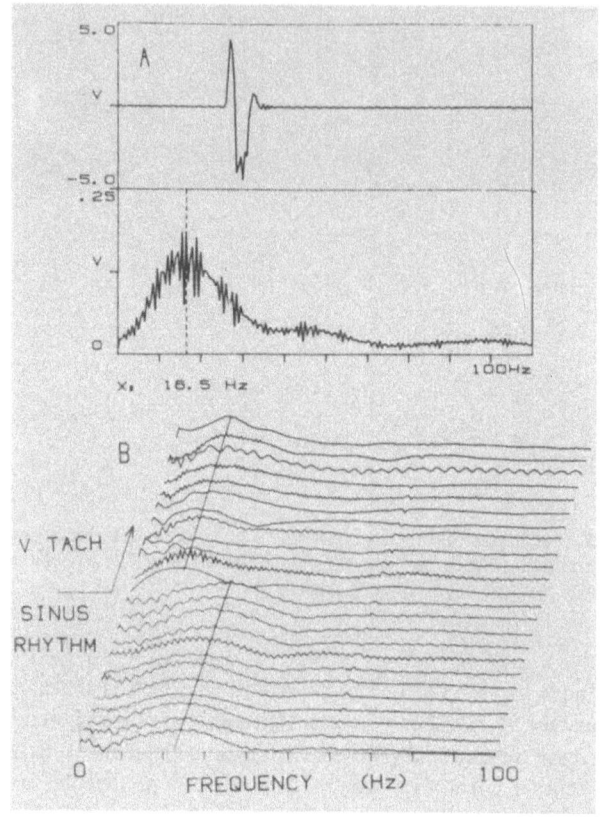

Fig. 3. Graph showing influence of VT on frequency spectra of ventricular potentials in eleven patients.

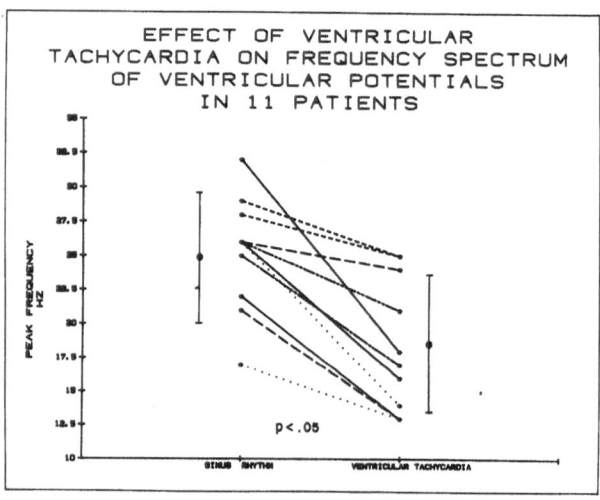

wideband recordings during sinus rhythm and VT yielded similar, although somewhat less pronounced, results.

Discussion

Physiological interpretation of frequency

The records analyzed herein, recorded with bipolar electrodes from the superficial layers of the subepicardium, may primarily represent myocardial activation wavefronts, with minimal contribution from specialized conduction fibers. The shape of the waveform recorded by bipolar electrodes depends upon the direction of wavefront propagation, its distance from the electrodes, as well as upon the wavelength and velocity of the wavefront. If the depolarization wavelength is constant, then the signal duration is inversely proportional to conduction velocity. Thus, for signals of similary morphology, signal frequency provides a relative measure of conduction velocity, and the spectra herein could provide a measure of conduction velocity within a small region of myocardium. The relationship between frequency of myoelectric potentials and conduction velocity has already been established for skeletal muscle (9).

The effect of filtering on ventricular potentials can be seen from Figure 1A. High pass filtering suppresses the T wave, and increases the frequency within the QRS by electronic differentiation. Furthermore, since the major frequency components of the signals recorded were below the cutoff frequency of 30 Hz, they are in a region of amplification where response declines with frequency. Assuming an amplifier roll-off of 6 dB per octave means that a pure signal of 15 Hz is amplified approximately half as much as a signal 30 Hz or greater. Filtering, therefore tends to exaggerate the spectral differences among patients.

Effect of cardiac rhythm on frequency of ventricular potentials

Our observations in sinus rhythm using direct myocardial recordings in patients with recurrent VT confirm and extend previous analyses of catheter endocardial recordings in patients undergoing pacemaker implantation (7). Our results show that VT is associated with a decline in frequency in 10 out of 11 patients examined. The effect was observed in both wideband and high-pass filtered recordings, although it was exagerrated in the latter. These results could suggest that ventricular conduction velocity, at sites distant from those of arrhythmogenesis, declines during VT. A decline would be related to altered directions of intraventricular impulse propagation during VT, or a decline in myocardial conduction speed. Alternatively, it is possible that the results represent prolonged or delayed activation at sites distant from or near to the recording electrodes. Further analysis, including correlation of frequency changes with signal morphology in various types of rhythms, may yield further clues to the mechanism.

References

1. Wit AL, Allessie MA, Bonke FIM, Lammers W, Smeets J, Fenoglio JJ: Electrophysiologic mapping to determine the mechanism of experimental ventricular tachycardia initiated by prematrue impulses. Am J Cardiol 1981; 49: 166–185.

2. Ideker RE, Smith WM, Wallace AG, Kasell J, Harrison LA, Klein GJ, Kinicki RE, Gallagher JJ: A computerized method for the rapid display of ventricular activation during the intraoperative study of arrhythmias. Circulation, 1979; 59: 449–458.
3. Josephson ME, Horowitz LN, Farshidi A, Spear JF, Kastor JA, Moore EN: Recurrent sustained ventricular tachycardia. 2. Endocardial mapping. Circulation, 1978; 57: 440–447.
4. El-Sherif N, Scherlag BJ, Lazzara R, Hope RR: Reentrant ventricular arrhythmias in the late myocardial infarction period. 2. Patterns of initiation and termination of reentry. Circulation, 1977; 55: 702–718.
5. Waldo AL: Seminar on surgical therapy for ventricular arrhythmias. Amer J Cardiol 1981; 49: 163–165.
6. Spach MS, Miller WT, Dolber PC, Kootset, JM, Sommer JR, Mosher CE: The functional role of structural complexities in the propagation of depolarization in the atrium of the dog. Circ Res 1982; 50: 175–191.
7. Myers GH, Kresh YM, Parsonnet V: Characteristics of intracardiac electrograms. Pace 1978; 1: 90–97.
8. Kleinert M, Elmquist H, Strandberg H: Spectral properties of atrial and ventricular endocardial signals. Pace 1979; 2: 11–19.
9. Stulen FB, DeLuca CJ: Frequency parameters of the myoelectric signal as a measure of muscle conduction velocity. IEEE Trans on Biomed Engr 1981; 28: 515–523.

Authors' address:
Sanjeev Saksena, M.D.
Cardiac Electrophysiology
Newark Beth Israel Medical Center
Newark, N.J. 07112

Left Ventricular Function During Ventricular Pacing and Ventricular Tachycardia in Man

S. Saksena, W. Craelius, D. Pantopoulos, S. T. Rothbart, R. Werres

Summary: We studied acute changes in left ventricular (LV) function during ventricular pacing (VP) and induced ventricular tachycardia (VT) in patients undergoing combined hemodynamic and electrophysiologic studies. Sixteen patients, 15 males, 1 female, with sustained VT and organic heart disease, age range 52–79 (mean 68 ± 8) years, were studied in the drug free state. Using fluid and catheter tip micromanometer systems, peak LV systolic pressure (LVSP), LV end-diastolic pressure (LVEDP), LV peak DP/DT and LV peak negative DP/DT were analysed. Data were obtained in sinus rhythm (SR), VP at 100/mm and 150/min and induced VT. Sequential changes were studied during the first 50 beats of VT and correlated with VT cycle length, VT morphology and VP. Within the first 5 beats of VT there is a decrease in LVSP ($p < 0.01$), LV peak DP/DT ($p < 0.01$), and LV negative DP/DT ($p < 0.01$) without significant alterations of LVEDP. These changes stabilize within the initial 20 VT cycles. Similar changes in LV function parameters were observed during VP at 100/min, 150/min and rapid VP and were pacing cycle length dependent. In 6 patients, there were no differences in LV parameters during VT and VP at identical cycle lengths.

We conclude that impaired LV relaxation occurs during ventricular pacing and ventricular tachycardia. This may lead to inadequate ventricular filling contributing to LV systolic dysfunction. LVEDP is maintained due to incomplete relaxation. Heart rate is major determinant of hemodynamic status during VT and VP.

Introduction

Hemodynamic deterioration is a well recognized accompaniment of ventricular tachycardia (VT), although hemodynamically stable VT has also been described (1). The factors determining hemodynamic stability during VT have not been extensively investigated. Isolated ventricular premature depolarizations have been reported to cause transient circulatory alterations due to a reduction in stroke volume (2). Experimental studies have demonstrated similar changes in sustained VT (3). Presently, there is no published information available on LV function during sustained VT in man. Herein we report observations on acute changes in LV function during induced sustained VT and high rate ventricular pacing in patients undergoing combined hemodynamic and electrophysiologic studies.

Methods:

a) Patient Selection

Patients with recurrent sustained VT were entered into this study. In this study, "recurrent" was defined as "3 or more spontaneous episodes" and "sustained" as an arrhythmia lasting more than 30 seconds or requiring electrical or pharmacologic termination for hemodynamic compromise in a shorter period of time. The subjects entered into this study fulfilled the following selection criteria:

683

1. Absence of recent myocardial infarction.
2. Reproducible induction of sustained monomorphic VT during electrophysiologic studies.
3. Complete hemodynamic evaluation prior to and during VT induction.

b) Techniques

Patients were studied in the nonsedated postabsorptive state. Informed consent was obtained. All antiarrhythmic drug therapy was discontinued for a period of five drug half lives prior to study. Other cardioactive medications were continued.

1. Electrophysiological Studies:

Standard venous and arterial catheterization techniques were used. A Berkovits-Castellanos hexapolar electrode catheter was used for atrial and ventricular pacing. A tetrapolar electrode catheter was used to record His Bundle electrograms. Additional tetrapolar electrode catheters were used to record multiple intracardiac electrograms. Three surface ECG leads (I, aVF, V1) were recorded simultaneously with the intracardiac electrograms. Systemic arterial blood pressure was monitored using an indwelling femoral arterial sheath. A multichannel display recorder (Electronics for Medicine VR-12, White Plains, N.Y.) was used to amplify and display the electrograms. Hard copy recordings were obtained at speeds of 50–250 mm/sec. All records were stored on magnetic FM tape. Programmed electrical stimulation (PES) was performed using a custom-made programmed stimulator (Bloom Associates, Ltd, Narberth, PA) which delivered rectangular pulses of 1 msec duration at twice diastolic threshold.

The PES protocol used for induction of VT included:

1. Single premature atrial extrastimuli during sinus and high right atrial drive rhythms at two or more cycle lengths.
2. Rapid atrial pacing with incremental rates until the Wenckebach phenomenon was observed.
3. Single premature ventricular extrastimuli in sinus rhythm.
4. One or two premature extrastimuli during ventricular drive rhythm.
5. Rapid ventricular pacing at cycle lengths of 400–250 ms or up to ventricular refractoriness, whichever was shorter.
6. Three or four extrastimuli during ventricular drive rhythm.

Extrastimuli were introduced late in diastole in the spontaneous or paced rhythm. Coupling intervals of the extrastimuli were reduced in 10–20 ms decrements until refractoriness was reached. Additional extrastimuli were introduced at coupling intervals 50 ms greater than the refractory period and the interval was gradually reduced. If arrhythmia induction was not achieved at the initial stimulation sites, alternative stimulation sites were used (right ventricular outflow tract, left ventricle) and the PES protocol repeated until reproducible arrhythmia induction was observed. After arrhythmia induction was achieved, the mechanism of the arrhythmia and the effect of various therapeutic modalities (pacing, antiarrhythmic drugs) was tested.

2. Hemodynamic and Angiographic Studies

Right and left heart catheterization was performed using standard arterial and venous catheterization techniques. Patients were fully anticoagulated with heparin. For left ventricular hemodynamic studies, a catheter tip micromanometer system (Millar Instruments) or a fluid filled catheter system (a 7 French Zucker multipurpose catheter connected to a Statham P23 electronic transducer) was used. The fluid filled system was calibrated against the catheter tip micromanometer and showed good correlation (r value 0.90) over a wide range of pressures. The catheter was introduced into the left ventricle and baseline right and left heart hemodynamics were obtained. Left ventricular pressures and the first derivative of the left ventricular pressures (dp/dt) were continuously recorded. Left ventricular hemodynamic parameters were obtained during sinus rhythm, atrial and ventricular pacing, programmed ventricular stimulation and after VT induction. After completion of hemodynamic studies the catheter system was withdrawn and electrophysiologic studies continued for arrhythmia management.

c) Study Parameters and Analysis:

The left ventricular parameters studied included:
1. Peak LV systolic and LV end-diastolic pressure.
2. Positive and negative LV dp/dt.
Parameters were analysed during sinus rhythm, ventricular pacing at 100/min, 150/min (600 and 400 msec cycle lengths) and more rapid pacing rates as well as acutely after VT induction. The first 50 VT cycles were analysed. The characteristics of the induced VT (morphology and cycle length) were also reviewed. Data were analysed for statistical significance using the paired Student t-test.

Results

1. Clinical Characteristics

Sixteen patients with ages ranging from 52–79 (mean 68 ± 8) years, 15 males, 1 female completed the study protocol. Thirteen patients had coronary artery disease and 3 patients had cardiomyopathy. Resting LV end diastolic pressure in sinus rhythm ranged from 15–28 (mean 22 ± 6) mm/Hg. LV ejection fractions ranged from 11–68%.
The induced ventricular tachycardia morphology was RBBB in 8 patients, LBBB in 5 patients and indeterminate in 3 patients. The arrhythmia cycle lengths ranged from 180–490 (mean 335 ± 86) ms.

b) LV Function during Ventricular Pacing

Left ventricular pressures and indices during sinus rhythm and ventricular pacing at cycle lengths of 600 and 400 msec are shown in Fig. 1A and 1B. Peak left ventricular systolic pressure, peak dp/dt and negative dp/dt showed a significant decrease during ventricular pacing as compared to sinus rhythm. Peak left ventricular systolic pressure declined from 122 ± 18 mmHg (sinus rhythm) to 99 ± 20 mmHg (VP 600 ms) and 81 ± 15 mmHg (VP 400 ms). Peak left ventricular dp/dt declined from 1532 ± 630 mmHg/sec to 884 ± 220 (VP 600) and 813 ± 202 mmHg/sec (VP 650 ms). Peak negative LV dp/dt declined from 1253 ± 465 mmHg/sec (sinus rhythm) to 843 ± 197 mmHg/sec (VP 600 ms) and 591 ± 140 mmHg/sec (VP 400 ms). Left ventricular end diastolic pressure was 22 ± 4 mmHg in sinus rhythm and did not change significantly during ventricular pacing at 600/ms (18 ± 4 mmHg) or 400 ms (20 ± 4 mmHg).

c) LV Function during Induced VT

As shown in Fig. 2A, mean LV peak systolic is significantly lowered by the fifth VT cycle (p < 0.01). Similarly, LV peak dp/dt and negative dp/dt are significantly decreased by the fifth VT cycle (Fig. 2B). LVEDP did not show a significant change although a trend towards higher values was noted early during VT. LV function parameters stabilized by the twentieth VT cycle.

Fig. 1. Left Ventricular Function during Ventricular Pacing; A: Left ventricular pressures during ventricular pacing. Effect of ventricular pacing at 100 beats/min and 150 beats/min on peak LV systolic pressure and LV end diastolic pressure. B: Left ventricular function indices during ventricular pacing. Effect of ventricular pacing (at same rates as in Fig. 1A) on peak LV dp/dt and negative dp/dt. Abbreviations: SR – Sinus rhythm; VP – Ventricular pacing.

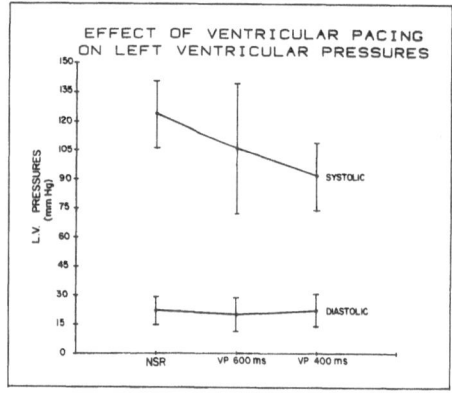

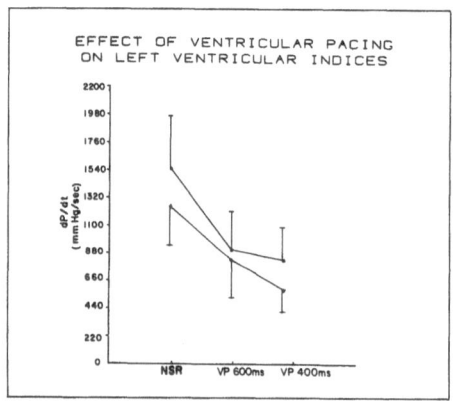

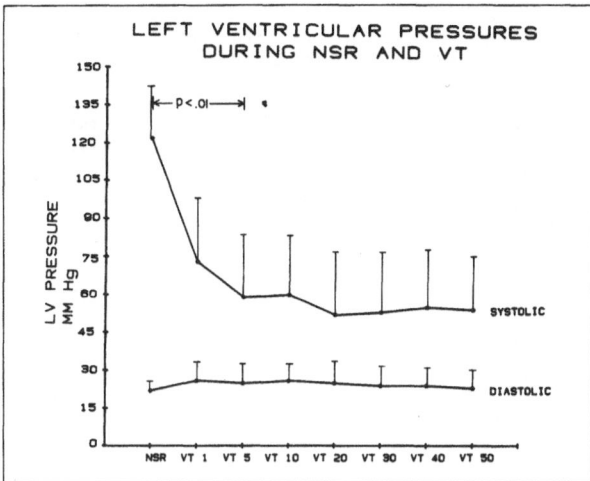

Fig. 2: Left Ventricular Function during Ventricular Tachycardia; A: Left ventricular pressures during onset of ventricular tachycardia (VT). Sequential VT beats (numbered 1 to 50) are shown with LV pressures as in Fig. 1A. B: Left ventricular function indices during onset of ventricular tachycardia. Sequential VT beats (numbered 1 to 50) are shown with LV function indices as in Fig. 1B. Abbreviations: As in Fig. 1.

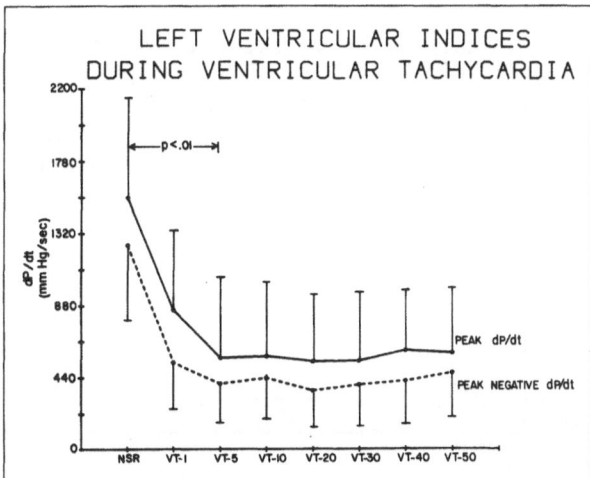

d) Comparison of LV Function during Ventricular Pacing and VT

Fig. 3A shows serial changes in LV pressures in one patient over a wide range of ventricular pacing cycle lengths, and at two induced ventricular tachycardias of similar morphology, but differing cycle lengths. LV peak systolic pressure declines with shortening of pacing cycle length, and roughly equivalent changes are noted for VT. LVEDP begins to increase at cycle lengths shorter than 400 ms. Similar observations were noted for LV peak dp/dt and negative dp/dt. Similar results were found in five other patients in whom ventricular pacing could be performed at cycle lengths identical to VT cycle length.

The cycle length dependency of LV parameters during VT is illustrated for another patient in Fig. 3B. Note the dramatic differences in hemodynamic function occurring in the two VT's, which differ in rate by only 20 msec.

Fig. 3: Comparison of Left Ventricular Function during Ventricular Pacing and Ventricular Tachycardia. A: Serial changes in LV pressures in a patient at different ventricular pacing cycle lengths (in msec). The crosses and squares represent two induced ventricular tachycardias in the same patient with similar morphologies but different rates.

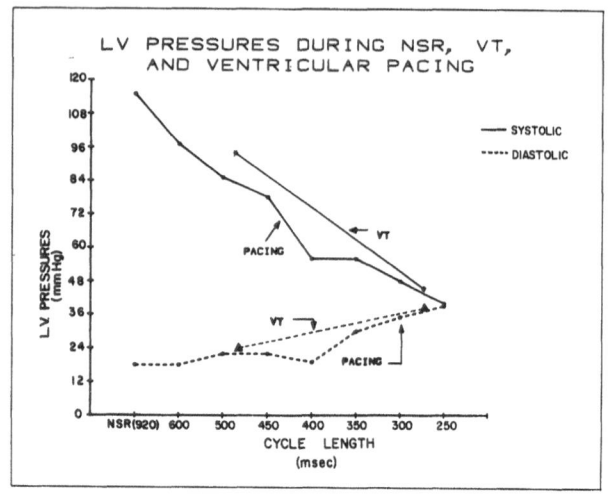

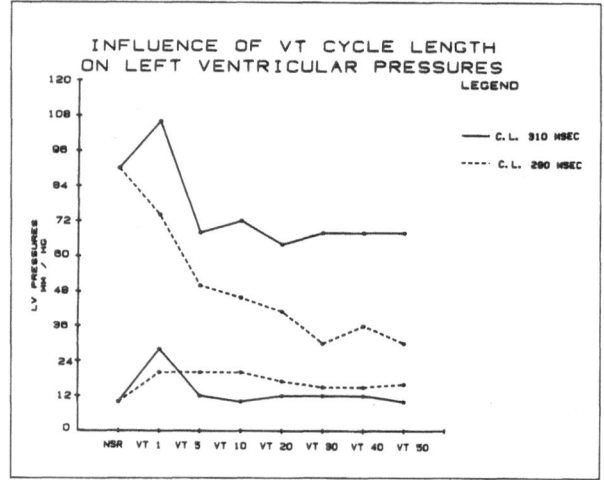

Discussion:

Early studies on the hemodynamic sequelae of cardiac arrhythmias attempted to characterize changes in cardiac function during atrial fibrillation (7, 8). With the advent of cardiac pacing, the hemodynamic effects of ventricular and later atrial and atrioventricular sequential pacing were studied (9–12). Sparse information was available on tachyarrhythmias in vivo since, until recently, they could only be studied when they occurred fortuitously in the clinical cardiac laboratory (3). With the availability of electrophysiologic procedures, controlled induction and termination of these arrhythmias is now possible. Hemodynamic studies in SVT with differing electrophysiologic mechanisms have been reported (4–8). Studies of cardiac function during VT have been largely confined to the experimental or noninvasive laboratory (6, 13, 14). To our knowledge, there is no systematic study available on LV function during sustained VT in man.

688

The onset of SVT is characterized by a decline in systolic blood pressure, systemic arterial pulse pressure and cardiac index coupled with an increase in pulmonary artery and right atrial pressures (4, 5). Subsequently, a reflex increase in systemic arterial resistance increases blood pressure. Our observations during the onset of VT show a fall in peak LV systolic pressure and consequent fall in systemic arterial pressure. LVEDP for the group did not change significantly. Similar changes were observed during asynchronous ventricular pacing. In fact, pacing at rates identical to VT rate produced an equivalent degree of depression of LV function.

The mechanisms of changes in LV function during tachyarrhythmias have not been fully elucidated. Several mechanisms have been suggested to account for changes observed in SVT (2, 3, 4). These include rate dependent abbreviation of ventricular filling, altered atrioventricular contraction relationships and atrioventricular valvular regurgitation during VT. An additional mechanism, altered ventricular contraction patterns in VT has received considerable attention (14–16). This study suggests that reduction in diastolic time is a major mechanism underlying hemodynamic impairment in VT. This leads to incomplete relaxation (manifest as reduction of negative dp/dt) and subsequently impaired contraction. Incomplete relaxation preserves LVEDP which may even increase at particularly fast cycle lengths. We have observed an improvement in LV function parameters during VT and AV dissociation when atrial contraction occurs in late diastole. The importance of ventricular filling is underlined by a recent report of significant hemodynamic improvement when atrial contraction is synchronised to enhance ventricular filling in VT (17).

Alteration of ventricular contraction patterns does not appear to be a major factor in hemodynamic function particularly in VT with short cycle lengths. Ventricular pacing with presumably a different ventricular activation pattern than the clinical VT produced identical pressure changes to the native VT in six of our patients. Our observations in patients with resting LV dysfunction and wall motion abnormalities differ from a previous report (16). The role of atrioventricular valvular regurgitation and resting LV function cannot be fully assessed from this study. Our observations suggest that symptomatic hemodynamic deterioration during VT is often determined by the arrhythmia cycle length. Interventions prolonging VT cycle length will limit or may even eliminate hemodynamic compromise during the arrhythmia.

References

1. Papadopoulos C, Blazek CJ: Ventricular tachycardia of 70 days duration with survival. Am J Cardiol 1963; 11: 107.
2. Cohn K, Kryda W: The influence of ectopic beats and tachyarrhythmias on stroke volume and cardiac output. J Electrocardiol 1981; 14: 207.
3. Nakano J: Effects of atrial and ventricular tachycardias on cardiovascular dynamics: Am J Physiol 1964; 206: 547.
4. Goldreyer BN, Kastor JA, Kerschbaum KL: The hemodynamic effects of induced supraventricular tachycardia in man. Circulation 1973; 54: 783.
5. Saunders DE, Ord JW: The hemodynamic effects of paroxysmal supra-ventricular tachycardia in patients with Wolff-Parkinson-White Syndrome. Amer J Cardiol 1962; 9: 223.
6. McIntosh HD, Momi JJ Jr: The hemodynamic consequences of arrhythmias: Progress in Cardiovascular Diseases. 1966; 8: 330.

7. Kory RC, McNeely GR: Cardiac output in auricular fibrillation with observation on the effect of conversion to normal sinus rhythm. J Clin Invest 1951; 30: 653.
8. Hecht H, Osher WJ, Samuels AJ: Cardiovascular adjustments in subjects with organic heart disease before and after conversion to normal sinus rhythm. J Clin Invest 1951; 30: 647.
9. Sowton E: Hemodynamic studies in patients with artificial pacemakers. Brit Heart J 1964; 26: 737.
10. Gilmore JP, Sarnoff SJ, Mitchell JH, Linden RJ: Synchronicity of ventricular contraction: observations comparing the hemodynamic effects of atrial and ventricular pacing: BREMS, Heart J 1963: 25; 299.
11. Samet P, Castillo C, Bernstein WH: Hemodynamic sequelae of atrial, ventricular and sequential atrioventricular pacing in cardiac patients. Am Ht J 1966; 72: 725.
12. Samet P, Bernstein WH, Levine S, Lopez A: Hemodynamic effects of tachycardias produced by atrial and ventricular pacing. Am J Med 1965; 39: 905.
13. Smirk FH, Nolla-Panades J, Wallis T: Experimental ventricular flutter and ventricular paroxysmal tachycardia. Am J Cardiol 1964; 14: 79.
14. Daggett WM, Bianco JM, Powell WJ, Austen WG: Relative contributions of the atrial systole – ventricular systole interval and of patterns of ventricular activation to ventricular function during electrical pacing of the dog heart. Circ Res 1970; 27: 69.
15. Eber LM, Berkovits BV, Matloff JV, Gorlin R: Dynamic characterization of premature ventricular beats and ventricular tachycardias. Am J Cardiol 1974; 33: 378.
16. Lima JA, Weiss JL, Guzman PA, Eaton LW, Reid PR, Traill TA: Incomplete filling and incoordinate contraction as mechanisms of syncope in ventricular tachycardia (abstr). Am J Cardiol 1982; 49: 917.
17. Hamer A WF, Zaher C, Peter CT, Mandel WJ: Hemodynamic benefits of sequential atrial pacing during ventricular tachycardia in man (abstr). J Am Coll Cardiol 1983; 1 (2): 636.

Authors' address:
S. Saksena, M.D.
Cardiac Electrophysiology
Newark Beth Israel Medical Center
201 Lyons Avenue
Newark, N.J. 07112 (USA)

690

Hemodynamics During Simulated Paroxysmal Ventricular Tachycardias in Valvular Aortic Stenosis: Role of the Transvalvular Systolic Gradient and Aortic Valve Area During Stress Conditions

J. Thormann, M. Schlepper, H. Neuss, W. Kramer, M. Kindler

Summary: Although of clinical significance, the influence generated by VT on varying degrees of AS has not been systematically investigated: this also applies to the residual TVG after aortic valve replacement (AVR). We, therefore, assessed changes of cardiac output (CO), LV- and pulmonary artery pressures (LVP, AOP, PAP) and of AVA during paced VT (110-, 140-, 170 bpm) in 49 pts, some of the subgroups being: 1) AS with "small TVGs" with an average of 19 mmHg (= AS 19) and 10 mmHg, respectively (= AS 10, i.e. residual TVG after AVR); 2) AS with "large TVGs" with an average of 74 mmHg (= AS 74).

As VT-rates increased, TVG and CO decreased; LV-efficiency correlated well with AVA size but inversely with TVG. As for differences in hemodynamic reactions to VT-stress AS 19 (and AS 10) vs. AS 74, the amount of developed LVP was established as the key determinant. In addition, the empirically recognized "phenomenon of apparent valve changes" (Circulation 44:1003, 1974) proved predictable: calculated AVA diminished with VT 170 and more so with Isoproterenol-stress (ISO), while ergometry caused AVA size to increase. During ISO in AS 10 the residual TVG rose 5.2-fold and AVA decreased by 50%, i.e. AVR leaves the pt with a negligible TVG which, during stress conditions, might well increase to levels of a moderate AS; this needs consideration regarding pt's activities after AVR.

Stress-induced hemodynamic changes may help evaluate AS and AVR. The inconsistency of determinants of AVA in their mathematical relationship for pts under stress results in the phenomenon of "apparent changes of valvular geometry". They seem to be predictable with regard to both direction and magnitude as they differ characteristically according to the type of stress used.

Although of clinical significance, the influence generated by ventricular tachycardia (VT) on varying degrees of aortic stenosis (AS) has not been systematically investigated: This also applies to the residual transvalvular gradient present after aortic valve replacement.

Rhythm disturbances in AS, other than in normal hearts, come upon a myocardium which is hypertrophied and dilated; this applies both, for normofrequent rhythm disturbances as well as for arrhythmias in the tachycardia range. Tachycardia-induced reduction of the diastolic period (the time of myocardial perfusion) is comparatively more pronounced in AS due to a prolonged systolic ejection time necessary for the built-up of a gradient. Furthermore, in AS a significant compensatory dilatation of the coronary capacitance vessels has become limited at best, since this reserve function has been used up at rest conditions already, owing to the advanced left ventricular (LV) hypertrophy (1). Thus, myocardial ischemia is imminent, involving the total LV-subendocardium in contradistinction to the only localized ischemia in coronary artery disease (CAD) (2).

In figure 1 (left part) there are the results of paced VT with a rate of 170 bpm (black columns) and the hyperemic reaction after the application of Dipyridamol (D) (crosshatched columns). These conditions are given: for a healthy control group (left), for a group with coronary artery disease (CAD) (middle), and a group with LV-hypertrophy in aortic stenosis (right). Alterations of arterial pressures (AOP) (upper level), both, tachycardia-induced and during drug-mediated vasodilation are in the same range for all 3 groups (p > 0.05). Total coronary perfusion (CS-flow) (3) during tachycardia (presented in the middle) increases by an average of +30% for all 3 groups. However, the capacity of coronary reserve, which is available for the healthy ventricle, as mobilized by Dipyridamol (represented as crosshatched column, on the left) ist not available for the impaired left ventricles of either CAD or LV-hypertrophy. Myocardial ischemia is not reflected by the tachycardia-induced alterations, either of the arterial pressures or of coronary blood flow. However, lactate production (4) (lower level) of – 40% for the CAD-group and – 50% for the LV-hypertrophy group identifies tachycardia-induced myocardial ischemia. Thus, hemodynamic changes of the determinants of LV-hypertrophy reliably become apparent under the well standardized conditions of paced ventricular tachycardia, both in valvular AS and for the residual gradients after aortic valvular replacement.

Figure 1 (middle part, upper level) demonstrates the pacing-induced hemodynamic alterations in a patient group with an average systolic transaortic gradient of 51 mmHg, using the rates 100-, 140- and 170 bpm, "R" stands for control conditions at rest. LV-pressure (AOP, LVSP), stroke work (LVSWI), stroke index and systolic gradients (SG), all fell pro-

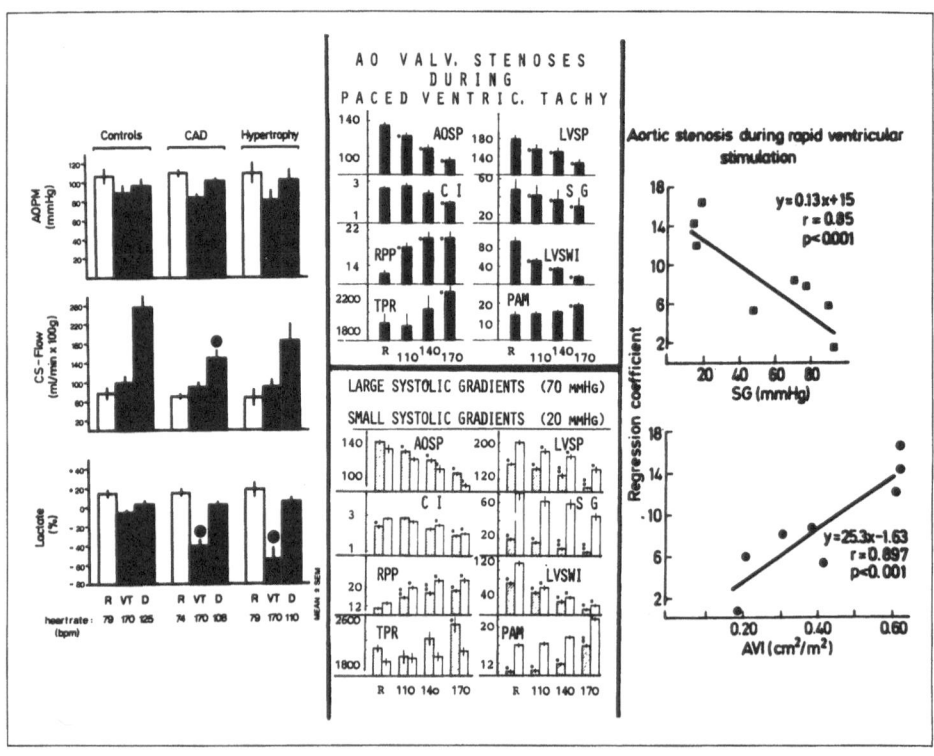

portionally with increasing heart rates, while tachycardia-induced changes of other parameters were significant only at maximal pacing rates; this applies for the decrease of aortic pressure, cardiac index (CI) as well as for the increase of diastolic aortic pressure, of the pulmonary artery pressure (PAM) and the total peripheral (TPR) and pulmonary vascular resistance.

In figure 1 (middle part, lower level) there is a demonstration of the comparison of hemodynamic alterations under the 3 steps of a paced tachycardia in AS with small systolic gradients (i.e. an average of 20 mmHg; depicted as white columns) and large systolic gradients (i.e. an average of 70 mmHg; depicted as crosshatched columns). Significant differences between the mean results are present for the LV-pressure (LVSP), for th AO-pressure (AOSP), the rate pressure product (RPP), and the peripheral vascular resistance (TPR), but at maximal pacing rates only.

Figure 1 (right part, upper level) represents the relation systolic transaortic gradient (SG) versus regression coefficient of the relation SG versus cardiac output (CO) alterations, during paced ventricular rates of 100-, 140- and 170 bpm in 8 patients with an average resting SG of 70 mmHg. The descent of these relations correlates well with the size of the SG. Thus, with rising paced rates, CO becomes diminished and with larger gradients this tendency is even more accentuated.

Figure 1 (right part, lower level) represents the relation aortic valvular area index (AVI) versus regression coefficients of the relations AVI versus cardiac output alterations during the 3 steps of ventricular stimulation. The ascent of the single relations in 8 patients correlates well with the size of the AVI. Thus, increasing pacing rates per se diminish CO but this tendeny is all the more pronounced the smaller a given aortic valvular area is.

In summing up the following resulted: 1) With large gradients there are lower CO values at rest and the decrease with rising rates is less rapid as compared to cases with lesser gradients where resting values are higher to start with and tachycardia-induced CO reduction is more rapid. 2) With increasing narrowing of the aortic valve area in aortic stenosis a more rapid decrease of the CO with rising rates can be expected.

In dealing with stress-induced changes of the determinants of the aortic valve area (which are part of the Gorlin formula (5)), it becomes apparent that this calculated area itself is variable, in other words, the aortic valve area does not behave like a fixed valvular orifice under altered hemodynamic conditions (6). The question arises whether this phenomenon might be relevant for patients with aortic stenosis and large or smaller gradients, or else for patients with a residual gradient following aortic valve replacement.

As shown in figure 2 (upper part) for 10 patients after aortic valve replacement a certain consistency of this phenomenon was demonstrated. During paced ventricular tachycardias with increasing rates between 110 and 170 bpm the residual transvalvular gradient (SG) progressively decreased, as could be also observed for the other determinants, that is for aortic préssure (AOMP) and cardiac output (CO). However, also the calculated aortic valve area (marked as AVA, bottom left) diminished. Thus, during pacing stress of 170 bpm the reduction in size of the SGs and of the AVA are most markedly apparent. However, AVA further reduces its size considerably, i.e. by an average of 50%, during inotropic stress condition by means of a brief infusion of isoproterenol (ISO); this is associated with a rise of the systolic gradient by an average of a factor 5.2. From this it might be deduced that there is a potential for the residual gradient after aortic valve replacement to rise ranging 50–60 mmHg during daily life stress conditions, that is to levels that are commonly present in moderate aortic stenosis.

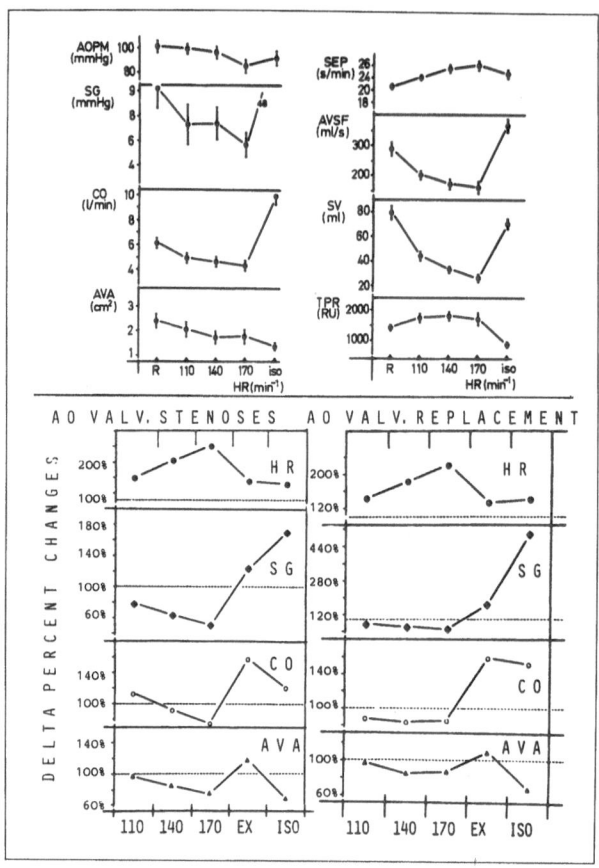

With regard to our findings that aortic valve area and their determinant parameters in aortic stenosis are subject to characteristic alterations, depending on the type of stress used, this also can be demonstrated from the analysis of the results of 28 investigations carried out between 1961 and 1979. The mean results are given in figure 2, bottom part left, for aortic valvular stenosis (AS), and on the right for patients after aortic valvular replacement (AVR). The average deviations from the control conditions at rest are given in per cent, from top to bottom for: the heart rate (HR), the transaortic systolic gradient (SG), the cardiac output (CO) and the aortic valve area (AVA). Alterations during rapid rate pacing in 3 steps appear on the left in each of the 2 graphs, changes during isoproterenol stress (ISO) on the right, respectively. The results are in accord with our own findings. The results of ergometric stress (marked EX) show an apparent deviation, in so far, as ergometry obviously rather induces an enlargement of aortic valve areas, and this in the presence of a comparatively moderate rise of transvalvular systolic gradients.

In summing up: Stress-induced hemodynamic alterations are useful as regards the assessment of the hemodynamic situation before and after aortic valve replacement. Changes of the determinant parameters of the aortic valve area, as well as the caluclated aortic valve area itself are predictable and consistent with regard to the direction and magnitude, depending on the type of stress used under well standardized conditions.

References

1. Buckberg G, Eber L, Herman M, Gorlin R. Ischemia in aortic stenosis: Hemodynamic prediction. Am J Cardiol 1975; 35: 778–784.
2. Flameng W, Schaper W, Lewi P. Multiple experimental coronary occlusion without infarction. Effects of heart rate and vasodilation. Am Heart J 1973; 85: 767–776.
3. Ganz W, Tamura K, Marcus HS, Donoso R, Yoshida S, Swan HJC. Measurement of coronary sinus blood flow by continuous thermodilution in man. Circulation 1971; 44: 181–189.
4. Trenouth RS, Phelps NC, Neill WA. Determinants of left ventricular hypertrophy and oxygen supply in chronic aortic valve disease. Circulation 1976; 53: 644–649.
5. Gorlin R, Gorlin SE. Hydraulic formula for calculation of the area of the stenotic mitral valve, other cardiac valves and central circulatory shunts. Am Heart J 1951; 41: 1–29.
6. Bache RJ, Wang Y, Jorgensen CR. Hemodynamic effects of exercise in isolated aortic stenosis. Circulation 1971; 44: 1003–1011.

Authors' address
Priv.-Doz. Dr. med. J. Thormann
Kerckhoff-Klinik der
Max-Planck-Gesellschaft
Benekestraße 4-6
6350 Bad Nauheim (FG)

Relative Contributions of Mitral and Pulmonary Venous Regurgitation to the Adverse Hemodynamic Consequences of Various Cardiac Arrhythmias

M. Naito, M. Miyairi, T. Asato, H. Nagoshi, M. Honda, E. L. Michelson, L. S. Dreifus

Summary: To compare the hemodynamic consequences of various cardiac arrhythmias, hemodynamic and angiographic studies were done on 20 open-chest, atrio-ventricular (A-V) heart-blocked dogs during various programmed pacing protocols. Cardiac output was determined during A-V pacing at A-V intervals of 100 msec, and –100 msec, ventricular pacing during A-V dissociation, and ventricular pacing during atrial fibrillation. In addition, cardiac output was measured during both regular and irregular ventricular pacing during each of the above rhythms. The presence of pulmonary venous and/or mitral regurgitation was evaluated during each pacing protocol.

During regular ventricular pacing, cardiac output was optimal at an A-V interval of 100 msec, but decreased by 25% at an A-V interval of –100 msec and by 18% during both A-V dissociation and atrial fibrillation. During atrial fibrillation, irregular rhythms imposed a further hemodynamic penalty in addition to the loss of active atrial transport. Pulmonary venous regurgitation was observed only during A-V dissociation and during regular pacing at A-V –100 msec. Mitral valvular regurgitation occurred only during irregular ventricular cycles, but not during regular ventricular pacing, even in the presence of A-V dissociation or atrial fibrillation.

Using these methods it was possible to resolve some previously reported controversies regarding the relative importance of A-V sequencing, atrial systole versus atrial fibrillation, regular versus irregular rhythms, as well as the importance of A-V sequencing, atrial systole versus atrial fibrillation, regular versus irregular rhythms, as well as the possible contribution of mitral and/or pulmonary venous regurgitation to the adverse hemodynamics of various cardiac arrhythmias.

The hemodynamic consequences of cardiac arrhythmias depend on numerous factors including the heart rate, the filling and emptying characteristics of the various chambers, the relative timing of atrial and ventricular systole, as well as effects of neurohumoral and vasomotor influences (1–4). Several previous investigators have considered the consequences of changes in atrial transport (1–4) and in the functional state of the heart (5–8) in the presence of various cardiac arrhythmias. However, the relative importance of rhythm regularity, the temporal relation of atrial and ventricular systole, and the role of active atrial transport have not been well defined. The purpose of this study was to further clarify the complex hemodynamic alterations resulting from cardiac arrhythmias using methods of programmed atrial and ventricular pacing, cardiac angiography and hemodynamic catheterization.

Methods

Twenty adult mongrel dogs weighing 11–18 kg were anesthetized with sodium pentobarbital (25–30 mg/kg, iv), and aortic pressure and lead II ECG were monitored continuously throughout the experiment. The chest was opened using a midline incision and

697

the pericardium was opened. Unipolar stainless steel wire electrodes were implanted into the left atrial appendage and the apex of the left ventricle for pacing purposes. These were connected to two programmable impulse generators (Bloom Associates) so that the atrium and ventricle could be paced separately. Then acute surgical heart block was produced by electrocoagulation of the atrio-ventricular node through a right atrial approach (9). ·

A # 7F Millar Dual Mikro-Tip catheter pressure transducer (PC-771) was inserted via the right carotid artery to record aortic and left ventricular pressures. A # 5F Millar Mikro-Tip catheter pressure transducer (PC-350) was introduced through a pulmonary vein to record left atrial pressure. Cardiac output was measured using a # 7F Swan-Ganz thermodilution cardiac catheter.

In 10 animals, left ventricular cineangiography was done using a # 8F short endhole Lehman angiographic catheter introduced from the right carotid artery and left atrial cineangiography was performed using a # 7F short Lehman angiographic catheter with sideholes near its tip. This catheter was inserted via one of the left or right pulmonary veins. For each angiogram, 8 to 10 cc of Renografin 76 was injected by hand and care was taken to inject the contrast material over 7 to 8 cardiac cycles.

Both atrial and ventricular pacing were done using a pulse width of 1.5 msec and twice diastolic threshold current. Four pacing modalities were studied both during regular ventricular pacing at a cycle length of 400 msec, and during irregular ventricular pacing at a mean cycle length of 400 msec. Irregular ventricular pacing was done by using the S_6 stimulator to introduce 5 extrastimuli at varying coupling intervals followed by a programmed pause of varying duration. The four pacing protocols were:

1. Atrial and ventricular pacing at an A-V interval of 100 msec.
2. Ventricular pacing only during sinus rhythm with A-V dissociation.
3. Atrial fibrillation with ventricular pacing. Atrial fibrillation was produced by stimulating the left atrial appendage at a cycle length of 50–90 msec.
4. Atrial and ventricular pacing at an A-V interval of –100 msec.

Results

Fig. 1 summarizes changes in cardiac output during various pacing protocols. During regular ventricular rhythms, cardiac output was maximum at an atrio-ventricular interval of +100 msec. During regular ventricular pacing, the difference between the cardiac output at an A-V interval of +100 msec and each of the other 3 pacing protocols was significant. Conversely, the cardiac output at an A-V interval of –100 msec was the lowest among the four regular ventricular pacing protocols, and there were significant differences between an A-V interval of –100 msec and each of the other 3 regular pacing protocols. However, there was no significant difference between regular ventricular pacing with random atrial systole (A-V dissociation) and regular ventriculr pacing with atrial fibrillation.

Among the four irregular ventricular pacing protocols the cardiac output was maximum at an A-V interval of +100 msec, and minimum at an A-V interval of –100 msec. However, during irregular pacing the cardiac outputs measured at an A-V interval of –100 msec and during atrial fibrillation with irregular ventricular pacing were indistinguishable. Cardiac output during irregular ventricular pacing was significantly

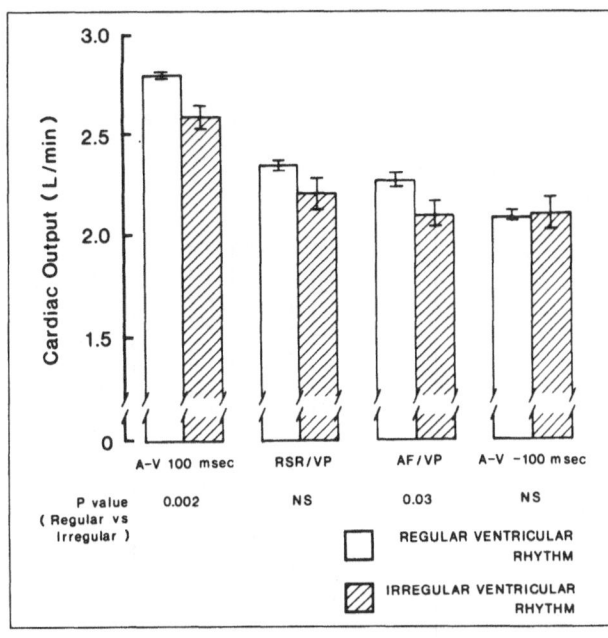

Fig. 1. Changes in cardiac output during regular (white bar) and irregular (crossed bar) ventricular rhythms. For both regular and irregular rhythms, cardiac output was maximum at an A-V interval of +100 msec, and minimum at an A-V interval of −100 msec. There was no significant difference between regular ventricular pacing (VP) with A-V dissociation (RSR/VP) and with atrial fibrillation (AF/VP). Cardiac output during irregular ventricular pacing was significantly lower than regular ventricular pacing both at an A-V interval of +100 msec, and during atrial fibrillation.

lower than regular ventricular pacing both at an A-V interval of +100 msec (−7%, p = 0.002), and during atrial fibrillation (−9%, p = 0.03).

During the various pacing protocols, changes in cardiac output were associated with concomitant changes in left ventricular and left atrial pressures. As demonstrated in Fig. 2, left ventricular systolic pressure was maximum during A-V pacing at an A-V interval of +100 msec for both regular and irregular ventricular rhythms. Compared to regular ventricular pacing, there was an approximately 3–7 mmHg reduction in left ventricular systolic pressure during irregular ventricular pacing for each of the four pacing protocols.

During both regular and irregular pacing left atrial pressure was minimum during A-V pacing at an A-V interval of +100 msec. However, increases in left atrial pressure during other pacing protocols were not statistically significant.

Table 1 summarizes the angiographic findings during various pacing protocols. Left atrial angiography revealed pulmonary venous regurgitation during A-V dissociation and during A-V pacing at an A-V interval of −100 msec. It was found that pulmonary venous regurgitation was associated with atrial contraction during the ventricular ejection period in each case. Mitral valvular regurgitation as revealed by left ventricular angiography occurred only in the presence of irregular ventricular cycles, and was not seen during rhythms with regular ventricular cycles.

Discussion

Although the present study was performed in an acute, openchest, anesthetized, canine model, we attempted to identify several hemodynamic factors which might be en-

Fig. 2. Left ventricular peak systolic pressure was maximum during A-V interval of +100 msec for both regular and irregular ventricular rhythms. Compared to regular ventricular pacing, there was an approximately 3–7 mmHg reduction in left ventricular peak systolic pressure during irregular ventricular pacing for each of the four pacing protocols.

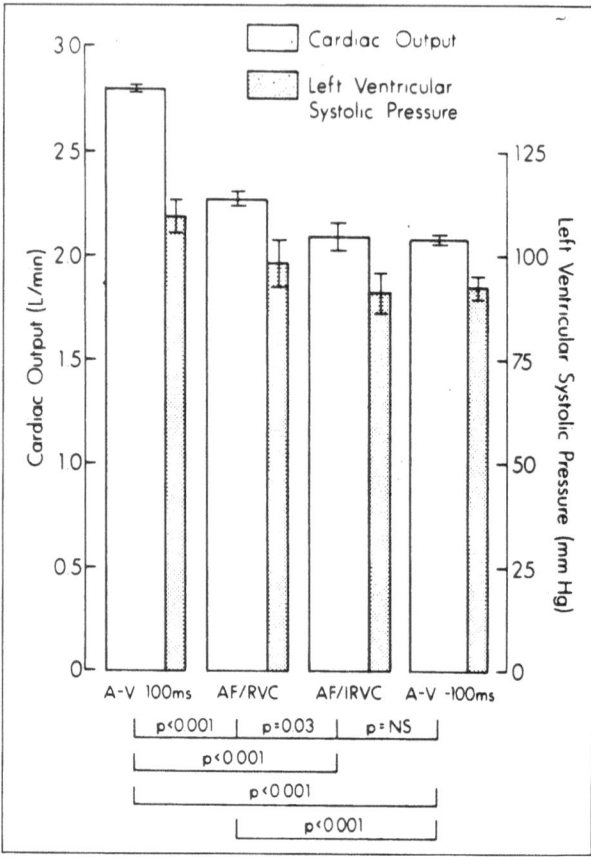

Table 1. Angiographic Findings During Various Pacing Protocols.

	A-V +100 msec		A-V dissociation RSR with VP		AF with VP		A-V −100 msec	
	R	IR	R	IR	R	IR	R	IR
Pulmonary Venous Regurgitation	−	+	+	+	−	−	+	+
Mitral Valve Regurgitation	−	+	−	+	−	+	−	+

Abbreviations: AF = Atrial Fibrillation
A-V = Atrio-ventricular
IR = Irregular ventricular pacing
R = Regular ventricular pacing
RSR = Regular sinus rhythm
VP = Ventricular pacing
− = Absent
+ = Present

countered in the clinical setting of cardiac arrhythmias. It has been generally accepted that the loss of atrial contraction may reduce cardiac output by as much as 25%. However, the precise role of atrial contraction during regular versus irregular ventricular rhythms, as well as the presence of atrial fibrillation, has not been fully elucidated.

Atrio-ventricular sequential pacing at an A-V interval of +100 msec resulted in optimal hemodynamics during both regular and irregular ventricular pacing. The most deleterious hemodynamics were observed during A-V sequential pacing at an interval of −100 msec. Since the mitral valve was closed during this pacing sequence, there was no active atrial transport to the ventricle, and worse, there was active atrial emptying retrograde into the pulmonary and systemic venous systems (Table 1) (1, 10, 11).

It has not been clear that the reduction in cardiac output during atrial fibrillation can be ascribed only to the lack of atrial contribution to ventricular filling (12, 13). In the present study observations were made in animals with intrinsically normal hearts. By comparing the cardiac output during regular pacing at an A-V interval of +100 msec with regular ventricular pacing during atrial fibrillation, we were able to isolate the net contribution of atrial systole in these normal hearts. The comparison of regular versus irregular ventricular pacing in the absence of active atrial transport enabled us to isolate the net effects of the irregular ventricular rhythms (Fig. 1). Cardiac output was reduced by approximately 9%. The results clearly indicate that the irregularity of the ventricular rhythm itself can have adverse hemodynamic consequences.

The contribution of mitral regurgitation to the adverse hemodynamic consequences of various arrhythmias has been controversial (13–16). In part, this has been related to limitations in quantifying the degree of A-V valvular regurgitation, and in the use of catheter techniques which may produce spurious regurgitation as visualized on routine angiograms.

Thus, the hemodynamic consequences of various cardiac arrhythmias are quite complex. Clinically, the potential adverse effects of abnormal A-V sequencing, irregular rhythms, atrial fibrillation, pulmonary venous regurgitation and rapid rates must all be considered. In addition, neurohumoral and vasomotor influences are also undoubtedly contributory in man, although those were not evaluated in the present study. Moreover, in patients with underlying cardiac dysfunction, the deleterious effects of any departure from normal rhythm may be even further exaggerated.

References

1. Gesell RA: Atrial systole and its relation to ventricular output. Am J Physiol 1911; 29: 32.
2. Burchell HB: A clinical appraisal of atrial transport function. Lancet 1964; 1: 775.
3. Mitchell JH, Gupta DN, Payne RM: Influence of atrial systole on effective ventricular stroke volume. Circ Res 1965; 17: 11.
4. Samet P, Bernstein WH, Nathan D, Lopez A: Atrial contribution to cardiac output in complete heart block. Am J Cardiol 1965; 16: 1.
5. Lendrum B, Feinberg H, Boyd E, Katz LN: Rhythm effects of contractility of the beating isovolumic left ventricle. Am J Physiol 1960; 199: 1115.
6. Koch-Weser J, Blinks J: The influence of the interval between beats on myocardial contractility. Pharmacol Rev 1963; 15: 601.
7. Edmands RE, Greenspan K, Fisch C: The role of inotropic variation in ventricular function during atrial fibrillation. J Clin Invest 1970; 49: 738.

8. Lab JPM, Elzinga SG, Papadoyannis D, Noble MIM: The contractile state of cat and dog heart in relation to the interval between beats. Circ Res 1980; 47: 559.

9. Starzl TE, Gaertner RA, Baker RR: Acute complete heart block in dogs. Circulation 1955; 12: 82.

10. Naito M, Dreifus LS, Mardelli TJ, Chen CC, David D, Michelson EL, Marcy V, Morganroth J: Echocardiographic features of atrioventricular and ventriculo-atrial conduction. Am J Cardiol 1980; 46: 625.

11. Naito M, Dreifus LS, David D, Michelson EL, Morganroth J, Mardelli TJ, Kmetzo JJ: Re-evaluation of the role of atrial systole to cardiac hemodynamics: Evidence for pulmonary venous regurgitation during abnormal atrioventricular sequencing. Am Heart J 1983; 105: 295.

12. Hecht HH, Lange RL: The hemodynamic consequences of atrial fibrillation. Mod Concepts of Cardiovasc Dis 1956; 25: 351.

13. Skinner NS, Mitchell JH, Wallace AG, Sarnoff SJ: Hemodynamic consequences of atrial fibrillation of constant ventricular rates. Am J Med 1964; 36: 342.

14. Daley R, McMillan IKR, Gorlin R: Mitral incompetence in experimental auricular fibrillation. Lancet 1955; 2: 18.

15. Skinner NS, Mitchell JH, Wallace AG, Sarnoff SJ: Hemodynamic effects of altering the timing of atrial systole. Am J Physiol 1963; 205: 499.

16. Sivaciyan V, Ranganathan N: Transcutaneous doppler jugular venous flow velocity recording: Clinical and hemodynamic correlates. Circulation 1978; 57: 930.

Authors' address:
Masahito Naito, M.D.
The 2nd Tokyo National Hospital
2–5–1, Higashigaoka Meguro-ku
Tokyo 151/Japan

Treatment of Ventricular Arrhythmias: Drugs

K. J. Frohner, K. Steinbach

The management of ventricular arrhythmias and the prevention of sudden death remain to be a major challenge for cardiologists. At present the major therapeutic approach to arrhythmias is pharmacological, although pacing techniques and surgery are used in an increasing number of patients.

Any antiarrhythmic therapy must be preceded by an exact quantitative and qualitative analysis of the arrhythmia in question. In the last decade in particular 24-h ECG monitoring has been used for this purpose. There is strong evidence from different studies that premature ventricular beats in the absence of significant heart disease do not identify a group of patients with an increased risk of subsequent cardiac death. In contrast to these "innocent PVC's" (Table 1) ventricular arrhythmias increase the risk of subsequent sudden death in patients with coronary heart disease. 8 of the 11 studies summarized by Winkle (1) concluded that arrhythmias identified on ambulatory ECG monitoring were important for predicting subsequent death. In addition, there is strong evidence from different studies that the extent of coronary heart disease and left ventricular dysfunction also play an important role in defining high risk groups. Schulze et al. (2) demonstrated that sudden death in patients after myocardial infarction occurred primarily in the group with both advanced grades of ventricular arrhythmias and an ejection fraction of less than 0.40. More recently Bigger (3) found a high mortality in patients with postinfarction ventricular tachycardia (38%, 1-year-mortality rate compared with a rate of 11,6% in the group of patients without tachycardia). He concluded that these patients should be considered for treatment with antiarrhythmic agents. Nevertheless management of left ventricular dysfunction and ischemia may also play an important role in treating these high risks patients.

Table 2 shows the increasing number of antiarrhythmic drugs now available in most European countries; some of them are still investigational in the United States. These newer agents are under intensive investigation and encouraging results have been published both for suppressing supraventricular and ventricular arrhythmias. Nevertheless these drugs should be used carefully, since adverse effects are not uncommon.

Before starting antiarrhythmic therapy it should be considered that there are no studies which validate the fact that antiarrhythmic treatment in high risk patients improves mortality. Therefore the potential advantages – prevention of sudden death and relief of symptoms – must be weighed against the risks.

Table 1. Innocent premature ventricular contractions.

1) Healthy individuals
2) Normal ECG, normal exercise test
3) Normal x-ray, TI-Scan
4) Normal angiogramm
5) no syncope

Table 2. Classification of antiarrhythmic drugs (modified from Harrison, Drugs – 1981).

Class	Subclass	"Standard" agents	Newer agents
I	A	Quinidine	Ajmaline
		Procainamide	Disopyramide
	B	Lidocaine	Aprindine
		Phenytoin	Ethmozin
			Mexilitine
			Tocainide
	C		Encainide
			Flecainide
			Lorcainide
II		Propranolol	Other Beta-blockers
III			Amiodarone
			Bretylium
			N–Acetylprocainamide
IV			Verapamil

Table 3. Benefits and risks of antiarrhythmic drug treatment.

Benefits	Risks
1. Prevention of sudden death	1. Side effects — cardiac / non cardiac / miscellaneous
2. Relief of symptoms	2. Cardiac decompensation
	3. Aggravation of ventricular arrhythmias
	4. Drug interactions

The benefits and risks of antiarrhythmic drug treatment are shown in Table 3. Side effects may occur frequently, especially when higher dosages are used and sometimes limit long-term antiarrhythmic therapy. Worsening of cardiac function is a second risk of antiarrhythmic drug therapy. In particular disopyramide exerts a profound negative myocardial inotropic effect and severe myocardial depression has been observed both in patients with and without preexisting congestive heart failure (4). A third problem, which should be considered before starting antiarrhythmic drug therapy, is the potential worsening of ventricular arrhythmias by antiarrhythmic agents. Precise ECG-monitoring and stimulation techniques demonstrate that this type of adverse reaction is of growing clinical importance. Using Holter-monitoring and exercise testing for evaluation of drug efficacy Velebit (5) observed a worsening of ventricular arrhythmias in 11% of the drug tests. Another phenomenon, the conversion of nonsustained to sustained ventricular tachycardia after administration of antiarrhythmic drugs was reported by Rinkenberger (6), who used programmed stimulation for the evaluation of drug efficacy. But it is noteworthy that most of the patients in this study who had nonsustained ventricular tachycardia during baseline study and sustained VT after drug administration had a history of sustained ventricular tachycardia or ventricular fibrillation. Drug interactions, which can provoke dangerous rhythm disorders, should also be taken into account before starting antiarrhythmic therapy (7, 8).

At present there is general agreement that programmed electrical stimulation and 24-hour ECG monitoring have led to new and important insights into the mechanisms and management of malignant ventricular arrhythmias. These techniques in combination with measurement of drug serum levels are very useful to test drug effectiveness in patients with life-threatening arrhythmias.

Programmed Electrical Stimulation

Programmed electrical stimulation is a very specific method (95–99%) for the detection of ventricular tachycardias (9, 10). The sensitivity ranges between 65 and 86% (11, 9). Therefore, Livelli concluded, "that ventricular tachycardia induced with programmed ventricular stimulation is an excellent basis for guiding the management of clinically significant ventricular tachyarrhythmias regardless of underlying heart disease". Previous studies (12, 13) have demonstrated, that suppression of the ability to initiate ventricular tachycardias by means of programmed stimulation predicts future protection from recurrent ventricular tachyarrhythmias.

Testing of an increasing number of drugs suitable for long-term therapy has been performed by different groups. For instance, quinidine was found effective by programmed stimulation in 34% of patients (14) and similar results have been reported from disopyramide (15). Podrid published a 46% response rate to tocainide (16), whereas mexiletine did not prevent inducibility in all of the 11 patients studied by Palileo (17).

By way of summary we may say that class I antiarrhythmic agents proved to result in an effective suppression of arrhythmias by means of programmed stimulation in 30–50% of the patients. As mentioned above there is general agreement in different studies that a drug which prevents induction of ventricular tachycardia during programmed stimulation will also result in long-term arrhythmia suppression, provided that the therapeutic blood serum concentrations are maintained. It is also well known that long-term antiarrhythmic drug therapy with drugs which had proved ineffective during programmed stimulation will lead to reccurrence of ventricular tachycardia in the majority of patients. This may be not apply to patients treated with amiodarone. Amiodarone, a class III antiarrhythmic drug with antianginal properties, is used increasingly in patients with malignant ventricular arrhythmias.

We have used serial programmed electrical stimulation for evaluation of drug effectiveness in 25 patients with sustained ventricular tachycardia and/or ventricular fibrillation (Figure 1). Our study protocol consists of 1 and 2 extrastimuli during spontaneous rhythm and at basic cycle lengths of 600, 500, 430 and 380 msec; in addition short bursts (180/min–200/min) were included. Serial testing was started with class I agents (1–4 trials) and when these drugs or combinations of them proved ineffective, amiodarone therapy was initiated. Programmed stimulation was repeated after 3–4 weeks of amiodarone therapy. Our results show that patients not inducible when on drugs, have no recurrences during long-term therapy. In 1 case the recurrence of VT during propafenone-therapy was due to non compliance (propafenon serum concentration at admission proved to be 0). A second programmed stimulation after resumption of propafenone therapy again

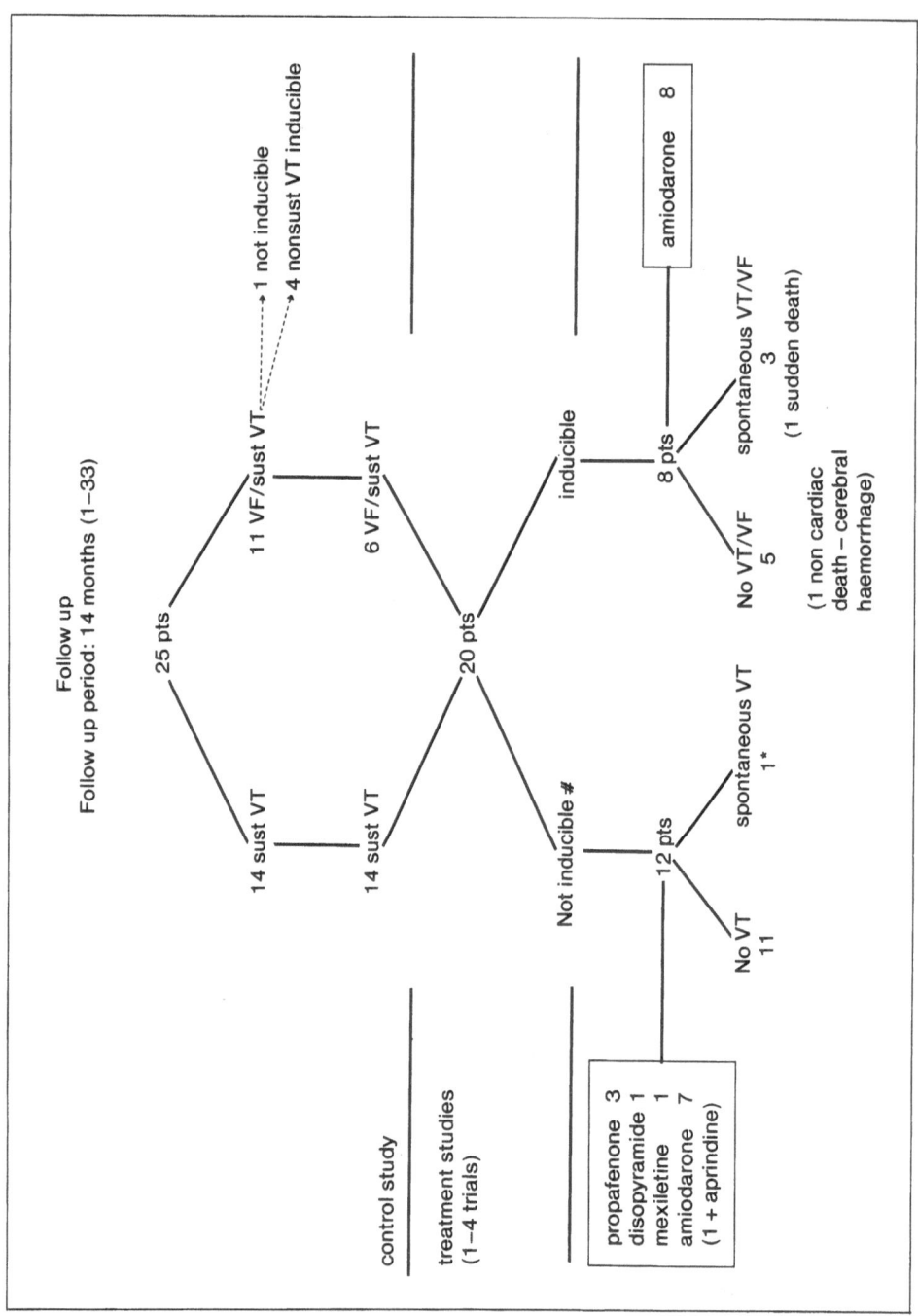

Figure 1. Results of programed stimulation and clinical follow-up of 25 patients with sustained ventricular tachycardia and/or ventricular fibrillation (see text).

\# not inducible (defined as 0–10 beats during programmed stimulation in patients with previous sustained VT).

* Recurrence of VT was due to non-compliance (propafenone serum concentration at admission 0 μg/ml).

showed effective arrhythmia suppression and no relapse occurred in this patient during long-term follow up.

In 25 patients treated with amiodarone Mc Govern (19) found similar results, which indicate that the response to programmed stimulation is highly predictive of long-term clinical outcome, even in amiodarone treated patients. However, Waxmann (18) found a dissociation between arrhythmia induction and clinical response. 38 of 43 patients were still inducible after administration of amiodarone but 50% of these patients had no recurrent ventricular tachycardia or ventricular fibrillation during follow-up. In our group of 15 amiodarone treated patients 8 were still inducible during programmed stimulation. 5 of these 8 patients had no recurrences of VT/VF during long-term follow up. However, amiodarone seems to be a very potent antiarrhythmic drug, but further studies are necessary to clarify the role of programmed stimulation in the evaluation of amiodarone efficacy.

Using programmed stimulation for evaluation of drug efficacy the route of drug administration may be of importance. There are three major limitations of drug testing with programmed stimulation using i.v. administration. First, no steady state is reached and high serum levels may not represent effective tissue concentrations. Tissue concentrations at specific sites, for instance in ischemic regions may be low. A third point is that metabolites formed during chronic therapy may contribute to the antiarrhythmic properties of the drug. The disadvantage of oral drug administration is the long duration of serial drug testing.

Ambulatory ECG-Monitoring

A second method for defining therapeutic efficacy is 24-h ECG monitoring. This method is very useful in patients with a high baseline PVC frequency. Nevertheless, the high rate of spontaneous variability (20) in ventricular ectopy must be taken into account before an effective response to drug administration is defined. Figure 2 illustrates an acute drug test with propafenone; 1 hour after administration of 450 mg propafenone complete abolition of PVC's and couplets occurs.

Graboys and coworkers (21) used ambulatory monitoring for the evaluation of drug effectiveness in patients who had experienced ventricular tachycardia or ventricular fibrillation. Long-term antiarrhythmic therapy was based on the results of acute drug testing. A positive response was defined as a 50% or greater reduction in the total number of PVC's, a reduction of more than 90% in grade 4 ventricular beats and complete ablation of grade 4 B and 5 PVC's. During follow up the mortality rate in those patients, in whom arrhythmia suppression could not be achieved was strikingly higher than in patients with well suppressed ventricular arrhythmias. However, acute drug testing cannot be performed in patients who do not have frequent and advanced grades of PVC's during Holter-monitoring. In addition, data from Platia (22) who compared the predictive value of programmed stimulation and Holter-monitoring in patients with ventricular tachycardia and ventricular fibrillation suggest that, although ventricular tachycardia on Holter is associated with a poor clinical outcome, the overall predictive accuracy of Holter-monitoring is of limited value in predicting those with a good clinical outcome. In contrast, programmed electrical stimulation was predictive of both good and poor clinical

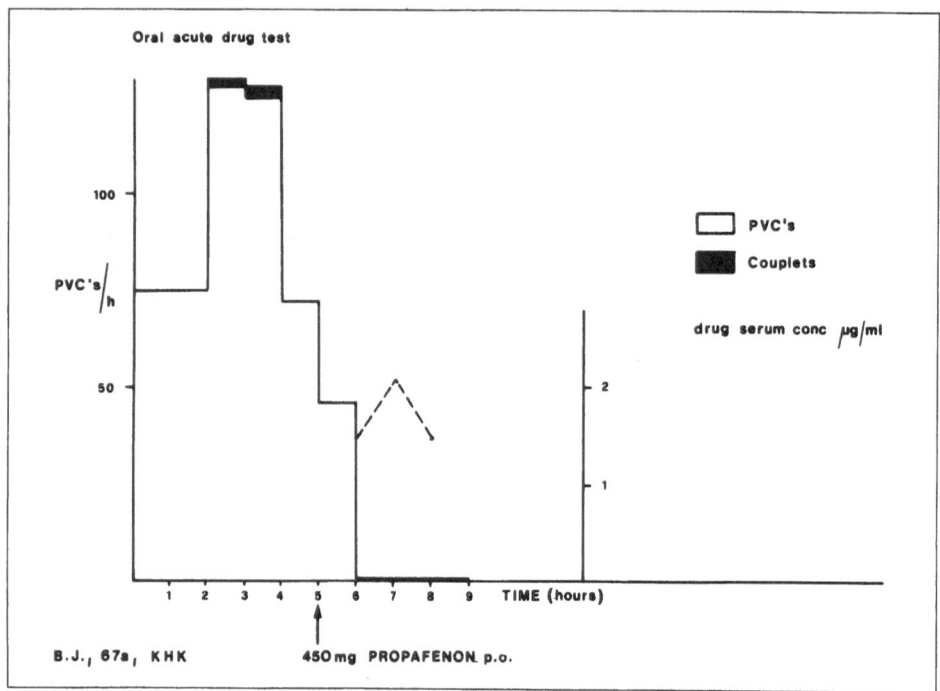

Figure 2. Acute drug test with propafenone in a 67-year old male with CHD. Note complete ablation of PVC's and couplets 1 hour after drug administration. Drug serum concentrations within the therapeutic range.

outcome. In 1979 Myerburg (23) reported the long term effects of class I drugs (Quinidine, Procainamide) on ventricular arrhythmias in survivors of prehospital cardiac arrest. In this study there was no significant difference in PVC frequency in patients with and without recurrent cardiac arrests. In contrast, all 8 patients with recurrent cardiac arrests during follow up had unstable plasma levels while 6 of 8 patients who have not had further episodes of VT or VF had consistently therapeutic drug serum concentrations. Myerburg concluded that clinical effectiveness of antiarrhythmic drugs may not be best measured by their effect on chronic PVC's.

Conclusions

Important advances in drug therapy of malignant ventricular arrhythmias have been made during the last years. However, the "perfect antiarrhythmic agent (i.e., high toxic to therapeutic ratio, long half-life time, minimal side-effects, availability of oral and intravenous preparations and high clinical efficacy) has yet to be introduced" (B. N. Singh). Programmed stimulation and 24-h ECG monitoring seem to be reliable methods to evaluate drug effectiveness. Nevertheless, further studies are necessary before these approaches can be recommended for routine use.

References

1. Winkle RA: Detection of patients at high risk for sudden death: the role of electrographic monitoring. In Kulbertus HE, Wellens HJJ, eds. Sudden death. The Hague: Martinus Niijhoff, 1980: 275–296.
2. Schulze RA, Strauss WH, Pitt B: Sudden death in the year following myocardial infarction: relation to ventricular premature contractions in the late hospital phase and left ventricular ejection fraction. Am J Med 1977; 62: 192–199.
3. Bigger JTh, Jr, Weld FM, Rolnitzky LM: Prevalence, characteristics and significance of ventricular tachycardia (three or more complexes) detected with ambulatory electrocardiographic recording in the late hospital phase of acute myocardial infarction. Am J Cardiol 1981; 48: 815–823.
4. Podrid PJ, Schoeneberger A, Lown B: Congestive heart failure caused by oral disopyramide. N Engl J Med 1980; 302: 614–617.
5. Velebit V, Podrid PJ, Lown B, Cohen BH, Graboys ThB: Aggravation and provocation of ventricular arrhythmias by antiarrhythmic drugs. Circulation 1982; 65: 886–894.
6. Rinkenberger RL, Prystowsky EN, Jackman WM, Naccarelli GV, Heger JJ, Zipes DP: Drug conversion of nonsustained ventricular tachycardia to sustained ventricular tachycardia during serial electrophysiologic studies: Identification of drugs that exacerbate tachycardia andn potential mechanisms. Am Heart J 1982; 103: 177–184.
7. Tartini R, Kappenberger L, Steinbrunn W, Meyer UA: Dangerous interaction between amiodarone and quinidine. Lancet 1982; 1: 1327–1329.
8. Steinbach K, Frohner K, Meisl F, Unger G: Interaction between propafenone and other drugs. In: Schlepper M, Olsson B, eds. Cardiac Arrhythmias. Proceedings 1st international Rytmonorm-Congress. Springer-Verlag 1983; 141–147.
9. Fisher JD: Role of electrophysiologic testing in the diagnosis and treatment of patients with known and suspected bradycardias and tachycardias. Prog Cardiovasc Dis 1981; 24: 25–90.
10. Vandepol CJ, Farshidi A, Spielman Sr, Greenspan AM, Horowitz LN, Josephson ME: Incidence and clinical significance of induced ventricular tachycardia. Am J Cardiol 1980; 45: 725–31.
11. Livelli FD, Bigger JTh, Reiffel JA, Gang ES, Patton JN, Noethling PM, Rolnitzky LM, Gliklich JI: Response to Programmed Ventricular Stimulation: Sensitivity and Relation to Heart Disease. Am J Cardiol 1982; 50: 452–458.
12. Horowitz LN, Josephson ME, Farshidi A, Spielman SR, Michelson EL, Greenspan AM: Recurrent sustained ventricular tachycardia. 3. Role of the electrophysiologic study in selection of antiarrhythmic regimes. Circulation 1978; 58: 986–997.
13. Mason J, Winkle RA: Electrode-catheter arrhythmia induction in the selection and assessment of antiarrhythmic drug therapy for recurrent ventricular tachycardia. Circulation 1978; 58: 971–985.
14. DiMarco JP, Garan H, Ruskin JN: Quinidine for Ventricular Arrhythmias: Value of Electrophysiologic Testing. Am J Cardiol 1983; 51: 90–95.
15. Lerman BB, Waxman HL, Buxton AE, Josephson ME: Disopyramide: Evaluation of Electrophysiologic Effects and Clinical Efficacy in Patients With Sustained Ventricular Tachycardia or Ventricular Fibrillation. Am J Cardiol 1983; 51: 759–764.
16. Podrid PJ, Lown B: Tocainide for refractory symptomatic ventricular arrhythmias. Am J Cardiol 1982; 49: 1279–1285.
17. Palileo EV, Welch W, Hoff J, Strasberg B, Bauernfeind RA, Swiryn S, Coelho A, Rosen KM: Lack of effectiveness of oral mexiletine in patients with drug-refractory paroxysmal sustained ventricular tachycardia. Am J Cardiol 1982; 50: 1075–1081.
18. Waxman HL, Groh WC, Marchlinski FE, Buxton AE, Sadowsky LM, Horowitz LN, Josephson ME, Kastor JA: Amiodarone for control of sustained ventricular tachyarrhythmia: clinical and electrophysiologic effects in 51 patients. Am J Cardiol 1982; 50: 1066–1074.
19. McGovern B, Garen H, Malacoff RF, DiMarco JP, Sellers TD, Ruskin JN: Predictive accuracy of electrophysiologic testing in the treatment of ventricular arrhythmias with amiodarone. Circulation 1982; 66: 11–223.
20. Morganroth J: Ambulatory monitoring: the impact of spontaneous variability of simple and complex ventricular ectopy. In: Donald C. Harrison, eds. Cardiac Arrhythmias – a decade of progress. Boston, Massachusetts: G. K. Hall Medical Publishers, 1980; 479–492.

21. Graboys TB, Lown B, Podrid PJ, DeSilva R: Long-term survival of patients with malignant ventricular arrhythmia treated with antiarrhythmic drugs. Am J Cardiol 1982; 50: 437–443.
22. Platia EV, Vlay Sc, Reid PR: A comparison of the predictive value of programmed electrial stimulation and Holter monitoring in patients with malignant ventricular arrhythmias. Am J Cardiol 1982; 49: 928.
23. Myerburg RJ, Conde C, Sheps DS, Appel RA, Kiem I, Sung RJ, Castellanos A: Antiarrhythmic drug therapy in survivors of prehospital cardiac arrest: comparison of effects on chronic ventricular arrhythmias and recurrent cardiac arrest. Circulation 1979; 59: 855.

Supported in part by "Jubiläumsfonds der Österreichischen Nationalbank; Projekt Nr. 1998" and Hochschuljubiläumsstiftung der Stadt Wien.

Authors' address:
Dr. K. J. Frohner
Wilhelminenspital
III. Med. Abteilung
Montleartstr. 37
A-1171 Wien

Role of Electrophysiologic Studies with Acute Drug Testing in Refractory Supraventricular Tachycardia

S. Saksena, J. Jacobs, S. T. Rothbart, K. Liptak

Summary: Twenty-two symptomatic patients with recurrent and refractory supraventricular tachy-arrhythmias (SVT) underwent electrophysiologic studies (EPS) to determine the precise mechanism of their arrhythmia, 13 patients had atrial fibrillation/flutter and 12 patients had reentrant PSVT. Sixteen of these pts had acute drug testing during programmed electrical stimulation (Group A) to select long term antiarrhythmic therapy and 6 patients had empirical selection of drug therapy based on the mechanism of SVT determined during EPS (Group B). Group A patients underwent 1–8 (mean 2.3 ± 1.8) acute drug tests. Group B patients were empirically treated with 1–3 (mean 2.2 ± 0.8) drugs per patient.

All 16 patients in Group A (100%) remained symptom-free on selected therapy without recurrent SVT during a follow-up period of 2–23 (mean 12 ± 7) months. In group B, 4 patients (66%) have had no recurrences of SVT or symptoms, while 2 patients have had recurrences during 15–24 (mean 18 ± 6) months of follow-up. We conclude that selection of chronic drug therapy based on SVT mechanism alone may be fairly successful in patients with refractory SVT but antiarrhythmic therapy on the basis of acute drug testing is superior and highly predictive of long-term response.

Introduction

Clinical electrophysiologic studies (EPS) using programmed electrical stimulation (PES) have been used to determine the precise mechanism of reentrant supraventricular tachycardia (1, 2, 3). Provocative drug testing using PES has been used to select effective long term antiarrhythmic therapy in patients with recurrent ventricular tachycardia (4, 5). This approach has been reported to be both clinically superior and cost-effective (6). Recent investigations have suggested that similar drug testing techniques can be applied to *selected subgroups* of patients with reentrant SVT and paroxysmal atrial fibrillation (7, 8, 9).

In this study we compared the long term clinical efficacy of antiarrhythmic therapy selected using serial drug testing with therapy selected empirically on the basis of the mechanism of SVT determined during EPS in *all types* of refractory SVT.

Methods

The selection criteria for entry into this study were:

1. Symptomatic patients with recurrent sustained SVT. "Recurrent" was defined as 3 or more episodes of SVT and "sustained" was defined as an arrhythmia of more than 30 seconds duration.
2. Electrocardiographic documentation of SVT.
3. Reproducible induction of SVT during EPS.

Electrophysiologic Study

All patients underwent baseline EPS in the nonsedated and post-absorptive state after obtaining informed consent. Antiarrhythmic therapy was discontinued at least five drug half-lives prior to the study. Standard venous and arterial catheterization techniques were utilized. A Berkovits-Castellanos hexapolar electrode catheter was used for atrial and ventricular pacing. A tetrapolar electrode catheter was used to record His Bundle electrograms. Additional tetrapolar electrode catheters were used to record multiple intracardiac electrograms. Recording sites included high, mid and low lateral right atrium, proximal and distal coronary sinus. Right ventricular recording sites included right ventricular apex, mid-septum and outflow tract. Three surface electrocardiographic leads (I, AVF, V1) were recorded simultaneously with intracardiac electrograms. Arterial blood pressure was monitored using an indwelling femoral arterial cannula. A multichannel display recorder (Electronics for Medicine VR-12, White Plains N.Y.) was used to amplify and display the electrograms. Hard copy recordings were obtained at speeds of 100–250 mm/sec. All data was stored on magnetic FM tape. PES was performed utilizing a custom-made programmed stimulator (Bloom Associates, Ltd., Narberth Pa.) which delivered rectangular pulses of 1 msec duration at twice diastolic threshold.

The PES protocol used for the induction of SVT included:

1. Single atrial premature extrastimuli during sinus and high right atrial drive rhythms at two or more cycle lengths;
2. Rapid atrial pacing with incremental rates until the Wenckebach phenomenon was observed;
3. Two premature atrial extrastimuli during atrial drive rhythm;
4. High rate atrial pacing up to rates of 800/minute for induction of sustained atrial flutter/fibrillation;
5. Single premature ventricular extrastimuli in sinus rhythm or ventricular drive rhythm at two or more cycle lengths;
6. Rapid ventricular pacing at cycle lengths of 400–250 ms or up to ventricular refractoriness, whichever was shorter.

Extrastimuli were introduced late in diastole in the spontaneous or paced rhythm. Coupling intervals of the extrastimuli were reduced in 10–20 ms decrements until refractoriness was reached. Additional extrastimuli were introduced at coupling intervals 50 msec greater than the refractory periods and the interval was gradually reduced. If PES from initial stimulation sites (high right atrium, right ventricular apex) was unsuccessful in arrhythmia induction, alternative sites (low right atrium, coronary sinus, left atrium) were used and the PES protocol repeated.

3. Serial EP Drug Testing

Consenting patients underwent follow-up EPS upon completion of drug administration. The stimulation protocol utilized in these studies was identical to the one used in control study in the same patient. Blood drug concentrations were obtained during follow-up EPS.

4. Selection of Chronic Oral Therapy

In patients completing drug testing (Group A), the drug/s noted to suppress induction of sustained SVT were continued. In patients who did not undergo drug testing (Group B), long-term antiarrhythmic therapy was empirically chosen on the basis of the mechanism of the SVT alone. The efficacy of such therapy was evaluated by clinical arrhythmia suppression as determined by symptoms, telemetry, 24 hour ambulatory ECG monitoring and exercise testing.

Non-invasive Studies

Patients showing successful arrhythmia suppression on drug therapy both spontaneously and during PES underwent a 24 hour ambulatory ECG recording and a symptom limited exercise test. The ambulatory ECG was analysed qualitatively. A modified Bruce protocol was used in the treadmill exercise test.

Clinical Follow-up

Patients were evaluated during the follow-up period with periodic clinical evaluations (3 month intervals), ambulatory 24-hour ECG recordings as well as through direct communication with either the patient or referring physician. No patient was lost to follow-up.

Data Analysis

Statistical comparison between patient groups was performed using a chi-square analysis.

Results

1. Clinical Characteristics (Table 1)

Twenty-two patients met the study inclusion criteria. There were 12 males and 10 females, age range 16–73 (mean 53 ± 17) years. Twelve patients had organic heart disease documented with invasive and noninvasive studies. Twelve patients presented with PSVT (reentrant) and 13 had paroxysmal atrial flutter/fibrillation. Three patients had both arrhythmias. Four patients had electrocardiographic manifestations of the preexcitation syndrome. The duration of the arrhythmia ranged from 1–480 (mean 89 ± 129) months prior to admission for EPS. The number of empirical drug trials prior to EPS was 1–5 (mean 2.8 ± 1.2) drugs. Rates of spontaneous SVT ranged from 100 to 300 (mean 196 ± 54) beats/min.

Table 1. Clinical characteristics of Patient Population.

	PT	Age	Sex	Diagnoses	SVT duration (months)	Rate (BPM)	Drug trials
1.	A.S.	57	M	NSHD/PAF	3	220	4
2.	L.S.	65	M	CAD/HTN/PAF	24	100	2
3.	M.O.	52	F	MVP/PSVT	216	200	2
4.	R.G.	67	F	NSDH/Preexcitation PSVT/PAF	12	300	3
5.	E.W.	59	M	Cardiomyopathy PAF	1	150	2
6.	C.O.	48	F	MVP/PSVT	216	180	2
7.	J.R.	48	F	NSHD/PSVT	36	160	2
8.	F.B.	38	F	NSHD/PSVT	216	225	4
9.	A.D.	61	F	RHD/PAF	3	150	2
10.	A.M.	67	M	IHSS/PAF	180	150	3
11.	P.G.	47	M	NSHD/Preexcitation PAF	4	250	3
12.	V.Z.	72	F	CAD/RHD/PAF	12	125	2
13.	J.G.	69	F	CAD/PAF	4	260	5
14.	J.T.	63	M	CAD/Preexcitation PSVT/PAF	180	300	5
15.	E.M.	69	M	CAD/PAF	2	220	3
16.	J.M.	67	F	HTN/PAF	24	250	4
17.	K.N.	17	M	NSHD/PSVT/PAF	24	200	4
18.	S.W.	39	F	MVP/Preexcitation PSVT	24	220	4
19.	A.P.	72	M	NSHD/PSVT	480	160	5
20.	A.P.	58	M	NSHD/PSVT	24	170	2
21.	E.B.	23	F	NSHD/PSVT	4	170	1
22.	L.R.	17	F	NSHD/PSVT	6	150	2

Abbreviations:
CAD – Coronary artery disease
IHSS – Idiopathic hypertrophic subaortic stenosis
HTN – Hypertension
MVP – Mitral valve prolapse
RHD – Rheumatic heart disease
PSVT – Paroxysmal supraventricular tachycardia
PAF – Paroxysmal atrial flutter/fibrillation.
NSHD – No significant heart disease.

2. Control EP Studies:

All patients had successful induction of sustained SVT during the control EP study. The arrhythmia mechanisms delineated at the time of this study are summarized in Table 2. Paroxysmal SVT was noted in 12 patients (55%). Six patients had A-V nodal reentry (Type I – 5 patients, Type II – 1 patient). Five patients had WPW syndrome with ortho-dromic PSVT being the most common arrhythmia. One patient had sinoatrial reentrant tachycardia.

714

Sustained atrial flutter/fibrillation was induced in 13 patients (59%). Concomitant ventricular preexcitation was present in 7 patients. Of these patients three had complete AV bypass tracts, three patients had partial AV nodal bypass or preferential AV nodal conduction and one patient had an atrio-His bypass tract.

3. Drug Studies

Sixteen patients underwent 1–8 drug tests (mean 2.3 ± 1.8) to identify suppressive antiarrhythmic therapy (Group A). Six patients did not undergo drug testing and selection of antiarrhythmic therapy was on the basis of SVT mechanism alone. One to 3 (mean 2.2 ± 0.8) drug trials were performed to identify a drug demonstrating arrhythmia suppression noninvasively.

Table 3 summarizes the drugs tested in Groups A and B. Chronic antiarrhythmic therapy selected in this patient population included digoxin (5 patients), propranolol (4 pa-

Table 2. Arrhythmia Mechanisms in 22 Patients with Paroxysmal SVT at Control EPS.

Reentrant Supraventricular Tachycardia	– 12 Patients
AV Nodal Reentry	– 6 Patients
– Type I	– 5 Patients
– Type II	– 1 Patient
Sinoatrial Reentry	– 1 Patient
Atrioventricular Reentry	– 5 Patients
– Orthodromic	– 4 Patients
– Antidromic	– 1 Patient
Paroxysmal Atrial Flutter/Fibrillation	– 12 Patients
– Absence of Ventricular Preexcitation	– 6 Patients
Atrial Flutter	– 3 Patients
Atrial Fibrillation	– 3 Patients
– Presence of Ventricular Preexcitation	– 7 Patients
Wolff Parkinson White Syndrome	– 3 Patients
Enhanced AV Conduction	– 3 Patients
Atrio-His Bypass Tract	– 1 Patient

Table 3. Drug Trials Performed in Study Groups.

Group A		Group B	
Digoxin	– 2 Patients	Digoxin	– 2 Patients
Procainamide	– 4 Patients	Quinidine	– 4 Patients
Disopyramide	– 1 Patient	Verapamil	– 3 Patients
Verapamil	– 11 Patients	Propranolol	– 3 Patients
Propranolol	– 3 Patients	Procainamide	– 1 Patient
Aprindine	– 2 Patients		
Amiodarone	– 6 Patients		
Quinidine	– 1 Patient		

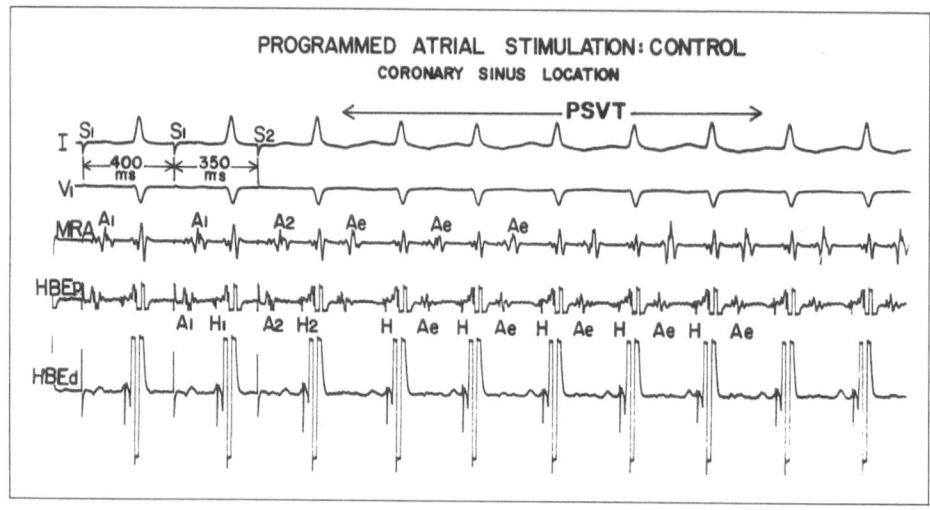

Fig. 1A. Induction of sustained atrioventricular reentrant tachycardia using programmed atrial stimulation from the coronary sinus. The tachycardia cycle length is 350 ms.

Abbreviations:

MRA – Mid right atrium

HBEp – Proximal His Bundle Electrograms

HBEd – Distal His Bundle Electrograms

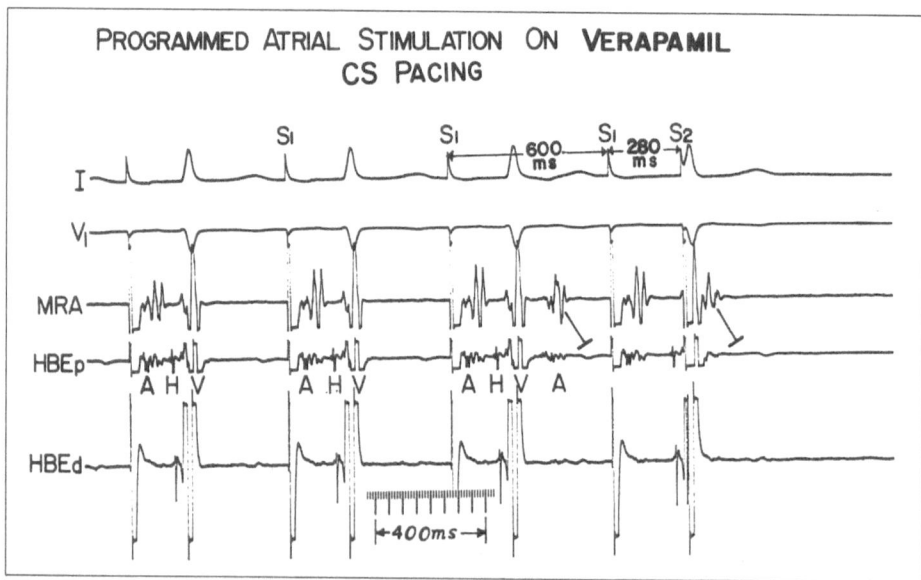

Fig. 1B. Programmed atrial stimulation from the coronary sinus after intravenous verapamil in the same patient as in Fig. 1A. Note single atrial echo beat during atrial pacing with AV nodal block.

Abbreviations: Same as in Fig. 1A.

tients), verapamil (9 patients), diisopyramide (1 patient), quinidine (3 patients), procainamide (4 patients), aprindine (1 patient) and amiodarone (1 patient). One patient underwent implantation of an antitachycardia pacemaker. Seven patients required combination therapy.

Fig. 1 shows induction of sustained AV nodal reentrant tachycardia during PES in a 22 year old female with symptomatic SVT. After administration of intravenous verapamil (10 mg) PES demonstrated inability to reinduce the sustained arrhythmia due to atrioventricular nodal block. Oral verapamil therapy has successfully suppressed the arrhythmia in this patient.

4. Clinical Follow-up

During the follow-up period of 2–23 (mean 12 ± 7) months for Group A, all 16 patients (100%) remained symptom free and with no evidence of recurrent SVT. Three patients (paroxysmal SVT – 2, atrial fibrillation – 1) experienced late side effects with diisopyramide (1), verapamil (1) and aprindine (1). All three patients experienced arrhythmias recurrences after discontinuation of therapy. Alternative EP based therapy was selected and tolerated by two patients who continue to show a favorable response. One patient who refused further EP evaluation continued to experience symptomatic recurrences. One patient in Group A died of an unrelated cause (chronic renal failure). In Group B, 4 patients (66%) had no recurrences of their arrhythmias, while 2 patients (33%) had documented recurrent episodes of SVT (atrial fibrillation with preexcitation – 1 pt, AV nodal reentry – 1 pt) during 7–24 (mean 18 ± 6) months of follow-up. There is a statistically significant difference in arrhythmia response between Groups A and B (P < 0.025).

Discussion

Previous clinical studies have demonstrated reproducible arrhythmia induction using PES in patients with paroxysmal SVT and paroxysmal atrial fibrillation (1, 2). Arrhythmia induction is used to analyse the mechanism/s of arrhythmogenesis and the electrophysiologic substrate/s involved in its maintenance (1, 2). Macro and microreentrant mechanisms may be operative in paroxysmal supraventricular tachycardia and paroxysmal atrial fibrillation (1, 2, 9). Programmed electrical stimulation may initiate these arrhythmias by creating conditions of slow conduction and unindirectional block in the electrophysiologic substrate. These techniques also provide an objective method to evaluate drug therapy. While drug therapy may be directed at suppression of the initiating event (premature depolarizations), it, more commonly, is effective by altering the electrophysiologic properties of the substrate for SVT (2, 3, 9). Our results would also confirm these observations.

Using these arrhythmia induction techniques, some investigators have reported a high predictive value of serial drug testing in paroxysmal SVT and atrial fibrillation (7, 8, 9). The number of patients in these reports has been small and follow-up limited in duration. It has also not been determined if successful drug therapy selection is related to elucidation of arrhythmia mechanism/s alone during EPS or serial drug testing of possibly effective antiarrhythmic agents. The results of this study indicate that drug therapy select-

717

ed on the basis of mechanism of SVT alone may be effective in some patients with refractory SVT. However, the long term clinical efficacy of therapy selected on the basis of drug testing is superior to that selected on the basis of mechanisms alone.

This study encompassed a wider variety of SVT and antiarrhythmic therapy than previous reports (7–9). The implications of these observations would be to advocate use of arrhythmia induction studies in patients with refractory SVT. With the safety of these procedures being established (10), these studies could prove to be cost effective in patients with SVT by avoiding multiple admissions for the same diagnosis. This has already been established for patients with recurrent ventricular tachycardia (6). While the details of stimulation and drug administration protocols for serial drug testing need further evaluation, preliminary data would support continuing clinical application of this technique.

References

1. Bigger JT, Goldreyer BN: The mechanism of supraventricular tachycardia. Circulation 1970; 42: 673.
2. Wu D, Denes P, Amat-y-Leon F, Dhingra RC, Wyndham CRC, Bauernfiend R, Latif P, Rosen KM: Clinical, electrocardiographic and electrophysiologic observations in patients with paroxysmal supraventricular tachycardia. Am J Cardiol 1978; 41: 1045.
3. Josephson ME: Paroxysmal supraventricular tachycardia. An electrophysiologic approach. Am J Cardiol 1978; 41: 1123.
4. Horowitz LN, Josephson ME, Farshidi A, Spielman S, Michelson EL, Greenspan AM: Recurrent sustained ventricular tachycardia 3. Role of the electrophysiologic study in selection of antiarrhythmic regimens. Circulation 1978; 58: 986.
5. Mason JW, Winkle RA: Electrode catheter arrhythmia induction in selection and assessment of antiarrhythmic drug therapy for recurrent ventricular tachycardia. Circulation 1978; 58: 971.
6. Ferguson D, Saksena S, Greenberg E, Craelius W: Clinical and economic impact of electrophysiologic evaluation of recurrent ventricular tachycardia: A three year study (abstr). PACE 1983; 6: 312.
7. Wu D, Amat-y-Leon F, Simpson RJ Jr, Latif P, Wyndham CRC, Denes P, Rosen KM: Electrophysiological studies with multiple drugs in patients with atrioventricular reentrant tachycardia utilizing an extranodal pathway. Circulation 1977; 56: 727.
8. Bauernfiend RA, Wyndham CR, Dhingra RC, Swiryn SP, Palileo E, Strasberg B, Rosen KM: Serial electrophysiologic testing of multiple drugs in patients with atrioventricular nodal reentrant paroxysmal tachycardia. Circulation 1980; 62: 1341.
9. Bauernfiend RA, Swiryn SP, Strasberg B, Palileo E, Scagliotti D, Rosen KM: Electrophysiologic drug testing in prophylaxis of sporadic paroxysmal atrial fibrillation: Technique, application and efficacy in severely symptomatic preexcitation patients. Am Ht J 1982; 103: 941.
10. Di Marco J, Garan H, Ruskin JN: Complications in patients undergoing cardiac electrophysiologic procedures 1982; 97: 490.

Authors' address:
S. Saksena, M.D.
Cardiac Electrophysiology
Newark Beth Israel Medical Center
201 Lyons Avenue
Newark, NJ 07112

Detection of Arrhythmias and Control of Efficacy of Antiarrhythmic Treatment – Role of Exercise Test and Long-Term ECG Monitoring

H. Weber, G. Joskowicz, Ch. Auinger

Summary: On the one hand arrhythmias occur asymptomatically. On the other hand they increase the risk of sudden death. Exercise stress test (ET) and longterm-ECG (LT-ECG) recordings are commonly used methods to detect arrhythmias and to evaluate antiarrhythmic therapy.

In normals exercise induced ventricular arrhythmias (VA) were present in 14–44%, whereas complex VA occur in 1–5%. The high sensitivity of LT-ECG led to a VA-detection rate between 41–77%, whereas 6–35% of the normals had complex VA. The detection rate depends on the monitoring duration. Comparing both methods, LT-ECG is more sensitive than ET in the VA-detection, but only if disregarding symptoms (angina) and ST-segment alterations. Post myocardial infarction exercise-induced angina and/or ST-depression stratifies the risk group more clearly than VA.

Otherwise many studies dealing with LT-ECG in the postinfarction period can demonstrate an increased risk of sudden death if complex VA could be found.

In the evaluation of an antiarrhythmic therapy ET was not used extensively. But it gives additional information in 15%, LT-ECG is limited by the spontaneous variability of infrequent arrhythmias, which can "mimick" a therapeutic success, Nevertheless a "drug effect" (i.e. statistically significant VA-reduction under prolonged monitoring duration) can be measured using LT-ECG. So both methods together have to be recommended to be used in the evaluation of therapy.

In conclusion ET and LT-ECG are valuable tools in the detection of VA, risk stratification and evaluation of antiarrhythmic treatment with the mentioned limitations. The application of both complementary methods will help us to evaluate our intentions to improve high-risk-patients' probability to survive.

Introduction

Arrhythmias and sudden death are a contemporary challenge (1). Arrhythmias per se can be lethal or are precursors of death. Risk profiles especially for the coronary heart disease (CHD) were developed for identification of high risk groups and for the evaluation of the efficacy of different therapeutic strategies used (2, 3).

While trying to solve these problems two noninvasive methods have passed methodological discussions and have approached today into the clinical routine: Exercise stress test (ET) and longterm-ECG (LT-ECG) (4–6).

This paper deals with the value of both methods ET and LT-ECG
- in the detection of arrhythmias in obviously healthy persons and in patients preferably with coronary heart disease (CHD);
- in the evaluation of the prognosis of ventricular-arrhythmias (VA) and
- in the evaluation of an antiarrhythmic treatment.

In such an attempt only rare selected papers can be discussed. But we cannot avoid mixing "apples and pears".

Detection of Arrhythmias:

– Normals:

Between 1966 and 1979 many studies dealing with ET in "Normals" (5, 7–14) were published. Primarily the definition of the different collectives used ranged from "obviously normals" over police-, air-, and businessmen to insurance-people. Also the ET-methods used were different.

However, premature ventricular contractions (PVC) were exercise-induced (EIVA) in 14–44%, whereas in 0–5% complex VA (> Lown 2) occurred (Table 1).

In LT-ECG 14–77% of healthy persons developed PVC and 6–35% CVA (Table 2) (15–21).

Differences in the definitions of "normal", the monitoring duration and the analysis methods used etc. limit the possibility of comparing the results with each other.

But it can be concluded that "obviously healthy" persons can develop VA and also CVA during ET and LT-ECG.

Table 1. Exercise-induced ventr. arrh. (EIVA) in "normals". Leg.: PVC% = percentage of "normals" who developed premature ventricular contractions during exercise. CVA% = Complex ventricular arrhythmias (> Lown 2).

		N	Population	PVC%	CVA%
Berkson	66	49	normals	14	–
Rodstein	71	333	insurance	19	–
McHenry	72	561	policemen	37	5
Beard	73	248	businessmen	44	3
Froehlicher	74	1380	airmen	35	3
Jelinek	74	163	normals	19	2
McHenry	76	285	policemen	16	1
Faris	76	462	policemen	36	–
Ekblom	79	163	normals	19	3

Table 2. Ventricular arrhythmias during LT-ECG in "normals". Leg.: LT-ECG = longterm ECG, PVC% = percentage of "normals" who developed premature ventricular contractions during LT–ECG, CVA% = Complex ventricular arrhythmias (> Lown 2).

Study		N	HR	PVC%	CVA%
Amsterdam	73	27	10	44	–
DeMaria	74	35	10	14	–
Clarke	76	86	48	73	8
Brodsky	77	50	24	50	6
Sobotka	81	50	24	76	12
Manger Cats	81	300	24	77	35
Bethge	82	170	24	41	18

720

Both methods were frequently used in patients with different diseases (22–26) to detect VA, predominantly in CHD (22, 23, 25, 26).

Comparing both methods it seems evident that LT-ECG has a higher VA-detection rate than ET (Table 3) (27–32).

From a detailed point of view (Table 4) ET failed in 6–24% of patients with arrhythmias detected by LT-ECG. The latter method used over 10 hours continuously could not detect EIVA in 10 and 19% (Table 4) (27, 28). A prolongation of the recording duration over 24 hrs reduced the percentage of maldetection to 2–7% (Table 4) (29, 32).

In conclusion LT-ECG seems to be more sensitive detecting VA than ET, but with disregard of the other parameters measured only during ET.

Prognostic value of VA in ET and LT-ECG

In ET the major interest was focused on symptoms and on the ST-T-segment during the past.

Only few studies deal with the prognostic value of EIVA post acute myocardial infarction (AMI) (33–41) with opposite results: Some studies demonstrate a 2–4 times enhanced risk of sudden death (SD), if EIVA could be detected early post AMI (34–37). Other authors could not confirm a predictive value of EIVA in accordance to SD (38–41).

Using ET, a prognosis after AMI can also be determined on the basis of symptoms, capacity and ST-segment response (33). Exercise induced angina and ST-depression provided accurate stratification of patients in a subgroup of relatively high and low risk for SD during the year after AMI (42).

Since 1973 the LT-ECG has been used in many postinfarction studies (Table 5) to evaluate arrhythmias as predictive risk factor for SD (43–54).

Despite many differences of the study design the risk of SD increased with the detection of CVA in LT-ECG:

The "Austrian Postinfarction Multicenter Study" (54), which includes only patients after the first penetrating myocardial infarction and younger than 70 years, shows a low inci-

Table 3. Exercise-Stress-Test vs. LT-ECG. Leg.: diff. = different underlying diseases, p. AMI = post acute myocardial infarction, CHD = coronary heart disease.

	Pat. N	Collect.	Exercise		LT-ECG	
			PVC%	CVA%	PVC%	CVA%
Kosowsky	71	66	diff.	39	26	27	14
Crawford	74	60	p. AMI	30	8	37	23
Ryan	75	100	CHD	56	20	88	40
Borer	80	45	p. AMI	38	5	79	42
Simon	80	41	CHD	61	–	59	23
Tiso	82	100	diff.	47	10	78	29
Weber	83	69	p. AMI	17	11	22	10

Table 4. Exercise stress test vs. LT-ECG.

		Kosowsky 71 (66 pts., diff.)					Crawford 74 (60 pts. p. AMI)	
		LT-ECG (10 hr) +	−				LT-ECG (10 hr) +	−
E.T.	+	14 (21%)	12 (19%)		E.T.	+	12 (20%)	6 (10%)
	−	4 (6%)	36 (54%)			−	10 (17%)	32 (53%)

		Ryan 75 (100 pts. CHD)					Tiso 82 (100 pts. diff.)	
		LT-ECG (24 hr) +	−				LT-ECG (24 hr) +	−
E.T.	+	44	2		E.T.	+	42	5
	−	24	30			−	18	35

		Weber 83 (69 pts. p. AMI)	
		LT-ECG (24 hr) +	−
E.T.	+	6 (8%)	5 (7%)
	−	10 (15%)	48 (69%)

dence rate of SD during the first year post AMI (Table 5). The risk for SD increased from 0.6% in patients with rare single PVC to 36% in patients with VT (> 3 consec. PVC) (54).

The probability to survive the first year decreased from 90% to 60% if VT could be detected in LT-ECG (55).

One study compared the results of ET and LT-ECG in CHD-patients with regard to the value of each method in risk group identification (37). Using a multivariate statistical analysis a higher risk group was characterized either by frequent EIVA and VA in LT-ECG or frequent EIVA and ST-segment depression in ET. On the other hand normal ET and LT-ECG stratified a low risk group after AMI (37).

In conclusion the more sensitive LT-ECG is superior to ET in the recognition of high risk patients after AMI, but if only EIVA were taken into account.

Including symptoms and ST-segment alterations ET seems to achieve a similar or better risk stratification than LT-ECG.

But now it is necessary to mention that other risk factors like left ventricular function, akinesia etc. were neglected.

Table 5. Ventricular arrhythmias detected by LT-ECG post AMI and the risk of sudden death. Leg.: Langzeit EKG = longterm ECG. Ueber (Std.) = recording duration (hrs). Wo post AMI = weeks after AMI (rec. date of LT-ECG), VES pos (%) = percentage of PVC detected during LT-ECG. VT = ventricular tachycardia. SCD = sudden cardiac death. Alter von bis (Jahre) = age (years). Monate = months. Oest. Inf. = "Austrian Postinfarction Multicenter Study".

Ref.	Pat. (N)	Follow up (Monate)	Langzeit-EKG über (Std.)	Wo post AMI	VES pos (%)	VT pos (%)	SCD (%)	Alter von bis	(Jahre) m̄
Kotler	73	160	30–54	12	12	80	3	9	<65	–
Moss I	74	100	20	6	3	72	4	4	33–78	57
Vismara	75	64	26	10	3	77	9	19	39–85	61
Moss II	76	272	12	6	3	50	1	5	<65	56
Van Durme	76	150	12	8	4	75	15	8	–	–
Rehnquist	77	160	12	6	3	39	3	6	<66	60
Ruberman	77	1739	24	1	3–6	51	10	5	35–74	–
Schulze	77	81	7	24	2	65	1	10	–	60
Bigger	78	100	12	24	3	80	13	12	25–90	61
De Soyza	78	56	19	24	3	70	4	2	24–73	54
De Busk	81	90	24	12	3	80	2	3	<70	52
Bigger	81	430	12	24	3	–	12	15	–	–
Öst. Inf.	81	216	10	24	3	32	5	5	<70	56
		(3618)	(7–54) m̄ 17	(1–24) m̄ 14	(2–36) m̄ 3.5	(32–80) m̄ 64	(1–12) m̄ 6	(2–19) m̄ 8	–	–

Evaluation of Therapy:

Today many placebo-controlled studies are running treating high risk patients (post AMI) either with antiarrhythmic drugs or with betablockers prophylactically. It is not the main topic of this paper to deal with this type of studies. They do not particularly focus on the treatment of arrhythmias themselves.

Another concept of antiarrhythmic therapy used in the daily routine is the drug induced suppression of VA.

ET was not extensively used for either systematic exposure of arrhythmias or assessment of antiarrhythmic drug efficacy (56).

Otherwise the evaluation of therapy is a domaine of the LT-ECG method: The quantification and qualification of arrhythmias during LT-ECG approached to new informations about the arrhythmias themselves, their behaviour under drug regimen and also to the limitations of the method (57): A prolongation of the monitoring duration up to 24 hrs excluded the circadian variability of arrhythmias. But the increasing spontaneous variability of infrequent arrhythmias particularly under antiarrhythmic therapy needs much more prolongation of the LT-ECG recording duration (> 24 hrs) to avoid a "mimicked therapeutic success" (57–59).

In LT-ECG a "drug effect" can be verified easily (60): under disopyramide treatment 13 (among 15) patients could be classified as responders, who did not develop CVA and the VA-rate decreased statistically significant. In only 5 patients the VA-reduction rate was more than 90%. In accordance to the above mentioned increasing variability of VA with decreasing VA-frequency the LT-ECG prolongation up until 48 hrs demonstrated a reproducible de facto abolition (no CVA, VA < 1%/24 hrs) of the VA under drug therapy only in 2 patients.

LT-ECG measures a "drug effect", but no conclusions can be drawn due to the prognosis of the patients until today.

So far both methods together have only be used in one study to evaluate the efficacy of therapy (61). In 15% LT-ECG and in 25% ET failed to demonstrate a drug induced suppression of CVA. If only LT-ECG was used, in 15% the outcome of drug therapy would be misclassified (61).

In conclusion both methods, ET and LT-ECG, are valuable tools in the detection of VA and risk-stratification, especially if the analysis of ET is not limited to EIVA but includes also other ET-parameters (symptoms, ST-T etc.).

Both methods identify risk groups of SD.

VA and CVA detected with ET and/or LT-ECG increase the risk of SD.

Antiarrhythmic drugs reduce VA, which can be evaluated by both mentioned and other methods.

But the basic question remains: Is the reduction or abolition of VA associated with a decrease of the SD-risk?

Only few data point out that a controlled antiarrhythmic treatment, including ET, LT-ECG, but also electrophysiological, invasive methods, lead to a significant increase of the probability to survive in patients with CVA (62). These data, however, are not uncontradicted (63).

Extensive follow up data have to be achieved under controlled conditions using both complementary methods, ET and LT-ECG, with the aim to reduce the risk of sudden cardiac death and to improve the probability to survive.

References

1. Lown B: Sudden cardiac death-1978. Circ 1979; 60: 1593.
2. Levy RI: Declining mortality in coronary heart disease. Arteriosclerosis 1981; 1: 312–325.
3. Moss AJ, Bigger T jr, Case RB, Gillespie J, Goldstein R et al: Risk stratification and prognostication after myocardial infarction. J A Coll Cardiol 1983; 1: 716 (abstr).
4. Barret PA, Peter T, Swan HJC, Singh BN, Mandel WJ: The frequency and prognostic significance of electrocardiographic abnormalities in clinically normal individuals. Progr Cardiovasc Dis 1981; 23: 299–319.
5. Berkson DM, Stamler J, Jackson W: The precordial electrocardiogram during and after strenuous exercise. Am J Cardiol 1966; 19: 43.
6. Winkle RA: Current status of ambulatory electrocardiography. Am Heart J 1981; 102: 757–770.
7. Rodstein M, Wolloch L, Gubner RS: Mortality study of the significance of extrasystoles in an insured population. Circ 1971; 44: 617.
8. McHenry PL, Fisch C, Jordan JW, Corya BR: Cardiac arrhythmias observed during maximal treadmill exercise testing in clinically normal men. Am J Cardiol 1972; 29: 331–336.
9. Beard EF, Owen CA: Cardiac arrhythmias during exercise testing in healthy men. Aerospace Med 1973; 44.
10. Froehlicher VF, Thomas MM, Pillow C et al: Epidemiologic study of asymptomatic men screened by a maximal treadmill testing for latent coronary artery disease. Am J Cardiol 1974; 34: 770.
11. Jelinek MV, Lown B: Exercise stress testing for exposure of cardiac arrhythmias. Progr Cardiovasc Dis 1974; 16: 479–522.
12. McHenry PL, Morris SN, Kavalier M, Jordan JW: Comparative study of exercise induced ventricular arrhythmias in normal subjects and patients with documented coronary artery diseases. Am J Cardiol 1976; 37: 609–616.
13. Faris JV, McHenry PL, Jordan JW, Morris SM: Prevalence and reproducibility of exercise induced ventricular arrhythmias during maximal exercise testing in normal men. Am J Cardiol 1976; 37: 617–622.
14. Ekblom B, Hartley LH, Day WC: Occurrence and reproducibility of exercise induced ventricular ectopy in normal subjects. Am J Cardiol 1979; 43: 35–40.
15. Amsterdam EA, Vismara L, Brocchini R et al: Ventricular ectopic beats. Relation to angiographically documented coronary artery disease. Clin Res 1973; 21: 399.
16. DeMaria AN, Amsterdam EA, Vismara LA et al: The variable spectrum of rhythm disturbances in the mitral valve prolaps syndrome. Circ 1974; 50: 111–222 (Suppl III).
17. Clarke JP, Shelton JR, Hamer J et al: The rhythm of the normal human heart. Lancet II: 1976; 508.
18. Brodsky M, Wu D, Denes P, Kanakis C, Rosen KM: Arrhythmias documented by 24 hour continuous electrocardiographic monitoring in 50 male medical students without apparent heart disease. Am J Cardiol 1977; 39: 390–395.
19. Sobotka PA, Mayer JH, Bauernfeind RA, Kanakis C jr, Rosen KM: Arrhythmias documented by 24 hour continuous ambulatory electrocardiographic monitoring in young women without apparent heart disease. Am Heart J 1981; 101: 753–759.
20. Manger-Cats V, Durrer D: Prevalence of cardiac arrhythmias in the normal active population. In: Roelandt J, Hugenholtz PG: Longterm ambulatory electrocardiography. Martinus Nijhoff Publ 1982; 123–132.
21. Bethge KP: Langzeit-Elektrokardiographie bei Gesunden und bei Patienten mit koronarer Herzerkrankung. Springer Verl 1982; p 26–33.
22. Wenger NK: Current use of ambulatory ECG recording. In: Wenger NK, Mock MB, Ringquist I: Ambulatory electrocardiographic recording. Year Book Med Publ 1980; p 5–19.
23. Winkle RA: Ambulatory electrocardiography and the diagnosis, evaluation and treatment of chronic ventricular arrhythmias. Progr Cardiovasc Dis 1980; 23: 99–128.
24. Mokotoff DM, Quinones MA, Miller RP: Exercise induced ventricular tachycardia. Chest 1980; 77: 10–16.
25. Udall JA, Ellestad MH: Predictive implications of ventricular premature contractions associated with treadmill stress testing. Circ 1977; 56: 985–989.

26. Bruce RA, DeRouen T, Peterson DR, Irving JA, Chinn N, Blake P, Hofer V: Noninvasive predictors of sudden cardiac death in men with coronary heart disease. Am J Cardiol 1977; 39: 833–840.

27. Kosowsky BD, Lown B, Whiting R, Quiney T: Occurrence of ventricular arrhythmias with exercise as comparing to monitoring. Circ 1971; 44: 826–832.

28. Crawford M, O'Rourke RA, Ramakrishna N, Henning H, Ross J jr: Comparative effectiveness of exercise testing and continuous monitoring for detecting arrhythmias in patients with previous myocardial infarction. Circ 1974; 50: 301–305.

29. Ryan M, Lown B, Horn H: Comparison of ventricular ectopic activity during 24-hour monitoring and exercise testing in patients with coronary heart disease. N Eng J M 1975; 292: 224–229.

30. Borer JS, Rosing DR, Miller RH et al: Natural history of left ventricular function during one year after acute myocardial infarction: Comparison with clinical, electrocardiographic and biochemical determinations. Am J Cardiol 1980; 46: 1–12.

31. Simon H, Gross-Fengels W, Schilling G, Schaede A: Ventrikuläre Rhythmusstörungen im ambulanten Langzeit-EKG in Abhängigkeit vom Befund im Belastungs-EKG. HerzKreisl 1981; 12: 103–110.

32. Tiso B, Fitscha P, Meisner W, Spitzer D: Comparison of 24 hour longterm electrocardiogram and exercise testing in detection of ventricular arrhythmias. Z Kardiol 1982; 71: 365–369.

33. Miller DH, Borer JS: Exercise testing early after myocardial infarction. Am J Med 1982; 72: 427–437.

34. Ericsson M, Granath A, Ohlsen P, Soedermark T, Volpe U: Arrhythmias and symptoms during treadmill testing 3 weeks after myocardial infarction in 100 patients. Brit Heart J 1973; 35: 787–790.

35. Granath A, Soedermark T, Winge T, Volpe U, Zetterquist S: Early work load tests for evaluation of longterm prognosis of acute myocardial infarction. Br Heart J 1977; 39: 758–763.

36. Theroux P, Waters DB, Halphen C, Debaisieux JC, Mizgala HF: Prognostic value of exercise testing soon after myocardial infarction. N Engl J Med 1979; 301: 341–345.

37. Ivanova LA, Mazur N, Smirnova TM, Sumarokov AB, Nazarenko VA, Svet EA: Electrocardiographic exercise testing and ambulatory monitoring to identify patients with ischemic heart disease at high risk of sudden death. Am J Cardiol 1980; 45: 1132–1138.

38. DeBusk RF, Davidson DM, Houston N, Fitzgerald J: Serial ambulatory electrocardiography and treadmill exercise testing after uncomplicated myocardial infarction. Am J Cardiol 1980; 45: 547–554.

39. Davidson DM, DeBusk RF: Prognostic value of a single exercise test 3 weeks after uncomplicated myocardial infarction. Circ 1980; 61: 236–242.

40. Smith JW, Dennis A, Gassmann A et al: Exercise testing three weeks after myocardial infarction. Chest 1979; 75: 12–16.

41. Gast D, Friedrich T, v. Leitner ER, Meister B, Andresen D et al: Wertigkeit der submaximalen Ergometerbelastung nach Myokardinfarkt. Z f Kardiol 1983, 72, Suppl 1, abstr 351.

42. Starling MR, Crawford MH, Kennedy GT, O'Rourke RA: Exercise testing early after myocardial infarction: Predictive value for subsequent unstable angina and death. Am J Cardiol 1980; 46: 909–914.

43. Kotler NM, Tabatznik B, Mower MM, Tominago S: Prognostic significance of ventricular ectopic beats with respect to sudden death in the late postinfarction period. Circ 1973; 47: 959–966.

44. Moss AJ, DeCamilla J, Engstrom F, Hoffmann W, Odoroff C, Davis H: The posthospital phase of acute myocardial infarction: Identification of patients with increased mortality risk. Circ 1974; 49: 460–466.

45. Vismara LA, Amsterdam EA, Mason DT: Relation of ventricular arrhythmias in the late hospital phase of acute myocardial infarction to sudden death after hospital discharge. Am J Med 1975; 59: 9–12.

46. Moss AJ, DeCamilla JJ, Davis HP, Bayer L: Clinical significance of ventricular ectopic beats in the early posthospital phase of myocardial infarction. Am J Cardiol 1977; 39: 635–640.

47. Van Durme JP, Pannier RH: Prognostic significance of ventricular dysrhythmias one year after myocardial infarction. Am J Cardiol 1976; 37: 178.

48. Rehnquist N, Sjoegren A: Ventricular arrhythmias prior to discharge and one year after acute myocardial infarction. N Engl J Med 1977; 297: 750–757.

49. Ruberman W, Weinblatt E, Goldberg JD, Frank CW, Shapiro S: Ventricular premature beats and mortality after myocardial infarction. N Engl J Med 1977; 297: 750–757.
50. Schulze RA, Strauss W, Pitt B: Sudden death in the year following myocardial infarction. Am J Med 1977; 62: 192–199.
51. Bigger JT, Heller CA, Wenger TC, Weld FM: Risk stratification after acute myocardial infarction. Am J Cardiol 1978; 42: 202–210.
52. DeSoyza N, Bennet FA, Murphy ML, Bissett JK, Kane JJ: The relationship of paroxysmal ventricular tachycardia complicating the acute phase and ventricular arrhythmias during the late hospital phase of myocardial infarction longterm survival. Am J Med 1978; 64: 377–381.
53. Bigger JT, Weld FM, Rolnitzky LM: Prevalence and significance of ventricular tachycardia in the late hospital phase of myocardial infarction. Am J Cardiol 1981; 47: 397 (abstr).
54. Weber H, Kaindl F, Steinbach K et al: Prävalenz und Signifikanz ventrikulärer Arrhythmien in der späten Spitalsperiode des Myocardinfarktes. Acta Med Austr 1981; 8: 187 (abstr).
55. Bigger JT, Weld FM, Rolnitzky LM: Prevalence, characteristics and significance of ventricular tachycardia (three or more complexes) detected with ambulatory electrocardiographic recording in the late hospital phase of acute myocardial infarction. Am J Cardiol 1981; 48: 815–823.
56. Graboys TB: The role of electrocardiographic monitoring, exercise stress testing and electrophysiological studies in the management of patients with malignant ventricular arrhythmias. In: Roelandt J, Hugenholtz PG: Longterm ambulatory electrocardiography. Martinus Nijhoff Publ, 1982; p 79–87.
57. Morganroth J, Michelson BL, Horowitz LN et al: Limitations of routine longterm electrographic monitoring to assess ventricular ectopic frequency. Circ 1978; 58: 408.
58. Steinbach K, Glogar D, Weber H, Joskowicz G, Kaindl F: Frequency and variability of ventricular premature contractions – the influence of heart rate and circadian rhythm. Pace 1982; 5: 38–51.
59. Winkle RA: Antiarrhythmic drug effect mimicked by spontaneous variability of ventricular ectopy. Circ 1978; 57: 1116.
60. Weber H, Glogar D, Joskowics G, Steinbach K: Quantitative evaluation of an antiarrhythmic therapy (disopyramide) in patients with frequent premature ventricular contractions using a computer assisted long-term ECG analysis system. Z Kardiol 1981; 70: 13–21.
61. Graboys TB: Limitations of ambulatory ECG-recording to assess therapy in the individual patient. In: Wenger NK, Mock NB, Ringquist I: Ambulatory electrocardiographic recording. Year Book Med Publ 1980; p 367–377.
62. Graboys TB, Lown B, Podrid PJ, DeSilva RA: Long-term survival of patients with malignant ventricular arrhythmias treated with anitarrhythmic drugs. Am J Cardiol 1982; 50; 437–443.
63. Bigger JT, Reiffel JA: Holter versus electrophysiologic studies in the management of malignant ventricular arrhythmias. Am J Cardiol 1983; 51: 1464–1465.

Authors' address:
H. Weber, M.D.
Kardiol. Univ. Klinik
Garnisongasse 13
A-1090 Vienna, Austria

Comparison of Clinical Significance of Programmed Stimulation Induced Ventricular Tachycardia and Fibrillation in Survivors of Acute Myocardial Infarction

L. K. Holley*, A. R. Denniss+, D. V. Cody+, S. M. Fenton+,
D. A. Richards+, D. L. Ross+, P. A. Russell+, A. A. Young+, J. B. Uther+

Summary: The clinical significance of ventricular tachycardia and ventricular fibrillation induced at electrophysiology studies was examined in 64 patients (pts) studied after transmural acute myocardial infarction. Ten patients had had documented late ventricular arrhythmias prior to the electrophysiology study. The stimulation protocol included 2 extrastimuli (S_1S_2, S_2S_3) delivered after a paced rhythm at 2 right ventricular sites (apex, outflow tract) and at 2 current intensities (2x threshold, 20 mA). Patients were followed for 6–18 months after the study.

Of the fiftyfour patients with no documented ventricular arrhythmia, 23 were induced into fibrillation (group 1), and 31 into tachycardia (group 2). All patients with documented ventricular arrhythmias were induced into tachycardia (group 3). There was no difference in patient age or infarct site amongst the three groups. Apart from two patients with an infarct age of greater than 1 year, infarcts to study time was greater than 1.5 weeks and less than 3 months S_1S_2 was not significantly different among the groups but S_2S_3 was significantly longer (242 msec $\pm$ 33) in group 3 than groups 1 and 2 (200 msec $\pm$ 40, 206 msec $\pm$ 41), $p < 0.05$. Minimum pacing amplitude to induce an arrhythmia was significantly lower in group 3 (10% at 20 mA) than in groups 1 and 2 (65% and 55%). None of the patients in group 1 died of cardiac causes while 27% of the patients in group 2 died of cardiac cause. The mean rate of the induced VT from the pts who died was slower, 244 $\pm$ 45 ppm than that of the VT in pts still alive 281 $\pm$ 44 ppm ($p < 0.05$). Fifty per cent of the patients in group 3 died of a cardiac cause.

The results indicate that after acute myocardial infarction (1) induced slow rate VT during an electrophysiology study is associated with a poorer prognosis than VF and fast VT; (2) induced VF may be of limited clinical significance. (3) VT is inducible with less aggressive stimulation in pts with documented ventricular arrhythmias.

Introduction

A recent study by Richards et al. (1) has shown that induction of ventricular tachyarrhythmias at electrophysiology study is a predictor of sudden death late after infarction. No attempt was made in this study to correlate arrhythmia morphology with prognosis. A recent computer model of induced ventricular tachyarrhythmias after myocardial infarction has indicated that there may be an underlying difference in the mechanism of induced ventricular tachycardia and fibrillation (2). This retrospective analysis was undertaken to investigate the relative clinical significance of programmed stimulation induced ventricular tachycardia and fibrillation in survivors of acute myocardial infarction. Patients have been drawn from the Richards study (1) together with early patients from a prospective study of Denniss (3).

+ Cardiology Unit, Westmead Centre, * Bioengineering Research Centre, Telectronics Pty. Limited, Sydney, Australia.

Study Methods

The patient population chosen for this study had been admitted to the Westmead Centre in 1980–81 following a myocardial infarction. They had been tested for inducibility of a tachyarrhythmia at electrophysiology study (EPS) following a transmural myocardial infarction. EPS was performed either because of a previous spontaneous tachyarrhythmia or because of research protocols (1, 3). None of the patients had had antiarrhythmic therapy or β-blockers for 5 days at the time of the study.

A USCI, quadrapole catheter with 12 mm² platinum electrodes located at 1 cm intervals from the distal end was placed in the right ventricle for the stimulation protocol. The protocol has been previously described by Richards et al. (4). A drive chain of 8 pulses at 500–600 msecs intervals was followed by a premature pulse. This pulse was introduced at successively decreasing intervals from 300 msecs until an arrhythmia was induced or refractoriness was encountered. In the latter case, the interval was set at 10 msecs longer that the effective refractory period and a second premature impulse was introduced at gradually decreasing intervals after each pacing cycle until refractoriness or an arrhythmia was induced. This procedure was carried out for all patients at the following sites and pacing amplitudes: right ventricular apex at twice diastolic current threshold, right ventricular outflow tract at twice diastolic current threshold, right ventricular apex at 20 mamps and right ventricular outflow tract at 20 mamps. The test was considered to be positive if a tachyarrhythmia of at least 10 seconds was inducible. The arrhythmias converted to sinus rhythm either spontaneously, after overdrive pacing or cardioversion. During the study the pacing procedure and subsequent ventricular response was monitored by a continuous paper recording by a Siemens Graf recorder at 25 mm/sec during pacing and at 100 mm/sec upon arrhythmia induction.

Classification of the induced arrhythmia morphologies after programmed stimulation was based upon the regularity of the rate and morphology. Tachycardia was defined as a regular rate, regular morphology signal while fibrillation was defined as irregular rate and irregular or chaotic morphology signal on the surface VCG.

None of the patients were placed on antiarrhythmia therapy after the study. Follow up of the patient was carried out at regular intervals up to 18 months after the study. In the case of the decreased patients, the nature of death was defined as accurately as possible by interview of witnesses, ECG documentation or post mortem examination.

Results

a) *Clincal Details and Morphology*

A total of 54 patients who had had no documented ventricular tachyarrhythmia between the time of the infarct and the time of the electrophysiology study, were included in this study. Twenty three of these patients were induced into ventricular fibrillation (Group 1), with the remaining 31 being induced into tachycardia (Group 2). A further 10 patients with previously documented late ventricular tachyarrhythmia were also included. A late ventricular tachycardia was defined as an arrhythmia occurring after the first 48 hours of the infarct. All of these patients were induced into tachycardia (Group 3).

A summary of the clinical details are shown in Table 1. There was no significant difference in the mean ages, the time between the infarct and electrophysiology study and the site of infarct between the first two groups. In the third group the mean patient age and infarct site were not statistically different from the first two groups. Two patients in this group had had an infarct more than one year prior to the electrophysiology study, with the remaining having an infarct age of greater than 2 weeks or less than 3 months.

b) *Stimulation Parameters and Morphology*

The stimulation parameters which were required to induce the ventricular tachyarrhythmia were also analysed and are summarised in Table 2. There was no significant difference in either the interval of the first or second premature pulses which induced an arrhythmia between the first two groups; there was also no difference in the pacing amplitude to induce either a tachycardia or fibrillation. However, a significantly lower amplitude and longer second premature stimulus induced a tachyarrhythmia in the group with previously documented tachyarrhythmia.

c) *Mortality and Morphology*

All the patients were followed up regularly after the electrophysiology study for at least 6 months with some up to 18 months. The incidence of cardiac death at follow up is shown in Table 3.

All the deceased patients in group 2 died of a sudden cardiac cause within one year after infarction. Four patients had documented tachycardia or fibrillation at the time of death while the sudden death of the other 4 patients was attributed to a cardiac cause. None of the fibrillation induced patients in this group have died (but one patient, in the prospec-

Table 1. Clinical details.

Induced Arrhythmia	Number	Age (yrs)	Infarct Site (% inferior)	Infarct Age (wks)
Fibrillation (no arrhythmias)	23	51 ± 9.2 ⎤	74 ⎤	1.9 ± 1.5 ⎤
			*	*	
Tachycardia (no arrhythmias)	31	54 ± 9.8 ⎦	61 ⎦	1.7 ± 0.8 ⎦
3. Tachycardia (documented tachyarrhythmia)	10	56 ± 10.8	56	18.8 ± 33.5**

* N.S.
** 2 pts with infarcts > 1 yr post infarct.

tive study, who had been induced into VF at electrophysiology study, has died suddenly). The group that, died had a significantly slower rate tachycardia induced at electrophysiology study ($p < 0.05$) (244 ± 45 ppm), than the tachycardia rate induced in the group still alive (281 ± 44 ppm). Fifty per cent of the patients who had had documented ventricular tachyarrhythmias also died of sudden cardiac cause.

Discussion

The fifty four patients without documented late ventricular arrhythmias chosen for this comparative study had similar clinical histories. At electrophysiology study, there was no difference in the pacing protocol used to induce either a sustained ventricular tachycardia

Table 2. Programmed stimulation results.

Induced Arrhythmias	S_1S_2 (msec)		S_2S_3 (msec)		Pacing Amplitude (% 20 mAmp current)	
Fibrillation (no arrhytmias)	220 ± 23	⎤	200 ± 40	⎤	65	⎤
		*		*		*
Tachycardia (no arrhythmias)	224 ± 28	⎦	206 ± 41	⎦	55	⎦
Tachycardia (documented tachyarrhythmia)	239 ± 37		242 ± 33		10	

* N.S.

Table 3. Mortality results.

	Alive	Dead	
Fibrillation (no arrhythmias)	23	0	23
Tachycardia (no arrhythmias)	23	8	31
Tachycardia (documented late tachyarrhythmia)	5	5	10
	51	13	64

$p < 0.01$

732

or ventricular fibrillation in these patients. These results would indicate that neither the clinical details nor the electrophysiology stimulus program used to induce an arrhythmia are indicative of poor prognosis. Furthermore, the results would also suggest that induced slow rate tachycardias are a more specific indicator of high risk of sudden death than fast tachycardia.

There was however a significant difference in cardiac related mortality between the tachycardia induced group and the fibrillation induced group ($p < 0.01$). This result suggests that the type of arrhythmia induced at electrophysiology study is a significant indicator of poor prognosis after infarction.

The results also indicate that patients who have had a late documented tachyarrhythmia are more likely to be induced into a tachycardia with low amplitude pulses and longer premature intervals than patients without documented ventricular arrhythmias.

Conclusions

This study investigated the clinical significance of programmed stimulation induced ventricular tachycardia and fibrillation in survivors of acute myocardial infarcts. An electrophysiologically induced slow rate, stable tachycardia is associated with a poorer prognosis than induced fibrillation or fast tachycardias. This result implies that an induced ventricular fibrillation may be of limited value in predicting patients at high risk of dying suddenly. In patients with documented late ventricular arrhythmias, ventricular tachycardia can be induced with less aggressive stimulation.

References

1. Richards DA, Cody DV, Denniss AR, Russell PA, Young AA, Uther JB: Ventricular electrical instability: a predictor of death after myocardial infarction. Am J Cardiology 1983; 51: 75–80.
2. Holley LK, Goodman AH, Richards DAB, Uther JB: Computer modelling of the electrical activation of the ventricular myocardium and re-entrant ventricular arrhythmias. Aust N Z J Med 1982; 12: 314.
3. Denniss AR, Richards DA, Farrow RH, Davison A: Use of the signal averaged vectorcardiogram to predict ventricular electrical instability after myocardial infarction. Circulation 1982; 66: II–16.
4. Richards DA, Cody DV, Denniss AR, Russell PA, Young AA, Uther JB: A new protocol of programmed stimulation for assessment of predisposition to spontaneous ventricular arrhythmias. Eur Heart J 1983 (in press)

Authors' address:
Dr. L. Holley
Bioengineering Research Centre
Telectronics Pty. Ltd.
14 Mars Road
Sydney 2066/Australia

Evaluation of Survivors of Pre-Hospital Cardiac Arrest

V. Hombach, H.-W. Höpp, A. Osterspey, H. Deutsch, U. Winter, H. H. Hilger

Summary: Sudden cardiac death is one of the unsolved problems in clinical cardiology. This syndrome has been reported to be associated in most cases (more than 80%) with underlying coronary heart disease, and in the remaining cases with cardiomyopathies, aortic stenosis, mitral valve prolapse, QT syndrome and WPW syndrome. From the experiences in the literature patients with severe coronary heart disease and with poor left ventricular function and complex ventricular arrhythmias carry a particularly high risk of sudden cardiac death. In addition, from recent studies the detection of (abnormal) ventricular late potentials within the ST segment of the high gain amplified, signal averaged surface ECG seems to provide a new marker of increased left ventricular irritability in CHD patients. One of the most important diagnostic goals in sudden death candidates is the assessment of ventricular vulnerability. This may be achieved by recording of complex ventricular arrhythmias, by detection of ventricular diastolic potentials within the ST segment, and by provocation of repetitive ventricular response with programmed ventricular stimulation. The identification and characterization of the risk of successfully resuscitated pre-hospital cardiac arrest victims to develop a new fatal event constitutes a major clinical problem. Based on the experiences from the literature and our own studies a high risk profile of those SD candidates to develop a new fatal event may be outlined as follows: Bradycardia of less than 60 bpm after successful resuscitation, atrio- or intraventricular block, severe coronary heart disease with triple vessel disease, low left ventricular ejection fraction and severe contraction abnormalities, complex ventricular arrhythmias, presence of ventricular late potentials, and inducibility of repetitive ventricular response.

Introduction:

From an estimated rate of sudden death victims of 400–600 000/year in the United States it becomes clear that sudden death constitutes a large quantitative problem with regard to the recognition of high risk individuals and prevention of the fatal event. Pathogenetically two major causes of sudden death (SD) have been elicited (1): In about 80% myocardial ischemia due to imbalance of myocardial oxygen support-demand ratio and additional aggravating factors (anemia, myocardial hypertrophy, hyperthyreoidism) are responsible for the initiation of fatal ventricular fibrillation. And in only 20% of cases extracardiac lesions, resulting from extracardiac complications of primary cardiac disease, exert negative reflexogenic influences on the heart followed by ventricular fibrillation. In a lot of papers SD has been reported to be related to Coronary Heart Disease (CHD) and to non-CHD diseases (hypertrophic cardiomyopathy, aortic stenosis, mitral valve prolapse, intraventricular conduction defects, QT syndrome, WPW syndrome, 2, 3, 4, 5, 6). However, CHD is by far the most frequent underlying heart disease in SD candidates. Acute myocardial infarction may be associated with 70–80% out-of-hospital SD, whereas SD rates in chronic CHD are at an average of 2–3% per year, and in unstable angina SD rates may amount to 18% per year (7). One of the most challenging problems in the management of SD victims is the recognition of predisposing factors and prevention of the fatal event.

Supported by the Deutsche Forschungsgemeinschaft, SFB 68, Cologne

Risk profile of SD candidates and predisposing factors:

Several electrocardiographic and hemodynamic indices, that might identify populations with a higher mortality risk than the normal age- and sex-matched individuals, have been discussed. Patients with intraventricular conduction disturbances, particularly with bifascicular blocks, had mortality rates of 23% to 43% between 1.5 to 3 years follow-up (8, 9, 10, 11), and the increased risk in these patients has been related to the underlying organic heart disease. Ventricular premature beats (VPB), as induced by ergometric stress tests, may indicate a higher incidence of latent CHD than in those individuals without VPBs during physical activity (12, 13, 14). This has been confirmed by follow-up studies, where those patients with exercise induced VPBs had an increased incidence of new coronary events like angina pectoris, myocardial infarction and SD (15). In addition, patients with various types of exercise induced VPBs in the post-myocardial infarction period (rare or frequent VPBs, multiform VPBs or couplets) had an increased mortality rate during one-year follow-up (16).

A stronger indicator of an increased risk of SD one year following myocardial infarction seems to be the spontaneous occurence of frequent or complex VPBs like bigeminies, couplets, salvos and ventricular tachycardias (17, 18, 19, 20, 21, 22, 23, 24, 25, 26). In 68% to 75% of SD patients ventricular couplets were recorded, and ventricular salvos were present in 26% to 75% of SD victims (25, 26). In contrast, complex and tachycardiac VPBs in apparently healthy individuals are reported to be harmless and seem not to impair short-term prognosis (25, 27). These conflicting data may be explained by normal left ventricular function in healthy subjects, since complex VPBs have been shown to occur most frequently in patients with poor left ventricular funcion (25, 28, 29, 30), and complex VPBs provided the highest significance in predicting SD when occurring in combination with severe left ventricular contraction abnormalities (31). Anyway, the role of complex VPBs as an independent predictor of SD risk seems to be well established in most of the studies reported so far, both in patients followed for one year after myocardial infarction (32) and in those with chronic CHD (33). In an excellent review of the literature, Winkle (34) summarized the role of VPBs as a risk indicator of SD as follows:

1. In populations frequent and/or complex VPBs on standard or Holter ECG seem to predict SD only in those with underlying heart disease.
2. Complex or frequent VBPs in the Holter ECG seem to be strong predictors of subsequent cardiac death.
3. The independent distribution of each type of complex VPBs and of frequent VPBs as predictors of SD is unknown
4. There appears to be a relationship between the occurrence of VPBs and the extent of CHD and left ventricular contraction abnormalities
5. Clinical factores, particularly those related to left ventricular function, seem to be of additional importance.

Since in most circumstances SD is caused by ventricular fibrillation, attempts have been made to assess ventricular vulnerability. Besides the spontaneous occurrence of complex VPBs and ventricular tachycardias, programmed ventricular stimulation has been introduced in order to test ventricular irritability, that may be indicated by the extrastimulus-induced repetitive ventricular response (35). This method proved to be useful in the serial control of antiarrhythmic therapy of ventricular tachycardias (36, 37, 38). In CHD patients with known ventricular tachycardia episodes programmed ventricular stimulation is able to provoke ventricular tachycardias in about 80% of cases (36, 37, 39), whereas these induction rates of ventricular tachycardias are considerably smaller in non-CHD patients (40, 41, 42). The prognostic signficance of extrastimulus-induced repetitive ventricular response in predicting SD in CHD patients is widely discussed (43, 44). In 22/61 patients surviving myocardial infarction Greene et al. (43) found positive ventricular response, whereas this phenomenon was negative in 39/61 patients. 8/22 patients with positive repetitive ventricular response died during follow-up of one year, in contrast to only 4/39 patients, in whom repetitive ventricular response could not be initiated, and this difference was statistically significant. However, the definite role of repetitive ventricular response as a prognostic factor that may predict the risk of SD, remains to be clarified, since these induction rates and the incidence of SD could not be confirmed by subsequent studies (44, 45).

Recently a newer electrophysiological parameter, the ventricular late potential within the ST segment, has been discussed as a marker of ventricular vulnerability and a possible predictor of patients at risk of SD, particularly in those with CHD. Experimental and clinical studies have shown that ischemic myocardium, e.g. at the border zone of an old myocardial infarction or of an aneurysm, may be later depolarized than normal perfused myocardial tissue, and this late activated tissue may be detected as electrical activity within the ST segment by intracardiac catheter electrodes or by endo- or epicardial direct registrations (46, 47), as well as by non-invasive high resolution surface electrocardiography (signal averaging technique: 48–56, beat-to-beat high resolution surface ECG: 57, 58). Such diastolic electrical activity might serve as a critical link for establishing re-entry circuits between normal and ischemic myocardium leading to short or long runs of ventricular tachycardias, that frequently may degenerate to ventricular fibrillation.

In clinical studies particularly with CHD patients, a high correlation could be found between the incidence of ventricular late potentials and the occurrence of VPBs (51, 52, 53, 54, 55) and the degree of left ventricular dysfunction (51, 54). Data on the prognostic significance of ventricular late potentials are sparse. In a study of Breithardt et al. (51) in patients with late potentials with a base width of more than 40 ms SD was more frequently observed than in those with shorter intervals to the QRS complex. The incidence of SD and of ventricular tachycardias was significantly lower in patients without ventricular late potentials or with diastolic potentiales of less than 20 ms duration, as compared to those with late potentials of more than 20 ms duration. 4 patients that developed sustained ventricular tachycardias following myocardial infarction had ventricular late potentials. In contrast, none of the patients without diastolic potentials developed ventricular tachycardias. Our own experiences with ventricular late potentials cover data of two groups of CHD patients, 50 patients followed from the first day of myocardial infarction by Holter ECG and by the signal averaging technique (in some also by programmed ventricular stimulation), and another 200 patients with chronic CHD, studied by Holter ECG, signal averaging technique and in a lot of patients by programmed ventricular stimulation. In the group of chronic CHD patients 108/200 had ventricular late potentials, 92/200 patients did not show late potentials within the averaged surface ECG. During follow-up of 20 ± 5 months 15/108 patients with late potentials died from sudden cardiac death, in contrast to 4/92 patients with non-arrhythmic death (3 from pump failure during myocardial infarction, 1 from neoplasm), the difference of sudden death rates being statistically significant (p < 0.01). The following values characterizing the diagnostic significance of complex VPBs and ventricular late potentials in the recognition of SD candidates were found: sensitivity: late potentials 100%, complex VPBs 60%, specificity: late potentials 56%, complex VPBs 80%, predictive value: late potentials 18%, complex VPBs 22%, late potentials plus complex VPBs 35%. In the group of patients with acute myocardial infarction 30/50 patients had late potentials at least 4 weeks after the acute stage of illness. 12/30 with late potentials died during follow-up of 18 ± 3 months, 7 during the first days after admission. On the other hand, only 1/20 AMI patients without ventricular late potentials died from pump failure during the acute phase of infarction. The difference in death rates again was statistically significant ($p < 0.01$). In these patients the following diagnostic criteria for characterization of SD patients was found from follow-up data: sensitivity: late potentials 100%, complex VBPs 60%, specificity: late potentials 62%, complex VPBs 86%, predictive value: late potentials 29%, complex VPBs 38%, combination of late potentials and complex VPBs 50%. Thus, from our experiences ventricular late potentials are a very sensitive marker of SD candidates in patients with acute myocardial infarction and with chronic CHD, but their specifity is relatively low. Predictive values of late potentials and of complex VPBs are of clinical significance in recognizing SD candidates, and their diagnostic impact can be considerably improved by combining both markers of ventricular vulnerability.

Diagnostic approach to patients prone to sudden death

From the experiences in the literature and our own data the following diagnostic goals should be approached, when trying to characterize patients prone to sudden cardiac death:

1. Diagnosis of underlying heart disease, particularly confirmation of CHD with overt or latent myocardial ischemia.
2. Assessment of left ventricular function or extent of dysfunction.
3. Evaluation of left ventricular electrical instability by
   a. recognition of complex VPBs (Holter ECG),
   b. detection of ventricular late potentials (signal averaging technique),
   c. provocation of ventricular repetitive response (programmed ventricular stimulation).

Myocardial ischemia and left ventricular dysfunction may be assessed by exercise ECG, exercise Tl-myocardial scintigraphy and radionuclide ventriculography and by coronary and left ventricular angiography as the "gold standard" of all the non-invasive methods currently used. The sensitivity of Tl-scintigraphy for recognition of myocardial ischemia is around 80–90% and may be relatively specific (60), and specificity of radionuclide ventriculography for assessment of left ventricular dysfunction may be in a similar range (60). Myocardial necrosis and infarct size may be properly evaluated by Tc-pyrophosphate scanning with a sensitivity of more than 90% (60). And one promising application of Tc-pyrophosphate scanning has been reported by Olsen et al. (61) for documentation of ongoing subclinical necrosis in patients with unstable angina and subsequent sudden cardiac death. These authors found in 67/199 patients with unstable angina without signs of overt infarction (ECG, enzyme pattern) an ongoing subclinical myocardial necrosis, and in 132/199 patients Tc-pyrophosphate scan was negative. Patients with negative scans had a 3% annual risk of subsequent myocardial infarction and a 6% risk of sudden death, in contrast to the infarction risk of 21% and sudden death risk of 22% in the group with positive scans.

Characterization of suvivors of Out-of-hospital cardiac arrest:

There are very few studies concerning the evaluation of successfully resuscitated SD victims (63, 64, 65, 66, 67, 68). The most important etiologic factor reported in these patients was CHD (70–79%), and in rare cases cardiomyopathy was found (3–16%) or valvular heart disease (7%). The history taken in these patients, was negative in 34% and positive for any symptom of heart disease in 66% (64), old myocardial infarction was reported in 52%, angina or chest pain in 50%, arterial hypertension in 35%, and smoking more than 10 cigarettes/day in 42% of cases (63). Ergometric exercise disclosed VPBs in 12/27 patients studied, and in 6 patients the exercise protocol had to be stopped because of malignant ventricular arrhythmias (multiform VPBs in 1 patient, ventricular tachycardia in 3, and ventricular fibrillation in 2 patients). A normal exercise capacity was found in 15/27 patients, and moderately to severely limited capacity in 9/27 patients. ST segment alterations were not mentioned (64). In another study of 36 successfully resuscitated SD victims radionuclide ventriculography disclosed a group of 18 patients with ejection fractions below 0.30, with diffuse wall motion abnormalities in 9/18 and regional contraction abnormalities in another 9/18 patients. During a 4-week-follow-up period mortality rates in the former group was 6/9 patients, and in the latter group 4/9 patients, a total of 13 deaths. In contrast, 18 patients had ejection fractions beyond 0.30, 4 with diffuse, 7 with regional, and 7 without any contraction abnormality. The subsequent mortality rates were 2/4 patients with diffuse, and 2/7 patients with regional contraction abnormalities, and none of the 7 patients with normal contraction pattern. These results clearly show that an ejection fraction below 0.30 and diffuse contraction abnormalities may be of considerable prognostic significance in SD candidates.

The most frequent electrophysiological mechanism of SD was ventricular fibrillation (62%), followed by bradyarrhythmias or asystole (31%), and by ventricular tachycardias (7%, 66). Patients with documented ventricular tachycardias had best prognosis of SD victims (59% of patients with ventricular fibrillation, and 76% of patients with ventricular tachycardias were discharged, 66). Complete left bundle branch block was found in 17% of 101 patients, and ventricular fibrillation recurred in 40–57% of the patients after admission (63, 66). Frequent VPBs were noted in 26% (63), and this number was greater in the other study (38/42 patients, 66). 10/38 patients with complex VPBs had recurrent cardiac arrest within the hospital, 28/38 remained free (66). 12/38 patients had an additional AV block, intraventricular conduction disturbance, or both, and 25/28 patients with no recurrence of cardiac arrest did not have AV conduction disturbances. In this study various conduction system abnormalities were considered as the better discriminating factor for recurrency of cardiac arrest than VPBs (66). In the study of Liberthson et al. (63) the chance of recurrent arrest after admission was greater (73%) in patients with post-resuscitation heart rates below 60 bpm, and the chance of not surviving was 95%. On the other hand, patients with post-resuscitation heart rates of more than 100 bpm did best with pre-hospital mortality of 17% and 57%-overall mortality from arrest through hospitalisation. Programmed ventricular stimulation was performed in only a small number of successfully resuscitated SD victims (66): 7/14 patients responded with repetitive response, 5/6 patients with ventricular tachycardias during resuscitation exerted sustained forms of ventricular tachycardia, and none of the patients developed ventricular fibrillation on the stimulation protocol.

We have studied a group of 21 patients with out-of-hospital documented ventricular tachycardia-fibrillation, and all of these patients had been successfully resuscitated by DC shock. This cohort consisted of 7 females and 14 males, with ages from 45–64 years (mean: 55.8 ± 5.8 years). CHD was confirmed in 20/21 patients (in 6 by non-invasive means, in 15 by coronary and left ventricular angiography), and in one patient hemodynamics and angiography were negative. The patients were studied by exercise ECG and Thallium-scintigraphy, and left ventricular vulnerability was tested by Holter ECG (complex VPBs or ventricular tachycardias), by signal averaging of high gain amplified surface ECG (ventricular late potentials), and by programmed right ventricular stimulation (repetitive ventricular response). Thereafter the patients were followed by 18 ± 3 months (example in Figs 1–3). The results obtained in this group of patients are listed in Table 1. Myocardial ischemia was detectable in 14/21 patients on exercise ECG (67%), and in 10/10 patients (100%) on Tl-myocardial scintigraphy. Left ventricular contraction abnormalities were present in 10/14 patients studied with left ventricular angiography (72%). VPBs of Lown's classes III, IVa and b and ventricular tachycardias were detected within the Holter ECG in 14/21 patients (67%), ventricular late potentials in 14/21 patients (67%), and repetitive ventricular response in 12/21 patients (57%). 4 patients died during follow-up. Because of the small number of cases there was no statistical difference between the presence or absence of ST segment depression, of Tl-scans, of left ventricular contraction abnormalities, of complex VPBs, of ventricular late potentials and of repetitive ventricular response in those patients that died and those that survived. The corre-

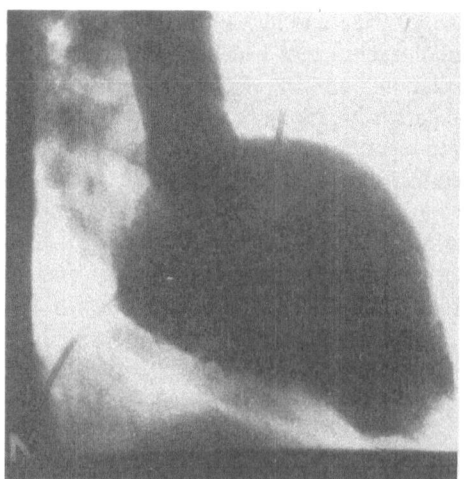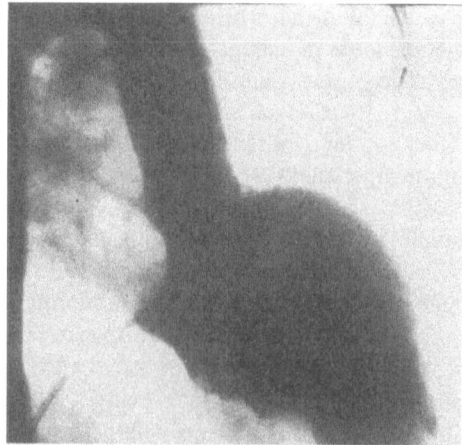

Fig. 1: Left ventricular angiogram of a 45 years old female with old anterior myocardial infarction, showing a large anterior wall aneurysm (left: diastole, right: systole). This patient had been successfully resuscitated from out-of-hospital ventricular tachycardia/fibrillation.

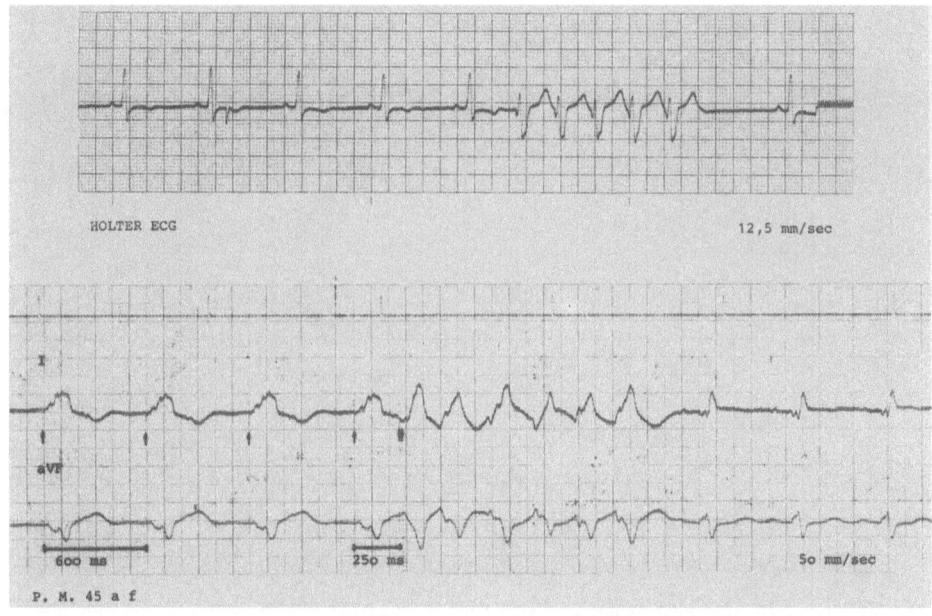

Fig. 2: Same patient as in figure 1. Holter ECG (top) revealed short runs of spontaneous ventricular tachycardias. During programmed ventricular stimulation (bottom) at basic driven rhythms of 100 stimuli/min (left panel) a short run of non-sustained ventricular tachycardia could be induced by one ventricular premature stimulus (center) with spontaneously recurring sinus rhythm (right panel).

Table 1. Diagnostic findings in 21 out-of-hospital resuscitated sudden death victims. Numbers in brackets: sensitivity in per cent, PV: predictive value in per cent (number of true positive results times 100, divided by the number of true positive plus false positive results). SD-PTS: Sudden death patients.

Method	Parameter	Total Group	SD-PTS	PV(%)
Exercise ECG	ST segment depression	14/21 (67%)	4/4 (100%)	29
	VEA-induction	2/21 (10%)	1/4 (25%)	50
TL-myocardial scintigraphy	perfusion defect	10/10 (100%)	2/2 (100%)	20
Left ventricular angiography	LV contraction abnormality	10/14 (72%)	3/3 (100%)	30
	LV-aneurysm	4/14 (29%)	1/3 (33%)	25
Holter ECG	VEA Lown classes III, IV a+b, VT	14/21 (67%)	2/4 (50%)	14
Signal Averaged ECG	Ventricular late potentials	14/21 (67%)	3/4 (75%)	21
Programmed ventricular stimulation	repetitive ventricular response	12/21 (57%)	3/4 (75%)	25

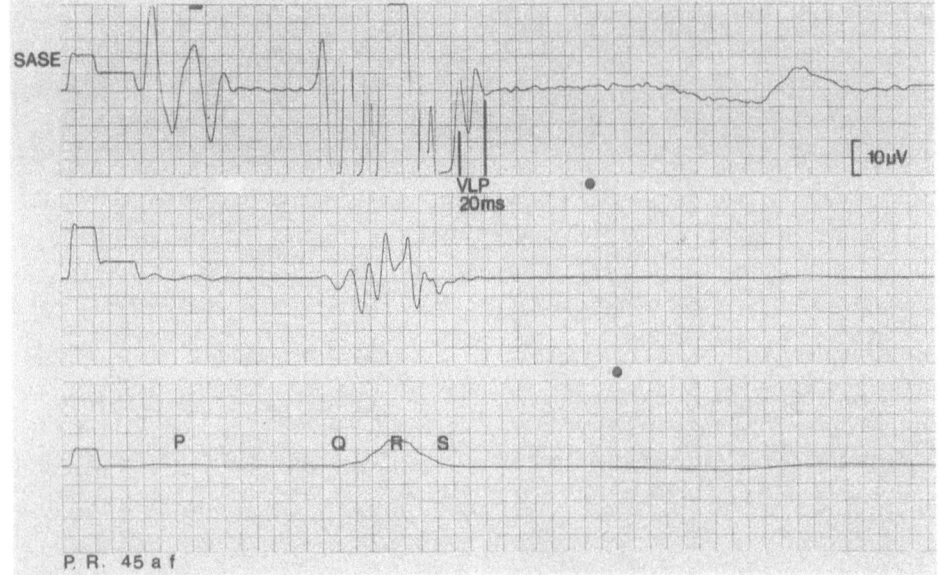

Fig. 3: High gain amplified signal averaged surface ECG (SASE) showed a ventricular late potential with a base width of 20 ms merging from the terminal portion of the QRS complex. VLP: ventricular late potential.

In this patient the three parameters of ventricular vulnerability were positive, i.e. presence of spontaneous ventricular tachycardia (complex VEA) within Holter ECG, presence of ventricular late potentials within the averaged surface ECG, and inducibility of repetitive ventricular response on programmed ventricular stimulation.

sponding predictive values with either method are summarized in Table 1. The highest predictive values were found with ST segment alterations (29%), left ventricular contraction abnormalities (30%), and with induction of repetitive ventricular response (25%). The high value with exercise induced VPBs (50%) has to be taken with caution, since there were only 2/21 patients with positive response, and one of these two patients was a SD candidate. One might expect that predictive impact of these parameters may be much stronger with larger SD populations to be studied as well as by longer follow-up periods.

If one tries to characterize a high risk profile of survivors of pre-hospital cardiac arrest to recurrency of a further fatal event, the following items may be of importance:

1. Bradycardia of less than 60 bpm immediately after successful resuscitation.
2. Atrio- or intraventricular block.
3. Severe Coronary Heart Disease (triple vessel disease, low left ventricular ejection fraction, severe left ventricular contraction abnormalities).
4. Complex ventricular ectopic beats or ventricular tachycardias.
5. Presence of ventricular late potentials within the high gain amplified signal averaged surface ECG.
6. Inducibility of repetitive ventricular response on programmed ventricular stimulation.

References

1. Baroldi G: Pathology and mechanisms of sudden death. In: Hurst JW (ed): The Heart. New York: McGraw Hill Book Company, 1982: 589–599.
2. Lown B: Cardiovascular collapse and sudden cardiac death. In: Braunwald E (ed): Heart Disease, A Textbook of Cardiovascular Medicine, Philadelphia–London–Toronto: WB Saunders, 1980: 778–817.
3. Epstein SE, Maron BJ: Sudden death in patients with hypertrophic cardiomyopathy. In: Kulbertus HE and Wellens HJJ (eds) Sudden Death, The Hague–Boston–London: Martinus Nijhoff Publishers, 1980: 347–357
4. Schwartz PJ: The long QT syndrome. In: Kulbertus HE and Wellens HJJ (eds): Sudden Death, The Hague–Boston–London: Martinus Nijhoff Publishers, 1980: 358–378.
5. Kulbertus HE, De Leval-Rutten F, Dubois M, Petit JM. Sudden death in subjects with intraventricular conduction defects. In: Kulbertus HE and Wellens HJJ (eds): Sudden Death, The Hague–Boston–London: Martinus Nijhof Publishers, 1980: 379–391.
6. Wellens HJJ, Bär FW, Farre J, Ross D, Vanagt EJ: Sudden death in the Wolff-Parkinson-White syndrome. In: Kulbertus HE and Wellens HJJ (eds): Sudden Death, The Hague–Boston–London: Martinus Nijhoff Publishers, 1980: 392–399.
7. Hurst JW: Prognosis of coronary heart disease. In: Hurst JW (ed) The Heart. New York: McGraw Hill Book Company, 1982: 1058–1068.
8. De Pasquale NP, Bruno MS: Natural history of combined right bundle branch block and left anterior hemiblock. Am J Med 1973: 297–303.
9. Narula OS, Gann D, Samet P: Prognostic value of HV intervals. In: Narula OS (ed) His Bundle Electrocardiography and Clinical Electrophysiology. Philadelphia: Davis Company, 1975: 437–449.
10. Denes P, Dhingra RC, Wu D, Wyndham CR, Amat-y-Leon F, Rosen KM: Sudden death in patients with chronic bifascicular block. Arch Int Med 1977: 137, 1005–1010.
11. McAnulty JH, Kauffmann S, Murphy ES, Kassebaum DG, Rahimtoola SH: Survival in patients with intraventricular conduction defects. Arch Int Med 1978: 138, 30–35.
12. Zaret B, Conti R: Exercise induced ventricular irritability: hemodynamic and angiographic correlations. Am J Cardiol 1972: 29, 298–299.
13. Chung EK: Exercise Electrocardiography. Practical Approach. Baltimore: The Williams and Wilkins Company, 1979.
14. Goldschlager N, Cake D, Cohn K: Exercise-induced ventricular arrhythmias in patients with coronary artery disease. Am J Cardiol 1973: 31, 434–440.
15. Udall JA, Ellestadt MH: Predictive implications of ventricular premature contractions associated with treadmill stress testing. Circulation 1977: 56, 985–989.
16. Wehd FM, Chen KL, Bigger JT, Rohnitzky LM: Risk stratification with low-level exercise testing 2 weeks after acute myocardial infarction. Circulation 1981: 64, 306–314.
17. Kotler MN, Tabatznik B, Mower MM, Tominaga S: Prognostic significance of ventricular ectopic beats with respect to sudden death in the late postinfarction period. Circulation 1973: 47, 959–966.
18. Luria MH, Knoke JD, Margolis RM, Hendricks FH, Kuplic JB: Acute myocardial infarction: Prognosis after recovery. Ann Int Med 1976: 85, 561–565.
19. Moss AJ, De Camilla J, Engstrom F, Hoffman W, Odoroff C, Davis H: The posthospital phase of myocardial infarction: Identification of patients with increased mortality risk. Circulation 1974: 49, 460–466.
20. Rehnquist N, Sjogren A: Ventricular arrhythmias prior to discharge and one year after acute myocardial infarction. European J Cardiol 1977: 5/5, 425–442.
21. Ruberman W, Weinblatt E, Goldberg J, Frank CW, Shapiro S: Ventricular premature beats and mortality after myocardial infarction. New Engl J Med 1977: 297, 750–757.
22. Schulze RA, Strauss HW, Pitt B: Sudden death in the years following myocardial infarction. Am J Med 1977: 62, 192–199.
23. Vismara LA, Amsterdam EA, Mason DT: Relation of ventricular arrhythmias in the late hospital phase of acute myocardial infarction to sudden death after hospital discharge. Am J Med 1975: 59, 6–12.

24. Lown B: Sudden cardiac death. In: Hombach V and Hilger HH (eds): Proceedings of the International Symposium on Holter Monitoring Technique, Cologne 11–13th May, 1983, Stuttgart–New York: FK Schattauer-Verlag, 1983, in press.

25. Bethge KP: Langzeitelektrokardiographie bei Gesunden und bei Patienten mit koronarer Herzkrankheit. Berlin–Heidelberg–New York: Springer-Verlag 1982.

26. Van Durme JP, Pannier RH: Prognostic significance of ventricular dysrhythmias 1 year after myocardial infarction. Am J Cardiol 1976: 27, 178.

27. Hinkle LE, Carver ST, Stevens M: The frequency of asymptomatic disturbances of cardiac rhythm and conduction in middle-aged men. Am J Cardio 1969: 24, 629–650.

28. Califf RM, Burks JM, Bhar VS, Margolis JR, Wagner GS: Relationship among ventricular arrhythmias, coronary artery disease and angiographic and electrocardiographic indicators of myocardial fibrosis. Circulation 1978: 57, 725–732.

29. Calvert A, Lown B, Gorlin R: Ventricular premature beats and anatomically defined coronary heart disease. Am J Cardiol 1977: 39, 627–634.

30. Sharma SD, Ballantyne F, Godstein S: The relationship of ventricular asynergy in coronary artery disease to ventricular premature beats. Chest 1974: 66, 358–362.

31. Lichtlen PR, Bethge KP, Platiel H: Inzidenz des plötzlichen Herztodes bei Koronarpatienten in Abhängigkeit von Anatomie und Rhythmusprofil. Z Kardiol 1980: 69, 639–648.

32. Bigger JT, Weld FM, Rolnitzky LM: Prevalence, characteristics and significance of ventricular tachycardia (three or more complexes) detected with ambulatory electrocardiographic recording in the late hospital phase of acute myocardial infarction. Am J Cardiol 1981: 48, 815–823.

33. Moss AJ, Davis HT, De Camilla J, Bayer LW: Ventricular ectopic beats and their relation to sudden and nonsudden cardiac death after myocardial infarction. Circulation 1979: 60, 998–1003.

34. Winkle RA: Detection of patients at high risk for sudden death: The role of electrocardiographic monitoring. In: Kulbertus HE and Wellens HJJ (eds): Sudden Death. The Hague–Boston–London: Martinus Nijhoff Publishers 1980: 275–296.

35. Greene HL, Reid PR, Schaeffer AH: The repetitive ventricular response in man. A predictor of sudden death. New Engl J Med 1978: 299, 729–743.

36. Pedersen DH, Troup PJ, Zipes DP: Prognostic significance of repetitive ventricular response using programmed ventricular pacing. Clin Res 1978: 26, 652 A.

36a Fisher JD, Cohen HL, Mehra R, Altschuler H, Escher DJW, Furman S: Cardiac pacing and pacemakers. II. Serial electrophysiological-pharmacological testing for control of recurrent tachyarrhythmias. Am Heart J 1977: 93, 658–668.

37. Mason JW, Winkle RA: Electrode-catheter arrhythmia induction in the selection and assessment of antiarrhythmias drug therapy for recurrent ventricular tachycardia. Circulation 1978: 58, 971–985.

38. Horowitz LN, Josephson ME, Farshidi A, Spielman SR, Michelson EL, Greenspan AM: Recurrent sustained ventricular tachycardia. 3. Role of the electrophysiologic study in selection of antiarrhythmic regimens. Circulation 1978: 58, 986–997.

39. Josephson ME, Horowitz LN, Farshidi A, Kastor JA: Recurrent sustained ventricular tachycardia. 1. Mechanisms Circulation 1978: 57, 431–440.

40. Wellens HJJ, Durrer DR, Lie KI: Observations on mechanisms of ventricular tachycardia in man. Circulation 1976: 54, 237–244.

41. Denes P, Dhingra RC, Amat-y-Leon F, Wyndham C, Mautner RK, Rosen KM: Electrophysiologic studies in patients with chronic recurrent ventricular tachycardia. Circulation 1976: 54, 229–236.

42. Prystowsky EN, Naccarelli GV, Herger JJ, Zipes DP: Elektrophysiologische Untersuchungen bei Patienten mit ventrikulären Tachykardien. In: Schlepper M and Olsson B (eds): Kardiale Rhythmusstörungen, Diagnose–Prognose–Therapie, Berlin–Heidelberg–New York: Springer-Verlag 1983: 67–75.

43. Greene HL, Reid PR, Schaeffer AH: Further evaluation of the repetitive ventricular response in man. In: Kulbertus HE and Wellens HJJ (eds): Sudden Death, The Hague–Boston–London: Martinus Nijhoff Publishers 1980: 251–274.

44. Mason JW: Repetitive beating after single ventricular extrastimuli: Incidence and prognostic significance in patients with recurrent ventricular tachycardia. Am J Cardiol 1980: 45, 1126.

45. Naccarelli GH, Prystowsky EN, Jackman WM, Heger JJ, Rinkenberger RL, Zipes DP: Repetitive ventricular response: Prevalence and prognostic significance. Br Heart J 1981: 46, 152.

46. Klein H, Werner P, Frank G, Bethge KP, Lichtlen PR: Value of left ventricular endocardiac catheter mapping in patients with ventricular arrhythmias. European Heart J 1981 (Suppl A), 2, 42.

47. Josephson ME, Horowitz LN, Farshidi A: Continuous local electrical activity: A mechanism of recurrent ventricular tachycardia. Circulation 1978: 57, 569–665.

48. Berbari EJ, Scherlag BJ, Hope RR, Lazzara R: Recording from the body surface of arrhythmogenic ventricular activity during the ST segment. Am J Cardiol 1978: 41, 697–702.

49. Fontaine G, Frank R, Gallais-Hammonno F, Allali I, Phan-Thue H, Grosgogeat Y: Electrocardiographie des potentiels tardifs du syndrome de post-excitation. Arch Mal Coeur 1978: 71, 854–864.

50. Uther JB, Dennett CJ, Tau A: The detection of delayed activation signals of low amplitude in the vectorcardiogram of patients with recurrent ventricular tachycardia by signal averaging. In: Sandoe E, Julian DG, Bell JW (eds): Management of ventricular tachycardia–Role of Mexiletine, Amsterdam–Oxford: Excerpta Medica 1978: 80–82.

51. Breithardt G, Borggrefe M, Karbenn U, Haerten K, Ostermeyer J, Seipel L: Die mögliche Bedeutung von Spätpotentialen für die Identifizierung von Patienten, die einer antiarrhythmischen Therapie bedürfen. In: Schlepper M and Olsson B (eds): Kardiale Rhythmusstörungen–Diagnose–Prognose–Therapie, Berlin–Heidelberg–New York: Springer-Verlag 1983: 39–55.

52. Hombach V, Höpp H-W, Braun V, Behrenbeck DW, Tauchert M, Hilger HH: Die Bedeutung von Nachpotentialen innerhalb des ST-Segmentes im Oberflächen-EKG bei Patienten mit koronarer Herzkrankheit. Deutsch Med Wochenschr 1980: 105, 1457–1462.

53. Rozanski JJ, Mortara D: Delayed depolarizations in patients with recurrent ventricular tachycardia and left ventricular aneurysm. In: Hombach V and Hilger HH (eds): Signal Averaging Technique in Clinical Cardiology, Stuttgart–New York: FK Schattauer-Verlag 1981: 205–218.

54. Höpp H-W, Hombach V, Braun V, Behrenbeck DW, Tauchert M, Hilger HH: Ventricular delayed depolarizations in patients with chronic stable coronary heart disease and with acute myocardial infarction. In: Hombach V and Hilger HH (eds): Signal Averaging Technique in Clinical Cardiology, Stuttgart–New York: FK Schattauer-Verlag 1981: 231–252.

55. Simson MB: Use of signals in the terminal QRS complex to identify patients with ventricular tachycardia after myocardial infarction. Circulation 1981: 64, 235–242.

56. Oeff M, v. Leitner ER, Brüggemann T, Andresen D, Staphit R, Schröder R: Methodische Probleme bei der Registrierung ventrikulärer Spätpotentiale. Z Kardiol 1982: 71, 204.

57. Hombach V, Kebbel U, Höpp H-W, Winter U-J, Braun V, Deutsch H, Hirche H, Hilger HH: Fortlaufende Registrierung von Mikropotentialen des menschlichen Herzens – erste Erfahrungen mit einem neuen, hochauflösenden EKG-Verstärkersystem. Deutsche Med Wochenschr 1982: 107, 1951–1956.

58. El-Sherif N, Mehra R, Gomes JAC, Kelen G: Appraisal of a low noise electrocardiogram. J Am Coll Cardiol 1983: 1, 456–467.

59. Höpp H-W, Hombach V, Osterspey A, Deutsch HJ, Winter U, Braun V, Hilger HH: Clinical and prognostic significance of ventricular arrhythmias and ventricular late potentials in CHD patients. In: Hombach V and Hilger HH (eds): Proceedings of the International Symposium on Holter Monitoring Technique, Cologne 11–13th May 1983, Stuttgart–New York: FK Schattauer-Verlag, In press.

60. Pitt B: Detection of high risk patients for sudden death: The role of myocardial imaging with radioisotopes. In: Kulbertus HE and Wellens HJJ (eds): Sudden Death, The Hague–Boston–London: Martinus Nijhoff Publishers 1980: 297–304.

61. Olsen H, Lyons K, Aronow WJ, Waters H: Identification of high risk unstable angina pectoris for mortality and myocardial infarction. Circulation 1977: 56, 669 (Suppl III).

62. Dewhurst NG, Muir AL: Comparative prognostic value of radionuclide ventriculography at rest and during exercise in 100 patients after first myocardial infarction. Br Heart J 1983: 49, 111–121.

63. Liberthson RR, Nagel EL, Hirschman JC, Nussenfeld SR: Prehospital ventricular defibrillation. Prognosis and follow-up course. New Engl J Med 1974: 291, 317–321.
64. Cobb LA, Baum RS, Alvarez HA, Schaefer WA: Resuscitation from out-of-hospital ventricular fibrillation: 4 years follow-up. Circulation 1975: 51/52 (Suppl III), 223–228.
65. Weaver WD, Lorch GS, Alvarez HA, Cobb LA: Angiographic findings and prognostic indicators in patients resuscitated from sudden cardiac death. Circulation 1976: 54, 895–900.
66. Myerburgh RJ, Conde CA, Sung RJ, Mallon SM, Sheps DS, Appel R, Castellanos A: Prehospital cardiac arrest: Early and long-term clinical and electrophysiological characteristics. In: Kulbertus HE and Wellens HJJ (eds): Sudden Death, The Hague–Boston–London: Martinus Nijhoff Publishers 1980: 219–236.
67. Goldstein S, Landis JR, Leighton R: Characteristics of resuscitated out-of-hospital cardiac arrest victims with coronary heart disease. Circulation 1981: 64, 977.
68. Ptacin MJ, Fresch DD, Soin JS, Brooks HL: Evaluation of left ventricular global and segmental function by radionuclide ventriculography in sudden coronary death survivors of pre-hospital cardiac arrest: Correlation to subsequent short-term prognosis. Am Heart J 1982: 103, 54–56.

Authors' address:
V. Hombach, M.D.
Medical Clinic and Policlinic III
and Department of Cardiology,
University of Cologne,
5000 Köln

The Role of Electrophysiologic Testing in the Therapy of Patients with Unexplained Syncope

A. J. Greenspon, R. M. Greenberg, W. S. Frankl

Summary: The role of electrophysiologic testing in the diagnosis and therapy of patients with unexplained recurrent syncope was evaluated in twenty-six patients. Abnormalities were detected during the electrophysiology study in 17 of 26 patients (65%). Ventricular tachycardia (VT) was induced in 6 patients while conduction defects were detected in 11 patients. Therapeutic decisions based on the findings of the electrophysiology study were made in the patients with abnormal studies. Fifteen of the 17 patients with laboratory directed therapy were free of recurrent syncope when followed for a mean 12.2 ± 7.9 months. Syncope recurred in 4 of 9 patients with a non-diagnostic study. One additional patient with a non-diagnostic study died suddenly.

Eleven of the 26 patients had bundle branch block (BBB) or interventricular conduction defect (IVCD). In this subgroup of patients 4 patients had VT, 4 had conduction defects and 3 had non-diagnostic studies.

Electrophysiologic testing in patients with recurrent unexplained syncope provides additional useful diagnostic information. Conduction defects and tachyarrhythmias are frequently found during electrophysiologic testing in these patients. Laboratory directed therapy is effective in preventing recurrent syncope. Finally, ventricular tachycardia is frequently induced, even in patients with underlying BBB or IVCD, highlighting the importance of programmed electrical stimulation in the evaluation of these patients.

Introduction

Sudden loss of consciousness or syncope is a common medical symptom. In most cases a specific cause can be identified by history, physical examination, and standard non-invasive laboratory tests (1–3). However, there remains a small group of patients in whom the cause of recurrent syncope is unknown despite extensive evaluation. In this group of patients cardiac arrhythmias and conduction disturbances are often suspected as the cause of syncope, but have not been documented due to the infrequent occurrence of these events. This study was designed to evaluate the role of electrophysiologic studies in the evaluation of this group of patients.

Material and methods

Twenty-six patients with recurrent unexplained syncope were referred to the Cardiac Electrophysiology Laboratory at Thomas Jefferson University Hospital. Previously, all patients had undergone complete history, physical examination, and routine laboratory testing which did not reveal any non-cardiac cause of syncope. Neurological evaluation including an electroencephalogram or computed axial tomography was performed in each patient. 48 hours of continuous inpatient or ambulatory monitoring off antiarrhythmic medication did not reveal any significant arrhythmias. Patients with sinus bradycardia less than 45 beats/min., SA block, Mobitz II second degree AV block, or greater than three spontaneous repetitive ventricular depolarizations were excluded from the study. No patient had obstructive, valvular heart disease. The clinical characteristics of the 26 patients are summarized in Table 1.

Table 1.

Patient	Age, Sex		Cardiac DX	ECG	Electrophysiologic Study Results	Treatment	Follow-up (mos)	Symp-toms
1	82	F	PCD	LBBB	↑ HV	pacemaker	32	no
2	64	F	CM	1° AVB, RBBB, LAFB	↑ HV, Mobitz II	pacemaker	27	no
3	36	M	NONE	WNL	CS hypersensitivity	pacemaker	23	no
4	72	F	NONE	LAFB	–	–	22	no
5	19	F	MVP	WNL	–	–	18	yes
6	72	M	CM	1° AVB, LIVCD, LAFB	sustained VT	Amiodarone	17	no
7	81	M	NONE	WNL	non-sustained VT	Procainamide	16	no
8	59	F	PCD	WNL	–	–	18	yes
9	78	F	NONE	WNL	↑ SACT, ↑ CSNRT	pacemaker	14	no
10	63	F	NONE	WNL	–	–	14	no
11	29	M	NONE	WNL	AV node dysfunction	–	12	no
12	49	M	AVR, MVR	1° AVB, LBBB	sustained VT	Amiodarone	11	yes
13	31	M	PCD	RBBB, LAFB	intra-His block	pacemaker	8	no
14	55	M	CAD	IMI	intra-His block	pacemaker	7	no
15	57	M	CAD	AMI	sustained VT	Amiodarone	7	no
16	73	M	CM	WNL	CS hypersensitivity	pacemaker	10	no
17	51	F	AI	RIVCD	non-sustained VT	Procainamide, pacemaker	8	no
18	65	M	NONE	WNL	–	–	10	no
19	35	F	CM	1° AVB, LBBB	–	–	10	yes
20	63	M	PCD	RBBB, LAFB	CS hypersensitivity	pacemaker	6	no
21	32	M	MVP	WNL	–	–	15	yes
22	67	F	CM	LBBB	sustained VT	Quinidine & Mexiletine	6	yes
23	81	F	NONE	WNL	↑ CSNRT	pacemaker	3	no
24	64	M	CM	1° AVB, LIVCD, LAFB	–	Procainamide	1	died
25	60	M	CAD	IMI	–	–	1	no
26	52	F	HCVD	1° AVB	AV node dysfunction	pacemaker	2	no

Definitions: PCD = primary conduction disease, CM = cardiomyopathy, MVP = mitral valve prolapse, AVR = aortic valve replacement, MVR = mitral valve replacement, CAD = coronary artery disease, AI = aortic insufficiency, HCVD = hypertensive cardiovascular disease, LBBB = left bundle branch block, AVB = AV block, RBBB = right bundle branch block, LAFB = left anterior fascicular block, LIVCD = left interventricular conduction defect, IMI = inferior myocardial infarction, AMI = anterior myocardial infarction, CS = carotid sinus, VT = ventricular tachycardia, CSNRT = corrected sinus node recovery time, SACT = sinoatrial conduction time.

The electrophysiology study was performed in the post-absorptive non-sedated state. All anti-arrhythmic medications were discontinued at least 48 hours prior to the study. Pacing catheters were inserted either percutaneously or via cutdown and positioned at multiple cardiac sites including the high right atrium, coronary sinus, right AV junction for recording of the His potential, and the apex of the right ventricle. Intracardiac recordings were filtered between 30 and 500 Hz and recorded with surface electrocardiographic leads I, AVF, and V_1 on a Electronics for Medicine VR-12 multichannel recorder.

Programmed cardiac stimulation was performed with a programmed digital stimulator (Bloom Associates) which delivered impulses of 2 msec. duration at twice diastolic threshold. The protocol for atrial and ventricular stimulation included the following:

1. Atrial pacing at incremental rates beginning just above the sinus rate and continuing until second degree AV block developed.
2. Premature atrial stimulation during spontaneous rhythm and following atrial pacing at multiple cycle lengths.
3. Ventricular premature stimulation from two right ventricular sites at multiple cycle lengths using one, two, and three premature stimuli.
4. Brief bursts of rapid ventricular pacing up to 250 beats per minute.
5. Carotid sinus massage for 5 seconds.

If ventricular tachycardia (VT) could be induced during the baseline study, the patients underwent serial electropyhsiologic testing to determine an effective anti-arrhythmic regimen (4, 5). If all available anti-arrhythmic agents failed to suppress induction of VT, the patients were placed on oral Amiodarone 400 mg daily, following a loading dose of 1200 mg per day for 10–14 days.

Corrected sinus node recovery times (CSNRT) were calculated according to the method of Narula (6). Values for sinoatrial conduction time were determined using the method of Strauss and associates (7). The normal values for AH and HV intervals and AV Wenckebach rate were taken from published data (8).

Prolongation of the HV interval was considered significant if it was greater than 70 msec.

If a specific electrophysiologic abnormality was demonstrated during the electrophysiology study it was presumed that this was diagnostic of an arrhythmic cause of syncope. Therapy was then directed by the results of the study.

Definitions:

1. SA node dysfunction- abnormal corrected sinus node recovery time and/or sinoatrial conduction time.
2. AV node dysfunction- prolonged AH interval and AV node Wenckebach at atrial pacing rate of less than 130 beats/min.
3. Infranodal conduction defect- HV interval greater than 70 msec, development of Mobitz II AV block with atrial pacing.
4. Carotid sinus hypersensitivity- greater than 3 seconds of asystole following carotid sinus massage.
5. Non-sustained VT- 6 or greater repetitive ventricular responses following premature ventricular stimulation.
6. Sustained VT- VT lasting longer than 15 seconds or requiring cardioversion for hemodynamic compromise.

Results

Electrophysiologic findings: The electrophysiologic abnormalities, subsequent treatment and follow-up of the 26 patients are outlined in Table 1. Seventeen of the 26 patients (65%) had abnormalities detected during the electrophysiology study which were considered to be the cause of their recurrent syncope. VT was induced in six patients. Two patients had rapid non-sustained VT while in four patients the VT was sustained. DC cardioversion was required in all four patients with sustained VT because of hemodynamic collapse.

Conduction defects were detected in eleven patients. Two patients had sinus node dysfunction and two had AV node dysfunction. Evidence of abnormal infranodal conduction was demonstrated in four patients. Prolongation of the HV interval (> 70 msec.) occurred in 2 of these patients. In one, Mobitz II second degree AV block was induced with atrial pacing. The two additional patients demonstrated intra-His block with atrial pacing. Three other patients showed evidence of carotid sinus hypersensitivity. The remaining nine patients had non-diagnostic electrophysiologic studies.

Bundle branch block (BBB) or interventricular conduction defects (IVCD) were seen in eleven patients. Four patients had left bundle branch block, 3 had right bundle branch block and left anterior fascicular block (LAFB), 1 had LAFB, 1 had right IVCD, and 2 had left IVCD plus LAFB. Abnormalities were detected during the electrophysiology study in 8/11 of these patients. Four patients had VT (3 sustained, 1 nonsustained) and four had conduction defects.

Treatment:

Therapeutic decisions based on the findings of the electrophysiologic study were made in the 17 patients with abnormal studies. The six patients with VT had serial programmed ventricular stimulation on various anti-arrhythmic drug regimens. A positive response was obtained in three of six patients. Both patients with non-sustained VT had a positive response to oral procainamide. One of the patients with sustained ventricular tachycardia responded to a combination of Quinidine and Mexiletine. The three patients with a negative response were placed on oral Amiodarone. Two of the patients with ventricular tachycardia subsequently received permanent pacemakers. One patient (# 12) developed symptomatic sinus arrest while on oral Amiodarone. The other patient on oral procainamide (# 17) had evidence of sinus arrest during contrast injection of the right coronary artery. The reason for insertion of a permanent pacemaker is not clear.

Ten of the 11 patients with conduction defects demonstrated during the initial electrophysiology study received permanent pacing. Patient # 11 had evidence of AV node dysfunction and was followed clinically.

None of the 9 patients with non-diagnostic studies received permanent pacemakers. One of these patients (# 24) was treated with anti-arrhythmic medication even though VT could not be induced during the electrophysiology study.

Clinical Follow-up

The 26 patients included in the study were followed for a mean of 12.2 ± 7.9 months (range 1–32 months). Fifteen of the 17 patients in whom therapy was directed by the results of electrophysiologic testing have been free of recurrent syncope during the follow-up period (Fig. 1). Both patients with recurrent syncope had inducible sustained VT during the initial study and were treated with anti-arrhythmic medication. Syncope recurred in patient # 12 one month following reduction of Amiodarone dosage. Patient # 22 developed nausea and unsteadiness during the first month of therapy with Quinidine and Mexiletine. Syncope recurred following discontinuation of Mexiletine. Since being placed on oral Amiodarone, the patient has had no recurrent symptoms.

Syncope continued to recur in four of the 9 patients with non-diagnostic studies (Fig. 2). An additional patient (# 24) died suddenly 1 month following initial study. A diagnosis for syncope was made in two of the four patients with recurrent events. One patient (# 8) had a transient ischemic attack 15 months following the initial study while the other (# 21) continues to have syncopal episodes despite treatment for non-sustained VT detected on later ambulatory monitoring. Syncope continues to be unexplained in the two remaining patients.

Discussion

The purpose of this study was to assess the role of electrophysiologic studies in the diagnosis and treatment of patients with unexplained syncope. The major findings of the study are:

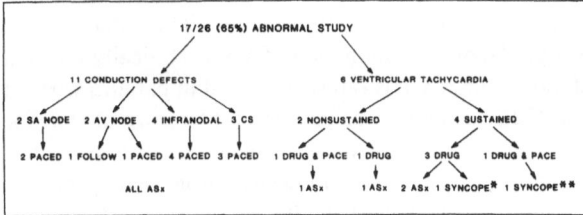

Fig. 1. The electrophysiologic findings and clinical follow-up of the 17 patients with an abnormal study. * Syncope occurred following discontinuation of Mexiletine. ** Syncope occurred 1 month following reduction of Amiodarone dosage. Abbreviations: CS = carotid sinus hypersensitivity; ASx = asymptomatic.

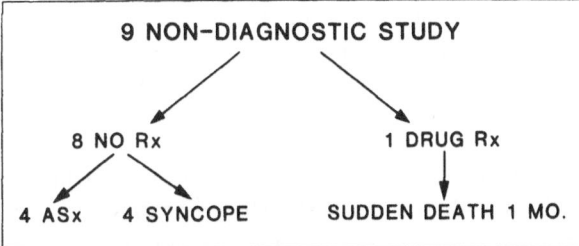

Fig. 2. The clinical follow-up of the nine patients with a non-diagnostic study.

1. conduction defects and tachyarrhythmias are frequently found during electrophysiologic testing in these patients;
2. therapy directed by the results of electrophysiologic testing is effective in preventing recurrent syncope;
3. VT was induced in 6/26 patients overall and 4/11 patients with BBB or IVCD highlighting the importance of programmed stimulation.

Cardiac electrophysiologic studies using intracardiac recordings and programmed electrical stimulation have been successfully applied to patients with known tachyarrhythmias and conduction defects (9–15). When these techniques were applied to our patients with unexplained recurrent syncope abnormalities were detected in 17/26 (65%) patients. Eleven patients had conduction defects and six patients had inducible VT. Other studies have shown that abnormalities are encountered during electrophysiologic study in a similar percentage of patients with unexplained syncope (16–19). By contrast, Gulamhusein and co-workers found that the electrophysiologic study was diagnostic in only 11.8% of their patients (20). Their study group consisted of patients with normal electrocardiograms and no clinical evidence of heart disease.

The differences in the diagnostic yield of the electrophysiologic study as well as the differing percentage of inducible VT may be explained by comparing the patient population of the various studies. Our patients had a high incidence of conduction system disease (42%) and underlying heart disease (69%). In our group of patients and those studied by others (16–19), the pre-test likelihood of a cardiac arrhytmia as the cause of syncope was high as opposed to the group of patients studied by Gulhamhusein and co-workers with no organic heart disease in whom the pre-test likelihood of a cardiac arrhythmia was much lower. Therefore, by applying Bayesian analysis electrophysiologic testing may have a high diagnostic yield in selected patients with unexplained syncope (21).

It is well established that prolongation of the HV interval in symptomatic patients is of prognostic importance (13–15). Our study and the observations of others (16–20) show that programmed stimulation gives additional diagnostic information. These data suggest that in patients with recurrent syncope, laboratory induction of VT is clinically relevant and not due to the stimulation technique. First, VT is rarely provoked in patients without a clinical history of the arrhythmia (22). Secondly, our patients with recurrent syncope have been free of recurrent symptoms when treatment was directed by the results of electrophysiologic testing. Thirdly, return of symptoms when effective drug therapy was reduced or discontinued is additional indirect evidence that VT was the cause of syncope. In our patients with conduction defects during electrophysiologic study it was presumed that transient bradyarrhythmias was the cause of syncope. It is impossible to be certain that these laboratory abnormalities were related to the patient's symptoms since abnormalities of sinus node and AV node conduction are sometimes encountered in asymptomatic patients (23, 24). However, our patient group was composed of patients with recurrent symptoms so that treatment could be adequately followed. None of the patients with conduction defects who had a permanent pacemaker inserted has had recurrent syncope.

Further evidence that laboratory abnormalities are useful in directing the treatment of patients with recurrent syncope is supplied by the patients with non-diagnostic studies. In these nine patients, syncope recurred in four patients and one patient died suddenly. Other studies have shown that patients with non-diagnostic studies continue to have symptoms (16, 18, 19). Programmed stimulation of the left ventricle and following isoproterenol may have increased the diagnostic yield of inducible arrhythmias in these patients.

Previous studies have shown that syncope and sudden death continue to occur in some patients with symptomatic bundle branch block despite permanent pacing (13, 25). This suggests that tachyarrhythmia rather than bradyarrhythmia is the cause of symptoms. Of our 11 patients with BBB or IVCD, four had conduction defects and four had inducible VT. Two of the four patients with inducible VT received permanent pacemakers in addition to drug therapy making it difficult to assess their therapy. However, in one of these patients syncope recurred when the anti-arrhythmic drug dose was reduced. The remaining 2 patients with BBB or IVCD and inducible VT are asymptomatic on anti-arrhythmic medication alone. This underscores the need for complete electrophysiologic studies, including programmed stimulation in patients with BBB and syncope.

In most patients a cause for syncope can be demonstrated by conventional techniques (1–3). This study demonstrates the additional value of electrophysiologic testing in the diagnosis and management of patients when the diagnosis is still unknown. Abnormalities were detected during the electrophysiology study in 17 of 26 patients. Fifteen of the 17 patients with laboratory directed therapy were completely free of symptoms when followed for a mean of 12.2 ± 7.9 months. It should be emphasized that false positive and false negative tests may occur. The finding of a non-diagnostic study does not exclude the possibility of a cardiac arrhythmia as the cause of symptoms as one of our patients died suddenly and one subsequently had non-sustained VT. However, in selected patients cardiac electrophysiologic studies provide additional important diagnostic and therapeutic information when the diagnosis cannot be made by other means.

Acknowledgement

We gratefully acknowledge the secretarial assistance of Karen Goldsmith.

References

1. Johansson VW: Long-term ECG in ambulatory clinical practice. Eur J Cardiology 1977; 5: 39.
2. Lipski J, Cohen L, Espinoza J, et al: Value of holter monitoring in assessing cardiac arrhythmias in symptomatic patients. Am J Cardiology 1976; 37: 102.
3. Boudoulas H, Schaal SF, Lewis RP, et al: Superiority of 24-hour outpatient monitoring over multi-stage exercise testing for the evaluation of syncope. J Electrocardiography 1979; 12: 103.
4. Mason JW, Winkle RA: Electrode catheter arrhythmia induction in the selection and assessment of anti-arrhythmic drug therapy for recurrent ventricular tachycardia. Circulation 1978; 58: 971.
5. Horowitz LN, Josephson ME, Farshidi A, et al: Recurrent sustained ventricular tachycardia 3. Role of the electrophysiologic study in selection of anti-arrhythmia regimens. Circulation 1978; 58: 986.
6. Narula OS, Samet P, Javier RP: Significance of the sinus node recovery time. Circulation 1972; 45: 140.
7. Strauss HC, Saroff AL, Bigger JT, et al: Premature atrial stimulation as a key for understanding sinoatrial conduction in man. Circulation 1973; 47: 86.
8. Josephson ME, Seides SF: Clinical cardiac electrophysiology: Techniques and interpretations. Lea & Febiger, Philadelphia 1979; 44.
9. Josephson ME, Horowitz LN, Farshidi A, et al: Recurrent sustained ventricular tachycardia 1. Mechanisms. Circulation 1978; 57: 431.

10. Wellens HJJ, Schulenburg RM, Durrer D: Electrical stimulation of the heart in patients with ventricular tachycardia. Circulation 1972; 46: 216.
11. Josephson ME, Horowitz LN: Electrophysiologic approach to therapy of recurrent sustained ventricular tachycardia. Am J Cardiology 1979; 43: 631.
12. Josephson ME, Kastor JA: Supraventricular tachycardia: Mechanisms and management. Ann Int Med 1977; 87: 346.
13. Dhingra RC, Denes P, Wu D et al: Syncope in patients with chronic bifascicular block. Annals of Int Med 1974; 81: 302.
14. Scheinman MM, Peters RW, Modin G, et al: Prognostic value of infranodal conduction time in patients with chronic bundle branch block. Circulation 1977; 56: 240.
15. Altschuler H, Fisher JD, Furman S: Significance of isolated HV interval prolongation in symptomatic patients without documented heart block. Am Heart J 1979; 97: 19.
16. DiMarco JP, Garan H, Harthorne JW, et al: Intracardiac electrophysiologic techniques in recurrent syncope of unknown cause. Annals of Int Med 1981; 95: 542.
17. Brandenburg RO, Holmes DR, Hartzler GO: The electrophysiologic assessment of patients with syncope. (Abst) Am J Cardiology 1981; 47: 433.
18. Hess DS, Morady F, Scheinman MM: Electrophysiologic testing in the evaluation of patients with syncope of undetermined origin. Am J Cardiology 1982; 50: 1309.
19. Akhtar M, Shenasa M, Denker S, et al: Role of cardiac electrophysiologic studies in patients with unexplained recurrent syncope. Pace 1983; 6: 192.
20. Gulamhusein S, Naccarelli GV, Ko PT, et al: Value and limitations of clinical electrophysiologic study in assessment of patients with unexplained syncope. Am J Med 1982; 73: 700.
21. Rifkin OR, Hood WB Jr: Bayesian analysis of electrocardiographic stress testing. NEJM 1977; 297: 681.
22. Vandepol CJ, Farshidi A, Spielman SR, et al: Incidence and clinical significance of induced ventricular tachycardia. Am J Cardiology 1980; 45: 725.
23. Brodsky M, Wu D, Denes P, et al: Arrhythmias documented by 24-hour continuous electrocardiographic monitoring in 50 male medical students without apparent heart disease. Am J Cardiology 1975; 39: 390.
24. Meytes I, Kaplinsky E, Yakini JH, et al: Wenckebach AV block: a frequent feature following heavy physical training. Am Heart J 1975; 90: 426.
25. Peters RV, Scheinman MM, Modin G, et al: Prophylactic permanent pacemakers for patients with chronic bundle branch block. Am J Med 1979; 66: 978.

Authors' address:
Arnold J. Greenspon, M.D.
Thomas Jefferson University Hospital
111 S. 11th Street
Suite 5611D
Philadelphia, Pennsylvania 19107

Effects of Intravenous Amiodarone on Refractory Periods of the His Purkinje System

B. Perrot, D. Zallot, N. Danchin, F. Cherrier, G. Faivre

Summary: In 4 patients an intrahisian second degree AV block occurred during oral amiodarone (Am) therapy (daily dose of 400 mg) and disappeared 3 months after the end of Am. To assess a relation between Am and intrahisian AV block, 150 mg of Am were injected in 26 patients (pts) with prolonged HV interval and/or infrahisian block induced by programmed atrial (A) extrastimulus technique. His Purkinje anterograde effective refractory period (HP ERP) was the longest H1 H2 interval in which conduction to the ventricles failed to occur (H1 = His bundle electrogram of the A paced rhythm, H2: His bundle electrogram after the extrastimulus); HP functional RP (HP FRP) was the shortest propagated V1–V2 interval and HP relative RP (HP RRP) was the longest H1 H2 interval with H2–V2 > H1–V1. The HP RP were studied before and after Am at the same A paced rhythm. HP–RP increased (2 to 12%) in 9pts; HP-AV-conduction was abnormal (spontaneous HV interval > 55 ms, HV interval after Ajmaline ⩾ 100 ms, intrahisian second degree AV block during A pacing a rate ⩽ 150 b/min) in 6 pts. HP-RP could not be calculated in 8 pts: an AV nodal block occurred after inj. of Am. The HP-AV-conduction was normal in these pts. HP RP were identical in 7 pts, shorter in 2 pts. In these pts the HP-AV-conduction was normal.

In conclusion, intravenous Am lengthened HP RP in 9 pts out of 26 (34%). This effect was more frequent in pts with abnormal HP-AV-conduction. Am should be used with carefulness in pts with abnormalities of HP-conduction. The occurrence of a second or third degree AV block with normal QRS during oral Am therapy indicates an electrophysiological study to determine the level of the block which might be within AV node or HP system.

Introduction

Amiodarone is a potent antiarrhythmic agent which is especially useful in controlling supraventricular tachycardias associated with the Wolff Parkinson White syndrome as well as refractory ventricular tachyarrhythmias (1, 2, 3). If the general adverse effects are frequent and known, the cardiovascular side effects of Amiodarone are rare (4).

Four patients reported cardiac adverse effects. A type II second degree AV block was recorded after 2–5 months of oral therapy in a dose of 400 mg/day. His bundle recording showed a conduction delay within His Purkinje system.

A permanent pacemaker was implanted in all of them but the resting ECG became normal within 3 months after the end of oral amiodarone therapy. Repeated electrophysiologic studies were not performed.

To assess a relationship between amiodarone and the His Purkinje System (HPS), between the HPS refractory periods (HPS RP) and the HPS conduction time and to show a depressive action on diseased conduction system, intravenous amiodarone was given to patients who had a prolongation of HV interval during atrial premature stimulation.

I. Patients and Methods

1. Population

26 patients who had a prolongation of the HV interval during single test stimulus method, were selected; in these patients the anterograde HPS RP could be measured. The ages of the patients ranged from 37 to 82 years.

An electrophysioloic study was performed to assess the causes of dizziness or syncope in 21 patients and to delineate the mechanism of tachycardias in 5 patients.

2. Electrophysiologic studies

- The study was performed in the fasting state and after all medications had been stopped for at least 72 hours.

Electrodes for stimulation and recording were positioned in the high right atrium, close to the septal cusp of the tricuspid valve and at the apex of the right ventricle. Surface ECG leads I, III, V1, V2, V6 and the intracardiac electrograms (right atrium, His bundle electrogram) were recorded using a Siemens IEKG 823 system at paper speed 100 mm/sec. Pacing was performed using a programmable stimulator (Medtronic 1325) delivering impulses of 1.8 ms duration at a current strength of 1 to 3 mA.

- The following electrophysiological measurements were made during the study:
  1. Basic intervals PA, AH and HV.
  2. Anterograde AV conduction assessed by atrial pacing at incremental rates until 2nd degree AV block occurred.
  3. Anterograde conduction system refractory periods determined by the extrastimulus technique: Atrial premature stimulation (A2) was introduced during sinus rhythm and driven atrial rhythm (A1 A1) after every 8 beats with a progressively shortened interval of prematurity until atrial refractoriness was reached. The driven atrial rhythm was made generally at the slowest paced rate producing stable atrial capture.
- After the control measurements had been recorded, Amiodarone was administered intravenously in a dose of 150 mg over a period of 1 min. Four minutes post injection the measurements of anterograde conduction system refractory periods were repeated.

In particular the His Purkinje system refractory periods were measured at the same cycle length of that for the baseline test.

- 15 minutes following the end of this study Ajmaline was administered intravenously in a dose of 1 mg/kg over a period of 1 min. 3 minutes later, HV interval was measured and the level and the rate of the second degree AV block was assessed by atrial pacing at incremental rates.

3. Definitions

A1 H1 and V1 represented the atrial, His bundle, and ventricular electrograms of either spontaneous or driven beats. A2, H2, V2 represented the atrial, His bundle, and ventricular electrograms in response to the extra stimulus (S2).

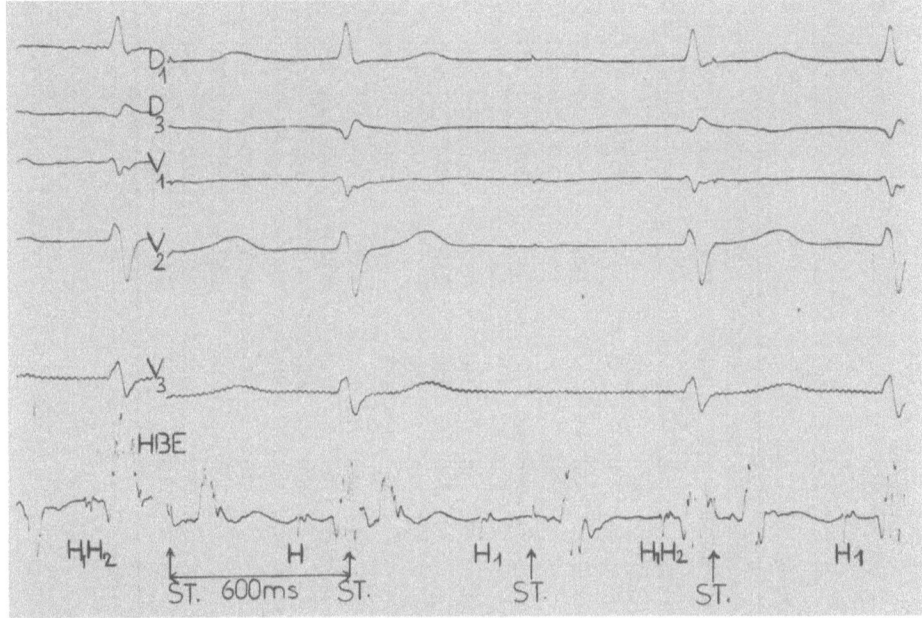

Fig. 1. Electrophysiologic study performed 15 days following arrest of oral amiodarone.
The Holter monitoring showed a second degree AV block (type Mobitz II). During electrophysiologic study there was just a first degree AV block due to an intrahisian AV block. (HI H2 = 25 ms, H1V1 = 60 ms, H2 V = 45 ms) and a suprahisian AV block (AH1 = 180 ms). During atrial pacing the second degree AV block was intrahisian and occurred at rate of 100 beats/min.

- The atrial effective refractory period (A. ERP) was the longest S1 S2 interval in which atrial capture failed to occur.
- The ERP of the His Purkinje system (HPS ERP) was the longest H1 H2 interval in which conduction to the ventricles failed to occur.
- The relative refractory period of the His Purkinje system (HPS RRP) was defined as the longest H1 H2 interval at which the H2 V2 interval becomes longer than H1 V1 interval of spontaneous or driven beats. Prolongation of H2 V2 could reflect conduction delays in the His bundle distal to the His bundle recording site and/or delays in both bundle branches.
- The functional refractory period of the His Purkinje system (HPS FRP) was the shortest V1 V2 interval achieved. All determinations could be not be obtained in all patients.

II. Results

A) Effect of intravenous amiodarone on the refractory periods of the His Purkinje system (HPS RP).

757

Table 1. Increase of the HP refractory period (c = control values, Am = values after Amiodarone).

	Age (years)	Sex	Resting ECG	AH int (ms)	HV int (ms)	A pacing Rate of 2nd AVB (beats/min)	Ajmaline (HV ms)	HPFRP (ms)	HPRRP (ms)	HPEPR (ms)	AERP (ms)	CL (ms)
1 C	75	F	LBBB	40	55	230 SupraH	InfraH 2/1	310	300	280	200	600
Am					55		Av block	340	320	320	210	600
2 C	37	M	RBBB + LAH	60	70	100 InfraH		630		580	250	800
Am				80	70			660		650	260	800
3 C	78	F	LBBB	90	40	100 InfraH		540		500	300	1300
Am				90	40			550		535	340	1300
4 C	69	M	Normal	50	40	220 SupraH	50	360	340	330	260	650
Am				65	40			370	350	360	260	650
5 C	66	F	RBBB	70	40	180 SupraH	70	410	320		200	700
Am				70	40			460	350		200	700
6 C	82	M	RBBB + LAH	55	70	80 InfraH		480		400	280	950
Am				60	70			550		430	290	950
7 C	56	M	RBBB + LAH + 1rstd AV block	50	95	140 InfraH		430	420	410	250	700
Am				55	95			445	435	430	260	700
8 C	76	F	Normal	45	30	180 SupraH	60	510	500	470	330	900
Am				45	30			540	510	480	300	900
9 C	71	M	RBBB + LPH	160	70	100 InfraH		670		660	300	900
Am				160	70			710		700	310	900

1. Increase of the HPS RP (Table 1):

HPS FRP, RRP and ERP were prolonged at comparable rates in 9 patients (group 1) (average 31, 6 ms ± 20 ms). Both RRP and ERP were prolonged (Fig. 2–3) but the mean increase of every refractory period was not always identical. HV interval was unchanged. The A-ERP was unchanged in 2 patients, prolonged in 6 patients and shortened in 1 patient.

2. Constancy or shortening of the HPS RP (Table 2):

The HPS RP were unchanged in 7 cases and were shortened in 2 patients (group 2). The mean shortening was 15 ms. The HV interval was unchanged.
The A ERP was prolonged in 3 patients, shortened in 2 patients and not calculated in 3 patients who developed atrial echo beats after amiodarone.

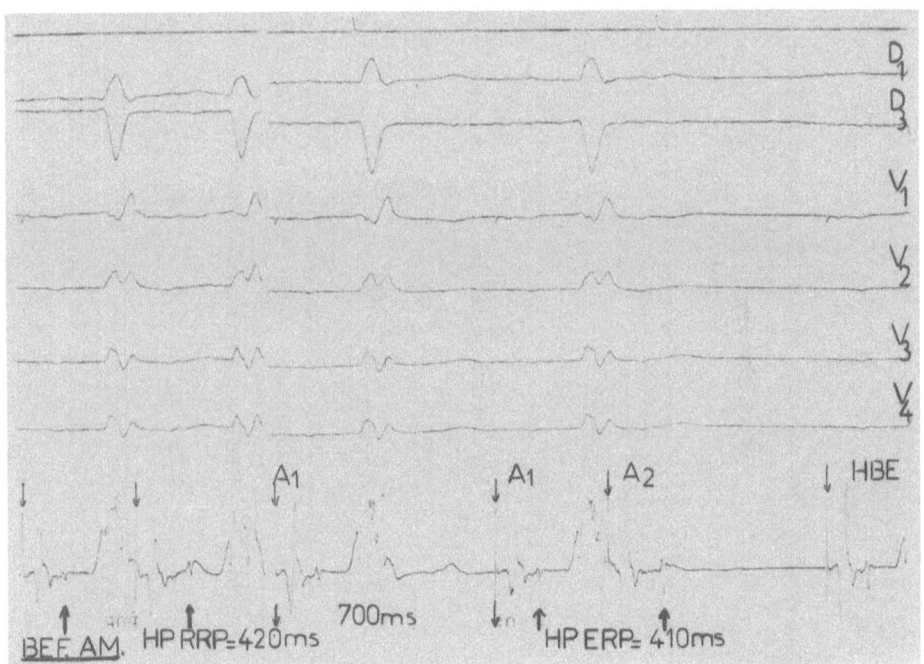

Fig. 2. Electrophysiologic study before amiodarone: the ECG showed a RBBB and LAH – HV was prolonged (HV = 70 ms).
With the method of atrial premature stimulation A2, introduced during driven atrial rhythm (A1 A1 = 700 ms), the value of HP RRP was 420 ms, HP ERP: 410 ms.

Table 2. Constancy of the HP refractory periods after Amiodarone (Am).

	Age (years)	Sex	Resting ECG	AH int (ms)	HV int (ms)	A pacing Rate of 2nd AVB (beats/min)	Ajmaline (HV ms)	HPFRP (ms)	HPRRP (ms)	HPEPR (ms)	AERP (ms)	CL (ms)
1 C	58	M	Normal	80	40	200 SupraH	60	420	380	370	210	800
Am					40			400	380		200	800
2 C	49	F	Normal	70	40	190 SupraH	60	420	420	390	230	900
Am					40			420	410			900
3 C	59	F	Normal	70	40	150 SupraH	60	410	400		250	700
Am					40			410	400		230	700
4 C	56	F	Sinus Brady-cardia	60	30	170 SupraH	40	460	450	445	320	1100
Am					30			460	450			1100
5 C	69	F	RBBB	50	50	160 SupraH	95	340		330	230	600
Am					50			340		330		600
6 C	28	F	RBBB + LPH	70	55	230 SupraH	90 + InfraH 2nd AVB (150b/min)	460		430	250	800
Am					55			460		430	260	800
7 C	43	F	Normal	60	40	180 SupraH	50	340	320		230	550
Am					40			340	300		235	550
8 C	56	M	RBBB + LAH	80	50	160 SupraH	90	480	450		280	1000
Am					50			500	440			1000
9 C	66	M	RBB	70	55	160 SupraH	60	480	420	410	280	900
Am					55			440	430		290	900

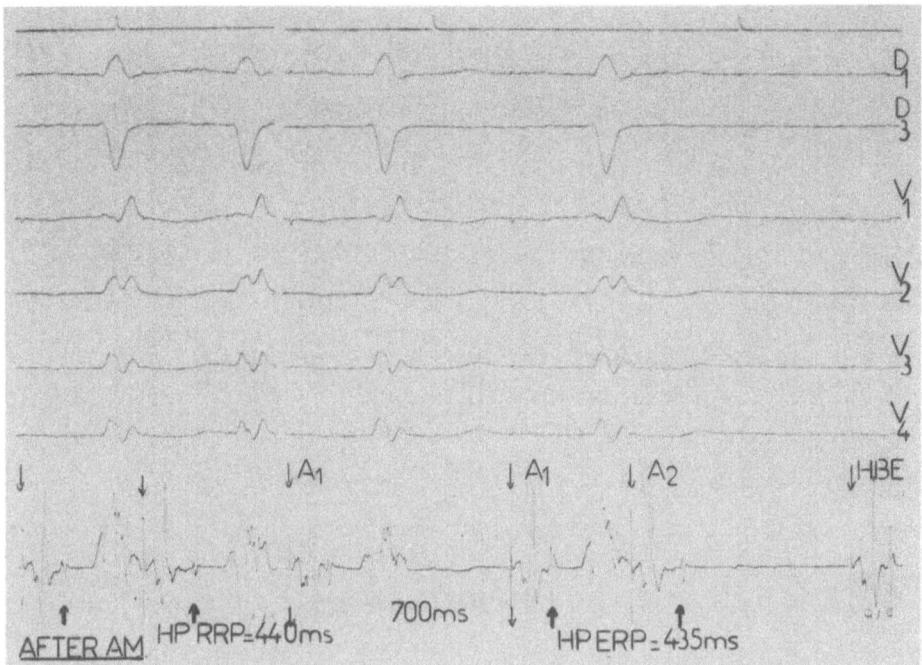

Fig. 3. Electrophysiologic study after injection of 150 mg Amiodarone in the same patient than on figure 2. During the identical driven atrial rhythm (A1-A1 = 700 ms) the value of HP RRP became 420 ms, HP ERP = 410 ms.

3. Occurrence of an AV nodal block with undetermined HPS RP (Table 3):

Prolongation of the AV node FRP masked any effect of amiodarone on the HPS in 8 patients (group 3). There was no change in HV interval. AH-interval was unchanged in 5 patients, prolonged in 2 patients, shortened in 1 patient.

B) Relationship between the action of amiodarone on HPS RP and basic AV conduction

AV nodal conduction was defined as abnormal when:
– Basic AH interval > 110 ms
– Onset of anterograde AV nodal Wenckebach block at rate ⩽ 130 beats/min.
HPS AV conduction was defined as abnormal when:
– Basic HV interval > 55 msec.
– Onset of an infrahisian AV block at rate of atrial pacing < 150 beats/min.
– HV Interval > 100 msec or occurrence of a second degree infranodal AV block following injection of Ajmaline.
1. In group I the HPS AV conduction was abnormal in 6 patients and normal in 2 patients. The AV-nodal conduction was normal except in a case with prolonged AH interval.

Table 3. Occurrence of a AV nodal block during premature atrial stimulation after Amiodarone.

	Age (years)	Sex	Resting ECG	AH int (ms)	HV int (ms)	A pacing Rate of 2nd AVB (beats/min)	Ajmaline (HV ms)	HPFRP (ms)	HPRRP (ms)	HPEPR (ms)	AERP (ms)	CL (ms)
1 C	73	M	RBB + LAH	110	50	140 SupraH	90	490	450	430	250	1050
Am				110	50							1050
2 C	68	F	LBBB	110	55	150 SupraH	70	490	480	470	260	1100
Am				120	55							1100
3 C	38	M	LBBB	45	55	250 SupraH	60	380		370	240	800
Am				50	55							800
4 C	74	F	Sinus Brady-cardia	120	50	160 SupraH	50	550	490	450	250	1100
Am				120	50							1100
5 C	70	M	RBBB	60	40	160 SupraH	60 + InfraH 2nd AVB (Rate 140b/min)	420		410	220	900
Am				60	40							900
6 C	67	F	Normal	60	30	220 SupraH	60	430	430	400	210	700
Am				60	30							700
7 C	39	M	Normal	80	40	180 SupraH	70	430	420		260	900
Am				80	40							900
8 C	77	M	Sinus Brady-Cardia	90	35	180 SupraH	70	480	440		250	1150
Am				80	35							250	·1000

2. In group II the HPS-AV conduction was normal in 8 patients and uncertain in 1 patient: in this case basic HV-interval (55 msec) and HV-interval following Ajmaline (90 ms) were normal, but an infrahisian second degree AV-block occurred during atrial pacing at rate of 150 beats/min after Ajmaline. The AV nodal conduction was always normal.

3. In group III the HPS-AV conduction was normal in 7 patients and uncertain in 1 patient: In this case basic HV-interval (40 msec) and HV interval following Ajmaline (60 msec) were normal but an infrahisian second degree AV block occurred during atrial pacing at rate 140 beats/min after Ajmaline.

The AV-nodal conduction was normal except in 1 patient with prolonged AH interval (120 ms).

The main difference between the three groups was the frequency (66%) of a pathological HPS-AV conduction in group I which had a prolongation of the HPS RP after amiodarone.

C) Relationship between the effect of amiodarone and the value of HPS refractory periods

– In group I the mean basic HPS-ERP was 453.75 msec. The mean HPS-ERP was 482.22 msec; individual values were very variable, due to important differences of the cycle length (600 to 1300 msec).

The mean cycle length was 833.33 msec.

– In group II the mean basic HPS ERP was 395.83 msec. The mean HPS FRP was 423.33 msec.

The mean cycle length was 816.66 msec.

– In group II the mean basic HPS ERP was 421.66 msec. The mean HPS FRP was 458.75 msec.

The mean cycle length was 962.5 msec.

For a similar mean cycle length the values of HPS-RP were longer in group I than in group II. They were difficult to compare with the group III which had a longer mean cycle length responsible for longer HPS-RP.

III. Discussion

Amiodarone is an antiarrhythmic agent of class III (Vaughan Williams) which has been shown to be effective in suppressing atrial and ventricular arrhythmias.

Both intravenous and oral forms of the drug are effective but their electrophysiological effects are not strictly similar (5) because of the extremely long and variable half life of the oral preparation; most studies are performed using the intravenous form; the antiarrhythmic effects of intravenous amiodarone begin between the first and the third minute following injection and are maximum ten minutes post injection (6).

1. Previous studies

– The major cellular electrophysiologic effect of amiodarone is uniform prolongation of action potential duration with little effect on the rate of rise of the upstroke; it may be related to a competitive inhibition of sodium, potassium dependent ATP ase activity (7, 8).

– In animals, intravenous use reduces the diastolic slope of the sinus node, increases the duration of the sinus node action potential, and prolongs the duration of the action potential in both the atrium and ventricle leading to prolongation of refractory periods (9).

– In man, intravenous amiodarone (5 mg/kg) has been shown to reduce the heart rate, lengthen the refractory periods in the atrium, AV node, His Purkinje System and ventricle and to depress AV-node conduction without any effect on infranodal conduction (10, 11, 12).

The effect of oral amiodarone are sligthly different but they have rarely been studied because of the very long half life of the drug (13).

Wellens (5) shows a prolongation of the effective refractory period of the atrium and ventricle and an increase of HV-interval after oral amiodarone while intravenous amiodarone does not change these values. The effective refractory period of the AV-node and the AH interval are prolonged both after intravenous and oral amiodarone.

Finerman (14) finds a prolongation in conduction time in the AV node (AH interval), HPS (HV interval) and an increase in the QRS width during atrial pacing after oral amiodarone. The increase of HV-interval was noted in same patients even in those with normal HV intervals prior to the drug. For this author, the prolongation of the His Purkinje system relative refractory period is not important enough to explain the prolongation of the HV-interval. This may be explained by the presence of some form of intraventricular conduction defect on the surface ECG. However the effects of amiodarone on the action potentials of diseased His Purkinje tissue is not known.

Rosenbaum (15) has drawn attention to the fact that chronic amiodarone therapy may exacerbate pre-existing right bundle branch disease in some patients. Since ischemia may convert the dependence of phase 0 depolarization of an action potential from a sodium mechanism to predominantly a calcium mechanism and since the effect of amiodarone on the isolated sinus node may be due to inhibition of calcium dependent mechanisms, a similar effect of amiodarone on diseased His Purkinje tissue may have a marked effect on conduction in the HPS.

– During the chronic use of amiodarone the cardiovascular side effects of the drug are rare. Fauchier (15) and Marcus (17) do not report worsening of patients with bundle branch block and infrahisian impairment. However, Rosenbaum (15) reported a widening of QRS complexes in 6 out of 68 patients with intraventricular conduction disturbances and the occurrence of 2 second degree AV blocks.

2. Present study

In 4 patients a second degree intrahisian AV block occurred during oral amiodarone therapy.

Although the effects of oral and intravenous amiodarone are different we have looked for a relationship between the known depressive action of intravenous amiodarone on the His Purkinje System refractory periods and the existence of a diseased AV conduction system.

In a previous study (18) we have shown a relationship between the values of HPS effective refractory period and the HPS AV conduction: HPS-ERP was longer than 400 ms for a cycle length < 1000 ms in patients with abnormal HPS-AV-conduction.

Beside the role of the HPS-AV-conduction, 3 other variables can change the HPS refractory periods, they depend on the value of the HPS RP themselves, of the cycle length and of the effective refractory period of the AV node (19).

When the cycle length increases, HPS-RP is prolonged; the AV-node ERP should be shorter than the HPS ERP to note HV-prolongation during atrial premature stimulation.

After amiodarone the prolongation of the AV-node refractory periods usually masks any effects on the HPS and it becomes difficult to study the value of the HPS RP.

In all patients of this study the HPS RP could be measured. Their changes have been compared to the AV conduction. It appears that intravenous amiodarone prolongs the HPS RP principally in patients with diseased HPS-AV-conduction; the HPS RP is unchanged in 9 cases, prolonged in 2 cases, and uncalculable in 8 patients.

Another relationship is noted between the initial value of HPS RP and the action of amiodarone. The drug prolongs the longer HPS RP. When the HPS ERP is > 400 ms for a cycle length < 1000 ms, HPS-AV-conduction is usually pathological and the use of amiodarone may be responsible for prolongation of the HP RP.

In conclusion, intravenous amiodarone lengthened the HPS refractory periods in 9 patients out of 26 (34.6%). This effect was found to be more frequent in patients with abnormal HPS-AV-conduction. There is a relationship between pathological distal AV conduction and a long initial value of HPS ERP. Intravenous amiodarone should be used with carefulness in patients with HP ERP > 400 ms for a cycle length < 1000 ms, lengthening of HPS ERP being possible.

In clinical use, although the effects of intravenous and oral amiodarone are sligthly different and because of the relationship between the prolongation of HPS-AV-conduction and HPS RP the drug should be used with caution in patients with abnormalities of HPS conduction. The occurrence of a second or third degree AV block with normal QRS during oral amiodarone therapy warrants an electrophysiological study to determine the level of the block which might be within AV node or HP system.

References

1. Podrid P, Lown B: Amiodarone therapy in symptomatic sustained refractory atrial and ventricular tachyarrhythmias. Am Heart J 1981; 101: 374–379.
2. Rowland E, Krikler D: Electrophysiological assessment of amiodarone in treatment of resistant supraventricular arrhythmias. Br Heart J 1980; 44: 82–90.
3. Ward DE, Camm AJ, Spurrell RAJ; Clinical antiarrhythmic effects of amiodarone in patients with resistant paroxysmal tachycardias. Br Heart J 1980; 44: 91–95.
4. Rotmensch H, Belhassen B, Ferguson R: Amiodarone – Benefits and risks in perspective. Am Heart J 1982; 104: 1117–1119.
5. Wellens H, Brugada P, Roy D, Heddle B, Bar F: A comparison for the electrophysiological effects of intravenous and oral amiodarone. Am J Cardiol 1982; 49: 1043.
6. Derrida JP, Chiche P: Pharmacocinétique des principaux antiarythmiques. Coeur Med Int 1978; 17: 79–88.
7. Sebag C, Motte G: Mécanismes d'action cellulaire des médicaments antiarythmiques. Coeur Med Int 1978; 17: 509–519.
8. Vaughan Williams EM: Intérêt des études expérimentales d'antiarythmiques et leur application clinique. Coeur Med Int 1978; 17: 471–489.
9. Puech P, Cabasson J, Mellet JP, Guimond L, Bachy C, Massine A: Analyse des effects électrophysiologiques de l'amiodarone par l'enregistrement simultané des potentiels d'action monophasique et du faisceau de His. Colloque sur l'amiodarone, Paris, nov 1977: 18–21.

10. Touboul P, Attalah G, Gressard A, Michelon G, Chatelain MT, Delahaye JP: Effets électrophysiologiques des agents antiarythmiques chez l'homme. Tentative de classification. Arch Mal Coeur 1978: 72–81.
11. Touboul P, Huerta F, Porte J, Delahaye JP: Bases électrophysiologiques de l'action anitarythmique de l'amiodarone chez l'homme. Arch Mal Coeur 1976; 69: 845–853.
12. Touboul P, Porte J, Huerta F, Delahaye JP: Electrophysiological effects of amiodarone in man. Am J Cardiol 1975; 35: 173.
13. Frank R, Fontaine G, Grosgogeat Y: Etude de l'effet antiarythmique de l'amiodarone per os par les méthodes provocatives. Colloque sur l'amiodarone, Paris, Nov 1977: 35–42.
14. Finerman W, Hamer A, Peter T, Weiss D, Mandel W: Electrophysiologic effects of chronic amiodarone therapy in patients with ventricular arrhythmias. Am Heart J 1982; 104: 987–995.
15. Rosenbaum MB, Chiale PA, Halpern MS, Nau GJ, Przybylski J, Levi RJ, Lazzari JO, Elizari MV: Clinical efficacy of amiodarone as an antiarrhythmic agent. Am J Cardiol 1976; 38: 934–944.
16. Fauchier JP, Brochier M, Raynaud R: Etude clinique des effets antiarythmiques ventriculaires de l'amiodarone (orale ou injectable). Ann Cardiol Angéiol 1973; 22: 427–435.
17. Marcus F, Fontaine G, Frank R, Grosgogeat Y: Clinical pharmacology and therapeutic applications of the antiarrhythmic agent, amiodarone. Am Heart J 1981; 101: 480–493.
18. Perrot B, Cherrier F, Faivre G: Valeurs de la période réfractaire antérograde effective du faisceau de His. Arch Mal Coeur 1981; 74: 381–389.
19. Denes P, Wu D, Dhingra R, Pietras R, Rosen K: The effects of cycle length on cardiac refractory periods in man. Circulation 1974; 49: 32–41.

Authors' address:
Dr. Beatrice Perrot
Cardiologie chu Brabuis
F-54500 Vandoeuvre
France

Effect of Antiarrhythmic Drugs on Ventricular Late Potentials at Sinus Rhythm and at Constant Atrial Rate

R. A. Jauernig, J. Senges, W. Lengfelder, I. Rizos, Ellen Hoffmann, J. Brachmann, W. Kübler

Summary: In 16 patients with documented sustained ventricular tachycardia and late potentials recorded by precordial signal averaging, the effects of various class I and III antiarrhythmic drugs on late potentials were examined during sinus rhythm and during atrial pacing at 100 or 120/min. During sinus rhythm, antiarrhythmic drugs produced no consistent change of late potential duration and no change of late potential amplitude: prolongation of late potentials ranged from 2 to 26 ms, shortening of late potentials occurred in 20% and ranged from 1–10 ms. During atrial pacing, the late potential duration was consistently prolonged, the mean from 42 ± 18 to 48 ± 20 ms ($p < 0.01$) after antiarrhythmic drugs. Shortening of late potentials did not occur. The late potential amplitude remained unchanged (4.7 ± 2.0 vs. 4.6 ± 1.5 μV). Changes in late potential duration induced by the antiarrhythmic drugs were not related to their antiarrhythmic efficacy assessed by programmed right ventricular stimulation. Thus, the effects of antiarrhythmic drugs on late potentials are dependent on atrial rate. The changes observed, however, are smaller than those reported from direct recordings in animal experiments and are not suitable for the guidance of antiarrhythmic drug therapy.

Introduction

Ventricular late potentials recorded from the body surface by signal averaging have been reported to occur in 50–90% of patients with sustained ventricular tachycardia and chronic myocardial infarction (1–4). They are thought to represent late depolarization of a mass of ventricular tissue after delayed conduction through depressed pathways and it has been demonstrated that late potentials can be altered or abolished by effective antiarrhythmic surgery (4, 5). The effects of antiarrhythmic drugs on late potentials have been studied in less detail and data were obtained only at sinus rhythm (6). In this study, the effects of class I and III antiarrhythmic drugs on duration and amplitude of ventricular late potentials were examined in patients with documented sustained ventricular tachycardia, 1) at sinus rhythm and 2) at constant atrial rate.

Methods and Patients

A Princeton Applied Research signal averager (model 4203) and preamplifiers (model 113) were used for recording at least three bipolar leads from four electrodes, two placed parasternally left and right between the first and second intercostal space, one approximately 6 cm medial to the apex and one in the posterior axillary line at the height of the fifth intercostal space. Total system amplification was 5×10^5, bandpass filter settings were between 100 and 300 Hz. The averaged signals were printed out using a Hewlett-Packard 7015B x-y pen recorder. The methods employed were adapted from those suggested by Breithardt et al. (1). The study group comprised 16 patients who fullfilled the following 2 criteria: 1) a history of documented sustained ventricular tachycardia and 2) late potentials in signal averaged precordial leads. They were between 36 and 82 years old (mean 58 ± 11, S.D.), one was female, 15 were male, 2 had no past history of myocardial infarction, 14 had suffered myocardial infarction between 1 month and 14 years prior to the study (mean 29 ± 46 months, S.D.), 2 patients had anterior, 10 posterior, and 2 both anterior and posterior myocardial infarction. The tracings were evaluated visually by two independent examiners. The end of a late potential was defined by retrograde analysis of the ST-segment to the point where the constant baseline noise level was clearly exceeded. From this point, the duration of the late potential was measured retrogradely to the onset of the first highfrequency deflection that exceeded twice the medium amplitude of the late potential. The late potential amplitude was measured from the maximum deflection of the signal.

From all patients, control recordings were obtained in the nonsedated, post-absorptive state after all antiarrhythmic therapy had been discontinued for at least two days. The following drugs were applied intravenously (dosage in brackets, mg/kg body weight; number of trials indicated before each drug):

5× Ajmaline (1.25 mg/kg); 5× Aprindine (3 mg/kg);
4× Disopyramide (2 mg/kg); 1× Flecainide (1.5 mg/kg);
3× Lidocaine (3 mg/kg); 1× Mexiletine (3 mg/kg);
2× Procainamide (15 mg/kg); 5× Propafenon (1.5 mg/kg);
2× Quinidine (10 mg/kg); 14× Sotalol (1.5 mg/kg).

The dose of oral Amiodarone was 800 mg daily for two weeks, followed by a maintenance dose of 400 mg/day. 6 recordings on oral Amiodarone were obtained, at least 6 weeks after initiation of the treatment.

In 9 patients, a hexapolar catheter electrode for both right atrial and ventricular stimulation was used. In those patients, the antiarrhythmic drugs were tested both for their ability to prevent induction of ventricular tachycardia and for their effects on late potential duration and amplitude during sinus rhythm and during atrial pacing at a higher rate, usually 100 or 120/min. Student's t-test was used for statistical evaluation. Values are given as means with standard deviations.

Results

During sinus rhythm, the mean late potential duration increased insignificantly from 38 ± 16 ms to 41 ± 20 ms. During 41 trials, a shortening of late potential duration ranging from 2 to 10 ms was observed in 20% of all cases (Fig. 1). There was no significant correlation between prolongation or shortening of late potentials and the antiarrhythmic efficacy of the drugs during programmed right ventricular stimulation. The mean action potential amplitude was 4.8 ± 1.3 μV under control conditions and 4.9 ± 1.6 μV after antiarrhythmic drug administration. Fig. 2 gives an example of antiarrhythmic drug effects on late potentials during sinus rhythm.

At constant atrial rate, 100 or 120/min, depending on heart rate during sinus rhythm and the rate of second degree AV-block, the mean action potential duration increased from 42 ± 18 ms to 48 ± 20 ms. This increase was statistically significant ($p < 0.01$), and in contrast to the effects seen at sinus rhythm, no shortening of late potential duration was observed after the administration of antiarrhythmic drugs (Fig. 3).

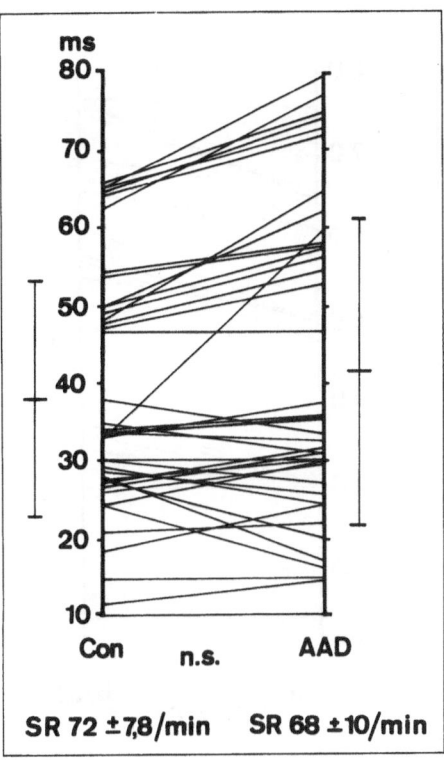

Fig. 1. Effect of antiarrhythmic drugs (AAD) on ventricular late potential duration during sinus rhythm. CON = Control. There is a nonsignificant trend towards longer late potential duration after antiarrhythmic drugs. A shortening of late potential duration occurred in 20% of all cases.

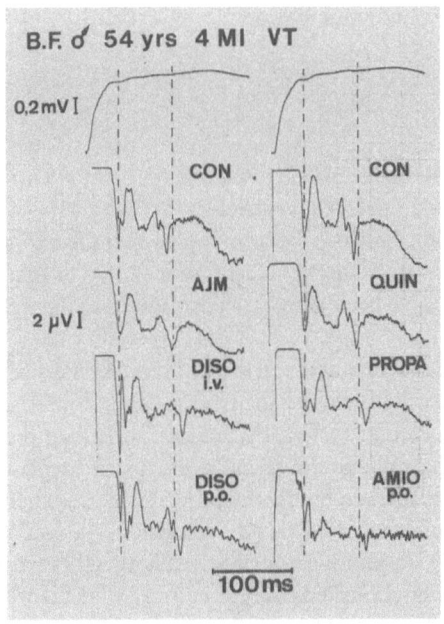

Fig. 2. Effect of various antiarrhythmic drugs on late potential duration during sinus rhythm in a 54 years old male patient with a past history of multiple myocardial infarctions (MI) and recurrent sustained ventricular tachycardia (VT). The two top tracings are reference curves at lower gain obtained under control conditions. CON = Control; AJM = Ajmaline; QUIN = Quinidine; DISO = Disopyramide; PROPA = Propafenon; AMIO = Amiodarone. Disopyramide both intravenously (i.v.) and orally (p.o.) and Amiodarone (p.o.) prevented induction of VT, the other drugs did not.

Fig. 3: Effect of antiarrhythmic drugs (AAD) on ventricular late potential duration at constant atrial rate. CON = Control. The late potential duration is significantly prolonged by the antiarrhythmic drugs. Note that in contrast to Fig. 1, a shortening of late potential duration was never observed.

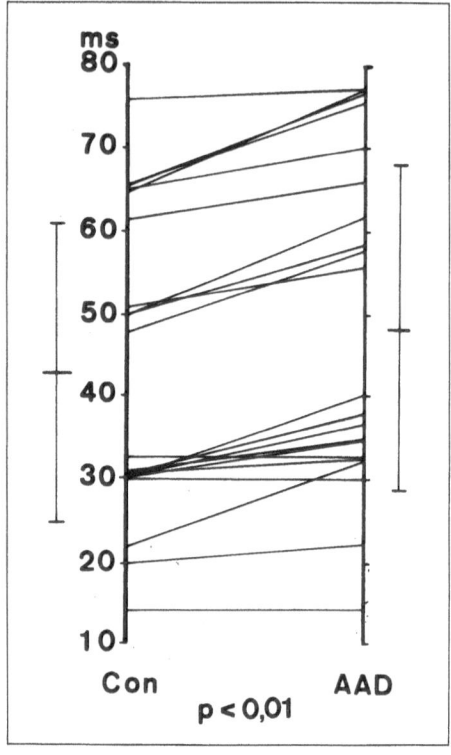

The mean amplitude of the late potentials was 4.7 ± 2.0 μV under control conditions and 4.6 ± 1.5 μV after administration of the antiarrhythmic drugs.

Discussion

Low amplitude late potentials recorded from the body surface in patients prone to ventricular tachycardia have been related to regional delayed ventricular activation (1–4). Experimental data suggest a positive correlation between late potentials recorded from the body surface and those directly measured from infarcted epicardium (7, 8). In man, late potentials recorded from the body surface have been shown to correspond to delayed fragmented endocardial electrographic activity (9).

Effective antiarrhythmic surgery guided by endocardial and epicardial mapping has been shown to abolish late potentials recorded precordially whilst their postoperative persistence indicated persistant ability to induce ventricular tachyarrhythmias (5). In one previous study, the absence of late potentials during precordial signal averaging in patients with ventricular tachycardia effectively controlled on antiarrhythmic drug treatment could have been interpreted to indicate a potential value of signal averaging for assessing the efficacy of antiarrhythmic drug therapy (1). In another previous study using precordial signal averaging, antiarrhythmic agents never abolished delayed activity whilst it was abolished by aneurysmectomy (4). In one report, the duration of the averaged highly amplified QRS-complex increased with Amiodarone, Quinidine and Procainamide, but the incidence of late potentials was unchanged (6). In a canine model of re-entrant ventricular arrhythmias, conduction in potentially re-entrant pathways evidenced by delayed epicardial electrical activity was slowed and eventually abolished by lidocaine and diphenylhydantoin (10, 11). In the same model, conduction disorders in ischemic myocardium varied with heart rate (12).

In this study, antiarrhythmic drugs did not affect late potentials in a consistent manner during sinus rhythm. When antiarrhythmic drug induced changes of sinus rate were eliminated and heart rate was kept constant by atrial pacing at 100 or 120 beats/min, antiarrhythmic drugs consistently produced a small but significant prolongation of late potential duration. These effects are, however, unsuitable to allow an assessment of antiarrhythmic drug efficacy in the prevention of ventricular tachyarrhythmias.

It has been speculated that this lack of effect of antiarrhythmic drugs on late potentials may indicate that antiarrhythmic drugs prevent ventricular tachyarrhythmias by acting on normal rather than damaged myocardium (6). This would, however, be in sharp contrast to experimental evidence (10, 11).

It could be speculated that more pronounced changes of late potentials might have been produced if atrial pacing had been done at a higher rate. There are, however, obvious limitations to further increase in heart rate, such as further impairment of compromised cardiac performance, reduced coronary perfusion, or early appearance of second degree AV-block after antiarrhythmic drug administration.

Thus, in spite of increasing evidence supporting the significance of late potentials as a marker for ventricular tachyarrhythmias, they do not appear to be of value for the prediction of antiarrhythmic drug efficacy.

References

1. Breithardt G, Becker R, Seipel L, Abendroth RR, Ostermeyer J: Non-invasive detection of late potentials in man – a new marker for ventricular tachycardia. Eur Heart J 1981; 2: 1–11.
2. Breithardt G, Borggrefe M, Karbenn U, Abendroth RR, Yeh HL, Seipel L: Prevalence of late potentials in patients with and without ventricular tachycardia: correlation with angiographic findings. Am J Cardiol 1982; 49: 1932–1937.
3. Simson MB: Use of signals in the terminal QRS complex to identify patients with ventricular tachycardia after myocardial infarction. Circulation 1981; 64: 235–242.
4. Rozanski JJ, Mortara D, Myerburg RJ, Castellanos A: Body surface detection of delayed depolarizations in patients with recurrent ventricular tachycardia and left ventricular aneurysm. Circulation 1981; 63: 1172–1178.
5. Breithardt G, Seipel L, Ostermeyer J, Karbenn U, Abendroth RR, Borggrefe M, Yeh HL, Bircks W: Effects of antiarrhythmic surgery on late ventricular potentials recorded by precordial signal averaging in patients with ventricular tachycardia. Am Heart J 1982; 104: 996–1003.
6. Simson MB, Waxman HL, Falcone R, Marcus NH, Josephson ME: Effects of antiarrhythmic drugs on noninvasively recorded late potentials. In: Breithardt G, Loogen F, eds. New aspects in the medical treatment of tachyarrhythmias. München–Wien–Baltimore: Urban & Schwarzenberg, 1983; 80–87.
7. Berbari EJ, Scherlag BJ, Hope R, Lazzara R: Recording from the body surface of arrhythmogenic ventricular activity during the S-T segment. Am J Cardiol 1978; 41: 697–702.
8. Simson MB, Euler D, Michelson EL, Falcone RA, Spear JF, Moore EN: Detection of delayed ventricular activation on the body surface in dogs. Am J Physiol 1981; 241: (Heart Circ Physiol 10) H363–H369.

9. Simson MB, Untereker WJ, Spielman SR, Horowitz LN, Marcus NH, Falcone RA, Harken AH, Josephson ME: Relation between late potentials on the body surface and directly recorded fragmented electrograms in patients with ventricular tachycardia. Am J Cardiol 1983; 51: 105–112.
10. El-Sherif N, Scherlag BJ, Lazzara R, Hope RR: Re-entrant ventricular arrhythmias in the late myocardial infarction period. Circulation 1977; 56: 395–402.
11. El-Sherif N, Lazzara R: Re-entrant ventricular arrhythmias in the late myocardial infarction period. Circulation 1978; 57: 465–472.
12. El-Sherif N, Scherlag BJ, Lazzara R, Hope RR: Re-entrant ventricular arrhythmias in the late myocardial infarction period. Circulation 1977; 55: 686–702.

Authors' address:
Dr. R. A. Jauernig
Medizinische Universitätsklinik (Kardiologie)
Bergheimer Straße 58
D-6900 Heidelberg

Drug-Induced Changes in the Duration of Ventricular Repolarization Evaluated by the Paced Endocardial Evoked Response

R. M. Donaldson, P. Taggart, F. Nashat, A. F. Rickards

Summary: The paced endocardial evoked response (PER) documents the dominantly local activation and repolarization which follows controlled (paced) depolarization from the same site. Duration of the PER at matched rates was used to assess the effects of drugs with class 3 mode of action on ventricular repolarization time in man. Amiodarone IV (5 mg/kg) prolonged PER duration from 258 ms to 297 ms (average 39.5 ms or + 15%) in 8 patients (pts) (p < 0.001). The AV nodal effective refractory period (ERP) increased from 276 ± 35 ms to 338 ± 60 ms (p < 0.01) but the ventricular ERP did not change, suggesting that early amiodarone activity favours changes in action potential duration. Sotalol IV (1 mg/kg) increased PER duration (average 32 ms or + 12%) in 7 pts (p < 0.005) and prolonged the ventricular ERP from 257 ± 5 ms to 276 ± 10.7 ms (p < 0.05). Oral bethanidine (5 mg/kg) increased PER duration at 4 hrs from 260 ms to 286 ms (average 25.8 ms or + 10%) in 6 pts (p < 0.005). Changes in PER correlated well with simultaneous MAP recordings in animal experiments and in man. The PER has the advantage of clinical simplicity, requiring only a conventional electrode.
The effects of drugs on the duration of the cellular action potential can be assessed indirectly by the PER, which constitutes a new tool in electrophysiological investigations.

Drug-induced changes in repolarization times in man have been documented using endocardial monophasic recordings with suction electrodes (1, 2) but most of the clinical studies have extrapolated the surface QT interval in the assessment of modifications of action potential duration. Though uniform prolongation of the ventricular action potentials can be detected as a lengthened QT interval, the QT itself represents the algebraic sum of millions of action potentials and its measurement is not a reliable index of the underlying transmembrane potential duration (3). Furthermore, correction of the QT interval to QTc by heart rate assumes a simple relationship between rate and QT interval; this assumption has been shown to be unjustified (4, 5, 6). A pharmacological decision based on a prolonged QTc can be misleading in instances where QT varies at the same heart rate or is invariant as heart rate changes. As many antiarrhythmic drugs induce heart rate changes, a rate-independent method using controlled depolarization would be of value in studying such agents.

The paced endocardial evoked response (PER) system has the advantage of clinical simplicity (7). The same electrode is used for pacing and sensing and it is possible to record the T wave which represents the dominantly local repolarization following a pacing-induced depolarization from the same site at a controlled heart rate. Measurements of the PER before and after drug administration should allow comparison of the effects of drugs on the duration of repolarization, studies which are only possible at present on a short term basis using endocardial suction catheters. The object of our investigation was to establish the potential clinical application of this method and to assess the acute effects of 3 antiarrhythmic drugs (amiodarone, sotalol and bethanidine) which are known to prolong action potential in tissue preparations.

Patients and Methods

The drugs were evaluated in 21 patients undergoing electrophysiological study in the non-sedated, post absorptive state. Cardio-active medications were stopped for at least three days before the study. Three or four pacing electrodes were introduced percutaneously into the right femoral vein and positioned in the heart. Recordings relevant to this study were made from a bipolar pacing electrode in the right ventricular apex.

The method of sensing and recording the paced endocardial evoked response has been described in detail (7). Basically the technique employs a conventional unipolar pacing electrode which delivers a pacing stimulus of approximately 2.5 mA for 0.5 ms to the ventricular endocardium, care being taken to ensure that only the cathodal current is applied. The PER is seen as a negative QRS wave reaching a nadir in approximately 40 ms after the pacing pulse; this is followed by a clearly defined positive T wave (Figs. 1 and 2). The

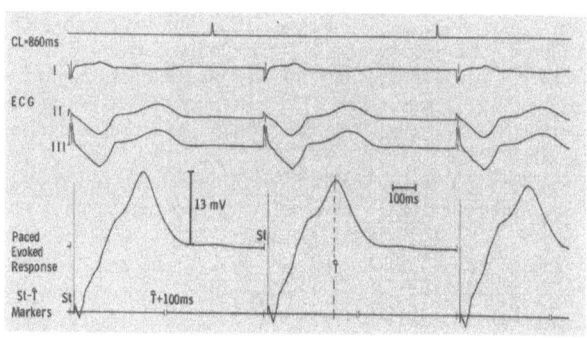

Fig. 1. The paced endocardial evoked response is seen as a negative QRS reaching a maximum amplitude approximately 40 ms after the pacing stimulus (St). The peak detector has an adjustable sensing window; this detector generates a marker pulse, 100 ms following detection of the peak of the evoked T wave (T̂). This marker is recorded together with St, and the St-T̂ interval measured automatically on a beat to beat basis by the pacing system. The St-T̂ time is corrected by subtracting the 100 ms imposed by the pacing system.

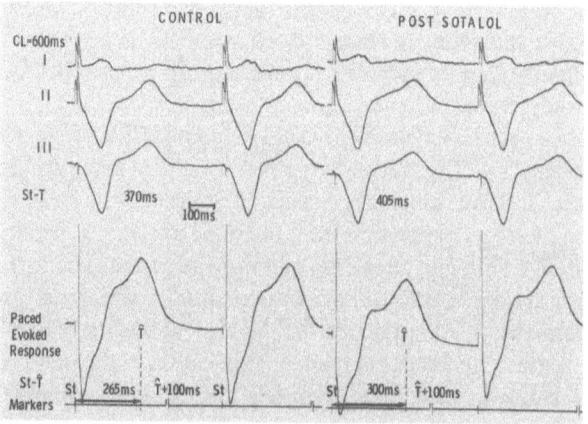

Fig. 2. Changes in the duration of the paced evoked response 10 minutes after intravenous sotalol. The PER increased 35 ms. Note also a similar change in the QT interval on the scalar ECG.

incorporation of a peak detector with an adjustable sensing window (Fig. 1) into the pace-maker permits measurement of the interval between the applied stimulus and the peak of the evoked T wave automatically on a beat to beat basis. The Stimulus-peak T wave interval was taken as the average of 30 consecutive cycles after subtracting the 100 ms imposed by the pacing system (Fig. 1). The distance between the pacing stimulus and the nadir of the negative QRS was deemed to represent activation time, while that between the stimulus and peak of the T wave provides a measurement of the local repolarization time.

Recordings of the ECG, the PER and the T wave timing markers were made at paced cycle lengths of 600 ms (100 beats per minute) and at a paper speed of 100 and 200 mm/s. The right ventricular effective refractory period (RV ERP) was documented before and on average 15 minutes after drug infusion using the extrastimulus technique. In 5 patients simultaneous right ventricular PER and monophasic action potentials were obtained and repolarization time measured by both methods.

Amiodarone was administered intravenously to 8 patients at a dose of 5 mg/kg over 10 minutes; sotalol was infused at a dose of 1 mg/kg in 7 patients; bethanidine administered orally to 6 patients at full adrenergic blocking doses (5 mg/kg).

Two-tailed paired t tests were utilized for data analysis.

Results

Amiodarone prolonged PER duration in all patients studied (n = 8) from a mean of $258 \pm$ (SD) 11.9 ms to 297 ± 8.9 ms (av 39.7 ms; 15% of control values) (p < 0.001). Maximum increase in PER was reached at 10 minutes post infusion coinciding with peak blood levels of the drug; at this stage the AV nodal refractory period was increased from 276 ± 35 ms to 338 ± 60 ms (p < 0.01) but the RV ERP had not altered significantly (Table). Local activation time as documented by the PER was also increased by a mean of 5 ms.

Bethanidine (n = 6) significantly prolonged the PER duration 4 hours after oral administration by an average of 25.8 ms (10% of control) (p < 0.005). The detailed results of the amiodarone and bethanidine studies have been published (7).

Table 1. Drug related changes in ventricular repolarization and refractoriness.

	Amiodarone (n = 8)			Sotalol (n = 7)		
	Before	After	Change	Before	After	Change
RV PER (ms)	258 ± 11.9	297 ± 8.9	39ms (+15%) p < 0.001	269 ± 18.6	301 ± 24.8	32ms (+12%) p < 0.005
RV-ERP (ms)	250 ± 12	265 ± 35	15ms p = NS	257 ± 5.7	276 ± 10.7	19ms (7.4%) p < 0.05

Cl = 600 ms

Sotalol (n = 7) increased the PER duration from 269 ± 18.6 to 301 ± 24.8 ms (av 31 ms, 12% of control values) (p < 0.005) (Fig. 2). In 5 of these patients simultaneous monophasic action potentials were obtained; the 90% repolarization time increased post sotalol infusion from 260 ± 18 ms to 291 ± 27.5 ms (p < 0.005). The RV ERP increased significantly at 10 minutes post sotalol infusion from 257 ± 5.7 ms to 276 ± 10 ms (p < 0.05).

Discussion

Knowledge of the electrophysiological effects of drugs in the intact beating heart can be obtained from measurement of the refractory periods; interpretation of the course and duration of repolarization in these conditions has been technically difficult, requiring the use of the monophasic action potential (MAP) recordings with suction electrodes. Only recently has this method been applied to the evaluation of drugs in man (1, 2). MAP recordings have technical limitations (8) and additional pacing is required to correct the changes in MAP duration produced by changes in the underlying heart rate.

By recording the local repolarization which follows a paced depolarization from the same site, the PER is suitable for the accurate assessment of the effects of drugs on the duration of myocardial repolarization. The incorporated peak detector assures reproducibility of the data; because the signal to noise ratio of the PER is tenfold that of the surface ECG (the average evoked T wave amplitude is 7 ± 3 mv), the peak of the T wave is easily visible even at very fast heart rates (Fig. 3). Furthermore, alterations in local activation time induced by drugs can only be documented by the PER.

We have previously demonstrated that drug-induced changes in the timing of local repolarization measured by the PER paralleled changes in duration of simultaneously recorded paced monophasic action potentials (7) and similar results were obtained during the sotalol study in the 5 patients in whom the PER and MAP D 90% was recorded. Both of these methods would thus appear to be complementary for the indirect assessment of the effects of therapeutic agents on the action potential duration of myocardial cells.

Fig. 3. Simultaneous recordings of the ECG, the PER and left ventricular monophasic action potential (LV MAP) in an open chested dog experiment. The 90% MAP repolarization time (D 90%) and the stimulus-T wave peak (St-T̂) are compared. As the paced cycle length (CL) decreases, there is a parallel decrease in the duration of myocardial repolarization time as assessed by both methods.

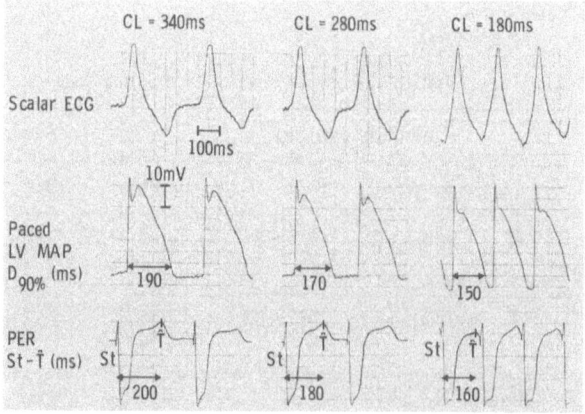

The current study confirms the clinical applications of this method in the assessment of the acute effects of drugs on action potential duration. The prolongation of the repolarization time by intravenous amiodarone as documented by the PER in man is of similar magnitude to that recorded in dogs using MAP (9). Amiodarone early activity at ventricular level appears thus to favour changes in action potentials duration as opposed to changes in refractoriness.

The sympathetic antagonist bethanidine prolonged the duration of the PER in similar magnitude to that produced by its analogue bretylium in tissue preparations (10). These changes in repolarization time probably account for the antiarrhythmic properties of bethanidine.

In addition to its intrinsic beta adrenoreceptor blocking properties, sotalol hydrochloride increases the duration of the cellular action potential in tissue preparations. Our studies using the paced endocardial evoked response method supports the data obtained by MAP in man (11) that sotalol causes acute prolongation of myocardial action potential in addition to prolonging ventricular refractoriness.

The effects of drugs on action potentials of various tissue models together with the clinical electrophysiological data obtained during the investigation of these agents have contributed to a clearer understanding of specific electropharmacological and antiarrhythmic actions and permit comparison with new drugs. Our studies suggest that the effects of "class 3" antiarrhythmic agents (12) on local myocardial repolarization can accurately be assessed by the paced evoked response and this new method should contribute to overcoming the many difficulties in comparing the results from in vivo experiments with the clinical effects of these drugs in man.

References

1. Olsson SB, Edvardsson W: Clinical electrophysiologic study of antiarrhythmic properties of Flecainide: acute intraventricular delayed conduction and prolonged repolarization in regular paced and premature beats using intracardiac monophasic action potentials with programmed stimulation. Am Heart J 1981; 102: 864–871.
2. Samuelsson EG, Harrison DC: Electrophysiologic evaluation of Encainide with use of monophasic action potential recording. Am J Cardiol 1981; 48: 871–876.
3. Vaughan Williams EM: QT and action potential duration. Br Heart J 1982; 47: 513–514.
4. Rickards AF, Norman J: Relation between QT interval and heart rate. New design of physiologically adaptive cardiac pacemaker. Br Heart J 1981; 45: 56–61.
5. Vaughan Williams EM, Hassan MO, Floras JS, Sleight P, Jones JV: Adaptation of hypertensives to treatment with cardioselective and non-selective beta-blockers. Absence of correlation between bradycardia and blood pressure control, and reduction in slope of QT/RR relation. BR Heart J 1980; 44: 473–487.
6. Milne JR, Camm AJ, Ward DE, Spurrell RAJ: Effect of intravenous propranolol on QT interval. A new method of assessment. Br Heart J 1980; 43: 1–6.
7. Donaldson RM, Rickards AF: Evaluation of drug induced changes in myocardial repolarization using the paced evoked response. Br Heart J 1982; 48: 381–387.
8. Olsson B, Varnauskas E, Korsgren M: Further improved method for measuring monophasic action potentials of the intact human heart. J Electrocardiol 1971; 4: 19–23.
9. Cabasson J, Puech P, Mellet JM, Guimond C, Bachy C, Sassine A: Analyse des effets electrophysiologiques de l'amiodarone par l'enregistrement simultane des potentials d'action monophasiques et du faisceau de His. Arch Mal Coeur 1976; 69: 691–699.
10. Bigger JT, Jaffe CC: The effect of bretylium tosylate on the electrophysiological properties of ventricular muscle and Purkinje fibers. Am J Cardiol 1971; 27: 82–92.

11. Edvardsson N, Hirsch I, Emanuelsson H, Ponten J, Olsson SB: Sotalol-induced delayed repolarisation in man. Eur Heart J 1980; 1: 335–343.
12. Vaughan Williams EM: Classification of anti-arrhythmic drugs. In "Symposium on Cardiac Arrhythmias". Sandøe E, Flensted-Jensen E, Olesen KH, eds. AB Astra Södertälje, Sweden, 1970: 449–472.

Authors' address:
Robert M. Donaldson
National Heart Hospital
Westmoreland Street
London W1M 8BA
U.K.

Treatment of Ventricular Tachyarrhythmias-Pacing

G. Steinbeck, Ch. Naumann d'Alnoncourt, B. Lüderitz

Summary: For termination of life-threatening, sustained ventricular tachyarrhythmias, both temporary pacing by intravenous insertion of pacing wires as well as permanent pacing by implantation of anti-tachycardiac pacemakers may be used. Pioneering work of Wellens and Josephson and associates has shown that in the vast majority of patients with recurrent sustained ventricular tachyarrhythmias, this arrhythmia can be both terminated and induced by programmed electrical stimulation of the heart under safe conditions in the catheterization laboratory. This method has gained rapid and widespread application for the following applications:
1. Termination of serious ventricular tachyarrhythmias otherwise difficult to manage,
2. Induction of tachyarrhythmias out of diagnostic reasons in patients in whom the spontaneous occurrence of these arrhythmias is suspected (unexplained syncope; sudden circulatory arrest). Serial electrophysiologic testing for assessment of antiarrhythmic drug efficacy in patients with recurrent sustained ventricular tachycardia or ventricular fibrillation.

In contrast to these frequently used applications of temporary pacing, only a small subgroup of selected patients should be treated chronically by implantation of anti-tachycardia pacemakers. Prerequisites of this therapeutic modality include:
1. Refractoriness of the arrhythmia to medical therapy;
2. antiarrhythmic surgery is not possible, the patient refuses surgery, or the risk seems to be high;
3. reliability of arrhythmia termination by pacing;
4. cooperation of the patient.

In this report we describe the results of implantation of anti-tachycardia pacemakers in six patients with recurrent sustained drug-refractory ventricular tachycardia. Based on these results, indications, risks, complications, and future trends of permanent anti-tachycardia pacing in ventricular tachyarrhythmias are discussed.

Pioneering work of Wellens (1) und Josephson and co-workers (2) has shown that in patients with recurrent sustained ventricular tachyarrhythmias this arrhythmia can be reproducibly terminated as well as initiated by programmed electrical stimulation of the heart under safe conditions in the catheterization laboratory. These findings can best be explained if one holds a reentry circuit responsible as mechanism of the tachycardia, although an automatic mechanism can hardly be excluded under clinical conditions. Whatever the electrophysiological mechanism of the tachycardia may be, pacing for the management of these patients may be used on a temporary basis by intravenous insertion of a pacing wire coupled to external programmable stimulators as well as on a permanent basis by implantation of anti-tachycardia pacemakers.

Temporary pacing

Today there are two major and widely used indications for temporary pacing in patients with ventricular tachyarrhythmias:
1. acute termination of serious sustained ventricular arrhythmias,
2. induction of tachyarrhythmias out of diagnostic reasons and serial electrophysiologic testing for assessment of antiarrhythmic drug efficacy.

779

ad 1.

Acute termination by programmed electrical stimulation via temporary pacing leads is most often used in the coronary care unit in patients with serious sustained ventricular tachyarrhythmias which are otherwise difficult to manage. The following pacing modes are used: Single premature stimuli, underdrive pacing, overdrive pacing, double, triple ... premature stimuli, burst pacing.

Exactly timed single premature stimuli, applied by an external programmable stimulator, may terminate ventricular tachycardias; also a pacing rate clearly below the rate of tachycardia may terminate the arrhythmia. Both methods, however, are usually only effective when the rate of the ventricular tachycardia is low (approximately below 180/min) (3). Overdrive pacing is understood as pacing the ventricles for a variable period at a rate up to 30 beats per minute faster than the rate of ventricular tachycardia. If this method fails, timed double or triple premature stimuli or, ultimately, burst pacing (pacing rate more than 30 beats per minute faster than tachycardia rate) may terminate the arrhythmia.

An example is shown in Fig. 1. Ventricular tachycardia is present. Single (left upper panel) and double premature stimuli (right upper panel) as well as overdrive pacing (not shown) do not terminate the tachyarrhythmia. Finally a short burst of rapid stimuli (interval 100 ms) is applied which ultimately stops the tachycardia. Recently it has been re-

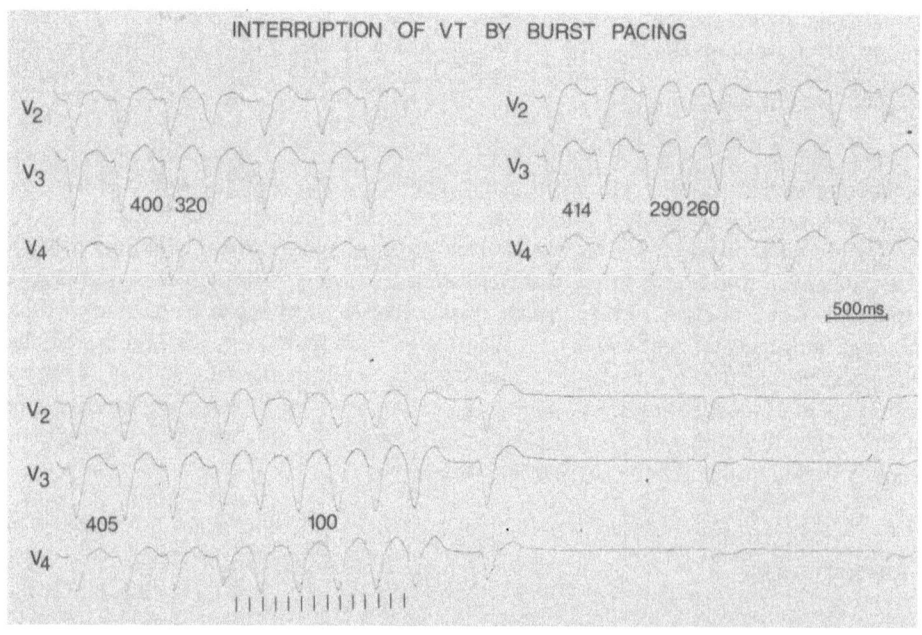

Fig. 1. Interruption of ventricular tachycardia by programmed ventricular stimulation. In all three panels unipolar leads V_2, V_3 and V_4 are shown.
To panel left: Single premature stimuli shorten the R-R interval, but do not stop tachycardia.
Top panel right: Douple premature stimuli are also ineffective.
Bottom panel: A series of 14 stimuli at an interval of 100 ms terminates the tachycardia.

ported that an increase of stimulus current strengths may increase the likelihood to terminate the arrhythmia (4) as well as one or two premature stimuli coupled to a series of overdrive pacing (5).

The more aggressive the stimulation protocol necessary for termination, the more it is likely that ventricular tachycardia does not stop, but degenerates into ventricular fibrillation. This is shown in Fig. 2.

Single premature stimuli (left upper panel) applied during ventricular tachycardia are ineffective, application of double premature stimuli (right upper panel) is followed by a ventricular echo. When the coupling interval of the premature stimuli is shortened further (bottom panel), ventricular fibrillation ensues so that the patient had to be DC-cardioverted. The incidence of acceleration of tachycardia rate and ventricular fibrillation while trying to interrupt the tachycardia by programmed stimulation, ranges between 7 and 50% (6, 7, 8).

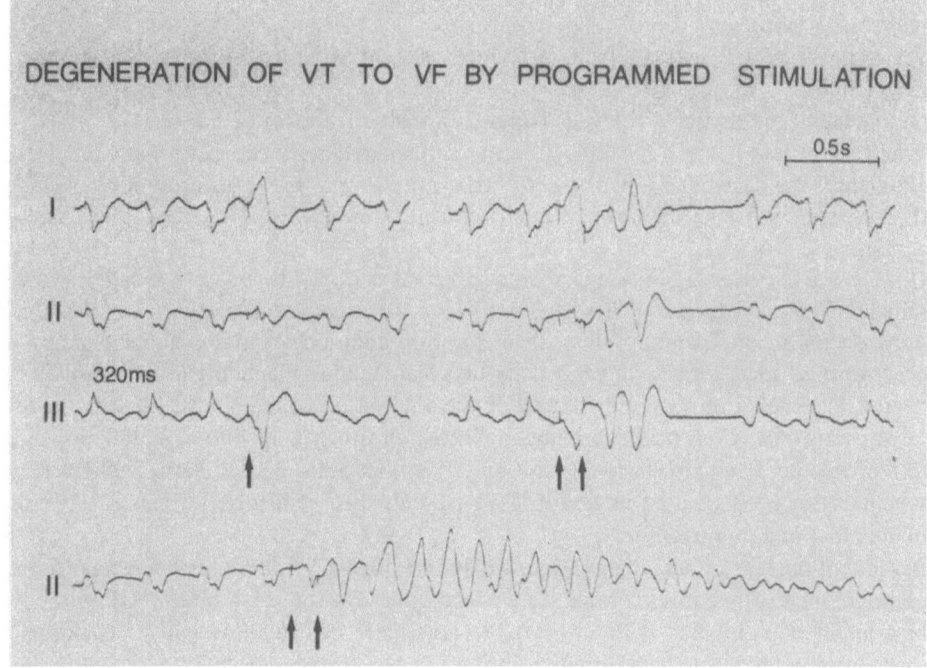

Fig. 2. Degeneration of ventricular tachycardia to ventricular fibrillation by programmed stimulation. Records of lead I, II and III are shown.
Top panel left: Application of single premature stimulus, ineffective.
Top panel right: Application of double premature stimuli, followed by one extra beat and, thereafter, persistence of tachycardia.
Bottom panel: Increasing the prematurity of the second premature stimulus, ventricular fibrillation is induced.

ad 2.

For the evaluation of patients with unexplained syncope or sudden circulatory arrest, induction of tachyarrhythmias may be of extreme diagnostic value (9). Furthermore, serial electrophysiologic testing in patients with recurrent sustained ventricular tachycardia or fibrillation may then be used for individual assessment of antiarrhythmic drug efficacy (10, 11).

Permanent pacing

In contrast to the frequently used applications of temporary pacing, implantation of anti-tachycardia pacemakers appears to be the therapy of choice only in a small, selected subgroup of patients with recurrent ventricular tachycardia.

Necessary prerequisites include refractoriness of ventricular tachycardia to medical therapy, reliability of tachycardia termination by pacing, cooperation of the patient; furthermore, antiarrhythmic surgery should either be not possible or the risk of operation high (12).

The following pacing modes may be used in anti-tachycardia pacemakers: underdrive, overdrive up to burst pacing, and extra-stimulus pacing. The pacemaker is activated either by the patient when he becomes symptomatic, or acts automatically when the tachycardia starts.

An example of the action of an implanted, patient-activated overdrive-pacemaker is shown in Fig. 3 (see also 13).

On the left of the rhythm strip, ventricular tachycardia is shown.

When the patient places a magnet above the implanted battery and starts an external trigger device, the pacemaker elicits a series of overdrive stimuli which promptly terminate the tachycardia. Using this principle, this patient terminated many attacks of his tachycardia.

Our general experience of antitachycardia pacemaker implantations in six patients is detailed in Table 1. The pacing mode chosen was underdrive in two, overdrive in three and burst pacing in one patient. All of them received additional antiarrhythmic therapy in order to slow down the rate of ventricular tachycardia and to facilitate its interruption by pacing. Pacemaker implantation turned out be of clear-cut benefit for all patients (see follow-up data); however, pacing became ineffective in two patients (no. 3 and 6), acceleration of rate occurred also in two (no. 3 and 4) so that anti-tachycardia pacemaker function later on was not used anymore. Two patients died suddenly, further two because of apoplexy and pump failure.

Because of the fear of rate acceleration, we, unlike others (12), have been reluctant to implant automatically-activated burst pacemakers intervening at high rate, which in the future might be combined with implantable automatic defibrillators (14) as back-up in case acceleration of rate or ventricular fibrillation occurs due to pacing.

Additional problems of permanent antitachycardia pacing include the fact that almost all patients need additional antiarrhythmic drug therapy. Furthermore, the antitachycardia pacemaker function may become ineffective due to a spontaneous change of the patient's tachycardia in rate and/or excitation pattern.

The latter problem may be partly overcome by a new generation of more sophisticated pacemakers, who allow to reprogram externally special antitachycardia pacemaker func-

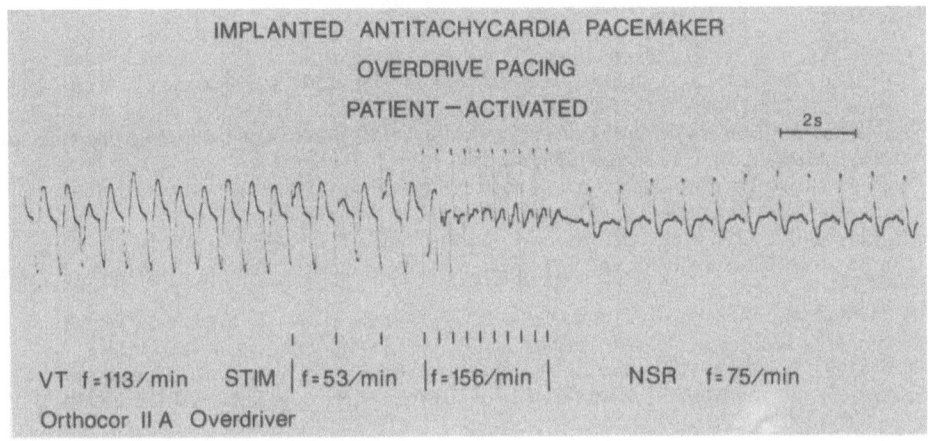

Fig. 3. Rhythm strip showing the application of an implanted, patient-activated anti-tachycardia overdrive pacemaker (Omni-Orthocor II A Overdriver). Further explanations see text.

Table 1. Implanted anti-tachycardia pacemakers.

Case	Age (yr) and Sex	Diagnosis	Antiarrhythmic Drugs	Pacing Mode and Activation	Follow up
1	50 M	CMP	mexiletine, propafenone	underdrive 90/min permanent (VOO)	Many Terminations of VT. † sudden (24 mo)
2	65 M	CAD, A	mexiletine	underdrive 70/min, Magnet	Many Terminations within 2 years; thereafter no VT anymore
3	66 M	CAD, A	disopyramide	overdrive 156/min patient-activated	Many Terminations; after 6 mo Reprogramming (burst pacing 210/min) After 12 mo VT-acceleration by pacing † apoplexy after 14 months
4	62 M	CMP	amiodarone, mexiletine	overdrive 170/min, patient-activated	10 Terminations. VT acceleration after 1 year † pump failure (23 mo)
5	75 M	CAD	propafenone	overdrive 155/min, patient-activated	3 Terminations Follow up 23 mo
6	60 F	CAD, A	aprindine	burst 210/min patient-activated	5 Terminations Pacing ineffective after 16 mo † sudden (17 mo)

Abbreviations: CMP = Congestive cardiomyopathy; CAD = Coronary artery disease; A = Aneurysm.

tions such as rate and duration of overdrive, coupling intervals of extra-stimuli etc. Preliminary results are promising further supporting the view that anti-tachycardia pacemakers will have their role for managing a small, but definite group of patients with ventricular tachycardia.

References

1. Wellens HJJ: Electrical stimulation of the heart in the study and treatment of tachycardias. Stenfort Kroese, Leiden, 1971.
2. Josephson ME, Horowitz LN, Farshidi A, Kastor JA: Recurrent sustained ventricular tachycardia. I. Mechanisms. Circulation 1978; 57: 431.
3. Wellens HJJ, Bär FW, Gorgels AP, Muncharaz JF: Electrical management of arrhythmias with emphasis on tachycardias. Am J Cardiol 1978; 41: 1025–1034.
4. Waxman HL, Cain ME, Greenspan AM, Josephson ME: Termination of ventricular tachycardia with ventricular stimulation: salutary effect of increased current strength. Circulation 1983; 65: 800–804.
5. Gardner MJ, Waxman HL, Buxton AE, Cain ME, Josephson ME: Termination of ventricular tachycardia. Evaluation of a new pacing method. Am J Cardiol 1982; 50: 1338–1345.
6. Roy D, Waxman HL, Buxton AE, Marchlinski FE, Cain ME, Gardner MJ, Josephson ME: Termination of ventricular tachycardia: role of tachycardia cycle length. Am J Cardiol 1982; 50: 1346–1350.
7. Josephson ME, Horowitz LN: Electrophysiologic approach to therapy of recurrent sustained ventricular tachycardia. Am J Cardiol 1979; 43: 631–642.
8. Fisher JD, Mehra R, Furman S: Termination of ventricular tachycardia with bursts of rapid ventricular pacing. Am J Cardiol 1978; 41: 94–102.
9. Ruskin JN, Di Marco JP, Garan H: Out-of hospital cardiac arrest: electrophysiologic observations and selection of long-term antiarrhythmic therapy. N Engl J Med 1980; 303: 607.
10. Horowitz LN, Josephson ME, Farshidi A, Spielman SR, Michelson EL, Greenspan AM: Recurrent sustained ventricular tachycardia. 3. Role of the electrophysiologic study in selection of antiarrhythmic regimens. Circulation 1978; 58: 986.
11. Mason JW, Winkle RA: Electrode-catheter arrhythmia induction in the selection and assessment of antiarrhythmic drug therapy for recurrent ventricular tachycardia. Circulation 1978; 58: 971.
12. Fisher JD, Kim SG, Furman S, Matos JA: Role of implantable pacemakers in control of recurrent ventricular tachycardia. Am J Cardiol 1982; 49: 194–206.
13. Lüderitz B, Naumann d'Alnoncourt, Steinbeck G, Beyer J: Therapeutic pacing in tachyarrhythmias by implanted pacemakers. Pace 1982; 5: 366–371.
14. Mirowski M, Reid PR, Mower MM, et al: Termination of malignant ventricular arrhythmias with an implanted automatic defibrillator in human beings. N Engl J Med 1980; 303: 322–324.

Authors' address:
Priv.-Doz. Dr. G. Steinbeck
Medizinische Klinik I der Univ.
Klinikum Großhadern
Marchioninistr. 15
8000 München 70

Treatment of Tachyarrhythmia by Implantable Devices: Patient Activated Pacemaker

W. Scheibelhofer, P. Probst

Summary: The ability to interrupt supraventricular and ventricular tachycardias in the catheterization laboratory is well established. During recent years, the use of implanted pacemakers, which are able to deliver programmed extrastimuli or bursts, has become available investigational tool. This study gives a comprehensive view into the stimulation patterns used to interrupt such tachycardias, and an in-depth description of the pacemakers currently available which can deliver such antitachycardic stimuli. In this study, the problems, indications, and contraindications of patient activated pacemakers are stressed. Our patient group consisted of 6 patients suffering from supraventricular (3 pts), ventricular (1 pt) and WPW (2 pts) tachycardia; the follow-up periods ranged from 6 to 29 months ($\overline{m}$: 17 months). We used the Cordis Omniorthocor system (4 pts) and the Medtronic SP 500 system (2 pts), 3 pts were paced from the atrium and 3 pts were paced from the ventricle. Burst pacing was used in 2 pts (atrium only) and PES was used in 4 pts. During the follow-up period the pt with VT, who suffered from dilated cardiomyopathy, died suddenly 6 months after implantation. All 6 pts were able to interrupt their frequent attacks of tachycardia successfully, but in almost every pt changing electrophysiologic properties necessitated reprogramming of the unit during follow up.
In selected cases, patient activated pacemakers may be beneficial in enhancing the quality of life of pts who were refractory to conventional drug treatment.

Electrical pacing for the treatment of tachycardias within the catheterization laboratory is well established (1). Permanently implanted pacemakers have been used for the same purpose since 1968, when Ryan first used a demand pacemaker which was converted to an asynchronous mode by the application of a magnet, in the treatment of WPW-syndrome (2). All systems which rely on the recognition of the tachycardia, and subsequent activation of the antitachycardic system by the patient, constitute the group of "patient activated systems" in contrast to permanent and automatic systems. This paper will provide an overview of the various pacing modes which have been shown to be effective in antitachycardia pacemakers. We will then present a compilation of patient activated pacemaker systems available today. Finally, we will present our own experiences with 2 slightly different systems of the most recent generation of antitachycardia pacemakers.

The first Table (1) illustrates the choice of pacing modes which may be used for the tachycardia termination. Underdrive was the first method used as mentioned above. This method is very simple: each conventional pacemaker can be converted to an asynchronous mode by magnet application and random capture will scan the whole diastole, if the tachycardia rate is not the exact multiple of the magnet rate. Only those tachycardias will respond to underdrive, however, in which one single capture is sufficient to interrupt the tachycardia circle, and it has been shown that only relatively slow tachycardias fulfill this condition (3). A much larger portion of patients will benefit from the application of several, mostly 1–3, critically timed extrastimuli (3). When more than one is used, the first serve to "peel back" the refractory zone while the last is able to permeate the tachycardia circle and to interrupt it. Systematic alteration of the coupling intervals, in order to find the termination zone, even in the presence of changing electrophysiologic circum-

Table 1. Pacing modes for tachycardia termination.

1. Underdrive (random single capture).
2. Programmed extrastimuli, PES (single or multiple captures), with or without scanning and rate adaptability.
3. Overdrive (multiple captures), with or without ramp technique and rate adaptability.
4. Burst (multiple captures), with or without rate adaptability.
5. Multimode pacing (multiple captures), e.g. burst followed by PES.
6. Early diastolic high frequency stimulation (single capture).
7. Dual chamber pacing.

Table 2. Patient-activated antitachycardic pacemakers.

A) SSI pacemaker activated by magnet: underdrive competion.
B) Custom magnetically activated burst pacemaker.
C) SSIM pacemaker programmable for: overdrive or burst (–400 ppm).
D) Inductive or radiofrequency pacemaker: overdrive or burst.
E) Radiofrequency pacemaker with sensing capability: PES.
F) SST pacemaker: burst, overdrive or PES.
G) SSI pacemaker, converted to SST by magnet.
H) SSI pacemaker with radiofrequency circuit (bidirectional): Burst, overdrive or PES.

stances, is referred to as "scanning". "Rate adaptability" means that the coupling intervals may be adjusted to the tachycardia cycle length by defining them as a function of this cycle length, rather than to give them fixed values in msec. A rate up to 30 beats per minute more than the tachycardia rate to overdrive the tachycardia, is a method most often used in the setting of the Coronary Care Unit. It may be a constant rate or an accelerating or decelerating rate. Higher rates to interrupt a tachycardia are used in burst pacing, a very efficient method for termination of both supraventricular and ventricular tachycardias but burdened with a much higher risk for acceleration of the arrhythmia than the aforementioned methods. Acceleration has been reported with programmed extrastimuli too, but it has been shown (4) that 53% of patients with recurrent ventricular tachycardias showed acceleration after burst pacing at least once. The fact that this was seen in only 4% of all episodes of burst treatment underscores the necessity for repetitive testing in patients considered for this form of treatment, in order to exclude all patients with a tendency for acceleration. It is also possible to combine some of the aforementioned pacing methods: so-called multimode pacing (3); or to achieve a single capture with very fast but short trains of stimuli (5). The use of dual chamber pacing has been covered by Doctor Curry (6).

The second Table (2), is a compilation of the hardware which is available either, off the shelf or custom made, and the various stimulation modes the units offer. Again, the simplest and easiest approach is the standard pacemaker together with a magnet for underdrive.

786

Custom, magnetically activated burst pacemakers have been used successfully to deliver a preset burst upon magnet application, while the pacemaker also works as a normal demand pacemaker the rest of the time (7).

Standard multiprogrammable pacemakers may be temporarily programmed to higher rates and one company sells a small battery driven patient unit which allows temporary reprogramming of up to 400 beats per minute.

A subcutaneous coil connected to an electrode and following the field fluxes of an induction coil (8) has a long history even for pacing for prolonged periods, and the contemporary radio frequency units are, up to now, the most widely used antitachycardic implantable devices. To initiate pacing, a handheld RF transmitter is applied to the chest wall, directly over the implanted receiver. It generates a pulse modulated RF signal that is demodulated by the receiver and converted to pacing pulses. Normally, only bursts can be applied, but a sensing capability may be included which allows for programmed extrastimuli to be applied (9). AAI and VVT pacemakers, with short refractory periods, have been used for stimulation of the heart, according to externally applied subcutaneous stimulation by a handheld activator (10). This activator may contain sensing circuitry to determine the tachycardia rate, and it may be able to deliver extrastimuli, as well as bursts. In order to prevent inadvertent triggering, the triggered mode may be activated by magnet application only, while the pacemaker is in the inhibited mode normally. Finally, a RF circuit, for interactive communication of the implanted pacemaker with an external activator may be incorporated into a standard pacemaker.

Methods

The demographic data, as well as the type of arrhythmias experienced by the 6 patients, who were treated with antitachycardia pacemakers in our own institution, are presented in Table 3. Two different antitachycardia pacemaker system were used: The Cordis Orthocor system, which consists of an implanted, programmable SSI pacemaker converted to SST mode by magnet application, and the handheld overdriver, which may deliver

Table 3. Patients and methods.

6 patients (3 female, 3 male)
Age: 44–69 a ($\overline{m}$: 56 a)
Arrhythmia: SVT 3 pts
WPW· 2 pts
VT 1 pt
Follow up: 6–29 M ($\overline{m}$: 17 M)

	Atrium	Ventricle
PES	1 Cordis Omniorthocor 234 A	2 Cordis Omniorthocor 234 A 1 Medtronic SP 0500
Burst	1 Cordis Omniorthocor 239 A 1 Medtronic SP 0500	O

787

bursts, or up to 3 critically timed stimuli, of which the number and coupling intervals can be changed after opening the overdriver. One of our patients was found to alter these values himself, using a screwdriver. This is no longer possible in the newer generation of Cordis overdrivers, which we are currently using. The Orthodriver III contains a microcomputer which is programmed by the Orthocor-Prescriber, a desk top computer which allows the physician to interact with the program, and verify parameter values that are placed into the overdriver. These values cannot now be changed by a patient. The implanted pacemaker, the Orthodriver II, and the Orthocor-Prescriber together are used for noninvasive electrophysiologic studies in the follow up of patients, and this new system is able to deliver bursts of up to 200 beats and as many as six programmed extrastimuli.

Our second system, the Medtronic SP 500-system, consists of an implanted demand-pacemaker with radio frequency telemetry of sensed events, a patient activator, which emits radio frequency signals that trigger the implanted pacemaker, and a prescriber for EP studies, pre- and postimplant, to define the optimal setting of the patient activator. You may use bursts or up to 3 independently programmed extrastimuli, which may be programmed in milliseconds or as a fraction of the sensed tachycardia cycle length. Furthermore a scan mode is included, which automatically reduces the coupling interval of the first or last stimulus by 8 msec after each unsuccessful treatment. Figure 1 demon-

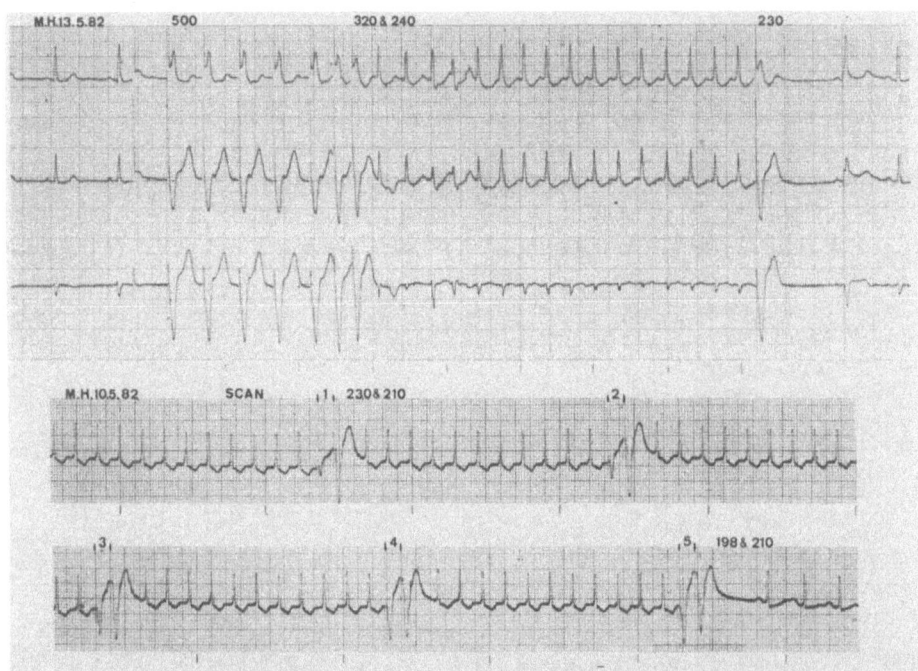

Fig. 1. Usefulness of "scan mode" in a pt with changeable electrophysiologic properties. While on some days one stimulus with a long coupling interval (upper pannel) is sufficient, at other times, two stimuli with short coupling of the first one are needed. The scan mode decreases the first coupling interval by 8 msec after each unsuccessful treatment (lower panel).

strates the usefulness of this feature in one of our patients with concealed retrograde conduction and extremly changeable electrophysiological conditions without apparent cause. While sometimes one stimulus, with a coupling interval of 230 msec was sufficient, and refractoriness occurred at 210 msec, it was necessary to use two stimuli on other occasions, with much shorter coupling intervals. The scan-mode is the only way to treat this condition.

Table 3 also characterizes the types of pacemakers used, as well as the mode of interruption of the tachycardias. You will notice that we did not use bursts in the ventricle.

Results

Case 1: In a patient with WPW-syndrome, the Cordis pacemaker is implanted with a ventricular lead; this patient has extremly changeable and very frequent attacks, in spite of cordarone therapy. Twice, a change in medication necessitated reprogramming of the overdriver, but even during constant, unchanged medication, there were two different types of tachycardia, and due to huge differences in electrophysiological properties, there was no one, single method that was able to interrupt all of the patients tachycardias. As the Cordis system does not incorporate a scan mode, we finally gave the patient two dif-

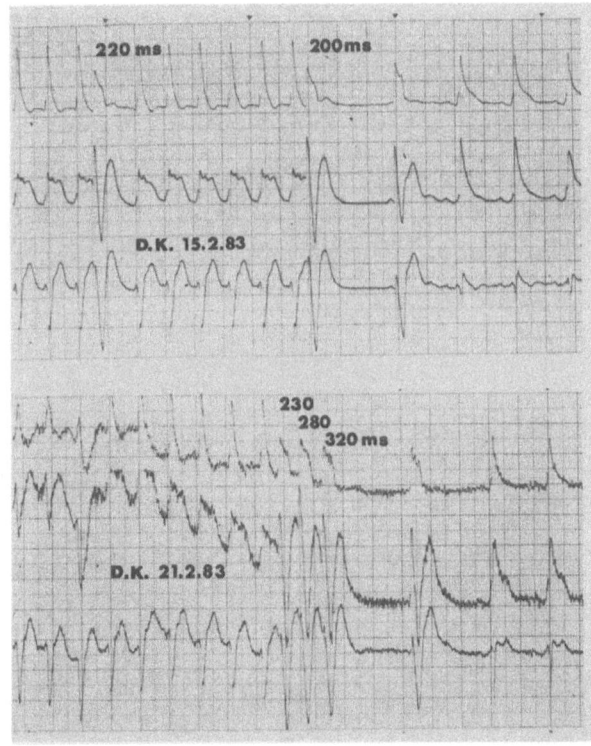

Fig. 2. Very changeable EP properties in a pt with WPW syndrome. As no single system was able to interrupt all tachycardias, and as no "scan mode" is presently available in the Cordis system, the pt was equipped with two overdrivers with different settings.

ferently programmed overdrivers, which he now uses one after the other, and with this arrangement, successful and reliable treatment has been achieved (Fig. 2).

Case 2: The patient with ventricular tachycardia suffered from severe dilated cardiomyopathy. He also received a Cordis system and was able to interrupt the tachycardia at home. After 6 months of follow-up, the patient died suddenly at home; his wife told us that he had successfully used the unit a few minutes before his death which was caused by pulmonary edema.

Case 3: In this patient, with supraventricular tachycardia, undersensing caused intermittent asynchronous stimulation and resulted in a tachycardia, which the patient was able to terminate herself, because sensing was normal during the tachycardia (Fig. 3). After a lead change, the unit worked properly. This patient now has almost no tachycardias, because she now tolerates higher doses of verapamil than before she received the atrial pacemaker.

Case 4: In this patient, with supraventricular tachycardia, the Cordis system, programmed to deliver bursts, apparently did not work reliably. It continually took the patient several attempts to terminate his tachycardia, and sometimes he had to come to hospital. An ECG, taken during such an attempt to interrupt the tachycardia (Fig. 4A) showed that the "malfunction" was related to bad positioning of the overdriver, which was not correctly placed above the implanted pacemaker. Therefore, the pacemaker was not converted to AAT mode, and it could not be triggered by the impulses from the overdriver. After training, the patient now was able to use the unit appropriately, and no more difficulties were encountered (Fig. 4B).

Case 5: This is the patient refered to previously (Fig. 1), who needed the scan mode because of very changeable electrophysiological conditions in a setting of concealed retrograde conduction. In this case the ventricles were paced and a Medtronic system was used. This patient has about three attacks per week, which are all converted, reliably.

Fig. 3. Undersensing of an atrial antitachycardic pacemaker during sinus rhythm leads to a tachycardia (upper panel), while normal sensing is present during the tachycardia (middle panel), so the patient can interrupt the tachycardia by using the pacemaker (lower panel; continuous recording).

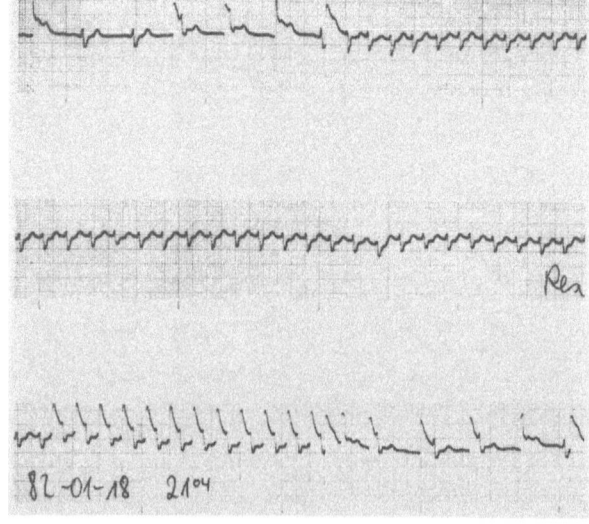

Fig. 4A. (upper panel): During a supraventricular tachycardia, the pt applies a burst of ineffective stimuli from the overdriver, which does not trigger the implanted pacemaker, because the pacemaker is not converted to the triggered mode. After correct positioning of the magnet over the pacemaker, the implanted unit is converted to AAT mode (**Fig. 4B**, lower panel), and is triggered by the burst from the overdriver, and successfully terminates the tachycardia.

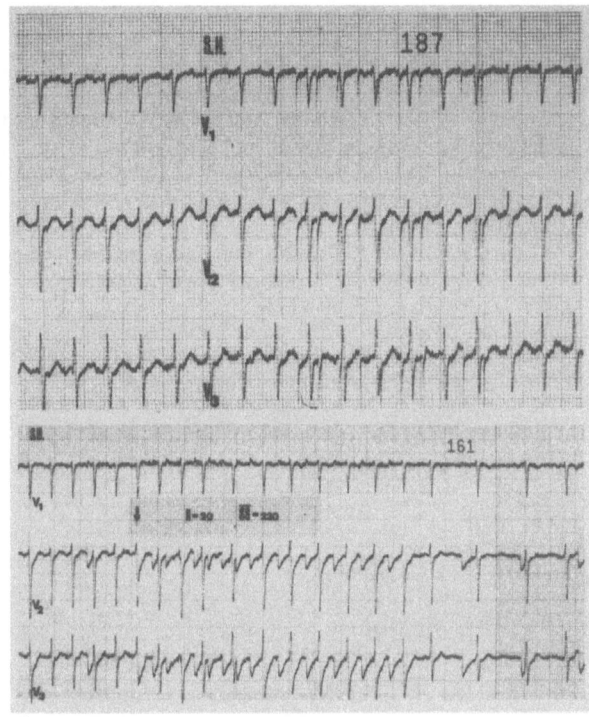

Case 6: In this patient, treated by atrial bursts, the Medtronic system was implanted because of atrial tachycardia. She had no problems during the follow-up period of fourteen months and now uses the unit from six to eight times each month.

In *Conclusion*, patient activated antitachycardic pacemakers are efficient and reliable. Due to changing electrophysiologic conditions, noninvasive reprogramming of the relevant parameters is often needed, and an automatic scan mode is very helpful. Currently their use is justified in selected patients who do not respond well to drug treatment, or are drug intolerant, if the tachycardia responds consistently to pacing, has no tendency for acceleration, does not lead to early syncope or confusion, and occurrs in a patient who is sufficently intelligent to use his unit appropriatly. Patient triggered systems are not meant to prolong life, but we have observed that our patients experience an enormous improvement in "quality of life" and that the antitachycardic systems give them a feeling of control over their illness.

References

1. Waldo AL, Wells JL, Cooper TB, MacLean WA: Temporary cardiac pacing: applications and techniques in the treatment of cardiac arrhythmias. Progr in Cardiovasc Dis 1981; 23: 451–474.
2. Ryan GF, Easley RM, Goldstein S: Paradoxical use of a demand pacemaker in treatment of supraventricular tachycardia due to the Wolff-Parkinson-White syndrome. Circulation 1968; 38: 1037–1943.

3. Fisher JD, Soo GK, Furman S, Matos JA: Role of implantable pacemakers in control of recurrent ventricular tachycardia. Am J Cardiol 1982; 49: 194–206.
4. Fisher JD, Mehra R, Furman S: Termination of ventricular tachycardia with bursts of rapid ventricular pacing. Am J Cardiol 1978; 41: 94–102.
5. Fisher JD, Ostrow E, Kim SG, Matos JA: Ultrarapid single-capture train stimulation for termination of ventricular tachycardia. Am J Cardiol 1983; 51: 1334–1338.
6. Berkovits B, Castellanos A, Dreifus LS, Lemberg L, Mandel W, Obel P: Double-demand sequential pacing for treatment of paroxysmal reentry tachycardias. Pacing and Clinical Electrophysiology 1980; 3: 364–377.
7. Coumel P, Mugica J: Treatment of tachycardias by pacing. In: Watanabe Y, ed Cardiac pacing, proceedings of the Vth International Symposium, Tokyo, March 14–18, 1976. Amsterdam: Excerpta Medica, 1977: 191–193.
8. Williams DO, Davison PH: Long-term treatment of refractory supraventricular tachycardia by patient-controlled inductive atrial pacing. Brit H J 1974; 36: 336–340.
9. Critelli G, Grassi G, Chiarello M, Perticone F, Adinolfi L, Condorelli M: Automatic "scanning" by radio frequency in the long-term electrical treatment of arrhythmias. Pace 1979; 2: 289–296.
10. Kappenberger L, Sowton E: Programmed stimulation for long-term treatment and non-invasive investigation of recurrent tachycardia. Lancet 1981; 1: 909–914.

Autors' address:
Dr. W. Scheibelhofer
Kardiologische Univ. Klinik
Garnisongasse 13
A-1090 Wien/Österreich

Automatic Implantable Devices for Termination of Tachycardia

A. J. Camm, R. A. J. Spurrell

Summary: For more than ten years manually activated pacemakers have been used to terminate tachycardia. More recently automatically activated systems have been introduced. Automatic activation ensures prompt initiation of therapy and can usually operate without an external device of any sort. The major disadvantage of automatic activation is provocation of unwanted arrhythmias with which neither the implanted device nor the patient can cope. There is now considerable encouraging experience with the use of automatic devices for the termination of supraventricular (and atrioventricular) tachycardias. Clinical reservations have ensured that ventricular tachycardias have not been extensively treated with automatically activated systems. However, the recent development of new tachycardia conversion pacing system with improved detection and termination algorithms, may allow their successful application to the treatment of a broader range of tachycardias.

Introduction

An automatic device for tachycardia termination does not require activation by the patient, his physician, his relatives or friends. External devices which contain pacemaker logic and which require the co-operation of the patient, and in some instances confirmation of the tachycardia by the external unit, are not considered automatic. Even though an external unit could be worn in readiness for "automatic" activation by tachycardia such devices are now superceded by totally implantable automatic units.

Automatic versus Manual Activation (Table 1)

The major advantage of an implanted automatic system is that tachycardia can be rapidly detected and terminated, perhaps before symptoms occur. Totally implanted systems also free the patient from the encumbrance of an external control or logic box.

Table 1. Advantages and disadvantages of automatic activation.

Advantages	Prompt initiation of treatment
	External device not necessary
	Seriously symptomatic tachycardias may be treated
Disadvantages	Accurate sensing essential
	Danger from provocation of unwanted arrhythmias
	Possibly unsuitable for ventricular tachycardia
	Potential repetition of unsuccessful pacing sequence

a) *Sensing of Tachycardia*

Until recently tachycardia has been recognised only in terms of the repetition frequency of sensed events. Obviously such a method does not necessarily distinguish between physiological and pathological tachycardia but several automatic devices can discriminate between these tachycardias simply by the use of numerous tachycardia trigger rates. Unfortunately there may be overlap between the rates of sinus and pathological tachycardia and more sophisticated sensing algorithms are necessary. Some investigational devices contain the optional requirement that the rate of tachycardia is rapidly achieved. This is a significant improvement but it is likely that, with the increasing use of two channel pacemakers and digital processing the recognition of particular pathological tachycardias will be easy to achieve by analysis of the timing and shape of tachycardia elelctrograms.

Automatic tachycardia terminating pacemakers should not be falsely triggered and "oversensing" of tachycardia must be avoided. Thus it is important that such devices are bipolar and possess a range of programmable sensitivities. It is also desirable that the pacemaker may be inactivated in the event of repeated unnecessary or ineffective pacing interventions.

b) *Tachycardia Termination Algorithms*

The major determinants of the ability of pacemakers to terminate tachycardia are the rate and location of tachycardia (1, 2). The tachycardia focus of circuit does not usually change position but the rate of tachycardia is very variable. Physiological and pharmacological interventions may effect the rate of tachycardia and influence the ability of a pacemaker to terminate it. Thus, particularly automatic pacemakers, must be sufficiently versatile to adapt to changing situations. Underdrive, overdrive and extrastimulus pacemakers operating with fixed or static values were used but these are less successful than newer devices which operate with automatically changing parameters. The simple scheme of orthorhythmic pacing (i.e. adapting the pacing interval in proportion to the tachycardia interval) has not been particularly successful and more versatile methods of varying pacing intervals and rates have been developed. These include scanning extrastimuli, and variable, accelerating or decelerating bursts. With the incorporation of such variable parameters the method of automatically changing the parameter has been approached imaginatively and various intriguing and elegant solutions have been devised (3, 4, 5). As yet the potential advantages and disadvantages of some of these modalities have not been established. If, despite the best adaptive changes, tachycardia continues, automatic disengagement of the pacemaker should occur. This option is available in several new investigational devices.

In most adaptive systems, in order to circumvent unnecessary searching for successful pacing sequences, a "memory" facility has been incorporated. The memory recalls successful pacing intervals for reapplication when tachycardia next occurs. Therefore, tachycardia termination must be accurately diagnosed or, otherwise the memory would be loaded with incorrect information and would recall unsuccessful sequences. When pacing algorithms are largely based upon this remembered information, eg. adaptive table scanning, accurate diagnosis of tachycardia termination is essential. This problem has not received sufficient attention.

c) *Absence of External Device*

When an external device is to be used to terminate tachycardia the device must often be worn or carried by the patient. Most external systems must be atcivated by the patient, or his representative, and, therefore, the tachycardia must be sufficiently prolonged to produce symptoms. However, symptoms such as confusion and syncope may prevent manual activation of the pacemaker by the patient. The majority of patients encounter substantial physical or psychological difficulties with external devices and prefer totally implanted automatic systems (6).

d) *Automatic Activation*

Even if tachycardia is correctly appreciated by an implantable device the operation of the pacemaker outside the relative safety of a hospital or doctor's office may risk the provocation of potentially fatal arrhythmias. Pacemaker treatment of ventricular tachycardia, especially of ischaemic origin, may be a particular risk. No modality of pacing is immune to this complication and other methods of tachycardia termination, such as vagotonic manoeuvres, drug therapy, chest wall thump and DC cardioversion may all provoke unwanted arrhythmias. If not promptly extinguished, tachycardia may become less easy to terminate because of compensatory autonomic adjustments (7) or may degenerate into more chaotic tachyarrhythmias not susceptible to pacemaker termination (8). If pacemaker treatment of possibly vulnerable tachycardias must be contemplated the relative risks of allowing tachycardia to continue whilst a hospital or physician is found, rather than prompt intervention by an automatic pacemaker must be considered. Although it is possible that future automatic antitachycardia systems will incorporate defibrillating modalities to cope with ventricular fibrillation provoked by pacemakers, a superior solution would be the development of safer pacing modalities or better methods of patient selection. Experience already gathered suggests that the large majority of tachycardias can be efficiently and safely controlled by tachycardia terminating pacemakers.

Automatic Modalities for Tachycardia Termination (Table 2)

1) *Underdrive Pacing* (Figure 1)

Automatic competitive pacing at a rate slower than the rate of tachycardia will theoretically result in the eventual delivery of a stimulus any "single beat tachycardia termination zone" that exists. There has been substantial clinical experience with the use of this modality in combination with bradycardia support pacing (dual-demand pacing). Whilst it is true that some patients are successfully treated with this technique the majority are not (9, 10). The reason for the failure of this form of pacing is that in everyday life single beat termination zones often do not exist or are very small. The somewhat haphazard scheme of "searching" is time consuming (11) and if tachycardia synchronization occurs a full scan will not be affected. Overall long-term results are poor but dual-demand units may be successfully used when the rate of tachycardia is suitable (less than 160 beats/minute but greater than the usual trigger rate of 137 beats/min and not harmonically re-

Table 2. Tachycardia termination pacing algorinthms.

---

c) Underdrive (upside-down pacing)
a) Underdrive and bradycardia support (dual-demand)
a) Dual chamber double demand
d) Marginal underdrive

a) Burst overdrive – synchronous (coupled)
a) Burst overdrive – synchronous
b) Scanning burst
b) Concertina burst
d) Marginal overdrive plus scanning extrastimulus
a) Decremental burst
a) Incremental burst

a) Linear decremental scan
c) Linear incremental scan
b) Bisectional scan
b) Geometric centrifugal scan
b) Ultra high frequency stimulation
b) Adaptive table pacing
c) High pulse energy scan

---

a) Commercially available algorithm
b) Available in investigational units
c) Previously available and possibly available by special order
d) In development

---

lated to the pacing rate), and involves a large and anatomically convenient circuit. Possibly two channel (dual chamber) automatic underdrive pacemakers are more successful (12). More versatile automatic underdrive systems with a range of trigger rates and pacing rates are now being evaluated.

2) *Burst Pacing* (Figure 2)

A train of stimuli at a rate faster than tachycardia may result in progressive capture (entrainment) and saturation (failure to support continued one way conduction) of the tachycardia circuit. Although the majority of experience with burst pacing has been achieved with external or manually activated systems automatic atrial burst pacing has undoubtedly been very successful in the treatment of paroxysmal junctional or atrial tachyarrhythmias. There is too little experience with automatic burst ventricular pacing for either junctional or ventricular tachycardia to be sure of the long-term efficacy of the technique. Some burst pacemakers for automatic tachycardia termination emit bursts precisely coupled to the tachycardia complexes thereby reducing the risk of initiating unwanted arrhythmias. Most presently available systems cannot distinguish pathological from physiological tachycardia and are further limited by the use of a single pre-programmed pacing sequence such that if pacing fails to terminate tachycardia the futile pacing sequence is repeated.

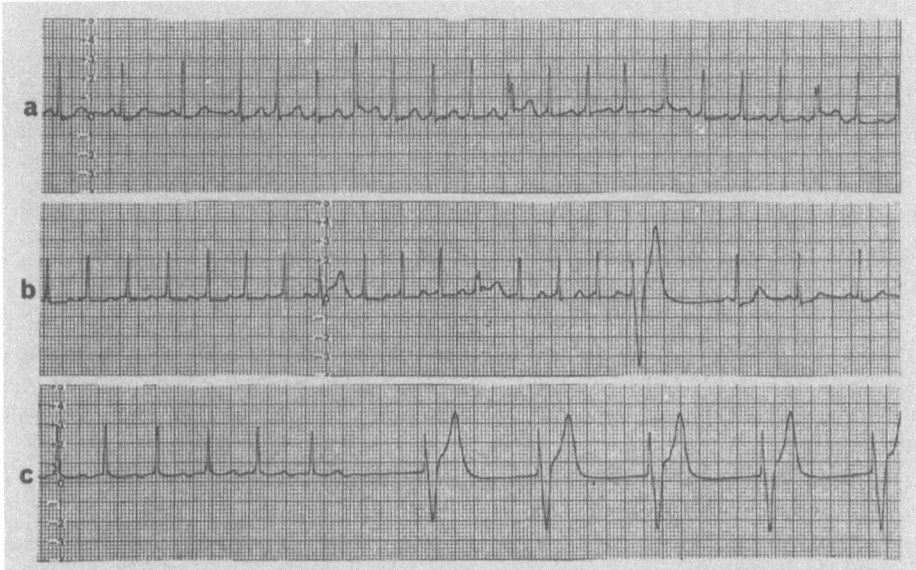

Fig. 1. Automatic underdrive pacing with a highly programmable dual demand pacemaker. The traces demonstrate:
a) sluggish "search" because of virtually exact harmonic relationship between the pacing rate (36 beats/minute) and tachycardia rate (145 beats/minute);
b) termination of tachycardia by a pacing induced ventricular premature systole; and
c) failure to activate tachycardia termination pacing when the rate of tachycardia is too slow (110 beats/minute).
Spontaneous tachycardia termination is followed by bradycardia support pacing (50 beats/minute).

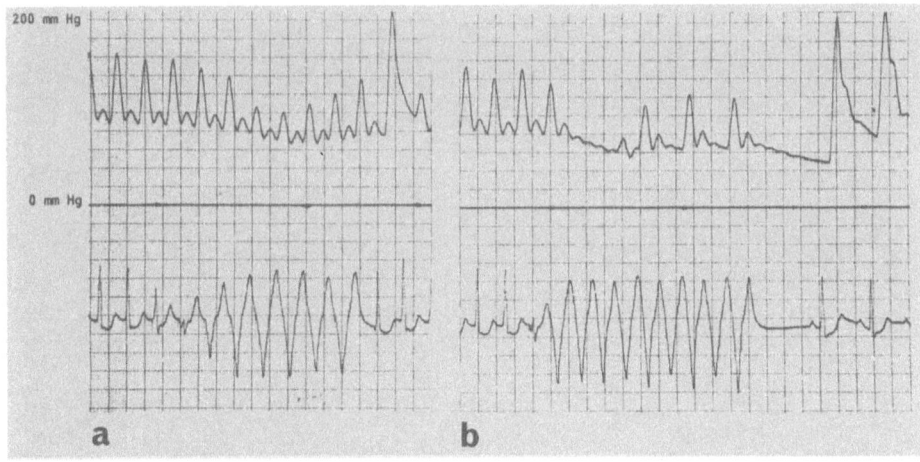

Fig. 2. Automatic overdrive pacing:
a) a burst of eight stimuli at a rate of 205 beats/minute fails to terminate tachycardia but results in significant hypotension (top trace);
b) change of burst characteristics to 10 stimuli at 235 beats/minute results in extinction of tachycardia and resumption of sinus rhythm.

3) *Extrastimulus Pacing* (Figure 3)

In recent years implantable automatic extrastimulus pacemakers have become availabe (13). Fixed coupling interval extrastimulus pacemakers were satisfactory for only a small number of patients but "scanning" systems are considerably more versatile. Simple linear scans (13–15) and more complex centrifugal scans or bisectional searches have been successfully developed and are used in automatically activated pacemakers.

The majority of paroxysmal tachycardias induced in the laboratory are susceptible to one or two appropriately timed premature beats. The timing of the first of two beats is more critical than the timing of the subsequent beat. Thus in the Telectronics 4151 PASAR (15), of which approximately 100 are implanted world-wide, the first premature stimulus automatically scans diastole (15 steps of 6 msecs) and the second stimulus is adjustable to a range of static coupling intervals. Our experience with this system, implanted in 19 patients, followed up for an average of 17 months has led to the following conclusions:

a) Reliable long-term single beat tachycardia termination is not usual – even when pre-implantation studies suggest that only one stimulus is required.

b) If at pre-implantation electrophysiological study tachycardia termination requires two stimuli successful long-term operation of the pacemaker may require additional drug treatment.

c) There is only occasional confusion between physiological and pathological tachycardia and this can usually be resolved by concomitant use of beta-blockers.

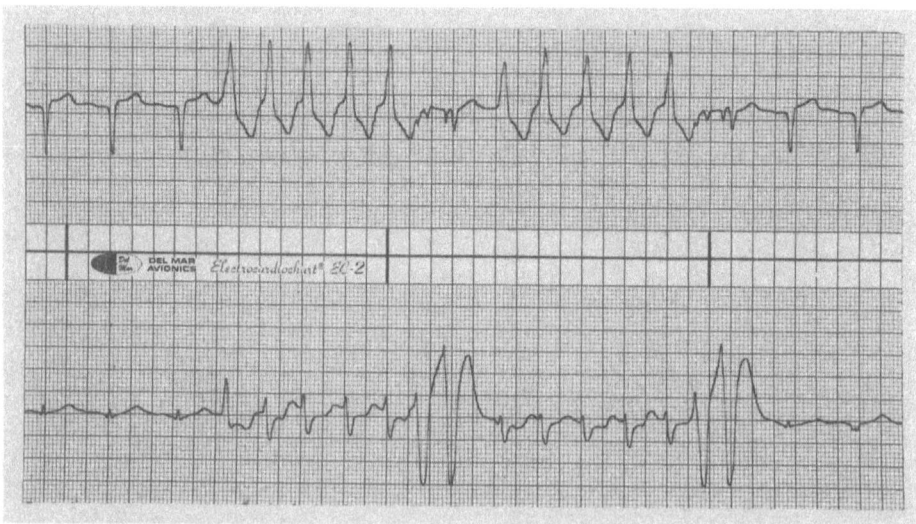

Fig. 3. Automatic extrastimulus pacing. Ambulatory electrocardiographic trace demonstrating spontaneous initiation of paroxysmal ventricular tachycardia. Double extrastimuli fail to terminate tachycardia at the first attempt but when the coupling interval between the tachycardia complex and the first of the extrastimuli is reduced by 6 msec (PASAR) the tachycardia is succesfully terminated.

d) Bradycardia support pacing is rarely essential when treating patients with paroxysmal junctional tachycardias (but may be more necessary for the treatment of patients with atrial or ventricular tachycardia due to underlying heart disease).
e) The memory function may prevent effective scanning.
f) Most, but not all, patients with susceptible tachycardias at initial study can be effectively treated in the long-term by implantation of this extrastimulus device.

New Automatic Implantable Devices for Tachycardia Termination

Many new tachycardia terminating pacing algorithms have been evaluated in the laboratory. Some are now embodied in implantable devices and are designed to operate automatically in response to tachycardia. Currently under evaluation are two systems which contain important new concepts: Siemens P43 and Telectronics 4171.

1) Siemens P43 (TACHYLOG)

This device utilizes "eprom" circuits and comprises:
a) An implantable stimulator for electrophysiology study;
b) An implantable device for monitoring the cardiac rhythm;
c) A conventional multiprogrammable bradycardia pacemaker; and
d) A tachycardia terminating pacemaker capable of utilizing one to four different algorithms including adaptive table scanning, bisectional searching, geometric centrifugal scans and highly specified but fixed bursts.

The implantation of this evaluation device will allow a comparison between various pacing methods for tachycardia termination. It will be possible to establish whether sophisticated and relatively complex pacing algorithms hold real advantage over simpler systems.

Telectronics 4171 (CONCERTINA)

This pacemaker is both an extrastimulus and a coupled burst (up to seven stimuli) pacemaker. It includes all the features of the Telectronics 4151 (PASAR) and also has optional bradycardia support pacing. In this pacemaker the burst may be programmed to adjust its characteristics if tachycardia is not successfully terminated. The entire burst may be scanned relative to the tachycardia complex. Alternatively the frequency of the burst may be changed in a way which simulates the action of a concertina. Our early experience with the system has revealed that almost all junctional tachycardias are amenable to termination by this extended PASAR algorithm (3).

Conclusion

Numerous pacing algorithms for tachycardia termination have been tried in the electro-physiology laboratory. In recent years underdrive, burst and extrastimulus modes have been developed as implantable pacemakers designed to recognize tachycardia and respond automatically. There is now sufficient clinical experience attesting to the short-term value of automatic implantable pacemakers for tachycardia termination but this use of pacemakers is not yet widespread because there is understandable concern about long-term efficacy and safety. Encouraging long-term follow-up of patients fitted with automatic systems is now emerging and new, sophisticated and ingenious pacing methods are potentially even more effective and safe. However, before endorsing the incorporation of a complex, automatic antitachycardia option within every multi-modal, multiprogrammable pacemaker, considerably more experience with the use of dedicated antitachycardia pacemakers is required.

It is likely that the ideal future tachycardia terminating pacemaker will be automatic and will utilize relatively simple pacing algorithms. Automatic systems should not be designed to rely on a complex, time-consuming and potentially dangerous multiplicity of responses, but should probably automatically disengage in the event of repeated failure to terminate tachycardia. Patients with tachycardias which are not amenable to safe and simple pacemaker termination are unsuitable for this form of therapy.

References

1. Ward DE, Camm AJ, Spurrell RAJ: The response of regular reentrant supraventricular tachycardia to right heart stimulation. Pacing and Clinical Electrophysiology 1979; 2: 586.
2. Naccarelli GV, Zipes DP, Rahilly T, Heger JJ, Prystowsky EN: Influence of tachycardia cycle length and antiarrhythmic drugs on pacing termination and acceleration of ventricular tachycardia. American Heart Journal 1983; 105: 1.
3. Nathan A, Hellestrand K, Bexton R, Nappholz T, Spurrell RAJ, Camm AJ: Clinical evaluation of an adaptive tachycardia intervention pacemaker with automatic cycle length adjustment. Pacing and Clinical Electrophysiology 1982; 5: 201.
4. Sowton E, Elmqvist H, Segerstad C: Two years clinical experience with a self searching tachycardia pacemaker. American Journal of Cardiology 1981; 47: 476.
5. Sowton E, Wainwright RJ, Schmidinger H: Clinical use of a new antitachycardia pacemaker. Proceedings of British Cardiac Society, Bristol 1983.
6. Nathan A, Hellestrand K, Bexton R, Ward D, Spurrell R, Camm J: Problems with patient-activated pacemakers for tachycardia termination. Proceedings of VIIth World Symposium on Cardiac Pacing, Vienna 1983.
7. Curry PVL, Rowland E, Fox KM, Krikler DM: The relationship between posture and electrophysiological properties in patients with paroxysmal supraventricular tachycardia. Arch Mal Coeur 1978; 71: 293.
8. Bauernfiend RA, Wyndham CR, Swiryn SP, Palileo EV, Strasberg B, Lam W, Westveer D, Rosen KM: Paroxysmal atrial fibrillation in the Wolff-Parkinson-White syndrome. American Journal of Cardiology 1981; 47: 562.
9. Krikler DM, Curry P, Buffet J: Dual-demand pacing for reciprocating atrioventricular tachycardia. British Medical Journal 1976; 1: 1114.
10. Curry PVL, Rowland E, Krikler DM: Dual-demand pacing for refractory atrioventricular reentrant tachycardia. Pacing and Clinical Electrophysiology 1979; 2: 137.
11. Sowton E, O'Keeffe DB, Curry PVL: Use of a multiprogrammable pacemaker in the dual-demand mode: influence of pacing rate on termination of tachycardias. European Heart Journal 1980; 1: 165.
12. Berkovitz B, Castellanos A, Dreifus LS, Lemberg L, Levy S, Mandel W, Obel P: Double demand sequential pacing for treatment of reentry tachycardias. Pacing and Clinical Electrophysiology 1980; 3: 364.
13. Spurrell RAJ: Artificial cadiac pacemakers. In DM Krikler and JF Goodwin (Ed): Cardiac Arrhythmias. Londen, WB Saunders, 1975; pp 238.

14. Spurrell RAJ: Future aspects of cardiac pacing. In B Luderitz (Ed): Cardiac Pacing. Springer Verlag, Heidelberg 1976; pp 235.
15. Spurrell RAJ, Bexton R, Nathan A, Hellestrand K, Nappholz R, Camm AJ: Implantable automatic scanning pacemaker for termination of supraventricular tachycardia. American Journal of Cardiology 1982; 49: 753–760.

Authors' address:
Prof. J. Camm
Cardiology Department
St. Bartholomew's Hospital
London EC1A 7BE
England

Programmable Implantable Automatic Pacemaker for Paroxysmal Tachycardia

J. K. Vohra, Diane M. Jackson, H. G. Mond, C.-W. Kong, A. M. Tonkin, D. Hunt

Summary: This paper presents our experiences with a programmable, automatic scannning, arrhythmia reversion pacemaker (PASAR 4151 Telectronics) in 15 patients with frequent, paroxysmal tachycardias refractory to standard anti-arrhythmic therapy. The age range was 19 to 73, five were males and ten females. All patients had detailed EP studies. An external PASAR 4400 stimulator was used to determine the site of stimulation and other parameters required to achieve reversion. During a follow-up of 1 to 15 months ($\overline{m}$ 9) ambulant monitoring was routinely performed.

Seven patients had AV node re-entry and six patients had AV re-entry tachycardia associated with pre-excitation. One patient each had sinus node re-entry and ventricular tachycardia. Right ventricle was the site of bipolar stimulation in eight patients, RA in five and coronary sinus in two patients. PASAR 4151 consistently reverted tachycardia in 13 out of 15 patients and provided a safe, totally implantable mode of tachycardia reversion. After PASAR 4151 implantation, at least during the first few months, patients require a careful follow-up. Concomitant drug therapy may also be required in some patients with frequent episodes of tachycardia.

This paper summarises our clinical experience with PASAR 4151 in 15 patients. Twelve of the 15 units were implanted at The Royal Melbourne Hospital and three at the Flinders Medical Centre. All patients had detailed electrophysiological (EP) studies (Table 1) and reversion of tachycardia with extrastimuli from various chambers of the heart was checked using PASAR stimulator (PASAR 4400). At the time of implantation, reversion was confirmed again from the site of electrode placement. Following implantation patients were carefully followed and pacemaker function was checked. Periodic 24 hour ambulatory monitoring was performed during the follow-up period. All patients in this series had a long history of paroxysmal tachycardias requiring repeated hospital admissions and had received treatment with various antiarrhythmic drugs.

Case histories of some of the patients in the series are outlined.

Case 1: P. K. A female, aged 54, had paroxysmal supraventricular tachycardia (PSVT) which satisfied all the criteria of sinus node re-entry (SNRTc). At EP study SNRTc at two different rates were induced. The slower tachycardia (130/m) which had not been symptomatic, became so after PASAR implantation. If the tachycardia detect rate was kept at 130/minute, the extrastimuli caused a faster tachycardia of between 160 and 170/minute which required different extrastimulus interval for reversion.

After several trials with drugs the slower tachycardia has been suppressed by 480 mg of verapamil per day. She has also had two episodes of unrelated paroxysmal atrial fibrillation and requires quinidine for prevention of this arrhythmia.

Case 2: M. M. A female, aged 54, had suffered from recurrent palpitations for over 20 years. She had required several cardioversions and hospital admissions for PSVT despite treatment with digoxin, verapamil, propranolol and quinidine in varying doses and drug combinations. A Radiofrequency pacemaker with electrode in the RA appendage was im-

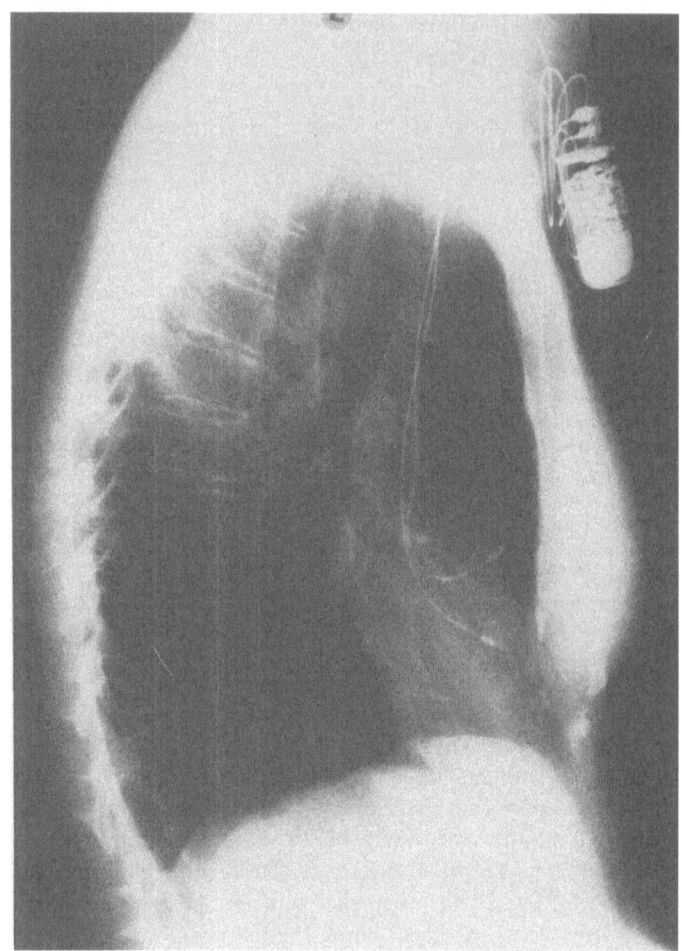

Fig. 1. Case 2, AVNRT.
Lateral chest X-ray showing two unipolar atrial electrodes. The upper electrode positioned in the RA appendage was originally used with a Radiofrequency pacemaker.
When PASAR 4151 was implanted the RA appendage electrode was used to sense atrial electrogram. The lower, Medtronic Bisping screw-in electrode was used for atrial stimulation.

Table 1. PASAR 4151. Total pts 15: Ages 19 to 73 yrs: 5m

Sinus node Re-entry	1
AVNRT	7
AVRT	6
Ventricular Tc	1

Table 2. PASAR 4151: Bipolar electrode positions.

SNR Tc	RA appendage	1
AVNRT	RA appendage + MID ANT RA	1
	Coronary sinus	2
	Low RA	3
	RV	2*)
AVRT	RV	6
VTc	RV	1

*) One patient, Case 4, had RV and subsequently coronary sinus electrode. See text for details.

planted in 1978 and had been very successful in terminating episodes of PSVT. Because of frequent episodes and practical difficulties of using a patient-initiated device, a PASAR 4151 was implanted in July, 1981. The RA appendage electrode was left in position while an endocardial screw-in (Medtronics Bisping) electrode was positioned in mid anterior RA. (Illustration No. 1)

PASAR 4151 has been successful in reverting all episodes of PSVT (up to 50 episodes per month, m = 29) within a few seconds. She has been maintained on digoxin and verapamil to reduce the frequency of tachycardia episodes.

Case 3: J. G. This 58-year-old male is the only patient who has had PASAR 4151 for ventricular tachycardia (VTc) which had proved refractory to antiarrhythmic drugs and was submitted to coronary artery bypass graft surgery. Epicardial mapping showed VTc arising from two different sites and surgical treatment for VTc was unsuccessful. Following surgery repeated episodes of VTc again proved refractory to drug therapy.

At repeat EP studies, VTc was easily reverted with RV underdrive and single and double RV extrastimuli. During spontaneous and induced VTc and rate never exceeded 150 to 160 beats/minute. There was also no acceleration of tachycardia rate or induction of ventricular fibrillation despite repeated reversions using RV extrastimuli (RVES).

Since implantation of PASAR 4151 in July, 1981 nearly 100 episodes of VTc have been successfully and promptly reverted by PASAR 4151. He has been maintained on antiarrhythmic drugs to reduce the frequency of tachycardias.

Recently an attempt was made to reduce his antiarrhythmic treatment but this resulted in an episode of VTc which was not reverted with PASAR 4151 and the drugs had to be reintroduced.

Case 4: E. S. in whom PASAR 4151 has failed is a female, aged 73, with recurrent and refractory PSVT. Double RVES were initially successful but a few weeks later she had episodes of PSVT which only responded to RVES when the tachycardia rate was slowed by intravenous administration of verapamil.

It was felt that proximal coronary sinus stimulation could be more effective by being closer to the tachycardia circuit; however, this too, was unsuccessful in the long-term. Various antiarrhythmic combinations to reduce the tachycardia rate were tried but she ultimately required amiodarone 200 mg per day and this drug has suppressed PSVT.

Case 5: B. G. This 55-year-old female had repeated episodes of PSVT for over 10 years. At EP studies PSVT was consistently and promptly reverted by proximal coronary sinus double extrastimuli. PASAR 4151 was implanted in September, 1981 and has consistently reverted all episodes within a few seconds. She has not required any antiarrhythmic therapy.

Table 2 gives details of bipolar electrode positions used in our 15 patients. We have used coronary sinus stimulation in only two patients and although in Case 4, coronary sinus stimulation was ineffective in reverting tachycardia, in both (Cases 4 and 5), long-term (15 and 14 months respectively) pacing has been possible without any sensing or threshold problems.

All six patients with atrioventricular re-entry tachycardia (AVRT) had paraseptal accessory atrioventricular connection (AAVC). In all these six patients, Medtronics bipolar electrode was positioned in the RV apex for tachycardia termination.

Fig. 2. Case 5, AVNRT.
Continuous ECG rhythm strips showing reversion of PSVT by proximal coronary sinus double extrastimuli.
The eighth pair of extrastimuli (marked with arrows) revert the tachycardia to sinus rhythm.

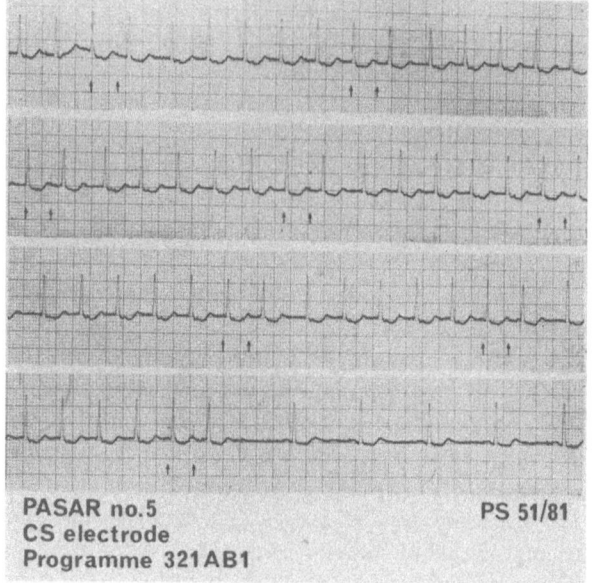

PASAR no.5   PS 51/81
CS electrode
Programme 321AB1

In patients with AVNRT, we have preferred atrial stimulation using a pulse width of 0.6 ms and sensitivity of 2 mV. In one patient (Case No. 11) two bipolar Bisping electrodes were implanted in the low RA. At follow-up examination the atrial signal was not consistently sensed during sinus rhythm despite increasing sensing to 1 mV. However, all episodes of PSVT have been successfully reverted using 1 mV sensing as the atrial signal is sensed better during PSVT than during sinus rhythm.

The patients have been followed up for three to 22 months (mean 14). As Case 1 presented with episodes of PSVT following implantation until the slower tachycardia was suppressed with high doses of verapamil, she has been classified as partial success. Case 4 has been classified as a failure. In the remaining 13 patients PASAR has been considered successful.

Nine patients out of 15 have required concomitant anti-arrhythmic therapy. The commonest indication has been frequent episodes of tachycardia. Some of these patients had as many as 30 episodes of PSVT per day and even though PASAR 4151 was successful in reverting the episodes, they found the sensation unpleasant and two patients (Cases 2 and 10) even experienced transient dizziness at the onset of tachycardia.

Another indication for continued drug therapy was reduction of the sinus rate. In two patients (Cases 3 and 11) sinus tachycardia approached the tachycardia detect rate and triggered the pacemaker. Both these patients responded to small doses of beta adrenergic blocking drugs (atenolol 25–50 mg per day). In two patients with AVRT (Cases 7 and 12), beta adrenergic blockers were required to prevent repeated re-induction of tachycardia after successful reversion. In these patients tachycardia was re-induced by the block of the AAVC by the second sinus beat following the pause induced after tachycardia reversion by RVES. In both patients, beta adrenergic blocking agents were successful in preventing re-induction.

Reprogramming of PASAR 4151 parameters in the early follow-up period was not uncommon and is considered a part of the follow-up. Extrastimulus interval (8 instances) and tachycardia detect rate (5 instances) were common indications. None of the patients in our series consistently reverted with single atrial or ventricular extrastimulus. Even in two patients with AVRT and paraseptal AAVC, where single RVES reverted PSVT during EP studies and early follow-up, second ES had to be programmed to achieve consistent reversion.

Discussion:

PASAR 4151 is the first programmable automatic implantable pacemaker for tachycardia reversion using extrastimulus technique (1). It has been successful in reverting episodes of tachycardia in 13 out of 15 patients. Patient No. 4, where this device has been unsuccessful, had AVNRT and presumably had a small re-entry circuit which made it difficult for the extrastimuli to penetrate the tachycardia circuit, particularly when the rate was faster during spontaneous, as opposed to the induced, episodes. Case 1, where the patient presented with repeated episodes of tachycardia until the slower of the two tachycardias was suppressed by quite high doses of verapamil (480 mg/day), has been classified as a partial success.

The relatively high incidence of concomitant drug therapy after PASAR implantation (9 out of 15 patients) is probably explained by our selection of patients who suffered from very frequent episodes.

We conclude that PASAR 4151 provides a safe, totally implantable mode of tachycardia reversion in adequately investigated and selected patients with PSVT. Its use in paroxysmal VTc should be confined to very carefully selected patients where the risk of tachycardia acceleration or induction of ventricular fibrillation by RVES is considered negligible.

After PASAR 4151 implantation, at least during the first few months, patients require a careful follow-up. Concomitant drug therapy may also be required in some patients with frequent episodes of tachycardia.

Reference:

1. Spurrell RAJ, Nathan AW, Bexton RS, Hellstrand KJ, Nappholz T, and Camm AJ (1982). Implantable automatic scanning pacemaker for termination of supraventricular tachycardia. Am J Cardiol 49: 753–760.

Authors' address:
J. Vohra, M.D.
Cardiology Department
The Royal Melbourne Hospital
Australia, 3050

Centrifugal Geometric Scanning – an Alternative Concept in Pacemaker Treatment of Tachycardias

H. O. Vallin, Ch. Hård af Segerstad, P. Insulander, K. O. Edhag, H. Lagergren

Summary: Short term efficacy and safety of a new scanning concept for termination of AV recipro-cating tachycardias were assessed in five patients, two with dual AV nodal pathways and three with an accessory AV connection. The concept includes geometric partioning of the scanning interval concentrating the attempts to its early part, a centrifugal search outwardly from a memorized extra stimulus delay and alternation of the number of extrastimuli. After initial definition of the termina-tion characteristics in each patient the system was found efficient during a 48-hours recorded period. No adverse effects were observed.

In optimizing pacemaker treatment of reciprocating tachycardias various problems have to be approached: 1. Although many tachycardias, especially those with a spacious reentry circuit as in the WPW-syndrome, permit termination with one extra stimulus (ES), two or three ES are often needed (1). 2. Lack of prompt termination may results in secondary autonomic acceleration of tachycardia (2) leading to more difficult interrup-tion. 3. A spontaneous variation occurs in the duration and position of the termination zone of the tachycardia i.e. the interval during which an extra stimulus has to fall to pro-duce termination (3).

A number of different stimulation concepts have been applied for pacemaker termination of tachycardias. In addition to periods of regular underdrive or overdrive stimulation also critically timed extra stimuli have been utilized either with a fixed coupling interval (4) or with the ES scanning through a defined part of the heart cycle (5). For a fixed coupling interval to be efficient either a stable or a wide termination zone is required to guarantee that the extra stimuli reliably stays inside the zone. Extra stimulus scanning improves the possibility to hit the termination interval when it is narrow or its position varies. Such scanning may be performed with a regular stepwise decrease from a memorized efficient stimulus delay down to a programmed minimum value and thereafter restarting late in the heart cycle (5). Termination will occur rapidly if the termination zone is unchanged or has moved to an earlier position in the heart cycle but will take a longer time when it was moved the other way.

Methods

Taking these considerations into account we have designed an alternative concept for ta-chycardia termination including the following features:
1. Scanning is performed starting with a memorized previously successful ES delay and if this is not efficient further delays are attempted alternatively earlier or later in a cen-trifugal fashion until the tachycardia is terminated or eight attempts are run through (figure 1).

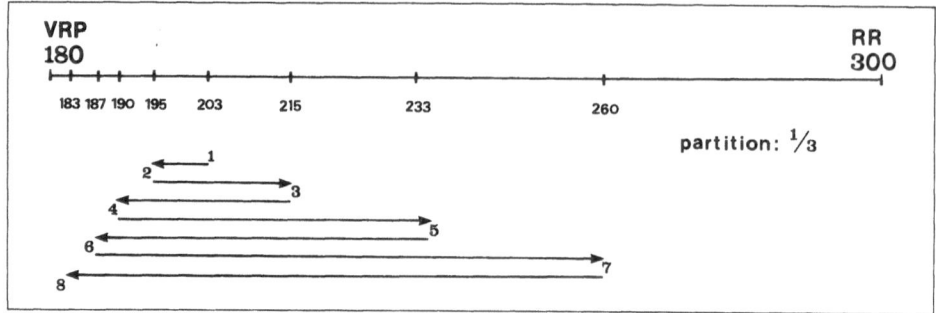

Fig. 1. The principles for centrifugal geometric scanning illustrated in a tachycardia with an RR-interval of 300 msec and a minimum delay of the extra stimulus programmed to the same value as the ventricular refractory period (VRP). See text for further explanation.

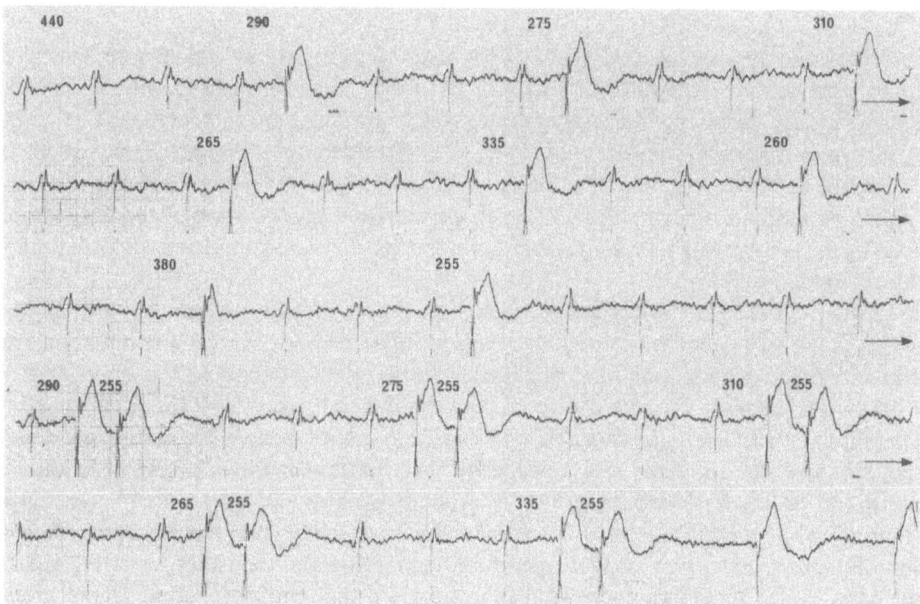

Fig. 2. Termination of tachycardia in patient no. 1 with WPW-syndrome and an RR-interval of 440 ms. A scanning of eight attempts with a single ES is performed, starting with a coupling interval of 290 ms and then alternately decreasing and increasing the delays until the minimum programmed value of 255 ms is reached. The tachycardia is remeasured and a second ES with a fixed coupling interval is added during the next scanning cycle.

2. As the termination zone is more often located soon after the refractory period than later in the RR-interval, the termination attempts are concentrated to this early part. A minimum delay is programmed, often close to the refractory period, and the interval remaining to the end of the RR-interval is partioned in eight steps according to a geometric series decreasing each step with one third of the remaining interval. The

RR-interval of the tachycardia is remeasured after a full scanning cycle of eight attempts and the delays adjusted.

3. To compensate for variation in the optimal number of extra stimuli automatic alternation between one and two or between two and three extra stimuli may be included in the program to occur after each scanning cycle of eight attempts. The coupling intervals to the second and third ES are fixed and identical. The characteristics of the program is illustrated by the ECG in figure 2.

The described program was applied in an external control box driving an implanted QRS-synchronous pacemaker with a short refractory period according to the system described by Kappenberger et al. (4). The control box is activated only when a preprogrammed tachycardia condition is fullfilled. In this investigation we used the control box for chest wall stimulation.

Short term efficacy and safety of this system were studied in five patients, two with AV-nodal and three with AV-reentry paroxysmal tachycardias. All patients had a right ventricular endocardial pacemaker lead. Initially an assessment was performed of the influence of changes in posture and physical activity on tachycardia cycle length, refractory period of the paced chamber, number of extra beats needed and the position and duration of the termination zone. The analyses were performed at three different hours of the day in each patient.

A 48-hrs ECG-recording was then performed and the termination characteristics of both spontaneous and induced tachycardias were studied, the latter being induced by synchronized ES transmitted to the patient's implanted pacemaker by chest wall stimulation. The number of attempts before termination of each tachycardia was determined and the coupling interval of the efficient combination of ES calculated.

Results

Variation in termination characteristics

The duration of both the RR-interval and the ventricular refractory period during tachycardia varied with posture and immediately after physical exercise (Fig. 3). Compared to the values in the supine position decreases were observed in all patients. The greatest shortening of the interval, 45 msec, corresponding to a rise in heart rate from 220 to 260 b/min was seen in patient no. 5 and a shortening of the ventricular refractory period of 25 msec occurred in patient no. 4, both patients with the WPW-syndrome.

Also the duration and position of the termination zones, as well as the number of ES needed, showed variation. The number of extra stimuli efficient in the different situations are shown in Table 1. In two patients single extra stimuli were sufficient to terminate tachycardia in all types of activities although in patient no. 1 the zone was very narrow, less than 5 msec after exercise. A second ES with a fixed coupling interval to the first one broadened the termination window and therefore the pacemaker was programmed to alternate between one and two extra stimuli.

In three patients two ES were needed already in the supine resting position increasing to three during activity. When patient no. 5 was on a low dosage of sotalol even three ES were not efficient after physical exercise but became reproducibly so when the dosage was increased to 160 mg b.d.

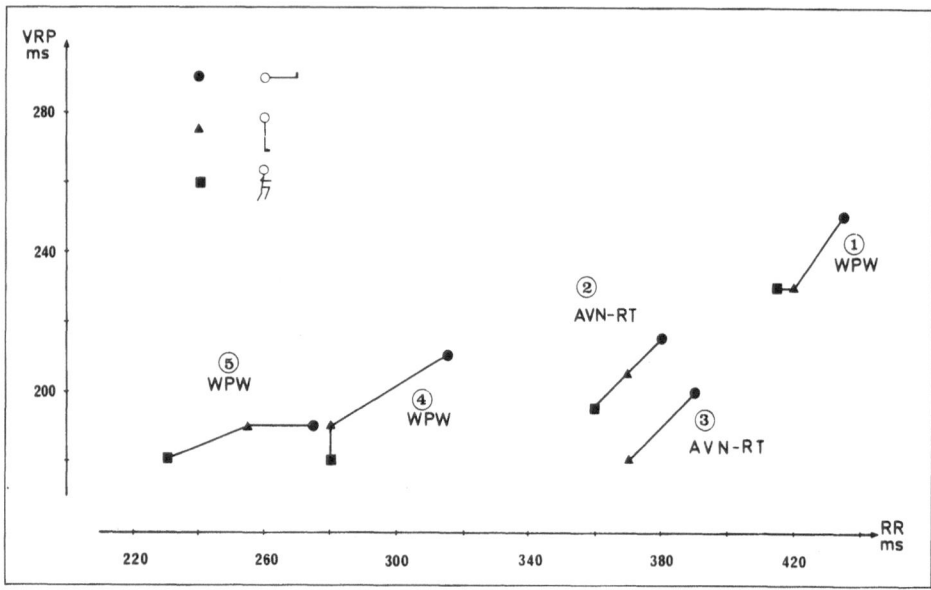

Fig. 3. Tachycardia RR interval and ventricular refractory period (VRP) during the initial evaluation of five patients in the supine and standing positions and immediately after exercise.

Table 1. Number of stimuli terminating tachycardia under different activities.

Pat no:	1. WPW sotalol 80 mg b.d.			2. AVN-RT			3. AVN-RT			4. WPW			5. WPW sotalol 40 mg b.d.		
No. of stim Posture	1	2	3	1	2	3	1	2	3	1	2	3	1	2	3
○—		+	+	+	+		−	+	−	−	+	−	−	+	+
🧍		+	+	+	+		−	+	−	−	+	+	−	−	+
🏃		(+)	+	+	+		−	−	+	−	−	+	−	−	−

Higher degrees of activity tended to require a higher number of extra stimuli. However, as was the case in patients no. 3 and 4, the higher number was not necessarily efficient at a lower degree of activity.

Results from 48-hrs ECG-monitoring

In addition to the induced tachycardias four patients had spontaneous attacks of reentry-tachycardias during the recorded period. In all patients the coupling interval to the efficient extra stimulus varied on different occasions. The program including alternation of

812

the number of ES after eight attempted coupling intervals was used and found to be of importance in the two patients in whom the number of ES was found to be critical at the initial evaluation. In these patients the efficient number of ES varied at different attacks. In the others the number of ES remained constant although the delays varied.

During the test period two patients were on drug treatment, both taking Sotalol, one patient as prophylaxis against atrial fibrillation and the other, patients no. 5, to slow down the maximal heart rate of the tachycardia.

During the monitored 48 hrs less than one complete scanning sequence (maximum 16 attempts) was efficient terminating all spontaneous or induced tachycardia in each patient. No ventricular tachyarrhythmias were induced or other adverse effects noticed during the recorded period.

Discussion

Many factors influence the possibility to terminate reciprocating tachycardias with electrical stimulation. For junctional tachycardias the type of the tachycardia (1, 6), its rate (7), the distance between the circuit and the stimulation electrode (6) are of importance. Different termination principles show varying degrees of efficacy (6). In addition considerable spontaneous variation in termination characteristics occure in the same patient with changes i posture and activity (3) probably related to variation in the autonomous tone.

Thus, a scanning principle as was described by Spurrell 1975 (5) offers considerable theoretical advantages and the results from a follow up study of an implantable automatic pacemaker with this system have been encouraging (8).

Prompt termination is advantageous not only to limit the patient's symptoms but may also be expected to increase termination efficacy as an acceleration or warming up of tachycardias involving the AV-node is often seen soon after its start (2) and as tachycardias with a high rate tend to have a narrow termination zone or require more than one extra stimulus for termination (7).

When tachycardia is not terminated by an ES with a previously efficient delay, the termination zone may have moved to either an earlier or later position in the heart cycle. The window will theoretically be found most rapidly again if the search is performed outwardly or centrifugally with alternately shorter and longer delays. When one of the outer limits of the scanning is reached, either the programmed minimum delay or the RR-interval, the remaining attempts of the search will be performed towards its other limit.

The finding in our series that a tachycardia with a higher rate generally required a higher number of ES agrees with previous experiences by Wellens et al. (7). The same tendency was also seen in most of our patients when the tachycardia rate increased as a result of changes in posture or activity (Table 1). With the present design, including a scanning first ES and fixed coupling intervals to the second and third ES, a higher number of ES was not always efficient at lower degrees of activity. Thus, although three ES were efficacious after exercise in patients no. 3 and no. 4, two but not three ES stopped tachycardia in the standing position. This finding is most probably explained by the last ES restarting the tachycardia.

Although the five patients included in this series had experienced frequent paroxysms of tachycardia, only spontaneous attacks occurring during the 48 hours recording period had been too few to allow evaluation of the termination concept. Thus tachycardias were also initiated by chest wall stimulation. The rate and configuration of these tachycardias were similar to those previously recorded. The termination characteristics agreed with those found at the initial electrophysiological assessment.

The patients were admitted to hospital during the recording period. To avoid a too artificial recording situation the patients were encouraged to exercise to at least the level of ordinary daily activities by taking walks, rapidly climb several flights of stairs etc.

During the evaluation period the control box remained connected with two leads for chest wall stimulation to permit immediate activation when tachycardia occurred. For subsequent clinical use, however, the patients were instructed to hold the two contact leads on the box between their hands when they experienced tachycardia. By necessity this leads to a delay before activation is possible and therefore a fully implantable version of our concept would represent an obvious improvement for long term tachycardia control.

References

1. Rowland E, Curry PVL, Krikler DM: The assessment of underdrive pacing in the early termination of reentrant atrioventricular tachycardia. In: Proceedings of the VI World Symposium on Cardiac Pacing, Pacesymp, Montreal 1979; Chapter 9–5.
2. Curry PVL, Rowland E, Fox KM, Krikler DM: The relationship between posture, blood pressure, and electrophysical properties in patients with paroxysmal supraventricular tachycardia. Archives des Maladies du Coeur et des Vaisseaux. 1978; 71: 293–299.
3. Crick J, Way B, Kappenberger L, Sowton E: Variation in tachycardia termination window with posture and exercise (Abstract). Pace 1981; 4: A–7.
4. Kappenberger L, Sowton E: Method for control of tachycardia by long-term programmed stimulation. Br Heart J 1979; 41: 371.
5. Spurrell RAJ: Artificial Cardiac Pacemakers. In: Krikler DM, Goodwin JF, eds. Cardiac Arrhythmias; The Modern Electrophysiological Approach. WB Saunders Company Ltd, 1975; 238–258.
6. Ward DE, Camm AJ, Spurrell RAJ: The response of regular re-entrant supraventricular tachycardia to right heart stimulation. Pace 1979; 2: 586–595.
7. Wellens HJJ, Bar FW, Gorgels AP, Muncharaz JF: Electrical management of arrhythmias with emphasis on the tachycardias. Am J Cardiol 1978; 41: 1025–1034.
8. Spurrell RAJ, Nathan AW, Bexton RS, Hellestrand KJ, Nappholz T, Camm AJ: Implantable Automatic Scanning Pacemaker for Termination of Supraventricular Tachycardia. Am J Cardiol 1982; 49: 753–760.

Author's address:
Dr. Hans Vallin
Department of Medicine
Huddinge Hospital
S-141 86 Huddinge
Sweden

Treatment of Ventricular Tachyarrhythmias with Implantable Automatic Cardioverter-Defibrillator

M. Mirowski, P. R. Reid, M. M. Mower, L. Watkins, Jr., E. V. Platia, L. S. C. Griffith, J. M. Juanteguy

Summary: The automatic implantable cardioverter-defibrillator is an electronic device designed to continuously monitor the heart, identify malignant ventricular tachyarrhythmias, and then to deliver effective countershock to restore normal rhythm. There are two defibrillating electrodes which are also used for waveform analysis; one is located in the superior vena cava, the other is placed over the cardiac apex. A third bipolar right ventricular electrode serves for rate counting and R-wave synchronization. When ventricular fibrillation occurs, a 25 joule pulse is delivered; when ventricular tachycardia faster then a preset rate is detected, the discharge is R-wave synchronized. The device can recycle three times if required. Special batteries can deliver over 100 shocks or provide a 3 year monitoring life. Implantation of the device is made either through a thoracotomy or by a subxiphoid approach. Thus far, the device has been implanted in over 100 survivors of a follow-up period up to 39 months (average 9 months). Acceleration of ventricular tachycardia to a faster rhythm or to ventricular fibrillation occurred only rarely and is dealt with most successfully through recycling. Actuarial analysis has indicated 22.9% one-year total mortality, a 52% decrease from the 48% mortality which would be expected in the same group of patients without the device; the mortality attributed to arrhythmias was only 8.5%. Thus, the automatic cardioverter-defibrillator can reliably identify and correct potentially lethal ventricular tachyarrhythmias, leading to a substantial increase in survival in properly selected high-risk patients.

The automatic implantable cardioverter-defibrillator is an electronic device designed to continuously monitor the electrical activity of the heart, identify malignant ventricular rhythms and then to deliver effective countershock to restore normal heart action (1, 2). The main purpose of this self-contained diagnostic-therapeutic system is to prevent sudden death in selected high-risk patients whenever and wherever they are stricken by a malignant arrhythmia. Because the device performs its functions promptly and automatically, the constraints of time and the need for trained personnel, the two major stumbling blocks in conventional pre-hospital resuscitation, are largely eliminated.

The original clinical model of the automatic implantable defibrillator was encased in titanium and hermetically sealed with a laser weld; it weighed 250 grams and occupied a volume of 145 milliliters. Specially designed lithium batteries provided a monitoring life of three years or the capability of delivering in excess of 100 shocks. There were two transcardial defibrillating electrodes which also served for sensing, one located on an intravascular catheter was designed for placement in the superior vena cava and the other, a flexible rectangular patch, covered the apex of the heart.

This model was basically designed to detect and treat ventricular fibrillation. The device identified the arrhythmia by continuously analyzing the probability density function of the cardiac electrical activity. This function defines the fraction of time spent by the input electrogram near the isoelectrical line with ventricular fibrillation being diagnosed by the striking absence of isoelectric potential segments.

Since the great majority of sudden cardiac death survivors suffer from hemodynamically unstable ventricular tachycardias rather than from ventricular fibrillation which is observed only at a later stage, if at all, the diagnostic-therapeutic spectrum of the device was soon extended to the entire range of ventricular tachyarrhythmias (3, 4).

This recent version of the device (Fig. 1), now in clinical use, detects and treats both ventricular fibrillation and ventricular tachycardias. The new design includes the addition of a bipolar right ventricular electrode which serves for reliable heart rate counting, R-wave synchronization and, eventually, will be used for pacing as well.

Some 20 seconds after a suitable arrhythmia is detected, the device delivers truncated exponential pulse of 25 joules; it can recycle as many as three times if the initial discharge is ineffective. After the last discharge, about 35 seconds are required to reset the counter and to allow a full series of pulses to be delivered again at the next episode. When ventricular tachycardia faster than a preset cut-off rate is recognized, the delivered discharges are synchronized with the R-wave. The device is thus no longer a defibrillator only, but rather a cardioverter-defibrillator.

Non-invasive testing of the device can be accomplished with an external analyzer. Transient placement of a magnet over the device initiates the capacitor charging cycle, with the charge being delivered into a built-in test-load resistor rather than through the leads to the patient. An electromagnetic transducer measures the capacitor charging time. Progressive increases in this time denote battery depletion, while failure to initiate the charging cycle indicates abnormal operation of the device. The analyzer also stores and telemeters out the total number of defibrillating pulses received by the patient. The cardioverter-defibrillator can be activated and deactivated at will by proper application of the magnet; it also contains a magnetically activated piezoelectronic transducer emitting coded audio signals indicating the various functional states of the device.

The initial implantees were required to have survived at least two episodes of cardiac arrest outside the setting of acute myocardial infarction; one such episode had to occur despite presumably effective drug therapy with the lethal arrhythmia documented at least once (5, 6). Subsequently, these criteria have been relaxed and presently implantation of the device is being considered in patients with episodes of ventricular fibrillation or hemodynamically unstable ventricular tachycardia not associated with acute M.I. and

Fig. 1. The automatic implantable cardioverter-defibrillator with its superior vena cava, bipolar right ventricular, and apical patch electrodes.

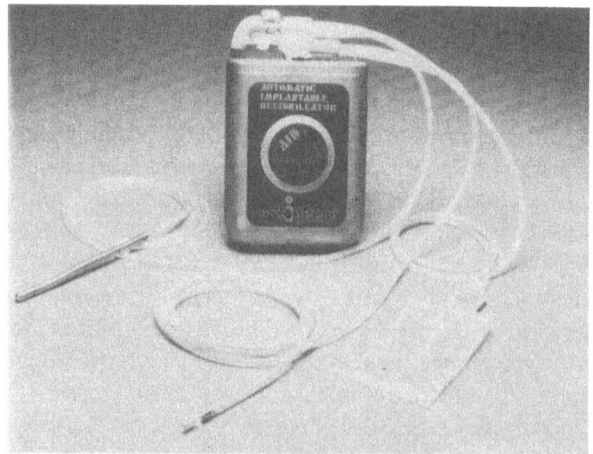

continued evidence of inducibility at electrophysiological studies in spite of antiarrhythmic therapy.

Initially, a left thoracotomy and medial sternotomy were used for implantation of the automatic defibrillator (7). More recently, a subxiphoidal approach obviating a thoracotomy became the routine implantation technique and has already been performed in some 20 cases (8). This procedure involves percutaneous insertion of the superior vena cava catheter into the left jugular vein and positioning it at the level of the right atrial junction. A small incision is then made below the xiphoid, the apical electrode introduced and sutured to the pericardium, the leads being tunneled under the skin and connected to the pulse generator implanted in a left para-umbilical pocket.

Over 1,000 defibrillator implant-months have thus far been accumulated during the clinical evaluation study of the device; the average implant time was 9 months with the longest being 39 months. The functional performance of the new cardioverter-defibrillator appears to be even better than that of the first generation device and the overall clinical results have been most encouraging (4–6). In the series of Hopkins implantees alone, over two hundred episodes of malignant ventricular arrhythmias activated the device in various settings with virtually all of the spontaneous and with the overwhelming majority of the induced rhythms being properly identified and converted to sinus rhythm by the implanted device (Fig. 2).

The phenomenon of acceleration of ventricular tachycardia into a faster rhythm or even into ventricular fibrillation occurred only three times in more than 130 episodes of the arrhythmia. The device handles this problem successfully through recycling, with the new malignant arrhythmia being detected by the sensing system and terminated with an additional countershock. In the recent model, the R-wave synchronization ensures the delivery of the countershock outside the vulnerable period of the cardiac cycle, increasing even more the considerable safety margin provided by the recycling approach. In absence of spontaneous arrhythmias, malignant rhythms were routinely induced following implantation to ensure that the device properly indentified and corrected them.

Following their return to the community, many patients reported episodes indicative of recurrent malignant arrhythmias automatically terminated by their implanted defibrillators. Because of the inherent difficulties in graphically documenting such episodes outside

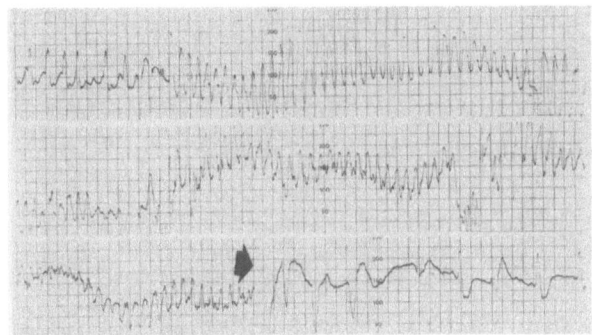

Fig. 2. ECG of an implantee who developed atrial flutter of 28 minutes duration during which the device remained quiescent. The last few beats of this supraventricular rhythm, seen in the left portion of the upper strip, are followed by two spontaneous premature ventricular contractions which induce ventricular flutter-fibrillation. Twenty-three seconds later (arrow) the malignant arrhythmia is automatically terminated with a single 25 joule discharge. The strips are continuous.

817

the hospital, the diagnosis is usually made on the basis of a characteristic sequence of events described by the implantees and/or bystanders. Typically, palpitations and weakness were initial symptoms, promptly accompanied by dizziness and/or collapse, followed by evidence of internal discharge consisting of diffuse muscle contraction and immediate recovery with a feeling of well-being. In several patients, documentation of the underlying events was obtained when they reached the hospital emergency room where their symptoms recurred and their arrhythmias were again terminated automatically (9).

The survival experience of the implantees was analyzed in the group of 52 initial patients who underwent implantation of the device through September 1982; 42 implantees were from Hopkins and 10 were from Stanford (10). The average ejection fraction in the total group was 33%. Twelve deaths have occurred in this series: Four patients died in end-stage heart failure, two from cardiogenic shock following endocardial resection and coronary artery bypass grafting, one from cerebral hemorrhage and another of pancreatic carcinoma. Four deaths were unwitnessed and we presume that they were sudden and arrhythmic.

This information was expressed in actuarial form using the Kaplan-Meier method (Fig. 3). It is apparent that the one-year mortality from all causes is 22.9%, the sudden death mortality is 8.5%, and the estimated mortality which would have occurred in the same group of patients if the automatic defibrillator had not been implanted was 48%. This represents a 52% decrease in total mortality during the year which followed implantation of the device (10).

Significantly enough, most of the deaths which occurred in this series were due to the patient's underlying disease process rather than to arrhythmias. Moreover, even though the arrhythmic mortality was only 8.5% at one year, 2 of the 4 patients whose deaths were unwitnessed and were presumed to be sudden, had defibrillation thresholds exceeding the energy output of the then-available devices. With higher energy pulse generators now

Fig. 3. Life-table survival experience in 52 patients after implantation of the automatic defibrillator. Upper curve (broken line) was derived from implantees whose death was unwitnessed and was presumably sudden. The middle curve (solid line) shows the total survival experience. The lower curve (dotted line) is an estimate of the survival that would have occurred in the entire group of patients without the implanted device. The difference between identical time points on the middle and lower curves is an estimate of the improved survival. The 95% confidence interval at 1 year for the total survival curve is shown (10).

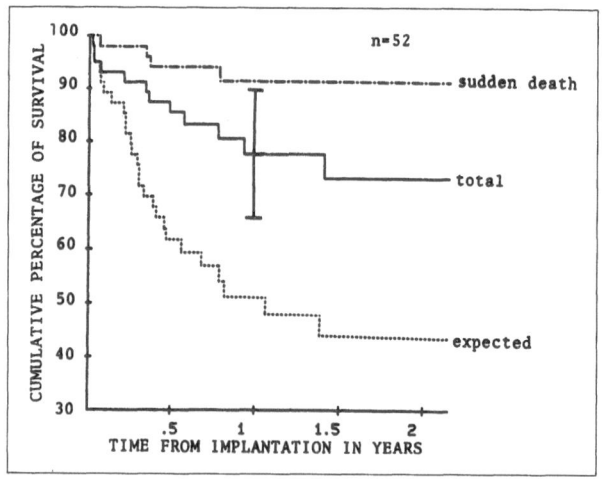

available for such patients, and with the development of more effective electrode systems, a further decrease in arrhythmic mortality rate is possible (10).

The observed improvement in total mortality and the virtual abolition of deaths due to arrhythmia are clearly related to the life-saving capabilities of the implanted automatic defibrillator. While a much larger and longer experience is needed to reach definite conclusions, it is evident that this new therapeutic modality is adding a new dimension to management of potentially lethal arrhythmias and to prevention of sudden cardiac death.

References

1. Mirowski M, Mower MM, Staewen WS, Tabatznik B: Standby automatic defibrillator: an approach to prevention of sudden coronary death. Arch Intern Med 1970; 126: 158–161.
2. Mirowski M, Mower MM, Langer A, Heilman MS, Schreibman JL: A chronically implanted system for automatic defibrillation in active conscious dogs: experimental model for treatment of sudden death from ventricular fibrillation. Circulation 1978; 58: 90–94.
3. Mirowski M: Prevention of sudden arrhythmic death with implanted automatic defibrillators. Ann Intern Med 1982; 97: 606–608.
4. Reid PR, Mirowski M, Mower MM, Platia EV, Griffith LSC, Watkins L Jr, Bach SM, Imran M, Thomas A: Clinical evaluation of the internal automatic cardioverter-defibrillator in survivors of sudden cardiac death. Amer J Cardiol 1983; 51: 1608–1613.
5. Mirowski M, Reid PR, Mower MM, Watkins L, Gott VL, Schauble JF, Langer A, Heilman MS, Kolenik SA, Fischell RD, Weisfeld ML: Termination of malignant ventricular arrhythmias with an implanted automatic defibrillator in human beings. New Eng J Med 1980; 303: 322–324.
6. Mirowski M, Reid PR, Watkins L, Weisfeldt ML, Mower MM: Clinical treatment of life-threatening tachyarrhythmias with the automatic implantable defibrillator. AM Heart J 1981; 102: 265–270.
7. Watkins L Jr, Mirowski M, Mower MM, Reid PR, Griffith LSC, Vlay SC, Weisfeldt ML, Gott VL: Automatic defibrillation in man. The initial surgical experience. J Thorac Cardiovasc Surg 1981; 82: 492–500.
8. Watkins L JR, Mirowski M, Mower MM, Reid PR, Freund P, Thomas A, Weisfeldt ML, Gott VL: Implantation of the automatic defibrillator: The subxiphoid approach. Ann Thorac Surg 1982; 34: 515–520.
9. Mirowski M, Reid PR, Mower MM, Watkins L: Successful conversion of out-of-hospital life-threatening arrhythmias with the implanted automatic defibrillator. Am Heart J 1982; 103: 147–148.
10. Mirowski M, Reid PR, Winkle RA, Mower MM, Watkins L Jr, Stinson EB, Griffith LSC, Kallman CH, Weisfeldt ML: Mortality in patients with implanted automatic defibrillators. Ann Intern Med 1983; 98: 585–588.

Authors' address:
M. Mirowski, M.D.
Sinai Hospital of Baltimore
Baltimore, Maryland 21215
USA

Ventricular Fibrillation Detection by Intramyocardial Pressure Gradients*⁾

B. G. Denys, A. E. Aubert, H. Ector, H. De Geest

Summary: Ventricular fibrillation recognition is a major problem before automatic implantable defibrillators (AID) will become useful on a large scale. In this work a pressure gradient measurement is proposed instead of using some kind of ECG processing. Endo- and epicardial pressures in the left ventricular wall were measured with high fidelity tip transducers. The intramyocardial wall gradient was determined by digital subtraction of these pressures.

Measuring endo- and epicardial pressures in the left ventricular wall permits to differentiate between ventricular arrhythmias with and without haemodynamic repercussion. During a normal sinus beat an intramyocardial pressure gradient exists with a maximum near the endocardium during systole and a maximum at the epicardium during diastole. This gradient decreases to a constant level without cyclic changes when left ventricular activity becomes uncoordinate. Our method permits to monitor left ventricular performance without an intraventricular transducer. Furthermore by using differential pressure measurements, the influence of transducer baseline drift is easily eliminated. Further study is needed to evaluate the system in long term experiments.

Introduction

Cardiac pacemakers are used world wide and became very sophisticated and miniaturized. An automatic implantable defibrillator (AID) on the contrary has been used in only a few clinical studies (1).

A demand pacemaker (DPM) and an AID show a great similarity. Both include a double circuit: one for sensing and one for pulsing. In a DPM sensing is rather easy: its basic concept is to detect asystole or the lack of electrical activity of heart muscle within a given time limit. The task of the AID is much more difficult. The electrical activity of the heart has not only to be sensed but also analyzed. The arrhythmias have to be recognized without false positive or false negative results. Indeed only ventricular fibrillation (VF) and malignant ventricular tachycardias should be allowed to trigger the signal for cardioversion.

AID sensing systems described up to now mostly use processing of ECG signals as input (2). Other systems include right ventricular pressure (3, 4), right ventricular impedance (5) or a combination of different parameters (6). This paper deals with the idea of a new approach to the detection of VF and malignant ventricular tachycardias by continuous measurement of subendocardial and subepicardial pressure in the left ventricular wall.

Methodology

Experiments were performed in 9 mongrel dogs of either sex weighing 18 to 28 kg. Anesthesia was induced with fluanisol (Hypnorm®) (0.5 ml/kg body weight S.C.) and main-

---

*⁾ Patent Nr. 8301582

tained with sodiumpentobarbital (Nembutal®). The dogs were intubated with a cuffed endotracheal tube and ventilated with a mixture of 50% O$_2$ and 50% room air by means of a Bird respirator. A left thoracotomy was performed in the fifth intercostal space. The pericardium was opened anteriorly and parallel to the left phrenic nerve and attached to the chest wall to form a pericardial cradle.

Left ventricular pressure (LVP) was measured with a high fidelity miniaturized pressure transducer (Gaeltac, Isle of Skye) introduced from the right carotid artery. Before introduction into the artery the baseline of the catheter was established in a 37 °C 0.9% saline solution. Mechanical calibration was performed in a pressure chamber (H. Gauer) by applying pressures between 0 and 100 mmHg and adjusting amplification. Gaeltec catheters have a very low temperature drift (0.2%/ °C) and a very high linear response (DC to 2.4 kHz).

Intramyocardial tissue pressure (IMP) was measured with a miniaturized transducer mounted on a 1.2 mm needle. This system was custom built by Gaeltec. The sensing portion of the transducer (dimensions 2 × 1 mm) was recessed in the needle 5 mm from the tip (Fig. 1). Connection of the needle to the amplifier was made of silicone tubing to minimize frictional forces. The needle transducers were firmly implanted directly in the anterior free wall of the left ventricle. Markers on the shaft indicated depth. Pressures were measured at two depths in the myocardial wall: one transducer was located approximately at the endocardial layer (ENDO) and one at the epicardial layer (EPI). Both were positioned at a distance of approximately 1.5 cm. Before introduction the transducer were calibrated the same way as the LV catheter.

Ventricular fibrillation (VF) was induced with a DC current impulse at 6 V and a current of 10 to 20 mA using a unipolar pacing catheter in contact with the right atrial wall in 9 experiments.

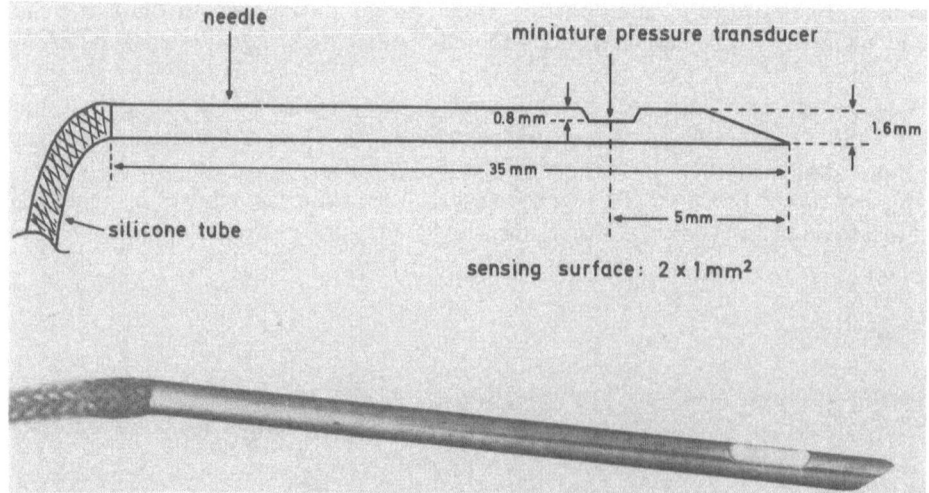

Fig. 1. Schematic drawing and picture of the needle mounted transducer.

Ventricular tachycardia (VT) and VF were induced in one experiment. A pacing electrode was positioned in the right ventricular apex under fluoroscopic control and a Janssens Scientific Instruments SU2 Programmable stimulator was used. The pacing frequency was increased to 300 pulses per minute. LVP, lead II of the ECG, subendocardial (ENDO) and subepicardial IMP (EPI) were recorded simultaneously on a direct writing ink-jet 16 channel recorder (Siemens-Elema Mingograph) at a paper speed of 100 mm/s and on a 12 channel FM tape recorder (Honeywell 101, Denver, USA) on one inch tape at a speed of 3.73 i/s.

Observations were made before and during VF and VT. Computer processing was performed on a DPO system (Digital Processing Oscilloscope, Tektronix, Beaverton, USA) (7) including a PDP 11/05 computer (Digital Equipment, Mass., USA) with 28K memory. ENDO and EPI were subtracted digitally to obtain the intramyocardial pressure gradient (ENDO-EPI curve). Peak-to-peak values were determined on LVP (end diastolic pressure to systolic maximum of LVP) and on the intramyocardial pressure gradient before and during ventricular fibrillation.

Results

During a normal heart beat an intramyocardial pressure gradient exists throughout the cardiac cycle as is shown on the first part of Fig. 2. The upper panel shows the ECG with a transition from sinus rhythm to VF. On the middle panel LVP, endo- and epicardial pressures are shown. The lower panel shows the intramyocardial pressure gradient defined as the ENDO-EPI curve. During systole maximal intramyocardial pressure, exceeding LVP, occurs at the endocardium: the ENDO-EPI curve shows a positive peak. During diastole however epicardial pressure is higher than endocardial pressure: ENDO-EPI has a negative peak. The second part of Fig. 2 shows the onset of VF. LVP decreases ra-

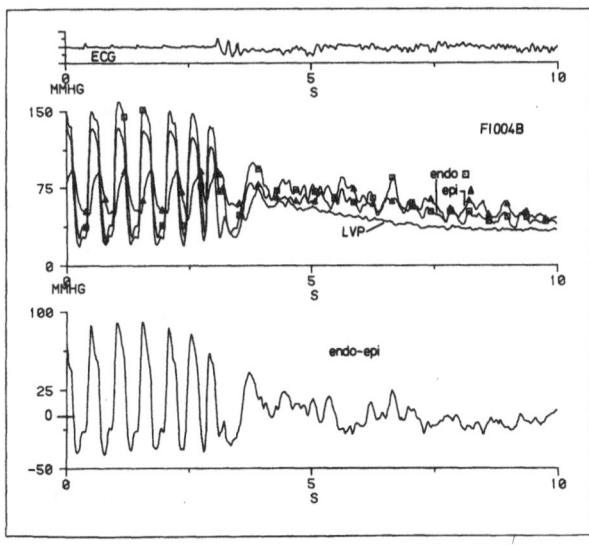

Fig. 2. *Upper panel:* ECG. *Middle panel:* left ventricular pressure (LVP), endocardial pressure □ (ENDO) and epicardial pressure (EPI) ■ during the transition of a normal sinus rhythm to ventricular fibrillation. *Lower panel:* endocardial minus epicardial pressure (ENDO-EPI) or the intramyocardial pressure gradient.

Table 1. Peak-to-peak values of the intramyocardial pressure gradient and LVP before and during ventricular fibrillation (mmHg).

Exp.	Before VF		During VF	
	ENDO-EPI	LVP	ENDO-EPI	LVP
1.	128.5	150.1	66.1	34.7
2.	31.1	73.2	19.8	14.6
3.	127.3	116.5	41.7	33.4
4.	50.1	57.7	16.1	13.6
5.	66.2	53.4	33.9	13.4
6.	77.8	98.7	18.9	14.8
7.	39.8	102.1	15.7	11.7
8.	77.2	88.8	26.3	5.7
9.	102.0	83.4	35.6	8.2
Mean ± 1 SD	77.8 ± 35.6	91.5 ± 30.0	30.5 ± 13.7	16.7 ± 10.3

N = 9

ENDO-EPI: intramyocardial pressure gradient, LVP: left ventricular pressure, VF: ventricular fibrillation, SD: standard deviation.

Fig. 3. *Upper panel:* ECG. The first part shows paced ventricular tachycardia, the second part ventricular flutter whereas the third part ventricular fibrillation. *Middle panel:* left ventricular pressure (LVP), endocardial pressure □ (ENDO) and epicardial pressure (EPI) ■. *Lower panel:* the intramyocardial pressure gradient.

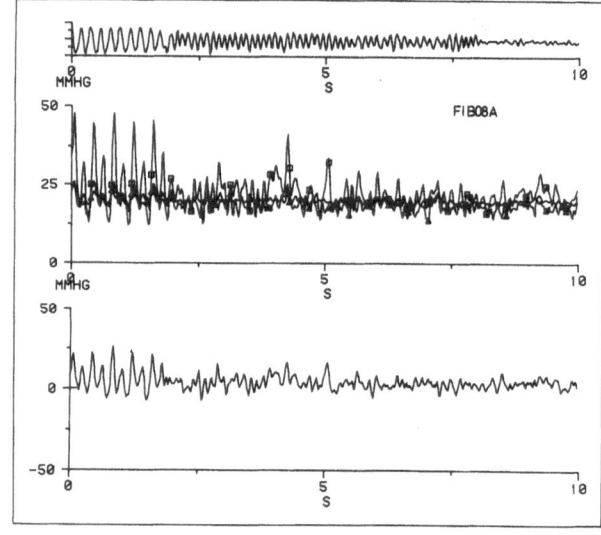

pidly. At the same moment the intramyocardial pressure gradient decreases to a constant value. Peak-to-peak values of ENDO-EPI and LVP before and during VF are shown on Table 1. Paired t-test, performed on the intramyocardial pressure gradient before and during VF and on LVP before and during VF, showed a significant decrease (p < 0.001). Fig. 3 illustrates the transition from paced tachycardia over ventricular flutter to VF. Although LVP was rather low it is seen that when ventricular flutter appears on the

ECG, LVP further decreases without obvious cyclic changes. This evolution is even more prominent on the intramyocardial pressure gradient. As soon as ventricular flutter occurs the pressure gradient falls rapidly and decreases further to a constant value. Thus the intramyocardial pressure gradient persists as long as ventricular arrhythmias have no haemodynamic repercussion as monitored by cyclic changes of LVP.

Discussion

Before the AID will be used on a larger scale, some main problems still have to be solved. The most critical point remains the sensing circuit. The problem is not only what to sense and how, but also what are the selectivity and the specificity required for this purpose.

Early systems were designed to detect only VF whereas the present tendency is to broaden the application to tachyarrhythmias with haemodynamic repercussion (8). Right ventricular pressure has been described as a possible parameter (3, 4). However this gives only information about right ventricular haemodynamics which has the inconvenience of being a low pressure system. Therefore the pressure transducer has to be extremely stable and sensitive. On the long term the covering of the transducer by connective tissue becomes a supplementary problem. ECG processing is a valid method for recognition of VF since the electrical fibrillation signal has some specific quantities (2). Recent developments in Mirowsky's concept enable the recognition of arrhythmias other than VF (8). Autocorrelation analysis of the ECG was proposed by Aubert et al. as an alternative method (9). These methods however give no information about the haemodynamic status. So it is extremely difficult to differentiate between arrhythmias with or without haemodynamic repercussion since the relation between the ECG and the mechanical heart activity is not absolute. A combination of ECG processing and right ventricular impedance monitoring has been proposed to avoid this pitfall (6). The authors claim that with this method malignant arrhythmias with important haemodynamic deterioration can be recognized selectively. This extra parameter would decrease false positive results and provide more safety.

We not only measured pressure but a pressure gradient in the ventricular wall. During the heart cycle a pressure gradient exists between the endo- and epicardium (10–12). During systole the maximal gradient is directed to the endocardium whereas during diastole the maximum is close to the epicardium. Whenever an organized heart contraction occurs this intramyocardial pressure gradient is built up. On the contrary, when heart muscle fibers show no simultaneous activity the ENDO-EPI difference becomes minimal without cyclic changes. This method offers several advantages. The intramyocardial pressure is related to some extent to LVP. Thus pressure information about the left heart is available without intraventricular device. The idea of monitoring LVP may be interesting but the risks of thrombosis caused by an intraventricular transducer on the left side of the heart are too high. Influence of drift of the baseline of the pressure transducers is minimalized as absolute peak-to-peak values are independent of DC levels. Problems by tissue growth are of less importance since the transducer are already implanted in heart muscle. The main advantage of this method is that ventricular arrhythmias with haemodynamic repercussion are recognized.

The needle mounted transducers used in this study are only an experimental set up. Other devices including the two pressure transducers and designed for chronic implantation are in construction. Although the system still has to be applied in long term studies, in conscious dogs the results clearly show that continuous measurements of intramyocardial pressure gradients add a new dimension to AID sensing and can broaden their indication and application.

References

1. Watkins LJr, Mirowski M, Mower MM, Reid PR, Griffith LSC, Vlay SC, Weisfeldt ML, Gott VL: Automatic defibrillation in man. The initial surgical experience. J Thorac Cardiovasc Surg 1981; 39: 492–500.
2. Mirowski M, Mower MM, Reid PR, Watkins L, Langer L: The automatic implantable defibrillation. New modality for treatment of life-threatening ventricular arrhythmias. Pace 1982; 5: 384–401.
3. Mirowski M, Mower MM, Staewen WS: Standby automatic defibrillator: an approach to prevention of sudden coronary death. Arch Intern Med 1970; 126: 158.
4. Mirowski M, Mower MM, Staewen WS: The development of the transvenous automatic defibrillator. Arch Intern Med 1972; 129: 773.
5. Bourland JD: Automatic detection of ventricular fibrillation for an implanted defibrillator. Abstract, Frontiers in Medical Signal Processing, Chicago, Ill, USA, Nov. 8–10, 1977.
6. Tacker WAJr, Bourland JD, Thacker JR, Babbs CF, Holmes HR, Fisher PG, Geddes LA: Optimal spacing of right ventricular bipolar catheter electrodes for detecting cardiac pumping by an automatic implantable defibrillator. Med Instrument 1980; 14: 27–29.
7. Aubert AE, Denys BG, Denef B, Van de Werf F, De Geest H, Kesteloot H: Computer processing of echo-mechanocardiograms. Methods and results. Comp Biomed Res 1982; 15: 57–75.
8. Mirowski M, Mower MM, Reid PR: The automatic implantable defibrillator. Am H J 1980; 100: 1089–1092.
9. Aubert AE, Denys BG, Ector H, De Geest H: Fibrillation recognition using autocorrelation analysis. IEEE Comp Cardiol, Seattle, Washington, 1982; 477–480.
10. Kreuzer H, Schoeppe W: Das Verhalten des Druckes in der Hewand. Pflügers Arch Ges Physiol 1963; 278: 181.
11. Baird RJ, Manktelow RT, Shah PA, Ameli FH: Intramyocardiac pressure. A study of its regional variations and its relationship to intraventricular pressure. J Thorac Cardiovasc Surg 1971; 174–950.
12. Stein, PD, Marzilli M, Sabbah HN, Lee T: Systolic and diastolic pressure gradients within the left ventricular wall. Am J Physiol 1980; 238: H625–H630.

Authors' address:
B. G. Denys, M.D.
Division of Cardiology
Department of Pathophysiology
K. U. Leuven, Campus Gasthuisberg
B-3000 Leuven, Belgium

Synchronized Low Energy Transvenous Cardioversion

Douglas P. Zipes, James J. Heger, Eric N. Prystowsky

Summary: In this study, we present one data on the use of transvenous cardioversion with synchronized shocks of low energies via a catheter electrode.

Animal studies: After a two hour occlusion of the LAD 35 dogs underwent programmed electrical stimulation. The induced VT was terminated with transvenous cardioversion using 10 F electrode catheters (Medtronic 6880) connected to a Medtronic 2316 cardioverter. This delivered a truncated exponential wave form, approximately 6 msec in duration with increasing energy levels from 0.0005–2.5 J.

Of the 30 sustained VT, cycle length $\geqslant$ 200 msec, 83% were terminated reproducibly by shocks of $\leqslant$ 1.0 and 67% $\leqslant$ 0.5 J.

For shocks introduced within the first 80% of the QRS, RVRs were rare and acceleration or degeneration to fibrillation never occurred. For shocks introduced within the vulnerable period (ST-T) energies of 0.008 J accelerated the VT or produced ventricular fibrillation.

Human studies were performed in 13 pts with coronary artery disease (55–72 y old). In 11 patients on one or more occasions the transvenous cardioversion terminated VT with energies of 0.025 to 2.0 J.

Including subthreshold attempts, a total of 196 shocks was delivered. Awake unsedated patients tolerated shocks of < 0.5 J without difficulty. Shocks > 0.5 J produced moderate skeletal muscle stimulation.

In the future the ideal implantable device will be capable of transvenous cardioversion and, if that fails or if ventricular fibrillation is precipitated, it will then deliver automatically a defibrillating shock.

For many years electrical transthoracic cardioversion and defibrillation have been used successfully and safely to terminate most tachyarrhythmias. Recently, Mirowski et al. (9, 10) after more than a decade of research and development, perfected an implantable defibrillator that delivers 25–30 joules to terminate ventricular fibrillation. Based on these concepts, we reasoned that the principles of transthoracic cardioversion could be adapted for use with an intracardiac device that could deliver *synchronized* cardioversion shocks of low energies via a catheter electrode to successfully and safely terminate sustained ventricular tachyarrhythmias (3, 15–17). This system might also terminate supraventricular tachyarrhythmias. In the following discussion we present our developmental animal studies and initial clinical experience with this concept.

Animal Studies (3)

Mongrel dogs underwent a 2-hour occlusion of the left anterior descending coronary artery (LAD) proximal to the main diagonal branches supplying the apical region using a

Supported in part by the Herman C. Krannert Fund; by Grants HL-06308, HL-07182 from the National Heart, Lung and Blood Institute of the National Institutes of Health, Bethesda, Maryland, and by the American Heart Association, Indiana Affiliate, Inc.

827

Harris two-stage procedure (2). Two hours after complete occlusion, arterial flow was reestablished. Three to 8 days after myocardial infarction, dogs were anesthetized and a median sternotomy was performed. A # 10F electrode catheteter, specially designed for cardioversion (Medtronic model 6880) was inserted through the right external jugular vein and advanced to the right ventricular apex (Fig. 1). The catheter consisted of four stainless steel electrodes: Two electrodes at the tip separated by 5 mm and two similarly spaced electrodes 13 cm from the tip. Each electrode had a surface area of 1.25 cm. The distal pair of electrodes located in the right ventricular apex was used for bipolar R-wave sensing to time cardioversion shocks. When a shock was delivered, the distal pair of electrodes was coupled together to form the cathode and the proximal pair of electrodes (located in the superior vena cava) was coupled together for the anode. In five dogs, a second 6880 electrode catheter was inserted into the left external jugular vein and advanced into the distal coronary sinus. The distal pair of electrodes of this catheter was used as the anode, with the cathode being the two electrodes of the first catheter located in the right ventricular apex. Finally, in three dogs, a 5 cm diameter cone electrode (11), composed of two stainless steel wire mesh sheets separated by a 5 mm Silastic band, was sutured onto the apex of the heart. The apex cone electrode was the cathode and the superior vena cava electrode formed the anode. Shocks were timed from the bipolar R-wave recorded

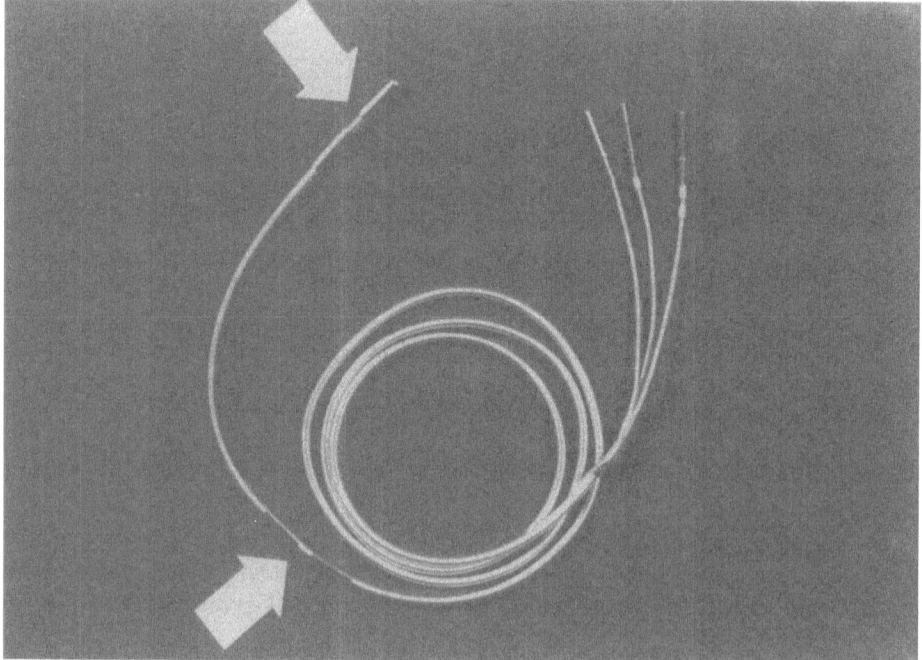

Fig. 1. Picture of electrode catheter. Arrows point to pairs of electrodes. Reproduced with permission from Zipes, D. P., Jackman, W. M., Heger, J. J. et al. Clinical transvenous cardioversion of recurrent life-threatening ventricular tachyarrhythmias: low energy synchronized cardioversion of ventricular tachycardia and termination of ventricular fibrillation in patients using a catheter electrode. Am Heart J 1982; 103: 789.

between the two wire mesh sheets. The cardioverter (Medtronic model 2316) delivered a truncated exponential wave form (13), 6 msec in duration, at nine energy levels: 0.0005, 0.001, 0.008, 0.025, 0.09, 0.5, 1.0, 2.0 and 2.5 J. A programmable stimulator (Medtronic model 5325) was interfaced with the pulse generator to provide the sensing function and timing for the cardioversion shocks.

Programmed electrical stimulation (1.8 msec rectangular stimuli at twice late diastolic current threshold) of the epicardial sites near the infarction border zone was used to induce sustained ventricular tachycardia (1, 4, 8). After induction of sustained ventricular tachycardia, shocks between the right ventricular apex and superior vena cava were introduced at a fixed time within the QRS complex. Beginning with 0.0005 J, shocks of progressively increasing energy were delivered until ventricular tachycardia was terminated. Ventricular tachycardia was reinitiated and the same sequence repeated two to five times to determine the minimum energy required to reproducibly terminate the tachycardia at that time in the tachycardia cycle. Shocks of greater energy (up to 2.5 J) were applied to determine the safety of higher energy pulses.

Similar testing was done at 5–20 msec intervals throughout the tachycardia cycle. This protocol was repeated with shocks delivered between the right ventricular apex and coronary sinus in five dogs and between the epicardial apex cone electrode and superior vena cava electrodes in three.

All dogs had sinus rhythm at the onset of study. Programmed electrical stimulation induced sustained ventricular tachycardia with constant cycle length, ventricular activation sequence and QRS morphology in 14 dogs. Two or more morphologically different forms of sustained ventricular tachycardia, each with a distinct cycle length and ventricular activation sequence, were induced in 12 of the 14 dogs, for a total of 35 different ventricular tachycardias. A mean of 17.9 ± 29.7 ($\pm$ SD) episodes of each tachycardia was induced, for a total of 627 episodes of sustained ventricular tachycardia tested by intracardiac DC shock. The mean ventricular tachycardia cycle length was 257 ± 63 msec.

Figure 2 shows the analog record of a successful termination of ventricular tachycardia by a shock delivered between the right ventricular apex and superior vena cava. Between 20 and 40 msec from the onset of ventricular activation, shocks of 0.09 J reproducibly terminated the ventricular tachycardia.

The maximum required termination energy (shocks between the right ventricular apex and superior vena cava) for each of the 35 ventricular tachycardias is plotted as a function of tachycardia cycle length in figure 3. Of the 30 sustained ventricular tachycardias with a cycle length $\geqslant$ 200 msec (mean 275 ± 46 msec), 25 (83%) were reproducibly terminated by shocks of $\leqslant 1.0$ J and 20 (67%) by shocks of $\leqslant 0.5$ J. Only one of the five tachycardias with a cycle length $<$ 200 msec (mean 145 ± 25 msec) was terminated reproducibly by shocks of $\leqslant 1.0$ J. There was no significant linear or log-linear relationship between the maximum required termination energy and the tachycardia cycle length.

The maximum required termination energy for shocks delivered between the right ventricular apex (cathode) and coronary sinus (anode) was not significantly different from that of shocks between the right ventricular apex (cathode) and superior vena cava (anode) for the seven tachycardias in the five dogs tested. For shocks delivered between the epicardial apex cone electrode (cathode) and the superior vena cava electrodes (anode), the maximum required termination energy was decreased by a factor of 20–250 for all six tachycardias in the three dogs tested (Fig. 3). Shocks of 0.008 J terminated five of six ventricular tachycardias using this electrode arrangement.

829

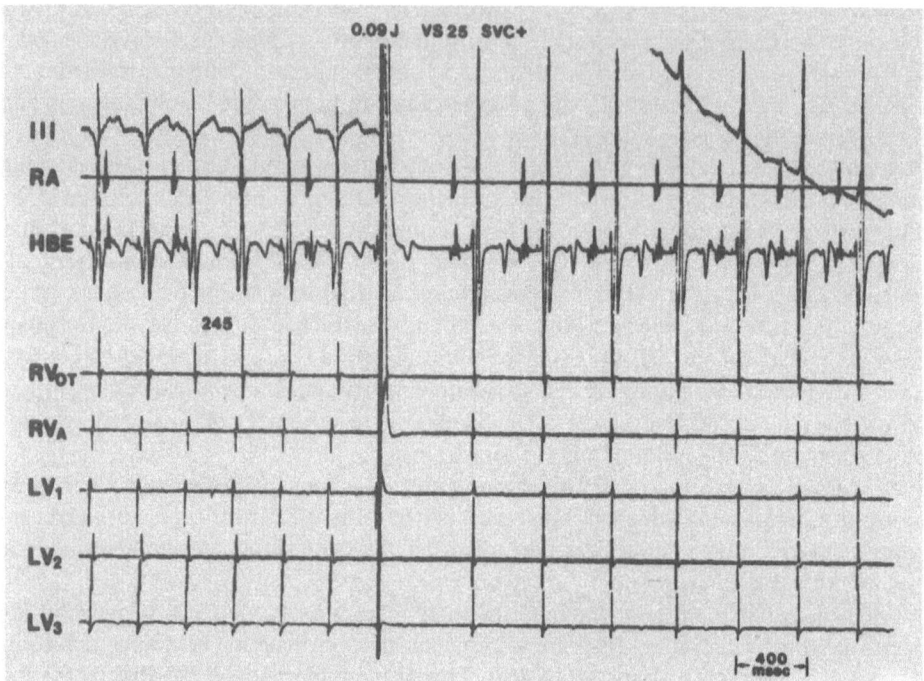

Fig. 2. Termination of sustained ventricular tachycardia (cycle length 245 msec) by a shock of 0.09 J delivered between the right ventricular apex and superior vena cava. ECG lead III, right atria (RA), His bundle (HBE) and epicardial electrograms were recorded from the right ventricular outflow track (RV_{ot}), right ventricular apex (RV_a), and the left ventricle (LV) around the border of the antero-apical infarction. The shock was introduced 25 msec after the onset of ventricular activation (VS25) which is recorded earliest in lead III. The shock restored sinus rhythm, evidenced by the narrow QRS complexes, preceding His bundle potentials (H) at a normal HV interval and fixed association with atrial depolarization. Reproduced with permission from Jackman, W. M., Zipes, D. P.: Low-energy synchronous cardioversion of ventricular tachycardia using a catheter electrode in a canine model of subacute myocardial infarction. Circulation 1982; 66: 187.

Of the 748 shocks of 0.008–1.0 J introduced within the first 80 percent of the QRS interval, only 12 (1.6%) produced repetitive ventricular responses and none accelerated the ventricular tachycardia or precipitated ventricular fibrillation (Fig. 4). For shocks of 2.0 and 2.5 J, there was an 11% incidence of repetitive ventricular response of four or more complexes. However, these repetitive responses began more than 400 msec after the shock, had a cycle length longer than that of the original tachycardia, slowed progressively and terminated spontaneously.

Shocks introduced during the last 20% of the QRS interval and within the ST-T interval resulted in repetitive ventricular responses. As the energy was increased progressively, multiple-beat repetitive ventricular responses or ventricular fibrillation occurred.

In the ventricular tachycardias with cycle lengths < 200 msec, the safety of shocks introduced during the QRS interval was inconsistent. Two of 17 shocks $\geq$ 0.5 J placed within the first 80% of the QRS interval resulted in ventricular fibrillation.

Atrioventricular dissociation occurred frequently during ventricular tachycardia. Therefore, shocks synchronized to the QRS interval fell randomly in the atrial cycle. Shocks in-

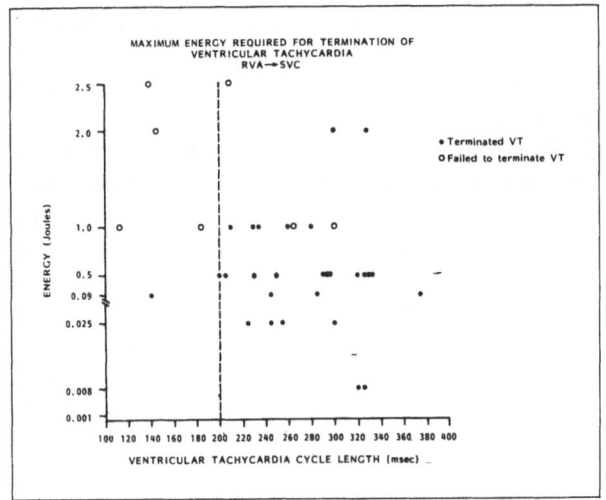

Fig. 3. Maximum required termination energy for shocks delivered between the right ventricular apex and superior vena cava for each of the 35 ventricular tachycardias (VT), plotted as a function of tachycardia cycle length. Open circles indicate ventricular tachycardias that were not reproducibly terminated by shocks applied within the QRS interval, plotted at the highest energy level at which shocks failed to terminate VT. Reproduced with permission from Jackman, W. M., Zipes, D. P.: Low-energy synchronous cardioversion of ventricular tachycardia using a catheter electrode in a canine model of subacute myocardial infarction. Circulation 1982; 66: 187.

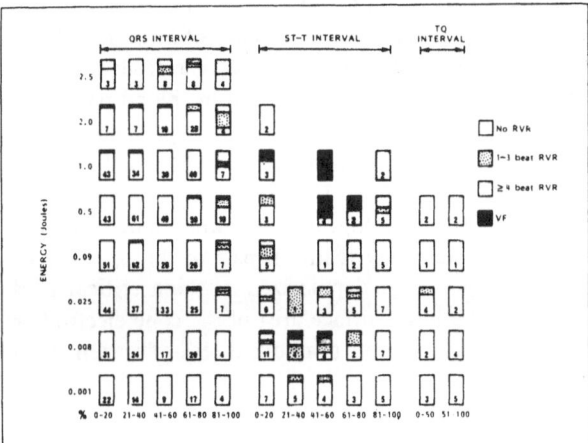

Fig. 4. Incidence of repetitive ventricular response (RVR) produced by shocks delivered between the right ventricular apex and superior vena cava, plotted as a function of energy level and timed within the tachycardia cycle at which shocks were applied. Data are cumulative for all tachycardias with cycle lengths exceeding 200 msec. Time is normalized to percent of the QRS, ST-T and TQ intervals. Numbers inside boxes indicate the number of shocks tested. The percent of each box that is unfilled represents the percent of shocks that produced no RVR. The percent of each box that is coarsely stippled, finely stippled, or solid black represents the percent of shocks that produced repetitive ventricular responses of one to three complexes, four or more complexes (including acceleration of ventricular tachycardia and ventricular flutter) or ventricular fibrillation (VF), respectively. Reproduced with permission from Jackman, W. M., Zipes, D. P.: Low-energy synchronous cardioversion of ventricular tachycardia using a catheter electrode in a canine model of subacute myocardial infarction. Circulation 1982; 66: 187.

troduced during the second quarter of the atrial cycle occasionally resulted in repetitive atrial responses, including atrial flutter or fibrillation. When induced, atrial flutter or fibrillation usually terminated spontaneously within 2–3 seconds after onset.

This study demonstrated that shocks of 1.0 J or less, delivered through transvenous intracardiac catheter electrodes and synchronized to the QRS complex, reproducibly terminated 83% of the sustained ventricular tachycardias with cycle lengths $\geqslant$ 200 msec that were induced in dogs 3–8 days after myocardial infarction. For shocks introduced within the first 80% of the QRS interval, repetitive ventricular responses were rare and acceleration of the ventricular tachycardia or degeneration to ventricular fibrillation never occurred. For shocks introduced during the ST-T interval, corresponding to the vulnerable period of the ventricular cycle (14), energies as low as 0.008 J accelerated the ventricular tachycardia or produced ventricular fibrillation. Since shocks were not synchronized to the atrial cycle due to the presence of atrioventricular dissociation, atrial flutter or fibrillation was precipitated in 9% of shocks $\geqslant$ 0.5 J, but usually terminated spontaneously within 3 seconds.

Only one of five ventricular tachycardias with cycle length < 200 msec (> 300 beats/min) was terminated by shocks $\leqslant$ 2.5 J. Also, in these more rapid tachycardias, shocks $\geqslant$ 0.5 J introduced within the QRS interval occasionally produced ventricular fibrillation. Since ventricular activation extended through most of the cycle length in these tachycardias, repolarization of some part of the ventricular myocardium (and therefore the vulnerable period) probably extended in to the next QRS interval. There may exist no discrete period in the QRS interval during which a low energy shock can safely terminate these very rapid tachycardias.

Placing the anode in the coronary sinus did not significantly decrease the energy requirement to terminate ventricular tachycardia or decrease the incidence of atrial fibrillation, and therefore appeared to offer no advantage over the single catheter electrode configuration. This result may be explained by a „short-circuiting" effect of the blood pool. Since the resistivity of blood is approximately one-third that of the total biologic media (blood, interstitial fluid and muscle) (6), much of the current was probably lost to the blood pool between the right ventricular apex and coronary sinus. In contrast, the large epicardial apex cone electrode reduced dramatically (20–250-fold) the maximum required termination energy. The decrese in energy requirement may relate in part to the pathway traveled by the current, so that shocks of less energy depolarized a region critical to the maintenance of tachycardia. More likely, the large surface area of the cone electrode reduced electrical resistance and the epicardial location minimized loss of current to the blood pool.

Human Studies (16, 17)

After written informed consent was obtained, the catheter was inserted in 13 patients percutaneously through an antecubital jugular or subclavian vein and its tip was positioned under fluoroscopic guidance at the right ventricular apex. Patients were men, 55 to 72 years old (mean 61 years), and had a history of a remote myocardial infarction. All patients were referred for evaluation and therapy of recurrent sustained ventricular tachycardia. Twelve patients were awake and nonsedated during all cardioversion attempts of ventricular tachycardia. One patient requested to be anesthetized when the energy of the shocks exceeded 0.5 J during the first two cardioversion procedures. For the third cardioversion procedure, the patient remained awake and unsedated. All patients were receiving cardioactive drugs.

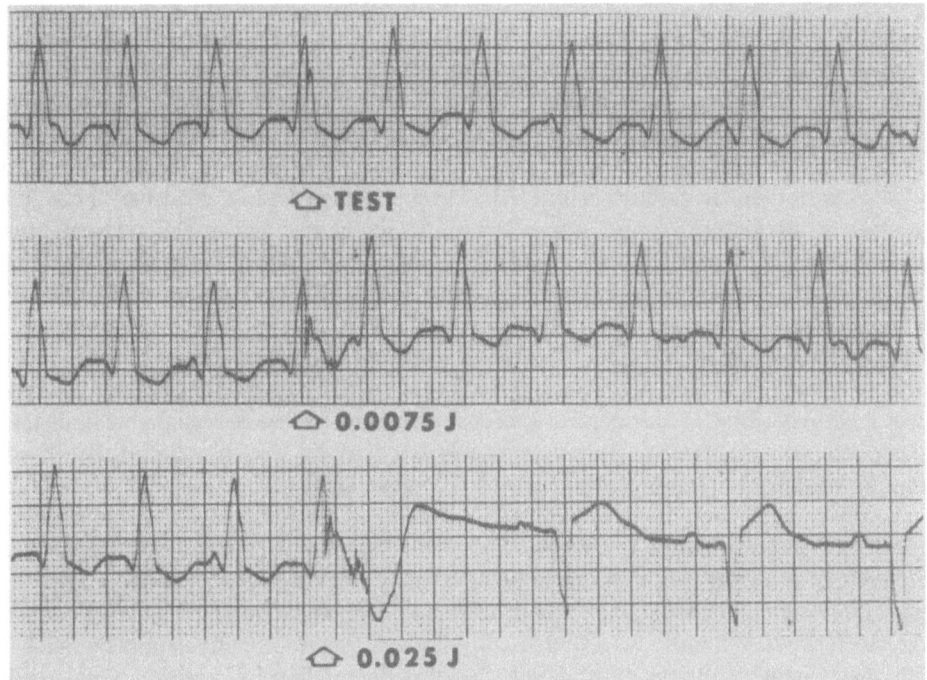

Fig. 5. Transvenous cardioversion. Top panel. Test stimulus delivered into QRS complex. Middle panel. Subthreshold shock shortened RR interval of ventricular tachycardia but did not terminate tachycardia. Bottom panel. Threshold shock terminated ventricular tachycardia. Lead II. Reproduced with permission from Zipes, D.P., Jackman, W. M., Heger, J. J. et al. Clinical transvenous cardioversion of recurrent life-threatening ventricular tachyarrhythmias: low energy synchronized cardioversion of ventricular fibrillation in patients using a catheter electrode. Am Heart J 1982; 103: 426.

Table 1

Patient	VT Episodes Terminated	Cardioversion Threshold (joules, mean, range)
1	18	0.13, 0.075–0.25
2	20	0.06, 0.025–0.1
3	6	1.17, 0.75 –2.0
4	2	0.16, 0.075–0.25
5	1	2.0, –
6	6	0.68, 0.1 –2.0
7	1	1.25, –
8*	311	5.7, 4–20
9	0	> 0.75
10	0	> 2.0
11	1	1.5
12	1	0.25
13	5	0.08, 0.05–0.1

* American Optical Cardioverter, see text.

Transvenous cardioversion terminated ventricular tachycardia in 11 of 13 patients on one or more occasions with energies of 0.025 to 2.0 J using a truncated exponential waveform (Fig. 5) and 4–20 J using a damped sine wave (see below) (Table 1). In two patients ventricular tachycardia was not terminated by shocks of up to 0.75 and 2.0 J, respectively. Ventricular tachycardia resulted in profound hypotension with loss of consciousness in these two patients and therefore testing was discontinued. The tachycardia was terminated by transthoracic cardioversion (320 J) in one patient and in the other, burst right ventricular pacing (six stimuli, cycle length 260 msec) produced a chaotic ventricular tachycardia (cycle length 280 msec) that spontaneously terminated after five complexes. Shocks of 25 J terminated three episodes of ventricular fibrillation in one patient (see below) (Fig. 6).

Including subthreshold attempts, a total of 196 shocks ranging between 0.0075 and 2.0 J was delivered. On several occasions, repetitive ventricular activity occurred. One patient, who had undergone 18 consecutive successful transvenous cardioversions wihtout incident, deteriorated clinically. Rapid ventricular tachycardia (200 beats/min) with hypotension was present almost continuously for 72 hours. During that time he received intravenously or orally bretylium, amiodarone, lidocaine and digoxin. Balloon counterpulsation was begun to provide hemodynamic support. Synchronized transvenous cardioversion (0.075 J) in this setting transformed the ventricular tachycardia (cycle length 315 msec) to ventricular flutter (cycle length 190 msec) that was terminated by at transthoracic shock of 320 J. Shortly thereafter, a conventional synchronized transthoracic shock of 50 J precipitated ventricular fibrillation that was then defibrillated with a 320 J transthoracic shock. Because this early cardioverter has a maximum output of 3.0 J, termination of ventricular flutter or ventricular fibrillation was not attempted transvenously during these episodes. Subsequently, the catheter electrode was connected to a standard cardioverter/defibrillator and the next three episodes of spontaneous ventricular fibrillation were terminated by a 25 J shock delivered transvenously (Fig. 6).

Another patient had six episodes of sustained ventricular tachycardia successfully terminated by 0.1 J (one episode), 0.25 J (one episode), 0.5 J (two episodes), 0.75 J (one epi-

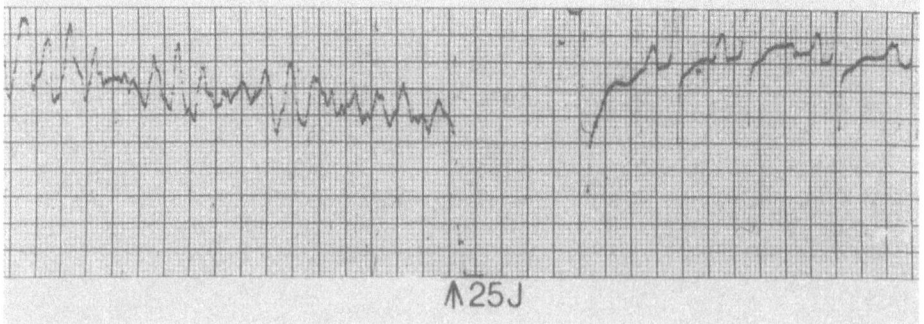

Fig. 6. Transvenous defibrillation. A 25 J shock (arrow) terminated ventricular fibrillation. Reproduced with permission from Zipes, D. P., Jackman, W. M., Heger, J. J. et al. Clinical transvenous cardioversion of recurrent life-threatening ventricular tachyarrhythmias: low energy synchronized cardioversion of ventricular fibrillation in patients using a catheter electrode. Am. Heart J. 1982; 103: 426.

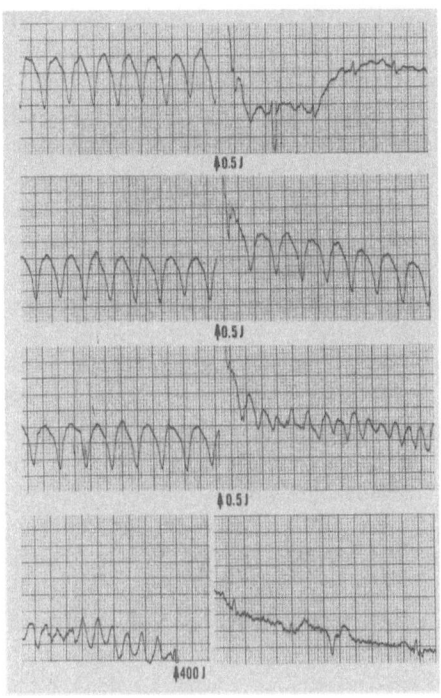

Fig. 7. ECG rhythm recordings from a patient showing termination of ventricular tachycardia with 0.5 J in panel A, failure to terminate ventricular tachycardia with a slightly greater shock in panel B, initiation of ventricular fibrillation with a still greater shock in panel C, and termination of the ventricular fibrillation with an external shock of 400 J in panel D. Reproduced with permission from Zipes, D. P., Prystowsky, E. N., Browne, K. F., et al.: Additional observations on transvenous cardioversion of recurrent ventricular tachycardia. Am. Heart J. 1982; 104: 163.

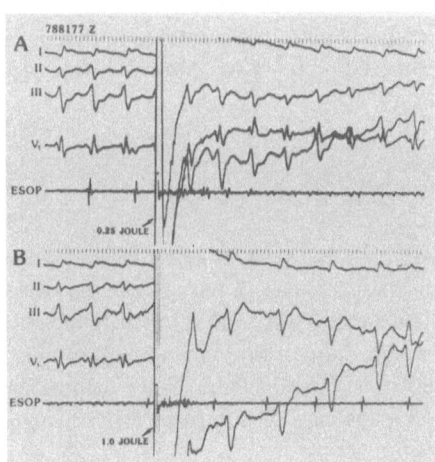

Fig. 8. Termination of atrial fibrillation. In the upper panel a 0.25 J shock is delivered synchronously into the QRS complex through a transvenous catheter. The stimulus fails to convert the ventricular rhythm but induces atrial fibrillation. In the lower panel a shock of 1.0 J is delivered synchronously into the QRS complex and the atrial fibrillation and ventricular tachycardia are both terminated to restore sinus rhythm.

sode), and 2.0 J (one episode). The catheter position was probably not stable (accounting for the changing thresholds) and the shock synchronized at different points in the QRS complex (Fig. 7). Shocks in the midportion of the QRS complex terminated the ventricular tachycardia with none or one repetitive response (panel A). Shocks of equal intensity in the latter portion of the QRS complex (panel B) sometimes failed to terminate the ventricular tachycardia. A shock delivered slightly later in the QRS complex, after termina-

835

tion of the absolute ventricular refractory period and during the early portion of the vulnerable period (panel C), initiated ventricular flutter/ventricular fibrillation that was promptly terminated by transthoracic cardioversion (panel D).

Despite the presence of AV dissociation during ventricular tachycardia in all patients and the resultant random delivery of the shocks in relation to atrial systole, repetitive atrial activity occurred after only five of the 196 shocks. A shock of 0.25 J did not terminate the ventricular tachycardia in one patient and produced atrial fibrillation that was then terminated, along with the ventricular tachycardia, by a subsequent shock of 1.0 J a few minutes later (Fig. 8).

One patient deserves special note. He was referred for treatment of drug-refractory recurrent ventricular tachycardia which occurred on the *precise* day that another patient presented. We connected the catheter electrode to a conventional external American Optical (AO) cardioverter through a junction box we had built previously, just in case we needed to treat two patients at the same time. He ultimately died with refractory cardiogenic shock in an agonal slow ventricular rhythm with electromechanical dissociation. Prior to his hemodynamic collapse, he had received 311 cardioversions in a 12-hour period. We synchronized the shock from skin electrodes through the AO cardioverter and delivered the shocks from the standard AO cardioverter through the transvenous catheter electrode. Naturally the precise voltage setting on the meter of the AO cardioverter cannot be determined with the degree of accuracy we were able to achieve using our specially made cardioverter. However, 245 episodes of ventricular tachycardia were terminated with 4 J, 45 episodes with 8 J, and 21 episodes with 20 J. One shock in the latter range accelerated the ventricular tachycardia from 140 to 210 per minute, but otherwise there were no problems.

Awake, unsedated patients tolerated shocks of $\leqslant 0.5$ J without difficulty. Shocks in this range were described as a "giant hiccough" or a light blow to the chest due to diaphragmatic or intercostal muscle contraction. Shocks exceeding 0.5 J were less well tolerated and produced moderate skeletal muscle stimulation.

Conclusions

Conventional synchronous transthoracic cardioversion is the most effective and safest form of electrical therapy to terminate ventricular tachycardia (7), but has obvious limitations for chronic application. The impetus for this study was to develop a therapeutic approach that was as safe and as effective as synchronous transthoracic cardioversion but could be used chronically, eventually as totally implanted system. Since completion of this study, such a system has been developed and has now been implanted in three patients (18).

Transvenous cardioversion terminates ventricular tachycardia in patients with very small amounts of energy. It is possible that antiarrhythmic drugs in these patients influenced the cardioversion thresholds to some degree. Quite possibly, ventricular tachycardia that failed to terminate in two patients with intracardiac shocks of 0.75 J and 2.0 J would have been terminated by higher energies, had they been tried. Thresholds may be influenced by the size of the heart, origin of the ventricular tachycardia in relation to electrode position, and other factors. Future developments in catheter electrode design and the waveform of the shock may reduce energy requirements further.

·Perhaps transvenous cardioversion may be used for some patients who have recurrent episodes of supraventricular tachycardia as well. In the animal study (3), we terminated several episodes of atrial flutter or atrial fibrillation by delivering a transvenous shock of 1.0 J. In the present study, 1.0 J terminated atrial fibrillation.

Transvenous cardioversion is not without some risk, but that is not suprising in light of the known potential arrhythmic complications of transthoracic cardioversion (5). Transvenous cardioversion may not be any different than transthoracic cardioversion regarding *safety*. All the precautions used with transthoracic cardioversion regarding a precisely synchronized shock should be employed. Delivering electricity to the ventricle is not totally without risk, regardless of how the technique is carried out.

Transvenous cardioversion has multiple potential applications. For example, the catheter electrode connected to an external unit can be used on a temporary basis for the patient who has frequent recurrences of ventricular tachycardia or ventricular fibrillation, thereby avoiding repeated chest trauma and the need of anesthesia for cardioversion if thresholds are low. The catheter electrode can be used to pace the heart. Thus, during electrophysiologic studies in patients, pacing-induced ventricular tachycardia or ventricular fibrillation can be terminated with the same catheter electrode. As a permanent implant, the size of the generator could be relatively small and longevity relatively long, compared to the automatic implantable defibrillator (9), because of the reduced energy requirements. A transvenous cardioversion system will have the additional advantage of not requiring a thoracotomy for implantation. It is also possible that transvenous cardioversion may be easier to test and use than pacing modalities. The latter generally require in-depth electrophysiologic evaluation of the patient to determine precise electrophysiologic parameters – i.e., number of stimuli, intervals, adjustment for cycle length of the tachycardia, and other factors necessary to terminate ventricular tachycardia by pacing. Also, cardioversion may be less influenced by physiologic changes or drugs that may alter the parameters of pacing-induced termination markedly. Finally, since in many patients, episodes of spontaneous ventricular fibrillation are preceded by ventricular tachycardia (12), the former may be prevented entirely by cardioverting the latter. Conceivably in the future the ideal implantable device will be capable of transvenous cardioversion and, if that fails or if ventricular fibrillation is precipitated, it will then deliver a defibrillating shock.

Acknowledgement

The authors thank Doctors W. Jackman, K. Browne, D. Chilson, G. Naccarelli, G. Rahilly*, B. Skale and Elizabeth Darling, R. N. for their contributions to this study. Modified from an article in Sudden Cardiac Death, Grune and Stratton, in press.

References

1. Garan H, Fallon JT, Ruskin JN: Sustained ventricular tachycardia in recent canine myocardial infarction. Circulation 1980; 62: 980.

---

* deceased

2. Harris AS: Delayed development of ventricular ectopic rhythms following experimental coronary occlusion. Circulation 1950; 1: 1318.
3. Jackman WM, Zipes DP: Low-energy synchronous cardioversion of ventricular tachycardia using a catheter electrode in a canine model of subacute myocardial infarction. Circulation 1982; 66: 187.
4. Karagueuzian HS, Fenoglio JJ, Jr, Weiss MB, Wit AL: Protracted ventricular tachycardia induced by premature stimulation of the canine heart after coronary artery occlusion and reperfusion. Circ Res 1979; 44: 833.
5. Kerber RE, Martins JB, Gascho JA et al: Effect of direct-current countershocks on regional myocardial contractility and perfusion. Circulation 1981; 63: 323.
6. Lesigne C, Levy B, Saumont R et al: An energy-time analysis of ventricular fibrillation and defibrillation thresholds with internal electrodes. Med Biol Eng 1976; 14: 617.
7. Lown B: Electrical reversion of cardiac arrhythmias. Br Heart J 1967; 29: 469.
8. Michaelson EL, Spear JF, Moore EN: Initiation of sustained ventricular tachyarrhythmias in a canine model of chronic myocardial infarction: importance of the site of stimulation. Circulation 1981; 63: 776.
9. Mirowski M, Reid PR, Mower M et al: Termination of malignant ventricular arrhythmias with an implanted automatic defibrillator in human beings. New Engl J Med 1980; 303(6): 322.
10. Mirowski M, Reid PR, Watkins L et al: Clinical treatment of life-threatening ventricular tachyarrhythmias with the automatic implantable defibrillator. Am Heart J 1981; 102: 265.
11. Rubin L, Hudson P, Snively S et al: Defibrillation threshold energy and epicardial electrode size (abstr.). Med Instrum 1980; 14: 58.
12. Ruskin JN, DiMarco JP, Garan H: Out-of-hospital cardiac arrest. Electrophysiologic observations and selection of long-term antiarrhythmic therapy. New Engl J Med 1980; 303: 607.
13. Schuder JC, Rahmoeller GA, Stoeckle H: Transthoracic ventricular defibrillation with triangular and trapezoidal waveforms. Circ Res 1966; 19: 689.
14. Wiggers CJ, Wegria R: Ventricular fibrillation due to single, localized induction and condenser shocks applied during the vulnerable phase of ventricular systole. Am J Physiol 1940; 128: 500.
15. Yee R, Zipes DP, Gulamhusein S et al: Countershock using an intravascular catheter in an acute care setting. Am J Cardiol 1982; 50: 1124.
16. Zipes DP, Jackman W, Heger JJ et al: Clinical transvenous cardioversion of recurrent life-threatening ventricular tachyarrhythmias: low energy synchronized cardioversion of ventricular tachycardia and termination of ventricular fibrillation in patients using a catheter electrode. Am Heart J 1982; 103: 789.
17. Zipes DP, Prystowsky EN, Browne K et al: Additional observations on transvenous cardioversion of recurrent ventricular tachycardia. Am Heart J 1982; 104: 163.
18. Zipes DP, Prystowsky EN, Miles W, Brown J, Heger JJ: Implantable transvenous cardioverter. J Am Coll Cardiol (abstract). In press 1984.

Authors' address:
Douglas P. Zipes, M.D.
Indiana University School of Medicine
1100 West Michigan Street
Indianapolis, Indiana 46223

Efficacy of a "Ramp Up" Protocol for Transesophageal and Intraatrial Stimulation in Patients with Drug-Resistent Supraventricular Tachyarrhythmias

K. Frohner, E. Gutierrez, N. Neubauer, F. Meisl, G. Unger, K. Steinbach

Summary: The efficacy of a "ramp up" protocol for transesophageal and intraatrial stimulation was evaluated in 20 patients with drug refractory atrial flutter and in 2 patients with atrial tachycardia. Transesophageal stimulation terminated atrial flutter in 12 of 20 patients (= 60%). Sinus rhythm could be achieved in 10 and atrial fibrillation occurred in 2 patients. Subsequent intraatrial stimulation was effective in the remaining 8 patients, in whom esophageal stimulation had been unsuccessful. In 2 patients with atrial tachycardia transesophageal pacing was ineffective. Intraatrial stimulation restored sinus rhythm in 1 and external electrical countershock had to be used in the other. Therefore the overall success rate of our stepwise stimulation protocol was 95%. Transesophageal stimulation is a safe and reliable technique with a considerable success rate in atrial flutter which justifies its being used before invasive procedures.

Digitalis alone or combinations with antiarrhythmic drugs are traditional therapeutic tools in the treatment of atrial flutter (1). Successful restoration of sinus rhythm has been reported in up to 80% of patients after digitalis therapy (2). Nevertheless, more aggressive methods have to be used in patients with drug-resistant atrial flutter or atrial tachycardia. External electrical countershock is the preferred treatment in urgent situations, but since the first report (3) of successful termination of atrial flutter by rapid atrial stimulation, pacing techniques are used in an increasing number of patients.

The purpose of our study was to evaluate the efficacy of a "ramp up" protocol for transesophageal and intraatrial stimulation in patients with atrial flutter or atrial tachycardia resistent to digitalis and antiarrhythmic drugs.

Materials and Methods

The study group consisted of 22 patients, 16 males and 6 females, aged between 36 and 86 years (mean 66 years); 11 patients had coronary artery disease, 5 patients had pulmonary disease, 1 patient dilative cardiomyopathy, 1 patient congenital heart disease and 1 patient uremic pericarditis. In 2 patients no underlying heart disease was detected. 20 patients presented with atrial flutter with a mean atrial cycle length of 240 msec ranging between 175 and 280 msec (mean atrial rate 252 beats/min). 2 patients had atrial tachycardia with rates of 166/min and 200/min respectively.

In all patients (n = 22) digitalis therapy or combinations with antiarrhythmic drugs (quinidine – 11 pts, disopyramide – 2 pts, propafenone – 1 pt) had failed to restore sinus rhythm. Drug therapy was continued or increased up to the stimulation and drug serum levels were obtained on the day of the study.

Stimulations were performed with a stimulator (Medtronic 5325) capable of delivering impulses of 1.8 ± 0.1 msec duration. In all patients a stimulus strength of 20 mA was used for transesophageal pacing. The esophageal lead (Vygon) with an interelectrode distance of 4.5 cm was introduced through the mouth.

Stimulation was performed at the point where the unipolar atrial electrograms exhibited the greatest amplitude and, if ineffective, at proximal and distal sites. Transesophageal stimulation was initiated at a rate about 10 beats slower than the spontaneous atrial rate and then increased in steps of 50–100 beats/min up to the rate of 800 beats/min.

Stimulation was maintained for 20–60 sec and was discontinued after every step and if sinus rhythm, atrial fibrillation or changes in F wave rate or configuration occurred. If transesophageal stimulation was ineffective, intraatrial stimulation was performed using the same protocol.

Results

The results of transesophageal and intraatrial stimulation are summarized in Table 1. Transesophageal stimulation terminated atrial flutter in 12 (Group I) of 20 patients (= 60%) and failed to terminate atrial flutter in the remaining 8 patients (Group II) and in 2 patients with atrial tachycardia (Group III). Therefore, the overall success rate was 54%.

Group I: Direct conversion to sinus rhythm occurred in 2 patients of Group I (Fig. 1). In 2 patients a change of the rate and configuration of the F-waves could be achieved (Fig.

Table 1. Results of transesophageal and intraatrial stimulation in 22 patients.

Group I Atrial flutter terminated by transesoph. stim.		Group II Atrial flutter terminated by intraatrial stim. (after ineff. transesoph. stim.)
12 pts 238 ± 33 msec 256 ± 38 beats/min	mean atrial cycle length mean atrial rate	8 pts 243 ± 25 msec 248 ± 24 beats/min
	Effect of "ramp up" stimulation	
2	direct conversion $\rightarrow$ sinus rhythm	3
2	change of rate and morphology of the F-waves $\rightarrow$ sinus rhythm	1
6	conversion to atrial fibrillation $\rightarrow$ sinus rhythm	4
1	$\rightarrow$ persisting atrial fibrillation	0
1	$\rightarrow$ atrial fibrillation and re-occurrence of atrial flutter	0

Group III (2 pts): Atrial tachycardia
1 pt = esoph. stim. ineff. $\rightarrow$ intraatrial stimulation restored sinus rhythm.
1 pt = esoph. and intraatrial stim. ineffective $\rightarrow$ sinus rhythm after external electrical countershock.

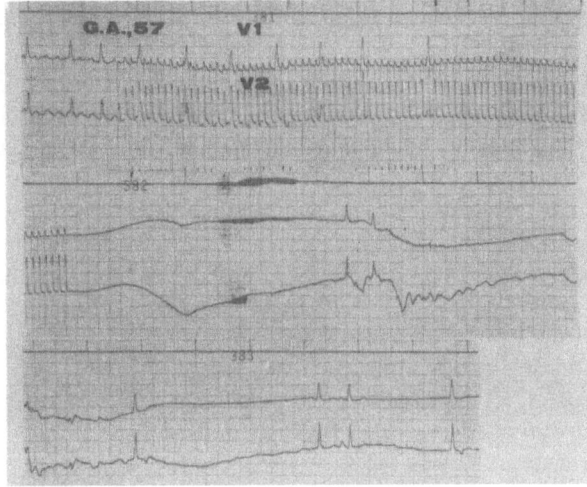

Fig. 1. Atrial flutter in a 57 year – old woman with coronary artery disease (type I atrial flutter, atrial cycle length 220 msec). Rapid transesophageal stimulation with 500 beats/min results in termination of atrial flutter followed by asystole. After some escape beats sinus rhythm occurred.

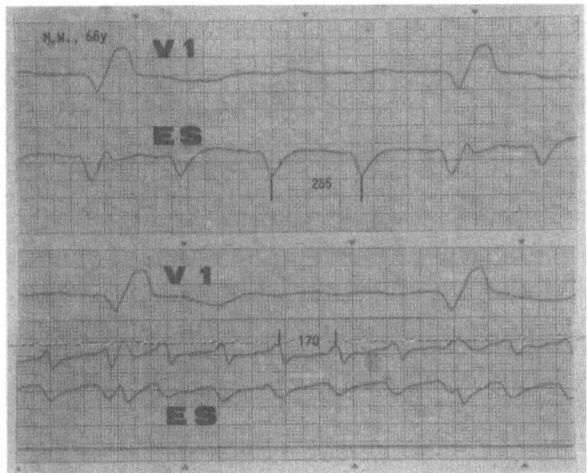

Fig. 2. Atrial flutter in a 66 year old man with CAD, previous MI and RBBB. The upper panel shows classical or type I atrial flutter with a cycle length of 265 msec (= flutter rate 226/min) and positive F waves in lead V1 (negative in lead I, II; not shown). After transesophageal pacing at a rate of 400/min a change of the rate (CL = 170 msec) and morphology of the F waves occurred (lower panel), suggesting type II atrial flutter. 4 minutes later type II flutter spontaneously converted to sinus rhythm. ES = unipolar atrial electrograms (esophageal lead). Paper speed 100 mm/sec.

2), which was followed by sinus rhythm after 2 and 4 minutes, respectively. In 8 patients transesophageal stimulation resulted in atrial fibrillation which converted to sinus rhythm in 6 patients between 2 minutes and 8 hours. In 1 patient atrial fibrillation persisted and in 1 patient atrial flutter re-occurred after 5 minutes. The stimulation rates, which proved effective in Group I patients were ≤ 400 beats/min in 7 patients (60%) and > 400 beats/min in 5 patients (40%).

Group II: In 8 patients, in whom transesophageal pacing had proved unsuccessful, subsequent intraatrial stimulation was performed. Direct conversion to sinus rhythm could be achieved in 3 patients and atrial fibrillation with subsequent conversion to sinus rhythm occurred in 4 patients. In 1 patient intraatrial stimulation resulted in an increase of the atrial rate (215/min to 280/min) with conversion to sinus rhythm after 60 minutes.

Stimulation rates of ≤ 400 beats/min terminated atrial flutter in 6 patients (75%) and rates of > 400 beats/min in 2 patients (25%).

Group III consisted of 2 patients with atrial tachycardia at atrial rates of 166 beats/min and 200 beats/min (cycle length 360 and 300 msec). The digoxin serum concentrations in these two patients were within the therapeutic range. In both patients transesophageal pacing proved ineffective and therefore intraatrial stimulation was performed. Direct conversion to sinus rhythm could be achieved in 1 patient and external electrical countershock had to be used in the other.

The mean atrial cycle length of group I patients was 238 msec (range 175–280 msec); the corresponding atrial rates ranged from 214 beats/min –342 beats/min (mean 256/min). In group II the mean atrial cycle length was 243 msec (range 220–280), the atrial rates ranged from 214–272 beats/min (mean 248 beats/min).

As can be seen in Table 2 the atrial rates, the amplitude of the unipolar esophageal electrograms and the serum concentrations of digoxin (n = 12), digitoxin (n = 8) and quinidine (n = 7) did not show any significant statistical difference. There was only a significant difference in age.

Discussion

Since Haft's (3) report on successful termination of atrial flutter by rapid atrial stimulation this method has been used extensively to treat supraventricular tachyarrhythmias. Nevertheless, intracavitary stimulation requires venous puncture, fluoroscopy and sterile conditions. These prerequisites are not necessary when using the esophageal route, which offers an ideal site of electrical stimulation due to its close relation to the posterior structures of the atria.

Our study – based on the stepwise use of transesophageal and intraatrial pacing – evaluated the efficacy of a fixed "ramp up" protocol in patients with drug resistant atrial flutter and atrial tachycardia.

The success rate of transesophageal stimulation in our group of patients with atrial flutter was 60%. If the two patients with atrial tachycardia are included the overall success rate was 54%.

Table 2. Comparison between effective (Group I) and ineffective (Group II + III) transesophageal stimulation.

Group I	22 patients	Group II + III
72 ± 9	AGE p < 0.005	58 ± 10
256 ± 38 beats/min	Atrial rate n.s.	248 ± 24 beats/min*)
1.1 ± 0.5 mV	Amplitude n.s.	1.1 ± 0.4 mV
2.3 ± 1.3 ng/ml	Digoxin n.s.	1.9 ± 0.3 ng/ml
18.6 ± 3 ng/ml	Digitoxin n.s.	23.8 ± 12 ng/ml
3.05 ± 1.05 μg/ml	Quinidine n.s.	3.18 ± 1.5 μg/ml

*) pts with atrial tachycardia excluded; student-t test.

Direct conversion to sinus rhythm after esophageal pacing was rare and occurred in only 2 patients. In one patient prolonged asystole occurred during and after cessation of rapid stimulation at a rate of 500 beats/min (Fig. 1). In this patient a permanent pacemaker had to be implanted later because of recurrent episodes of dizziness due to sick sinus syndrome.

In 2 other patients with classical or type I atrial flutter transesophageal pacing at rates of 400 beats/min and 800 beats/min respectively resulted in a change of the rate and morphology of the F-waves, suggesting development of type II atrial flutter (Fig. 2). Similar observations have been made by Wells and Waldo who used fixed atrial electrodes in patients with atrial flutter after open heart surgery (4).

In both patients type II atrial flutter spontaneously converted to sinus rhythm within 4 minutes. In 6 of 12 successful treated patients conversion to sinus rhythm was preceded by atrial fibrillation. Montoyo (5) used transesophageal pacing in 6 patients with atrial flutter without restoration of sinus rhythm, but atrial fibrillation was achieved in 4 cases. Stimulus duration and stimulus strength were similar to those used in our study. Recently Gallagher (6) published stable atrial pacing in all 39 patients using pulse durations of 9.9 msec and a mean threshold of 11 ± 5 mA, whereas in only 33 or 39 patients capture occurred with a pulse duration of 2.0 msec as was used in our study. The same author reported successful restoration of sinus rhythm in 11 of 17 patients with atrial flutter, 4 patients developed atrial fibrillation and in 2 patients atrial flutter was unaltered by transesophageal pacing (7). The higher success rate may be due to a longer pulse duration of 9.9 sec used in Gallagher's study. Nevertheless the study populations are not comparable, because our patients presented with established drug refractory atrial flutter, whereas more than half of Gallagher's patients had induced atrial flutter.

However new inflatable balloon electrodes (8) which provide closer contact to the atria may improve the results of transesophageal stimulation in atrial flutter even using short impulse durations.

Only few data exist concerning effective stimulation rates in transesophageal pacing. In 1978 Sterz (9) reported successful termination of supraventricular tachyarrhythmias including atrial flutter using transesophageal stimulation and suggested that stimulation rates of > 400 beats/min may be ineffective. However, rapid stimulation at rates between 400 and 800 beats/min terminated atrial flutter in 5 of 12 patients of our study group. Thus, we would also recommend the use of such higher stimulation rates.

In the two groups treated for atrial flutter atrial rates and the amplitudes of the unipolar esophageal electrogram were comparable (Table 2) and therefore had no predictive value in assessing the outcome of transesophageal stimulation.

Esophageal and intraatrial pacing produced only mild discomfort in most of the patients. In only 1 patient dizziness occurred during asystole after cessation of pacing.

During transesophageal stimulation no ventricular pacing occurred and our results demonstrate, that rapid atrial stimulation can be performed safely in patients treated with digitalis and antiarrhythmic drugs.

Conclusions

Ramp up transesophageal stimulation is a safe and reliable technique for the treatment of patients with drug resistent atrial flutter. Termination of atrial flutter could be achieved in 60% of the patients. In 83% of them sinus rhythm could be restored. Atrial fibrillation with slower ventricular response occurred in 17%. In 2 patients with atrial tachycardia esophageal stimulation was ineffective.

Subsequent intraatrial pacing in patients in whom transesophageal pacing had proved unsuccessful increased the overall success rate of our protocol to 95%.

The considerable success rate of transesophageal stimulation in atrial flutter justifies its being used before invasive procedures.

Supported in part by "Jubiläumsfonds der Österreichischen Nationalbank; Projekt Nr. 1998" and Hochschuljubiläumsstiftung der Stadt Wien.

References

1. Lindsay J, Hurst JW: The clinical features of atrial flutter and their therapeutic implications. Chest 1974; 66: 114–121.
2. Fowler NO, Gueron M: Conversion of atrial flutter with digoxin alone. Circulation 1962; 26: 712.
3. Haft JI, Kosowsky BD, Lau SH, Stein E, Damato AN: Termination of atrial flutter by rapid electrical pacing of the atrium. Am J Cardiol 1967; 20: 239–244.
4. Wells JL, MacLean WAH, Hames TN, Waldo AL: Characterization of atrial flutter. Studies in man after open heart surgery using fixed atrial electrodes. Circulation 1979; 60: 665–673.
5. Montoyo JV, Angel J, Valle V, Gausi C: Cardioversion of tachycardias by transesophageal atrial pacing. Am J Cardiol 1973; 32: 85–90.
6. Gallagher JJ, Smith WM, Kasell J, Cook L, Reiter M, Sterba R, Harte M: Esophageal pacing: A diagnostic and therapeutic tool. Circulation 1982; 65: 336–341.
7. Kerr CR, Sterba R, German LD, Gallagher JJ: Management of atrial flutter by transesophageal atrial pacing. Circulation 1981; Abstracts 54th scientific session IV – 297.
8. Andersen HR, Pless P: Trans-esophageal pacing. Pace 1983; 6: 674–679.
9. Sterz H, Prager H, Koller H: Transösophageale rasche Stimulation des linken Vorhofes zur Elektrotherapie ektoper, tachykarder Vorhofrhythmusstörungen. Z Kardiol 1978; 67: 136–138.

Authors' address:
Dr. Klaus Frohner
Wilhelminenspital
III. Med. Abteilung
Montleartstr. 37
A-1171 Wien/Österreich

Cardioversion of Atrial Tachyarrhythmias by Low-Energy Transvenous Technique

D. G. Benditt, J. M. Kriett, H. G. Tobler, D. W. Benson, Jr., J. Fetter, P. A. Chevalier

Summary: This study assessed the feasibility of terminating atrial tachyarrhythmias by low-energy DC shock delivered through an electrode catheter positioned within the right atrial appendage. A modified defibrillator provided low stored-energy levels (0.16–6.1 joules) in calibrated increments of 0.1–0.2 joules. Six chloralose anesthetized open chest dogs were studied using four standard electrode catheters with differing stimulation surface electrode areas (SEA), or electrode configurations, but with similar ring-to-tip interelectrode (R/T) distances: (1) Medtronic 5816 (SEA 85 mm² R/T 16 mm), (2) Medtronic 5818 (SEA 53 mm², R/T 16mm), (3) Medtronic 6904A (SEA 20 mm², R/T 22 mm), and (4) USCI quadpolar with the two proximal terminals and the two distal terminals paired (approximate SEA 26 mm², approximate R/T 20 mm). Efficacy of each electrode configuration for cardioversion of pacing-induced atrial tachyarrhythmias (atrial cycle lengths 120–200 ms) was assessed sequentially. Shocks were delivered at random during the atrial cycle, and in 16/70 (23%) trials, the atrial tachyarrhythmia was terminated. In 7/16 successful trials termination was successful at stored energies less than 0.3 joules (approximately 0.2 joules delivered energy). Leads 6904A and USCI quadpolar failed to terminate tachyarrhythmias. Successful termination was associated with shocks delivered within 40 ms of the preceding atrial electrogram, while failure to terminate tachycardia was associated with arrhythmia present for longer than five minutes. Thus, if relatively large surface area electrodes are employed, transvenous cardioversion of atrial tachyarrhythmias is feasible and may be useful during recent onset tachyarrhythmias such as occur postoperatively or during invasive electrophysiological testing.

Introduction

Transient atrial tachyarrhythmias (atrial fibrillation or flutter) occur commonly during the course of invasive electrophysiological studies or following cardiac surgery, and occasionally therapeutic intervention is necessary. In the case of electrophysiological studies, if pacing techniques (1) are ineffective in terminating the arrhythmia, administration of general anesthetic prior to conventional DC cardioversion, or infusion of antiarrhythmic medication, may impair the validity of further testing. In the post-operative patient, it may be desirable to avoid both anesthetic and antiarrhythmic agents.

Recently, a method for low-energy synchronous cardioversion of ventricular tachyarrhythmias using a catheter electrode has been proven effective both in animals (2, 3) and in man (4–6). Consequently, this study was designed to determine whether an analagous cardioversion technique using a transvenously positioned electrode catheter may be applicable for treatment of atrial tachyarrhythmias.

This work was supported in part by grants HL-29460, HL-06097, HL-06593 from the National Heart, Lung and Blood Institute, Bethesda Maryland and by a Grant-In-Aid from Medtronic, Inc., Minneapolis, Minnesota.

Methods

Experimental Preparation and Recordings

Six chloralose anesthetized mongrel dogs (20–35 kg) of either sex, were intubated and mechanically ventilated with room air (Harvard Model 607 Respirator). The heart was exposed through a left thoracotomy and two bipolar electrodes (1 mm interelectrode distance) for electrogram recording and pacing were carefully sutured to the right atrium. In a few experiments, a similar bipolar electrode was sutured to the epicardial surface of the right ventricle.

The right femoral vein was exposed surgically in order to permit introduction of electrode catheters. Catheters were tested in random order. In each case, the catheter to be tested was advanced transvenously into the right atrium and manipulated to lie within the right atrial appendage. It was not possible to test all catheters in every dog. The mechanical and electrical specifications of each catheter examined are listed on Table 1, and the stimulating electrode configurations are shown in Figure 1.

Atrial tachyarrhythmias were initiated by means of rapid atrial pacing (pulse width 2–3 ms, cycle lengths 90–120 ms) using a custom designed optically isolated stimulator. Electrograms and surface electrocardiograms were amplified and filtered (40–500 Hz for electrograms, 0.08–50 Hz for electrocardiograms) using Hewlett-Packard 8811A amplifiers. Analog recordings were obtained using a Hewlett-Packard Sanborn 770 recorder.

Cardioversion Technique

This study employed an existing external defibrillator modified to provide low-stored energy levels (0.16 to 6.1 joules) in calibrated increments of 0.1–0.2 joules. The waveform was a rapidly decaying truncated exponential pulse of variable amplitude. The distal electrode pole was electrically negative with respect to the proximal pole.

Following initiation of sustained atrial tachycardia (Definition: atrial cycle length $\leq$ 200 ms with duration $\geq$ 30 seconds) by rapid atrial pacing, shocks of progressively greater en-

Table 1. Electrode catheter specifications

Catheter	Body diameter mm	F*	Tip diameter mm	F*	Stimulating electrode area mm²	Inter-Electrode distance mm
Medtronic 5816	3.8	12	4.0	12	85	16
Medtronic 5818	3.2	10	3.2	10	53	16
Medtronic 6904A	3.12	10	3.2	10	20	22
USCI quadpolar**	2	6	2	6	approximately 26	approximately 20

* F = French size
** Proximal two terminals paired, distal two terminals paired

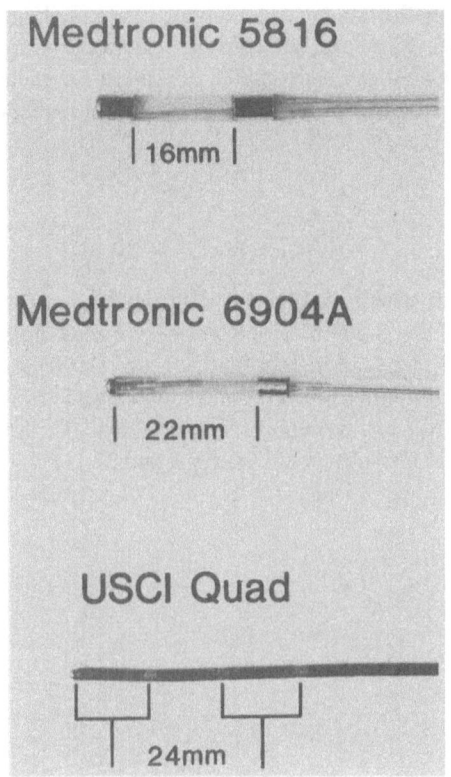

Fig. 1: Photograph illustrating stimulating electrode configurations in three of the four electrodes used in this study. Medtronic Model 5818 electrode is not shown, but is similar in configuration to Model 5816 except for a smaller body diameter and stimulating surface electrode area (see Table 1).

Medtronic 5816

| 16mm |

Medtronic 6904A

| 22mm |

USCI Quad

| 24mm |

ergy were delivered at random during the atrial cycle. After successful termination of an induced atrial tachycardia, the electrode catheter type and energy level were recorded. The study was repeated two or more times prior to exchanging catheters.

Results

Energy Requirements and Electrode Configurations

In this study pacing-induced atrial tachyarrhythmias usually exhibited a distinct, relatively regular atrial electrogram with a cycle length 120–200 ms (Figure 2). However, tachyarrhythmias exhibiting more highly disorganized atrial electrogram patterns also occurred (Figure 3).

Seventy transvenous cardioversions were attempted. In each instance, the initial attempt utilized the lowest available stored-energy (0.16 joules). If the initial cardioversion attempt failed, stored energy was gradually increased by 0.1–0.2 joules increments and shocks were repeated. In 16/70 instances (23%), termination of the atrial tachyarrhythmias was successful, and in 7 attempts less than 0.3 joules stored energy (approximately 0.2 joules delivered energy) was required. In no instance did stored-energy greater than 0.6 joules succeed when lesser energy levels had failed.

Termination of tachycardia was achieved only with test electrodes having relatively large stimulation electrode areas (Medtronic models 5816 and 5818). Both electrodes were equally effective. On the other hand, the two electrodes with smaller stimulating surface areas (Medtronic model 6904A and the modified USCI quadpolar catheter) were ineffective in all trials.

Mode of Tachycardia Termination

Successful conversion of atrial tachycardia was usually associated with delivery of the shock within 40–60 ms of the preceding atrial electrogram. Two termination sequences tended to occur. In the majority of successful tachycardia terminations, the shock appeared to modify the atrial tachycardia rate, with either acceleration or slowing of atrial electrical activity for 5–14 cycles (Figure 2) prior to reversion of sinus rhythm. Abrupt termination with restoration of sinus rhythm was also observed (Figures 2 and 3).

Fig. 2: Recordings illustrating termination of atrial tachyarrhythmia by transvenous technique using a Medtronic Model 5818 catheter electrode. In both panels, traces from top to bottom are ECG leads I and aVF, and an atrial electrogram (At EG). Stored energy of each shock is indicated. In both panels the atrial tachyarrhythmia exhibits a relatively regular atrial electrogram. However, in Panel A the tachyarrhythmia terminates abruptly with the shock, while in Panel B the rate of atrial electrical activity is altered by the shock and tachycardia terminates within a few atrial cycles.

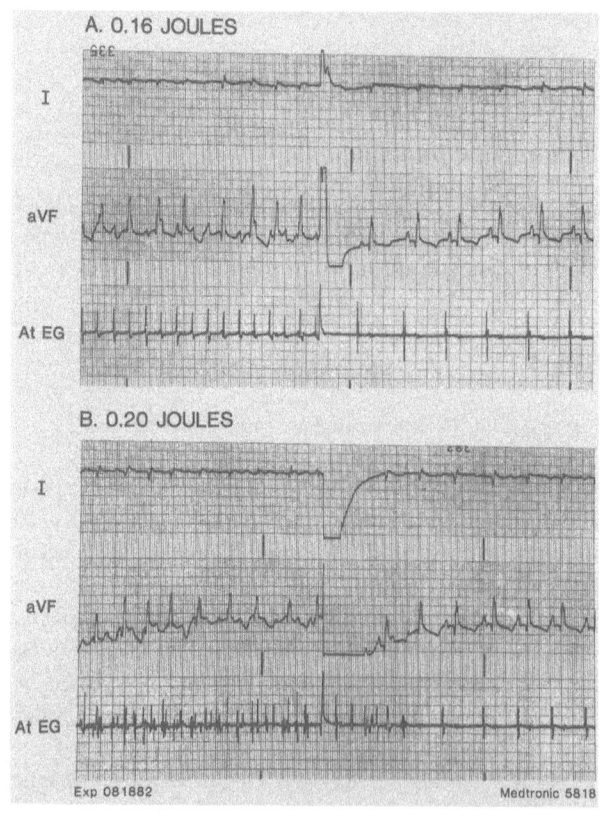

848

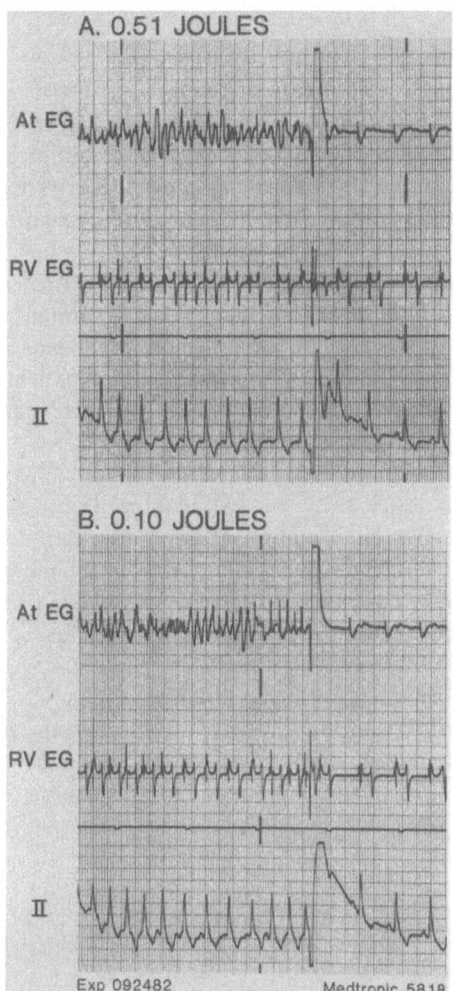

Fig. 3: Recordings illustrating termination of atrial tachyarrhythmia by transvenous shock. The traces top to bottom are an atrial electrogram (At EG), a right ventricular electrogram (RV EG) and surface ECG lead II. The tachyarrhythmia exhibits rapid disorganized atrial electrical activity. Abrupt tachycardia termination is observed following shock. Stored energy of shock is indicated in each panel.

Limitations

Ability to terminate atrial tachycardia in this study was adversely influenced by the duration of the arrhythmia. Tachycardia present for greater than 5 minutes was highly resistant to termination.

On two occasions, cardioversion attempts resulted in development of ventricular fibrillation. In one instance the electrode catheter had migrated from the right atrial appendage to the right ventricle, and an asynchronous 1 joule shock resulted in ventricular fibrillation which required conventional DC countershock to terminate. The second episode of ventricular fibrillation occurred with a 0.6 joule shock despite the electrode catheter being in an appropriate position within the right atrial appendage.

849

Discussion

Findings in this study indicate that low-energy cardioversion of recent onset atrial tachyarrhythmias is feasible provided relatively large surface area stimulating electrodes are employed. Although detailed studies are required to optimize both electrode surface areas and interelectrode spacing for application in man, this technique may prove useful during electrophysiologic testing procedures or in post-operative patients where development of atrial tachycardias is relatively common.

Recently, the development of intravascular catheter techniques for termination of ventricular tachyarrhythmias has drawn considerable attention. The ability to deliver intracardiac shocks safely through an electrode catheter has not only been demonstrated experimentally (2, 3), but has also had practical application for the treatment of patients (4–6). Consequently, adaptation of this technique for termination of atrial tachyarrhythmias seemed reasonable.

The consistency with which atrial tachyarrhythmias were terminated in this study (23%) was considerably less than the 83% success reported by Jackman and Zipes (3) in the treatment of ventricular tachycardia in dogs. The latter study employed a custom designed 10 French electrode catheter (Medtronic Model 6880) with an effective stimulating surface electrode area of 2.5 cm². Most likely the choice of catheter electrodes with smaller surface area for this study accounted for the lower success rate. However, our objective was to determine whether standard electrode catheters similar to those used for cardiac pacing or electrophysiological testing, could be effective for this application.

In summary, we have demonstrated the feasibility of employing transvenous catheter techniques for treatment of atrial tachyarrhythmias, and have provided an initial assessment of electrode catheter design requirements. Optimization of catheter configuration in further studies is necessary prior to considering clinical evaluation of this technique in man.

Acknowledgement

The authors would like to thank Barry L. S. Detloff and Thomas Gohman for assistance with the experiments, and Frances Wallace and Wendy Markuson for preparation of the manuscript.

References

1. Waldo AL, MacLean WAH, Karp RB, Kouchoukos NT, James TN: Entrainment and interruption of atrial flutter with atrial pacing. Studies in man following open heart surgery. Circulation 1977; 56: 737–745.
2. Schuder JC, Stoeckle H, West JA, Keskar PY: Relationship between electrode geometry and effectiveness of ventricular defibrillation in the dog with catheter having one electrode in right ventricle and other electrode in superior vena cava, or external jugular vein, or both. Cardiovas Res 1973; 7: 629–637.
3. Jackman WM, Zipes DP: Low-energy synchronous cardioversion of ventricular tachycardia using a catheter electrode in a canine model of subacute myocardial infarction. Circulation 1982; 66: 187–195.
4. Mirowski M, Mowen MM, Gott VL, Brawley RK: Feasibility and effectiveness of low-energy catheter defibrillation in man. Circulation 1973; 47: 79–85.

5. Zipes DP, Jackman WM, Heger J, Chilson D, Browne KF, Nacarelli GV, Rahilly GT, Prystowsky EN: Clinical transvenous cardioversion of recurrent lifethreatening ventricular tachyarrhythmias: Low-energy synchronized cardioversion of ventricular tachycardia and termination of ventricular fibrillation in patients using a catheter electrode. Am Heart J 1982; 103: 789–794.
6. Yee R, Zipes DP, Gulamhusein S, Kallok M, Klein GJ: Low energy countershock using an intravascular catheter in an acute cardiac care setting. Am J Cardiol 1982; 50: 1124–1129.

Authors' address:
David G. Benditt, M.D.
University of Minnesota Medical School
Box 341 – Mayo Memorial Building
Minneapolis, MN 55455

Low Energy Transvenous Intracavitary Cardioversion of Tachycardias

G. O. Hartzler, M. J. Kallok

Summary: Ninety intracardiac direct current shocks ranging 0.1–5.0 joule were administered to 12 awake patients utilizing a unique transvenous electrode catheter. Fifty-one of 73 (70%) of all ventricular tachycardia episodes and 2 of 2 supraventricular tachycardia episodes were effectively terminated. Atrial flutter, atrial fibrillation and ventricular fibrillation were not terminated. Ventricular fibrillation resulted from 2 unsynchronized intracardiac discharges. We conclude that low energy transvenous intracardiac cardioversion can effectively and safely terminate a majority of ventricular tachycardia episodes.

Recurrent ventricular tachycardia, particularly in patients with coronary artery disease and compromised left ventricular function remains a major cause of morbidity and mortality. Traditional therapies of antidysrhythmic drugs, pacing techniques, coronary revascularization, and attempted surgical ablation may be ineffective, inappropriate or contraindicated in many patients. The permanently implantable defibrillator is an alternative therapy for fortunate survivors of malignant arrhythmia but at the present time has limited availability, requires a major operation for electrode attachment and implantation, and cannot be utilized for temporary management of patients with recurrent ventricular tachycardia and fibrillation within the Intensive Care Unit setting.

We report an initial clinical experience with a transvenous electrode catheter system and a modified external cardioverter capable of delivering low energy intracardiac direct current shocks for termination of tachyarrhythmias.

Methods

Technical Aspects

An especially designed 9.5 French transvenous pacing/cardioverting/defibrillating electrode (Medtronic model 6880*) was utilized for all studies (figure 1). Two stainless steel or platinum alloy tip electrodes allow for bipolar endocardial pacing and sensing while providing relatively large surface area (250 mm²) for internal cardioversion. A proximal electrode pair serves as the anode during cardioversion and is located 125 cm from the tip, generally being positioned near the junction of the right atrium with the superior vena cava when the tip electrodes are positioned within the right ventricular apex. When manually activated, the external cardioverter delivers an R-wave synchronized 0.1 to 5.0 joule discharge having a 4 to 6 msec truncated exponential wave form.

---

*) Medtronic, Inc., Minneapolis, Minnesota, USA.

Fig. 1. Frame from cinefluoroscopy during electrophysiologic study of patient with recurrent ventricular tachycardia. Distal electrode pair (arrow) of 6880 cardioverting catheter in right ventricular apex. Proximal electrode pair near right atrial-superior vena cava junction. Additional electrode catheters in right atrial appendage, region of His bundle and left ventricle (2).

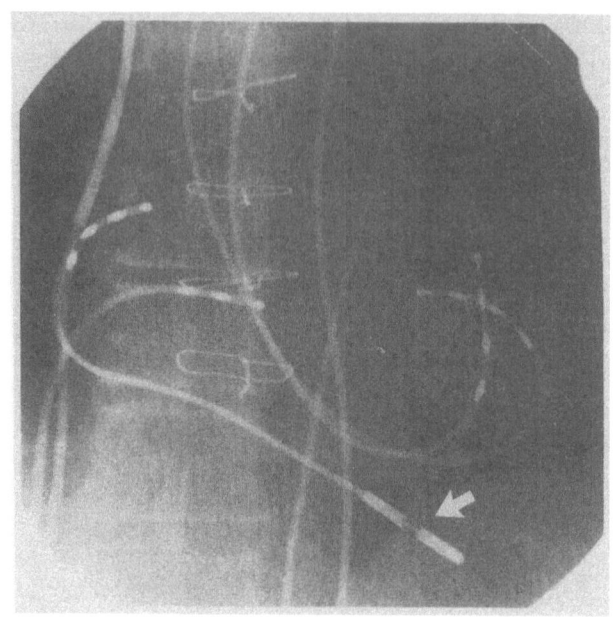

Patient Population

Patient studies were conducted under the guidelines of a protocol approved by our Institutional Review Board. Twelve patients (10 males and 2 females), ages 27 to 70 years, comprised the study population. Each was awake, alert but mildly sedated. In 9 instances the internal cardioverter or ICS was placed during elective invasive electrophysiologic study. In 3 instances the ICS was placed to facilitate management of refractory recurrent ventricular tachycardia occurring in critically ill patients within the Medical Intensive Care Unit. Eight of 9 patients with ventricular tachycardia experienced prior anteroseptal myocardial infarctions and 7 patients had an overt left ventricular aneurysm. A single patient had ventricular tachycardia complicating his idiopathic congestive cardiomyopathy in the absence of coronary artery disease. All patients with ventricular arrhythmias were receiving antidysrhythmic drugs at the time of this study with 7 of 9 patients receiving 2 or more drugs simultaneously. The ICS was assessed in 3 patients with supraventricular arrhythmias including one with the Wolff-Parkinson-White syndrome and a typical macro-reentrant, retrograde accessory pathway tachycardia, a second patient with chronic atrial flutter and a third patient with chronic atrial fibrillation.

In all but one patient with ventricular tachycardia, the electrode catheter was placed by percutaneous puncture of the right internal jugular vein. The retrograde femoral vein route was utilized in one patient with ventricular tachycardia and 2 patients with supraventricular arrhythmias. During electrophysiologic study, a Medtronic 5325 stimulator was utilized for pacing and induction of sustained tachycardia by programmed stimulation.

Table 1. Ventricular tachycardia 9 Patients.

VT Cycle length (msec)	#1 340–500	#2 280	#3 280	#4 380–440	#5 370	#6 260–380	#7 280–400	#8 500	#9 350
0.1	SSSSS SSFF			FF	F		SSSSS SSSF	S	
0.25					S	F	SSSS	S	
0.5		F		SFF	S		SF	SSSSSS SS	SS
Joules 0.75				F		F			
1.0		FF	F	SS		S	SF		SS
2.0		F	S						
3.0		F*							
5.0						SSSSS FF	S		

S = successful termination;
F = failed termination;
* = induction ventricular fibrillation (non-synchronized)
Patient # 4 had transfemoral catheter placement.
Patients # 6 and 8 received 4 and 2 additional shocks respectively for attempted termination of ventricular fibrillation.

Results (Table 1)

Acute pacing thresholds ranged 1 to 7 milliamperes with a mean of 5.0 milliamperes. Sensing thresholds were not systematically assessed.

Ninety shocks were delivered for 73 episodes of ventricular tachycardia, 7 episodes of ventricular fibrillation and 10 episodes of supraventricular tachycardia including 2 macro-reentrant tachycardias, 2 episodes of atrial fibrillation and 6 episodes of atrial flutter. Subjective acceptance of shocks was greatest for 0.75 joules or less with most patients objecting to shocks of 1.0 joules or greater.

Atrial flutter and fibrillation. All discharges ranging to 5.0 joules proved ineffective for termination of atrial flutter and fibrillation.

Reentrant supraventricular tachycardia (Wolff-Parkinson-White syndrome). Two of 2 induced macro-reentrant (retrograde accessory pathway) supraventricular tachycardias terminated with 0.5 joule discharges.

Ventricular fibrillation. No episode of ventricular fibrillation terminated with discharges to 5.0 joules.

Ventricular tachycardia (Figures 2 and 3). Seventy-three shocks ranging 0.1 joule to 5.0 joule converted 51 (70%) episodes of sustained ventricular tachycardia. Of episodes not terminating by intracardiac shocks, 6 of 22 (27%) failed at an energy level of 0.1 joule. Fourteen of 22 (67%) failed at energy levels of less than or equal to 1.0 joules. All remaining failures occurred at greater than 1.0 to 5.0 joule discharges for tachycardias of cycle length less than or equal to 320 msec.

855

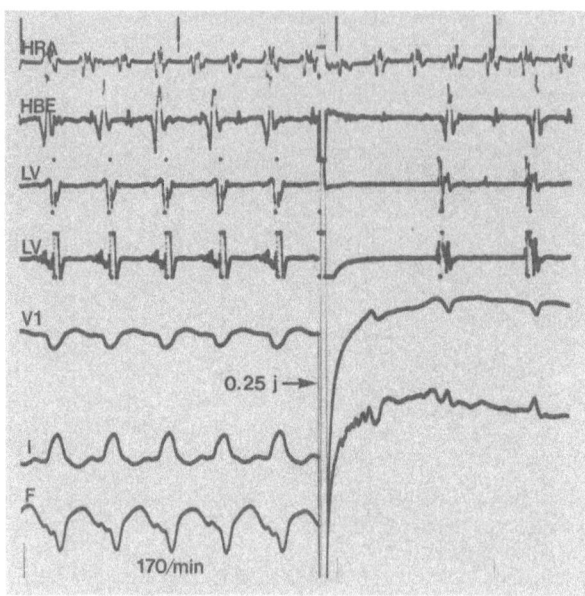

Fig. 2. Ventricular tachycardia 170/minute terminated by single 0.25 joule shock. Superimposed atrial flutter was induced by previous 0.1 joule shock but failed to convert with 0.25 joule discharge. Conducted responses following VT cardioversion. HRA – high right atrium; HBE – recording from His bundle region; LV – 2 electrograms from different left ventricular sites; VI, I, F – standard surface electrocardiograms.

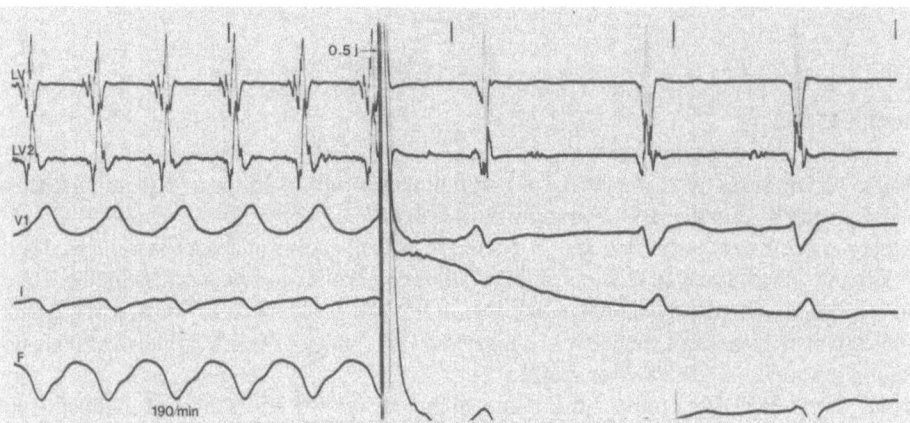

Fig. 3. Cardioversion of ventricular tachycardia 190/minute with 0.5 joule shock. LV1 and LV2 – left ventricular electrograms; VI, I, F – surface electrocardiograms.

Complications

Ventricular fibrillation was induced by a non-synchronized 3.0 joule discharge delivered during atrial flutter with the catheter tip anomalously positioned within the coronary sinus. A second episode of ventricular fibrillation was induced by a single 3.0 joule discharge from an appropriately positioned catheter during rapid ventricular tachycardia (280 msec cycle length). Because of a technical malfunction, the accuracy of R-wave synchronization cannot be determined for the shock although it is suspected that the discharge was random and inappropriately coupled to the preceding R-wave.

Atrial flutter was induced by two 0.1 joule discharges in two separate patients. Conducted responses to atrial flutter reinduced ventricular tachycardia on two occasions in a single patient. Spontaneously terminating AV nodal reentrant supraventricular tachycardia was induced by a single 0.5 joule shock in a patient with coincidental dual AV nodal pathways undergoing electrophysiologic study of recurrent ventricular tachycardia.

Observations and Discussion

Our experience with low energy intracardiac shocks for conversion of atrial flutter and fibrillation is limited. Consequently it is premature to conclude that low energy transvenous intracardiac shocks may not play a useful role in the future management of patients with these arrhythmias. Intuitively and based on external energy requirements for elective cardioversion, atrial fibrillation would be expected to require higher energy shocks than those investigated in this study. An additional factor increasing the likelihood of failure for both atrial fibrillation and flutter may be the electrode catheter location with direction of current flow excluding a large area of left atrial muscle mass. Low energy discharges (5.0 joules or less) did not terminate ventricular fibrillation. However, this was not unexpected in view of previously reported human data indicating a requirement for intracardiac shocks ranging 5 to 40 joules for termination of ventricular fibrillation using the 6880 catheter (1 and 2).

The finding that relatively low energies (5.0 joules) and on occasion extremely low energies (0.1 joule) terminated 70% of ventricular tachycardia episodes is extremely important. Similarly, analysis of failures is critical to the assessment of this technique. Fourteen of 22 failures occurred in the setting of ventricular tachycardia cycle lengths less than 320 msec. With the custom cardioverter utilized for this study, accurate R-wave synchronization was not assured at cycle lengths less than 340 msec because of an inappropriately long system refractory period. Consequently, improper synchronization may have played a role in the failure to terminate rapid ventricular tachycardias. Alternatively, increased rates may require higher energies or different shock wave-forms for more consistently successful termination. An additional 5 of 22 failures to terminate ventricular tachycardia occurred in a single patient in whom the electrode catheter had been placed by the transfemoral route. Consequently, the proximal or anodal electrode pair was located near the junction of the inferior vena cava with right atrium, altering the direction of current flow during discharge and potentially reducing the ICS effectiveness. The remaining 3 of 22 failures occurred at very low energy discharges of 0.1 joule. Further investigation of transvenous cardioversion of rapid ventricular tachycardias is warranted utilizing cardioverters having lesser refractory periods and greater energy outputs with variable wave forms and pulse durations.

Placement of the ICS greatly facilitated management of 3 patients with drug-refractory ventricular tachycardia within the Medical Intensive Care unit. Although elective manual activation was required by nursing personnel, the system could be rapidly charged and discharged, resulting in ventricular tachycardia termination before loss of consciousness in a majority of cases. Consequently, the need for high energy transthoracic direct current shocks was greatly diminished.

857

Placement of the ICS is now a "routine" feature of our invasive electrophysiologic studies in patients with ventricular tachycardia and fibrillation. When ventricular tachycardia is induced for drug testing or endocavitary mapping, termination by low energy shocks has proven to be an effective and more humane technique than transthoracic shock, particularly when burst pacing and programmed ventricular stimulation fail.

The technique of transvenous cardioversion and the results of this study have significant future implications. The ICS appears safe, reasonably effective and practical, particularly as a temporary adjunct to the performance of an invasive electrophysiologic study and for the management of malignant ventricular arrhythmias occurring within the Intensive Care unit. A simple yet fully automatic cardioverter providing back-up defibrillating energies in the 25 to 40 joule range should be developed for temporary bedside use. Similarly, the ideal permanently implantable system would also provide back-up defibrillating energies as well as automatic recognition and discharge modes. The added features of optional burst pacing for tachycardia termination and demand ventricular pacing would increase the unit's versatility and safety.

In conclusion, low energy transvenous cardioversion can effectively terminate a majority of ventricular tachycardia episodes. With further refinement of the technique and development of an appropriate implantable cardioverter, this mode of therapy will assume a major role in the management of patients with recurrent life-threatening ventricular arrhythmia.

References

1. Zipes DP, Jackman WM, Heger JJ et al: Clinical transvenous cardioversion of recurrent life-threatening ventricular tachyarrhythmias: Low energy synchronized cardioversion of ventricular tachycardia and termination of ventricular fibrillation in patients using a catheter electrode. Am Heart J 1982; 103: 789.
2. Yee R, Zipes DP et al: Low energy countershock using an intravascular catheter in an acute care setting. Am J Cardiol, Nov. 1982; 50: 1124–29.

Authors' address:
Dr. G. Hartzler
Mid-America Heart Institute
St. Luke's Hospital
4320 Wornall Road
Kansas City, Missouri 64111
USA

Internal "Microshock" for Arrhythmia Termination

A. W. Nathan, R. S. Bexton, K. J. Hellestrand, R. A. J. Spurrell, A. J. Camm

Summary: To test the efficacy of low-energy endocardial cardioversion, 14 patients, with 18 arrhythmias, were investigated. 4 had atrial flutter, 4 atrial fibrillation, 2 AV nodal reentrant tachycardia, 2 atrioventricular reentrant tachycardia and 6 ventricular tachycardia. A lead with a total electrode surface area of 500 mm^2 (100 mm separation) was placed in the right atrium or ventricle and used with an attenuated QRS synchronous defibrillator. 24 shocks were delivered to the atrium (4-1430, mean 294 mJ) and 34 to the ventricle (4-6700, mean 557 mJ). 1 patient with atrial flutter was successfully treated as were both patients with atrioventricular tachycardia and 4 with ventricular tachycardia. Atrial fibrillation and AV nodal tachycardia were not terminated. Atrial fibrillation was produced in 2 patients. Nonsustained ventricular tachycardia occurred in 1, and ventricular fibrillation in another, both with poor synchronization. Pacing terminated all episodes of AV nodal and atrioventricular tachycardia, and 4/6 episodes of ventricular tachycardia. No pain was felt by 1 patient, but pain was mild in 1, moderate in 3 and severe in 9. Low energy endocardial cardioversion is not universally successful even at the highest tolerable energies and timing is critical. Using the present pulse waveform and electrode, considerable discomfort may result.

Direct current external cardioversion is an effective method for treating tachyarrhythmias. Mirowski et al. introduced the concept of an implantable defibrillator in 1970 (1), initially using an endocardial electrode catheter within the right ventricle, but subsequent clinical work has made use of an epicardial patch electrode (with an indifferent electrode in the superior vena cava) delivering 25 to 30 J (2). In 1981, Jackman and Zipes reported on the use of very low energy discharges, of 8 to 2000 mJ, delivered using an electrode catheter, to cardiovert ventricular tachycardia in a canine model (3), and have recently reported on a similar technique in man (4).

To evaluate the effectiveness, safety and patient tolerance of low energy catheter cardioversion ("microshock"), a group of patients suffering from a wide variety of arrhythmias was studied.

Patients

Fourteen patients, 11 male and three female, aged 22 to 70 (mean 46) years, with a total of 18 different arrhythmias, were studied. Patient data are summarized in Table 1. Only two patients were receiving antiarrhythmic medication (quinidine in patient 1 and amiodarone in patient 12).

Catheter and Defibrillator

The electrode catheter (Medtronic 6880) is a purpose built lead, of 100 cm length, with two pairs of stainless steel electrodes (Fig. 1), capable of being used for pacing as well as for cardioversion. The two parts of each pair have a separation of 5 mm, and the two pairs are separated by 100 mm (150 mm in the electrode used in patient 14). Each electrode has a surface area of 125 mm²: thus the total area of each pole is 250 mm² when used for cardioversion. The two distal electrodes each have a separate conductor coil terminating in separate connector pins, connected in parallel when used for cardioversion, but the two proximal electrodes are interconnected and have a common conductor coil and connector pin.

A conventional direct current, surface R wave synchronous, defibrillator was used (delivering a damped sinusoidal, "Lown", waveform) together with a purpose built matched resistive attenuator, which, at a typical load of 100 Ohms, provided attenuation of 60 : 1.

Table 1. Patient data.

Case No	Age (y)	Sex	Arrhythmia	Mode of Induction	Drugs	Route of Insertion	TCL (ms)
1	70	M	AFl	Spontaneous	Quinidine	Subclavian	210
2	36	M	VT	Induced	–	Femoral	310
3	69	M	AF	Spontaneous	–	Subclavian	550
4	26	M	AFl/AF	Induced	–	Subclavian	195/395
5	61	F	AFl/AF	Induced	–	Subclavian	200/420
6	22	M	AVRT/AFl	Induced	–	Femoral	280/185
7	50	F	AVNRT/AFl	Induced	–	Subclavian	240/340
8	60	M	VT	Induced	–	Subclavian	380
9	53	F	AVNRT	Induced	–	Femoral	510
10	24	M	AVRT	Induced	–	Femoral	320
11	47	M	VT	Induced	–	Femoral	335
12	53	M	VT	Spontaneous	Amiodarone	Femoral	355
13	54	M	VT	Induced	–	Femoral	340
14	23	M	VT	Induced	–	Femoral	255

Abbreviations:
AF = Atrial fibrillation, AFl = Atrial flutter, AVNRT = Atrioventricular nodal reentrant tachycardia, AVRT = Atrioventricular reentrant tachycardia, F = female, M = male, ms = milliseconds, TCL = tachycardia cycle length (mean ventricular response in patients with atrial fibrillation), VT = ventricular tachycardia, y = years.

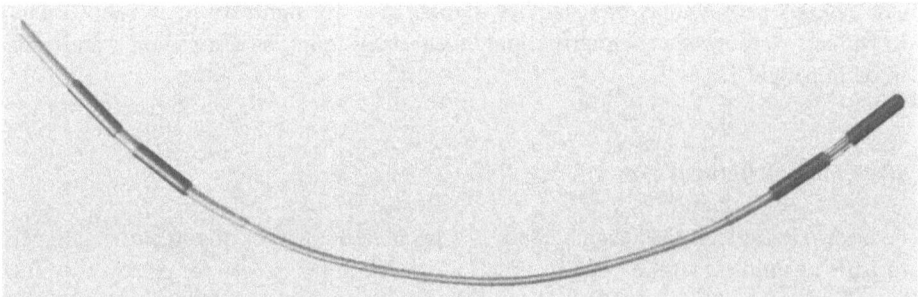

Fig. 1. Medtronic 6880 "microshock" electrode.

To measure the actual voltage and current delivered, output waveforms were recorded on an X-Y plotter (Fig. 2) using a specially constructed isolated amplifier and a transient recorder.

Protocol

The arrhythmias were induced in 11 patients during electrophysiological studies and were spontaneous in three. Prior to cardioversion, standard methods of pacing were employed to attempt termination in order to provide comparative data (except in patients with atrial fibrillation).

The catheter was introduced into a subclavian or femoral vein. Atrial stimulation, with the distal electrode on the atrial septum (and also on the lateral right atrial wall in patient 1), was attempted in patients with atrial arrhythmias and in patients with AV nodal reentrant tachycardia and atrioventricular reentrant tachycardia, and ventricular stimulation, with the distal electrode in the right ventricular apex, was only used if atrial stimulation was ineffective or intolerable. In patients with ventricular tachycardia, only ventricular stimulation was used. A low energy of 3.4 to 200 (mean 55) mJ was used for the first attempt at cardioversion, and the energy was increased until success was achieved or until stimulation became intolerable.

After cardioversion patients were asked to describe any discomfort that they had suffered during the procedure, and to grade it as absent, mild, moderate or severe discomfort. No sedation was used in 11 patients.

Results

A total of 24 shocks (3.4 to 1430, mean 294 mJ) were delivered to the atrium and 34 (4 to 6700, mean 557 mJ) to the ventricle. Data are summarized in Table 2.

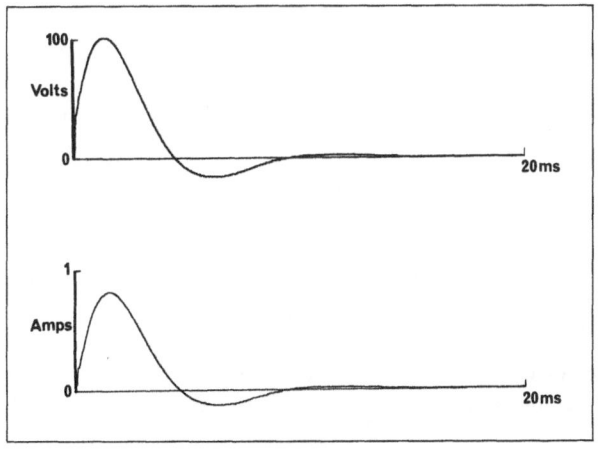

Fig. 2. Typical pulse waveform recorded on X-Y plotter.

Table 2. Overall results.

	Number of arrhythmias	Overall successes	Terminations/Attempts		Termination by pacing
			Atrium	Ventricle	
AFl	4	1	0/14	1/3	0/4
AF	4	0	0/3	0/9	NA
AVNRT	2	0 ·	0/2	0/5	2/2
AVRT	2	2	5/5	3/3	2/2
VT	6	4	–	4/14	4/6

Abbreviations:
AF = atrial fibrillation, AFl = atrial flutter, AVNRT = atrioventricular nodal reentrant tachycardia, AVRT = atrioventricular reentrant tachycardia, NA = not attempted.

Atrial flutter was treated in four patients. Shocks were delivered to the atrium in all four patients, a total of 14 times (4 to 1340, mean 382 mJ) and to the ventricle in patient 6 only (three shocks, 18, 97 and 198 mJ). In the remaining three patients there was degeneration into atrial fibrillation in two (cases 4 and 5), and one patient would not accept further cardioversion because of pain (case 1). Conversion to sinus rhythm only occurred in patient 6, with a ventricular shock of 18 mJ, but although this occurred eight beats after the shock had been delivered, the atrial flutter had been quite stable before this. However, when flutter was reinduced, ventricular shocks of up to 198 mJ were ineffective, although the arrhythmia eventually reverted to sinus rhythm spontaneously. External cardioversion was needed in one patient during atrial flutter (case 1), and in another after conversion to atrial fibrillation (case 4). Atrial fibrillation, induced in patient 5, reverted to sinus rhythm spontaneously after one hour.

Atrial fibrillation was present in four patients. Direct atrial stimulation was only performed in patient 3 (shocks of 11, 130 and 1390 mJ), and these shocks were all unsuccessful. The other three patients (4, 5 and 7) had previously received atrial discharges for other arrhythmias, and further atrial stimulation was not performed because these previous shocks had caused undue pain. Ventricular shocks were used in all four patients (nine discharges, 11 to 1390, mean 732 mJ), but were unsuccessful in terminating these arrhythmias. There was spontaneous reversion in two patients, but patients 3 and 4 both required external cardioversion.

Both patients with AV nodal tachycardia received atrial and ventricular discharges. Neither the two atrial (17 mJ), nor the five ventricular (17 to 200, mean 80 mJ) shocks caused termination of tachycardia in either patient. Burst pacing was effective for terminating both tachycardias, but extrastimulus pacing was only effective for terminating tachycardia in patient 9.

Internal cardioversion was effective in both patients with atrioventricular tachycardia. Patient 6 had five episodes of tachycardia induced, and all were terminated (3.4 and 5 mJ in the atrium; 8.5, 15 and 18 mJ in the ventricle). Atrial discharge alone was employed in patient 10, and all three episodes of tachycardia were successfully stopped with 20 mJ (Fig. 3). Extrastimulus and burst pacing were effective in terminating tachycardia in both patients.

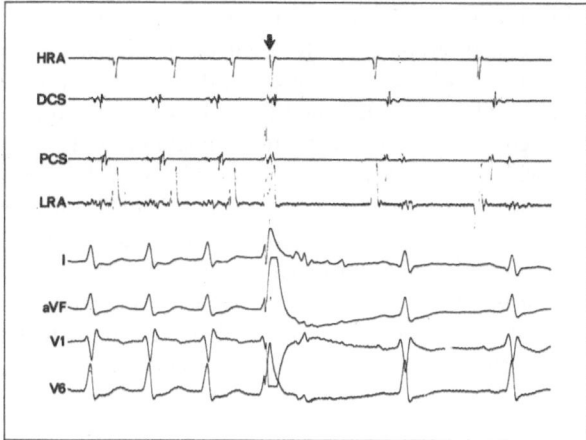

Fig. 3. 20 milliJoule shock delivered to the right atrium in a patient with an atrioventricular reentrant tachycardia due to a left lateral accessory pathway. The arrow indicates the timing of the discharge. High right atrial electrograms (HRA), distal coronary sinus electrograms (DCS), proximal coronary sinus electrograms (PCS) and low right atrial electrograms (LRA) are shown, together with four surface leads. The paper speed is 100 mm/second.

A total of 14 ventricular shocks (17 to 6700, mean 828 mJ) were delivered to the six patients with ventricular tachycardia. Termination was successful on the final attempt in four patients, but was unsuccessful in two (patients 12 and 14) who required external cardioversion, the latter because of ventricular fibrillation induced by the internal microshock. Overdrive or extrastimulus pacing was successful in causing termination in patients 2, 8, 13 and 14, but was unsuccessful in patient 12, and when attempted in patient 11 caused acceleration of tachycardia, which then responded well to internal microshock. Four proarrhythmic effects occurred. Atrial fibrillation was produced from atrial flutter in patient 6 (94 mJ to the atrium) and from AV nodal tachycardia in patient 7 (83 mJ to the ventricle). More importantly, there were eight beats of ventricular tachycardia produced in patient 7 after a ventricular discharge of 170 mJ for atrial fibrillation, and ventricular fibrillation was induced from ventricular tachycardia in patient 14 using a shock of only 150 mJ. Both of these were associated with poor synchronization to the QRS complex.

One patient did not complain of any pain or discomfort (20 mJ) but one patient complained of mild discomfort (200 mJ), three complained of moderate discomfort (6 to 6700 mJ) and nine complained of severe discomfort (patients 4 to 500 mJ). There was undoubtedly more pain caused by atrial discharges and discomfort was generally related to the energy delivered. Patient 5 described a shock of only 4 mJ as severely painful when delivered in both the atrium and the ventricle and several others described shocks of only 17 to 20 mJ as severely painful in both chambers. The patients described the pain as "a giant hiccup", "like electrocution" or "like being kicked by a mule" and most of the patients who described severe discomfort declined to have the procedure repeated.

Discussion

Our overall results are disappointing. Internal cardioversion was successful in four of six patients with ventricular tachycardia, but pacing was also effective in four.

863

The lack of response in atrial fibrillation and very limited response in atrial flutter is also disappointing. The active electrode was positioned on the right atrial septum, which might be thought to be an ideal position. In addition, in patient 1, the lateral right atrial wall was used without success. The use of shocks, delivered from the coronary sinus to give a different field of discharge, was considered. However, Bradman and Fisher reported coronary sinus rupture using shocks within the coronary sinus in a canine model designed to test a technique for ablation of anomalous conduction pathways (5), which mitigated against this. Even when using larger epicardial "paddles" (which should require less energy than a catheter electrode for successful conversion) energies of 10 J are frequently needed for the treatment of atrial fibrillation occurring during open heart surgery, and this may explain the lack of success when using smaller energies delivered from smaller electrodes. In the patients with atrial flutter, synchronization to the atria might have been more effective and less likely to cause atrial arrhythmias than a shock synchronized to the ventricles. However, even with an atrial electrode some energy will be delivered to the ventricles and this might cause ventricular fibrillation if delivered during the ventricular vulnerable period.

The failure of response of the two patients with AV nodal tachycardia is difficult to understand, but both patients with atrioventricular tachycardia responded to very low energy shocks (3.4 mJ in patient 6 and 20 mJ in patient 10).

Considerable discomfort was reported by many patients. In the patients who were successfully treated, cardioversion was associated with severe discomfort in two, with moderate discomfort in two, with mild discomfort in two (one of whom later described severe discomfort when a larger shock was used, unsuccessfully, for a different arrhythmia)·and with no discomfort in only one. A total of nine of the 14 patients experienced severe pain after at least one shock during the evaluation. Cine-radiographs were recorded during several of the discharges and these show diaphragmatic stimulation in some of the patients and the description of a giant hiccup, suggested by many, substantiates this. However, even with the proximal electrode in the superior vena cava or below the diaphragm in the inferior vena cava, despite using a widely separated electrode (150 mm) as used in patient 14, severe pain was described by many and this must prove limitation to the widespread use of the present technique.

Of even more importance however, were the four proarrhythmic effects seen. The development of atrial fibrillation from atrial flutter using an atrial stimulus is not particularly sinister, although the development of atrial fibrillation from AV nodal tachycardia using ventricular stimulation is more intriguing. However, non-sustained ventricular tachycardia after ventricular stimulation for atrial fibrillation gives rise to concern as does to induction of ventricular fibrillation in a young patient with ventricular tachycardia using only 150 mJ. Both these latter two arrhythmias were associated with technical problems causing a lack of synchronization, with the shock being delivered on the peak of the T wave. Sensing problems are not rare in patients with implantable pacemakers, and presumably malsensing might occur with either external or implantable microshock systems, giving rise to potentially disastrous results.

Heilman et al. (6), and Jackson and Zipes (3) have shown that energy requirements for cardioversion or defibrillation may be drastically reduced (up to 100 fold) by the use of high surface area epicardial electrodes in comparison with endocardial catheter electrodes. However, even when using large surface area epicardial electrodes, for instance during thoracic surgery, energy requirements may be as high as 2 to 30 J, and therefore energies in excess of this may be needed in conjunction with catheter electrodes. Mirowski et al. have changed from using an catheter electrode (in canine work), which was relatively easy to place. to an epicardial system in conjunction with a transvenous electrode (in clinical practice), which requires more substantial surgical intervention for implantation (2). This system has been used for treating ventricular tachycardia as well as ventricular fibrillation, using energies of 25 to 30 J for both.

Because of both the considerable discomfort that many occur and the possible dangers of internal microshock, its use is likely to be restricted to those with serious ventricular arrhythmias. However, these patients may be liable to spontaneous ventricular fibrillation as well as ventricular tachycardia. In addition, ventricular tachycardia may degenerate into ventricular fibrillation if not successfully treated or may be converted to fibrillation, even when using a properly synchronized microshock (4, 7). Therefore, it seems that although the present concept may be suitable for short term coronary care unit or electrophysiology laboratory use, before it is extended to long term use as an implantable device, a backup defibrillator capacity must be available to treat ventricular fibrillation. Whether or not a suitable device capable of both microshock cardioversion and larger energy defibrillation (together perhaps with bradycardia support pacing) can be constructed within reasonable size constraints is not certain.

Patients with ventricular tachycardia present a difficult therapeutic challenge and the ideal implantable device may consist of a bradycardia support pacemaker together with a tiered arrangement of burst or extrastimulus pacing, microshock and defibrillation.

References

1. Mirowski M, Mower MM, Staewen WS, Tabatznik B, Mendeloff AI: Standby automatic defibrillator. An approach to prevention of sudden coronary death. Arch Intern Med 1970; 126: 158–161.
2. Mirowski M, Mower MM, Reid PR, Watkins L, Langer A: The automatic implantable defibrillator. New modality for treatment of life-threatening ventricular arrhythmias. PACE 1982; 5: 384–401.
3. Jackman WM, Zipes DP: Transvenous, low energy cardioversion of ventricular tachycardia in a canine model of subacute myocardial infarction. Circulation 1981; 64 (Supp IV): 171.
4. Zipes DP, Jackman WM, Heger JJ, Chilson DA, Browne KF, Naccarelli GV, Rahilly GT, Prystowsky EN: Clinical transvenous cardioversion of recurrent life-threatening ventricular tachyarrhythmias: low energy synchronized cardioversion of ventricular tachycardia and termination of ventricular fibrillation in patients using a catheter electrode. Am Heart J 1982; 103: 789–794.
5. Brodman R, Fisher JD: Technique for ablation of anomalous conduction using catheter placed in coronary sinus: canine studies. Circulation 1982; 66 (Supp II): 217.
6. Heilman MS, Langer A, Mower MM, Mirowski M: Analysis of four implantable electrode systems for automatic defibrillator. Circulation 1975; 52 (Supp II): 194.
7. Waspe LE, Fisher JD, Kim SG, Matos JA: Reliability of transvenous shocks for termination of ventricular tachycardia and ventricular fibrillation. J Am Coll Cardiol 1983; 1: 595.

Authors' address:
A. W. Nathan, M.B.
West Smithfield
St. Bartholomew's Hospital
London EC1A 7BE
England

Electrophysiological Mapping as a Guide to Arrhythmia Surgery

J. A. Reiffel, J. T. Bigger, Jr., J. I. Gliklich, H. M. Spotnitz, F. D. Livelli, Jr., K. Ferrick

Summary: This manuscript reviews electrophysiological mapping as it is used to guide surgical ablation of arrhythmogenic areas, particularly in patients with Wolff Parkinson White Syndrome or with ventricular tachycardia. Discussed are techniques for an interpretation of: preoperative mapping of bypass tracts (antegrade and retrograde) and ventricular tachycardia, as well as intraoperative epicardial and endocardial mapping of bypass tracts (antegrade and retrograde) and ventricular tachycardia. Representative figures are shown and references to other detailed reviews are provided.

Introduction

Cardiac electrophysiologic mapping as a prelude to surgery (1–3) consists of recording multiple electrograms to geographically localize an arrhythmic focus or define its pathway. In this review, we will discuss the techniques for and interpretation of epicardial and endocardial mapping. We will emphasize applications in the Wolff-Parkinson-White syndrome (WPW) and in ventricular tachycardia (VT), the two major patient groups in which mapping guided surgical ablative therapy is used.

Techniques and Interpretation

Preoperative mapping (genral comments)

Endocardial mapping is always performed preoperatively since the feasibility and risks of surgery may depend upon the arrhythmia site. Septal bypass tracts, for example, are more difficult to approach and carry a higher risk of surgical heart block than free wall tracts. Similarly, surgical feasibility, risks, and success for VT are in part related to its site of origin. Moreover, the arrhythmia may be inducible or tolerated only in the catheterization laboratory, in which case the only arrhythmia map available will be the preoperative one. (See below for possible adjunctive intraoperative techniques). Preoperative mapping is done with standard electrode catheters (bipolar, interelectrode distances of ≥ 1 cm), paper speeds of ≥ 100 mm/sec, and band pass filters 10 to 30 Hz at the low end. Biplane fluoroscope is mandatory for VT, and helpful for bypass tracts.

Preoperative mapping (bypass tracts, preliminary comments):

Multiple atrial regions are mapped in W.P.W. (Table 1). The left atrium is mapped with a catheter in the coronary sinus. Coronary sinus length will determine whether the

867

anterolateral left atrium can be recorded. Approximation of the anterior left atrium can be achieved via the left pulmonary artery, but actual mapping of the anterior and antero-lateral left atrium can only be done transseptally. Both antegrade and retrograde maps are made as bypass tracts may be unidirectional, bidirectional, and multiple.

Preoperative mapping (bypass tracts with antegrade conduction)

Antegrade mapping (Fig. 1) is performed by pacing both the right and left atrium sequentially (11). At equal pacing rates preexcitation will be more complete with tracts ipsilateral rather than contralateral to the stimulus and, within the ipsilateral chamber, at the catheter site closest to the tract. Reasonable localization of the anticipated site can also be made by careful study of the delta wave vector on the ECG prior to electrophysiological study (11).

Preoperative mapping (bypass tracts with retrograde conduction)

Retrograde mapping is performed by determining atrial activation sequencing during PSVT and/or fixed rate ventricular pacing (Fig. 2). The timing of retrograde atrial depolarization (determined by the first baseline crossing of the rapid intrinsic deflection (8)) is noted at each recording site. V-A conduction normally occurs via the His bundle and A-V node; hence, initial atrial activation is recorded on the His bundle electrogram. The atrial activation sequence is eccentric, however, for most retrogradely conducting bypass tracts with the atrial segment near the mouth of the tract activating before the atrium on the His bundle electrogram. Anterior septal tracts have normal rather than eccentric retrograde activation sequences, but may be demonstrated by finding non-decremental (thus, non A-V nodal) V-A conduction and/or by demonstrating retrograde conduction from a VPD induced at a time when the A-V node is still refractory from antegrade conduction. Lastly, for free wall tracts, the site of earliest retrograde activation should be bracketed by later sites (5).
Prior to surgery retrograde bypass tracts defined by the above must be proven to participate in the genesis of the PSVT. Prolongation of the tachycardia cycle length and/or V-A conduction with ipsilateral but not contralateral bundle branch block during PSVT (11) or advancement of the tachycardia without sequence alteration following a VPD (4) may offer such proof.

Table 1. Mapping sites for Wolff Parkinson White syndrome.	Right atrium	Left atrium:
	anteromedial	posteromedial
	anterior	mid posterior
	anterolateral	posterolateral
	lateral	lateral
	posterolateral	anterolateral
	posterior	anterior
	posteromedial	

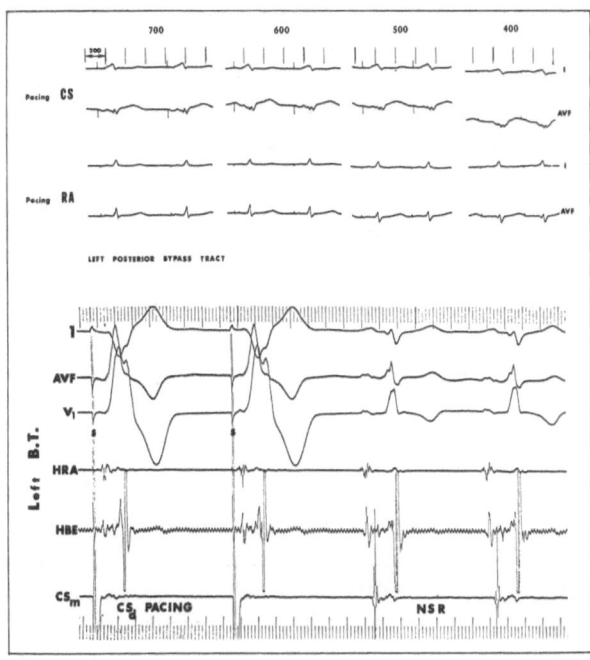

Fig. 1. Antegrade mapping in 2 patients with Wolff Parkinson White Syndrome with left sided bypass tracts. In the upper panel are seen ECG leads 1 and AVF as recorded during both coronary sinus (CS) and right atrial (RA) pacing at 4 paced cycle lengths: 700, 600, 500 and 400 msec. This patient had a left posteromedial bypass tract. Note that at any paced rate the presence of the short PR and delta wave are more apparent with CS than with RA pacing. Note also that manifestations of pre-excitation are present despite slow pacing rates (cycle length 700 msec) at a site near the tract (CS) but that they are seen only at more rapid pacing rates at a site remote from the tract. The lower panel, taken from a patient with a left posterolateral bypass tract, further exemplifies some of these points. ECG leads I, AVF and V1 are recorded simultaneously with high right atrial (HRA), His bundle (HBE), and mid coronary sinus (CSm) electrograms during the last 2 beats of distal coronary sinus pacing and the recovery of sinus rhythm. The pacing stimuli are labeled (S). Note that during pacing near the tract (cycle length 800 msec) pre-excitation (short PR and delta wave) is marked while during sinus rhythm, despite an even shorter cycle length (680 msec), preexcitation is much less marked.

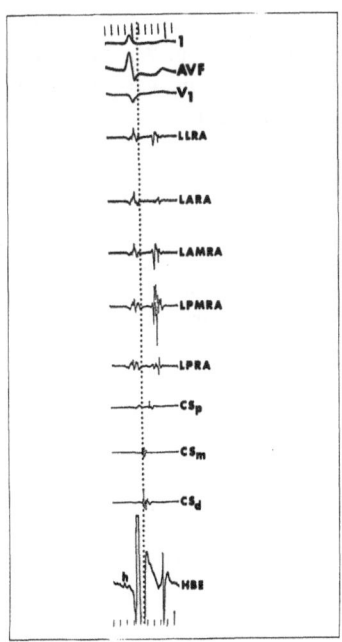

Fig. 2. Retrograde atrial activation sequencing during PSVT in a patient with a left sided bypass tract (Kent Bundle). ECG leads I, AVF and V1 as well as a His bundle electrogram (HBE) (with the His deflection denoted by an h) are recorded simultaneously with atrial electrograms from the following sites: low lateral right atrium (LLRA), low anterior right atrium (LARA), low anteromedial right atrium (LAMRA), low posteromedial right atrium (LPMRA), low posterior right atrium (LPRA), and 3 coronary sinus (CS) sites – proximal (p), mid (m), and distal (d). One representative beat during the PSVT is shown. Note that atrial activation following the QRS appears first on the CSd and CSm tracings and then spreads elsewhere. In this figure the amplification on the CS channels is low and only the high frequency atrial electrogram is seen well, although preceeding low amplitude ventricular depolarization is visible. See text for further discussion.

Preoperative mapping (ventricular tachycardia, preliminary comments)

Localization of VT requires mapping multiple, often biventricular, endocardial sites (2, 22, 26) (Table 2). Right ventricular mapping is essential with Uhl's disease, cardiomyopathy, and arrhythmogenic right ventricular dysplasia (28). At least 3 orthogonal ECG leads (usually I, AVF, V1) must be recorded in VT to catagorize tachycardia morphology. In patients with more than one clinically relevant tachycardia (1), each must be mapped separately. We, and others (1-2), have found that varying VT morphologies may arise from a single site (the result of different exit pathways) or from quite disparate loci. On each electrogram we determine local activation times in the same manner as with bypass tracts.

Preoperative mapping (ventricular tachycardia, activation sequencing)

At each site the timing of local activation during induced VT relative to both the onset of the surface QRS and a stable right ventricular electrogram is determined (Fig. 3). The earliest activating site is taken as the site of interest (2-3) re: surgical ablation. Typically, local activation proceeds from slightly before the QRS, throughout the QRS and occassionally the ST-T segment, followed by a diastolic pause. If the tachycardia is very rapid the diastolic pause may be absent and the relationship of local activation to preceeding versus subsequent QRS may be unclear unless a VPD is placed during the tachycardia. This produces a single long cycle during which the relative timing of the local electrograms to QRS becomes evident. The earliest site always occurs before the inscription of the QRS on the body surface (1). Occasionally with septal sites of origin, activation appears equally early on both right and left ventricular septal electrograms and/or after the onset of the QRS (2). If so, the catheter is either near but not quite at the earliest site or there is an intraseptal intramural origin (2). Lastly, continuous electrical activity at one site throughot systole and diastole (usually in an aneurysm) may be seen. Whether this is a site of reentry (27) from which activation spreads preferentially to one edge of the aneurysm or whether this is not electrogenically related to the tachycardia is still debated (2, 3).

Table 2. Mapping sites for ventricular tachycardia.	Right ventricular:	Left ventricular:
	inflow tract	anterior septum
	anterior wall	mid septum
	apex	posterior septum
	outflow tract	apex
	septal sites	base
		high anterior
		low anterior
		high anterolateral
		low anterolateral
		high posterolateral
		low posterolateral
		inferior
		aneurysm

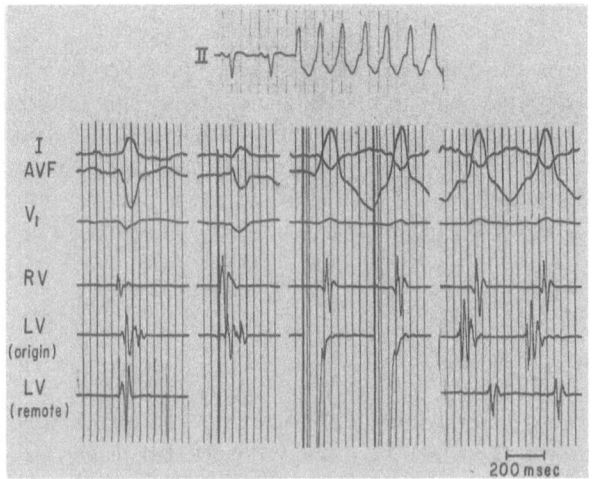

Fig. 3. Preoperative mapping of ventricular tachycardia (VT). ECG leads I, AVF, and V1 are recorded with an RV reference electrogram in each panel. In each panel an electrogram recorded from the region of the LV in which the VT is felt to arise is shown (LV origin). In the left hand and right hand panels, a second LV electrogram at a site remote from the site of origin is also recorded (LV remote). From left to right there are 4 panels: sinus rhythm, right ventricular apical pacing, left ventricular pacing during pace mapping, and sustained ventricular tachycardia. Above these 4 panels is a lead II ECG rhythm strip taken during the spontaneous start of the patient's VT. During NSR (left hand panel), note the wide (150 msec), fractionated electrogram at the LV origin, but the narrow (80 msec) electrogram at the remote LV site. In this patient, fractionation did not increase at the site of origin during RV pacing though it does in some. Note that during LV pace mapping at this same LV site, the configuration of the paced QRS is identical to that during the ventricular tachycardia. In this patient this was the only LV paced site which yielded this QRS configuration. Note during sustained VT that activation at the LV origin preceeds the inscription of the QRS on the body surface while the remote LV site and RV reference activate late. These are typical findings – see text for further discussion.

Preoperative mapping (ventricular tachycardias, adjunctive techniques):

When VT is not reliably induced or hemodynamically tolerated, other mapping techniques have been proposed.

Sinus Rhythm maps (2, 8):

Since conduction delay and block are necessary substrates for reentry, it has been assumed that areas in which local electrograms are prolonged and fractionated (Fig. 3) or several late (post QRS) or double potentials are seen may be sites of VT origin. This is the case for non infarction RV tachycardia (8, 16–18) and may be the case for LV post infarction VT. In our last seven cases of drug refractory, post infarction VT, we correlated the site of origin determined by VT mapping with the sites in which fractionated electrograms of ≥ 100 msec duration were recorded during NSR. In all seven the origin by VT mapping was a site which had prolonged fractionated sinus rhythm electrograms. Spielman et al. reported similar results (22). However, since there were typically several sites with abnormal sinus rhythm electrograms, operative resections based on this would be more extensive than if guided by VT mapping. Similar conclusions have been reached (3, 10) using intraoperative sinus rhythm mapping.

871

Pace mapping:

It has also been assumed that if the tachycardia morphology can be produced by local ventricular stimulation, then the site stimulated must be the site of origin. This has been termed pace mapping (Fig. 3) (2, 18). Although occassionally useful, pacing at several sites often gives complexes resembling those of the VT (using 3 ECG leads) and, both we and others (21) have found that changes in catheter position as little as a 1 cm can result in markedly different paced morphologies. We believe that at best, pace mapping is a corroborative technique.

Intraoperative mapping (preliminary comments)

Intraoperative mapping (3), uses the same principles as above, but special probes rather than catheters (3, 8, 9). In addition to the exploring probe (5), epicardial plaque electrodes, needle electrodes, or temporary pacing wires (3, 8) are used to record stable reference electrograms and for atrial and/or ventricular stimulation. Epicardial mapping is attempted prior to cardiac cooling (8) and cardiopulmonary bypass but hemodynamic compromise during VT may necessitate cardiopulmonary bypass or diastolic counterpulsation. Endocardial mapping is done during total cardiopulmonary bypass, preferably prior to cooling (1). The standard recording probes (8) have been bipolar or tripolar hand held stalk or ring electrodes which allowed single site recording. Because both tolerance of the tachycardia and surgical morbidity are time dependent, we and others (3, 9, 13, 14, 31) have developed multipoint recording probes to decrease data acquisition and processing time. For example, our surgeon now uses a glove which has tripolar electrodes on each of the 4 finger tips (9, 31) (Fig. 4), thus providing four simultaneous electrograms. Only the earliest point on each set of 4 tracings usually needs to be analyzed immediately, thus reducing mapping time by a factor of 16. Ultimately, mapping of the entire heart simultaneously on one beat will be feasible, using epicardial sock or endocardial contour arrays of multipoint electrodes connected via multiplexer to computerized date processors that we and others are developing (3, 13, 14, 28).

For VT the entire epicardium must be mapped; for bypass tracts both sides of the A-V ring and those areas that reflect early spread of septal activation are explored (8). A cardiac schematic with an overlaid numerical grid (4) (Fig. 4) is used for referencing. The epicardium is mapped at sites corresponding to each location on the grid (50–70 points total). Similarly, endocardial mapping is performed according to anatomical regions of interest in defined sequences (see below).

Intraoperative epicardial mapping (bypass tracts)

Both antegrade mapping utilizing atrial pacing and retrograde mapping during PSVT or ventricular pacing are performed intraoperatively (Fig. 5). The sites for atrial or ventricular pacing and for the reference electrodes are chosen to maximize tract detection (4). With antegrade mapping, the site of earliest activation during the delta wave is sought. Location specific details of data analysis can be found elsewhere (4, 5) but certain principles will be addressed here. With free wall tracts, the site of earliest epicardial activation

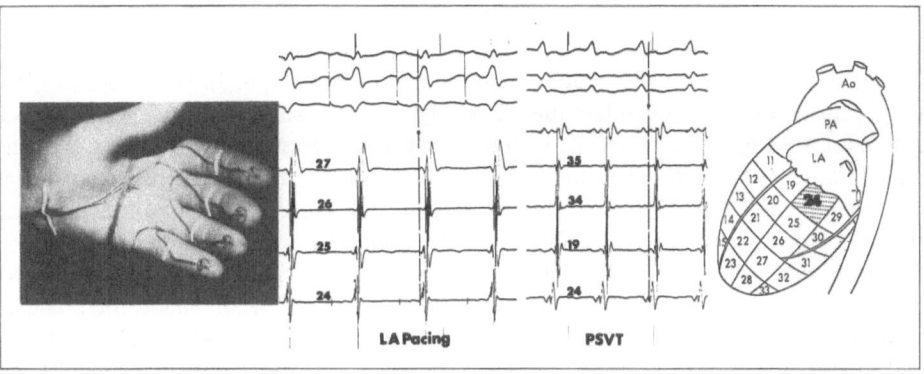

Fig. 4. Intraoperative mapping.
This figure consists of 4 panels. From left to right are: our 4 point mapping glove (9), antegrade mapping of a bypass tract, retrograde mapping of a bypass tract, and a lateral view of the mapping grid we used (derived from the Duke University grid). The grid and 2 middle panels are taken from a patient with a left sided tract at site 24 (highlighted on the grid). On both mapping panels ECG leads I, AVF and V1 are simultaneously displayed with a reference electrogram and four exploring electrograms – one from each recording finger. The antegrade map is performed during left atrial pacing; the retrograde map is performed during PSVT. Not shown are grids of the anteromedial and posterior views which contain the rest of the numerically identified sites used for mapping (see text). The retrograde map is performed with the exploring electrodes placed on the atrium adjacent to the numerically identified ventricular sites. Note that the earliest antegrade ventricular activation during left atrial pacing is at site 24 and the earliest retrograde atrial activation site is on the atrial side of the A-V ring adjoining site 24.

during antegrade conduction is simultaneous with or slightly before the onset of the delta wave. With septal tracts, because of the delay from septal activation to epicardial breakthrough, the earliest epicardial site is always after the onset of the delta wave and the area of earliest epicardial activation does not immediately overlie the tract (4). The same comments apply to retrograde mapping except that it is now the region of earliest atrial activation which is sought. Unipolar electrograms (4, 8) or transmyocardial multi-pole needle electrodes (3) can be used if necessary to assess tract depth.

Intraoperative endocardial mapping (bypass tracts)

For endocardial mapping, the A-V ring(s) of interest is viewed as if a clock face. During atrial stimulation, the ventricular endocardium around the underside of the ring, and during PSVT or ventricular pacing, the atrial endocardium around the upper side of the ring is recorded at sites corresponding to each hour, with the site of earliest antegrade and retrograde activation being sought. Multiple, non-contiguous sites of early activation suggest preferential spread via the specialized conduction system or more than one tract.

Intracardiac epicardial mapping (ventricular tachycardia)

Operative mapping is usually performed during induced VT (2, 8, 9). Sinus rhythm mapping is clearly useful in non infarction related right ventricular tachycardias where sites of delayed or split potentials correlate with regions which successfully identify areas for surgical ablation (8, 16, 18). The utility of sinus rhythm mapping for post infarction VT is not yet established (22), though both epicardial and endocardial intraoperative sinus rhythm mapping has been used with limited experience yet, some success (8, 10). Criteria for identifying areas of interest in sinus rhythm maps, especially epicardial, are not yet standardized. Because the tachycardias are almost invariably of endocardial and/or myocardial origin there is no role for epicardial pace mapping (1), and the earliest epicardial site is never as early as the earliest endocardial site determined preoperatively (1), or in the O. R. (3, 23). When there is a free wall site of origin, the discrepancy is less than with septal or papillary muscle origins (2, 23) (analogous to septal bypass tracts). Moreover, the presence of diseased subendocardial or myocardial tissue (1) and the associated likelihood of non-perpendicular epicardial breakthrough further affects the timing of epicardial recordings. Nonetheless, because VT is often not inducible once the ventricle has been opened, we consider epicardial, like cath lab, mapping to be necessary.

Intraoperative endocardial mapping (ventricular tachycardia)

Intraoperative endocardial mapping during VT is performed as during the preoperative map. Ventriculotomy is usually through the infarct scar or aneurysm and the oval opening is viewed as a clock face. Again, electrograms are recorded at each hour on the clock starting at the edge of the ventriculotomy or aneurysmectomy and moving deeper into the ventricle in successive rings 1 cm farther from the edge (1). Additionally, recordings, are made from the papillary muscles when they are visibly involved by scar. The site of the earliest local electrogram in sought.

Ventricular tachycardia, three additional considerations:

1. Occasionally patients are encountered in whom the spread of activation is circumferential around the edge of the aneurysm or scar, rather than radial from an early site (1), and continues around with no diastolic pause (even with an induced VPD). Some have speculated that this represents recording over an entire macroreentrant pathway (2). In these cases, pressure anywhere around the ring often, but not always (3) terminates the tachycardia and incision in or excision of part of the loop often prevents its recurrence.
2. If a VT is still inducible after ventriculotomy, its configuration and rate are often different that the clinical VT(s). It is not always certain that a tachycardia so encountered is the one of interest and hence, ablative surgery must be guided by the epicardial and preoperative map or by sinus rhythm mapping. Pace mapping is uninterpretable under these circumstances.
3. In some patients, especially those with posterior, inferior, non-aneurysmal scars, endocardial mapping may more easily be performed using a probe across the mitral

valve than via retrocardiac ventriculotomy. The advantages of the extremely flexible glove probe we use are highlighted in such instances.

Concluding remarks

Although brief, the discussion above should provide the reader with a reasonable picture of current techniques for electrophysiological mapping. Additional information, if necessary, can be found among the cited references. With this knowledge, we would hope that mapping as described will be used whenever ablative surgical therapy is considered. Mapping guided surgery offers the patient the opportunity to have therapeutic success at the lowest risk, since it allows identification of the minimal area of ablation necessary. With continued advances in technique, speed, and knowledge, we anticipate mapping will assume even wider applicability with enhanced certainty and safety. This should ensure even further success and utility of arrhythmia surgery.

References

1. Horowitz LN, Josepshon ME, Harken AH: Epicardial and endocardial activation during sustained ventricular tachycardia in man. Circulation 1980; 61: 1227–1238.
2. Josephson ME, Horowitz LN, Spielman SR, Waxman HL, Greespan AM: Role of catheter mapping in the preoperative evaluation of ventricular tachycardia. Am J Cardiol 1982; 49: 207–220.
3. Gallagher JJ, Kasell JH, Cox JL, Smith WM, Ideker RE, Smith WM: Techniques of intraoperative electrophysiologic mapping. Am J Cardiol 1982; 49: 221–240.
4. Gallagher JJ, Kasell J, Sealy WC, Pritchett EL, Wallace AG; Epicardial mapping in the Wolff Parkinson White Syndrome. Circulation 1978; 57: 854–866.
5. Gallagher JJ, Sealy WC, Kasell J: Intraoperative mapping studies in the Wolff Parkinson White Syndrome. Pace 1979; 2: 523–537.
6. Mason JW: The role of surgery in the treatment of arrhythmias. Hosp Pract 1981; 16 (12): 66–74.
7. Kastor JA, Horowitz LN, Harken AH, Josephson ME: Clinical electrophysiology of ventricular tachycardia. N Engl J Med 1981; 304: 1004–1020.
8. Waldo AL, Arciniegas JG, Klein H: Surgical treatment of life threatening ventricular arrhythmias: The role of intraoperative mapping and consideration of the presently available surgical techniques. Prog Cardiovasc Dis 1981; 23: 247–264.
9. Spotnitz HM, Gliklich JJ, Ross S, Reiffel JA, Malm JR, Bigger JT Jr, Hoffman BF: Four contact glove probe method for rapid recording of cardiac electrograms during surgery. Ann Thorac Surg 1982; 33; 403–405.
10. Kienzle MG, Falcone RA, Kempf FC, Miller JM, Harken AH, Josephson ME: Intraoperative endocardial mapping: Relation of fractionated electrograms in sinus rhythm to endocardial activation in ventricular tachycardia – surgical implications (abstr). J Am Coll Cardiol 1983; 2: 582.
11. Gallagher JJ, Pritchett ELC, Sealy WC, Kasell J, Wallace AG: The preexcitation syndromes. Prog Cardiovasc Dis 1978; 20: 285–327.
12. Rossi P, Massumi A, Gilette P, Hall RJ: Arrhythmogenic right ventricular dysplasia: clinical features, diagnostic techniques, and current management. Am Heart J 1982; 103: 415–420.
13. Wit AL, Allesse MA, Bonke FIM, Lammers W, Smeets J, Fenoglio JJ: Electrophysiologic mapping to determine the mechanism of experimental ventricular tachycardia initiated by premature impulses. Am J Cardiol 1982; 49: 166–185.
14. Downar E, Parson I, Cameron DC, Waxman MB, Mikelborough LL: On line mapping of ventricular arrhythmias – initial clinical experience (abstr). J Am Coll Cardiol 1983; 1: 621.

15. Ostermeyer J, Breithardt G, Kolvenbach R, Korfer R, Seipel L, Schulte HD, Bircks W: Intraoperative electrophysiologic mapping during cardiac surgery. Thorac Cardiovasc Surg 1979; 27: 260–270.
16. Fontaine G, Guiraudon G, Frank R, Coutter R, Cabrol C, Grosgogeat Y: Intraoperative mapping and surgery for the prevention of lethal arrhythmias after myocardial infarction. Ann NY Acad Sci 1982; 392: 396–410.
17. Fontaine G, Guiraudon G, Frank R, Vedel J, Grosgogeat Y, Cabrol C: Modern concepts of ventricular tachycardia. The value of electrophysiological investigations and delayed potentials in ventricular tachycardia of ischaemic and non-ischaemic aetiology. 31 operated cases. Eur J Cardiol 1980; 8: 505–580.
18. Fontaine G, Guiraudon G, Frank R, Fillette F, Tonet J, Grosgogeat Y: Correlations between latest delayed potentials in sinus rhythm and earliest activation during chronic ventricular tachycardia. In: Bircks W, Loogen F, Schulte HD, Seipel L, Eds, Medical and Surgical Management of Tachyarrhythmias. Berlin, Heidelberg: Springer-Verlag 1980; 138–54.
19. O'Keefe DB, Curry PVL, Prior AL, Yates AK, Deverall PB, Sowton E: Surgery for ventricular tachycardia using operative pace mapping. Br Heart J 1980; 43: 116–122.
20. Curry PUL, O'Keeffe DB, Pitcher D, Sowton E, Deverall PB, Yates AK: Localization of ventricular tachycardia by a new technique – Pace mapping (abstr). Circulation 1979; 60: II-25.
21. Josephson ME, Waxman HL, Cain ME, Horowitz LN, Kastor JA: Endocardial pace mapping to localize the origin of ventricular tachycardia (abstr). Am J Cardiol 1981; 47: 488.
22. Spielman SR, Horowitz LN, Greenspan AM, Unterecker WJ, Simson MB, Kastor JA, Josephson ME: Activation mapping in sinus rhythm in patients with ventricular tachycardia relationship to cycle length and site of origin (abstr). Am J Cardiol 1981; 47: 497.
23. Spielman SR, Michelson EL, Horowitz LN, Spear JF, Moore EN: The limitations of epicardial mapping as a guide to the surgical therapy of ventricular tachycardia. Circulation 1978; 57: 666–670.
24. Josephson ME, Horowitz LN, Spielman SR, Greenspan AM, Vanderpol C, Harken AH: Comparison of endocardial catheter mapping with intraoperative mapping of ventricular tachycardia. Circulation 1980; 61: 395–404.
25. Wittig JH, Boineau JP: Surgical treatment of ventricular arrhythmias using epicardial, transmural, and endocardial mapping. Ann Thorac Surg 1975; 20: 117–26.
26. Josephson ME, Horowitz LN, Farshidi A, Spear JF, Kastor JA, Moore EN: Recurrent sustained ventricular tachycardia. 2. Endocardial mapping. Circulation 1978; 57: 440–447.
27. Josephson ME, Horowitz LN, Farshidi A: Continuous electrical activity: a mechanism of ventricular tachycardia. Circulation 1978; 57: 659–666.
28. Iwase T: Study of computer display of epicardial map. Part II. Epicardial map in the Wolff Parkinson White Syndrome. Nippon Kyobu Geka Gakkai Zasshi 1981; 29: 1345–1358.
29. Iwa T, Kawasuji M, Misaki T, Iwase T, Magara T: Localization and interuption of accessory conduction pathway in the Wolff Parkinson White Syndrome. J Thorac Cardiovasc Surg 1980; 80: 271–279.
30. Iwa T, Iwase T, Kawasuji M, Magara T, Kobayashi H, Watonabe Y: Epicardial mapping. Surgical management and epicardial mapping in Wolff Parkinson White Syndrome. Nippon Rinsho 1979; 37: 3038–3644.
31. Gliklich J, Reiffel J, Spotnitz H, Gang E, Livelli F Jr, Malm JR, Bigger JT Jr, Hoffman BF, Ross S: Simplified technique for arrhythmia mapping during open heart surgery (abstr). Circulation 1981; 64: IV-290.

Authors' address:
James A. Reiffel, M.D.
Department of Medicine
Division of Cardiology
Columbia University
630 West 168th Street
New York, N.Y. 10032
USA

876

Intracardiac Cardioversion for Ablation of the Atrioventricular Conduction System in Patients with Drug Resistant Atrial Flutter

T. Pop, W. Kasper, T. Meinertz, A. Rückel, N. Treese, C. J. Schuster, C. Pfeiffer

Summary: The technique of intracardiac cardioversion for the ablation of the atrioventricular conduction system was used in three male patients (65, 53 and 57 years of age) with atrial flutter unresponsive to medical management. In the first patient a DC current of 80 J was applied while the other patients required 300 and 400 J respectively. In the first patient a transient third degree AV-block was induced enabling the ventricular rate to be easily controlled with drugs. This patient died 5 months later of resistant congestive heart failure. Autopsy revealed no gross evidence of myocardial damage in the tricuspid valve area or in the interventricular septum. In the other two patients a permanent third degree AV-block was induced, necessitating the implantation of a pacemaker. CK and CK-MB releases of moderate degree were observed in these two patients but no Tc pyrophosphate was stored.
We conclude that intracardiac cardioversion for ablation of the AV-conduction system is a safe and efficient procedure in selected patients with drug resistant supraventricular arrhythmias.

In 1982 Gallagher et al (1) and Scheinman et al (2) reported a catheter technique for closed-chest ablation of the atrioventricular conduction system. Using this technique it was possible to control refractory supraventricular arrhythmias withouut resorting to electrosurgical cardiac procedures. In this report we have summarized our initial experience in three patients with drug resistant atrial flutter.

Patients and Methods

The catheter technique for closed-chest ablation of the atrioventricular conduction system was used in three patients with atrial flutter and 2/1 AV-conduction which had proved refractory to adequate dosage of antiarrhythmic drugs, high-rate atrial stimulation and cardioversion (Table 1). Digitalis in high doses and verapamil also proved ineffective in reducing the ventricular rate. Beta-blockers could not be used, because all three patients suffered from a chronic obstructive pulmonary disease. In all patients the arrhythmia aggravated their disabling dyspnoea. After giving informed written consent, the patients were taken to the catheterization laboratory. A No 6 F bipolar electrode catheter was inserted into the left subclavian vein and positioned at the apex of the right ventricle to serve as temporary pacemaker. An additional conventional 6 F quadripolar electrode catheter was inserted via the right femoral vein and positioned across the tricuspid valve to record the His-bundle-electrogram. The catheter was so positioned that a maximal deflection in the His-bundle was recorded from an unipolar lead, from the distal electrode ring in all cases (Fig. 1). This electrode was connected to the cathode of a conventional defibrillator. The anodal paddle covered with conductive jelly was firmly positioned against the left lateral wall of the chest.

Table 1. Clinical and electrophysiologic data.

Patient No.	Age years	Sex	Cardiac Diagnosis	Internal Shocks, J	Peak Total CK and CK–MB, U/l	Spontaneous Pacemaker Rate, Beats/min
1	61	M	Coronary Heart Disease	80	56 4	54
2	53	M	Coronary Heart Disease	200 300 300	237 22	40
3	57	M	Dilative Cardiomyopathy	300 400	153 12	33

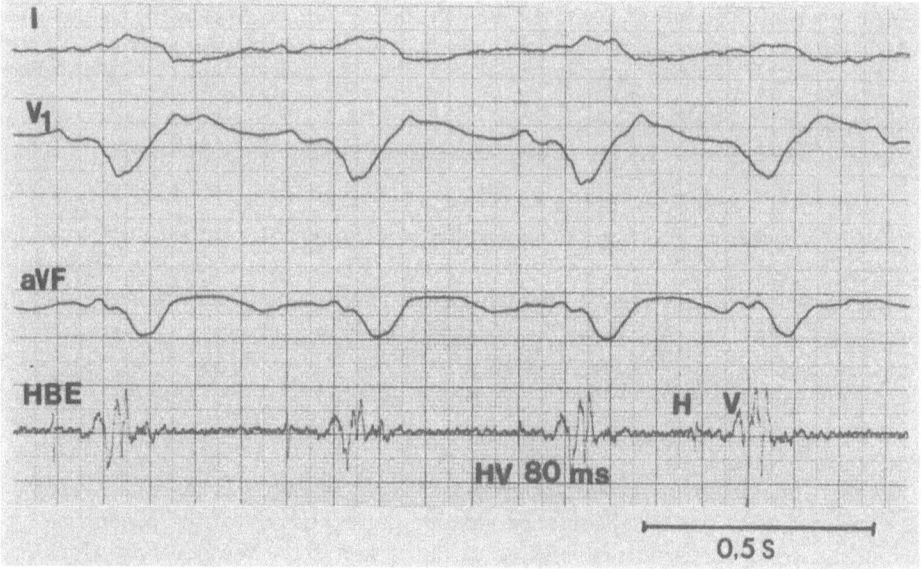

Fig. 1. Patient No. 1. Simultaneous recordings on surface ECG leads I, aVF and V₁ and His-bundle-electrogram (HBE) with largest His-bundle-potential (H).

The patients were anaesthetized with intravenous Etomidate in preparation for the delivery of electric shocks. A series of DC defibrillatory shocks, synchronized to the R wave of the surface ECG, were administered through the femoral catheter. After induction of complete AV-block (Fig. 2) ventricular pacing was initiated using the electrode catheter previously inserted into the apex of the right ventricle. The patients were monitored for 60–90 min, then transfered to the coronary care unit. Serial creatinine phosphokinase determinations were obtained up to 48 hours after cardioversion. A technetium (Tc 99 m) pyrophosphate scan was performed 1 or 2 days after the procedure in patients No. 2 and 3. In the same two patients, 48 hours after the induction of complete AV-block, a permanent pacemaker was implanted.

878

Results

In patient No 1 a single DC shock of only 80 J was delivered. Patient No 2 needed 3 shocks (200, 300, and 300 J, respectively), while in patient No 3 two shocks (300 and 400 J) where neccessary to induce a persistant AV-block. The shocks were delivered in all three patients during atrial flutter giving complete AV-block and reversion to sinus rhyhtm (Fig. 2).

In patient No 1 although AV-conduction resumed after 20 hours sinus rhythm persisted until his death 5 months later. The other two patients reverted after 1 and 2 days, respectively to atrial flutter, which persisted during the follow-up period. In patient No. 1 the electrophysiologic investigation performed 4 days later, showed an impaired conduction in the AV-node (3/1 to 4/1 AV conduction at a driving rate of 250/min, previously 2/1 AV-conduction). But the AV-block induced was stable. The mean rates of escape rhythm were 54 beats/min, 40 beats/min and 33 beats/min, respectively. His-bundle potential could not be recorded after induction of the AV-block. The QRS configuration resembled right bundle-branch block in the first patient and vacillated between a right- and a left-bundle-branch appearance in the other two patients. In patient No 1, no ventricular premature beats were observed after cardioversion. The other two patients showed ventricular extrasystoles in the first 3 hours following the application of direct current. In patient No 3 bigeminal beats could be observed for a short period.

Creatine phosphokinase values did not increase in the first patient. In the other two patients maximal levels of 237 U/l (after 24 hours) and 153 U/l after 12 hours, were observed. Accordingly CM-MB levels increased to 22 U/l and to 12 U/l, respectively. In these two patients the technetium (Tc 99 m) pyrophosphate scan revealed no areas of abnormal uptake.

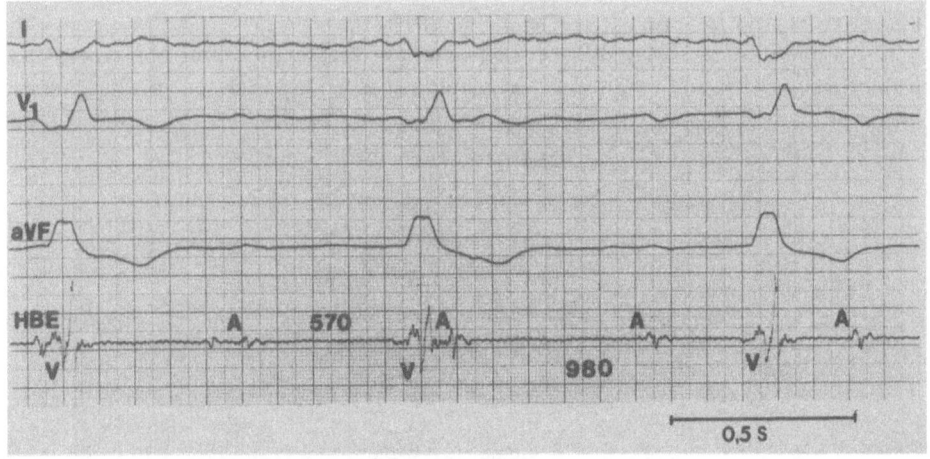

Fig. 2. Same patient after DC-application (80 J). There is a complete AV-block with right bundle-branch-block resembling ventricular beats. No His-bundle potential is observed.

Follow-up (Table 2)

The first patient remained in sinus rhythm during a follow-up period of 5 months. He died of therapy-resistant congestive heart failure. Postmortem examination revealed biventricular hypertrophy and dilatation. There was no gross evidence of myocardial damage in the region where the current was applied. Detailed histological studies of the conduction system are in progress.

During a follow-up period (6 and 4 1/2 months, respectively) in patients No 2 and 3 the AV-block persisted. Patient No 2 is as yet without any medication and in fair condition. Patient No 3 died suddenly 4 1/2 months after the catheterization ablation of the atrioventricular conduction system. A postmortem examination was not obtained.

Discussion

Previous reports concerning ablation of the atrioventricular conduction system in patients with supraventricular arrhythmias were published only by Gallagher et al (1), Scheinman et al (2) and more recently, by Manz et al (3). Gallagher et al (1) were able to induce a persistent AV-block in 9 out of 10 patients using energy levels from 200 to 300 J. Scheinman et al (2) were successful in 4 out of 5 patients using 400 to 500 J, whiled Manz et al (83) induced a stable AV-block in only one out of four patients. The level of energy they used lay between 150 and 300 Joule.

The success of the ablation procedure depends on the proper placing of the electrode and the level of energy used (1). Our failure to induce a persistent third degree AV-block in the first patient is probably due to the rather low levels of energy applied. In the series of Gallagher et al (1) and Scheinman et al (2) the only unsuccessful cases were those in whom very low energy levels were employed. Nevertheless, application of direct current shock can modify the conduction properties of the AV-node to such an extent that either the patients remain quite free from arrhythmias, or the ventricular rate during supraventricular tachycardia can easily be controlled with drugs (1, 2, 3). When the main therapeutic goal is the induction of a stable and persistent AV-block, then energy levels of 200 J or more must be used.

In the previous reports and in our patient group, no complications were observed. In the postmortem examination reported by Scheinman et al (2), and that of our first case no gross morphologic damage in the tricuspid valve area or the interventricular septum could be demonstrated. The CK and CK-MB levels increased moderately in our patients

Table 2. Follow-Up Data.

Pat. No.	Follow-Up Period Months	AV-Conduction	Present Status
1	5	1/1	Deceased (Heart failure)
2	6	Complete AV-Block	Alived
3	4½	Complete AV-Block	Deceased (Sudden death)

No 2 and 3, as in all patients of Gallagher et al (1). This probably reflects the fact that the electric current induces some myocardial damage. It must however be negligible because neither Scheinman et al (2) nor we ourselves were able to disclose any abnormal up-take of technetium Tc 99 m pyrophosphate. In Gallagher's patient group, the myocardial scanning was positive in only one patient and equivocal in another. In our patients No 2 and 3 ventricular extrasystoles were recorded immediately after application of current. Nevertheless they disappeared without any medication in the following 3 hours. We used in diverging from other reports a left lateral, a not a posterior position for the anodal paddle. This seems to have no influence on the success of closed chest ablation of the atrioventricular conduction system. We conclude from our preliminary results that the catheter technique for closed-chest ablation of the atrioventricular conduction system is a safe and effective procedure for the successful treatment of patients with drug-refractory supraventricular arrhythmias.

References

1. Gallagher JJ, Svenson RH, Kasell JH, German LD, Bardy GH, Broughton A, Critelli G: Catheter technique for closed-chest ablation of the atrioventricular conduction system. A therapeutic alternative for the treatment of refractory supraventricular tachycardia. New Engl. J. Med. 1982; 306: 194–200
2. Scheinman MM, Morady F, Hess DS, Gonzalez R: Catheter-induced ablation of the atrioventricular junction to control refractory supraventricular arrhythmias. JAMA 1982; 248: 851–855.
3. Manz M, Steinbeck G, Lüderitz B: His-Bündel-Ablation. Eine neue Methode zur Behandlung bedrohlicher supraventrikulärer Herzrhythmusstörungen. Internist 1983; 24: 95–98.

Authors' address:
Prof. Dr. T. Pop
II. Medizinische Klinik
der Universität
Langenbeckstr. 1
D-6500 Mainz

Closed-Chest Ablation of His Bundle: A New Technique Using Suction Electrode Catheter and DC Shock

P. Polgár, P. Molnár*, F. Wórum, Sz. Békássy**, P. Kovács, I. Lörincz

Summary: The purpose of this paper is to describe a new technique for closed-chest ablation of His bundle. Ten mongrel dogs were generally anesthetized. A bipolare suction electrode catheter was introduced through the femoral vein into the right heart and positioned to the His bundle. When a large His potential appeared, – 100 mmHg suction was applied. In this way the electrode was well fixed on the His bundle. The central terminal of the suction electrode was connected by a switching device to the cathodal output of standard cardioversion unit. A back paddle was positioned adjacent to the left scapula and connected to anodal output of the cardioversion unit. The defibrillator was discharged synchronously with the QRS complex. Using this technique we were able to induce heart block in 9 of 10 dogs by passing an average of 150 J one time through the suction electrode. At the end of the procedure we implanted a used demand pacemaker into the dogs. In 9 of 10 dogs the total AV-Block persisted at the end of the third week. After 3 weeks the dogs were killed and their hearts were investigated histologically.

This technique is an improvement of the method for electric His bundle ablation. Using this method the dislocation of the catheter – which could have serious consequences – can be avoided.

Patients with recurrent supraventricular tachyarrhythmias in some cases cannot be managed adequately by either pharmacologic or pacemaker techniques. For such patients, interruption of atrioventricular (AV) conduction followed by implantation of a permanent ventricular pacemaker has been shown to provide effective therapy (1–5). Previous attempts to ablate AV conduction in clinical and experimental situations have included ligation of tissue near the AV node (7), injection of formalin into the tissue surrounding the His bundle (8), surgical transection of the His bundle (1), mechanical crushing (9) and electrocautery of the AV node-His bundle (5, 18, 19). The catheter technique for ablation of the His bundle does not require open-heart surgery, with its attendant risks (5).

The purpose of this paper is to describe a new catheter technique for closed-chest ablation of His bundle, using suction electrode catheter and direct current (DC) shock. This technique is the modification of the method for electrocautery of the AV node-His bundle (5).

Methods

Ten mongrel dogs, 15–20 kgs, were anesthetized by 30 mg/kg intravenous sodium pentobarbital. After endotracheal intubation, the dogs were ventillated by a respirator, and repeated doses of pentobarbital sodium were infused as necessary throughout the experi-

) I. Department of Medicine, Department of Pathology and II. Surgical Clinic**, Medical University of Debrecen, Hungary

ment. The upper back of each dog was shaved, and a metal plate – ten cms in diameter – covered with conducting jelly was placed over the shaved area. The animals were immobilized so that there was firm pressure between the plate and the shaved area. Control 6-lead electrocardiograms were recorded. A bipolare F6 electrode catheter (United States Catheter Instruments), two F4 electrode catheters (Cordis Co.) and one self devised and made bipolare (or unipolare) suction electrode catheter were inserted percutaneously into the dog's heart, via the femoral veins. The F6 catheter was inserted for His bundle potential recording. One of the F4 electrodes was placed into the right atrium for recording the atrial signal, the other one was used for stimulating the right ventricle. The suction electrode catheter was positioned, under fluoroscopy and ECG control, very close to the F6 catheter, for recording the His bundle potential as proximal as possible. When an appropriately large His bundle deflection was recorded by the suction electrode, – 100 mmHg suction was applied through the catheter. In this way the suction electrode was well fixed on the His bundle (Fig. 1). The central terminal of the suction electrode was connected to the cathodal output of a standard cardioversion unit. The back paddle was connected to the anodal output of the cardioversion unit. A single direct current pulse from a standard cardioversion unit was delivered between the central terminal of suction electrode and the back paddle. The delivered impulse was 4 ms in duration and the delivered energy was 150 J. The DC shock was synchronised to the surface electrocardiogram.

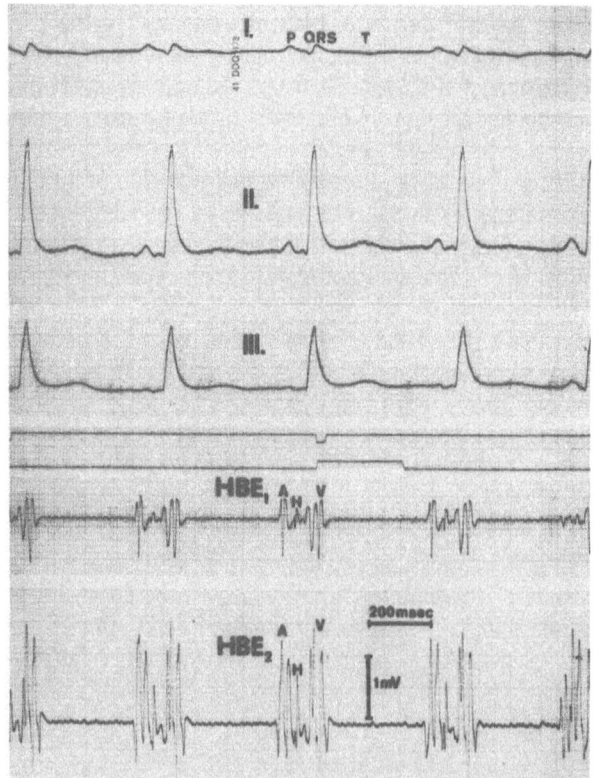

Fig. 1. His bundle recordings used to positioning the suction electrode catheter before ablation. Recordings (from the top down) are from standard electrocardiographic Leads I., II., III. and the two His bundle recordings. HBE₁ is recorded with bipolare F6 electrode. HBE₂ is recorded by bipolare suction electrode catheter under suction of – 100 mmHg. The recording was made with a paper speed of 100 mm/sec.

After appearance of an escape rhythm the dogs underwent continuous electrocardiographic monitoring for a period of 4 hours. After 4 hours of stable atrioventricular block, a used permanent transvenous programmable ventricular pacemaker was implanted. Routine ECG and external chest wall stimulation were repeated daily during the 3 weeks follow-up period. On the last day of the follow-up period the dogs were again anesthetized and a bipolare F6 catheter electrode was appropriately positioned to record His bundle or fascicular potentials.

The animals were sacrificed by bleeding to death via the femoral canules under anesthesia. The hearts were quickly removed and opened in the conventional method. The chambers were packed with cotton and the hearts were fixed in 10% neutral formalin for 48 hours. Twelve blocks of the myocardium harbouring the area of the macroscopic lesions and the His bundle were cut according to the method of Lev et al. (6) and routine paraffine embedding was followed by subserial sectioning. The different parts of the lesions and of the His bundle were easily identified.

Results

Electrophysiologic studies

In all animals complete heart block with a stable subsidary rhythm was achieved (Fig. 2a). Heart block remained complete and permanent in all dogs except one, in whom conduction resumed after 1 hour, with evidence of impaired conduction in the AV node. Table 1 demonstrates the results of studies performed in 10 animals 4 hours after the His bundle ablation. Prior to induction of AV block, all of them had QRS complexes ranging from 40–60 msec in duration (av = 48 msec). Following induction of AV block, the QRS of the escape rhythms ranged from 60–120 msec in duration (av = 95.5 msec). In all cases there was complete AV block, with escape rhythms ranging in cycle length from 670–2000 msec (av = 1464 msec). One dog had complete AV block only in the first hour, after then the conduction resumed.

Three weeks after induction of complete AV block His bundle deflection could be obtained in two dogs from the eight. In these two cases the H-V interval was 20 msec (Fig. 2b).

Pathology

Particular care was taken in the gross examination of the hearts. No perforation of the septum or tricuspid valve was observed.

In two of the animals, sacrificed one day after application the suction and DC shock, the gross alterations included foci of hemorrhage localized along the septal wall of atria. Minimal fibrinous deposition accompanying the hemorrhage was present. The hemorrhage was the most intensive close to the junction of the septal wall.

When looking at the chronic phase of lesion (3 weeks after the suction and DC shock) the marked reduction of acute reaction was evident leaving a rather circumscribed area of granulation with slight discoloration at the latter place.

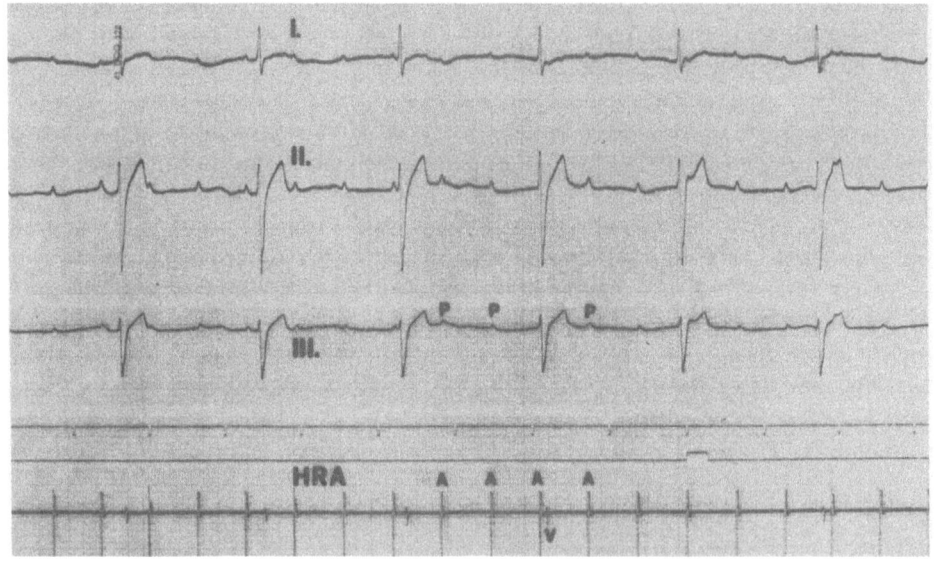

Fig. 2. a) Recording of surface electrocardiogram Leads I.–III. (top) and high right atrial (HRA) electrogram, demonstrating complete heart block (Atrial rate 94 beats/min, ventricular rate 33 beats/min). Paper speed 25 mm/sec.

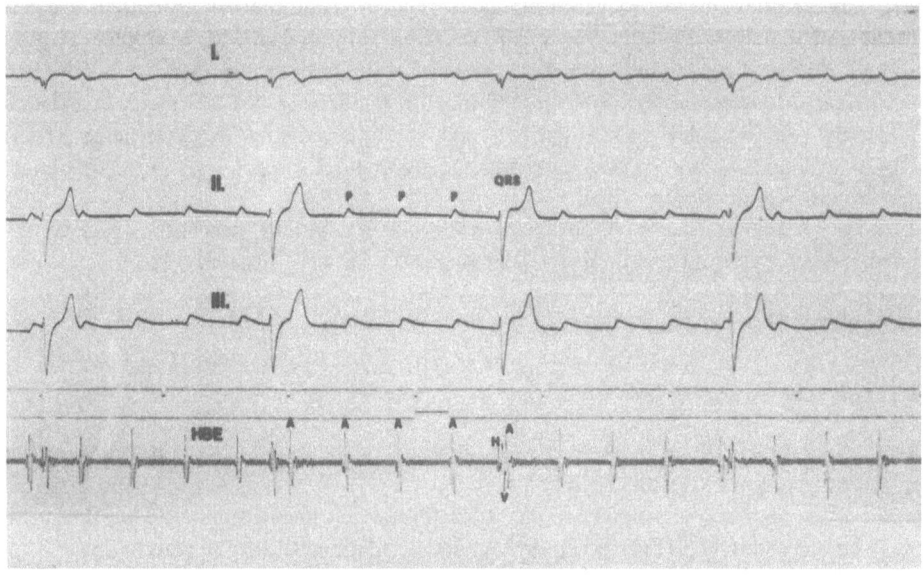

b) His bundle recording after catheter ablation of proximal part of His bundle. There is complete atrioventricular block. Each QRS complex is preceded by a His potential. Recordings (from the top down) are from standard electrocardiographic Leads I.–III. and bipolare recording of distal His bundle potential (HBE). Atrial cycle length: 420 msec ventricular cycle length: 1800 msec, H-V = 20 msec. Paper speed: 50 mm/sec.

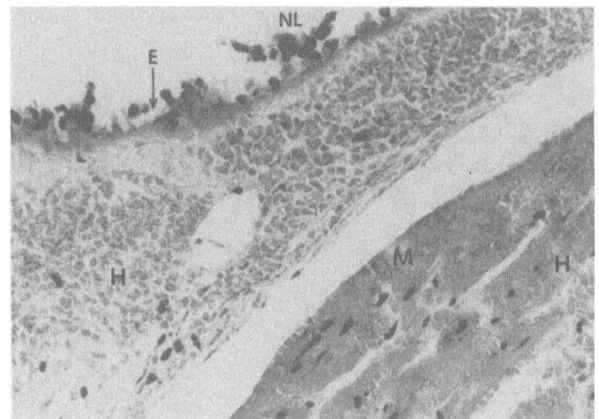

Fig. 3. a) Endocardium (E) of the right atrium with subjacent muscle (M) 2 hours after suction and electrocoagulation. Neutrophile leukocytic (NL) reaction with fibrinous exudation is evident on the surface. Note extensive hemorrhage (H). The gap between subendocardial hemorrhage and muscle is artefactual (HE stain, orig. magn. × 160).

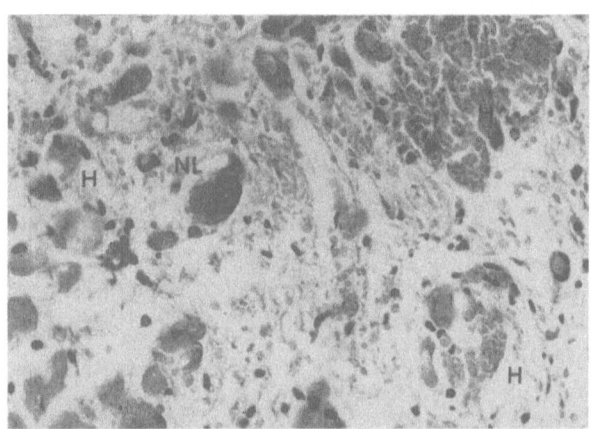

b) His bundle from the same animal. Hemorrhage (H) is accompanied by inflammatory reaction. NL = neutrophile leukocytes. Fragmentation and/or floccular degeneration of the fibers are obvious (HE stain, orig. magn. × 400).

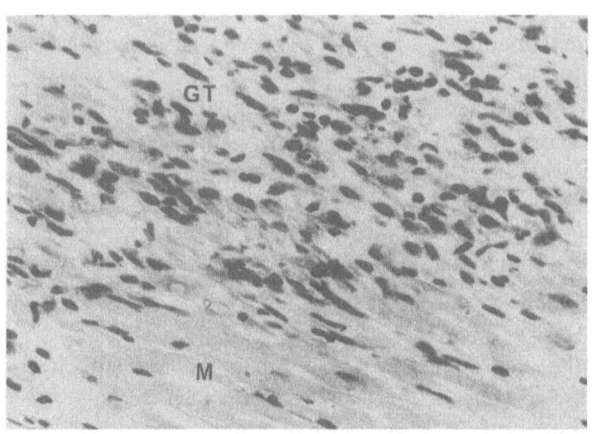

c) Chronic effect of coagulation. Three weeks following coagulation induced the same way as above. Marked lymphocytic, histiocytic and fibroblastic infiltration is shown. The granulation tissue (GT) replaces muscle fibers (M) (HE stain, orig. magn. × 160).

Table 1. Electrophysiological parameters before and after induction of complete AV block in dogs. Animal No. 10 had complete AV block only for one hour.

Dog	Spontaneous rhythm			
	QRS duration		ACL	VCL
	msec			
	A	B	B	B
1.	40	60	385	2000
2.	45	90	428	925
3.	40	120	640	1800
4.	50	70	480	670
5.	45	105	435	1175
6.	60	110	425	1765
7.	45	100	455	1330
8.	50	90	420	1800
9.	55	115	460	1715
10.	50	–	–	–

Abbreviations: A = before His bundle ablation; B = after His bundle ablation; ACL = atrial cycle lenght; VCL = ventricular cycle length.

Microscopically the lesion showed hemorrhage with inflammatory reaction (Fig. 3a). Fragmentation and/or floccular degeneration of the fibers was obvious (Fig. 3b). After 3 weeks marked lymphocytic, histiocytic and fibroblastic infiltration was shown. The granulation tissue replaced muscle fibers (Fig. 3c).

Discussion

On rare occasions, patients with recurrent supraventricular tachycardia remain disabled because available antiarrhythmic agents are ineffective or poorly tolerated. Interruption of the AV node-His bundle with implantation of a permanent ventricular pacemaker provides an alternative mode of therapy (1–5, 7, 10–13).

The need for complete heart block has resulted in the developement of several open-chest techniques to interrupt atrioventricular conduction at the His bundle or atrioventricular node (14–16). In an effort to achieve closed-chest ablation of the His-bundle, Beazell et al. attempted to deliver pulsed electrical energy from a cardioversion unit to the region of His bundle (17, 18). In 1981 Gonzales et al. described the closed-chest electrode-catheter technique for His bundle ablation in dogs (19). Recently Gallagher et al. reported the application of catheter technique for closed-chest ablation of the atrioventricular conduction system in humans (5).

The catheter technique for ablation of the His bundle does not require open-heart surgery, with its attendant risks (5). Malpositioning of the catheter could have serious consequences, potentially resulting in dysfunction of tricuspid valve or producing a focus of arrhythmia in the atrium or ventricle. We therefore used a self devised and made suction electrode catheter for His bundle ablation.

Within the past decade the suction electrode technique has become a simple, safe and easily reproducable method for recording the monophasic action potential of the intact human heart (20). We also have gained ample experience with this technique and construction of special suction electrodes (21, 22). We succeeded in the destruction of the AV node-His bundle region and in producing complete AV block by using only the suction technique without DC shock (23). Application of suction through the catheter fixes the electrode in a stable position on the His bundle and the dislocation can be avoided.

The described technique proved to be successful in 9 of 10 dogs. Only one shock was required, and chronic stable atrioventricular block persisted for the duration of the 3 week follow-up period in 8 dogs. The dogs appeared healthy, the implanted pacemakers were well tolerated.

The electrophysiological characteristics of the escape rhythm suggest a distal His bundle or fascicular origin. The QRS complex was always broad, the spontaneous heart rate varied between 30 and 87 beats/min and a His bundle deflection could be recorded before the QRS complex only in two cases.

Gross postmortem examination revealed no evidence of valvular scars. In addition, no perforation of the septum or tricuspid valve was observed.

This technique is an improvement of the method for electric His bundle ablation (5). Using this method the dislocation of catheter – which could have serious consequences – can be avoided. The technique is simple, safe and quick, requires no special apparatus, and can produce stable chronic atrioventricular block with a high degree of consistency.

We are greatful to János Szakácsi and János Koroknai for technical assistance.

References

1. Gianelli S Jr. Ayres SM, Gromprecht RF, Conkli EF, Kennedy RJ: Therapeutic surgical division of the human conduction system. JAMA 1967; 199: 155–160.
2. Harrison L., Gallagher JJ, Kasell J, et al: Cryosurgical ablation of the A-V node-His bundle: a new method for producing A-V block. Circulation 1977; 55: 463–470.
3. Gallagher JJ, Sealy WC, Anderson RW, et al: The surgical treatment of arrhythmias. In: Kulbertus HE, ed. Re-entrant arrhythmias; mechanisms and treatment. Baltimore: University Park Press, 1977; 351–366.
4. Sealy WC, Gallagher JJ, Kasell J: His bundle interruption for control of inappropriate ventricular responses to atrial arrhythmias. Ann Thorac Surg. 1981; 32: 429–438.
5. Gallagher JJ, Svenson RH, Kassel JH, German LD, Bardy GH, Broughton A and Critelli G: Catheter technique for closed-chest ablation of the atrioventricular conduction system. New Engl J Med 1982; 28: 194–200.
6. Lev M, Midran J, Erikson EE: A method for the histopathologic study of the atrioventricular node, bundle and branches. Arch Pathol 1951; 52: 73–83.
7. Dreifus LS, Nichols, H. Morre D, Watanabe Y, Truex R: Control of recurrent tachycardia of Wolff-Parkinson-White syndrome by surgical ligature of the A-V bundle. Circulation 1968; 38: 1030–1036.
8. Randall OS, Westerhof N, Van den Bos GC and Sipkema P: Production of chronic heart block in closed-chest dogs: an improved technique. Am J Physiol 1981; 241: H279–H282.
9. Meakins J: Experimental heart block with atrio-ventricular rhythm. Heart 1913; 5: 281–286.
10. Sealy WC, Anderson RW, Gallagher JJ: Surgical treatment of surpraventricular arrhythmias. J Thorac Cardiovasc Surg 1977; 73: 511–522.

11. Dunaway MC, King SB Jr, Hatcher CR Jr, Louge RB: Disabling supraventricular tachycardia of Wolff-Parkinson-White syndrome (type A) controlled by surgical A-V block and a demand pacemaker after epicardial mapping studies. Circulation 1972; 45: 522–528.

12. Edmonds JR Jr, Ellison RG, Crews TL: Surgically induced atrioventricular block as treatment for recurrent atrial tachycardia in Wolff-Parkinson-White syndrome. Circulation 1969; 39 (suppl I) 105–111.

13. Coumel P, Waynberger M, Fabiato A, Slama R, Aigueperse J, Bouvrain Y: Wolff-Parkinson-White syndrome. Problems in evaluation of multiple accessory pathways and surgical therapy. Circulation 1972; 45: 1216–1230.

14. Baum T, Peters JR, Butz F and Much DR: A method for the placement of His bundle electrodes and production of atrioventricular block in dogs. J Appl Physiol 1975; 38: 932–933.

15. Schlang HH, Kupersmith J, Weiman GF, Rhee C and Litwak RS: Creating permanent complete heart block by indirect cauterization without atriotomy. Am J Physiol 233 (Heart Circ Physiol) 1977; H723–H726.

16. Klein GJ, Sealy WC, Pritchett ELC, Harrison L, Hackel DB, Davis D, Kassel J, Wallace AG, and Gallagher JJ: Cryosurgical Ablation of the Atrioventricular Node-His Bundle: Long-term Follow-up and Properties of the functional Pacemaker. Circulation 1980; 61: 8–15.

17. Beazell J, Tan K, Criley J, Schulman J: The electrosurgical production of heart block without thoracotomy. Clin Res 1976; 24: 137A.

18. Beazell JW, Tan KS, Fewkes JL, Furmanski M, Fisher DA: Technique for the production of permanent lesions in the intracardiac conduction system. Clin Res 1977; 25: 141A.

19. Gonzales R, Scheiman MM, Margaretten W, Rubinstein M: Closed-chest electrode-catheter technique for His bundle ablation in dogs. Am J Physiol 1981; 241: H283–H287.

20. Olsson B., Varnauskas E., and Korsgren M: Further Improved Method for Measuring Monophasic Action Potential of the Intact Human Heart. J Electrocardiology 1971; 4: 19–23.

21. Polgár P, Wórum F, Kovács P, and Lörincz I: Improved Suction Electrode Catheter for Recording Monophasic Action Potentials and Stimulation of the Heart. In: Claude Meere ed Proceedings of the VIth World Symposium on Cardiac Pacing, Montreal 1979; Chap. 4–7.

22. Polgár P, Kovács P, Wórum F, and Lörincz I: The prognostic value of right atrial monophasic action potential after conversion of atrial fibrillation. In: Antalóczy Z, Préda I, eds. Electrocardiology '81, Budapest: Publishing House of the Hungarian Academy of Sciences, 1982; 549–552.

23. Polgár P, Molnár P, Békássy Sz, Kovács P, Lörincz I, and Wórum F: A new technique for His bundle ablation using suction electrode catheter. In: Proceedings of 10th International Congress on Electrocardiology 1983, Bratislava, VEDA, Publishing House of the Slovak Academy of Sciences, In Press.

Authors' address:
Dr. Péter Polgár
I. Dept. of Medicine
University Medical School
P.O. Box 19
H-4012 Debrecen
Hungary

Transvenous Ablation of Atrioventricular Conduction by High Energy Shock – a New Method of Tachycardia Control

D. E. Ward, K. Hellestrand, A. Nathan, A. J. Camm

Summary: Six patients were referred for investigation and treatment of refractory arrhythmias. Each patient had failed to respond to antiarrhythmic drugs and transvenous ablation of atrioventricular conduction was thought appropriate. With a temporary ventricular pacing system in situ, a second electrode was used to record His and atrial electrograms. A 270–300 watt-second shock was delivered through this lead when the His potential was maximised. The tachycardia was controlled in 5/6 patients and the procedure was without deleterious effects.

Currently, there are three basic approaches to the treatment of tachycardias; drug therapy, pacemaker therapy and surgery. The last two methods are usually considered only if drug therapy has been ineffective or is inappropriate. Pacemaker treatment is most applicable to tachycardia which may be terminated by properly timed electrical stimuli (1). Surgery is considered in patients with tachycardias which cannot be reliably and effectively controlled by antiarrhythmic drugs and for which pacemaker treatment is either not applicable or ineffective (2). In patients with refractory supraventricular or junctional tachycardias not associated with anomalous atrioventricular connections the operation of choice is ablation of AV conduction by controlled selective damage to the AV node-His bundle region (2, 3) thus eliminating the ventricular response to the tachycardia. This has been achieved by localised cryothermal injury with the patient on normothermic cardiopulmonary bypass. Recently, Scheinman et al. (4) described a technique of producing AV block in dogs using a high energy transvenous shock. The same group have recently reported there experience with the technique in five patients (5) and Gallagher et al. have reported on 9 patients (6). In this report we describe our results in six patients with supraventricular tachycardias which had proved difficult to treat with antiarrhythmic drugs.

Patients and methods

Six patients, 3 men and 3 women, aged between 37 and 80 years were referred for investigation and treatment of refractory tachycardias. The clinical information is summarised in Table 1. All patients had been treated with at least 2 antiarrhythmic drugs including amiodarone in five patients. Four patients had associated illnesses which made surgery a high risk procedure. Pacemaker therapy was inappropriate in those patients with incessant atrial tachycardia or recurrent atrial fibrillation and was unsuccessful in the patients with atrial flutter or AV nodal tachycardia. No patient had evidence of recent myocardial infarction.

Table 1. Clinical data. Abbreviations: PSVT = persistent supraventricular tachycardia; PAFL = paroxysmal atrial flutter; CAF = chronic atrial fibrillation; AM = amiodarone; DG = digoxin; DS = disopyramide; BB = beta blocker; VE = verapamil; PH = phenytoin; QU = quinidine; CRF = chronic renal failure; CVD = cerebrovascular disease; MI = myocardial infarction; MR = mitral regurgitation; MVR = mitral valve replacement, PHT = pulmonary hypertension.

Patient	Age	Sex	Clinical arrhythmia	Drugs	Associated illness	Previous DC shocks
1	62	F	PSVT–5 days 10 years	Am, Dg, BB, Ve, Ds	CRF, hypertension CVD, chest infection	10
2	51	M	PSVT–7 days 1 week	Dg, Am	Poor LV function Old MI	0
3	54	F	PSVT–6 mths + 15 years	Dg, Am, BB, Ve	Thoracoplasty Breast carcinoma	3
4	37	F	SVT 5 years +	Dg, Ve, BB, Ds	None	0
5	80	M	PAFL, PAT 5 months	Dg, Ve, Am, BB, Ds	Pericardial disease	4
6	55	M	PAF 5 years +	Dg, Am, Ve, BB, Ds	None	0

All patients underwent an electrophysiological study prior to transvenous shock. The methods of processing and recording signals have been described previously (7). The results together with the electrocardiographic appearances are summarised in Table 2. A pacing electrode was positioned in the right ventricle prior to transvenous shock in all patients. After the tachycardia had been characterised, attention was focused on the recordings from the His bundle catheter. A new 6 or 7F gauge woven dacron bipolar electrode (USCI) was used in each patient. The electrode catheter was manipulated to record the largest possible bipolar His potential. Unipolar signals were then recorded between each electrode pole and a skin electrode in the region of the left scapula. The aim of these manoeuvres was to record as large a unipolar His potential as possible while preserving a large atrial electrogram as suggested by Gallagher et al. (6). When this was achieved the patient was anaesthetised with intravenous methohexitone.

Using specially constructed adaptors, the pole exhibiting the largest amplitude His deflection was connected to the output of a standard direct current cardioverter with the other terminal connected to a backplate in the region of the left scapula. Using ECG synchronisation, approximately 275–300 watt-seconds of energy was delivered to the catheter.

Results

The results are shown in Table 2. Three patients developed sustained AV block after one shock. Three patients had two or more shocks. Two of these (nos. 4 and 5) AV block lasted for several hours before conduction resumed. Despite further shocks on a separate occasion sustained AV block could not be produced. One patient (no. 1) maintained AV

Table 2. Electrocardiographic and electrophysiological data. AT = atrial tachycardia; SR = sinus rhythm; PAVNT = paroxysmal AV nodal tachycardia; PAFL = paroxysmal atrial flutter; AF = atrial fibrillation; JER = junctional escape rhythm; 1 = first degree AV block; NR = not recorded; RBBB = right bundle branch block; (V) = ventricular rate.

| | Initial ECG and EPS data | | | | | Final ECG and EPS data | | | | | |
Pt	Rhythm	Rate (V)	QRS	Axis	HV	Rhythm	Rate (V)	QRS	Axis	HV	No. shocks
1	AT 1:1	140–160	N	0°	60	AT	140	RBBB	+110°	Nr	2
2	AT 1:1	130–180	N	−30°	55	AT, AVB, JER	60	N	0°	55	1
3	AT 1:1	140–180	N	+70°	50	AT, AVB, JER	60	N	+70°	25	1
4	AVNT SR	180	N	0°	40	SR	70	RBBB	−45°	40	2,3
5	PAFL 2:1	160–185	N	0°	45	SR, 1° AVB	72	RBBB	−15°	45	1,2
6	PAF	100–180	N	+30°	40	JER	50	N	+30°	NR	1

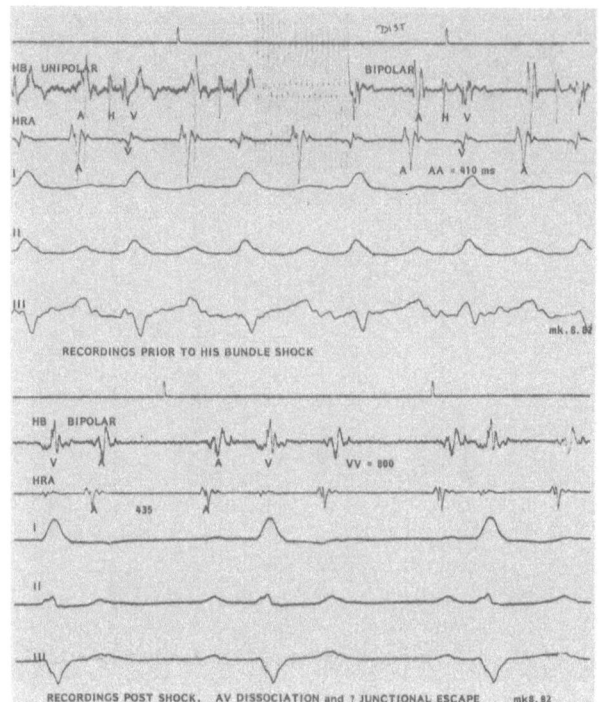

Fig. 1. Upper panel: simultaneous recordings of surface ECG leads I, II, III with intracardiac recordings from the His bundle (HB) and high right atrial (HRA) regions during chronic atrial tachycardia in patient 3.
A = atrial electrogram
H = His bundle electrogram
V = ventricular electrogram
Lower panel: recordings immediately after transvenous ablation of AV conduction. Atrial tachycardia continues.
Paper speed in figures 1 and 2 = 100 mm/second.

conduction after 2 shocks which had caused right bundle branch block and right axis deviation. Two days later she developed complete AV block but died as a result of bronchopneumonia. Of the three patients with incessant atrial tachycardia, the arrhythmia was terminated in one but recurred 24 hours later. Five patients developed a spontaneous escape rhythm after shocking. In all of these the escape rhythm appeared after a latent period of 2 to 10 minutes after the shock procedure (Figure 1). In no patient could a His potential be recorded immediately after the shock regardless of the presence or absence of AV conduction or an escape rhythm. Prior to implantation of a pacemaker in four patients, intracardiac recordings were repeated (Figure 2). A His potential could be recorded in all four patients (Table 2). In three patients the HV interval was identical to that recorded prior to shock. Two patients had escape rhythms at the time of restudy. The characteristics of the escape rhythm are summarised in Table 3A. Junctional recovery times were performed in these patients as described elsewhere (8) (Fig. 3). In one patient (no. 2) the escape focus was above the His bundle with a normal HV interval. In another patient, the escape beats were not preceded by a normal His spike but a small right bundle branch potential or distal His potential was recorded. The QRS complexes were identical in axis and morphology to conducted beats prior to shock. This escape rhythm probably arose high in the fascicular system or the distal His bundle. Atropine 1.2 mg intravenously did not result in significant increases in the escape rate in these patients but a shortening of the junctional recovery time was noted. Attempts to provoke AV nodal tachycardia in patient 4 were unsuccessful despite the return of AV conduction.

894

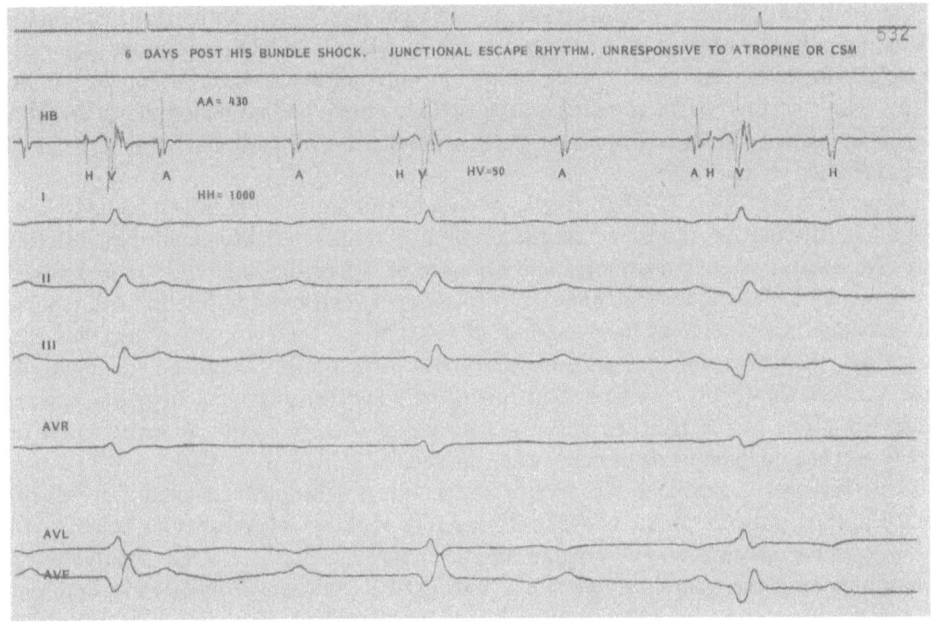

Fig. 2. Escape rhythm arising above the His bundle 6 days after shock in patient 2. Note that left atrial tachycardia continues.

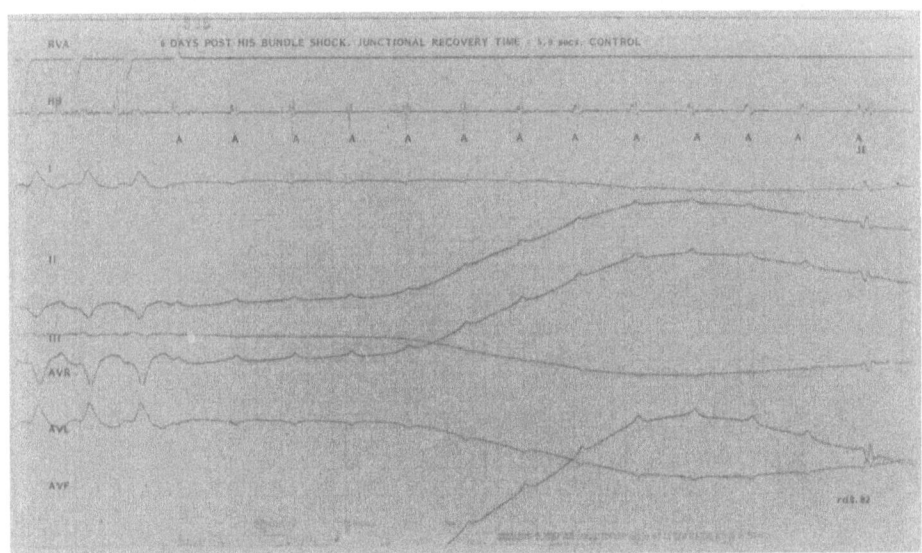

Fig. 3. Suppression of the junctional escape rhythm by right ventricular pacing in patient 2. Atrial tachycardia (A) continues.

Changes in the QRS axis or the appearance of right bundle branch block of conducted beats after shock occurred in all three patients in whom conduction returned. One patient developed marked right axis deviation and one had left axis deviation. In the patients with "narrow" QRS complex escape rhythms, there was no major change in QRS axis. One patient (no. 2) had transient tachycardia-dependent left bundle branch block of the junctional escape rhythm.

Cardiac enzyme (CPK and HBD) rises were noted in all patients but in two patients, conventional external DC shocks within the previous 48 hours may have contributed to this rise. No clinical or electrocardiographic evidence of myocardial infarction was observed in any patient. One patient (no. 3) had two episodes of ventricular fibrillation 4 days after transvenous shock. The serum potassium at this time was 3.0 mmol/l. When this was corrected, there was no recurrence of ventricular arrhythmias. Another patient (no. 4) had transient sinus tachycardia after the procedure. No other unwanted arrhythmias were observed. None of the patients had any evidence of tricuspid valvular malfunction or other new haemodynamic disturbance after the shock.

Five patients had permanent pacemakers implanted. A ventricular demand unit was selected in three patients. In the patient with severely impaired left ventricular function, an AV sequential pacemaker was programmed to trigger on alternate atrial signals during continuing atrial tachycardia giving him a ventricular rate varying from 60 to 90 bpm.

Table 3. A) Characteristics of the junctional escape rhythm. CL = cycle length; C = control; A = atropine. B) Follow-up data. CK = creatine kinase; HBD = hydroxybutyric acid dehydrogenase; GOT = glutamate-oxalate transaminase; AV = atrioventricular; V = ventricular; FI = flecainide; Other abbreviations as in tables 1–3.

A

Pt	Site	HV	QRS	CL msec		JRT msec	
				C	A	C	A
2	nodal	55	narrow	1040	990	5920	1660
3	?fascicular	25	narrow	1080	1050	2250	1620

B

Pt	Drugs	ECG/tape	Max enzyme rise			Pyro scan/echo	FU months
			CK	HBD	GOT		
1	–	–	39	211*	–	–	died
2	nil	AV pacing	35	196*	–	negative	5
3	nil	V pacing	403*	261*	–	negative	6
4	BB	SR	–	362*	58	negative	7
5	FI	SR	43	172	–	negative	3
6	nil	V pacing	–	137	45	negative	3

* = significant elevation

Real-time two dimensional echocardiograms were performed before and after the shock in 4 patients. There was no echocardiographic evidence of tricuspid valvular malfunction. Amplitude-processing (9) of echocardiographic signals in 2 patients did not reveal any change in echo "density" in the region of the inlet septum. A pyrophosphate scan (10) revealed positive uptake in the septal region in one of two patients.

The patients have been followed for 2 to 9 months. There has been no recurrence of conduction in four patients and no recurrence of junctional tachycardias in patient 4 (see Table 3B). One patient (no. 5) continues to have paroxysmal atrial arrhythmias. Another patient (no. 2) died 6 months later as a result of left ventricular disease. Detailed histological studies of the AV conduction system are in progress.

Discussion

Surgical ablation of AV nodal-His bundle conduction is a recognised approach to the treatment of atrial and junctional tachycardia which cannot be controlled by drug treatment (2, 3). Until recently this could be reliably achieved only by open heart surgery with the patient on cardiopulmonary bypass. Various methods of inflicting damage, including incision, diathermy and cryosurgery have been used. The latter method has been popular because of the ability to cause reversible damage by limited cooling, thus improving the accuracy of the procedure (2, 3). However effective the direct approach, the risks of open heart surgery are a disadvantage. These risks may be prohibitive in very sick patients as was the case in four of our patients. A transvenous method of ablating AV conduction is therefore a major advance in the management of refractory supraventricular tachycardias. Previous experimental attempts to produce AV block using "closed-chest" methods have included injection of formalin (11) and electrosurgery (12). Each of these methods is unreliable and in addition requires specialised equipment. They are, therefore, unsuitable for use in human patients. This new method introduced after detailed animal studies by Gonzalez and colleagues (4), requires adaptation of standard DC cardioversion apparatus. In addition, the same electrode may be used to deliver the shock and record signals immediately before and after the shock procedure. This is a considerable advantage because it appears that correct positioning of the electrode before delivery of the shock is critical. Gallagher (6) has emphasised the importance of recording a good sized atrial electrogram as well as His potential before shocking. It may be that the method is more likely to induce complete AV block if the high-energy shock is delivered in the region of the atrionodal rather than the AV node-His junction. Failure to achieve optimal positioning of the electrode may explain why one patient did not develop immediate AV block. Subsequent electrocardiograms exhibited right bundle branch block and marked right axis deviation suggesting damage to the fascicular system as well as the right bundle. Such damage could have been caused if the catheter was advanced some way into the right ventricular inlet although His bundle lesions could produce these changes (13, 14). It is interesting to note that marked changes in QRS axis or the appearance of fixed bundle branch block occurred only in those patients in whom AV block was not sustained or could not be induced. It is probable therefore that a more distal position of the electrode delivering the shock is less likely to cause sufficient, appropriately sited injury to result in permanent AV block. The reasons for failure to achieve complete AV block in patient with AV nodal tachycardia are not clear. However, and "ideal" result was achieved in that tachycardias did not recur and AV conduction was preserved. This has also been documented in one of the patients in Gallagher's series (6). A similar result has also been reported following direct cryosurgical ablation of the AV node-His bundle (15).

The approximate delivered energy used in our patients is intermediate between that used by Scheinman et al. (5) and Gallagher et al. (6). We, like each of these groups, had several instances where more than one shock was necessary. On no single occasion was more than three shocks delivered.

The escape rhythm observed in our patients is similar to that described in the series of Gallagher et al. (6). However, Scheinman et al. (5) documented only slow, wide QRS escape rhythms and could not record either distal or proximal His potentials suggesting a low escape focus. Differences in technique may account for the difference between these results and those of Gallagher (6) and our own which suggest that the characteristics of the escape rhythm after transvenous His bundle shock are very similar to those observed after direct cryosurgical ablation (8, 16, 17). The site of block, the nature of the subsidiary escape focus and the response to atropine are presumably determined by the extent and location of damage.

The indications for transvenous His bundle ablation are not yet clearly established. However, we feel it reasonable to consider this new technique in any situation where surgery would be considered appropriate. An additional group of patients are those in whom surgical ablation is electrophysiologically appropriate but in whom the risk of operation is high because of general debilitation or associated disease. The safety of the technique is reaffirmed by our results. However, it must be appreciated that malpositioning of the catheter may lead to extensive trauma due to dissipation of high energies within the chambers and vessels of the heart. Success of the method is critically dependent on electrode position and high quality electrograms are therefore essential.

The mechanism by which AV block is produced is not known. Our observations (unpublished) with isolated hearts suggest that a large pressure wave is developed within the heart causing an explosion. Thus, localised barotrauma may be the mechanism of disruption of electrical continuity of the AV node-His bundle. Tidd et al. (18) investigated the effects of a surgical electronic lithoclast capable of delivering up to 18 watt-seconds over a few microseconds. They documented the formation of a high pressure wave and concluded that this alone was sufficient to fragment calculi. They suggested that the time-integral of pressure rather than the maximum developed pressure was the main instrument of damage. They emphasised the potential hazards of this effect. A similar mechanism is probably responsible for damage to conducting tissues. It seems likely therefore that the muscular and fibrous wall of the heart (pericardium and myocardium) and the surrounding thoracic contents are important in the dissipation of energy. For this reason it is probably unwise to attempt transvenous ablation in patients with conditions which may impair safe dissipation of energy (eg, total pericardiectomy, pneumonectomy) until further information is available.

As yet, the method has been used only to ablate the AV conduction over the normal conduction pathway. Gallagher et al. (6) inadvertently interrupted conduction in a septal accessory pathway but we do not recommend the technique for this application at present. Although potentially useful for abolition of ventricular tachycardias (especially if the right bundle branch is involved in a reentry circuit), we feel that present information is insufficient to support the use the technique for this purpose.

Conclusion

The technique of ablation of AV conduction by high-energy shock delivered to the region of the His bundle is safe and effective. We believe that this method, properly employed, is an important advance in the managment of refractory supraventricular tachycardias. In particular, it avoids the risk of surgery which would have been the only alternative in these patients. The technique should only be performed in centres with the equipment and experience of clinical cardiac electrophysiological methods.

Acknowledgements

We would like thank Drs A Leatham, RV Gibson and DG Gibson for allowing us to report their patients. We are very grateful to the Medical Electronics Departments of the Brompton Hospital and St Bartholomew's Hospital for preparing and testing the equipment.

References

1. Ward DE, Camm AJ, Spurrell RAJ: The response of regular reentrant supraventricular tachycardias to right heart stimulation. PACE 1979; 2: 586–595.
2. Gallagher JJ: Surgical treatment for arrhythmias: current status and future directions. Am J Card 1978; 41: 1035–1044.
3. Camm AJ, Ward DE, Spurrell RAJ, Rees GM: Cryothermal mapping and cryoablation in the treatment of refractory cardiac arrhythmias. Circulation 1980; 62: 67–74.
4. Gonzalez R, Scheinman MM, Margaretten W, Rubinstein M: Closed-chest electrode catheter technique for His bundle ablation in dogs. Am J Physiol (H) 1981; 241: 283–287.
5. Scheinman MM, Morady F, Hess DS, Gonzalez R: Catheter-induced ablation of the atrioventricular junction to control refractory supraventricular arrhythmias. JAMA 1982; 248: 851–855.
6. Gallagher JJ, Svenson RH, Kasell JH, German LD, Bardy GH, Broughton A, Critelli G: Catheter technique for closed-chest ablation of the atrioventricular conduction system. A therapeutic alternative for the treatment of refractory supraventricular tachycardia. N Engl J Med 1982; 306: 194–200.
7. Ward DE, Camm AJ: Methodologic problems in the use of atrial pacing studies in the assessment of AV conduction. Clin Card 1980; 3: 155–162.
8. Bexton RS, Ward DE, Camm AJ: Electrophysiological characteristics of junctional pacemakers in congenital AV block and following His bundle cryoablation. Clin Card 1982.
9. Logan-Sinclair RB, Wong CM, Gibson DG: Clinical application of amplitude processing of echocardiographic images. Br Heart J 1981; 45: 621–627.
10. Dymond DS, Jarritt PH, Britton KE, Langley D, Spurrell RAJ: Positive myocardial scintigraphy at the bedside – evaluation using a portable gamma camera. Postgrad Med J 1978; 54: 641–648.
11. Fisher VJ, Lee KJ, Christianson LC, Kavaler F: Production of chronic atrioventricular block in dogs without thoracotomy. J Appl Physiol 1966; 21: 1119–1121.
12. Beazell J, Tan K, Criley J, Schulman J: The electrosurgical production of heart block without thoracotomy. Clin Res 1976; 24: 137A.
13. Narula OS: Longitudinal dissociation in the His bundle. Bundle branch block due to asynchronous conduction within the His bundle in man. Circulation 1977; 56: 996–1006.
14. El-Sherif N, Amat-y-Leon F, Schonfield C, Scherlag B, Rosen KM, Lazzara R, Wyndham C: Normalization of bundle branch block patterns by distal His bundle pacing. Clinical and experimental evidence of longitudinal dissociation in the pathologic His bundle. Circulation 1978; 57: 473–483.
15. Pritchett ELC, Anderson RW, Benditt D, Kasell J, Harrison L, Wallace AG, Sealy WC, Gallagher JJ: Reentry within the AV node: surgical cure with preservation of atrio-ventricular conduction. Circulation 1979; 60: 440–446.

16. Klein GJ, Sealy WC, Pritchett ELC, Harrison L, Hackel DB, Davis D, Kassell J, Wallace AG, Gallagher JJ: Cryosurgical ablation of the atrio ventricular node – His bundle: long term follow-up and properties of the junctional pacemaker. Circulation 1980; 61: 1–15.
17. Gonzalez R, Scheinman MM, Thomas A, Desai J, Peters R, Dzindzio B: Electrophysiologic characterization of surgically induced His bundle rhythm in man. PACE 1981; 4: 152–160.
18. Tidd MJ, Webster J, Cameron Wright H, Harrison IR: Mode of action of a surgical electronic lithoclast – high speed pressure, cinematographic and Schlieren recordings following an ultra-short underwater electronic discharge. Biomed. Engin 1976; 14: 5–24.

Authors' address:
D. E. Ward, M.D.
Cardiology Department
ST George's Hospital
London SW17

Creation of Experimental Atrioventricular Block using DC Shock via a Percutaneous Transaortic Electrode Catheter

O.-J. Ohm, L. S. Dreifus, H. Mitamura, Ch. Sauermelch, H. Haupt, S. Vail, M. Schaffenburg, E. L. Michelson

The need to develop an experimental model in the closed chest animal for the study of hemodynamic and electrophysiologic effects of various physiologic and pharmacologic interventions has led several investigators to develop means for ablating the atrioventricular (AV) node and/or bundle of His. In addition, the potential clinical utility of such a method has also been apparent (1, 2).

Previous experimental procedures including blunt dissection (3, 4), formaldehyde injection (5–8), cauterization (9, 10), cryo-ablation (11) and recently, pulsed electrical coagulation (12–15) of the AV node have been only partially successful in producing permanent AV block.

Recently, pulsed electrical coagulation for His bundle ablation produced by a 30–100 Watt DC shock delivered through an insulated pacing catheter passed percutaneously, transvenously to the atrioventricular junction in the right ventricle, has been described. This technique appeared superior to other methods since it could be performed rapidly in a closed chest animal or individual; however, the technique was occasionally inconsistent or required multiple shocks due to catheter mobility in the vicinity of the His bundle and tricuspid valve.

This study describes pulsed electrical disruption of the His bundle using a percutaneous, retrograde arterial, aortic approach, with positioning of the catheter tip in the region of the non-coronary cusp of the aortic valve.

Methods

A standard commercially available, unaltered 6 or 7 French (USCI, 5655, 5656) tri- or quadripolar catheter was introduced via the left carotid artery. The electrode tips were positioned without fluoroscopy above the aortic valve until a maximum bipolar His bundle electrogram was recorded (Fig. 1). The heart contractions were then usually transmitted through the catheter and indicated that the electrode tip was placed near one of the aortic cusps. Unipolar His bundle electrograms were usually unsatisfactory due to electromagnetic interference. Since our technique for placing the electrode catheter indi-

Dr. Ohm is supported in part by grants from the Rebekka Ege Hegermanns Legaey to the University of Bergen, Norway and the Royal Norwegian Council for Scientific and industrial Research.
Dr. Michelson is recipient of Clinical Investigator Award 5K08 HL00709-03 from the National Heart, Lung and Blood Institute, National Institutes of Health, Bethesda, MD

901

Fig. 1. His bundle recording from the aortic root at the non-coronary cusp. Electrograms from A-atrium, H-His bundle, and V ventricle.

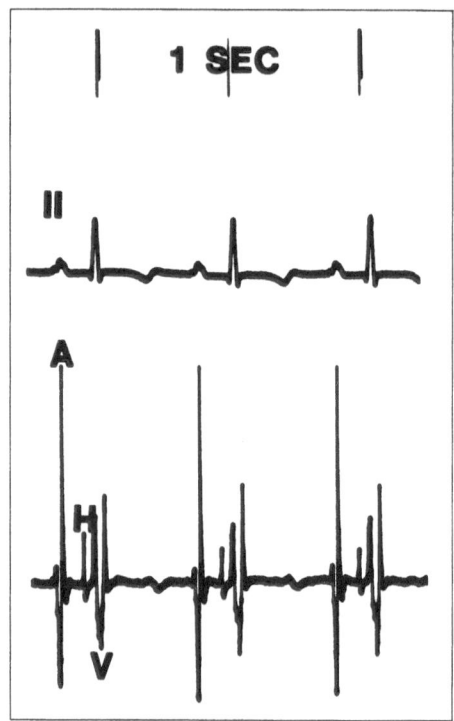

cated that the electrode tip was always in good contact with the tissue, this electrode was kept connected to the electrogram switch box. The other poles of the catheter were then disconnected. A separate indifferent electrode lead from the switch box to a ground plate was placed under the back of the dog. One pole from a defibrillator was then connected to the His catheter through the switch box and the other pole to the common ground plate. Standard ECG lead II was monitored on an oscilloscope, recorded on tape and used to synchronize the DC shock from the R-wave.

Material

Two groups of animals were investigated.

Group I

Preliminary studies were done in 9 chronic myocardial infarction dogs to determine the feasibility of the technique and the energy requirements for producing permanent atrioventricular block. These dogs were studied open chest through a midsternotomy. In all animals, DC shocks from 20 to 80 watt seconds were sufficient for producing atrioventricular blocks. In 5 animals one DC shock from 20 to 40 watt seconds; in 3 animals two DC shocks from 20 to 80 watt seconds and in one animal three DC shocks from 20 to 80 watt seconds were applied to produce complete atrioventricular block, lasting throughout the observation period of up to 7–8 hours.

Group II

A second group, also consisting of 9 dogs, to be utilized in a study of AV synchronous pacing, was prepared in the following way: 10 days before the study a limited left-side thoracotomy was done and temporary pacing wires were attached to the left ventricle and the left atrial appendage and tunneled subcutaneously to exit through the nape of the neck for subsequent study. Based on the data in the pilot study shocks of 80 to 100 watt seconds were used for ablation.

Results

Group I

From 1 to 3 shocks were necessary to establish permanent atrioventricular block (Table 1). Permanent atrioventricular block lasted for the duration of each experiment.
The baseline sinus cycle length ranged from 310 to 575 msec with a mean of 431 msec. Since these animals were utilized for experiments using type I antiarrhythmic drugs, the QRS duration was abnormally long prior to the induction of DC shock. The escape rhythm at the end of the study following the creation of AV block showed a mean of 1045 msec with a range of 465 msec to 1400 msec. In each case AV block was produced demonstrating the feasibility of this method in this group of open-chest animals.

Group II

From 1–4 shocks were necessary to establish permanent atrioventricular block in this group (Fig. 2) (Table 2). The QRS width increased in all but one dog from initial values of 40 to 62 ms, mean 50 ms to 45 to 120 ms, mean 80 ms at the end of the experiment. Fig. 2A shows the time course of events following an 80 watt-second shock. Immediately following an 80 watt-second DC shock atrial fibrillation occurred with the first escape ventricular beat occurring after a 6-second pause. At the end of the experiment, 7 hours

Table 1. Number of DC Shocks and energy requirements in 9 open chest dogs.

Number of DC Shocks	Number of Animals	Energy Watt-sec
1	5	20 (1), 40 (4)
2	3	20 + 80 (2) 40 + 80 (2)
3	1	20 + 80 + 80 (1)

Table 2. Number of DC Shocks and energy requirements in 9 closed chest dogs.

Number of DC Shocks	Number of Animals	Energy Watt-sec
1	5	80 (2); 100 (3)
2	1	80 × 2
3	2	80 × 3; 80 × 1 + 100 × 2
4	1	80 × 3; 100 × 1

Fig. 2A. An 80 watt-second DC shock producing complete AV block. Aortic root blood pressure (Ao). Large time lines = 200 msec.

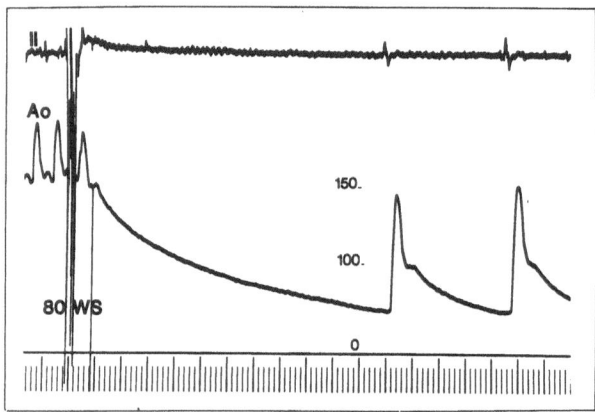

Fig. 2B. Persistence of complete AV block.

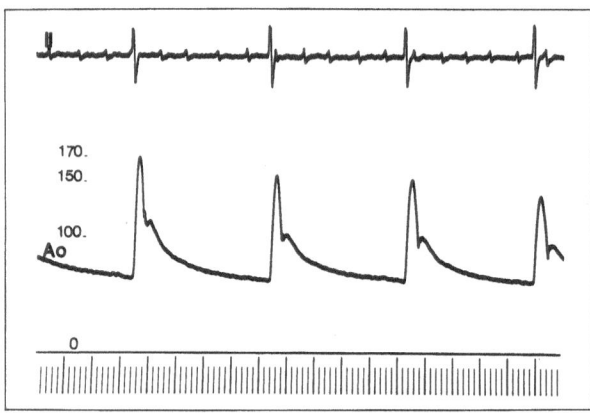

later, there was still total atrioventricular block with a ventricular escape interval of 2500 ms (Fig. 2B). The QRS width was 120 ms compared to 80 ms during sinus rhythm.

Atrial tachycardia occurred in one dog, atrial fibrillation in 3 and ventricular fibrillation in 3 dogs, with atrial fibrillation and ventricular fibrillation both occurring in 1 dog. In 2 dogs the ventricular fibrillation was treated with external DC shocks. The other arrhythmias reverted spontaneously to total atrioventricular block.

In one dog an 80 watt-second DC shock was introduced inadvertently from the proximal rather than distal electrode resulting in transient atrial tachycardia. A second 80 watt-second shock from the distal electrode was immediately followed by total atrioventricular block.

The baseline sinus cycle lengths in the 9 dogs ranged from 315 ms to 390 ms with a mean of 352 ms. At the end of the experiments the sinus cycle lengths varied from 255 to 432 ms with a mean of 349 ms. The cycle length was decreased in 4, increased in 4 and was unchanged in 1 animal.

The escape rhythm at the end of the experiment was a mean of 1374 ms with a range of 865 to 2220 ms. In 5 dogs the QRS was narrow (< 80 ms) and in 4 dogs wide (> 80 ms) after induction of AV block.

The dogs were sacrificed at the end of the experiments.

Areas of hemorrhagic injury were verified in all animals by dissection, and were localized predominantly to the non-coronary cusp in 14 dogs and in both the non-coronary and right coronary cusps in 4 dogs.

A typical lesion localized to the non-coronary cusp is shown in a dog in which a single shock of 80 watt-second resulted in total atrioventricular block (Fig. 3A). The needle is placed in the left coronary ostium. Note the destruction of the AV node with associated hemorrhage and edema (Fig. 3B).

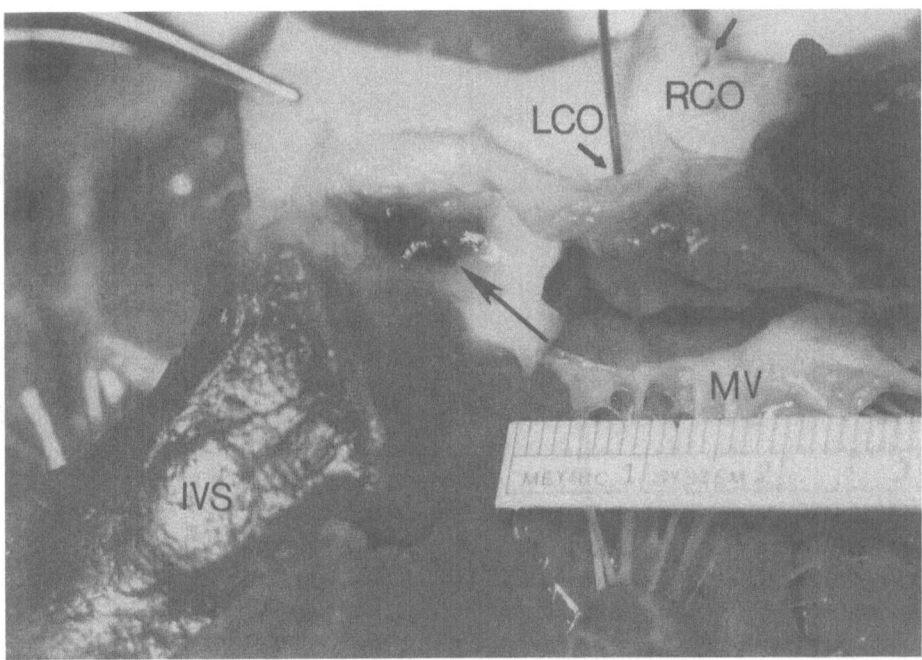

Fig. 3A. View of aortic valve below the non-coronary cusp (arrow), hematoma of the aortic valve. LCO = Left coronary ostium; RCO = Right coronary ostium; MV = Mitral valve; IVS = Interventricular septum.

Fig. 3B. Photomicrograph of the penetrating of the AV node showing severe destruction of normal architecture. Note dark large pleomorphic cells showing swelling and coagulation necrosis. Small dark cells are of inflammatory origin. AT = Atrial tissue; AVN = Compact portion of AV node; RB = Right bundle; LB = Left bundle.

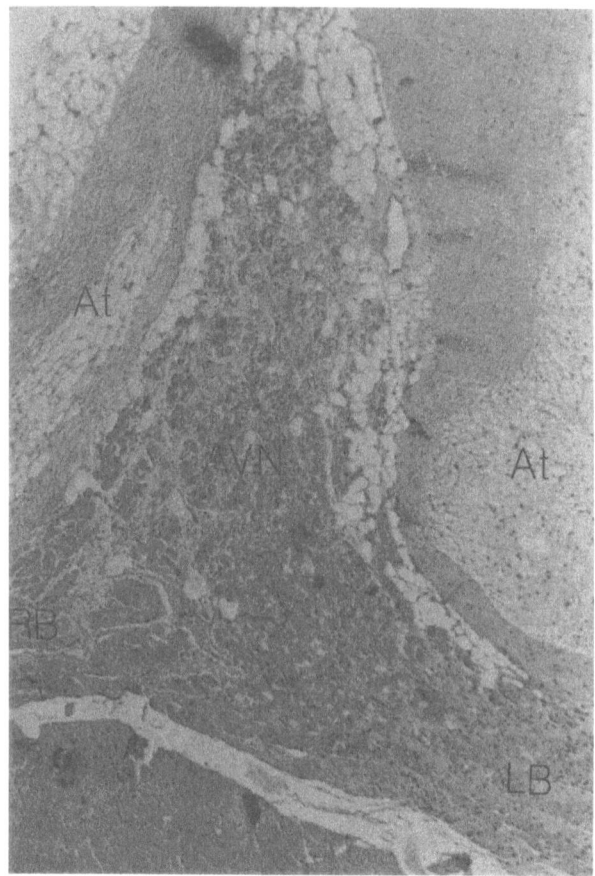

Discussion

Recently, pulsed energy electrical ablation of the His bundle as well as accessory bypass tracts and areas of ventricular ectopic impulse formation have been successful in patients (13). An effective and consistent method to produce AV block in closed chest dogs is also important and useful in developing experimental research models.

Since the non-coronary cusp of the aortic valve lies behind the His bundle, we considered that a DC shock delivered in the region of the non-coronary cusp as evidenced by an optimal His bundle recording, would be effective in producing a permanent AV block.

Our studies requiring heart block dogs to study the hemodynamic effects of synchronous and asynchronous atrioventricular pacing mandated that a quick effective method be developed to establish AV block prior to the initiation of our hemodynamic experimental protocol. Previous methods of positioning the electrode catheter in the region of the His bundle and tricuspid valve on the right side of the heart were inconsistent and produced only transitory atrioventricular block even after repeated DC shocks (9, 10, 12, 14, 15).

Previous studies have reported the induction of various cardiac arrhythmias including atrial and ventricular fibrillation, and ventricular tachycardia using various ablative methods (12, 14, 15). Ventricular fibrillation in the closed chest dog was produced in three instances in our limited series. In one dog ventricular fibrillation reverted to sinus rhythm and AV block spontaneously while two other animals required DC shock. Atrial fibrillation was produced in three instances and reverted to sinus rhythm and complete AV block in all cases.

The advantages of the aortic root approach to produce chronic AV block appears related to the rather precise positioning of the electrode catheter tip at the site of either the non-coronary or occasionally the right coronary sinus. In either of these positions, the catheter tip is not displaced due to the mechanical motion of the heart, at the time of the DC shock. Hence, this positions appear to be useful in producing atrioventricular block.

The pathology produced by electroshock shown in Fig. 3 indicates an area of injury in the region of the penetrating portion of the AV node. A wide QRS complex following DC shock was obtained in this animal, indicating an idioventricular escape rhythm. Escape rhythms were apparently idioventricular in approximately one-half of the animals and were proximal in origin in the other half. Accordingly, hemorrhagic areas indicated rather marked destruction of the His bundle region in juxtaposition to the non-coronary cusp. However, damage to either the non-coronary or right coronary cusp, as well as minor cusp perforation, was also observed.

Since these studies were performed in acute animals, long-term follow-up for the persistency of the AV heart block or complications such as rupture of the coronary cusp or aorta could not be ascertained. Consequently, long-term follow-up observations will be necessary to establish the long-term sequelae of this approach. Thus, this percutaneous transaortic catheter technique can be used to produce experimental AV block in the closed chest experimental animal. The method is rapid, practical and effective for this purpose. This method as presently used, however, is not suitable for human application.

References

1. Cobb FR, Blumenschein S, Sealy WC, Boineau JP, Wagner GS, Wallace AG: Successful surgical interruption of the bundle of Kent in a patient with Wolff-Parkinson-White syndrome. Circulation 1968; 38: 1018–1029.
2. Dreifus LS, Nichols H, Morse D, Watanabe Y, Truex RC: Control of recurrent tachycardia of Wolff-Parkinson-White syndrome by surgical ligature of the AV bundle. Circulation 1968; 38: 1032–1036.
3. Starz, TE, Gaertner RA: Chronic heart block in dogs. Method for producing experimental heart failure. Circulation 1955; 12: 259–270.
4. Starzl, TE, Gaertner RA, Baker RR: Acute complete heart block in dogs. Circulation 1955; 12: 82–89.
5. Turina M, Babotai I, Wegmann W: Production of chronic atrioventricular blocks in dogs without thoracotomy. Cardiovasc Res 1968; 4: 389–393.
6. Williams JCP, Lambert EH: Production of heart block in dogs without thoracotomy. Federation Proc 1964; 23: 413.
7. Steiner C, Kovalik AT: A simple technique for production of chronic complete heart block in dogs. J Appl Physiol 1968; 25: 631–632.
8. Babotai I, Brownlee R: Experimental atrioventricular block without thoracotomy: a new instrument. Cardiovasc Res 1971; 5: 416–418.
9. Pruett JK, Woods EF. Technique for experimental complete heart block. J Appl Physiol 1967; 22: 830–831.
10. Wieberdink J: Experimental production of permanent heart block (total or bundle branch block) without circulatory arrest or extracorporeal circulation. Thorax 1966; 21: 401–404.

11. Klein GJ, Sealy WC, Pritchett EL, Harrison L, Hackel DB, Davis D, Kasell J, Wallace AG, Gallagher JJ: Cryosurgical ablation of the atrioventricular node-His bundle: Long-term follow-up and properties of the junctional pacemaker. Circulation 1980; 61: 8–15.
12. Gonzalez R, Scheinman M, Margaretten W, Rubinstein M: Closed-chest electrodecatheter technique for His bundle ablation in dogs. Am J Physiol 1981; 241: H283–287.
13. Gallagher JJ, Svenson RH, Kasell JH, German LD, Bardy GH, Broughton A, Critelli G: Catheter technique for closed-chest ablation of the atrioventricular conduction system. A therapeutic alternative for the treatment of refractory supraventricular tachycardia. N Engl J Med 1982; 300: 194–200.
14. Beazell JW, Adomian GE, Furmanski M, Tan KS: Experimental production of complete heart block by electrocoagulation in the closed chest dog. Am Heart J 1982; 104: 1328–1334.
15. Gonzalez R, Scheinman M, Bharati S, Lev M: Closed chest permanent atrioventricular block in dogs. Am Heart J 1983; 105: 461–470.

Authors' address:
Leonard S. Dreifus, M.D.
Lankenau Hospital
Lancaster Avenue & City Line Avenue
Philadelphia, PA 19151

Treatment of Ventricular Arrhythmias: Surgery

J. L. Cox

Summary: During the past five years, the surgical approach to the treatment of ventricular arrhythmias associated with coronary heart disease has undergone a dramatic change in terms of patient selection, surgical indications, and the specific surgical techniques employed to alleviate these life-threatening arrhythmias. Because of the dismal results obtained using indirect surgical techniques for the treatment of refractory ischemic ventricular tachycardia prior to 1978, three new direct endocardial surgical procedures guided by intraoperative electrophysiologic mapping were introduced. The encircling endocardial ventriculotomy (EEV) of Guiraudon, the endocardial resection procedure (ERP) of Harken and its modification of "extended" ERP by Moran, and endocardial cryoablation introduced by our group at Duke University have all proven to be superior to the previous indirect surgical procedures. The operative mortality rate has been decreased from 27% to approximately 10% and the overall success rate has been increased from 50% to 90% with the introduction of the direct surgical procedures. Although each of these direct endocardial techniques is effective, the selection of the appropriate procedure for a given patient depends upon the electrophysiologic characteristics of the ventricular arrhytmia and on its anatomic "site of origin" in the left ventricle. As these procedures have been shown to be safer and more effective than the previous indirect operations, the indications for surgical therapy of refractory ischemic ventricular tachycardia have been expanded.

Introduction

Prior to 1978, several surgical procedures were employed for the treatment of ventricular tachyarrhythmias that were unresponsive to all types of medical therapy (Table 1) (1). Thoracic sympathectomy, coronary artery bypass grafting, heart wall resection including either myocardial infarctectomy or ventricular aneurysmectomy, and a combination of coronary artery bypass grafting and heart wall resection were employed in 171 patients with an operative mortality rate of 27%, a failure rate of 17%, and an overall success rate of 56%. The unsatisfactory results attained by these indirect surgical procedures coupled with the increasing knowledge and understanding of ischemic ventricular tachyarrhythmias led to the development of electrophysiologic techniques that could be applied both preoperatively and intraoperatively to better characterize individual arrhythmias. This, in turn, provided the stimulus for the development of more direct surgical approaches to their treatment.

Electrophysiologic Characterization of Refractory

Ischemic Ventricular Tachyarrhythmias

Ventricular tachyarrhythmias associated with coronary heart disease may occur on the basis of three etiologic mechanisms: an automatic ventricular focus, a reentrant circuit, and triggered automaticity. Although for many years, ventricular arrhythmias associated with ischemic heart disease were felt to occur primarily on the basis of an automatic fo-

909

cus resulting from "irritable" myocytes located in the marginally perfused border zones of myocardial infarctions, both experimental and clinical studies during the 1970's indicated that the majority of ventricular tachyarrhythmias associated with coronary heart disease occurred on the basis of a reentrant mechanism (2). The reentrant circuits responsible for refractory ischemic ventricular tachyarrhythmias may be micro-reentrant circuits that theoretically involve only a few myocardial cells or they may occur on the basis of macro-reentrant circuits involving the bundle branches of the specialized conduction system and the free-wall of the left ventricle. Whether or not triggered automaticity plays a role in the development of refractory ischemic ventricular tachyarrhythmias is as yet undetermined. Thus, from a practical standpoint, the clinical classification of the etiologic types of refractory ischemic ventricular tachyarrhythmias may be divided into automatic arrhythmias and reentrant arrhythmias. On a strictly empiric basis, automatic arrhythmias are defined as those that cannot be induced or terminated by programmed electrical stimulation and/or burst pacing techniques and reentrant arrhythmias are defined as those that can be induced and terminated by these pacing techniques. Although the differential response of these two types of arrhythmias to programmed pacing does not prove that they are either automatic or reentrant, this clinical classification has proven to be extremely helpful in selecting patients who will respond favorably to surgical treatment. In general, surgical therapy is more effective for the treatment of reentrant ventricular tachyarrhythmias than for those that occur on the basis of an automatic focus. Since automatic arrhythmias do not respond to pacing protocols and tend to be easily suppressed by general anesthesia, they are extremely difficult to induce and therefore to localize in the operating theater. Although general anesthesia, alterations in myocardial temperature and cardiac hemodynamics, and surgical manipulation combine to increase the difficulty of induction of reentrant arrhythmias, experience has proven that most reentrant arrhythmias can be induced intraoperatively, thereby allowing their region of origin to be localized and approached surgically.

Preoperative Electrophysiologic Evaluation and Patient Selection for Surgery

Patients who present with refractory ischemic ventricular tachyarrhythmias have significant coronary artery disease, a history of at least one myocardial infarction, and usually a left ventricular aneurysm. The addition of ventricular tachyarrhythmias to these serious anatomic abnormalities results in a constellation of problems that are among the most difficult encountered by cardiac surgeons. Although left ventricular dysfunction is a common associated finding in patients with refractory ischemic ventricular tachyarrhythmias, it rarely constitutes a contraindication to surgical therapy. Instead, the feasibility of surgical treatment in these patients is usually based upon the patient's history and the electrophysiologic characteristics of the dysrhythmia as determined by a preoperative endocardial catheter electrophysiology study. Such a study is mandatory in patients selected for surgery in order to:
1. confirm that the dysrhythmia is ventricular rather than supraventricular in origin,
2. document that the dysrhythmia can be induced and terminated by programmed electrical stimulation techniques thus establishing its reentrant basis,
3. confirm that the ventricular tachyarrhythmia originates from the region of the myocardial infarction or aneurysm, and

4. perform catheter mapping to localize the specific region of origin of the ventricular tachyarrhythmia.

Preoperative electrophysiology studies in patients with refractory ischemic ventricular tachycardia usually demonstrate the dysrhythmia to be ventricular tachycardia of a single morphologic type, indicating that it is originating from a single region within the left ventricle. Following induction, these monomorphic ventricular tachycardias are usually sustained for a sufficient period of time to allow endocardial catheter mapping to determine their site of origin. However, on occasion, monomorphic ventricular tachycardia is non-sustained and thus cannot be mapped during the preoperative electrophysiologic study. A second of type of ventricular tachycardia that is frequently associated with coronary heart disease is polymorphic ventricular tachycardia. This term is applied not only to ventricular tachycardia that originates from several different regions of the left ventricle giving rise to different morphologic types of tachycardia, but it is also applied to tachycardia that originates from one general region of the left ventricle but is characterized electrophysiologically by excessive fragmentation such that individual depolarization complexes may be difficult to identify. Polymorphic ventricular tachycardia may also be either sustained or non-sustained, but it commonly deteriorates rather quickly into ventricular fibrillation. Electrophysiologic deterioration to ventricular fibrillation may be the result of primary electrical instability or it may occur because of hemodynamic compromise associated with the onset of polymorphic ventricular tachycardia. The third type of refractory ischemic ventricular tachyarrhythmia is primary ventricular fibrillation which is identified during the preoperative electrophysiology study by the absence of any type of induced ventricular tachycardia prior to the onset of ventricular fibrillation following programmed electrical stimulation and/or burst pacing.

Surgical Indications and Contraindications

The major indications for surgery in patients with ischemic ventricular tachyarrhythmias are: 1. medical refractoriness to ventricular tachycardia, 2. patient intolerance to effective medical treatment, and 3. poor patient compliance. Surgical therapy is also indicated in patients with intractible angina pectoris requiring coronary artery bypass grafting who have *associated* ventricular tachycardia and in patients with congestive heart failure due to a left ventricular aneurysm requiring resection who have *associated* ventricular tachycardia. The major contraindications to surgery for refractory ischemic ventricular tachyarrhythmias are determined by the preoperative electrophysiology study and include: 1. non-inducible ventricular tachycardia, 2. non-sustained polymorphic ventricular tachycardia, 3. automatic ventricular tachycardia, and 4. primary ventricular fibrillation. Regardless of the patient's history of documented ventricular tachycardia, if the dysrhythmia cannot be induced at the time of the endocardial catheter electrophysiology study, surgery is not feasible since the induction of the dysrhythmia intraoperatively would be extremely unlikely. Likewise, if the patient is found to have non-sustained polymorphic ventricular tachycardia during the preoperative electrophysiology study, it is highly unlikely that the arrhythmia could be induced intraoperatively so that its origin could be localized. It should be mentioned, however, that if the non-sustained polymorphic ventricular tachycardia has proven to be life-threatening, one of the direct endocardial surgical procedures that does not absolutely require intraoperative electrophysiologic mapping may be indicated in these patients. As mentioned previously, the surgical results of treatment of automatic ventricular tachyarrhythmias has been notoriously unsuccessful. Likewise, there is currently no surgical procedure available for the treatment of primary ventricular fibrillation.

Direct Surgical Procedures for the Treatment of Refractory Ischemic Ventricular Tachycardia

Because of the unsatisfactory results of the indirect procedures for the treatment of refractory ischemic ventricular tachyarrhythmias (Table 1), several direct techniques have been devised for the treatment of these life-threatening dysrhythmias during the past 5 years. The direct surgical treatment of any arrhythmia may be successful by either to two means: isolation or ablation. An isolation procedure alleviates the detrimental effects of an arrhythmia by limiting its exit conduction pathways, but it does not alter the presence, frequency, or electrophysiologic characteristics of the arrhythmia. If confined to a relatively localized region of the heart, an arrhythmia may continue to occur unabated, but since the abnormal electrical activity cannot escape the confines imposed by the surgical procedure, the remainder of the heart is unaffected. An ablative procedure destroys the arrhythmia either by surgical resection, thermal ablation, or interruption of reentrant circuits responsible for the arrhythmia.

In 1978, Guiraudon introduced the encircling endocardial ventriculotomy (EEV) for the surgical treatment of refractory ischemic ventricular tachycardia (Fig. 1) (3). Guiraudon has suggested that the encircling endocardial ventriculotomy may either isolate arrhythmogenic myocardium from the remainder of the heart or ablate ventricular tachycardia by surgical division of at least one limb of the reentrant circuit responsible for the arrhythmia. Although experimental studies in our laboratory have demonstrated that the EEV is capable of isolating arrhythmogenic myocardium under certain experimental conditions (4), neither isolated, nonpropagated dysrhythmic activity nor local parasystole has been demonstrated clinically following the procedure. Whether or not the incision itself may divide a reentrant circuit has not been established either experimentally or clini-

Table 1. Results of indirect surgical procedures for refractory ischemic ventricular tachycardia. CABG = coronary artery bypass grafting; Resection = myocardial infarctectomy or aneurysmectomy.

Procedure	Patients	Operative Mortality	Failure	Success
Sympathectomy	12	25%	17%	58%
CABG	37	27%	27%	46%
Resection	95	24%	17%	59%
CABG and Resection	27	41%	4%	55%
Total	171	27%	17%	56%

912

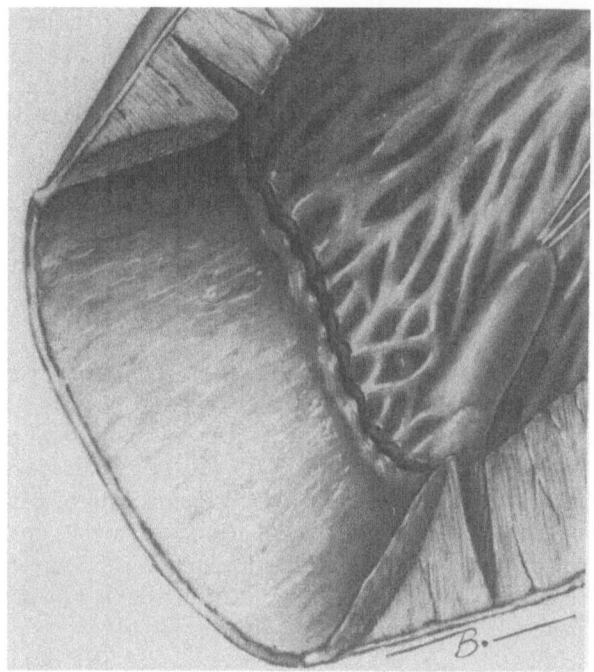

Fig. 1. Encircling endocardial ventriculotomy (EEV). A standard aneurysmectomy is first performed, leaving a 1 cm cuff of fibrous-tissue aneurysm wall with which to close the ventricle after completion of the procedure. The border between endocardial fibrosis at the base of the aneurysm and surrounding normal myocardium is identified. An incision perpendicular to the plane of the left ventricular wall is placed just outside the border of endocardial fibrosis and is continued around the entire base of the aneurysm. The depth of the incision of the left ventricular free-wall is such that only a narrow bridge of subepicardium, the epicardium, and the overlying coronary vessels are spared. The incision is made approximately 1 cm deep on the septal side of the aneurysm. The endocardial incision is then closed with a continuous 3–0 non-absorbable suture followed by closure of the left ventricular aneurysm in the routine manner.

cally. Our experimental studies have shown that the EEV causes a profound decrease in regional blood flow in the encircled myocardium, especially the subendocardium (5). This surgically induced regional ischemia results in ablation of much of the normal and abnormal intramural electrical activity in the encompassed myocardium (4). These findings suggest that the EEV alters local conduction characteristics in the region of arrhythmogenesis such that the conditions necessary for regional reentry are ablated. Although such a mechanism of action is quite effective from an electrophysiologic standpoint, the decreased regional myocardial blood flow results in a concomitant depression of the regional myocardial function of any non-fibrosed tissue that is encircled (6). The alteration in regional function may be of little consequence if the associated aneurysm or infarction is small, but if the encompassed region of the myocardium is large, left ventricular power failure can result from the procedure (7).

In 1979, Harken and Josephson introduced the endocardial resection procedure (ERP) for the treatment of refractory ischemic ventricular tachycardia (8). In order to perform the local endocardial resection procedure, it is necessary to obtain an intraoperative isochronous endocardial electrophysiologic map that is capable of localizing the arrhythmogenic area to at least one quadrant of the base of the infarction or aneurysm. Such extensive intraoperative mapping may preclude the application of this procedure if only short, non-sustained runs of ventricular tachycardia can be induced intraoperatively. However, if sustained ventricular tachycardia can be induced in the operating room to allow suffi-

913

cient time for appropriate mapping procedures to be performed, the localized endocardial resection procedure is an excellent technique for ablating these tachyarrhythmias. The exact mechanism of action of the endocardial resection procedure is unknown, but it is likely that the entire microreentrant circuit responsible for the ventricular tachycardia is resected with the surgical specimen. Because of the demonstrated effectiveness of the endocardial resection procedure, Moran has modified it for application in patients who cannot be mapped intraoperatively. In such patients, Moran resects all of the endocardial fibrosis around the base of the left ventricular aneurysm or infarction, thus precluding the necessity for intraoperative endocardial mapping. He has termed this procedure the "extended" endocardial resection procedure and has now applied it in 37 patients with satisfactory results (9).

The direct endocardial surgical procedures for the treatment of refractory ischemic ventricular tachycardia have proven to be much more effective than were the previously employed indirect procedures (Table 2). One hundred and sixty patients have now been reported to have undergone either and EEV, ERP, or extended ERP with an overall operative mortality rate of 12%, a failure rate of 1%, and an overall success rate of 87%. "Overall success" is defined in this group of patients as the total number of patients operated upon minus the operative deaths, minus the late deaths due either to the surgical procedure or to recurrent ventricular tachycardia, minus those patients who have recurrent ventricular tachycardia that cannot be controlled medically.

Despite these improved results, neither the EEV, the ERP, nor the extended ERP can be applied safely and effectively in all patients. For example, if ventricular tachycardia arises from the anterior or posterior papillary muscle or from the region of the posterior interventricular septum at the junction of the aortic and mitral valve anuli, several problems may arise that preclude application of an EEV, ERP, or extended ERP. Resection of endocardial fibrosis extending onto either papillary muscle usually results in the necessity for replacement of the mitral valve, although the valve apparatus itself might have been normal preoperatively. Moran has now replaced the mitral valve in 7 such patients as a result of the extended endocardial resection procedure (10). There are two technical problems associated with ventricular tachycardia arising from the high posterior interventricular septum near the junction of the aortic and mitral valves. The first involves the difficulty in mapping these patients even with a sustained ventricular tachycardia because of the necessity to retract the ventricular apex out of the pericardial sac. A longitudinal

Table 2. Results of direct surgical procedures for refractory ischemic ventricular tachycardia. EEV = encircling endocardial ventriculotomy; ERP = endocardial resection procedure; EERP = extended endocardial resection procedure.

Procedure	Patients	Operative Mortality	Failure	Success
EEV	47	17%	0%	83%
ERP	76	9%	1%	89%
EERP	37	11%	0%	89%
Total	160	12%	1%	87%

914

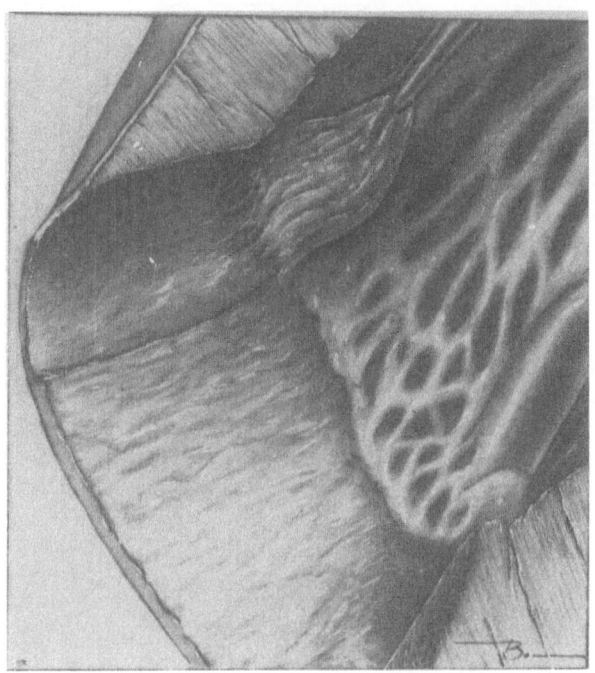

Fig. 2. Endocardial resection procedure (ERP). Following identification of the region of arrhythmogenesis, the endocardial fibrosis in the area of arrhythmogenesis is undermined and excised. In this fashion, an 8–25 cm² piece of endocardium extending 2–3 cm beyond the edge of the aneurysm is removed. In each case, this involves removal of 25–40% of the circumference of the base of the aneurysm. In patients without left ventricular aneurysms but with myocardial infarctions, a ventriculotomy is placed through the center of the infarction and endocardial resection of local areas of the infarction or of the posterior septum is accomplished. The area of tissue removed in these patients is usually less than 10 cm².

left ventriculotomy must be placed between the base of the posterior papillary muscle and the posterior interventricular septum and the endocardium of the posterior septum must then be mapped through this posterior ventriculotomy. Such retraction of the heart frequently induces significant aortic insufficiency which may preclude one's ability to identify accurately the site of origin of the arrhythmia. The second technical problem with employing endocardial resection for the treatment of arrhythmias arising in this region involves the potential disruption of either the aortic or mitral valve apparatus by the resection procedure itself. It has been our experience that these tachyarrhythmias usually originate extremely close to the junction of the aortic and mitral valves and that the resection of endocardial fibrosis to within 3–5 mm of the valve anuli frequently does not interrupt the tachycardia.

As a result of this inability to employ the EEV, ERP, or extended ERP safely and effectively for the treatment of all refractory ischemic ventricular tachycardia, we have employed endocardial cryoablation as the primary treatment of choice for tachycardia arising from the anterior or posterior papillary muscles and for tachycardia originating in the high posterior interventricular septum. This technique utilizes a 1.5 cm diameter cryoprobe with internally expanding nitrous oxide as the coolant. Following localization of the site of origin of the ventricular tachycardia, the cryoprobe is applied to the arrhythmogenic site for a period of 3 minutes at −60 °C (Fig. 3). A needle electrode with contacts every millimeter along the needle shaft is placed transmurally at the site of earliest endocardial activation during ventricular tachycardia. By monitoring the intramural electrograms during application of the endocardial cryothermia, the progression of the lethal

Fig. 3. Endocardial cryoablation. Once the area of earliest endocardial activation during ventricular tachycardia has been identified, an intramural plunge needle containing electrode contacts every millimeter along its shaft from endocardium to epicardium is placed at that site. A 1.5 cm diameter cryoprobe cooled with internally expanding nitrous oxide to $-60\,°C$ is placed over the site of earliest endocardial activity. The depth of the ultimate cryolesion can be controlled by on-line monitoring of intramural electrograms recorded from each of the electrode contacts along the needle shaft.

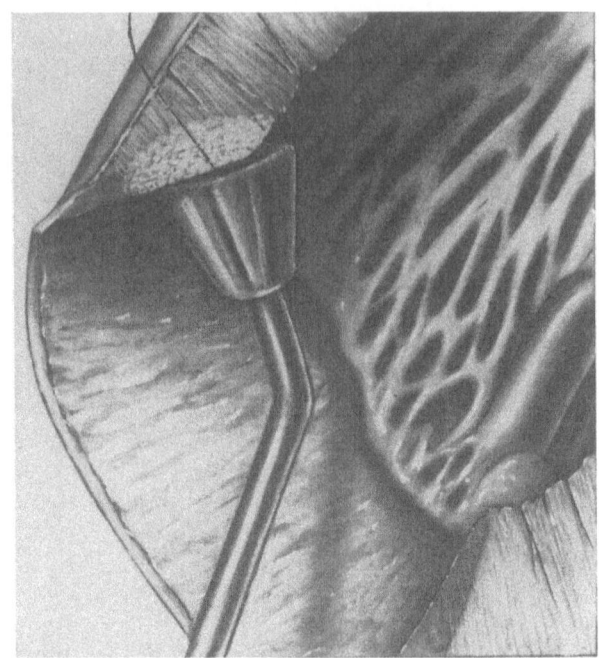

edge of the cryolesion can be monitored so that non-arrhythmogenic tissue surrounding the arrhythmogenic site can be spared (11).

Although we consider the localized endocardial resection procedure to be the treatment of choice in all cases of refractory ischemic ventricular tachycardia when it can be employed, our surgical approach depends upon two factors: 1. the intraoperative electrophysiologic characteristic of the ventricular tachycardia, and 2. the anatomic site of origin of the ventricular tachycardia (Table 3). If the patient has been selected for surgery properly on the basis of a preoperative electrophysiology study, the intraoperative manifestation of the tachycardia is usually one of three types: 1. sustained monomorphic ventricular tachycardia, 2. non-sustained monomorphic ventricular tachycardia, or 3. polymorphic ventricular tachycardia. Sustained monomorphic ventricular tachycardia can be mapped easily intraoperatively and its site of origin can be identified without difficulty. Proper localization of the site of origin of non-sustained monomorphic ventricular tachycardia may be very difficult intraoperatively unless an electrophysiologic mapping system capable of recording multiple electrograms simultaneously is available. In general, these types of arrhythmias must be treated with a less localized procedure than those employed for tachycardias that are sustained long enough for accurate intraoperative localization of the arrhythmogenic site. Likewise, polymorphic ventricular tachycardia essentially always requires one of the less localized procedures.

If the anterior left ventricular septum is found to be the arrhythmogenic site and the tachycardia is sustained and monomorphic, the localized endocardial resection procedure is employed. If the tachycardia cannot be mapped sufficiently because it is non-sustained, we perform an extended ERP to avoid the likelihood of recurrence postoperatively. If the tachycardia arising from this region is polymorphic, we have found it necessary not only

Table 3. Direct procedures of choice for refractory ischemic ventricular tachycardia (RIVT). EEV = encircling endocardial ventriculotomy; ERP = endocardial resection procedure; EERP = extended endocardial resection procedure; ECA = endocardial cryoablation; LV = left ventricle; VT = ventricular tachycardia.

Anatomic Site Of VT Origin	Sustained VT	Non-Sustained VT	Polymorphic VT
Anterior LV Septum	ERP	EERP	EERP + ECA
Anterior LV Free-wall	ERP	EERP	EERP + ECA
Anterior Papillary Muscle	ECA	ECA	EERP + ECA
Lateral LV Free-wall	ERP	EERP	EERP + ECA
Posterior LV Free-wall	ERP	ERP or EEV + ECA	EEV + ECA
Posterior Papillary Muscle	ECA	EEV + ECA	EEV + ECA
Posterior LV Septum	ERP + ECA	EERP + ECA	EERP + ECA

to resect all of the endocardial fibrosis associated with the left ventricular aneurysm but also to perform endocardial cryoablation in the area that shows the greatest degree of fragmentation during normal sinus rhythm mapping. Tachycardias arising in the anterior free-wall and in the lateral free-wall are appraoched in exactly the same manner.

If the anterior papillary muscle can be demonstrated to be the arrhythmogenic site of either a sustained or non-sustained monomorphic tachycardia, we perform endocardial cryoablation of the lower two-thirds of the papillary muscle. If the tachycardia appears to be arising from the anterior papillary muscle but is polymorphic, we resect all of the endocardial fibrosis associated with the aneurysm and cryoablate the lower two-thirds of the papillary muscle. We have not had to replace a mitral valve because of cryoablation of the papillary muscle. If the arrhythmogenic site can be localized to the posterior papillary muscle, we prefer to perform endocardial cryoablation. However, if the tachycardia is non-sustained so that we cannot be absolutely certain that the arrhythmogenic site is in the posterior papillary muscle, we perform an EEV around the entire border of fibrosis on the posterior free-wall, papillary muscle, and posterior LV septum. The EEV incision is based medially on the aortic valve anulus and laterally on the mitral valve anulus and is carried to within 5 mm of each anulus. An endocardial cryolesion is placed at either end of the EEV incision to complete the "encirclement" of the fibrotic myocardium containing the posterior papillary muscle (7).

Polymorphic ventricular tachycardia arising from the posterior LV free-wall is handled in an identical manner. However, if the arrhythmogenic site can be localized accurately to the posterior LV free-wall, we prefer to perform an ERP. In the case of non-sustained tachycardia arising from this region, we perform either an ERP or an EEV as the primary procedure with endocardial cryoablation being applied near the aortic and/or mitral valve anulus. If tachycardia arising from the posterior LV septum can be localized adequately, one may perform an ERP but cryoablation near the aortic anulus is usually indicated as well. If the tachycardia cannot be localized satisfactorily within the posterior LV septum because it is either non-sustained or polymorphic, we resect all of the fibrosis associated with the posterior LV septal infarction followed by application of endocardial cryothermia along the aortic and mitral valve anuli.

It is apparent that the specific surgical procedure applied in a given patient with refractory ischemic ventricular tachycardia must be tailored to the anatomic and electrophysio-

917

logic characteristics presented by each individual case. We believe that it is extremely important to perform these surgical procedures during induced ventricular tachycardia when the arrhythmia is sustained or to perform the procedures in the beating non-working heart in the case of non-sustained ventricular tachycardia. Immediately after performing the specific endocardial surgical procedure, we repeatedly attempt to reinduce the arrhythmia until we are convinced that it can no longer be induced. By performing the procedures without utilizing cardioplegic arrest, the potential temporary salutary effects of hypothermia and of the cardioplegic solution itself can be eliminated. It is our feeling that the 20% reinducibility rate of ventricular tachycardia during the postoperative study in most reported series is related to the fact that these surgical procedures are commonly performed during cardioplegic arrest and that the temporary effects of hypothermia and/or cardioplegia result in the lack of inducibility in the operating room immediately following surgery despite the fact that the tachycardia can be induced 7–10 days later in one of every five patients. By employing the surgical procedures as outlined in Table 3 without instituting cardioplegic arrest, we have had no postoperative recurrences of ventricular tachycardia and only one patient has had inducible ventricular tachycardia at the time of the postoperative study. That particular patient had polymorphic ventricular tachycardia with four separate morphologic types of tachycardia documented preoperatively and intraoperatively. He underwent an extended endocardial resection procedure for an anterior left ventricular aneurysm that involved the base of the papillary muscle. We did not cryoablate the base of the anterior papillary muscle at the time of surgery because of technical difficulties. Postoperatively, only a single morphologic type of tachycardia could be induced and it appeared to be arising from the base of the anterior papillary muscle. The patient was placed on Amiodarone and has had no further episodes of tachycardia during a 6-month follow-up period.

In summary, during the past 5 years, it has become possible to treat refractory ischemic ventricular tachycardia in a safe, effective, and predictable fashion due to the development of new direct endocardial surgical procedures. All of these surgical procedures are effective in a given situation and if applied in a logical manner based upon preoperative and intraoperative electrophysiologic data, they are almost uniformly successful.

References

1. Boineau JP, and Cox JL: Rationale for a Direct Surgical Approach to Control Ventricular arrhythmias. American Journal of Cardiology 1982; 49: 381.
2. Boineau JP, and Cox JL: Slow Ventricular Activation in Acute Myocardial Infarction – A Source of Re-entrant Premature Ventricular Contractions. Circulation 1973; 48: 971.
3. Guiraudon G, Fontaine G, Frank R, Escande G, Etievent P, and Cabrol C: Encircling Endocardial Ventriculotomy: A New Surgical Treatment for Life-Threatening Ventricular Tachycardias Resistant to Medical Treatment Following Myocardial Infarction. Annals of Thorac Surgery 1978; 26: 438.
4. Ungerleider RM, Stanley TE, Lofland GK, Williams JM, Ideker RE, Quick G, and Cox JL: Encircling Endocardial Ventriculotomy (EEV) for Refractory Ischemic Ventricular tachycardia: I: Electrophysiologic Effects. Journal of Thoracic and Cardiovascular Surgery 1982; 83: 840.
5. Ungerleider RM, Stanley TE, Lofland GK, Williams JM, Quick G, and Cox JL: Encircling Endocardial Ventriculotomy (EEV) for Refractory Ischemic Ventricular Tachycardia: II: Effects on Regional Myocardial Blood Flow. Journal of Thoracic and Cardiovascular Surgery 1982; 83: 850.

6. Ungerleider RM, Calcagno D, Stanley TE, Lofland GK, Williams JM, and Cox JL: Encircling Endocardial Ventriculotomy (EEV) for Refractory Ischemic Ventricular tachycardia: III: Effects on Regional Left Ventricular function. Journal of Thoracic and Cardiovascular Surgery 1982; 83: 857.
7. Cox JL, Gallagher JJ, and Ungerleider RM: Encircling Endocardial Ventriculotomy (EEV) for Refractory Ischemic Ventricular Tachycardia: IV: Clinical Indications, Surgical Technique, Mechanism of Action, and Surgical Results. Journal of Thoracic and Cardiovascular Surgery 1982; 83: 865.
8. Josephson ME, Horowitz LN, and Harken AH: Endocardial Excision: A New Surgical Technique for the Treatment of Ventricular Tachycardia. Circulation 1979; 60: 1430.
9. Moran JM, Kehoe RD, Lichtenthal P, Sanders JH, Jr, and Michaelis LL: Surgical Control of Malignant Ventricular Arrhythmia. Presented at 18th Annual Meeting of the Society of Thoracic Surgeons, New Orleans, Louisiana, January 11, 1982.
10. Moran JM, Kehoe RF, Loeb JM, Frederiksen JW, Tommaso CL, Sanders JH, and Michaelis LL: Role of Papillary Muscle Resection and Mitral Valve Replacement in Control of Refractory Ventricular Arrhythmia. Presented at 55th Scientific Sessions of the American Heart Association, Dallas, Texas, November 17, 1982.
11. Holman WL, Ikeshita M, Douglas JM, Jr, Smith PK, Lofland GK, and Cox JL: Ventricular Cryosurgery: Short-Term Effects on Intramural Electrophysiology. Annals of Thoracic Surgery (In Press).

Authors' address:
J. L. Cox, M.D.
Professor of Surgery
Chief, Division of Cardiothoracic Surgery
Washington University School of Medicine
Barnes Hospital
St. Louis, Missouri

Surgically Induced A-V Block by Means of Laser Beam: A Preliminary Feasibility Study

S. Erdman, L. Levinsky, J. Raiff, M. Aygen, M. J. Levy

Summary: Cardiac rhythm disorders are commonly encountered problems in cardiology. In pathological cardiac diseases where antiarrhythmic drugs have been ineffective, surgical interruption of the conduction system and implantation of a pacemaker are accepted therapeutic procedures.

We have developed an experimental method to block the conduction system utilizing the laser beam. A specially designed laser beam apparatus with energy source of CO_2 is able to produce complete A-V block in animals without the use of extra-corporeal circulation or entering the heart. In some of the experimental animals pacemakers were implanted following the procedure. It appears that the present model for producing A-V block may have certain advantages over the other techniques although more extensive work, with improved instrumentation and techniques, is needed before using the method in man.

The current indications for surgical treatment of supraventricular tachycardia are disabling and life-threatening tachycardia, which are resistant to drug treatment and to various pacing techniques.

Satisfactory surgical techniques, namely surgical section, thermocoagulation and cryocoagulation (1, 2), have been developed for the interruption of anomalous pathways or the bundle of His, or both.

The purpose of this experimental study is to test the feasibility of producing A-V block by means of a carbon dioxide laser (3, 4). The application of the laser beam (5), through a specially designed needle which can be inserted from the right atrium, may eliminate the need for extracorporeal circulation. In addition to being a non-electrical energy source, the CO_2 laser beam has an advantage over cautery, which may cause ventricular fibrillation.

Material and Methods

The instruments used included:
1. A Sharplan 791 CO_2 surgical laser (Fig. 1) (Laser Industries, Israel).
2. A special 17 gauge needle, gold plated inside with lens inserted at its top (Fig. 2).
3. Temporary epicardial leads (Medtronic model 5802-SS).
4. An external demand pacemaker (Medtronic model 5880-A).
5. A Sanborn 4-channel polygraph.

The experiments were performed on ten cats (3.5–4.5 kg) and on ten dogs (8–16 kg).

The animals were anesthetized with Pentobarbiton (25–30 mg/kg), following endotracheal intubation with Halothane (0.5–1%) through a Harvard respirator. The blood pressure was registered using a transducer connected to a femoral catheter. A right or left thoracotomy was performed at the fourth intercostal space, determined by the approach utilized to produce A-V block. The thoracotomy was performed by means of CO_2 laser

Fig. 1. The Sharplan CO$_2$ Laser for surgery. The 720 and 791 models were used in this experiment. Produced by Laser Industry, Israel.

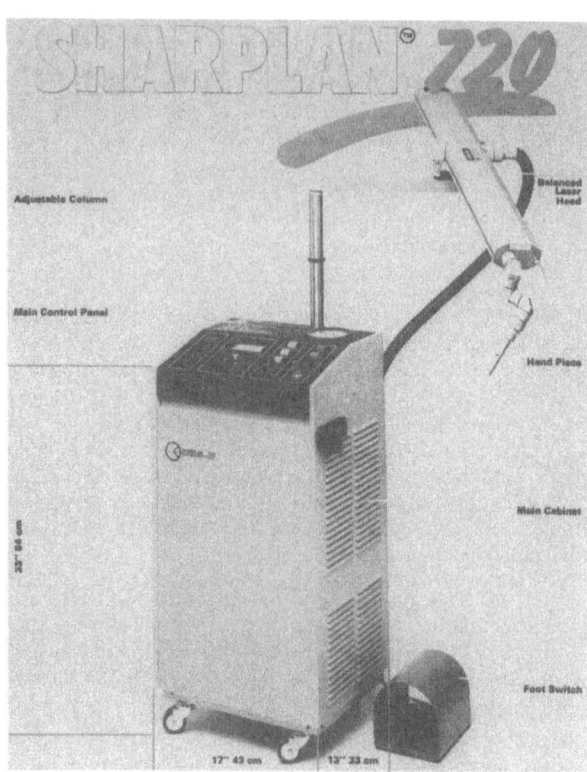

Fig. 2. The special 17 gauge needle produced especially for this experiment by Laser Industry, Israel.

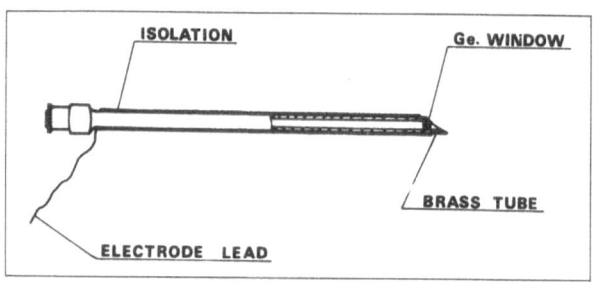

beam. There was hardly any bleeding at the incision margins; only larger vessels had to be ligated.

Heart wires were sutured on the atrial wall and on the right ventricle to provide temporary pacing after the heart block was created and to test the transmission of electrical impulse through the conduction pathway in both directions.

In the case of right thoracotomy (Fig. 3), a purse string suture was placed in the atrium at a point ventral to the superior vena cava (in five cats) or at a point ventral to the inferior vena cava (in five cats). The "special" needle was introduced through the purse string.

922

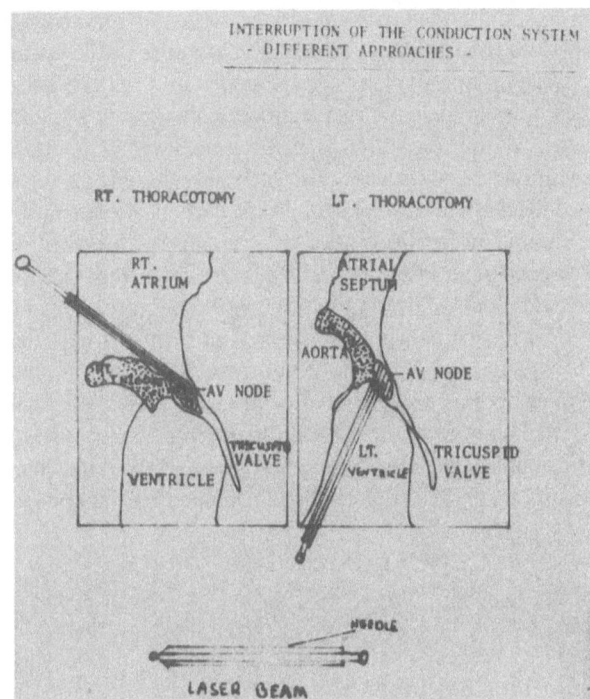

Fig. 3. This figure shows in diagramatic representation the method used to achieve heart block by right or left thoracotomies.

The coronary sinus and the tricuspid valve were used as anatomical reference points, and the needle was advanced towards the His bundle by using it as an explorative electrode, and then activated.

When a left thoracotomy was performed (Fig. 3), the purse string suture was placed in the wall of the left ventricle, close to the bifurcation of the circumflex artery. The laser beam needle was inserted through the purse string until it touched the wall of the aorta, 2–3 mm distal to the confluence of the right coronary artery leaflet and the non coronary leaflet, then moved over the surface of the septum, where the CO_2 laser beam was activated. After the heart block had been achieved, the purse string was closed. Electrocardiographic recordings were made during pacing alternately from the atrium and from the ventricle, to prove that the A-V block had been achieved. In case of impulse transmission in either direction through the A-V His pathways, the process was repeated until complete A-V block was established.

Technical Information on the Carbon Dioxide Laser and the Transmitting Needle

The Sharplan surgical laser is a 50 Watt carbon-dioxide laser which emits a highly collimated beam of infrared radiation at 10.6 microns. This radiation is directed along an articulated arm by a series of mirrors, to a focusing lens. The carbon-dioxide laser consists of a water-cooled plasma tube made of glass and an optical resonator. The active medium

923

is a flowing gas mixture of nitrogen, helium and carbon-dioxide which is maintained at a pressure of about 25 mmHg. The plasma tube has three electrodes, an anode in the center and a cathode at each end. High voltage is applied between the anode and the two cathodes to ionize the gas. Nitrogen molecules are excited by electronic collisions to a higher vibrational state from which ordinary dipole radiation to the ground level is quantum mechanically prohibited. This excitation energy is very efficiently transferred via super elastic collisions to an energetically adjacent vibrational state in the carbon-dioxide molecules. An excess of excited carbon-dioxide molecules is built up, creating the "population inversion" condition which is the essence of all laser action. When decaying from this excited state, the carbon dioxide molecules emit infrared radiation at 10.6 microns. This radiation is amplified through an optical resonator which consists of two mirrors clamped to individual water-cooled holders at each end of the tube. For maximum output, the mirrors are adjusted to be parallel to each other and perpendicular to the axis of the plasma tube. The rear mirror is coated for maximum reflection while the front one transmits 15 percent of the incident radiation, thus constituting the useful output of the laser. This highly collimated beam can be focussed to a small spot of about 100 micron diameter depending on the lens used.

The CO_2 Laser as a Surgical Tool

The basis of the CO_2 laser as a surgical tool lies in the fact that 10.6 micron radiation is highly absorbed by water which constitutes 80–90 percent of the body tissue. The high absorption coefficient of about 200 cm^{-1} facilitates heat delivery to highly localized tissue area with minimal thermal effect on adjacent tissue due to the low thermal conductivity of the water. The effect achieved on the irradiated tissue depends mainly on duration and total energy density delivered, and can be characterized as follows:

a) Evaporation – effective when energy delivered suffices to raise water temperature to 100 °C and causes evaporation (latent heat of 540 cal/gr).
b) Irreversible thermal damage – when tissue temperature is raised above 60–70 °C.
c) Reversible thermal damage.

Due to its high absorption by body tissue the CO_2 laser is most effective for tissue incision. When used in this mode thermal damage is limited to a tissue layer of 150 micron beneath the evaporated layers.

Adaptation of the Laser System for A-V Blocks

In normal surgical procedures the laser beam is applied on uncovered body tissue, either through a hand-held end-piece or through a standard operating microscope. Delivery of this radiation to internal tissues can be achieved by one of the following methods:

a) Transmission through rigid metal tubes (needles).
b) Transmission through flexible metal tubes.
c) Transmission through infrared fibers.

Research for the development of these transmission techniques is being currently conducted in various research centers around the world but none of them are as yet commercially available. The most promising recent development has been in the field of infrared flexible fibers with present power handling capability limited to about 2 watts. These will probably be commercially available in the near future.

The 17 gauge needle contains a brass tube and its distal end is closed by an infrared transparent window. The tube is covered by a plastic insulating sheath and soldered at its proximal end to an electrical output cable (Fig. 2). The laser radiation is focussed onto the orifice of the needle and then conducted along the needle partly through wall reflections and partly through waveguide effects. Transmission is accompanied by non-negligible heating of the brass tube.

The main problem encountered in the production of the needle, has been the end window, whose function is to block passage of blood into the needle. Most of the materials available to fashion an infrared window have been found unsuitable for this purpose due to hygroscopic properties of these materials or because of technical construction problems. The only readily available material, germanium, has the problem of thermal runaway. This phenomenon is evident in germanium at temperatures above 40 °C, turning it almost opaque to the infrared radiation (Fig. 4). The initial window temperature when inserted into the heart is around 37 °C; therefore, effective transmission was limited to a single short laser pulse. The laser power delivered in this manner was limited to about 2 watt at a pulse duration of $1/20-1/10$ sec. Spot size was 1.6 mm. At this power and spot size, onset of tissue evaporation is achieved with a pulse duration of

$$t = 3.18 \times 10^3 \, \frac{w^2}{p} = 50 \text{ msec}$$

w: Spot radius

p: Power

˙: Absorption coefficient (200 cm^{-1}).

The thermally destructed tissue layer, at this stage, is of approximately 150 microns thickness. Further radiation will evaporate the tissue layer at a range given approximately by:

$$Z (n) = 490 \, t \text{ (sec)}$$
$$\text{for } t = 0.5 \text{ sec } Z = 245 \text{ n.}$$

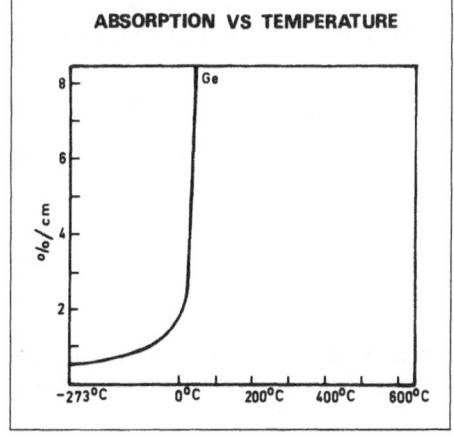

Fig. 4. Graph showing absorption vs temperature. The germanium allows us to work up to 40 °C at which point the germanium window becomes completely opaque to the laser beam.

Results

The many technical difficulties related to instrumentation included difficulties in applying the laser beam to one third of the animals. In 6 cats and 7 dogs, A-V block was obtained, but in half of them A-V conduction returned either spontaneously or when they were paced through the atrial or ventricular electrodes.

At the end of the experiments all of the animals were sacrificed and macroscopic anatomopathological examination was done. The point lesions, which represented the areas destroyed by the laser beams, were found situated in the right side of the atrial septum close to the entrance of the coronary sinus and close to the area of attachment of the septal leaflet of the tricuspid valve.

Discussion

Cardiac rhythm disoders are among the most commonly encountered problems in cardiology. Despite considerable progress in the understanding of basic mechanisms involved in the genesis and perpetuation of arrhythmias and in the action of antiarrhythmic drugs, therapeutic interventions are often empirical. Prolonged arrhythmia results from non-uniform characteristics of cardiac cells in regard to conduction velocity, duration of refractory period, automaticity and excitability. Antiarrhythmic drugs are effective in so far as they have the ability to prevent arrhythmia and to correct these irregularities. The search for drugs with antiarrhythmic properties continues because the ideal antiarrhythmic agent is not yet available.

Chronic antiarrhythmic prophylaxis is limited by the high incidence of side effects that occur with prolonged drug administration, and by the high failure rate of the drugs currently available. Failure to control some of the malignant arrhythmias (6) by medical means, has led to a search for alternative approaches. Various surgical means are being evaluated in patients with life threatening ventricular and supraventricular tachyarrhythmias (7, 8) which have been uncontrollable by medical measures.

The surgical procedures most frequently performed for the treatment of ventricular tachycardia are:

1) Coronary bypass graft, 2) infarctectomy, 3) aneurysmectomy, 4) stellate ganglionectomy in cases of prolonged Q-T syndrome, 5) mitral valve replacement in patients with ballooning of the mitral valve, and 6) section of reentrant V T pathways in the left and right ventricles.

The surgical approach to the treatment of supraventricular tachyarrhythmias consists of:

1. Interruption of the accessory pathways (9, 10, 11, 12), 2. interruption of the AV-His conduction system (13, 14), 3. or both (15).

Sealy and associates in 1969 reported successful surgical treatment of an intractable and life-threatening supraventricular tachycardia in a patient with pre-excitation syndrome. In this patient, division of the bundle of Kent prevented further bouts of tachycardia which were due to re-entry mechanism. Re-entry results from non-uniform conduction and excitation capabilities of cardiac cells. When atrial and ventricular myocardium communicate by more than one conducting pathway with such different electrical characteristics, an appropriately timed atrial premature beat may transverse one pathway and arrive at ventricular muscle and then echo back to the atrium via an alternate pathway (16). Reciprocal beats or echo beats involving a circus pathway in A-V node is another common example of re-entry. Baird and others reported successful division of the bundle of His and implantation of a permanent pacemaker in patients with supraventricular tachycardia.

Disabling and life-threatening supraventricular tachycardia may also occur as a result of an enhanced ectopic automatic activity with rapid atrioventricular conduction.

We are concerned with developing a method to produce conduction pathway surgery without extra-corporeal circulation. Many difficulties were encountered with instrumentation, especially with the malfunction of the needle, and in applying the laser beam to the appropriate anatomical region.

We were successful in applying it to two thirds of the animals. In 6 cats (60%) and 7 dogs (70%), A-V block was obtained, but in half of them, A-V conduction returned, either spontaneously or when they were paced through the atrial or ventricular electrodes. The return of normal conduction after producing A-V block, was undoubtedly due to failure to destroy and interrupt completely the His bundle. We are also not certain whether the animals which sustained A-V block, would retain it on long follow-up. In such acute experiments, the production of permanent complete A-V block, in our opinion, should at least be substantiated by histologic proof of complete interruption of the conduction pathways. At this stage such studies have not yet been performed.

We may conclude that a laser beam transmitted through a needle may be used to interrupt the A-V conduction. Further application of this technique, may be, the interruption of the atrioventricular accessory pathway and re-entrant pathways over the left and right ventricles.

Before any attempt can be made to use this method on man, more extensive work, with improved instrumentation and techniques, has to be peformed. The recently developed flexible infrared fibers could provide a technical solution.

References

1. Sealy WC, Gallagher JJ, Kasell, J: His bundle interruption for control of inappropriate ventricular responses to atrial arrhythmias. Ann Thorac Surg 1981; 32(5): 429–438.
2. Guirrandon G, Fontaine G, Frank R, Leanari R, Barra J, Cabrol C: Surgical treatment of ventricular tachycardia guided 34 ventricular mapping in 23 patients without coronary artery. Ann Thorac Surg 1981; 32(5): 439–450.
3. Wolbarsh ML ed: Laser application in medicine and biology, Vol 1–111, Plenum Press, 1971–1977.
4. Erdman S, Peled I, Gasner C, Kaplan I: A unique application of the carbon dioxide Laser in cardiac surgery. In: Laser Surgery, Jerusalem, Academic Press, 1976; pp 28–30. (First International Symposium on Laser Surgery, 5–6 Nov, 1975.)
5. Alden H: Horizons in electrical surgery. Ann Thorac Surg 1981; 32(5): 425–426.
6. Gallagher JJ, Svenson RH, Sealy WC et al: The Wolff-Parkinson syndrome and preexitation dysrhythmias, In: The Medical Clinics of North America, Symposium on Cardiac Rhythm Disturbances, I Vol 60 No 1, Jan 1976, Philadelphia WB Saunders, 1976; pp 101–123.
7. Gillette PC, Gallagher JJ, John J, Sealy WC: Concealed anomalous cardiac conduction pathways: an operable cause of supraventricular tachycardia. J of Pediatr (St Louis) 1977; 90(3): 427–430.
8. Kaplan BM: The tachycardia-bradycardia syndrome, In: The Medical Clinics of North America, Symposium on Cardiac Rhythm Disturbances, IV Vol 60 No. 1, Jan 1976, Philadelphia, WB Saunders, 1976; pp 81–99.

9. Sealy WC, Gallagher JJ et al: The surgical anatomy of Kent bundles based on electrophysiological mapping and surgical exploration. J of Throac & Cardiovasc Surg 1978; 76(6): 804–815.
10. Sealy WC, Gallagher JJ, Pritchett EL, Wallace AG: Surgical treatment of tachyarrhythmias in patients with both and Ebstein anomaly and a Kent bundle. J of Thorac & Cardiovasc Surg 1978; 76(6): 847–853.
11. Sealy WC, Gallagher JJ, Wallace AG: The surgical treatment of Wolff-Parkinson-White syndrome: evolution of improved methods for identification and interruption of the Kent bundle. Ann of Thorac Surg 1976; 22(5): 443–457.
12. Sealy WC, Wallace AG, Ramming KP et al: An improved operation for the definitive treatment of the Wolff-Parkinson-White syndrome. Ann Thorac Surg 1974; 17(2): 107–113.
13. Sealy WC, Anderson RW, Gallagher JJ: Surgical treatment of supraventricular tachyarrhythmias. J of Thorac & Cardiovasc Surg 1977; 73(4): 511–522.
14. Sealy WC: Surgical treatment of supraventricular tachyarrhythmias associated with the Wolff-Parkinson-White syndrome. The Heart 1977; 2388–2394.
15. Sealy WC, Hacker DB, Seaber AJ: A study of methods for surgical interruption of the His bundle. J of Thorac & Cardiovasc Surg 1977; 73(3): 424–430.
16. Harrison L et al: The shock electrode array: a tool for determining global epicardial activation during usable arrhythmias. Pace 1980; 3: 531–540.

Authors' address:
Dr. S. Erdman
Department of Cardiac Surgery
Beilinson Medical Center
Petah Tiqva 49 100
Israel

928

Long-Term Comparison of DVI and VVI Pacing in Carotid Sinus Syndrome

C. A. Morley*), E. J. Perrins, S. L. Chan, R. Sutton

Summary: Twenty-one patients treated with DVIM pacemakers for carotid sinus syndrome were entered into a double blind randomised trial of DVI versus VVI pacing. Daily symptoms were recorded on a diary card and overall preference for either treatment period reported blindly at the end of the trial. Six patients could not tolerate the change from DVI to VVI mode and were withdrawn from the trial. All had pacemaker syndrome related to ventriculo-atrial conduction. Of the fifteen patients who completed the trial, seven reported a preference for DVI pacing. There was no significant difference for symptom scores for dizziness with either pacing mode. DVI preference related to presence of VA conduction, but it did not correlate with the magnitude of the vasodepressor response or pacemaker induced hypotension. The high incidence of pacemaker syndrome makes DVIM pacing superior to VVI pacing in carotid sinus syndrome.

Introduction

Ventricular demand pacing will successfully alleviate syncope in patients with carotid sinus syndrome (1, 2, 3). However, less severe symptoms may recur in these patients after pacing (4). These may be due to either pacemaker syndrome (5, 6), or due to episodic hypotension. The latter symptoms are more common in patients with a large vasodepressor component to their hypersensitive carotid sinus reflex (4, 7, 8).

This study was undertaken to establish whether DVI pacing can prevent these problems and whether those patients benefiting from DVI pacing can be identified prior to pacemaker implantation.

Patients

Twenty-one patients treated with DVIM pacemakers for carotid sinus syndrome were studied. Eighteen were male and three female. Their mean age was 68 years (range 42–82 years). Seventeen had had primary DVI implants. These patients had been selected for DVI pacing on the basis of a prepacing arterial study showing > 50 mmHg systolic hypotension in response to carotid sinus massage combined with onset of temporary ventricular pacing or reproduction of symptoms during this manoeuvre. Four patients had been converted from VVI to DVI pacing. One had overt pacemaker syndrome and three had apparent vasodepressor symptoms. The mean duration of DVI pacing prior to trial entry was 3 months (range 1–17 months). None of the patients had been symptomatic during this period.

---

*) Supported by the British Heart Foundation.

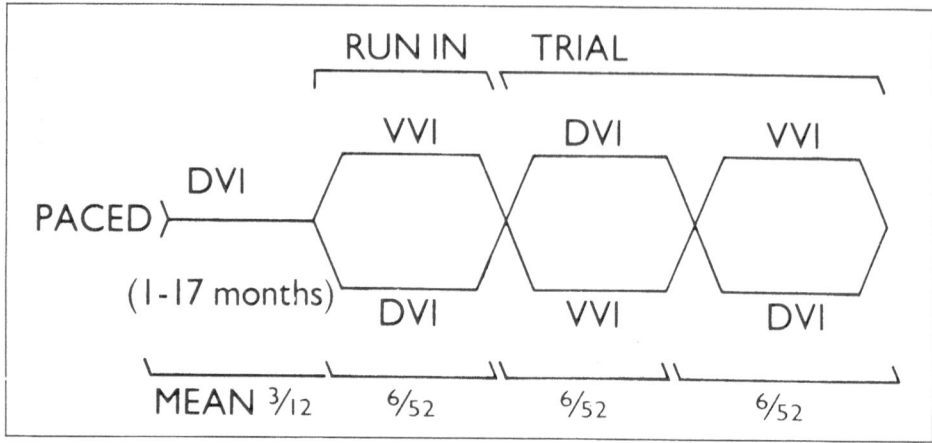

Fig. 1. Flow diagram summarising trial protocol.

Methods

The trial was a double blind, randomised study of DVI and VVI pacing. Each patient was 6 weeks in each mode, preceded by a 6 week run-in period also randomised for pacing mode. The paced rate was 60/min throughout the trial and all patients were observed to pace intermittently at this rate at rest. Patients recorded symptoms of minor or severe dizziness or syncope daily on a diary card. These symptoms were defined to the patients and the definitions printed on the cards as follows:

Mild Dizziness: Lightheadedness, unassociated with a sensation of rotation or sudden change of posture and insufficient to interfere with activity.

Severe Dizziness: As above but requiring patient to change posture or preventing activity.

Blackout: Sudden and unexplained loss of consciousness.

At the end of the trial the patient reported, blindly, overall preference for either treatment period. Symptoms were recorded during the 6 weeks run-in period in order to accustom patients to the diary card, but these were not used in the final analysis of the results.

Prepacing Assessment

All patients were assessed during pre-implantation electrophysiological study for ventriculo-atrial (VA) conduction, using ventricular paced rates of 50–150/min and right atrial recording.

Twenty of the patients had an arterial study at the time as the electrophysiological study to measure the hypotensive response to carotid sinus massage (vasodepressor response), to onset of ventricular pacing (pacemaker effect) and combination of these (Vasodepressor response and pacemaker effect). Symptoms reproduced by these manoeuvres were documented. Measurements of either brachial or radial intra-arterial pressure were taken

930

using 30–40° head up tilt to control the effect of posture on arterial pressure. Phasic arterial pressure was recorded using a Statham P23ID transducer. The mid-axilla was used as the zero reference point.

Definitions

Pacemaker Syndrome

Side effects caused by adverse haemodynamic consequences of pacing consisting of either dizziness, syncope, venous throbbing usually in the neck or dyspnoea and observed to occur during pacing and remit during sinus rhythm.

Vasodepressor Response (VDR)

Maximum fall in systolic blood pressure following carotid sinus massage during DVI pacing at a rate just sufficient to overdrive sinus rate.

Pacemaker Effect

Maximum fall in systolic blood pressure with onset of VVI pacing at a rate just sufficient to overdrive sinus rate.

Combined Vasodepressor Response and Pacemaker Effect (VDR + PME)

Maximum fall in systolic blood pressure following carotid sinus massage with onset of pacing at a rate just below sinus rate.

Results

Fifteen patients completed the trial. Results of total symptoms scores in either pacing mode, incidence of observed VA conduction, overt pacemaker syndrome and pacemaker mode preference are shown in Table 1. This shows no significant differences in symptom scores for dizziness in either mode. The majority of patients had fewer than one episode of minor dizziness throughout the study. The patient with most severe symptoms had aortic stenosis, ventricular tachycardia subsequently documented and died suddenly within three months of completing the study.

Seven patients preferred DVI mode and none preferred VVI mode. Two showing DVI preference had overt pacemaker syndrome, one with dyspnoea and venous pulsation and the other severe throbbing in his neck. The five other patients showing DVI preference were less aware of pacing in DVI mode and possibly had a minor degree of pacemaker syndrome.

Table 1. Results of symptom scores and pacing mode preference.

Patient	Symptom scores (total no. events)						VA conduction	Clinically overt pacemaker syndrome	Pacing mode preference
	Mild dizziness		Severe dizziness		Syncope				
	DVI	VVI	DVI	VVI	DVI	VVI			
1	0	0	0	0	0	0	+	–	DVI
2	16	20	2	12	0	0	+	–	DVI
3	0	2	0	0	0	0	+	–	DVI
4	4	4	0	0	0	0	+	+	DVI
5	1	0	0	0	0	0	+	–	DVI
6	4	7	0	0	0	0	+	–	DVI
7	5	0	0	0	0	0	+	+	DVI
8*	5	3	9	0	1	1	nil	–	Neither
9	0	0	0	0	0	0	+	–	Neither
10	0	0	0	1	0	0	nil	–	Neither
11	1	0	0	0	0	0	nil	–	Neither
12	1	0	0	0	0	0	nil	–	Neither
13	0	0	0	0	0	0	+	–	Neither
14	0	0	0	0	0	0	+	–	Neither
15	0	0	0	0	0	0	nil	–	Neither
Total	37	36	11	13	1	1			
	NS		NS						

* This patient had Aortic Sterosis and subsequently documented VT and sudden death.

Withdrawals

Six patients were withdrawn at their own request. All were unable to tolerate VVI pacing. Three were withdrawn during the run-in phase and three during the initial treatment period. The mean duration of ventricular pacing prior to withdrawal was 6 days (range 1/2–23 days). All these patients were asymptomatic prior to being programmed to VVI mode. All had pacemaker syndrome associated with 1 : 1 VA conduction with visible cannon a-waves. The details of their symptoms are summarised in Table 2. None of these patients reported symptoms, however, during brief temporary VVI pacing at pre-implantation electrophysiological study.

Pre-Implantation Assessment

VA conduction was present in 76% of all the patients during ventricular paced rhythm. The mean vasodepressor response was 33 mmHg. The mean pacemaker effect was 41 mmHg and combined hypotension was 60 mmHg. Symptoms were reproduced in 71% of patients overall during these manoeuvres.

Table 3 shows the results of a retrospective comparison of factors associated with subsequent DVI preference. VA conduction was the only parameter to correlate with DVI preference.

Table 2. Results due to pacemaker syndrome in the 6 patients withdrawn.

Mild dizzinesss	Severe dizziness	Dyspnoea	Venous throbbing (Associated with Cannon Waves)	VA Conduction
+	–	+	+	+
–	–	+	+	+
+	–	+	+	+
+	–	+	+	+
+	+	+	–	+
+	+	–	–	+

Table 3. Factors associated with DVI preference.

Preimplantation assessment	DVI preference including withdrawals n = 13	No mode preference n = 8	Fisher exact probability test
Mean VDR mmHg	34 ± 13	31 ± 12	NS
Mean PME mmHG	41 ± 10	43 ± 13	NS
Mean VDR + PME mmHG	58 ± 13	62 ± 11	NS
Symptoms reproduced by VDR + PME	7 (54(%)	8 (100%)	NS
VA Conduction	13 (100%)	3 (38%)	p = 0.003

Discussion

DVI pacing has been shown to be the preferred mode of pacing in the majority (62%) of patients studied. There was a high incidence of VA conduction (76%) and pacemaker syndrome (38%).

The very high incidence of pacemaker syndrome in this study may not reflect the true incidence of pacemaker syndrome in ventricular paced carotid sinus syndrome, as the patients studied were selected for DVI pacing on the basis of adverse haemodynamic parameters. Of 94 patients paced for carotid sinus syndrome at our centre a further 2 are known to have severe pacemaker syndrome (unpublished data). The overall incidence of clinically significant pacemaker syndrome in carotid sinus syndrome is therefore about 10%. The incidence of VA conduction in this study was however identical to that in our total series (4). It is therefore apparent that the majority of patients may tolerate VA conduction during VVI pacing.

The retrospective comparison of haemodynamic data with DVI preference showed that the magnitude of the vasodepressor response and pacemaker induced hypotension or symptoms reproduced by these manoeuvres did not predict subsequent DVI preference.

The presence of VA conduction was the only parameter to correlate with DVI preference. The presence of VA conduction cannot be used to predict an adverse outcome from VVI pacing as 38% of patients showing no preference for either pacing mode also had VA conduction, and none of the patients was symptomatic during brief temporary VVI pacing prior to implantation.

Symptoms scores for mild and severe dizziness were not significantly different in either pacing mode. Mild dizziness occurred in the majority of patients and this symptom is clearly not relieved by pacing, and may be vasodepressor in origin.

The high incidence of pacemaker syndrome and the difficulty in predicting patients at risk of this complication makes DVI pacing superior to VVI pacing in carotid sinus syndrome.

References

1. Walter PF, Crawley IS, Dorney ER: Carotid sinus hypersensitivity and syncope. Am J Cardiol 1978; 42: 396–403.
2. Davies AB, Stephens MR, Davies AG: Carotid hypersensitivity in patients presenting with syncope. Br Heart J 1979; 42: 583–6.
3. Peretz DI, Gerein AN, Miyagishima RT: Permanent demand pacing for hypersensitive carotid sinus syndrome. Can Med Assoc J 1973; 108: 1131–4.
4. Morley CA, Perrins EJ, Grant R, Chan SL, McBrien DJ and Sutton R: Carotid sinus syncope treated by pacing. Analysis of persistent symptoms and role of atrioventricular sequential pacing. Br Heart J 1982; 47: 411–418.
5. Morley CA, Perrins EJ, Chan SL, Sutton R: The role of hysteresis pacing in the hypersensitive carotid sinus syndrome. PACE 1983 in Press.
6. Alicandri C, Fouad FM, Tatazi RC, Castle L, Morant V: Three cases of hypotension and syncope with ventricular demand pacing. Possible role of atrial reflexes. Am J Cardiol 1982; 42: 137–142.
7. Sklaroff H: Carotid sinus hypersentivity asystole and hypotension in the same patient. Am Heart J 1978; 97: 815.

8. Patel EK, Yap VU, Fields J, Thonsan JH: Carotid sinus syndrome induced by malignant tumours in the neck. Emergence of vasodepressor manifestations following pacemaker therapy. Arch Intern Med 1979; 139: 1281–4.

Authors' address:
Dr. C. A. Morley
Cardiac Department
Westminster Hospital
Horseferry Road
London SW1P 2AP

935

Effect of Carotid Sinus Massage (CSM) on Arterial Blood Pressure in Patients with Hypersensitive Carotid Sinus Reflex and Syncope

A. Podczeck, G. Unger, F. Meisl, K. Frohner, K. Steinbach

Summary: In 19 patients with hypersensitive carotid sinus reflex and syncope, the arterial pressure was measured directly during sinus rhythm with VVI-pacing before and during CSM, and DDD-pacing before and during CSM. With VVI-pacing, the blood pressure decreased between 0 and 38% (mean 17%) in comparison to sinus rhythm. During VVI-pacing and CSM blood pressure decreased between 12 and 60% (mean 33%). During DDD-pacing and CSM in 2 patients the decrese of arterial blood pressure was in the same range as in VVI-pacing (20%), in 1 patient 10%, whereas decreased during VVI-pacing more than 30%. There was no correlation between the extent of arterial blood pressure decrease during CSM and clinical symptoms. With PM-implantation due to frequent syncopes patients experienced no further syncope during follow-up. This study indicates that DDD-pacing is not superior to VVI-pacing in patients with hypersensitive carotid sinus reflex and syncope.

Introduction

Carotid sinus syndrome (CSS), as indication for PM-implantation is still controversial (1, 2, 3, 4, 5, 6). This is due to the fact that, on the one hand no further syncopes were observed during follow-up in patients with hypersensitive carotid sinus reflex even without PM-implantation, on the other hand, patients experienced further syncopes even after PM-implantation. It is assumed that these patients suffer from a so called "mixed" type of CSS, where further syncopes are caused by vago-vasal reaction and blood pressure drop even if asystole is prevented by cardiac stimulation. So an evaluation of arterial blood pressure behaviour during CSM is of practical value to decide on PM-treatment and to select the pacing mode.

The present study was undertaken to evaluate:
– blood pressure behaviour during the transition from sinus rhythm to VVI-pacing
– blood pressure behaviour during VVI-pacing and CSM
– blood pressure behaviour during AV-sequential pacing and CSM
The follow-up served to evaluate CSM reproducibility and correlation with cardiovascular symptoms (CVS).

Patients and Methods

19 patients (14 males, 5 females), age between 49 and 91 years (mean age 65 y), with histories of syncopes were evaluated according to the following protocol:
1. 2 CSM tests at interval of 1–3 days: The test was classified as positive whenever asystole of more than 3 sec occurred during CSM. Only patients with a positive reaction on 2 occasions were included in the study.

2. Arterial pressure measurement:

Arterial blood pressure was recorded directly from the radial artery during sinus rhythm and VVI-pacing with a frequency of 2 beats/min above the frequency of the sinus rhythm before and during CSM.

Arterial blood pressure was measured both during CSM of the left and of the right side.

In 3 patients, blood pressure was also measured before and during AV-sequential pacing and CSM. Atrial and ventricular stimulation were performed with bipolar electrodes, with an electrode distance of 1.0 cm. Patients were stimulated with an external current PM, with an output 100% above threshold.

Results

1. Arterial pressure during sinus rhythm, VVI-pacing and VVI-pacing + CSM, DDD-pacing and DDD-pacing + CSM

The blood pressure behaviour of the 19 patients are shown in Table 1. In patients with a systolic blood pressure below 200 mmHg before CSM, the extent of blood pressure drop is independent of the value before the test. In contrast to this, patients with a blood pressure above 200 mmHg before CSM show a significantly higher drop in arterial pressure.

The patients were divided in three groups, according to their arterial blood pressure behaviour during VVI-pacing and CSM (Table II).

1/3 of the patients showed a decrease in arterial blood pressure by more than 30% during vagal stimulation, compared to the value before this manoeuvre. It is remarkable that the decrease of arterial blood pressure during the transition from sinus rhythm to VVI-pacing was in the same range for all 3 groups.

In 2 out of 3 patients with AV-sequential pacing and CSM the extent of arterial blood pressure drop was the same as during VVI-pacing (20%). In the third patient the blood pressure decreased only 10% during AV-sequential pacing, whereas during VVI-pacing a decrease of 31% was observed.

In 15 patients the blood pressure behaviour was identical during right- and left-side CSM. In 2 patients with right-side CSM, in 2 patients with left side CSM the decrease of blood pressure was more prominent.

Table 1. Behaviour of blood pressure during sinus rhythm, VVI-pacing and VVI-pacing + CSM.

SR	VVI	% fall of BP	VVI + CSM	% fall of BP
125–270 mmHg (Ø 172,7)	90–240 mmHg (Ø 144,5)	0–38% (Ø 17)	60–180 mmHg (Ø 122,4)	12–60% (Ø 33)

Table 2. Classification of the patients according to the arterial blood pressure behaviour during the transition from sinus rhythm to VVI-pacing

∅ BP	SR	VVI	VVI + CSM
group I (11 pts.) fall of BP < 20%	∅ 165,5 mmHg	∅ 150,0 mmHg	∅ 130,5 mmHg (–0-17%, ∅–4,7)
group II (3 pts.) fall of BP 20–30%	∅ 168,3 mmHg	∅ 151,6 mmHg	∅ 113,3 mmHg (–20-24%, ∅–22,3%)
group III (6 pts.) fall of BP > 30%	∅ 165,0 mmHg	∅ 151,0 mmHg	∅ 86,0 mmHg (–37-53%, ∅–41,6%)

2. AV-conduction

In 13 patients, AV-block was observed during left- as well as during right-side CSM, in 4 patients only during right-side CSM, in 2 patients only during left-side CSM (8).

3. Treatment and Follow-up

8 out of 19 patients received a PM because of frequent syncopes (6 patients VVI-mode, 2 patients DDD-mode). During a follow-up period of 2–14 months no patient in this group experienced a further syncope.

During the follow-up period 4 patients died, 2 of them had an implanted PM. 3 patients died of a stroke, 1 patient of an acute myocardial infarction. Of the other 15 patients, 10 were asymptomatic during follow-up (Group I: 6 patients, 4 with implanted PM; Group II: 1 patient; Group III: 3 patients). 5 patients suffered from dizzy spells (Group I: 3 patients, 2 patients with implanted PM; Group II: 1 patient; Group III: 1 patient). CSM was negative during follow-up in 10 patients, still positive in 5 patients. The reaction to CSM did not correspond to clinical symptoms.

Discussion

The percentage of patients with an implanted PM because of CSS varies from country to country. Canada e.g. reports in 1982 a percentage of 0.5%, in some countries of Europe the figure is between 4 and 6% (9). It is unknown if this disease is more frequent in Europe or if CSS is not considered as indication of PM-treatment in Canada. Some controversies concerning the indication of PM-treatment could be explained by an abnormal decrease of arterial blood pressure in addition to cardiac arrest during CSM. These patients still experience CVS, even if the cardiac arrest is prevented by PM-implantation.

The present study demonstrates that arterial blood pressure behaviour in patients with CSS is different from that of the normal population (6, 7). In contrast to the normal population, the arterial blood pressure decreases in 10 out of 19 patients by more than 50 mmHg (52–110 mmHg, mean 72.2 mmHg). For the time being there are no generally accepted criteria on what percentage of decrease in arterial blood pressure is indicative of a so called vago-vasal type of CSS; in particular whether the absolute blood pressure drop or the percentage of decrease in relation to the pretest values should be used. This demonstrates the difficulty to classify the different types of CSS. 57% of the patients in this study group showed a decrease in blood pressure during CSM of less than 20%. They can perhaps be classified as patients with an isolated cardiac type of CSS.

In most of the patients left-side as well as right-side CSM caused a blood pressure drop which was in the same range. This was also true for the influence of CSM on AV-conduction.

For the treatment of cardiac type of CSS, the implantation of a VVI-PM seems to be adequate. In these patients, where the PM is necessary to prevent an asystole for a short period of time, AV-sequential pacing is probably not superior. This recommendation is also based on the experience that the VVI-paced patients of this study had no further syncope during follow-up.

The results in 3 patients provide no clear indication whether AV-sequential pacing in mixed or vago-vasal type has any advantages (1). This finding is in agreement with Morley et al. who found that DDD-pacing has no advantages in patients with CSS. The uncertainty could be due to the fact that in the moment clear criteria for the different types of CSS are not yet established.

Even retrograde conduction is not considered as indication for DDD-pacing, whenever rate-programmable units are used.

AAI-pacing should not be used in CSS. In most patients CSM causes AV-block II° or III°. Although CSM, as an unphysiological test, does not reflect AV-conduction during a spontaneous vagal reaction, it is likely that AV-block can occur also under this condition and that AAI-pacing is then ineffective (10).

Clinical Implications

1. PM-implantation in patients with CSS is indicated whenever frequent syncopes occur and other reasons for CVS can be excluded.
2. In these patients PM-treatment is effective, even if arterial blood pressure decreases more than 30% during CSM.
3. It has not been established whether physiological pacing has advantages over VVI-pacing.
4. CSM was not reproducible in 50% of the patients during follow-up (11).

References

1. Morley CA, Perrins EF, Grant P, Chan SL, McBrien DJ, Sutton R: Carotid sinus syncope treated by pacing. Br Heart J 1982; 47: 411–418.
2. Büchner C, Thierfelder K: Die klinische Relevanz des Carotisdruckversuchs bei der Indikation zur Schrittmacherbehandlung. Herzschrittmacher 1982; 2: 25–28.
3. Leatham A: Carotid sinus syncope. Br Heart J 1982; 47: 409–410.
4. Merx S, Effert S, Hanrath P, Pop T, Rehder W, Schweizer P: Hyperaktiver Carotissinusreflex. DMW 1981; 106: 135–140.

5. Strauer BE, Brunner L, Dehne N: Die Behandlung des Carotissinussyndroms mittels kardialer Schrittmacherstimulation. DMW 1973; 98: 558–560.
6. Gadermann E, Heinz N, Saegler J: Die Synkopen des Carotissinussyndroms und ihre Behandlung. Internist 1973; 14: 502–510.
7. Franke H: Über das Karotissinussyndrom und den sogenannten hyperaktiven Karotissinus-Reflex. Schattauer-Verlag, Stuttgart 1963.
8. Morley CA, Perrins EJ, Sutton R: Pharmacological intervention in the carotid sinus syndrome. PACE 1983; 6: A-16.
9. Feruglio GA: World survey on cardiac pacing. Pace 1983; 6: A-157 – A-172.
10. Probst P, Mühlberger V, Kaliman J, Pachinger O, Steinbach K, Kaindl F: Electrostimulation in carotid sinus syndrome. PACE 1983; 6: 689.
11. Podczeck A, Frohner K, Meisl F, Unger G, Steinbach K, Significance of carotid sinus massage in patients with cerebrovascular symptoms. PACE 1983; 6: A-17.

Supported in part by "Jubiläumsfonds der Österreichischen Nationalbank; Projekt Nr. 1998" and Hochschuljubiläumsstiftung der Stadt Wien.

Authors' address:
Dr. A. Podczeck
Wilhelminenspital
III. Medical and Cardiac Dept.
Montleartstr. 37
A-1170 Wien/Österreich

Emergency Pacing Using the Fluid Column of a Cardiac Catheter

G. T. Meester, M. L. Simoons, C. J. Slager, P. P. Kint, W. Spaa,
P. G. Hugenholtz

Summary: The fluid column of a haemodynamic monitoring catheter can be used as a conductor for emergency cardiac pacing. For this purpose a special fluid column pacemaker, the FCP was designed. The pacemaker generates a current pulse of 0.1 to 7 mA at fixed rates. It was tested in animals and patients. In all instances cardiac capture through the fluid column of a flow-directed balloon catheter was achieved within a few seconds. The FCP was also effectively used in one emergency patient in cardiogenic shock with sudden total AV block. The FCP seems an ideal standby device for emergencies in intensive care areas, catheterization laboratories and operating rooms, where right heart catheters are often already inserted.

In the coronary and other intensive care units, cardiac pacing is used as an effective therapy for many forms of acute cardiac conduction disturbances (1, 2, 3). In an emergency the introduction of a stimulation catheter or the exchange of a haemodynamic monitoring catheter is essentially a relatively simple procedure (4). In the clinical setting, however, this intervention requires special expertise and materials and, most of all, extra time, while risks of infection are enhanced. The possibility of being able to pace the heart immediately and without an extra catheter exchange or intervention is therefore of a great practical advantage, especially in an emergency situation.

In intensive care units and other similar areas, many patients already have an indwelling right heart catheter, usually of the flow-directed ballon type without pacing electrodes, with its tip in the pulmonary artery. The electrode version of the floating catheter is not indicated for routine purposes, because it is more expensive than the non-electrode type and, secondly, because the necessity for emergency cardiac pacing occurs only in 1 or 2% of the patients in a Coronary Care Unit. In another approach to this problem, we have investigated whether the fluid column in a conventional catheter, when filled with saline, could be used as an electrical conductor to form a connection between the myocardium of the right ventricle and an external pacemaker.

When this is realized, the complete procedure to start ventricular pacing will take no more than the few seconds, necessary for connecting the external pacemaker to the fluid column of the catheter and next to pull back the cathetertip from the pulmonary artery into the right ventricle.

Methods

The main problem for the design is the high electrical impedance of the fluid column in a monitoring situation. For the fluid column in a flow-directed balloon catheter the electrical impedance is approximately 1 megOhm, depending to some extent not only on the model and size of the catheter, but also on the type of fluid in the lumen, which is

943

usually saline. A special pacemaker was therefore developed, which was able to overcome this high electrical resistance of the fluid column. The designed pacemaker circuitry is of the "fixed rate" and "constant current" type. It incorporates a feed back control circuit which maintains its 1 msec pulse at the adjusted current level, within a given range of external loading conditions. It is battery operated.

Results

In figure 1 the maximum output characteristics of the fluid column pacemaker are shown. The instrument is designed so that maximally 7 mA can be provided against a resistance of 1 megOhm with a pulse width of 1 msec.

This level has been shown to be, in our animal and patient experience, more than adequate for pacing the heart. Several experiments were carried out to test the pacemaker and the catheter connector assembly. First the pacemaker was tested in 30 piglets who were under general anaesthesia for various other experiments. All animals were in sinus rhythm. A balloon catheter was placed with its tip in the pulmonary artery and, for the pacing experiment, temporarily pulled back into the right ventricle. Ventricular capture at a rate just above the resting heartrate could be easily obtained in all animals. The mean current setting was 1.1 mA. The same experiment was performed in 2 dogs, also successfully.

Pacing of the left ventricle is also possible as demonstrated in three other piglets which had a Sones coronary angiography catheter in the left ventricle, and in two others with a pigtail angiography catheter, also positioned in the left ventricle. The mean current for consistent capture of the left ventricle was 0.3 mA in these five animals.

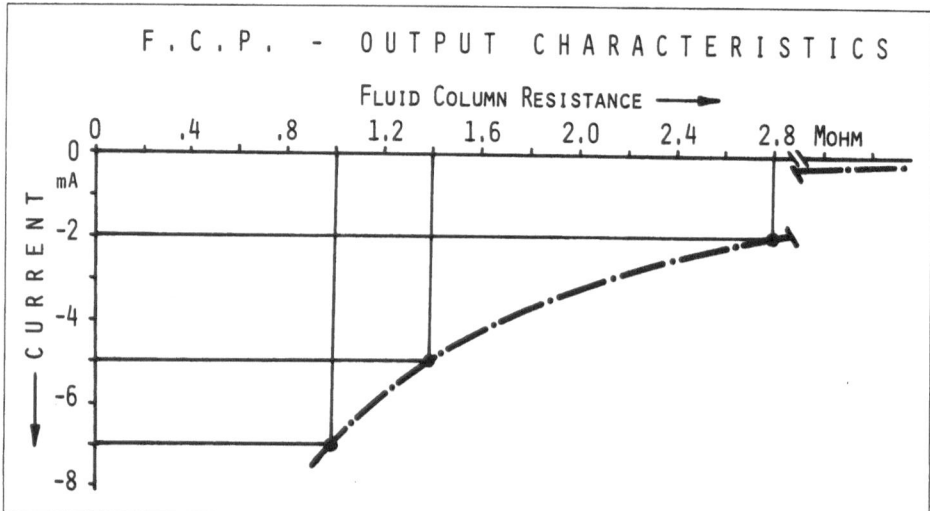

Fig. 1. FCP output characteristic.
Maximum current output as obtained during increasing load.

Next, the pacemaker was tested in 42 patients admitted to the CCU with a fresh myocardial infarct. All patients were in sinus rhythm and had an indwelling balloon catheter for monitoring purposes.

Prior to routine removal of this catheter and two days after admission, the FCP was tested in these patients with informed consent. In all patients pacing could easily be carried out. Ventricular capture was achieved within a few seconds in all patients. Pacing thresholds were between 0.3 and 4.5 mA, with a median value of 1.8 mA. After further pullback of the balloon catheter from the right ventricle into the right atrium, also right atrial pacing could be performed in 24 of 28 patients. Thresholds for the right atrium were between 0.3 and 3.8 mA with a median value of 1.5 mA.

The catheter was usually pulled back over a trajectory of 10 to 12 cm from the pulmonary artery into the outflow tract of the right ventricle to enable ventricular capture. The distance in an individual patient depends partly on the original position of the catheter tip and partly on possible slack. The leeway in the right ventricle was usually 5 to 7 cm before ventricular pacing was discontinued, due to the cathetertip entering the right atrium.

Finally, the FCP was used in a real emergency, in the Coronary Care Unit. During the testing period in the CCU, a 35 year male patient was admitted with a fresh anterior wall myocardial infarct. He was in cardiogenic shock and an intra aortic balloonpump was introduced.

A few hours later he suddenly developed total atrioventricular block with extremely low heart rates and consequent failure of the intra-aortic balloon assist device. To further aggravate the situation, the pacing leads of the already inserted multipurpose catheter proved to be defective and did not conduct the pacemaker pulses. Emergency pacing then was carried out using the FCP prototype through the fluid column of that same catheter over a period of approximately 15 minutes, until another conventional electrode catheter was introduced.

After some experience it became clear that a special design was needed for the connector between the FCP and the fluid column of the catheter. Figure 2 shows a diagram of this connector. The connector assembly also serves as an skin contact and is kept with fastening strips on the arm of the patient. The pacemaker operates with a voltage between 1 and 5 kVolt, depending on fluid column resistance and current setting. Accidental contact with one or both electrodes of the functioning pacemaker by the medical staff is harmless, because of the limited amount of energy involved, the pulse width being limited to 1 msec. Because of the emergency situations in which this pacemaker is designed to be used, the connector incorporates maximum contact and mechanical reliability. Incomplete connection between the catheter and the pacemaker is detected. Also, leakage of blood or other fluids or loosening of the fastening strips will give a visual and audio alarm, and pacing is discontinued automatically.

Conclusion

We have developed and tested an external pacemaker, the FCP, which is able to pace the heart through the fluid column of a cardiac catheter, when filled with saline or another conducting fluid. The device has been shown to be effective and safe, both in animals and patients, while it proved its value in one real emergency occurring during the testing

945

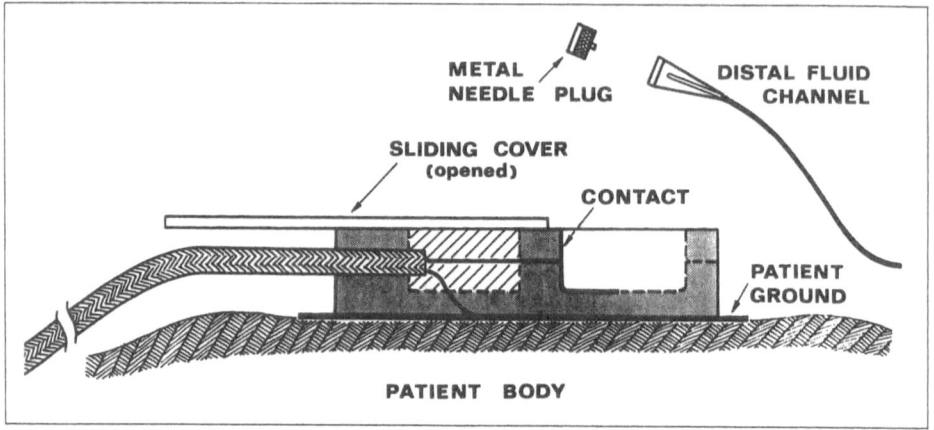

Fig. 2. Diagram of the pacemaker connector.
The connector has a metal base plate for skin contact and is fastened to the arm of the patient. On top a sliding cover over a slot dimensioned for the external end of a cardiac catheter when closed with a metal cap.

period. Finally, we feel it to be ideally suited for emergency situations in intensive care units, operating theaters or catheterization laboratories, where a cardiac catheter with a fluid column is already inserted.

References

1. Javier RP, Maramba LC, Hildner FJ, Cohen LS, Korn M, Schoenfeld CD, Samet P: Temporary cardiac pacing: technique and indications. Chest 1971; 59: 498–500.
2. Furman S, Escher DJW, Schwedel JB, Solomon N: Transvenous pacing. A seven year review. Am Heart J 1966; 71: 408–416.
3. Waldo AL, Wells JL Jr, Cooper TB, MacLean WA: Temporary cardiac pacing: applications and techniques in the treatment of cardiac arrhythmias. Prog Cardiovasc Dis 1981; 23: 451–474.
4. Furman S, Schwedel JB: An intracardiac pacemaker for Stokes-Adams seizures. N Engl J Med 1959; 261: 943–948.

Authors' address:
Dr. M. Simoons
Thoraxcenter
ARZ DIJKZIGT, University
P.O. Box 1783
NL-3000 DR Rotterdam
The Netherlands

Temporary Pacing in AMI Complicated by A-V Block: Hemodynamic Changes During VVI, DVI, VDTI Pacing with External Sorin BMMP 80 Pacer

L. Sernesi, R. Valentini, E. M. Greco, M. Arlotti, A. Lotto

Summary: A-V block may significantly decrease cardiac output (CO) in AMI through the loss of atrial contraction hence adding to the effects of bradycardia and myocardial damage. In this study we evaluated the effects of restoring the A-V synchronism using a Sorin BMMP 80, shifting sequentially form DVI or VDTI to VVI pacing. Twenty-six patients with transmural AMI (two anterior and 24 postero-inferior) complicated within the fourth day by A-V block and a low CO were investigated. Compared to VVI pacingrestoration of the normal A-V conduction resulted in an increase of CI ($2.16 \pm 0.43 \rightarrow 2.85 \pm 0.54$ l/min/m², $p < 0.001$, $+31\%$), of SI ($26.8 \pm 6.98 \rightarrow 35.0 \pm 8.0$ ml/min/m², $p < 0.001$, $+30\%$), of LVET ($+15\%$), of TTI ($+20.6\%$), a slight increase of BP, a reduction of TSR ($1707 \pm 331 \rightarrow 1414 \pm 188$ dyne/sec/cm⁻⁵, $p < 0.01$, -17.1%), of $\overline{CVP}$ ($7.9 \pm 2.6 \rightarrow 4.5 \pm 2.4$ mmHg, $p < 0.001$, -41.4%), of $\overline{WP}$ ($17.4 \pm 4.69 \rightarrow 13.20 \pm 1.78$ mmHg, $p < 0.01$, -20.6%). The best hemodynamic results were obtained with an A-V interval of 150 msec. DVI pacing evocated a temporary atrial fibrillation in two patients and the necessity to use an atrial overdrive determined a slight increase of TTI ($+20.6\%$). Two patients died in CCU from cardiogenic shock and pulmonary embolism, the others were discharged in a good hemodynamic state. In conclusion, DVI and VDTI pacing give better hemodynamic results as opposed to VVI pacing. DVI pacing seems to be indicated only in A-V block with atrial bradyarrhythmias.

Acute myocardial infarction (AMI) complicated by second to third degree A-V block often indicates a bad prognosis, not only for the ventricular hyperkinetic arrhythmias, enhanced by the low heart rate, but especially for the low cardiac output (CO), due to the loss of atrial systole and for the myocardial damage and bradycardia. It is not always possible to improve the hemodynamic pattern by increasing the ventricular rate with drugs or temporary ventricular pacing. In fact, the myocardium, with a low compliance due to the ischemia, can critically worsen its hemodynamics from the loss of atrial systole.

The purpose of this study is to evaluate the effects of restoring the A-V synchronism using a Sorin BMMP 80 external pacer, shifting sequentially from DVI or VDTI to VVI pacing in patients with transmural AMI, complicated by A-V block with a critical low CO.

We studied 26 patients (24 males, 2 females) affected by AMI (two anterior and 24 post-inferior) complicated within the fourth day by A-V block and a low cardiac output (cardiac index (CI) < 2.2 l/min/m²). Six of these patients had a second degree A-V block, Mobitz type I, two had a 2 : 1, 3 : 1 A-V block, and 18 had a third degree A-V block. His bundle recordings showed 24 suprahisian A-V blocks and two infrahisian A-V blocks. The ventricular rate averaged between 35 and 60 bpm, while the atrial rate varied between 55 and 100 bpm. We used two USCI 6F bipolar catheters in the right atrium and at the apex of the right ventricle in 19 patients, by the percutaneous technique, through a femoral vein. In the other seven patients we used only one USCI 6F esapolar catheter introduced percutaneously through the left cubital vein, so that the four proximal electrodes were in contact with the right atrium side and the two distal at the apex of the right ventricle. We used an external Medtronic 5330 pacer for ventricular and DVI pacing in the unipolar mode. The pacing rate was selected at five or 10 bpm over sinus rate to obtain a stable atrial overdrive. We used a new SORIN pacer type BMMP 80 for DVI and VDTI pacing. It was noted, in the first six patients studied, that the best hemodynamic results were with an A-V interval of 150 msec. All the patients were monitored with a Swan-Ganz catheter in a pulmonary artery and CO was calculated by termodilution method; we have evaluated the following parameters: systemic blood pressure (BP), central venous pressure ($\overline{CVP}$), cardiac index (CI), systolic index (SI), total systemic resistance (TSR), pulmonary wedge pressure ($\overline{WP}$); we have also evaluated LVET and TTI in all patients; the data were obtained after 30 min from the beginning of VVI, DVI, and VDTI pacing. We did not use any drugs in these patients before the study, except those patients in the fourth hemodynamic class, where we used vasodilatators and inotropic drugs . We excluded from this study all patients who needed ventricular pacing rates over 100 bpm, to avoid pacing with too elevated heart rate. It was impossible to complete the study in two patients because of the onset of atrial fibrillation during DVI pacing. In 24 of the 26 patients, we compared the VVI with the DVI and VDTI pacing.

After VVI pacing, according to the Forrester and Swan hemodynamic classification, 11 patients were in the second class, 3 were in the third class, and 10 were in the fourth class. After the DVI and VDTI pacing, only two patients remained in the fourth class while the other four passed in the second and four in the first; all the others in the second and third classes passed in the first one.

DVI and VDTI pacing, compared with VVI pacing induced (Fig. 1):

A) An increase in CI of 34%, from 2.16 ± 0.43 to 2.85 ± 0.54 l/min/m² (p < 0.001). In particular, the physiological pacing determined a significant increase of CI (mean

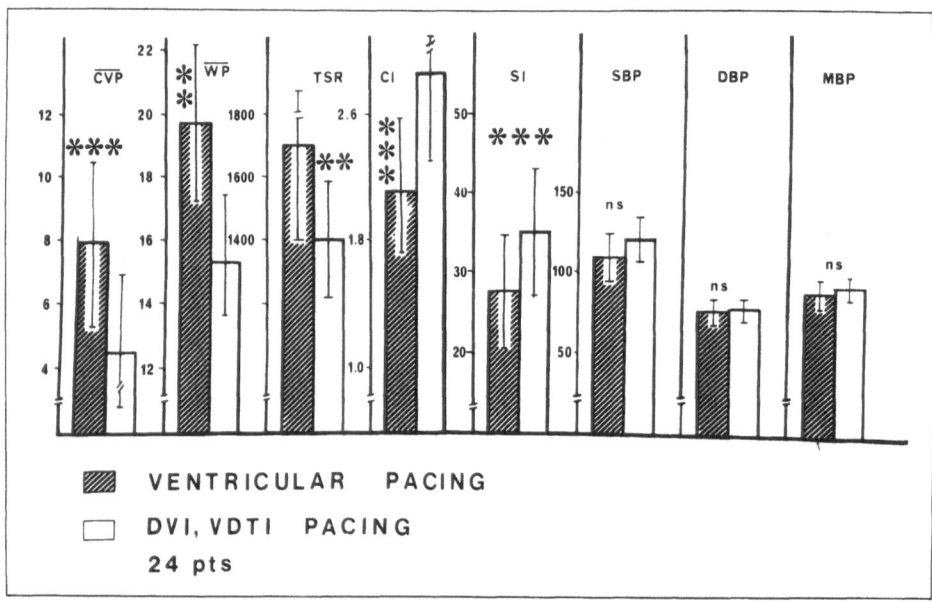

Fig. 1. Hemodynamic comparison between DVI and VDTI pacing with VVI pacing.

948

2.40 ± 0.30 l/min/m², p < 0.001) in six patients with a CI below 2 l/min/m²
(p < 0.001);

B) A significant increase of systolic index (SI) of 30%, from 26.8 ± 6.98 to 35.0 ± 8.01
ml/min/m² (p < 0.001);

C) An increase, but not statistically significant, of systolic blood pressure of 11.8%, from
107 ± 15 to 120 ± 13 mmHg of diastolic blood pressure, from 75 ± 8.0 to 77 ± 6.0
mmHg and of mean blood pressure. Nevertheless, in four patients with a critical hemodynamic pattern, we noted a significant increase of systolic, diastolic, and mean blood
pressure;

D) A decrease of total systemic resistance (TSR) of 17.1% (p < 0.01);

E) A decrease of central venous pressure (CVP) of 41.4%;

F) A decrease of wedge pressure (WP) of 20.6%;

G) An increase of LVET of 15%;

H) An increase of TTI of 20.6%.

Considering the two types of pacing, DVI and VDTI, the statistical analysis did not demonstrate statistical differences between them (Fig. 2).

In the patients submitted to VDTI pacing we noted a progressive and spontaneous decrease of atrial rate and subsequently of ventricular rate (about 5–10%), secondary to the
improved hemodynamics.

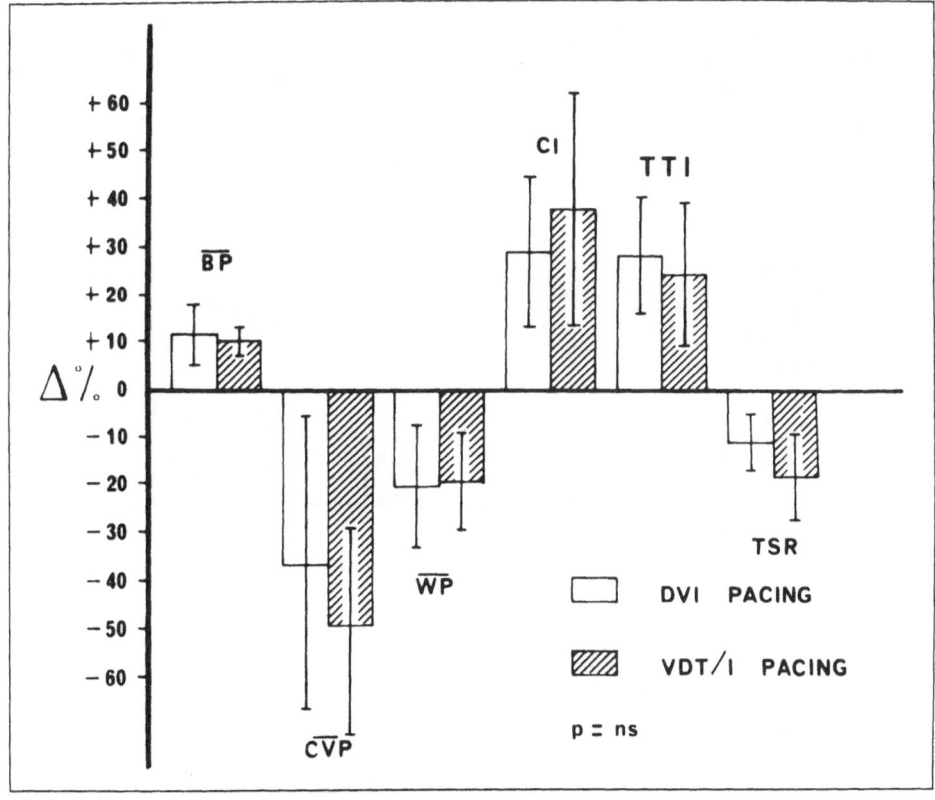

Fig. 2. Statistical analysis between DVI and VDTI pacing.

The follow-up was between six and 36 months. One patient affected by AMI, complicated by third degree A-V block, died on the first day of cardiogenic shock. Twelve patients restored their normal A-V conduction between 12 and 48 hours: one of them, with an inferior myocardial reinfarction complicated by third degree A-V block, died six months later, out of hospital, of unknown causes. Six patients were paced for two to five days: one of them, affected by an infero-posterior-lateral AMI and second degree A-V block, needed a permanent pacemaker five weeks after the acute ischemic phase, because of the persistence of a stable infrahisian first degree A-V block with LBB and left axis deviation. This patient died one month after the implant of sudden death. Another patient, with inferior AMI complicated by third degree A-V block, died of unknown causes, two years later. Three patients were paced for six to nine days: one of them, affected by antero-septal AMI and infrahisian A-V block, died on the ninth day of cardiac rupture, the second patient was paced for ten days, for a reinfarction on the seventh day; the third patient, with inferior and lateral AMI, died in CCU after ten days of pacing of pulmonary embolism.

Discussion

Many authors have pointed out the importance and the hemodynamic advantages in restoring the atrial contraction with physiological pacing, in contrast to VVI pacing, in those patients affected by AMI complicated by second or third degree A-V block (1, 2, 3, 4, 5). In our study, we have also evaluated the metabolic cost, with TTI, of physiological pacing, looking at the protection of ischemic myocardium. Our data have demonstrated that physiological pacing increased CI (31%), SI (30%), BP and reduced TSR (17.1%),

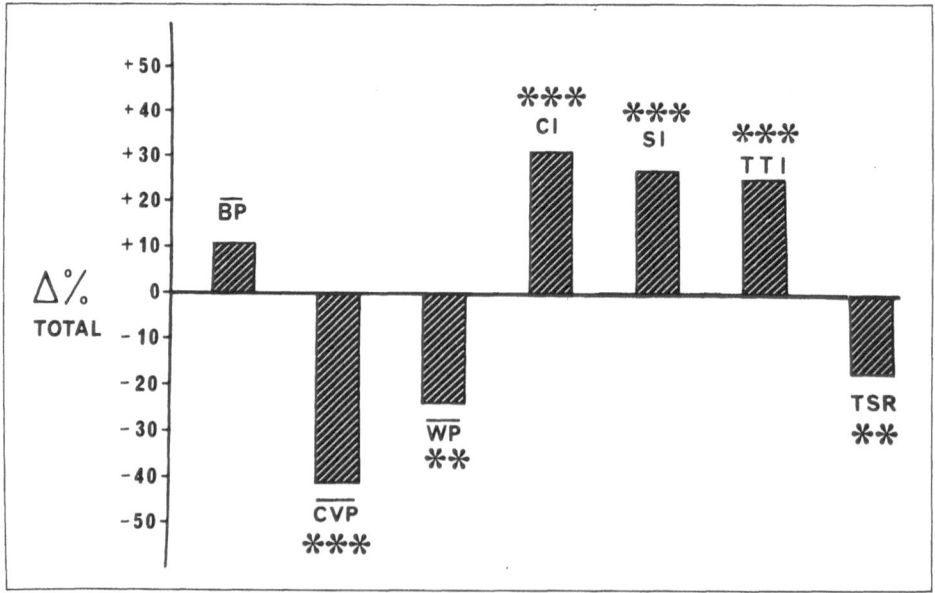

Fig. 3. Hemodynamic benefit of physiological pacing.

$\overline{WP}$ (20.6%), and $\overline{CVP}$ (41.4%) (Fig. 3). As DVI and VDTI pacing were performed in each patient at the same rates, it is obvious that the increase of CI is due to the increase of SI. So, this increment is the direct expression of the restored physiological A-V contraction, which is able to displace the preload at a more responsive point on the Frank Starling curve of the ischemic ventricle. The increase of TTI could be disadvantageous for the protection of the ischemic myocardium. If we consider, however, that DVI and VDTI pacing determine a greater increase in CI (31%) (Fig. 3) than in TTI, an increase of BP, and a decrease in ventricular filling pressures with a better coronary perfusion, it is clear that this mode of pacing is more functional.

Now, we want to examine the differences between DVI and VDTI pacing. In DVI pacing it is necessary to maintain atrial overdrive with an expensive O_2 myocardial consumption, while VDTI pacing allows not only ventricular pacing at atrial isorhythmic rates, but also utilizes the spontaneous heart rate decrease, secondary to the better hemodynamics so induced. In DVI pacing, atrial asynchronous pacing can determine the onset of atrial fibrillation, as we have noted in two of our patients.

We conclude that DVI pacing is an easy pacing technique; it is especially useful and necessary in patients presenting a low cardiac output. The increase in TTI, induced by this technique, is advantageously compensated for by a greater increase in coronary perfusion. VDTI pacing offers the best performance in contrast with DVI pacing, which is indicated only in A-V block complicated by atrial bradyarrhythmia.

References

1. Samet P, Bernstein, WH, Nathan DA, et al: Atrial contribution to cardiac output in complete heart block. Am J Cardiol 1965: 16: 1–10.
2. Leinbach RC, Chamberlain DA, Kastor JA, et al: A comparison of the hemodynamic effects of ventricular and sequential atrioventricular pacing in patients with heart block. Am H J 1969; 78: 502–508.
3. Gillespie WJ, Greene DG, Karatzas NB, et al: Effects of atrial systole on right ventricular stroke output in complete heart block. Brit Med J 1967; 1: 75–79.
4. Ruskin J, Harley A, Rembert J, et al: Contribution of atrial systole to ventricular stroke volume in man. Circulation 38, 1969; Suppl 6: 168.
5. Lotto A, Greco EM: La funzione cardiovascolare con i vari tipi di pacemakers. Estratto da: Il cardiopatico operato, Atti del Corso di aggiornamento Cardiologico tenuto a Milano nel Settembre 1973.

Authors' address:
Dr. Laura Sernesi
Cardiology Dpt. Ospedale Maggiore Policlinico
Via F. Sforza, 35
20100 Milano

Pacing in the World Today. World Survey on Cardiac Pacing for the Years 1979 to 1981

G. A. Feruglio[1]), K. Steinbach[2])

Summary: The state of the art of cardiac pacing in the world, in the early '80s, has been surveyed by the questionnaire technique with the assistance of national contact persons.

Data from 56 countries were collected, concerning over 220,000 new PM implants, nearly 63,000 replacements and over 340,000 patients in follow-up. Of the 5711 implanting centers, the majority use from 50 to 200 PM per year and only 1/10 perform prepacing electrophysiological studies. The age of patients at first implant was 12 y in less than 2% of cases and 80 y in up to 26% (Sweden). A-V block and sinoatrial disease are still the leading causes for permanent pacing; pacing in tachycardias is becoming relatively more common (3.5% in Australia; 9% in Finland). Lithium batteries are the most common power source today; in some European countries, however, HgZn batteries are still used (88.8% in Czechoslovakia). Multi-programmable generators are used in up to 74.2% of cases in the USA but, in the majority of countries, they represent 0–20% of the units at first implant. Epicardial leads are used in up to 21.8% of cases (Japan), atrial transvenous leads in up to 15.8% (USA); percutaneous insertions of transvenous leads are performed in up to 60% of cases (UK). Death from unknown causes is still an important cause for file closure (34.6% of cases in Austria). Cost of short/long-life PMs has increased in the last few years; still the total cost of pacing per month has decreased up to 40% in the last decade.

Introduction

Cardiac pacing is entering its third decade of continuous and vigorous growth in all aspects: clinical, technological and organizational ones. In the last twenty years, in fact, the spectrum of clinical applications has continuously widened and now extends from symptomatic bradycardias to recurrent, paroxysmal tachycardias. The magnificent advance of pacemaker technology has fostered a large array of sophisticated pulse generators including multiprogrammable, dual chamber, multimodal, interrogatable devices, far more specific in their clinical applicability. Organizational progress is reflected in the development of pacemaker centers for implantation and/or evaluation, national and international pacing societies and registries, and an increasing roster of meetings and congresses.

No doubt that we are now on the verge of a new era in cardiac pacing! This has prompted us to review the state of the art and to perform a new extensive survey, also in coincidence with a major event such as the VII World Symposium on Cardiac Pacing, in Vienna.

Continental Coordinators: A. F. Rickards (Europe); B. S. Goldman, V. Parsonnet (North America); A. Dussault (South/Central America); T. Iwa, G. Sloman (Asian-Pacific); I. W. P. Obel (Africa).
[1]) Istituto di Cardiologia, Ospedale Regionale, Udine (Italy).
[2]) Kardiologische Universitätsklinik, Vienna (Austria).

Previous organized surveys were carried out on various occasions: Montecarlo (September, 1970), Groningen (April, 1973), Tokyo (March, 1976), Montreal (October, 1979) (1–4). All these reviews provided considerably information on epidemiology, implantation criteria and techniques, evaluation methodology, follow-up technology and reliability of cardiac pacemakers. Such information appears to be of importance not just to manufacturers and distributors but to governments, health ministries, insurance carriers and especially to those most concerned with patient care and well-being, the physicians committed to cardiac pacing.

In undertaking this new extensive survey we intended not only to keep up with a tradition of the World Symposium on Cardiac Pacing, but also, by taking advantage of the previous experiences, to provide a common data base, with comparable information for etiology, pathophysiology, major clinical indications, complications, device reliability and socioeconomic impact in order to allow the rapidly growing local, national and continental organizations to discuss and compare their results in a meaningful and productive manner.

We are aware of the major limitations of all extensive reviews of this kind, due to the incomplete data, misunderstandings on questioned items, extrapolation of data and, not least, the rapid changes of the pacemaker scene. However, we believe in the value of such an effort which, in addition to the fascinating medico-social commentaries it can produce, gives testimony to the large amount and high quality of work performed throughout the world (Fig. 1).

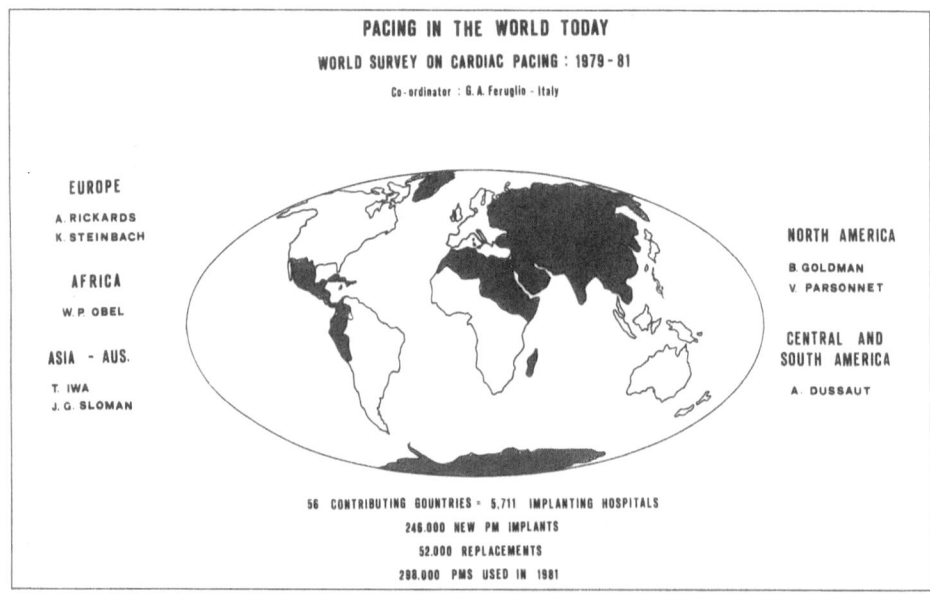

Fig. 1. The map of the survey.

954

Methods and Material

Like the previous survey of Montreal (4) this World Survey was carried out by the questionnaire technique and with the assistance of national contact persons. A comprehensive questionnaire, suitable for computer analysis and designed on the basis of a previous personal experience (Europacing '81) (5), was distributed to all countries of the world, where pacing activities were known to be present. The questionnaire was prepared to collect data on epidemiology, indications, patient follow-up and complications of cardiac pacing, as well as pacemaker hardware and organizational aspects of pacing in each country during the years 1979–1981.

The questionnaire concerned nearly 150 items, grouped under 18 headings including general information (country, number and practice, size of implanting hospitals, national data base and failure monitoring system, costs, etc.); prepacing electrophysiological studies; follow-up methods; total number of first implants and replacements; number of pacemakers re-used; age of patients at first implant; clinical indications for pacing; aetiology; pre-pacing ECG; pacemaker hardware and modes of pacing; leads; causes for file closure.

Despite some difficulties with data collection (credit must be given to the continental co-ordinators for their valuable assistance in this phase of the Survey), a response was obtained from 56 separate countries with 5711 implanting hospitals, where nearly 300,000 pulse generators were implanted in 1981 (Fig. 1). The contributing countries and co-ordinators are listed in Table 1.

In many instances the contributors did not designate whether their report contained data from all hospitals in their countries of origin or only from the major centers with some extrapolation. Time did not allow us to re-check some problematic data with the contact persons; this may reflect some errors in the interpretation of the questionnaires.

Some data has been re-interpreted to simplify presentation, without compromising the integrity of submitted information.

With the exception for the first implants and replacements reported in detail for each country or groups of countries (when numbers were too small to be analysed separately), in this paper the data are presented mostly consolidated by continent. Detailed information on the various items for any one country, has been tabulated in the abstract book of the VIIth World Symposium on Cardiac Pacing (6).

Results

The total number of first implants and replacements per country and per year of the Survey, are reported in Table 2. These numbers, consolidated per continent, are presented in Table 3. For the year 1981, a total of 227,023 first implants and 62,878 replacements were reported throughout the world, with a ratio first implants/replacements of 3.6.

Of the total number of pulse generators used in 1981 (289,901) the largest share belongs to North America (51%), followed by Europe (44%), while the rest of the world used only 5% of the total units (Fig. 2).

Considering the first implants only, as reported in Table 4, the annual increment is decreasing in North America (from 20.6% to 11.4% in three years) while it is increasing in Europe.

955

Table 1. 1983 world survey on cardiac pacing: contributing countries and coordinators.

Europe: (23 Countries)		North/Central/South America: (11 Countries)	
Co-ordinator: A. F. Rickards, K. Steinbach		Co-ordinators: B. Goldman/V. Parsonnet/ A. Dussaut	
Austria	(K. Steinbach)		
Belgium	(H. Ector)	Argentina	(A. Dussaut)
Bulgaria	(J. Markov)	Bolivia	(J. Barrenechea)
Czechoslovakia	(Z. Naprstek)	Brazil	(F. Lucchese)
Denmark	(J. Fabricius)	Canada	(B. Goldman)
Finland	(G. Häertel)	Chile	(A. Edwards)
France	(J. Torresani)	Honduras	(P. Fiallos Medina)
G.D.R.	(J. Witte)	Panama	(R. Blandon-D. Leon)
G.F.R.	(W. Irnich)	Paraquay	(J. Balansa)
Great Britain	(A. Rickards)	U.S.A.	(V. Parsonnet)
Greece	(J. Gialafos)	Uruguay	(H. Artucio)
Holland	(S. Hoorntse)	Venezuela	(A. Bello)
Hungary	(Z. Szabo/P. Kovacs)		
Iceland	(G. Oddsson)		
Ireland	(C. McCarthy)	**Australia: (2 Countries)**	
Italy	(G. Feruglio)		
Norway	(H. Grendahl)	Co-ordinator: G. Sloman	
Poland	(M. Stopczyk)	Australia	(G. Sloman)
Portugal	(S. Amram Sequerra)	New Zealand	(S. Yarrow)
Spain	(S. Botella Solana)		
Sweden	(O. Edhag)		
Switzerland	(I. Babotai)	**Africa: (13 Countries)**	
Yugoslavia	(M. Djordjevic)		
		Co-ordinator: I.W.P. Obel	
		Benin	(E. Bertrand)
		Centreafrique	(ID.)
		Ghana	(ID.)
Asia: (7 Countries)		Haute Volta	(ID.)
		Ivory Coast	(ID.)
Co-ordinator: T. Iwa		Mali	(ID.)
Hongkong	(S. Kong)	Mauritania	(ID.)
Indonesia	(B. Trisnohadi)	Niger	(ID.)
Israel	(S. Feldman)	Nigeria	(ID.)
Japan	(T. Iwa)	Senegal	(ID.)
Philippines	(A. Aventura)	South Africa	(I.W.P. Obel)
Singapore	(B. Chia	Togo	(E. Betrand)
Thailand	(P. Sakiyalak)	Zaire	(ID.)

With reference to the first implants per million inhabitants per country, a detailed report is given in Table 5. In Figure 3, the lowest and highest implantation rates in each continent are presented. The highest rate of new implants per million population was 518 as reported from the United States and Germany (FR). Such rate, in South America and Asia, was three times lower and extremely limited in Africa/(11/million in S. Africa).

The percentage of patient distribution according to age at first implant in 1981, is given in Table 6. In 1981, youngsters less than 12 y.o. represented up to 22% (Japan) of all newly implanted patients, while the elderly, over 80 years of age, represented up to 26%

956

Table 2. Pacing activities in all surveyed countries.

Country	Total number of first implants			Total number of replacements			Total number of pacemakers reused		
	1979	1980	1981	1979	1980	1981	1979	1980	1981
Canada	4 244	4 415	5 369	1 981	2 456	1 449	0	0	0
Unites States	94300	106 500	117 800	28 200	26 200	23 300	NA	NA	±750
Rep. of Panama	204	198	170	91	73	66	15	8	12
Argentina (2)	3 900	4 200	4 500	2 400	2 600	2 900	100	200	150
Chile	316	341	408	96	144	165	10	3	4
Other South Amer.	295	270	363	113	128	194	30	20	25
Black Africa	23	25	28	4	1	1	–	2	–
South Africa	290	267	337	297	245	217	15	30	25
Austria	1 602	1 661	1 780	863	761	556	60*)	60*)	60*)
Belgium	1 913	2 402	2 583	550	709	524	11	12	14
Bulgaria	186	174	277	58	64	58	12	9	13
Denmark	437	552	624	517	366	202	20	44	62
Finland	530*)	550*)	630*)	360*)	370*)	323	–	–	45*)
France	NA	NA	18 500*)	NA	NA	6 000*)	NA	NA	NA
Czechoslovakia	1 010	1 263	1 409	1 365	718	1 093	15	10	12
Greece	774	840	944	285	247	296	0	1	0
Germany (G.D.R.)	2 803	3 010	3 571	1 914	2 146	2 490	412	456	419
Germany (F.R.G.)	26 800*)	27 700*)	31 600*)	13 400*)	12 400*)	10 700*)	520	496	558
Hungary	786	910	1 067	393	475	532	53	100	104
Italy	7 980	8 824	9 500	5 052	4 234	4 702	86	95	140
Iceland	19	28	28	22	16	10	0	4	5
Norway	654	649	776	603	255	219	77	81	79
Poland	1 085	1 286	2 279	724	693	759	NA	NA	NA
Portugal (1)	264	312	409	198	258	180	17	23	3
Spain	3 050	3 275*)	3 550*)	1 350	950*)	825*)	25	75*)	100*)
Sweden	1 781	1 681	1 782	1 846	1 345	853	NA	NA	200*)
Switzerland	1 011	1 197	1 234	344	348	353	0	0	20*)
Netherlands (The)	2 421	2 639	2 876	1 568	899	536	86	95	140
United Kingdom	6 200*)	6 350*)	6 400*)	2 387	2 342	1 920	34	109	51
Yugoslavia	438	875	955	378	396	308	10	16	18
Israel	457	515	591	332	215	165	53	58	31
Japan	2 407	2 530	2 984	648	587	717	84	64	92
South Asia	250	248	299	85	111	80	1	5	8
Australia	747	742	811	244	267	192	49	50	34
New Zealand	171	153	224	74	74	83	12	5	3

*) Estimated; (1) Data from 4 centers out of 7; (2) Information from pacemaker companies.
NA = Not available.

957

Table 3. First implants and replacements (total number of PMs used) consolidated per continent.

Continent	1979	1980	1981	1979	1980	1981
N. America	98 544	110 515	123 169	30 181	29 256	24 749
C/S America	4 715	5 009	5 441	2 700	2 945	3 225
Africa	313	292	365	301	246	218
Europe	66 674	76 733	93 139	34 031	32 795	33 449
Asia	3 114	3 293	3 874	1 065	913	962
Australia a. New Zealand	918	895	1 035	318	341	275

Fig. 2. The largest share of the total number of PMs used in 1981, belongs to North America (51%), followed by Europe (44%). The rest of the world used only 5% of the total units implanted.

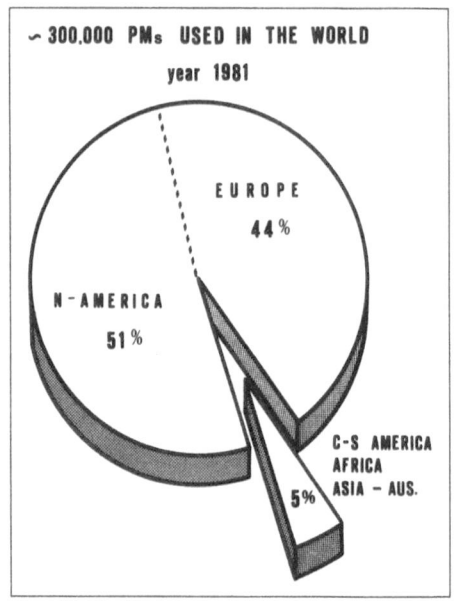

≈ 300.000 PMs USED IN THE WORLD
year 1981

EUROPE 44%

N-AMERICA 51%

C-S AMERICA
AFRICA
ASIA – AUS.
5%

Table 4. Annual percentage variation for total first implants in North America and Europe.

Years	N. America	Europe
1978–79	+20.6%	+17.1%
1979–80	+12.4%	+15.1%
1980–81	+11.4%	+21,3%

Table 5. Total number of first implants and implantation rates per million population in the surveyed countries.

Country	Population mid 1980 (000)*)	Total No of first implants in 1981	No of first implants per million population 1981
Canada	23.937	5.369	224.3
United States	227.323	117.800	518.2
Rep. of Panama	1.335	170	92.6
Argentina	27.740	4.500	162.2
Chile	11.104	403	36.7
Other South Amer. (1)	26.486	363	13.7
Black Africa (2)	99.030	28	0.3
South Africa	29.285	337	11.5
Austria	7.481	1.780	237.9
Belgium	9.833	2.533	262.7
Bulgaria	9.007	277	25.2
Denmark	5.122	624	121.8
Finland	4.863	630	129.5
France	53.508	18.500**)	345.7
Czechoslovakia	15.336	1.409	91.9
Greece	9.329	944	101.2
Germany (G.D.R.)	16.854	3.571	211.9
Germany (F.R.G.)	60.931	31.600**)	518.6
Hungary	10.754	1.067	99.2
Italy	56.940	9.500	166.8
Iceland	231	28	121.2
Norway	4.079	776	190.2
Poland	35.805	2.279	63.7
Portugal	9.836	409	41.6
Spain	37.378	3.550**)	95.0
Sweden	8.274	1.782	215.4
Netherlands (the)	14.079	2.786	197.9
Switzerland	6.466	1.234	190.8
United Kingdom	55.886	6.400**)	114.5
Yugoslavia	22.328	955	42.8
Israel	3.876	591	152.5
Japan	116.551	2.984	25.6
South Asia (3)	248.076	299	1.2
Austrialia	14.488	811	56.0
New Zealand	3.268	224	68.5

*) World Bank
**) Estimation
(1) Venezuela – Bolivia – Uruguay – Paraguay; (2) Senegal – Ivory Coast – Nigeria; (3) Indonesia – Singapore – Thailand – Philippines – Hong Kong

(Sweden). The great majority of patients (70% in German FR) was as usual, in the range of 61–80 years of age.

The main clinical indications for pacing in 1981 are presented in Table 7 and in Figure 4 a comparison between the two major areas of pacing in the world: North America and Europe, is attempted. Syncope was the most common pre-pacing clinical manifestation occurring in almost the same percentage of cases in North America (35%) and Europe

Fig. 3. Lowest and highest implantation rates in the various continents. In the US and Germany FR, the new implants reached the top number of 518 per million population.

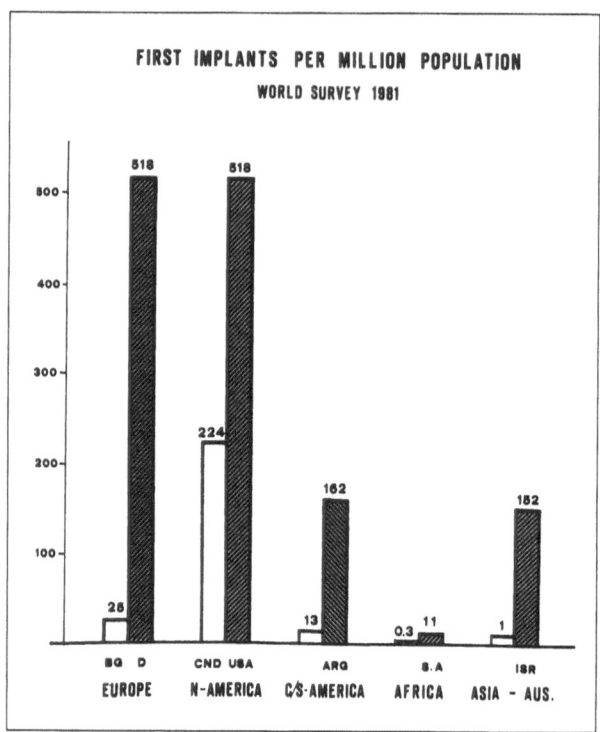

Table 6. Age distribution of patients.

Age of Pts. at first implant	
< 12 Yrs.	Up to 2% (Japan)
13–40 Yrs.	Up to 15% (Spain)
41–60 Yrs.	Up to 36% (Czechoslovakia)
61–80 Yrs.	Up to 70% (D.F.R.)
> 80 Yrs.	Up to 26% (Sweden)

Table 7. Clinical indications for pacing (% of first implants).

	N. America	Europe	C/S America	Africa	Asia-Aus.
Syncope	35	36	45	51	36
Dizzy spells	20	16	10	17	22
Bradycardia	12	21	20	11	16
Tachycardia	6	3	4	2	3
Prophylactic	7	3	11	6	5
Heart failure	10	8	3	8	7
Others	10	13	7	5	11

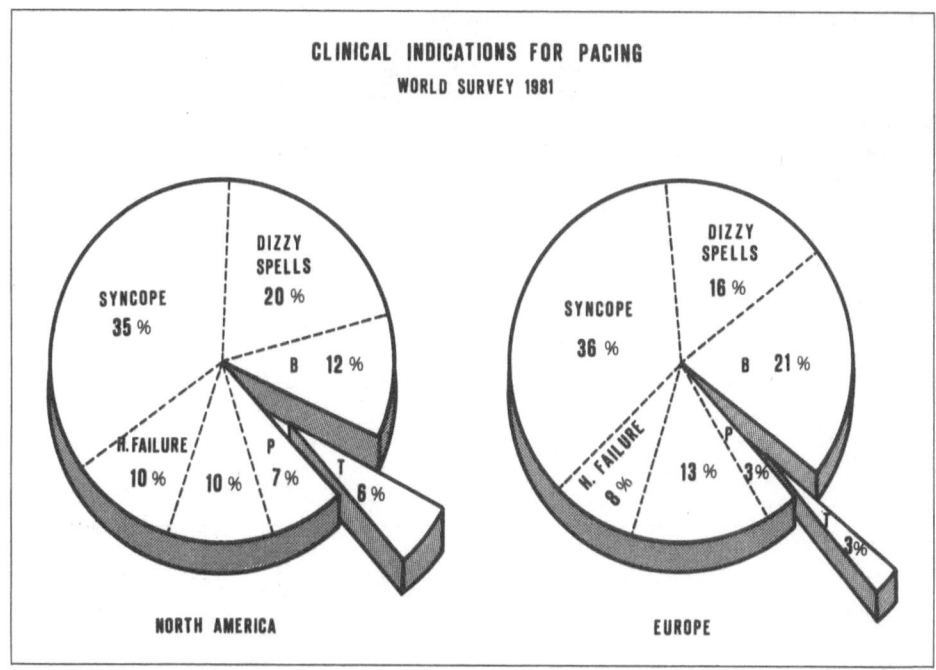

Fig. 4. The main clinical indications for pacing: a comparison between the two major areas of pacing in the world.

(36%). Dizzy spells and bradycardia run second and third respectively. Tachycardia as an indication for permanent pacing was 6% in North America, twice as frequent compared to Europe. Very similar data were reported for prophylactic pacing.

The most common ECG findings at first implant are given in percentages in Table 8. As expected, AV conduction disturbances and sinus node disfunctions were, by and large, the most frequent abnormalities. However, it is interesting to notice that the SSS as an indication for pacing was more frequent (46% of cases) compared to advanced AV block (31%) in the US. The reverse was reported for Europe and for all other countries. Furthermore, in Europe pacing for supraventricular and ventricular tachycardias occurred slightly more frequently compared to North America (1% versus 0.8% of cases).

Patient selection for permanent pacing has become more and more efficient and accurate in recent years. As reported in Figure 5, in 1981 up to 80% of patients underwent electrophysiological studies before implant, in Europe (Denmark) and in Japan. This figure was reported much lower for the US (21%) and other areas of the world.

Data concerning pacing modes in some representative countries and pacemaker hardware are reported in Tables 9–11. Simple ventricular demand pacing (VVI, VVT) was by far the most commonly used mode of pacing in 1981: 86.6% in the US; from 90 to 96% in Europe; over 98% in Australia and Argentina. Dual chamber pacing however was applied in a consistent percentage of cases in the US (8.8%), United Kingdom (6.7%) and Japan (3.6%).

Table 8. Pre-pacing ECG findings (% of first implants).

	N. America	Europe	C/S America	Africa	Asia-Aus.
Atrial rhythm disturbances and bradycardia	46	30	18	17	36
1st and 2nd degree AV-block	12	11	13	13	11
3rd degree AV-block	31	45	47	63	44
BBB and all forms of hemiblock	4	8	12	7	6
Supraventricular tachycardia	0.8	1	3	0	2
Ventricular tachycardia	0.8	1	2	1	0.7
Others	5.4	4	5	9	0.3

Fig. 5. The highest percentutages of patients undergoing prepacing electrophysiological studies were reported from Europe (Denmark) and Japan (80%). In the US only one patient out of five underwent such investigation.

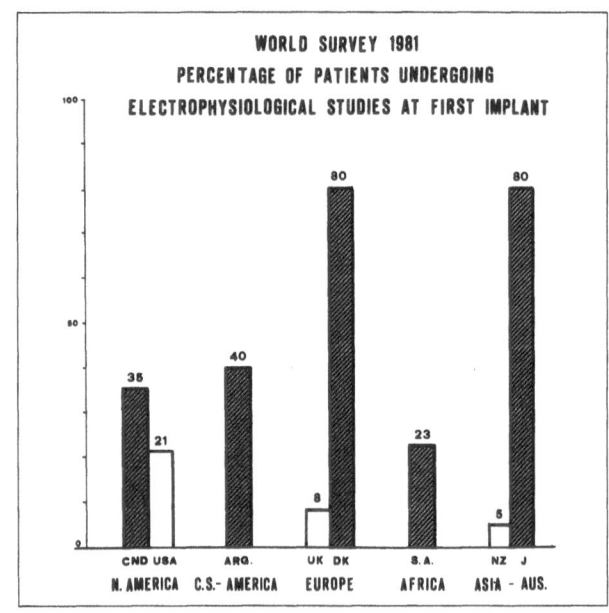

Programmable units accounted for 90% of the total used in US and Japan, while in some other countries their use was rather limited (20% in England) or inconsistant (German FR 1%) (Tab. 10). In those countries where programmability was commonly used, multiprogrammable units were the choice.

962

Table 9. Pacing modes in some countries (% of first implants).

	*) VOO	*) VVT	*) VVT	*) VAT	*) DVI	*) VDD	*) AOO	*) AAI	*) AAT	*) DDD	*) DC	Based on Cases
U.S.A.	0.8	86.6	1.5	0.4	6.9	1.1	0.9	1.2	0.2	0.4	8.8	114.855
Holland	0.0	96.5	0.3	1.0	0.5	0.1	–	1.6	0.0	0.0	1.6	2.876
U.K.	0.2	90.8	0.3	2.2	4.0	0.5	0.0	1.7	0.2	0.0	6.7	8.320
Italy	0.5	94.3	0.0	1.0	1.2	0.5	0.2	0.8	2.0	0.0	2.7	14.200
G.D.R.	1.1	19.8	74.8	0.5	0.3	0.1	0.0	3.4	0.0	0.0	0.9	3.548
Argentina	0.0	99.8	0.0	0.0	0.2	0.0	0.0	0.0	0.0	0.0	0.2	4.500
Japan	0.2	90.7	1.9	0.7	2.0	0.7	0.1	3.5	0.2	0.0	3.6	3.577
Australia	0.0	98.8	0.3	0.0	0.0	0.6	0.0	0.3	0.0	0.0	0.6	914

Table 10. Programmability in some countries (% of PMs used).

	Non progr. units	Progr. rate and/or output	Multi-progr.	Special tachyc. mode	Based on cases
U.S.A.	9.9	15.9	74.2	0.8	114.855 F.I.
Holland	24.2	28.2	47.6	0.5	2.876
U.K.	80.0	8.0	12.0	0.5	8.320
Italy	71.0	23.0	6.0	0.1	14.200
G.D.R.	99.1	0.5	0.4	0.2	3.548
Argentina	88.9	7.1	4.0	0.0	4.500
Japan	10.0	15.5	74.5	0.3	·3.577
Australia	60.2	27.7	12.1	1.3	914

Table 11. Pacemaker hardware – power source.

HgZn batteries are still used only in a few countries:

Czechoslovakia	88.8%
G.D.R.	83.7%
Poland	41.6%

In the rest of the world lithium batteries are the power source of choice.

Lithium cells were reported as the power source of choice throughout the world with the exception of some countries in Eastern Europe where HgZn batteries were still in use in 1981 (German FR 83.7% of cases). Only 4 new implants of radioisotopic units were reported in 1981 (Belgium) while, throughout the world, nearly 700 such units were still in use (most of them in US and German FR).

In Table 12, the type of catheter-electrode used and the techniques of introduction are given for a few representative countries. The transvenous insertion, as expected, was the method of choice in 1981; however, in Japan, one patient out of five received epicardial leads that year. The percutaneous puncture was quite frequently used in North America (in over 40% of cases) and was the preference in England (60% of cases). Active fixation electrodes were rather poorly used with the exception of German FR where they accounted for up to 22.1% of all electrodes used.

Information on the follow-up of pacemaker patients was limited to nearly 350,000 patients and was satisfactory only for some centers in Europe which controlled 104,211 patients in 1980 (5). About one third of these centers reported 250–600 patients in regular follow-up; however, in some countries, such as France, there were centers with very large numbers (over 2000 patients in follow-up). Almost 40% of centers in Europe used computerized patient files and 61% were linked to a national data base or to some kind of multicenter registration system. Nearly all patients in Europe were followed-up in dedicated pacemaker clinics; transtelephone impulse and ECG monitoring, and self-check techniques were consistently in use only in a few countries (UK).

The indications for generator and/or electrode changes were reported as in Table 13. Elective replacement of the pulse generator was very common in most countries eventhough a good percentage of units were removed at the end of battery life (38.4% of cases in Italy; 33.4% in Japan). Electrode problems were reported in up to 9% of cases in the UK and premature battery depletion in up to 6.2% in Italy. All types of generator failures accounted for up to 15.5% of cases in the US while failures of programming were reported to cause less than 1% of generator replacements throughout the world.

Eighteen cases of neoplasm arising from tissues surrounding the generator and/or the lead were reported from the six countries listed in Table 14 and referred to several years of pacing activity.

Among the indications for file closure, "death cause unknown" was reported quite frequently (about 30% of cases) (Table 15). Death was sudden in 8.4% of cases in Europe (%) and it was attributed to generator failure in 0.2% of cases in the US and 0.3% of cases in Europe.

Table 12. Electrodes – leads and way of insertion in some countries (% of total implants).

	Transvenous	T. percutaneous	Active fixation A + V	Epicardial
Canada	100.0	43.4	NA	0.0
U.S.A.	93.3	40.5	2.6–5.2	6.7
U.K.	97.4	60.0	NA	2.6
G.D.R.	99.8	9.8	= –0.3	0.2
G.F.R.	100.0	NA	9.4–22.1	0.0
Japan	78.2	12.9	0.3–4.3	21.8

Displacement (17%), conductor breakage (13%), exit block (11%), connector failure (9%), infection (8%), insulation break (5%) are the most common indications for electrode changes in the U.S.A.
NA = Not available

Table 13. Indications for generator change (%).

	U.S.A.*)	U.K.	Italy	Japan*)
Elective	26.6	28.2	38.2	27.9
For system change	3.8	2.7	4.4	3.4
For electrode problems	4.6	9.0	2.6	3.9
Mechanical protrusion	3.0	2.0	0.4	1.6
Infection	3.4	13.5	2.8	5.7
Failure slow rate	8.3	1.3	0.8	3.2
Failure fast rate	0.7	0.5	0.3	0.7
Failure sensing ($\pm$)	5.7	2.1	0.9	2.6
Failure programming	0.8	0.2	0.6	0.3
Battery depletion (premature)	4.0	4.9	6.2	5.8
Battery depletion E.O.	19.1	20.8	38.4	33.4

*) Largest users of programmability

Table 14. Cases of neoplasma arising from tissues in contact with either the generator and/or the lead.

Belgium	3 Cases
Greece	5 Cases
Italy	5 Cases
U.K.	1 Case
Hungary	2 Cases
Australia	2 Cases

Table 15. Death-cause unknown as an indication for file closure.

	% of file closure
U.S.A.	29.8
Chile	50.0
Austria	34.6
Italy	32.1
Portugal	33.3
U. K.	32.8
Japan	21.6

Table 16. PM re-use in 10 countries on 1981.

Country	First implants	Replacements	Total PMS used	Total PMS re-used	%
Norway	776	219	995	79	7.93
Sweden	1.782	853	2.635	200 (E)	7.59
Finland	624	202	826	62	7.50
G.D.R.	3.571	2.490	6.061	419	6.91
Hungary	1.067	532	1.599	104	6.50
Austria	1.780	556	2.336	60(E)	2.56
G.F.R.	31.600	12.400	44.000	558	1.26
Argentina	4.500	2.800	7.300	150	2.05
Australia	811	192	1.003	34	3.38
Israel	591	165	756	31	4.10

The fate of the explanted units is known only for some countries and for a limited number of cases. In the US about 70% of these units were returned to the manufacturer for verification while in Europe this percentage was less than 30% in 1980. The early explanted well-functioning units were refurbished and re-utilized in many countries (Table 16). These units represent nearly 8% of the total pacemakers used in the Scandinavian countries.

A tentative evaluation of the cost of an average pacemaker throughout the world, based on the information derived from the survey questionnaires, is given in Fig. 6. An average unit including lead(s), costs up to 2300 US dollars in Europe, 3500 US dollars in the US and 4200 US dollars in Japan. Large differences in average unit prices were encountered even in very close and similar countries such as Canada and the United States.

A comparison between 1981 and 1978 costs indicate that a primary implant went up 100% in Japan while it remained about the same in the US and throughout Europe. However, taking into account the increased average longevity of more recent units and the reduced cost of annual follow-up, the total cost of pacing per month has decreased in many countries in the world (US, UK, Italy) by up to 40% in the last decade.

Comments and Conclusions

The tabulation of this world survey and the commentaries of the Correspondents, that could not be reported here mainly for reasons of space, provide a fascinating picture of the world's medical and socio-economic scene. In analyzing the results we were impressed, even more than in past surveys, by the diversification of implantation rates, indications, methodology, complications, hardware, costs, etc. of cardiac pacemaker within any one continent let alone within the whole world. We were puzzled by the incredible

Fig. 6. Minimum and maximum costs for an average pacemaker in the various parts of the world.

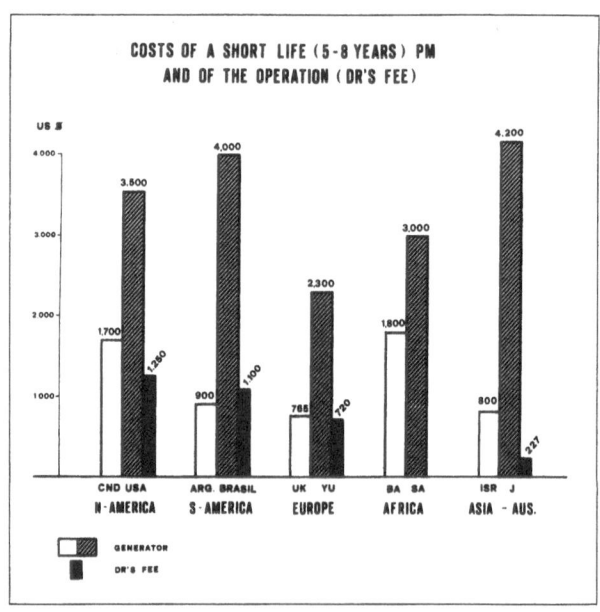

volume of pacemaker usage in some countries with implantation rates over 500 per million population, still we wonder whether for the countries lagging behind, it is just a matter of time before they reach such high implantation rates. In this respect, many countries in the world are now where the US and German FR were a few years ago, with implantation rates of 250–300 per million inhabitants, but also with similar "density" of pacemaker centers, prevalence of elderly people, health care system, the latter being important factors conditioning the growth of cardiac pacing in any country.

Important differences among countries are also evident in the use of programmability and dual chamber pacing (apparently due to socioeconomic reasons) while differences in indications, methodology and complications are more attenuated than in previous surveys.

Interest in the clinical applications of atrial or AV sequential pacing is apparently growing while, at this point in time, there is still very little interest for antitachycardia devices. Reliability of pulse generators and leads was generally improved. It is interesting to note that failures of programming were reported to cause less than 1% of generator replacements throughout the world.

Little progress in the follow-up of patients has been accomplished. Still one out of three cases of file closure, is due to death of the patient "cause unknown".

To close this commentary we would like to stress the need for surveys on smaller scales but aiming collecting hard data on all aspects of cardiac pacing, although much more expensive than the present one. As already pointed out on other occasions (4) the cost for such acquisition of solid information could be largely covered by saving money through pacemaker re-implantation. In 1981, in the Scandinavian countries, nearly 8% of pacemakers employed were units explanted within the first year, refurbished and re-used. If this survey has called attention, again, to nothing more than this last issue, it certainly has accomplished a great deal.

References

1. Survey of the Long-Term Stimulation Techniques all over the World. Symposium sur les Pacemakers, Monaco 17–19 September 1970. Annales Cardiolog. Ageiol 1971; 20: 285.
2. World Survey of Cardiac Stimulation. Cardiac Pacing: Proceedings of the IV International Symposium, Gröningen, April 17–19, 1973. HJTh Thalen Editor, Van Gorcum, Assen 1973: pag 41.
3. World Survey on Long-Term Follow-up of Cardiac pacing. Cardiac Pacing: Proceedings of the V International Symposium. Tokyo, March 14–18, 1976. Y Watanabe Editor, Excerpta Medica, Amsterdam 1977, pag 555.
4. World Survey on Cardiac Pacing. Cardiac Pacing, State of the Art 1979: Proceedings of the VI World Symposium on Cardiac Pacing, Montreal, October 2–5, 1979, C Meer Editor, Montreal 1979, Section 41.
5. Feruglio GA, Steinbach K: Cardiac pacing in Europe after two decades: A Comprehensive Survey. In Feruglio, GA (ed): Cardiac Pacing, Electrophysiology and Pacemaker Technology; Piccin Medical Books, Padua 1982: page 1–13.
6. Feruglio GA: Pacing in the World Today. Abstracts of the VIIth World Symposium on Cardiac Pacing. Pace 1983; 6: A149: A157–172.

Authors' address:
Prof. G. A. Feruglio
Ospedale Civile
33100-Udine (Italien)

Parametric Statistics for Performance Analysis

J. Dussel

Summary: The complicated nature of pacemaker performance may be explained by applying a classical method of product quality assessment to performance results. This shows that pacemakers may be distinguished into two populations. The one population, not necessarily always present, fails by infant mortality (im) and is superimposed onto the other population, failing by competing component failure (cf) and natural battery exhaustion (nbe). This permits to outline a general formula for mathematically describing the overall pacemaker failure probability in terms of its constituents. Application of the method to pacemaker performance data permits more accurate understanding and management of cardiac pacemakers. It additionally permits computer-assisted, simulated performance studies for anticipating problems, before these manifest themselves.

Introduction

Application of a classical method for product quality assessment to pacemaker results has shown, that pacemakers fail because of competing component failure (cf) or natural battery exhaustion (nbe)[1]. The overall probability of pacemaker failure, i.e. the Probability Density Function PDF (t) is given by:

$$PDF(t) = pdf_{cf}(t) \cdot csr_{nbe}(t) + pdf_{nbe}(t) \cdot csr_{cf}(t) \tag{1}$$

in which $pdf_{cf}(t)$ and $pdf_{nbe}(t)$ are the probabilities of cf and nbe respectively, while $csr_{cf}(t)$ and $csr_{nbe}(t)$ express that for the validity of $pdf_{cf}(t)$ and $pdf_{nbe}(t)$ the other event may not have occurred. In words, a pacemaker is exposed to a cf probability for as long as its battery has not failed. Under the assumption of normal distributions for the two failure modes, PDF(t) may be calculated and plotted graphically together with its constituents. This graph, at first view, differs considerably from the previously advocated bath-tub curve and the constant failure rate for early failures. Application of the method to further data confirmed the existence of a further cause of pacemaker failure, to be refered to as infant mortality (im).

Method

Following an actuarial survey for removing the bias unrelated to pacemakers from the data, the resulting cumulative survival rate CSR(t) is plotted on a normal probability graph.

Results

In Fig. 1, the CSR(t) of two series of cardiac pacemakers is plotted graphically on a normal probability graph. The data points indicate three straight line segments, related to im, cf and nbe respectively. Fig. 2 indicates that the upward kink in the composite data

969

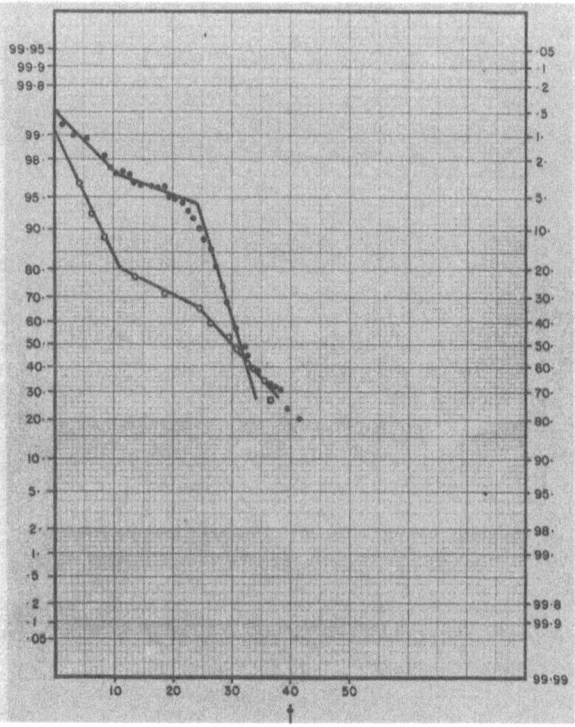

Fig. 1. The Cumulative Survival Rate CSR(t) of two series of cardiac pacemakers plotted on a normal probability graph.

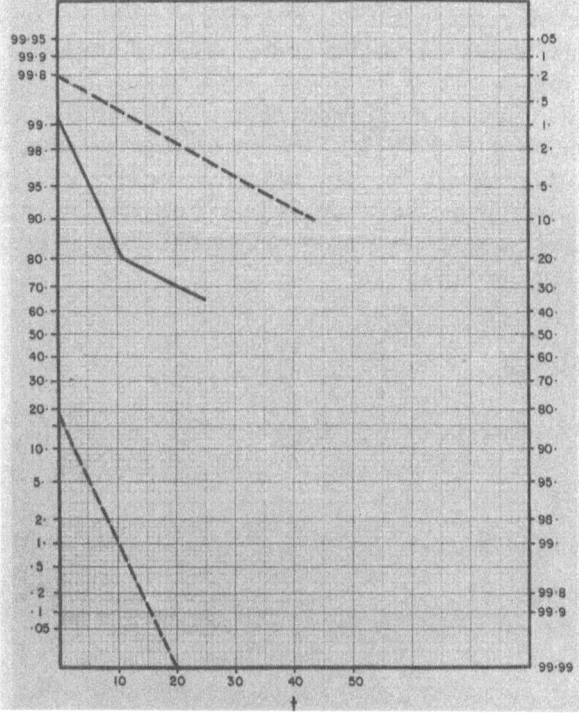

Fig. 2. The resolution of the composite data line of one of the series in Fig. 1 into its constituent parts for early failures.

970

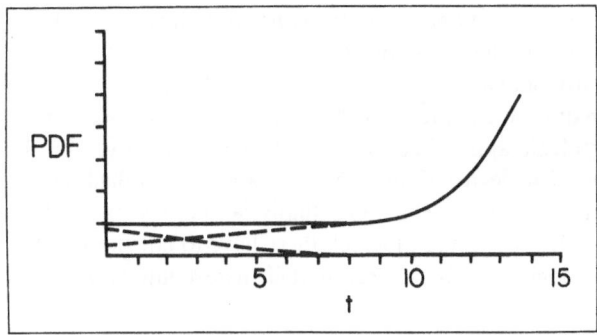

Fig. 3. The overall probability of early pacemaker failure arises from a combination of a down-sloping infant mortality and an upsloping component failure probability.

line, as arising from im and cf, should be resolved into the constituent lines representing cf and im individually.

In Fig. 3, the PDF(t) has been calculated for early failures of one of the series of Fig. 1, after extending formula (1) for incorporating a $pdf_{im}(t)$.

Discussion

Comparison of the previously reported results with those presented here shows, that not all pacemaker models suffer im. The results presented here should indicate how pace-maker failure probability actually relates to the bath-tub curve and the constant failure rate for early failures.

It appears that im-failures pull the cf data line down for as long as im-failures occur during early pacemaker life. This results into a later upward kink in the composite data line. Such upward kink can, for mathematical reasons, not occur in the same population of competing cf and nbe, as otherwise, because im acts early on pacemaker life, all pace-makers would fail because of im and never reach the stage of either cf or nbe. Thus, im-failures constitute a separate population, superimposed onto the population of cf and nbe. This indicates how formula (1) should be extended for incorporating a $pdf_{im}(t)$:

$$PDF(t) = (1-A) \cdot pdf_{im}(t) + A \cdot \{pdf_{cf}(t) \cdot csr_{nbe}(t) + pdf_{nbe}(t) \cdot csr_{cf}(t)\} \tag{2}$$

in which $(1-A)$ denotes the fraction of the im-failures in the series, and the remainder A is the fraction of the other population (cf + nbe) in the series. This indicates further, that the composite data line (Fig. 1) may be resolved into its constituents (Fig. 2).

Normal distributions are assumed for all three failure modes, such in first order approximation, which may be supported by the straightness of the line segments. Estimating a value for A from the data, and graphical determination of the parameters permits to calculate and graphically display PDF(t) and its constituents for early failures (Fig. 3). The calculated PDF(t) appears to be very constant until the upslope caused by the onset of nbe. This agrees with the constant failure rate for early failures, but this is reached only for pacemakers exposed to cf and im according to two superimposed populations. The constant failure rate does not apply to pacemakers not suffering im, and may thus not be applied generally. For longer life pacemakers suffering im, the constant failure rate will also not apply beyond the point, where im has lost its influence.

A true bath-tub curve may evidently only arise in case of an extremely high incidence of im, together with a low incidence of cf. It appears that the model as represented here by Formula (2) constitutes a more realistic approximation than the bath-tub curve and the constant failure rate, as it contains some degree of physical motivation. A production line of pacemakers may produce good pacemakers, which eventually fail because of either cf or nbe, and bad ones, containing a defect because of which these have to fail shortly after implantation. The challenge to distinguish early failures by their nature into two categories (im and cf), presents itself.

Resolution of the composite data line into its constituents encounters considerable mathematical problems. The best approach seems to be a computer-assisted optimisation procedure. For practical purposes, the CSR(t)-plot on a normal probability graph suffices, but further research on the true shape of each failure pattern is extremely important for computer-assisted simulated performance studies. The nbe-pattern has, most likely, a normal shape of which the standard deviation will increase with increasing longevity, as many factors like the load on the pacemaker, are permitted a longer period to act on the actual longevity. The true shape of the cf-pattern is less certain, as only a very first part of the pattern is observed. It may have a normal shape, but other like the Poisson-shape may prove to provide a better fit in the future. In this respect, performance data of nuclear-powered pacemakers are invaluable, as these should not present nbe-problems and reveal the true pattern of cf.

Simulated performance studies are invaluable for checking, for instance, whether there is a mismatch between pacemaker quality as reflected by the incidence of cf, and its projected longevity. Such simulated performance studies may thus be of great assistence for understanding situations, which have already occurred, or may be foreseen in the future. At this stage, a plot of the CSR(t) on a normal probability graph constitutes a powerful means for more accurate follow-up and performance assessment, such to the benefit of pacemaker patients.

Conclusions

Cardiac pacemakers may be distinguished into two superimposed populations. In the one population, all pacemakers fail eventually because of competing cf and nbe, while in the other population (which is not always present), all pacemakers fail because of im.

The presentation of the CSR(t) on a normal probability graph may be interpreted in terms of an underlying composite statistical pattern, and enables a more accurate follow-up and assessment of pacemaker performance.

The statistical pattern may be mathematically described in terms of its constituent patterns, which permits computer-assisted simulated performance studies. Such studies are invaluable for detecting a mismatch between pacemaker quality and its projected longerity, and for explaining further performance phenomena. Verification of the actual patterns of the constituents requires more information and data for further, in-depth analysis.

References

1. Of Pacemakers and Statistics; The Actuarial Method Extended. Jan Dussel, Anthony B. Wolbarst, Robert N Scott-Millar and Israel W. P. Obel. Pace – Vol. 3, January/February 1980, page 8–16.
2. Grunkemeier, GL, Thomas, DR, Starr, A: Statistical Considerations in the Analysis and Reporting of Time-related Events. Amer J Cardiol 1977; 39: 297.
3. Hald A: Statistical Theory with Engineering Applications. Book; New York, John Wiley and Sons, 1952; p 132.

Authors' address:
Jan Dussel, Drs.
Dept. Medical Physics
Johannesburg Hospital
P.O. Box 70002
Bryanston 2021
South Africa

Use Patterns of Permanent Cardiac Pacemakers

M. Bilitch, B. S. Goldman, R. G. Hauser, V. Parsonnet, S. Furman

Summary: Patterns of pacemaker implantation have changed significantly during the past eight years. A five-center North American Registry has compiled pacemaker data continuously since mid-1974. The data permit an evaluation of the changes in power sources, programmability, chambers paced and sensed and modifications in pacing mode at the time of pulse generator replacement. Comparison of data for 1975 and 1982 show a decrease from 58.4% to 24.0% in pulse generator replacement and a 100% increase in the use of programmable lithium powered units. Between 1980 and 1982 there was an increase from 11.3% in the use of communicating (telemetry) units and an increase from 7.8% to 29.2% in the implantation of dual chamber pacemakers.

Overall data indicate, 1) a significant difference in pulse generator actuarial survivial with different lithium chemistries; lithium iodide and lithium cupric sulfide units have the best seven-year performance. 2) Multiprogrammable pacemakers have become the standard unit for North America. Communicating units will be the predominant forms of multiprogrammable pacing for the foreseeable future. 3) The ratio between initial and replacement implantation continues to increase. The majority of replacements are, however, now for lithium units. 4) Replacement is often accompanied by an upgrade of the pacing mode to a dual chamber state.

Use Patterns of Permanent Cardiac Pacemakers

Five pacemaker centers in the United States and Canada have combined and reviewed their permanent pacemaker implantation experience continuously since July 1st 1974. Many variables have been recorded and have permitted an assessment of, amongst other things, the dynamics of pulse generator use. The increasing sophistication of pulse generators, improved power supplies, and more reliable leads have resulted in significant changes in use patterns. We report here portions of our data from the period July 1, 1974 through December 31, 1982. Other data are reported at regular intervals (1).

Methods

Data was collected from Newark Beth Israel Medical Center in Newark, New Jersey, Montefiore Hospital and Medical Center in New York City, Toronto General Hospital, Toronto, Ontario, Canada, Rush Presbyterian-St. Luke's Medical Center in Chicago, Illinois, and the University of Southern California Pacemaker Center, Los Angeles, California.

Patient and hardware information were transmitted to the University of Southern California. Data was compartmentalized into pulse generator, lead, and patient ledgers. This information was then stored on a computer system at the Newark Beth Israel Medical Center. Computer outputs were analyzed and used to prepare a series of reports. Between 1974 and 1981, selected data were transmitted to the United States Food and Drug Administration. Since 1978, pulse generator performance data has been regularly published in PACE (1).

Results

Implantation by power source reflects changes from the mercury zinc to lithium era. The last mercury zinc implantation was in 1979 and the last nuclear unit was implanted in 1980.

We have had experience with five lithium chemistries. Actuarial survival with lithium lead, lithium silver chromate, lithium thionyl chloride, lithium iodide, lithium cupric sulfide and nuclear plutonium 238 chemistries is shown in Fig. 1. Over a six year period, the performance of lithium cupric sulfide and lithium iodide powered pulse generators was equal. There was a reduced performance level of lithium thionyl chloride, lithium silver chromate cells, and lithium lead a power source no longer in commercial use. There was a slightly higher but significant actuarial survival performance of nuclear powered units.

Fig. 1. Actuarial surivial by lithium chemistry.

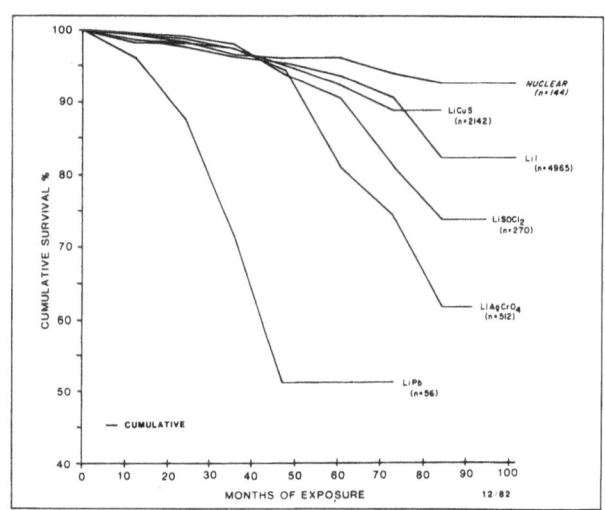

Fig. 2. Programmability – lithium units.

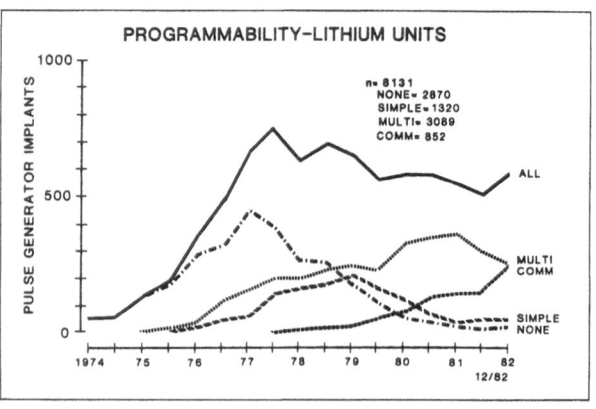

976

All centers have used noninvasively programmable units since the inception of the study. Since 1979, the use of multiprogrammable units has exceeded the implantation of simple programmable units. These data are shown in Fig. 2.

A review of the implantation of programmable and nonprogrammable units for the calendar year 1982, showed a steady and low level use of nonprogrammable units being, 1.9% for first six months and 2.6% in the second six months. There was a slight decrease in the number of simple programmable units being used from 8.1% to 6.8%. There was a substantial change in the use of communicating multiprogrammable units over noncommunicating, that is to say, nontelemetry units. Telemetry units were implanted 29.2% of the time between January and June 1982, but increased to 44.2% of all implantations between July and December of 1982.

The replacement rate of pulse generators steadily declined from 1974 through 1982 (Fig. 3). This was in contrast to the numbers of initial implantations which have held at a constant level. These data are presented as a percentage of initial implantations versus replacements. The total number of initial implantations was 5,950 and of replacements 4,335.

Data from the last six months of 1982, showed that of a total 577 pulse generator implants, 447 or 77.5% were initial implantations and 130 or 22.5% replacements. It is important to note that the majority of the replacements, 113 of the 130, were lithium powered units and only 17 were from the small number of mercury zinc units still left in service in our series.

A subset of replacements having a significant associated mode change were evaluated. During the study period 141 patients had 148 pulse generator replacements representing 148 mode changes. One hundred and thirty-three had one mode change, six two modes changes and two three changes (Table 1).

The particular changes have reflected the availability of various pieces of hardware including both single and dual chamber pulse generators and atrial and ventricular leads and electrodes. The data show (Table 2) that there was a steady increase from 0.4% in 1974 to 15.5% in 1982 of the replacements which were also accompanied by a mode change. Prior to 1980, the majority of changes were from one single chamber mode to another single chamber mode. However, from 1980 through 1982, the increasing availability of dual chamber pacemakers was accompanied by a steady increase in changes

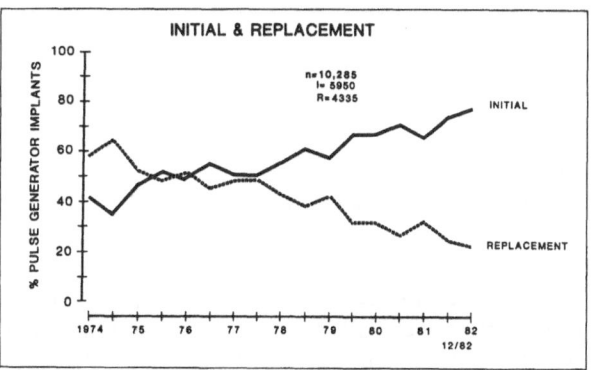

Fig. 3. Initial & replacement.

Table 1. Pacing mode changes July 1974–Dezember 1982.

141 Patients – 148 mode changes
133 – one mode change
  6 – two mode changes
  2 – three mode changes

Table 2. Pacing mode changes

Type	Year									
	1974	1975	1976	1977	1978	1979	1980	1981	1982	Total
Single chamber to single chamber	1	1	3	11	12	8	7	1	2	46
Single chamber to dual chamber			1	2	3	5	13	28	26	78
Dual chamber to single chamber		1				1	2		2	6
Dual chamber to dual chamber					1	1	2	3	11	18
Total	1	2	4	13	16	15	24	32	41	**148**
% of all replacements	0.4	0.3	0.8	1.9	2.3	2.6	6.1	9.0	15.5	

Table 3. Source of single chamber change

From	To				
	VVI	VOO	AAI	Other	Total
VOO	7	0	0	0	7
VVI	0	8	11	1 – Radio frequency	20
AAI	17	0	0	1 – Radio frequency + AAI	18
VAT	4	0	1	0	5
DOO	1	0	0	0	1
Radio frequency	1	0	0		1
Total	30	8	12	2	**52**

from single chamber to dual chamber function. Of 32 mode changes in 1981, 28 were from single to dual chamber and in 1982, 26 of 41 changes were from single chamber to dual chamber. Eleven of the 41 changes were from dual chamber to a different type of dual chamber mode.

The dual chamber mode changes represented primarily changes from VAT to either DDD or DVI and of the DVI mode to DDD (Table 3). Thus, it can be seen that of 10 changes from the VAT mode to another dual chamber mode that 4 were to DDD and 5

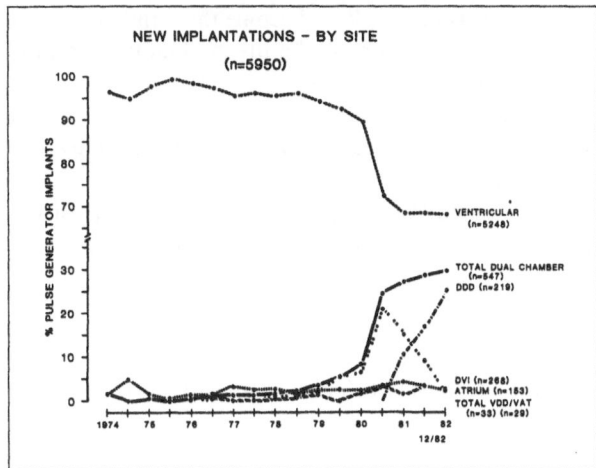

Fig. 4. New implantations – by site.

to DVI and of 9 DVI mode changes, 8 were to DDD and 1 to VDD. The greater availability of, at first DVI and then DDD pulse generators, undoubtedly accounted for the increase of these mode changes at the time of pacemaker replacement.

The rate of initial implantation of pacemakers held constant throughout our study (Fig. 4). The apparent smaller number of initial implantations between 1974 and 1977 represented a change in 1977 from an initial 3-centers to 5-centers. At that time, data from the two additional centers was incorporated from 1974 for lithium pulse generator implantations; the added data excluded mercury zinc implantations. Since 1979, there has been a steady increase in the use of dual chamber units and a concomitant fall in the number of ventricular units implanted. Activity during the last half of 1982 reflected an overall increase in the numbers of initial implantations and was accompanied by an increase in *both* exclusively ventricular *and* dual chamber pacing. The availability of investigational dual chamber pulse generator resulted in an initial increase in the use of DVI units and then following the latter half of 1981 through 1982, a sharp declined in DVI units accompanied by a steady and rapid increase in the use of DDD pulse generators.

The data in Fig. 4 are plotted as a percentage of pulse generator implantations; it can be seen that the comparative implantation rates of single chamber ventricular units and dual chamber implantations were in an approximate ratio of 70% to 30% respectively. The slight continuing increase in total dual chamber implantations was due to a decrease in the numbers of purely atrial procedures. The principle types of implanted pulse generators continued to be ventricular with the preponderance of dual chamber implantations being DDD.

Conclusion

The data indicate that,

a) there is a significant difference in actuarial survival of pulse generators with various types of lithium chemistry; lithium iodide and lithium cupric sulfide units have the best seven year performance.

979

b) In North America, multiprogrammable pacemakers have become the standard form of pulse generator. Communicating units will undoubtedly be the predominant form of multiprogrammable pacemaker in the calender year 1983.
c) The ratio between initial implantations and pulse generator replacements continues to increase. A significant replacement market has not as yet appeared. At the same a majority of replacements now represent lithium powered units.
d) When pulse generators are replaced a significant proportion involve the use of upgraded pacing modes. It is anticipated that this practice will continue to increase.

Reference

1. Bilitch M, Hauser RG, Goldman BS, Furman S, Parsonnet V: Performance of Cardiac Pacemaker Pulse Generators. PACE 1983: 6: 306–308.

Authors' address:
Dr. M. Bilitch
USC Pacemaker Center
1420 San Pablo Street, C-201
Los Angeles, CA. 90033
USA

Excessive Permanent Pacemaker Utilization in the State of Maryland
A Fallacy of the Hospital Record Face Sheet

L. Scherlis, D. H. Dembo

Summary: Recently, Public Citizen, a consumer advocate, reported on the basis of hospital record face sheet data alone that 33% of permanent pacemakers inserted in Maryland during 1979 and 1980, were unnecessary or questionable. The Maryland Society of Cardiology in cooperation with thirty-two hospitals in Maryland, reviewed 610 of 817 patients so classified. Although coded as having received permanent pacemakers, 16% received only a temporary pacemaker or generator change. The proper diagnosis justifying a pacemaker was omitted in 53% of face sheets, and coding errors were found in 39%. A review of the complete medical record demonstrated valid indications in 95% of hospital records reviewed. Hospital record face sheets are inadequate for assessing the appropriateness of permanent pacemakers.

In the State of Maryland, legislation establishing a hospital Cost Containment Commission provides for a state-wide health data system. Information is derived from the face sheet of hospital medical records and includes identification, billing information, diagnostic and procedure data. Patient and physician confidentiality is maintained by each hospital assigning code numbers for patients and physicians. The International Classification of Disease, Ninth Revision, Clinical Modification (ICD-9-CM) (1) is used to encode diagnoses and procedures. Such data are used by health planners, cost containment commissions and utilization review organizations for purposes including the determination of cost effectiveness of health care, the appropriateness of procedures, mortality, quality of care and hospital funding.

Public Citizen Health Research Group, a Ralph Nader affiliated consumer advocate organization reported (Table 1) to Richard S. Schweiker, Secretary of the United States Department of Health and Human Resources, in July of 1982, that 23% of pacemakers inserted in the State of Maryland were unnecessary, and that another 13% were questionably indicated. It was suggested that if this was representative of national trends, $ 280,000,000 per year are wasted on unnecessary pacemakers in the United States (2). They reviewed information derived from face sheet data on 2,222 patients in Maryland

Table 1. Permanent Pacemaker Implantations in Maryland.

	1979	1980	Total
Appropriate	626 (60.5%)	795 (66.9%)	1421 (64.0%)
Unnecessary	256 (24.8%)	248 (20.9%)	504 (22.7%)
Questionable	151 (14.6%)	146 (12.3%)	297 (13.4%)
Total	1033	1189	2222

Hospitals reported as having had permanent pacemakers inserted in 1979 and 1980. The Health Research Group selected a list of allowable indications (Table 2 and 3) and based on those criteria determined which diagnoses justified implantation of permanent pacemakers.

The present study was initiated by the Maryland Society of Cardiology to ascertain the validity of the Health Research Group report in using only face sheet data. The statewide data base for 1979 and 1980 was obtained providing the listing of all diagnoses for patients who received permanent pacemakers in Maryland during that period. All Maryland Hospitals inserting more than three pacemakers during 1979 and 1980 were contacted and through the Maryland Health Services Cost Review Commission, were provided with a computer printout listing the patients who did not have the necessary criteria for permanent pacemaker implantation. In each hospital a review of the complete medical record was undertaken, usually by Quality Assurance Committees, Utilization Review Committees or in some instances, teams of cardiologists, or Department of Medicine chiefs. A standard questionnaire was developed for providing detailed analysis of each complete medical record. The reviewers were asked to copy verbatim the diagnosis and codes as well as procedures and codes from face sheet and to record other specific diagnosis and procedures from the complete medical record. Any errors in charting were recorded, and the source of additional data was listed. The completed forms were review-

Table 2. Appropriate Indications.

426.0	– AV block complete (third degree AV block)
426.12	– Mobitz II AV block (incomplete AV block: Mobitz II; Second degree, Mobitz II)
426.54	– Trifascicular block
426.6	– Other heart block (Intraventricular block: not otherwise specified, diffuse, myofibrillar; sinoatrial block: Sinoauricular block)
426.9	– Conduction disorder, unspecified (Heart block not otherwise specified)
427.81	– Sinoatrial node dysfunction (Sinus bradycardia: persistent, severe; Syndrome: sick sinus, tachy-brady)
780.2	– Syncope and collapse (Blackout, fainting, vasovagal attack)

Table 3. Proper Indications Under Appropriate Circumstances (Questionable).

426.3	– Other left bundle branch block (LBBB: not otherwise specified, anterior fascicular with posterior fascicular, complete, main stem)
426.50	– Bundle branch block, unspecified
426.51	– Right bundle branch block and left posterior fascicular block
426.52	– Right bundle branch block and left anterior fascicular block
426.53	– Other bilateral bundle branch block (Bifascicular block not otherwise specified, bilateral bundle branch block not otherwise specified, right bundle branch with left bundle branch block (incomplete) (main stem)
426.89	– Other conduction disorders (Dissociation: AF, interference, isorhythmic; Nonparoxysmal AV node tachycardia)
427.1	– Paroxysmal ventricular tachycardia (Ventricular tachycardia (paroxysmal))
427.9	– Cardiac dysrhythmia, unspecified (Arrhythmia (cardiac) not otherwise specified)
746.86	– Congenital heart block (Complete or incomplete AV block)

ed in detail and formed the basis for this report. Public Citizen found 801 pacemaker insertions alleged to be inappropriate or questionable compared to the Maryland Society of Cardiology total of 817 insertions utilizing the same criteria. A total of 610 or 75% of the charts were reviewed in detail. Thirty-two hospitals participated in the study out of a total of 54 hospitals in Maryland. Zero to eight pacemakers were inserted in 13 hospitals. On review, only 514 or 84% of the patients had actually received a permanent pacemaker on the admission reviewed. 2% were pacemaker replacements, 10% had received only a temporary pacemaker and 4% had a history of pacemaker having been inserted on a previous admission.

A number of general coding problems were identified and are listed in Table 4. Specifically, coding problems include correct diagnosis listed, wrong code assigned; only five diagnoses accepted for data base purposes, diagnosis ≠/ 6 or ≠/ 7, listed the proper justifi-

Table 4. Coding Problems General.

1. Use of ICD-9 began in 1979
2. Lack of standard front sheet in Maryland
3. Coding may be completed before discharge summary or operative note is available
4. Coding may be completed before diagnoses are written on the front sheet
5. Copy of front sheet may go to billing department before coding & record room. Coding done in billing department for Medicare may be different from record room coding
6. Coding may involve highly technical terminology as with arrhythmias
7. Lack of precise diagnoses by physician
8. Physicians unaware of ICD-9 nomenclature
9. Coding may include chart review or be confined to diagnoses on front sheet
10. Different levels of training of record room personnel

Table 5. Charting Problems.

	≠/	%
A. Diagnosis Errors on Front Sheet		
1. Omission in recording diagnosis or diagnoses	303	52.6
2. Vague diagnosis subject to misinterpretation by coder	119	20.7
3. Other	31	5.4
B. Operation		
1. Omission in recording operation	33	5.7
2. Vague description of operation	14	2.4
3. Other	2	0.3
C. Coding Errors		
1. Misinterpretation errors		
a. Vague or unclear diagnosis/operation miscoded by coder	59	10.2
b. Diagnosis/operation affected by other diagnosis and miscoded	4	0.7
2. Wrong diagnosis coded	67	11.6
3. Wrong procedure coded	74	12.8
4. Other coding error	23	4.0
D. Other Errors	28	4.9

cation; combined diagnosis with only the first part of the diagnosis coded, i.e., AV block with profound bradycardia, and only coding AV block; lack of specificity in listing arrhythmia diagnosis; coding problems due to non-specific diagnosis; omission by physician of diagnosis on front sheet; failure to list the type of pacemaker correctly; and the wrong number assigned to a procedure. Charting errors found in the present study are summarized in Table 5.

As an example, in one patient, the only diagnosis on the face sheet was aortic stenosis. An aortic valve prosthesis was inserted as well as a permanent pacemaker. Chart review revealed the presence of complete heart block.

In another example, the face sheet recorded mature cataract as the only diagnosis but in a review of the complete medical record, complete heart block with multiple episodes of syncope was recorded.

As an example of error in coding, the diagnosis of Mobitz II arrhythmia was properly recorded in one patient and assigned ICD-9 code 428 which is for congestive heart failure and not Mobitz II arrhythmia which is 426.12.

Utilizing the same criteria as the Public Citizen Report, 31 pacemaker implants were characterized as questionable or unnecessary, i.e., 5.1 of 610 charts reviewed. The remaining 94.9% wree classified questionable or unnecessary in the Public Citizen Report because of fallacies inherent in their study methodology.

The Maryland Society of Cardiology utilizing similar criteria found 1.9% as questionable or unnecessary. Utilizing criteria which include ventricular overdrive as a valid indication, 23 implants were classified as questionable or unnecessary, i.e. 1.4% of the total 2,222 pacemakers inserted.

The accuracy of the coding of face sheet diagnoses and procedures is best when these are essentially simple and straight forward and not subject to misinterpretation. They are more difficult when diagnoses and procedures are complex, vague and technical and when fine distinctions must be made between almost identical terminology. Selected reviews by the Baltimore City Professional Standards Review Organization in Maryland have revealed coding error rates of 5–24% for hospitals in Baltimore City in the designation of a diagnosis to the wrong diagnostic related group. Cardiac arrhythmias probably represent the one discipline of cardiology which is most technical in its terminology. In completing the face sheet the physician may not mention the specific arrhythmia or may state it vaguely. Coding personnel are then faced with making distinctions in this selection in order to assign a specific four or five digit code.

The thrust of this study is to define the limitations of face sheet data in health planning in determining the appropriateness of procedures and accuracy of diagnoses. The allegations of the Health Research Group are not substantiated by this study. There is a need for educational programs to improve the accuracy and completeness of diagnosis and procedures on the face sheet to enhance accurate coding of these data if face sheets are to be used for health care planning, peer review and hospital funding.

References

1. International Classification of Diseases, 9th revision, Clinical Modification. Commission on Professional and Hospital Activities, 1968 Green Road, Ann Arbor, Michigan 48105, 1979.

2. Greenberg A, Kowey PR, Bargmann E, Wolfe SM: Permanent pacemakers in Maryland, Report by Health Research Group, 2000 P Street, NW Washington, DC 20036, July 7, 1982.

Authors address:
Dr. L. Scherlis
Maryland General Hospital
827 Linden Avenue
Baltimore, Maryland 21201
USA

Subject Index

988

Authors' Index